Aspinall's Complete Textbook of Veterinary Nursing

For Elsevier
Content Strategy Director: *Robert Edwards*
Content Development Specialist: *Nicola Lally/Katie Golsby*
Project Manager: *Andrew Riley*
Designer/Design Direction: *Miles Hitchen*
Illustration Manager: *Brett MacNaughton*
Illustrator: *GW India/MP*

Aspinall's Complete Textbook of Veterinary Nursing

Third Edition

Edited by

Nicola Ackerman

BSc(Hons) RVN CertSAN CertVNECC
VTS(Nutrition) V1 A1 C-SQP HonMBVNA
Head Medical Nurse, The Veterinary Hospital
Group, Plymouth, Devon, UK

Foreword by

Victoria Aspinall

BVSc MRCVS
Former Senior Lecturer in Veterinary Nursing,
Hartpury College, Gloucester, UK

ELSEVIER

Edinburgh London New York Oxford Philadelphia St Louis Sydney Toronto 2016

ELSEVIER

ISBN 978-0-7020-6602-3

Notices

Knowledge and best practice in this field are constantly changing. As new research and experience broaden our understanding, changes in research methods, professional practices, or medical treatment may become necessary.

Practitioners and researchers must always rely on their own experience and knowledge in evaluating and using any information, methods, compounds, or experiments described herein. In using such information or methods they should be mindful of their own safety and the safety of others, including parties for whom they have a professional responsibility.

With respect to any drug or pharmaceutical products identified, readers are advised to check the most current information provided (i) on procedures featured or (ii) by the manufacturer of each product to be administered, to verify the recommended dose or formula, the method and duration of administration, and contraindications. It is the responsibility of practitioners, relying on their own experience and knowledge of their patients, to make diagnoses, to determine dosages and the best treatment for each individual patient, and to take all appropriate safety precautions.

To the fullest extent of the law, neither the Publisher nor the authors, contributors, or editors, assume any liability for any injury and/or damage to persons or property as a matter of products liability, negligence or otherwise, or from any use or operation of any methods, products, instructions, or ideas contained in the material herein.

your source for books,
journals and multimedia
in the health sciences

www.elsevierhealth.com

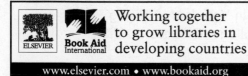

Printed in Great Britain
Last digit is the print number: 10

CONTENTS

*Additional chapters available online at
http://evolve.elsevier.com/Ackerman/vetnursing*

*Access our free student resources including
Multiple Choice Questions for each chapter,
extra chapters and the images from the book at
http://evolve.elsevier.com/Ackerman/vetnursing*

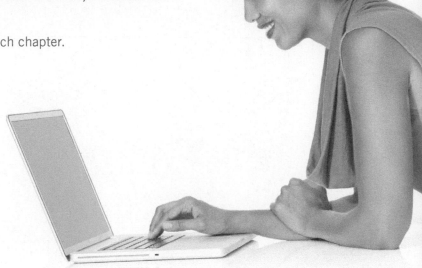

FOREWORD

To my amazement I find that it is more than 10 years since the first edition of *The Complete Textbook of Veterinary Nursing* was published. During those years veterinary science has developed and more significantly, the roles and responsibilities of the veterinary nurse have changed and increased. With these changes comes the need to update and reformulate the textbook. I am, however, now nearing retirement and my daily contact with student nurses, RVNs and even with veterinary practice is not as it used to be, so it was with some sadness that I made the decision to hand the task on to someone with much more current and extensive experience. I am certain that with Nicola Ackerman as editor, the book will continue to go from strength to strength. In addition the team at Elsevier have decided to rename the book *Aspinall's Complete Textbook of Veterinary Nursing* and I hope that as in the last 10 years, 'Aspinall's' will form part of the range of standard texts used by both student and qualified nurses for the whole of their working lives.

Victoria Aspinall 2016

Nicola Ackerman BSc (Hons) RVN Cert SAN AI MBVNA
BSc(Hons) RVN CertSAN CertVNECC
VTS(Nutrition) V1 A1 C-SQP HonMBVNA
Head Medical Nurse, The Veterinary Hospital Group,
Plymouth, Devon, UK

Lorraine Allan BVSc MRCVS PGCE MIfL
Team leader for veterinary nursing
Myerscough College
Preston, Lancashire, UK

Lisa Ashton MBA PGCE BA (Hons)
Equitation Science Coach and Consultant
EquiSci
Staffordshire, UK
Equitation Science International Tutor
Australian Equine Behaviour Centre
Melbourne, AUS
Former Education Officer
International Society for Equitation Science
UK
HE Equine and Animals Manager
Equine, Rodbaston College
Staffordshire, UK

Victoria Aspinall BVSc MRCVS
Former Senior Lecturer in Veterinary Nursing,
Hartpury College, Gloucester, UK

Sam Bell BSc(Hons) DipHE CVN Dip AVN (small animal)
Head Veterinary Nurse
Rowe Veterinary Group
Bradley Stoke, UK

Sally Bowden BSc (Hons) Cert Ed RVN
Writtle College
Chelmsford, Essex, UK

Emma Brooks VN
Veterinary Nurse
Bristol, UK

Gillian Calvo BSc (Hons), Dip AVN, Dip HE CVN, CCRP, RVN
Queen Mother Hospital for Animals
The Royal Veterinary CollegeHawkshead
LaneHatfieldHertfordshire, UK

Claire Cave VN
Freelance Lecturer in Veterinary Nursing
Woolavington, Bridgwater, Somerset, UK

Sarah Cottingham BSc (Hons) PG Dip CABC PGCE RVN
Course Leader in Veterinary Nursing
Animal Care Department
Plumpton College
East Sussex, UK

Sue Dallas VN
Freelance Lecturer in Veterinary Nursing
Great Ryburgh
Norfolk, UK

Suzanne Easton MSc BSc
Lecturer in Diagnostic Imaging
University of the West of England
Bristol, UK

Kristie Faulkner RVN Cert VBM
Business Development Director
Onswitch Ltd
UK

Maggie Fisher BVetMed CBiol MSB MRQA DipEVPC MRCVS
Shernacre Enterprise
Malvern, Worcester, UK

Cecilia Gorrel BSc MA Vet MB DDS Hon FAVD DEVDC
Director
Veterinary Oral Health Consultancy
Lymington, UK

Helen Harris Cert Ed
Team Leader
Veterinary Nursing
Duchy College
Camborne, UK

Paula Hotston Moore MEd RVN
Teaching Fellow
School of Veterinary Science
University of Bristol
Bristol, UK

Alison Jones BVetMed MRCVS
Principal 'Vets on the Park'
Lyndale, Moorend Grove
Cheltenham, Gloucestershire, UK

Lucy Kells RVN Dip AVN (Surgical)
Veterinary Nurse (current), Vale Wildlife Hospital, Beckford,
Gloucestershire, UK
Hospital Manager (2010-2015), The Wildlife Aid Foundation,
Leatherhead, Surrey, UK

Alison Lambert BVSc
Managing Director
Onswitch Ltd
UK

Jocelyn Lander RVN DipCABT
Behaviour Advisor
Thula Animal Behaviour and Training, UK

Catherine Lane MRCVS FdSc DipHECVN REVN
Head Nurse
Western Counties Equine Hospital Ltd
Devon, UK

Gareth Lawler BSc (Hons) PGCE
Lecturer in Animal Care
Pencoed College
Bridgend, South Wales, UK

Jessica Maughan BSc VN
Locum Nurse
Ruardean Woodside
Gloucestershire, UK

Suzanne May RVN
Head of Centre and Senior Lecturer in Veterinary Nursing
Harper Adams University College
Shropshire, UK

Samantha McMillan VTS (Anaesthesia) DipAVN DipHE RVN
Lecturer for Advanced Veterinary Nursing
The College of West Anglia/Anglia Ruskin University
Cambridge, UK

Pip Millard VN
Farm Manager
Badgeworth
Cheltenham, UK

Louise Minshell
Gloucestershire Wildlife Rescue\ Oak and Furrows Wildlife Rescue
Gloucestershire, UK

Helen Moreton BSc PhD
Senior Lecturer
Royal Agricultural University
Cirencester, Gloucestershire, UK

Louise O'Dwyer MBA BSc (Hons) VTS (Anaesthesia and ECC) DipAVN (Medical and Surgical) RVN
Clinical Director
PetMedics Veterinary Hospital
Manchester, UK

Julie Ouston MA VetMB MRCVS
Director
MYF Training Ltd
Hampshire, UK

Catherine Phillips RVN, REVN, CertEd, PgCert (VetEd), FHEA HonAssocRCVS
Head of Department of Veterinary Nursing
University Centre
Hartpury College
Hartpury
Gloucestershire, UK

Corinna Pippard MSc PhD
Visiting Lecturer
Anglia Ruskin University
Cambridge, UK

Michelle Richmond DipAVN (Medical) DipAVN (Surgical) Cert VN ECC RVN
The Veterinary Nursing Consultancy
Lymington, UK

Amanda Rock BVSc MRCVS
The Veterinary Hospital
Plymouth, UK

Trish Scorer VN
Internal Verifier for Abbeydale Vetlink Veterinary Training Ltd
Ashcott, Somerset, UK

Beverly Shingleton VN Cert Ed
Programme Manager for ND in Animal Management
Plumpton College
Plumpton, Nr Lewes
Sussex, UK

Sharon Smith RVN
University of Glasgow Small Animal Hospital
Glasgow, UK

Dorothy Stables MSc BA (Hons)
Former lecturer in Applied Biology
St Bartholomew's College of Nursing and Midwifery
City University
London, UK

Anja Walker BSc BVS MRCVS
Director of Western Counties Equine Clinic
Culmstock, Nr Cullumpton
Devon, UK

Juliet Whatley VN Cert Ed
External Verifier
RCVS
London, UK

Jane Williams VN Cert Ed
Lecturer in Veterinary Nursing
Buckfastleigh, Devon, UK

James Yeates BVSc PhD Cert WEL MRCVS
Chief Veterinary Officer at RSPCA
UK

Aspinall's Complete Textbook of Veterinary Nursing is a textbook that has really evolved alongside the profession. Written (mainly) by veterinary nurses for veterinary nurses that are working on the 'front line' in first and second opinion practices, the aim was to try and encompass the many different aspects that veterinary nurses currently undertake, from client communication in clinics through to emergency critical care and everything in-between. The role of aspects such as nursing clinics and emergency and critical care (ECC) nurses has shown how greatly the profession has changed, even since the last edition, and I have tried to reflect this in the additional chapters that have been included and the 'Emergency and Intensive Critical Care' chapter that has greatly evolved from the original First Aid chapter. The importance of fluid therapy and nutritional support of the critical patient has also developed into a chapter of its own. The importance of bandaging and different techniques has also been included in order to help serve as a reminder, or teaching aid, for VNS.

As a regulated profession it is vital that we undertake regular continued professional development (CPD) in the various areas in which we work. This textbook will serve as a ground basis and beyond for all areas. Recommended reading has been given in chapters so that additional advanced nursing techniques can be sought if required.

The book will hopefully serve as a 'go to reference' for all veterinary nurses (and others) within the profession. The digital elements of the textbook enable the reader to self-assess with multiple questions and observe some of the practical elements described in the text. By accessing the website you will also find additional chapters that complement the book, and ensure that the whole Veterinary Nursing syllabus has been covered.

Nicola Ackerman 2016

ACKNOWLEDGEMENTS

The development of *Aspinall's Complete Textbook of Veterinary Nursing* has been complex with many excellent authors all contributing towards the end goal. I would like to personally thank all of the authors for their help in reviewing and updating their chapters, but especially Sam McMillan and Louise O'Dwyer for their help and support with the book, and with additional new material.

Personally I would like to thank my husband, Chris, who has had to endure me dedicating the last year to reviewing, writing and editing the book. A vast amount of work has gone into the book, and it would not have been possible without his support. Thanks also to Ellena for her motivating chats and help with selection of the images for the front cover.

Lastly, I would like to personally thank Katie Golsby for her excellent guidance in the development and production of the book.

1 Ethics and Animal Welfare

JAMES YEATES

What are ethics and morality?

Each individual, society and profession has a way of making decisions about how to act and how other people should act. Individual veterinary nurses have a personal way of making decisions, which they reveal in what they do and what they say. The veterinary nursing profession also has its way, which it describes in the Royal College of Veterinary Surgeons (RCVS) *Guide to Professional Conduct*. A society has its way, which leads to its laws.

Ethics is the study of these ways of making decisions. It can be studied by sociologists, such as a survey of whether people approve of tail docking – this is called **descriptive ethics**. It can be studied by philosophers, who try to decide the best way to make decisions in general. This is called **normative ethics** and is discussed later; however, normative ethics is not limited to philosophers. It is done whenever one considers the ethics of a person, a profession or a society. People can then decide how to make decisions in real-life cases – this is called **applied ethics**. Applied ethics is an important part of many scientific and medical professions, and recently, the veterinary profession has begun to consider applied ethics in more depth.

Ethical conflicts

For much of the time, one obvious ethical responsibility must be followed, and in these situations, a nurse may not need to think about how to act, let alone have any complicated theories about it; however, at other times, nurses have conflicting ethical responsibilities. An **ethical conflict** is a situation in which a person has two or more ethical pressures that cannot both be fulfilled.

It is worth looking out for ethical conflicts that you deal with each day. Common ones include decisions about:
- Balancing an animal's quality of life and its quantity of life
- Balancing an animal's welfare and the owner's or practice's finances
- Being asked to assist in a procedure that you think is unethical for any reason
- Situations where the 'best option' is illegal
- Possibly reporting a colleague or owner to authorities
- Being given contradictory instructions by different vets or employers.

There are several ways to solve an ethical conflict. Two common methods are asking someone else or relying on 'gut feeling'. Both are quick and easy and involve a minimum of thought, and these characteristics make them useful for situations where a nurse has to act fast. However, just as such methods might not always reach the best solution in clinical issues, so too are they likely to be ethically less accurate than decisions that are better thought out.

It is worth following a rough procedure for dealing with an ethical conflict such as the one shown in Box 1.1. It is not necessary, and sometimes impossible, to follow this order rigidly, but the scheme lists important steps and describes them in more detail.

THINK ABOUT THE PREDICTABLE PROBLEMS IN ADVANCE (BOX 1.1)

Many conflicts can be predicted and anticipated.
- Some problems are created by the owners, e.g. some dog breeders breed bulldogs but the puppies often need to be delivered by Caesarean section. Some veterinary nurses consider it unethical to breed bulldogs because of the health problems that they have and unethical to help to perform a Caesarean, or think that one should insist on neutering the bitch at the same time.
- Other dilemmas are caused by the vet, e.g. when a nurse sees a vet acting unethically, there is a dilemma as to whether to 'whistle-blow'.
- Other dilemmas are caused by the law, e.g. in the UK non-native species such as grey squirrels cannot be released back into the wild after treatment.
- Many dilemmas depend on the owner, the law and the vet, e.g. nurses can expect many different cases of euthanasia. Some animals brought for euthanasia are completely healthy and might have a good life if the owner and vet did not agree to euthanise it. Others have been suffering for some time but their owner does not want them euthanised. Some do not have owners. Each case causes a different ethical dilemma.

BOX 1.1   A RATIONAL APPROACH TO ETHICAL CONFLICTS

- Think about the predictable problems in advance
- Describe the question and your choices
- Identify the choices that you have available physically
- Identify the choices that you have available legally
- Identify the stakeholders and predict how each one might be affected
- Choose a school of thought or a framework
- Identify choices you think are ethically acceptable
- Discuss your decision with other stakeholders
- Act
- Reflect on the decision and outcomes
- Prepare for next time

BOX 1.2   COMMON OPTIONS WHEN FACED WITH A CASE OF EUTHANASIA

- Kill the animal
- Let the animal die naturally
- Try to cure the animal's disease
- Palliate any suffering
- Rehome the animal with the owner's consent
- Take the animal and rehome it against the owner's wishes
- Do nothing
- Report the owner for cruelty

Thinking about these issues in advance allows you time to think when you are relaxed and not pressured by other people. It gives you time to get more information and discuss matters with other people. For example, you may need to discuss with an owner whether to resuscitate an animal if it crashes under anaesthesia *before* the animal crashes, as there is no time when it does. If you have some idea in advance that you might not be happy to assist a vet with a procedure, then it is useful to say so *before* the animal is admitted because:

1. It may avoid the vet trying to do the procedure on his or her own because you refused to help after the vet had committed himself or herself.
2. You may end up helping with the procedure to prevent the vet doing it on his or her own and then feeling inconsistent and weak.
3. Your decision might make the vet change his or her mind before committing himself or herself.

DESCRIBE THE QUESTION AND YOUR CHOICES

You cannot make a decision without knowing what that decision concerns. It is useful to describe the question as neutrally as possible so that it does not determine your answer in advance. For example, questions such as 'Should I fail to care appropriately for this animal?' or 'Should I act uncharitably to this owner?' will be answered by 'No', even though there might actually be very good reasons not to care for the animal, e.g. because it would cause danger to your colleagues, or to act uncharitably to the owner, e.g. because it would cost the practice money.

It is useful to separate the question you have to answer from the situation. Often situations could and should have been avoided, and it is very easy to moan about the situation and fail to make a decision. For example, if an animal is aggressive because it has been poorly trained or is unsuitable for the owner, then this is a situation that should have been avoided, but you still have to make a decision now about what you are going to do.

Once you have phrased the question, you can consider the possible answers. Some options are not immediately obvious and are revealed only by reflection. Doing nothing is always a choice but often not the right one. As an example, your choices when faced with a decision about euthanasia are listed in Box 1.2. It is useful to think of all these choices at this point, however imperfect or silly they seem, because you may find that the sensible options are not possible in some cases.

IDENTIFY THE CHOICES THAT YOU HAVE AVAILABLE PHYSICALLY

Very often you will find that some choices are physically impossible. For example:

- Treating an aggressive dog may be much more difficult than treating a nicer dog because you may be unable to get close to it.
- Some diseases may not be treatable because a cure has not yet been discovered.
- Sometimes you are limited by your own competence levels or available time.

It is psychologically important not to feel guilty for not achieving the impossible, and in some cases it may be better to be realistic.

IDENTIFY THE CHOICES THAT YOU HAVE AVAILABLE LEGALLY

Legal rules and the rules in the RCVS *Guide to Professional Conduct* are based on the official ethics of your profession and of society. Following the law is generally the right thing to do, and breaking the law is not usually an ethical option.

The law is discussed in more detail in Chapter 5, but here it is worth noting that the law often agrees with one's own ethics, e.g. allowing unreasonable suffering is illegal, unprofessional and unethical. Similarly, there are some ethical arguments as to why it is a good thing that owners own their pets and why informed consent is important – imagine what it would be like if other people could just decide whether your pet is killed or rehomed.

It is important in ethical decision making to see the difference between options available to you as a nurse and options available to other people. Nurses do not have all the legal options available to the owner and the vet. If these other people will not do what is right, this limits the options open to the nurse. In these cases, nurses must choose the best from the options they do have – which may be a less than ideal treatment or even euthanasia. They should then not feel guilty for the poor ethics of other people.

IDENTIFY THE STAKEHOLDERS AND PREDICT HOW EACH ONE MIGHT BE AFFECTED BY EACH CHOICE

Any decision in practice will involve a 'cast' of people or animals involved, referred to as *stakeholders*. Common stakeholders are:

- The patient
- The owner
- The nurse's colleagues

- The practice
- The profession
- The public
- The environment
- The nurse.

The stake for each person or animal may be different and may create conflicting duties. It is useful to consider how each stakeholder may be affected by each available option.

The patient

This is probably the most important stakeholder; however, an animal cannot be asked what it wants and it cannot make veterinary decisions for itself because it does not understand medical treatment, e.g. if hospitalised, animals cannot decide when to go to the toilet outside or whether to receive visitors. This means the nurse has to make these decisions.

A popular way to think about how animals are affected is in terms of animal welfare. You can think about animal welfare in terms of inputs and outcomes. **Inputs** are things provided for animals in terms of their environment, medical treatment, husbandry, and the animal's condition and genetics. **Outcomes** are the effects of those inputs on the animal's quality of life. This is classically defined as 'the state of the animal as it attempts to cope with its environment' (Fraser and Broom 2007), but there is disagreement about which outcomes are important.

Some argue that you should only look at **physical welfare**. You can assess how well an animal functions by looking at its biology. Biological assessments look at how well the animal is functioning as an organism. You can measure its levels of substrates such as stress hormones or cortisol and/or look for signs of pathology such as stomach ulcers. Clinical assessments, such as palpation, temperature, capillary refill time, biochemistry, radiography and so on, are examples of biological assessments.

Many argue that welfare is about the **feelings** of animals. Welfare scientists have been surprisingly resistant to such ideas, mainly because they are not measurable from the outside – no person can ever know *for sure* whether an animal is feeling pain; however, welfare science has begun to recognise that it can guess an animal's feelings from its behaviour. Firstly, it looks at what animals choose. Secondly, it looks at behaviours that show negative feelings such as pain, stress, fear, malaise, boredom and lethargy or positive feelings such as in play and company. Pain may be shown by increased sensitivity in the area local to an injury or an altered posture and also in general behavioural signs such as quietness or inappetence. Many of these factors have been incorporated into protocols such as pain scoring systems. Similarly, stereotypes such as feather plucking in parrots or pacing in a caged zoo animal can suggest anxiety or boredom.

Assessment of feelings can be done in practice through simple observations and empathy; however, it must be remembered that animals experience the world and illness in a very different way to a human in an equivalent situation. This means you cannot merely ask whether *you* would want to be treated in this way. You should try to imagine what it might be like to be, say, a *dog* in the situation, knowing what you know about canine brains. For example, unlike a person, a dog is unlikely to want to survive until Christmas or worry about its diagnosis; however, like a person, it may dislike being in a strange place (especially in a strange-smelling hospital surrounded by strangers) and without any control over its treatment.

Assessment in practice can be assisted by using a formal tool or framework. Frameworks such as the Five Freedoms, shown in Box 1.3, combine inputs and outcomes of animal welfare.

Often the best assessment is one that combines the abilities of the nurse, owner and veterinarian. Owners usually see the animal far more than you, often every day for many years, but owners might not have much experience of assessing welfare. They might have had bad previous experiences or personal feelings that may affect their judgement. The nurse and the vet can help the owners to be more objective. Owners usually do not know about the clinical facts and may also be unable to perceive future problems. The vet may have a great deal of knowledge and experience, but still only sees the animal for a few minutes and may try not to get too close to the animal in order to remain objective. The assessment of a nurse, especially one that is experienced and empathetic, is a useful addition to the assessment of the owner and veterinarian.

An animal might also be affected in other ways. Being dead does not involve suffering, but it does deprive the animal of good welfare and/or avoid future bad welfare. An animal may have **rights** that can be broken such as a right to life or liberty, e.g. killing a grey squirrel might breach its right to life; keeping it captive deprives it of a basic right to live as a wild animal (and causes poor welfare too).

An animal may also be affected in terms of whether its **integrity** is damaged. If an animal is mutilated, such as being declawed, this damages its integrity on top of any pain or other problems caused. The same is true if animals are deprived of living naturally. If a dog is prevented from performing certain species-specific behaviours (its '*telos*'), then it loses some of its 'doggyness'. It might also be harmful to make animals live in an unnatural way. Taking a parrot from its natural environment and making it live in a house is unnatural, *as well as* possibly being bad welfare.

The owner

Owners are important stakeholders who may be seriously affected by the different outcomes. Owners may be heavily involved with the animal, sharing in its suffering and feeling grief, guilt and loss at its death. Treatment can cost the owners time or money. Owners legally prosecuted might get a criminal record or large monetary fine.

As you may not know the owner very well, the best way to find out what is in owners' interests is to ask them what they want. This is important not only legally but also ethically because going against owners' wishes can be traumatic for them. It is unpleasant to be told by someone else what to do with your beloved pet, and some owners think it important that *they* fulfil their responsibility to their pet and want to be involved in all decisions. Feeling judged or bullied might even lead to owners being less keen to bring animals to your practice, or to veterinary practices at all.

Sometimes owners might not know all the choices available or the clinical facts about a decision. They may not know what happens to an animal in an operation or that there are effective treatments for conditions such as incontinence. Owners may be embarrassed or scared to say what they really want, such as if they cannot afford treatment. Owners may feel cruel for asking for euthanasia too early or for not asking early enough – and their idea of cruel can be very different from yours. Some owners find talking to nurses easier than to veterinary surgeons. In all these cases, effective communication can help owners make informed, reflective decisions.

Bereavement is an important aspect of how an owner may be affected. Research suggests that bereavement is experienced by about two in three clients and is severe in one in three (Adams et al. 2000). Grief can range from numbness to hysteria, from self-blame to anger. The well-known five stages of grief are shock and disbelief; anger and guilt; bargaining; depression; and finally, acceptance. They will vary in duration, severity and order. Sometimes stages occur before the animal is dead. These can be quite unpredictable, but still, anticipation and preparation can help in dealing with them. There is widespread recognition that appropriate grief is normal and emotionally useful, but also that every person deals with grief differently (Kubler-Ross 1969). Nurses can help with an owner's grief by letting the owner know it is acceptable and healthy to grieve and by not belittling it, e.g. by saying 'it's only a dog!'

The nurse's colleagues

Nurses work under the direction of a veterinary surgeon. The veterinary surgeon will have an interest in the case that may be personal, academic and financial and often bears full responsibility for the animal's treatment. The vet may suffer sadness, disappointment, loss of respect and anxiety if a case does not go well and may resent too much interference or feel in need of help or sympathy. The personality of the vet and the nurse–vet relationship will make each nurse's duties to the vet very different. A nurse will have different duties if she or he is a dogsbody, boss, colleague, friend or partner.

Other colleagues also count in everyday decisions, e.g. whether to do some work or just laze about is an ethical decision. It is an ethical duty not to speak badly of colleagues without good reason, or to put colleagues in difficult situations, including placing them in ethical conflicts.

One difficult ethical decision can be whether or not to pass a responsibility onto another colleague. Sometimes they are in a better position to decide than you are, or sometimes it is a decision that concerns them, e.g. it is their case. However, at other times, 'passing the buck' can actually make matters worse for the animal, and should not be used as a way to avoid making a decision yourself. A nurse should generally try to avoid placing colleagues in ethically tricky situations, e.g. by booking euthanasia in for a vet in a busy consulting period or when it is another vet's case.

The practice

The practice can be considered to be a stakeholder in two ways, either as a boss who makes money or as a society who work together. A practice boss is sometimes the vet involved in the case as well, but increasingly often, the boss (e.g. practice manager or corporate owner) has no veterinary training and may not even be known personally by the nurse. Bosses can have control over various aspects of practice (e.g. by limiting options) and authority (e.g. by paying wages).

In contrast, a practice can be considered as a small society that benefits all its members and local community. Whether helping the practice is seen as helping the practice owner or all of the staff may depend on whether the boss is more concerned about making money than about the staff or patients.

In most cases, money made by the practice is money paid by the pet owners, and any money that the pet owner is 'let off' paying comes out of the practice's budget. This leads to conflicts between the interests of the practice, of the pet owner and of the animal. For example, if a pet owner cannot pay for the best treatment, then the animal may have to have a less efficacious treatment. If the pet owner will not pay for any treatment, the practice may have to either refuse to treat the animal or work for free.

As a society, a practice can have a societal ethic. It can be easier to make ethical decisions if all staff help each other and 'sing from the same hymn sheet'. If one nurse refuses to assist in bulldog Caesareans but another one does it unthinkingly, all that has been achieved is that the first nurse has made a stand – it could be better if all refused. Sometimes practices try to achieve a societal ethic by having standard operating procedures (SOPs) that advise nurses to make a certain type of decision in a certain way, which may be to maximise welfare and/or maximise profit. Nurses are still morally responsible for deciding to follow an SOP, and they should not follow one that they think is immoral.

Profession and public

All Registered Veterinary Nurses (RVNs) are representatives of all nurses in general. This adds a further responsibility for nurses to act well because their actions reflect on all nurses, and they may also reflect on vets. As for a practice, 'singing from the same hymn sheet' can have benefits for all members. For these reasons, the RCVS has written down rules about what is professional conduct in its *Guide to Professional Conduct*.

The wider public might also be affected by some of the choices, e.g. humans or animals might be harmed if an animal with a notifiable disease is at large or benefitted by a free neutering clinic. In general, the public also benefit from knowing that they can rely on the nursing profession to treat their animals well; thus harming the profession may also harm the public and vice versa.

Some everyday decisions even have to consider the environment, e.g. leaving a light on in the premises overnight will have environmental effects; the cost of recycling must be balanced with the costs for the practice; and the release of non-native animals such as grey squirrels can have an effect on the native species, as well as being illegal.

Nurse

On the one hand, nurses should not be too selfish and should rule out any irrational or overly selfish motivations; on the other hand, nurses should recognise their own values and biases. Contrasting these with those of the other stakeholders may help identify disagreements and resolve conflicts because you can see how your own interests and values differ from those of others.

CHOOSE A SCHOOL OF THOUGHT OR A FRAMEWORK

There are many schools of thought about the different ways to make ethical decisions, and in general terms, we can divide these into two types:

1. Those that are mainly concerned with the nurse's actions
2. Those concerned with the stakeholders.

Often people 'mix and match', but being able to roughly separate the different schools of thought can be useful in conflicts.

1. Schools of thought concerned with the nurse

These examine the rules that nurses should follow in terms of their actions or in terms of the virtues that they should have. The terms 'morality' or 'immoral' usually refer to this kind of school of thought.

Rules. A moral theory that is primarily concerned with rules that people have a duty to follow is called a **deontology**. In these theories, it is the rules that are important and not the consequences of following them, e.g. 'Do not kill' should be followed even if killing would help you or others or even if the victim would die anyway.

Many modern philosophers argue for a deontological approach based on the writings of Immanuel Kant (1963, 1996). Kant argued that moral rules could be worked out by considering what would be acceptable if everyone did the same thing. Others have argued that duties can be worked out by imagining that everyone has to sign a contract agreeing on what morals to follow. Rules that are considered **absolute** should never be broken for any benefit. This means that no two rules could conflict (otherwise a nurse would have to break one of them). To prevent rules from conflicting with each other, Kant argued that absolute moral duties always say 'Do *not...*', which leaves the option of doing nothing.

Deontological theories could include animals, but most do not. Kant argued that only animals that appreciate moral rules can have moral status. This means that humans should never be killed or exploited but non-human animals can be exploited. In a similar way, animals cannot sign a contract. Animals (and humans who cannot reason or sign contracts) may still have an indirect moral status based on the psychological worry that being cruel to them might make one cruel to humans or because other people love them, but this is a lesser status.

Virtue ethics. The Ancient Greek teacher Aristotle argued that people should try to be virtuous, and his philosophy has been revived by modern writers. Virtues might include compassion, generosity, integrity, charity, humility, loyalty and so on. A moral person is one who balances these virtues correctly in the right character.

One 'virtue' that may be important in veterinary nursing is to be **caring**. Caring involves personal, committed relationships between nurses and the animals for which they have responsibilities (Donovan and Adams 1996). One problem for care-based ethics is that it is unavoidably biased to the animals we love. It might allow us to cause a lot of suffering to large numbers of battery chickens or lab rats in order to help our own dear pet a little.

Respectfulness is another virtue. One might think that dressing animals up or making them do party tricks does not respect their dignity even when it does not actually cause bad welfare. Respect for animals may require giving ethical conflicts at least some thought, whatever is decided in the end. Nurses may sometimes feel bad for thinking about a decision too little as if it was unimportant. Disrespect can also extend to treatment of animal corpses.

Another important virtue is **moral integrity**. This involves not sacrificing one's own morality too easily just because of the situation, e.g. a nurse who believes that bulldogs should not be bred might be faced with a decision whether to help in a Caesarean on a bulldog. Looking only at the single case, it might be thought that the nurse should help; however, if the nurse believes that bulldogs should not be bred at all, the nurse risks sacrificing his or her integrity in helping with something the nurse thinks is wrong.

Taking **responsibility** is also a virtue. Nurses should be able to take responsibility for when they have to make a decision and act. They should also take responsibility for what they have done. This may mean 'owning up' to things that they have done wrong, but it can also involve feeling legitimate self-satisfaction for having done something right (indeed feeling pleased is often worth missing out on the benefits of a more selfish option).

2. Schools of thought concerned with the stakeholders

These are concerned with how people and animals might be affected by any decision or action. They consider the effects of what people do usually in terms of harms and benefits, rights or fairness. These schools of thought can be used to formulate rules or virtues, but they are primarily concerned by the outcomes. Some of these frameworks are described next.

Animal rights. Rights theory is one of the most popular theories in modern ethics when considering humans. A person can have a positive right to have or do something, or a negative right to be left alone, e.g. a positive right to life means other people should help a person stay alive, a negative right not to be killed means only that other people should not kill the person. Rights theories usually exclude non-human species from having rights, especially positive rights; however, people such as Hermann Daggett, Henry Salt and Tom Regan have argued that animals do have some negative rights.

Consequence-based theories. Some people argue that one stakeholder can be harmed if this is sufficiently useful for other stakeholders. 'Utilitarians' argue that the correct way to make ethical decisions is to add up the 'utility' or 'usefulness' of each option for all stakeholders. The right option is the one that causes 'the greatest good for the greatest number'.

This sounds very sensible, but there are problems with **utilitarianism**. It misses the distinction between letting someone die and murdering the person because the consequences are the same in each (ignoring indirect considerations, such as the harm of being arrested, etc.). By allowing some stakeholders to be harmed to benefit others, utilitarianism could, at least in theory, allow some extreme harms for minimal benefits. It could allow exploitation of poor ethnic minorities or animals in order to benefit the rich, so long as the rich benefit more than the poor suffer. It could allow a cruel blood sport if the enjoyment it created was greater than the fear and suffering of the animals.

There are many different ways that ethicists have defined 'utility'. A founder of utilitarianism, the Reverend Jeremy

Bentham, argued that morality should maximise pleasure and minimise pain. You literally add up the total pleasure and subtract the total pain that would result from each available option and the right action is the one where this number is highest. Clearly, animals should count in this equation. Bentham famously asserted that the morally relevant question is not 'Can they *reason*?' nor 'Can they *talk*?' but 'Can they *suffer*?' (Bentham, 1789). Bentham's successor J.S. Mill thought that some enjoyments such as relationships and poetry were more valuable than the pleasures that animals experience, thus a human is more valuable than an animal; however, Mill still thought animals counted and their pain should be minimised (Mill, 1987).

As well as being a science, animal welfare can also be considered as a type of utilitarianism that aims to minimise animals' pain and suffering, e.g. the '3Rs' is an ethical framework to minimise the suffering of laboratory animals. Suffering can be decreased by *reduction* of the number of animals used, *replacement* of animals with alternatives and *refinement* of procedures to cause less suffering.

Naturalness. As previously described, some people argue that animals should be allowed to live natural lives. Animals should be allowed to have natural breeding, natural environments and natural interactions with other animals and to be free from mutilations 'as nature intended'. A related school of thought is **environmentalism**. The environment should be protected or left alone, and we should avoid exploiting it (too much). Sometimes these schools of thought disagree with animal welfare, e.g. some people think wild animals should be left to live their natural lives entirely unaffected by human interference, which means that humans should not get involved even when a wild animal is injured and in pain.

Justice. Others have argued that the outcome of any action should be just. You might be able to avoid pain for many animals by doing lots of painful experiments on just one, but this might seem unjust on that one animal. Justice can be considered in terms of legal justice, in terms of rights or in terms of fairness to all the different stakeholders – and these may disagree. For example, it might be thought unfair that the law says you have to kill a grey squirrel because it is grey, when red squirrels are not killed – it is not the squirrel's fault which colour it is.

Frameworks

Some ethicists have thought that no single theory or school of thought is correct, and they have come up with ethical frameworks to help analyse a problem without having to decide on just one ethical theory. Such frameworks do not always automatically generate an answer about how to act, but they help identify the different issues to consider and the different views of the stakeholders.

The Five Freedoms (Box 1.3) can be thought of as an ethical framework that combines different theories as well as being a framework for welfare assessment. A nurse can try to act so that the animal is as free from hunger, thirst, discomfort and so on as much as possible. In many European countries, they replace the 'Freedom to Perform *Normal* Behaviour' with 'Freedom to Perform *Natural* Behaviour'.

A common framework in medical ethics is based on **four principles** shown in Table 1.1. This approach combines elements of theories on rights, utilitarianism and justice.

Food ethicist Ben Mepham devised an '**ethical matrix**' framework that applies the four principles to each stakeholder. This is a tool that helps people look at all the angles on a decision and helps different people communicate their views in the same framework. Table 1.2 is an adapted example.

Religious ethics

Religious ethics are also often a combination of ethical approaches. The Jewish, Christian and Islamic faiths have been important in forming the ethics of much of Western society. For example, Jesus laid down some specific rules, e.g. 'love thy neighbour', and also provided a role model for how to be virtuous. Western religions are often thought to be against animal welfare, e.g. in ritual slaughter, but each religion has rules against cruelty and there are many different opinions

TABLE 1.1	Four principles and what they mean	
Principle (Beauchamp and Childress 1979)	**Meaning**	**Equivalent principle in the ethical matrix**
Respect for autonomy	Respecting the decisions that patients or owners make	Autonomy
Non-maleficence	Not making animals worse off	Well-being
Beneficence	Making animals better off	
Justice	Fairness and respect for rights	Fairness

TABLE 1.2	Generic ethical matrix		
	Principles*		
Stakeholders	**Well-being**	**Autonomy**	**Fairness**
THE ANIMAL	Animal welfare	Respect for telos (e.g. doggyness)	Intrinsic value
THE VET	Peace of mind; job satisfaction	Clinical freedom; conscientious objection	Professional and legal roles and responsibilities
THE CLIENT	Owner quality of life; money, time, convenience; enjoyment of pet	Respecting owner's wishes; informed consent	Outcome appropriate to their situation; getting the best service they can afford
THE PROFESSION	Maintain professional privileges	Maintain self-regulation	Not having overly large influence on public opinion of profession
THE PRACTICE	Public relations	Practice policies and SOPs	Need to keep business going

*As shown in Table 1.1.

within each religion. For example, many Christians preach the importance of caring for animals. In fact, the symbol of the British Veterinary Nursing Association (BVNA) is Francis of Assisi, a Christian saint, who preached to the animals and told people to care for all life.

Other religions such as Buddhism and Jainism vary in their respect, but some forms argue for complete avoidance of even accidental killing. Hinduism and Hare Krishna afford special respect to cows. All of these can affect how people think about animals and can even lead to legal battles when parties disagree, especially when people fail to appreciate the strength or logic of others' convictions.

IDENTIFY CHOICES YOU THINK ARE ETHICALLY ACCEPTABLE

Using the range of ethical schools of thought, you can try to work out which of the choices is ethically the best one for you and the situation. In some cases, several options are acceptable and you can choose the best among them.

You may think that one option should not be done, because:
- It would be wrong if everyone did it (a deontological position).
- It suggests a less caring nurse (a virtue ethics position).
- It breaches someone's right (a rights position).
- It causes unnecessary pain to animals (an animal welfare position).
- The harm is not outweighed by a greater good to another stakeholder (a utilitarian position).
- It is unnatural (a naturalist or environmentalist position).
- It is unfair (a justice position).
- Or a combination of any of the above, e.g. in a framework.

DISCUSS YOUR DECISION WITH OTHER STAKEHOLDERS

The different stakeholders might have different views. For example, in a decision on euthanasia, an animal's owners might want their animal kept alive at all costs because they want to avoid grief, because they are scared to make the decision, because they think killing an animal is cruel even if it is suffering, or because they may feel guilty for the animal's situation. Alternatively, they might want their animal killed because they cannot reasonably afford treatment, because it is aggressive or incontinent, or because they think that rehoming is less caring or less responsible than euthanasia. Some owners might want to be persuaded or given other options; others will have already made up their mind and resist challenges, such as the idea that their animal might be owned by someone else.

Talking to the other stakeholders as part of your decision making can be useful to:
- Help you test your own position by hearing it said out loud
- Give a chance for them to notice weaknesses in your argument
- Find out more information about how they would be affected
- Help you understand their position
- Help them understand your position
- Identify disagreements
- Help with resolving disagreements.

You might disagree for several different reasons. You might have different ethical principles, be less or more willing to take responsibility for the decision, or have different factual beliefs, such as a different assessment of the animal's quality of life. Identifying any or all of these can help to resolve the disagreement; good communication is therefore essential. Being overly argumentative, judgemental or not showing understanding, compassion or flexibility can be offensive and can make people less likely to reach the best decision.

Good communication can also help a nurse recognise other people's conflicts. Often when one feels that someone has done something wrong, the person who did it may have been in an ethical conflict. He or she may have decided to do the harm because it was the 'lesser of two evils', e.g. a vet might have struggled with a decision whether to perform a bulldog Caesarean, and decided it was better than letting the animal suffer or killing it. Similarly, some employers require their nurses to inform them as soon as they know that they are pregnant. This may require nurses to inform their employer before they would want to, but it may be necessary to avoid the greater harm to the foetus being exposed to harmful gases and radiation, and to the mother under health and safety requirements.

Euthanasia

As an example, one important case in which discussion is useful is in making a choice about the use of euthanasia or of life-saving treatment. Owners and vets might be experiencing ethical dilemmas and need help to make decisions. In addition, euthanasia usually cannot be done legally without the owner's consent and veterinarian's direction.

Getting the owner to make a good decision about euthanasia can be difficult, especially with a grieving client, and an understanding of the five stages of grief, described previously, may be useful. Shock may prevent owners being able to make any decision, and disbelief may make owners question your or the veterinary surgeon's advice. Others may resist understanding, e.g. by misunderstanding phrases like 'put to sleep', so these should be avoided. Anger and guilt occur in at least 50% of clients (Adams et al. 2000). Both may bias their decision making, e.g. guilt for not seeking veterinary advice earlier can make owners less keen to seek it now. Anger and guilt can also strain client–nurse relationships, tempting you to blame clients when you are angry, but this can inflame their anger and/or their guilt and is usually not productive. Guilt can also prevent owners from asking for euthanasia, or make them ask in a veiled way.

Bargaining involves the owner trying to alter the facts or your decision making, or trying to get some concessions. When this stage occurs at the time of the euthanasia decision (e.g. owners bargaining to delay euthanasia), compromising with the owner can be useful (e.g. using your discretion about matters such as payment and disposal). The owner's depression should be taken into account in euthanasia decisions; however, this is quite usual whenever a pet dies, so delaying euthanasia to avoid owner depression is not necessarily beneficial except where it may help the owner to make a more rational decision.

Disagreements between stakeholders

It may be the case that the different people involved will think that different things should be done. A nurse may disagree with an owner, a veterinary surgeon, an employer or all three. A major part of ethical thinking involves coming up with methods to resolve or avoid these conflicts. Nurses have a spectrum of options, from doing just what they are told to doing just what they want.

1. **Do what other people want.** Doing whatever the owner, vet or employer wants is, in general, a good way to keep within the law and to maintain good public and work relations. In this way, the vet's ethics becomes the nurse's (deontological) ethics. The risk is that owners, vets and bosses have no more training in ethical reasoning than nurses and may well make wrong decisions, however qualified/old/experienced/wage-paying they may be. When they do makes bad choices, this may harm the animal, nurse, owner and vet (even the person making the decision), and the nurse who has carried out their wishes is still morally blameworthy for deciding to do so.

2. **Make joint decisions.** It is helpful to remember that your assessment may not be perfect and that you can learn from other people. Discussion can help you improve your position and help the other stakeholders reflect on theirs. Wherever possible, this is likely to be the best decision, but where stakeholders cannot agree, constructive discussion may be difficult and other methods might be sought.

3. **Influence the owner or vet.** A nurse might try to influence the owner or vet. Legally, the owner's decision should be informed and not unduly influenced but there is a very fine line between 'neutral' advice and undue influence.

There are legitimate and acceptable ways to influence clients. Generally, owners rely on the veterinary team to provide advice and give recommendations and often ask directly, 'What is the best course of action?' or 'What would you do?' Even once they have been informed by the vet, owners may still need guidance in deciding between options, and the nurse can give useful advice on the decision-making process as well as providing the information. Similarly, vets may benefit from advice on certain issues – they are not always as sure as they may appear. With effective communication and empathy, nurses can provide education and advice about both the clinical issue and the welfare concepts and their ethical implications. So long as care is taken not to *unduly* influence the owner, this can legitimately achieve the nurse's goals. There are no such legal limits on influencing the vet, beyond professionalism and common decency.

4. **Direct opposition.** Sometimes it may be necessary for a nurse to tell the owner or vet that she or he disagrees with their choice. It is tricky to know when such comments are appropriate. Clearly, when nurses witness something they feel is unethical, they should not feel obliged to remain silent out of deference or out of fear of the personal consequences. On the other hand, comments may be inappropriate if the owner's or vet's decision is different from the nurse's but still perfectly reasonable or if the disagreement is too trivial to make it worth any ensuing unpleasantness. Criticisms from the benefit of hindsight are especially risky, as people can be very touchy about cases where the outcomes were not what they hoped.

Conscientious objection. In addition to nurses stating their disagreement with a decision, they can also decide not to be involved. This is called 'conscientious objection'. Even if nurses cannot force owners or vets to do the right thing, they can maintain their integrity by refusing to be involved. As with influencing, this has its ethical limits and a nurse should not refuse to do reasonable options just because there is an even

better option available. In cases where both vet and nurse may object to the owner's requests, communication between vet and nurse can help each other to check the reasonableness of their position and strengthen their resolve. In cases where the vet is compliant with the owner and where conscientious objection might harm the animal, nurses may have to reconsider their own position bearing in mind that two other people agree; but if they feel sure that they are right, then they may still wish to refuse to help.

Direct action. In some cases, a nurse might actively act without other people's consent, e.g. treating an animal without consent or without the veterinary surgeon's directions or refunding money against the boss's instructions. This is legally safer when the owner's/boss's wishes are unknown and the nurse acts reasonably. It is legally more risky when the nurse's actions affect other people's property against their wishes.

Whistle-blowing. 'Whistle-blowing', actively reporting the owner or vet, is a step further than direct action. You can report a colleague to the employer or line-manager (although this will not work if the problematic person *is* your employer). You can report veterinarians and RVNs to the RCVS professional conduct department by making a formal complaint. Employers can be reported to bodies such as the Health and Safety Executive, the Office of Fair Trading, Veterinary Medicines Directorate (VMD) or the police for contravening laws, such as fraud or misuse of drugs. Anyone who harms an animal or fails to provide for its needs – including owners, veterinarians and RVNs – can be reported to the police or Royal Society for Prevention of Cruelty to Animals (RSPCA) (Scottish Society for Prevention of Cruelty to Animals [SSPCA] in Scotland). The law governing these offences is covered in Chapter 5.

The ethical reasons to report someone can be based on avoiding certain consequences that cannot be legally achieved otherwise, e.g. preventing continued abuse, future harm to other animals or even children, where a nurse has additional concerns that a child might also be likely to be abused. They might also be based on justice, in that wrongdoers should not be allowed to get away with their misdeeds.

At the same time, there are ethical reasons *against* reporting. As well as being a legal and professional matter, respect for confidentiality has ethical bases. For example, the owner or other clients might be less keen to get their animals treated if they fear being reported. The person reported may suffer enormously. If the person is found guilty, this can lead to the person being struck off from working as a vet or RVN. If not, then it is a source of embarrassment and antagonism for the nurse who reported the person. So the option of reporting should not be taken lightly. One general rule might be to report only if a person has acted *unreasonably* and the whistle-blowing is likely to have a desirable effect overall.

ACT

The final act is often the hardest bit. Many philosophers have written about **weakness of will**, where people make decisions but then somehow do not quite put them into practice. Sometimes we forget to do things or wrongly assume that a colleague will do it. It can be useful to put a system such as care plans in place to help people remember and communicate better. Sometimes selfishness can stop a nurse from enacting his or her decision – a nurse might resolve to be more helpful or be less irritable but then feels tired or poorly and does not do it.

At other times, it is hard to complete a plan that harms one of the stakeholders. It can be very hard to kill an animal even when you think it is the right thing to do. When thinking about an imaginary animal suffering, it is easy to say 'Yes I would kill it', but with the animal and owner in front of you, it can be much harder. It is especially hard if it is your own animal. Such feelings are natural and they should not make you feel guilty or embarrassed. It can be good to remind yourself that you are doing what you think is right. Remember that owners face this problem as well, so you may need to help them carry out their decisions.

REFLECT ON THE DECISION AND OUTCOMES AND PREPARE FOR NEXT TIME

One of the most important stages is to think back over a decision. Reflective practice is a good way to develop one's ethical reasoning skills and improve as a nurse. It also helps prepare for next time, so this step and thinking about ethical problems before they occur may be combined.

Firstly, reflective practice can help you avoid future conflicts. Just as owners can learn to recognise early signs of ear or anal gland disease and avoid it flaring up, so you can get better at avoiding awkward situations. You can warn owners or vets in advance that you will not help with a bulldog Caesarean. You can tell members of the public not to bring healthy grey squirrels into the practice.

When a decision has gone well, one usually does not think to reflect on it, but reflecting on good decisions is useful. It can be a 'reward' that might help you act well next time. It can also help you see ways in which a decision could be improved; so next time, it is even better. It may help identify *why* a decision was good (e.g. was it down to good communication, empathy, integrity, animal welfare assessment, fairness, etc.) so that you can make sure you do the same next time. Reflecting that you did the right thing can reduce the guilt felt at the final act. The same goes for the vet and the owner, and it can be good to remind them that they did the right thing.

When a decision has gone badly, you may not want to think about it because you feel guilty, but this only makes matters worse. It can be better to bring this guilt out into the open; indeed this is one of the main aspects of psychotherapy. Reflecting on decisions that have gone wrong can help identify why they went wrong (e.g. was it down to not enough information, bad reasoning, weakness of will, etc.) in preparation for next time.

Reflection after the event is dangerous if done wrong. It is very easy to spot mistakes *after* they have been made. You forget that at that time you did not have the knowledge and experience that you do now that it is all over. This is true for clinical decisions as well. It is easy for a team or owner to think that one should, or should not, have operated once the dog is dead, but it may be that at the time, operating was, or was not, the best thing to do however it turned out. In reflecting on one's own decisions, it is wrong to feel guilt if the decision was right at the time, even if it turned out badly. Thus, you should not feel bad and you may also have a role in helping owners and vets avoid guilt for good past decisions. Conversely, in reflecting on other people's decisions, you should consider what they knew at the time. Judging people after the event can cause enormous offence and annoyance. This 'moralising' is one danger of ethical reasoning that you should make sure you avoid: ethics should be a constructive exercise helping everyone to make better decisions and achieve desirable outcomes in practice.

BIBLIOGRAPHY

Adams, C.L., Bonnett, B.N., Meek, A.H., 2000. Predictors of owners' response to companion animal death in 177 clients from 14 practices in Ontario. J. Am. Vet. Med. Assoc. 217, 1303–1309.

Bentham, J., 1789. Introduction to the Principles of Morals and Legislation. Clarendon Press, Oxford.

Donovan, J., Adams, C.J. (Eds.), 1996. Beyond Animal Rights: A Feminist Caring Ethic for the Treatment of Animals. Continuum, New York.

Farm Animal Welfare Council, 1993. Second Report on Priorities for Research and Development in Farm Animal Welfare. FAWC, London.

Kant, I., 1963. Lecture in Ethics (L. Infield, Trans.). Harper & Row, New York.

Kant, I., 1996. Metaphysics of Morals (M. Gregor, Trans.). CUP, Cambridge, pp. 192–193.

Kubler-Ross, E., 1969. On Death and Dying. Collier Books/Macmillan, New York.

Mill, J.S., 1987. In: Ryder, A. (Ed.), Utilitarianism and Other Essays. Penguin, New York, pp. 272–338.

RECOMMENDED READING

Animal Ethics Dilemma. Available from: <http://www.aedilemma.net/>.
A fun interactive tool that challenges you in a number of cases. It gives you an indication of your own underlying moral theories, but you should be careful not to pigeonhole yourself and then try to live up to that classification (remember it is only a tool).

Beauchamp, T., Childress, J., 1979. Principles of Biomedical Ethics. Oxford University Press, Oxford.
The original book describing the Four Principles, updated several times since. It uses medical cases, which makes it less directly relevant.

DeGrazia, D., 2002. Animal Rights: A Very Short Introduction. Oxford University Press, Oxford.
A brief and readable guide to animal ethics from a prominent philosopher. It is useful for considering the 'bigger picture' issues, rather than veterinary matters.

Fraser, A.F., Broom, D.M., 2007. Domestic Animal Behaviour and Welfare. CAB International, Oxford.

A good general review of welfare issues of different animals, this latest edition contains sections on companion animals.

Mepham, B., Kaiser, M., Thorstensen, E., et al., 2006. Ethical Matrix Manual. LEI, The Hague.
A brief guide to making and using ethical matrices.

Pullen, S., Gray, C., 2006. Ethics, Law and the Veterinary Nurse. Butterworth-Heinemann, Oxford.
A collection of essays on aspects of ethics and law for veterinary nurses. It is well written and focuses on nurse issues. It does have a high variation in quality of chapters, and some overlap.

Rollin, B., 2006. An Introduction to Veterinary Ethics. Wiley-Blackwell, Oxford.
This has been the main textbook on veterinary ethics. It is divided into a theoretical introductory part and a discussion of specific cases. The cases relate to real life, and Rollin writes engagingly and passionately.

Stewart, M.F., 2003. Companion Animal Death. Butterworth-Heinemann/Petsavers, Oxford.
A simple and short book on bereavement in pet owners.

Yeates, J., 2013. Animal Welfare and Veterinary Practice. Wiley/UFAW, Oxford.
A brief book for veterinary surgeons and nurses covering all aspects of welfare-based practice.

Yeates, J.W., 2014. The role of the veterinary nurse in animal welfare. Vet. Nurs. J. 29 (7), 150–251.
A short analysis of nurses' and others' responsibilities.

Yeates, J.W., Main, D., 2009. Assessment of companion animal quality of life in veterinary practice and research. J. Small Anim. Pract. 50 (6), 274–281.
Practical recommendations for QOL assessment in veterinary practice.

2 Customer Care and Communication

ALISON LAMBERT

KEY POINTS

- Communication is one of the most important aspects of customer care.

- Understanding the customer journey will enable you to help support your customers in the care of their pet.

- The telephone is the most important aspect of clients' communication with your practice.

Introduction

CUSTOMER CARE IS EVERYONE'S JOB

More and more practices and veterinary professionals are acknowledging the crucial role of the customer experience in the success of the practice. You might think, as a veterinary nurse, that your influence is fairly minimal here – after all, all the 'customer service' stuff happens at the reception desk; your role is to care for the animals, not the owners.

In fact this could not be further from the truth. Everyone at the practice is responsible for shaping the customer experience, and everyone must be equally good – what's the point in having a friendly and efficient check-in if the consultation is rushed, vague and running very late? You might have developed a relationship of trust with your client, but if the products you recommend are bundled at her with a surly grunt and a hefty bill back at reception, then the lasting impression of your practice is not good.

Consistently high quality is key.

IT'S NO LONGER GOOD ENOUGH TO BE JUST GOOD ENOUGH

Not so long ago, if an owner had a sick animal she would call the local practice.

That's *practice* – singular.

Nowadays, there are several practices in her town to choose from, all competing on price, quality and convenience. An owner is just as likely to search online and come to her own conclusions before buying some cut-price medication on her favourite shopping website. Or she may ask fellow dog walkers for advice, or speak to her groomer, kennel hand or that nice woman at the rescue centre who gave her mobile number and said to call any time with any queries.

The fact is that with far more options available to the average pet and horse owner, practices must work hard to show potential clients why they are the obvious, and best, choice. It means that everyone at the practice must convey the same message, in the same professional and friendly way. In the last few years the number of UK practices has more than doubled – chances are that you now have several competitors just a stroll away:

- 2000 – 2200 UK practices
- 2014 – 4723 UK practices.

Of course there's the Internet. In your own life away from work, you probably use your smartphone or computer to check out what people think about that new restaurant in town, to find out what time the hairdresser closes on Saturdays or to order your shopping for home delivery. It will therefore come as no surprise to learn that this is exactly what your potential clients are doing too. Google 'vets in [your town]' and see just how many options there are. You'll also be able to see what people are saying about the place where you work, as well as about other practices in the area. In just a few clicks you'll be able to get a fair idea of which are the good practices. Perhaps yours is even one of them.

In the face of so much choice, and with access to so much information, increasingly owners tell us that their practice choice is made according to what they hear about it. This does not come down to how many operating theatres you have, or whether your complication rates are the lowest in the area – it comes down to how your practice 'feels'.

IT'S NOT WHAT YOU HAVE, IT'S HOW YOU HAVE MADE THE CLIENT FEEL

When we ask owners to name three things that they associate with their vet practice, they don't mention awards, equipment and the number of registered veterinary nurses. They use words associated with their customer experience – friendly, caring, good, helpful and so on. The Wordle (Fig. 2.1) illustrates the words used, taken from Onswitch's extensive national database; the size of each word is determined by its frequency of use. You'll notice that 'expensive' is there. Of course. Except that this is almost certainly also related to customer care, or rather a lack of it.

Owners rarely mention price as a consideration when choosing and staying with a practice, because for them it's not so much about the numbers at the bottom of the bill, but all the care, help and concern that has gone into it. 'Value for money' is paramount – if you have spent time explaining options to a client, making clear recommendations that are clearly in the best interests of the animal and interacting both with her and her pet/horse in a genuinely warm fashion, then she will happily pay whatever you charge and view it as fair. If, however, she has been presented with a large and unexpected bill without explanation, after feeling rushed through the appointment by a nurse who never made eye contact and did not know the animal's name, then she will view that same bill as expensive.

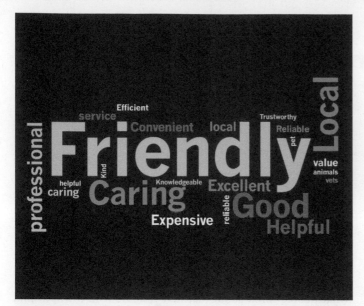

Fig. 2.1 'Describe your practice in three words.' (Onswitch qualitative research to March 2015)

Great customer care makes everything better. In this chapter we'll explore just why it's so important, and look at tips and techniques to help you deliver it consistently.

Customer experience is the key to business success

Research carried out in 2013 by independent research company Opinion Matters for New Voice Media found that an estimated £12 billion is lost by UK companies each year following an inadequate customer experience. Two thousand thirty-four UK adults were asked if they had switched to a different business as a result of poor customer service:

- 50% said yes.
- 28% said they switched because they did not feel appreciated.
- 22% moved because staff were unhelpful or rude.
- 16% switched because the buck had been passed.

While this is not uniquely veterinary sector data, these are also your customers – they have the same high standards for every company they deal with, be it a department store or a veterinary practice.

'In a fragile economy there is growing evidence of the link between customer satisfaction and business performance' (Institute of Customer Service, 2014). The Institute's latest report finds that:

- Customer service drives recommendation. When an organisation raises a customer's satisfaction by 3 points (out of 10) the likelihood of that customer recommending the organisation more than triples, from 17% to 56%.
- 60% of customers want a balance between price and service.
- A sizeable segment of customers have a preference for excellent service and are prepared to pay a premium for it.
- Just 15% are highly motivated to find the cheapest deals.
- The trust benefits of improving customer satisfaction are substantial and quantifiable. By delivering an increase of 10 points (out of 100) in its satisfaction index score, an organisation will receive on average an increase of 13 percentage points in the trust rating from its customers (The Institute of Customer Service, 2014).

The word 'trust' is key here – we all choose to use companies and services that we know will take good care of us, exceeding our expectations rather than simply meeting our needs. This is because great customer care is not about giving clients what they need; it's about treating them how they want to be treated – over the phone, at the reception desk and in the consulting room. George 'needs' a flea treatment, but his owner 'wants' to be treated with respect – for someone to take the time to check George over, talk to his owner and make clear recommendations as to which products are best suited to them, with explanations as to why.

You can't get that on Internet sites.

Communication first requires understanding

In this chapter we'll look at the various touch points where your clients interact with the practice, creating a 'customer journey' that extends way beyond her time in the building or on the yard. Before we can learn how best to communicate with our clients at each stage of their journey, we need to understand their expectations, and put their contact with you and your practice into context.

Most of you will have pets or horses yourself – you understand the immense joy and occasional moments of anguish that they bring to our lives. Sometimes this basic premise may get forgotten at the end of a busy day, when your nemesis appears at the consulting room door with a face like thunder. Re-setting your expectation that the next 10 minutes are inevitably going to be torture will help ensure that they are not. Mrs Brown is agitated, but you can turn this around. Perhaps she is unsettled simply because she is worried about the fact that her beloved Sooty isn't eating normally?

Great communication actually starts with saying nothing – let your body language do the talking (look your client in the eye, keep your posture open [no crossed arms], don't hide behind the table, nod and smile as she speaks) and listen to what she says. Really listen.

How she is feeling right now is directly related to how her animal is doing:

- When the pet/horse is well, she is calm.
- When the pet/horse is sick, she is worried and upset.
- When it is an emergency (even if it is only an emergency in her mind!), she will be very stressed.

Your communication style therefore needs to be able to flex according to her mood state. You have to acknowledge this and understand the background in order to communicate effectively. Pressing ahead with your own predetermined agenda for the consultation will undoubtedly lead to a breakdown in communication, an even more frustrated Mrs Brown and an unrewarding end to the day for you.

Let's take a moment to go back to basics and understand just who this person is that you're being asked to communicate effectively with.

Who is the 'average' pet owner?

Onswitch have undertaken plenty of research across the UK and throughout Europe, and we have built up a fairly consistent

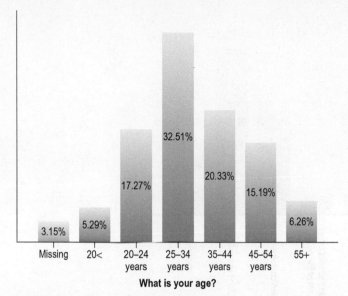

Fig. 2.2 Age of pet owners (Onswitch qualitative research to March 2015)

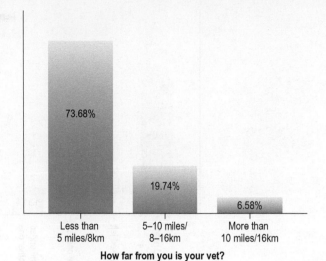

Fig. 2.3 Convenience is key (Onswitch qualitative research to March 2015)

picture of the average pet owner – who she is and how she thinks. The key observations are:

- Pets are viewed as a family member, not 'just' a dog.
- Anthropomorphic behaviour is common – owners overlay human characteristics and emotions onto their pets' actions and responses.
- Premiumisation of pet care is evident – hand-baked cat treats, extravagant accessories and dog food with human recipes in foil trays are all out there, and many owners are more than happy to pay for them.
- Half of dogs, 25% of rabbits and up to a fifth of cats are now classed as obese (Mintel data).
- Half of UK pets are not in a routine of preventative pet care (vaccinations, wormers, etc.). Owners love their pets, but many have not fully bought into the idea that these things are worth their time and money. Clearly we have some work to do here.
- The number of one-person households is rising – and while many are keeping pets as company, older people may choose not to keep pets either because they can't take care of them or are worried about the pet outliving them.
- Relative to the rest of the UK population, the over-45 age group is experiencing growth – at this stage of life pet ownership often shrinks; children leave home and family pets die and are not replaced.

AGE OF UK PET OWNERS

When we plot the age of the thousands of owners in our national database, the picture currently looks like that shown in Figure 2.2.

So your 'average' pet owner is likely to be middle-aged (between 25 and 45) and female (68% of the Onswitch database).

Research among 1200 riders by the British Horse Society finds that the demographics of horse owners are not that dissimilar – they are older (a third are aged over 45) but are also predominantly female (90%). We also know that three

quarters of pet owners live within 5 miles of their chosen practice (Fig. 2.3).

As we have seen, the 'average' owner also has more choice when it comes to veterinary care for her pets and horses. She is also more likely than her parents would have been to switch practices, rather than stay with the same vet for life. Crucially, this switching is often down to the customer experience received – when we asked owners to tell us why they had moved to another practice, over a quarter said that it was because they didn't like the clinical care, while just under a fifth said that it was down to poor customer service (Fig. 2.4).

'WHY DID YOU SWITCH PRACTICE?'

The bottom line is that if nurses, vets and receptionists are not treating the owner with respect, then we cannot rely on keeping their business. Which is why it is so important that we understand how best to meet our clients' needs through effective communication at every stage of their customer journey.

UNDERSTANDING THE CUSTOMER JOURNEY

Perhaps you have never given much thought to your customer's journey. You may even be wondering why this fancy marketing concept applies to veterinary practice at all – your clients don't 'go on a journey', they just bring their animals to you for treatment.

Well, maybe that was true 20 years ago – when the number of practices in the UK was half what it is now, when the Internet did not exist and when customer expectations were not nearly so high. Today, however, your customers are most definitely on a journey, and the truth is that if you don't recognise that, they will almost certainly be leaving you and heading for a practice that demonstrably does.

If you don't know where you're going, how are you going to know when you get there?

The term 'customer journey' simply describes the different points of interaction that an owner has with your practice. It's a really useful exercise to map out these various touch points, as you'll see that they often occur before an owner (and potential new client) has even set foot in your building.

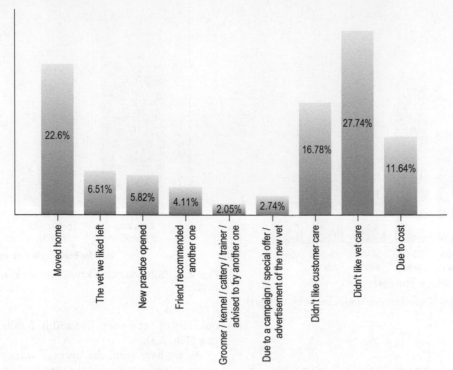

Fig. 2.4 'Why did you switch practice?' (Onswitch qualitative research to March 2015)

As you can probably guess, the phone is the first direct contact that the majority of owners have with your practice. They may have already come into contact with you virtually, either by doing some online research, talking to their friends and family or hearing about the practice from a local business or service (dog walkers, farriers, catteries etc.). Even if these businesses don't use your practice themselves, they will have an opinion on it, shaped by their own clients' feedback, both good and not so good. Google data suggest that 88% of consumers research before they buy, consulting on average 10.4 sources. That's a lot of potential competition.

This stage of awareness, precontact, is known as the Zero Moment of Truth.

The owner may then choose to make contact, almost certainly by phone – the First Moment of Truth – after which she will have formed an opinion of your practice based entirely on the person she spoke with. It may be while you're covering the reception desk at the end of your shift, tired and looking forward to going home. So it may not exactly be a fully representative picture of your practice, but it has made an impression nonetheless.

Assuming she liked what she heard, and felt good about your practice, the owner will then make an appointment to come and see you. This is where the Second Moment of Truth takes place – in the consulting room, when your delivery of both clinical and customer care is being subconsciously measured. Let's hope you're on form!

A customer journey map for the 'average' practice might look something like this (Fig. 2.5):

Awareness – Zero Moment of Truth.

Enquiry – First Moment of Truth. Having seen you on Google, or heard good things about you, the owner will call the practice. Maybe she will ask the price of your vaccinations, or whether you are taking on new clients at the moment – but whatever she asks, it's not *what* you say, but *how* you

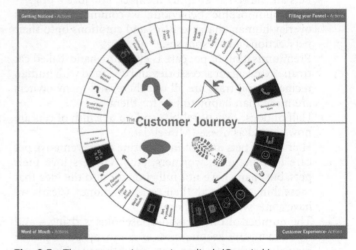

Fig. 2.5 The customer journey is cyclical. (Onswitch)

say it that will make the biggest impression at this crucial stage of her journey. If you are warm and friendly, provide plenty of information tailored to her circumstances and her pet or horse, and offer her an appointment, she will leave the call feeling that your practice is a place that cares for her as well as for her animal.

Selection – She has called a few practices, and the prices quoted are all pretty similar. She's going to choose the practice that she felt best about, and this could even be the most expensive one. Onswitch research shows that price alone drives just 10% of initial practice choices.

Visit – Second Moment of Truth. You have now gained a client! There are so many points of interaction involved in visiting a practice, all of them equally important in terms of the impression they create. If any one of these interactions is disappointing, it will colour her perceptions of the whole practice. What the owner sees, smells, hears, touches and feels at each stage counts:

- Signage close to the practice
- Car park
- Entrance
- Reception desk
- Waiting area
- Being called for appointment
- Consultation
- Collecting prescriptions
- Paying the bill
- Saying goodbye.

Repeat visit – Assuming her experience of your practice was wonderful at every stage, your client may choose to return. Never forget that she does have choices, and her journey can easily fork off towards another provider if your standards slip.

Recommend – This is, in some ways, the end of the journey. Your delighted client tells others about you, so that you gain new ones without having to spend a penny on marketing. And yet it's not the end of the journey at all, because just as those new clients may go on to recommend you to others, the one who brought them here in the first place will continue to use you – visiting more often and spending more as you earn her trust with an excellent customer experience that runs through every point of interaction.

Mapping the customer journey for your practice allows you to measure what happens at each stage. Put yourself in your clients' shoes and take the journey yourself – go outside and look at the building from the road, have a walk round the car park, take in the view from the doorway:

- What is your web presence like?
- How easy is it to find your practice?
- What do you see when you walk through the door?
- What does the waiting room smell like?
- Are the team wearing name badges, uniforms, smiles?

Every one of these seemingly small things combines to represent your practice, and any one of them can send a potential client headed for the competition.

The veterinary business model – five key steps to continued success

Having mapped out the customer journey, we can provide some signposts at key stages to turn callers into clients. Ultimately there are five crucial steps where your excellent communication and customer care can influence this circular customer journey:

a. Make the phone ring. This is all about building awareness in your area. It can be done through social media, door drops, sponsorship of local events, working closely with key opinion leaders in related animal care businesses and so on.

b. Convert the caller into a paying client – through the enquiry and selection stages discussed previously.

c. Convert the consultation into further treatment and care.

d. Charge correctly and fairly for all work done.

e. Get recommended (which in turn makes the phone ring, and so it goes round again…).

RAISING AWARENESS LOCALLY

Perhaps as a veterinary nurse, marketing does not feature in your job description, but there's no reason why it can't. If it isn't currently being managed by anyone at the practice, marketing is a great area to get your teeth into and one where you can really make a difference. After all, it's in everyone's interests to get the phone ringing with new clients wanting to register.

Getting that Zero Moment of Truth isn't just reliant on a potential client finding you online; you can actively communicate with local pet and horse owners to let them know just why your practice is so special. Pick a unique selling point to talk about – every small animal practice offers dietary management advice, for example, but you might be the only one who does it at a community centre drop-in session.

Routes you might consider include any or all of the following, depending on the time and budget available:

- Local radio
- Regional TV
- Adverts of flyers in local free press/dailies/weeklies
- Direct mail or email campaigns (the latter are much cheaper but need email addresses)
- Hoardings/bus stops/roundabout posters
- Posters in local businesses (where your target audience also shop) – takeaways, pet shops, library etc.
- Sponsoring and attending community events–dog walkathons, horse shows, village fetes
- Giving out branded merchandise (bags/pens/fridge magnets/dogdanas etc.)
- Attending shops, parks and places with a small stall or flyers, the places where pet and horse owners hang out
- Organising open days.

If you do take responsibility for managing this crucial line of client communications, it is important to ensure that the rest of the team know what you're doing. All that goodwill can easily be undone when an owner calls to take advantage of a special offer for new clients, except that the reception team don't know anything about it.

TELEPHONE CUSTOMER CARE – THE FIRST MOMENT OF TRUTH

Your landline is your practice lifeline

You may not give much thought currently to your practice phone – when it rings, someone answers it. The customer service team, or you if you happen to be at the reception desk, give advice, answer queries and book requested appointments, then get off the phone as quickly as possible. That's efficient, it works, it's what we've always done.

Except that today's pet and horse owner doesn't want to be treated like everyone else and given minimal time and attention. They expect (quite rightly) to be treated with interest, respect, enthusiasm and care, even on a short phone call. In fact, *especially* on a short phone call – an owner rings to ask the price for a vaccination, but what she is really looking for is an idea of what it feels like to be a client. If you are warm, welcoming and interested then she is highly likely to choose you ahead of the practice that simply said '£35' and hung up.

Let's say a new owner calls asking for the price of a vaccination. You could just tell her £35, or you could use the opportunity to ask after the animal, use its name, and engage the owner in a genuine warm dialogue discussing the services your practice offers in addition – a free health check, for example. You choose to do the latter, and she feels good about your practice, so she registers and books a vaccination consultation (£35) where you discuss diets and worming. In addition to the consultation and vaccination fee, she goes on to purchase a wormer (£15) and a premium life-stage diet (£30). She then comes back every 3 months to do more of the same, and has told her friends about the great service, so two of them register with you too.

Conservative estimates have the lifetime value of a pet to a practice at anywhere upward of £3,000 – a fantastic return on those 5 minutes you spent with the client on the phone.

Suddenly it's not just a phone call; it's an income stream. We already know that 90% of primary client contact is over the telephone, which means that the phone is instrumental in bringing in additional revenue by:

- Driving new client registrations
- Converting price checkers into clients (successful small animal practices convert 40% of calls into consultations, and successful equine practices can be up at 80%)
- Boosting compliance with routine preventative health care
- Turning consultations into additional investigations and procedures (successful practices convert a quarter of all primary calls into procedures).

When you think that the average practice receives 1000 calls per vet per month, suddenly the phone becomes a crucial stage on the customer journey. Every call needs to deliver an excellent customer experience, regardless of who is answering it and at what time of day.

The 'five steps' to success on the telephone

Perhaps you're thinking, 'It's all very well telling us we have to deliver excellent care consistently on every call, but we get so many phone calls, and so many of them just wanting basic information – how on earth am I supposed to do all this as well as my day job?'

If so, there's good news – a simple but highly effective five-step process will help you deliver an excellent customer experience every time. And it takes just a few minutes:

a. Use your name. Clarify a practice protocol that everyone uses for greeting callers: 'Hello, AnyVets, Sarah speaking, how can I help?'

b. Use the pet's or horse's name. Establish some personal details early on and repeat them back to the caller throughout; this is a great way to build rapport and trust.

c. Answer the price question at the end. If the caller has asked how much vaccinations are, let her know that they are administered in a double appointment with the veterinary surgeon, they carry out a full health check, with free nurse clinics/puppy parties, etc. Add value to your service, and never apologise if the price seems high – it is a fair reflection of everything else that goes with it and is unlikely to be significantly higher than elsewhere.

d. Provide practice information. Tell the caller if you offer late-night hours or have a large car park to make visiting easier. Direct her to your website for more information.

e. Always offer an appointment. Don't leave it for the owner to call back – ask whether tomorrow afternoon is convenient, for example, and offer to make a booking now.

Without face-to-face contact and in just a few minutes, it's more challenging to make a good first impression. Using these simple five steps, not only does the caller experience a glimpse of how it feels to be a client, but also you have an effective process to follow which makes it easy to provide great customer care even if you may be feeling tired, stressed or distracted.

Taking telephone customer care to the next level

Forward-thinking practices don't just wait for owners to ring, they manage calls proactively:

- Calling clients when booster vaccinations and dental checks are due
- Phoning the owner with updates following surgery (how many of you still advise owners to 'ring anytime after 2'?)
- Booking follow-up appointments at the time of the visit rather than saying 'give us a call if there are any problems'.

The telephone is a vital tool in client communication and customer care, and this aspect should be a part of all veterinary nurse training and continued professional development (CPD). If your managers need persuading that this is a good use of your time, remind them that the average lifetime value of a pet is £3,000. If your new skills bring in even just a handful, that course will have been an amazing investment.

FACE-TO-FACE CLIENT INTERACTION – THE SECOND MOMENT OF TRUTH

We've all had them – those clients that cause us to grit our teeth and assume the brace position as they approach. Yet in the vast majority of cases, it's actually not the client that is 'difficult', rather the situation, with emotions running high. The client's ability to think and act rationally may be affected by fear or uncertainty, so that any misunderstanding can easily become magnified into a conflict.

Communicating is not just about speaking

Mehrabian's model is a much-quoted insight into the communication process, showing that only a very small amount of what people express is done so through the words used:

- 7% of meaning is in the words that are spoken.
- 38% of meaning is paralinguistic (the way that the words are said).
- 55% of meaning is in facial expression.

It is therefore crucial to be aware of the importance of your body language and non-verbal cues when interacting with clients. We need to pick up on these cues given by our clients too, as these give a much better understanding of how they are really feeling.

BUILDING RAPPORT

Rapport happens when you and the owner are synchronised, and when you have reached this state you can be more direct, leading the conversation with clear recommendations. Conversely, if you have not established a rapport with the client, your assertiveness may well be interpreted as aggression.

The key here is to practise 'match, pace and lead' with your client:

Match:

- Mirror her body language (subtly of course).
- Match her words (don't use jargon and scientific terminology when she uses layman's terms).

- Repeat her words and play them back during the conversation (e.g. if she has told you she is worried about her dog's dry skin, then bring your recommendations back to this).

Pace:
- Take the conversation along at the same speed that your client sets.
- Check her understanding before moving on to new topics.

Lead:
- Move the consultation where you want it to go – she may have come in worried about dry skin, but if it indicates other things, move your recommendations towards the underlying issue once you have established rapport and understanding.

PROCESSES PREVENT ISSUES

In the consulting room, a breakdown in communication between nurse and client is the most common reason for problems. This will most likely be because of poor estimating (e.g. the owner receives a far higher bill than expected, for treatment the owner does not understand) or a lack of clarity and explanation (pets are hospitalised and the owner does not understand length of stay, what will happen or why).

Such breakdowns can be avoided by following a seven-step, tried-and-tested process:

a. Be prepared. Make sure you have read through the patient's notes and have all the relevant equipment and paperwork to hand. If you're giving vaccinations, have the vials in the room ready.

b. Greet and acknowledge the animal directly. Make eye contact, use your own name, talk to the pet/horse and use its name.

c. Establish the owner's priority through open questions. Open questions are those that do not have a 'yes' or a 'no' answer. Asking, 'How are you getting on, Misty?' will generate more information than 'So we're doing Misty's vaccinations today?'

d. Undertake an obvious examination. Remember we talked about owners wanting value for their money? This may be the only time you see the animal all year – carry out a thorough check from nose to toes and explain to the owner what you're looking for and what you've found along the way.

e. Make clear recommendations (academic studies find that owners are seven times more likely to comply with follow-up treatment when the word 'recommend' is used). Don't say things like 'I think we should', 'I'm just going to' or 'I'd like to try this' – they sound vague at best and unprofessional at worst. You are the expert; the owner is paying for your expertise, so give it.

f. Clarify and check that the owner understands, and is happy with, next steps.

g. Book the next appointment. Even if the patient is discharged there will be preventative health care and annual health checks to book, so don't wait for the owner to call – she may forget or go elsewhere.

WHEN PREVENTION FAILS, THERE IS A CURE

Sometimes, despite your best efforts, there are still difficult situations to deal with. Common causes for customer complaints include:

- Consultations starting or finishing late
- Nurses leaving the room midconsult (prepare yourself, remember?)
- Appearing rushed/distracted/unsympathetic
- Value perceptions:
  - 'I was only in for a few minutes'
  - 'It's how much?'

Fortunately, most situations can be resolved by using KLARDOC:

Keep calm.

Listen – Put assumptions aside and really hear what the client is telling you.

Acknowledge – Repeat what you have just heard, for clarity.

Refine and **D**efine – Summarise the key facts, aside from the emotion.

Overcome – Present possible solutions and alternatives.

Close – Thank the client and detail the timings of any further action.

The trick is to acknowledge that the client has her own frame of reference, her own background to the events unfolding in front of us; it then becomes far easier to take the emotion out of the situation by sympathising. As mentioned previously, a 'difficult' client is simply a frustrated, confused, worried or distracted client. Using the five-step telephone process and the seven-step consultation skills to manage communications effectively will greatly reduce both the frequency and pain of those difficult encounters (also see Chapter 3).

Once you have resolved a tricky situation, follow-up will be crucial in order to prevent recurrences. Communication breakdowns are another common reason for complaints so manage this by keeping in touch with your anxious owner in a pre-agreed way. Determine how you will contact her – phone, texts, emails – and let her know when to expect contact. If you know that her pet is listed for surgery at the end of the day, it doesn't help to say that you'll call in the afternoon after the operation – she'll be waiting for your call from 2pm onwards. If it won't be until 6pm that you can call, tell her, and let her know that by this time you'll be able to give her a full picture of how her beloved pet is doing.

Similarly, most payment issues can be avoided by providing detailed information in advance. When talking to your clients about fees and charges:

- Don't apologise.
- Itemise or summarise everything that's included.
- Be confident about your fees (make sure that you understand the pricing structure and have details to hand; don't be vague).
- Display prices clearly at reception.
- Give written estimates in advance.

If it sounds straightforward, it is! There's nothing mysterious or complicated about providing a great customer experience – we simply have to treat our clients how we expect to be treated as clients ourselves. Ultimately, if you are open and friendly, the rest will follow.

ONLINE COMMUNICATION: WEBSITES AND SOCIAL MEDIA

If your practice is not using social media to connect and communicate with your clients, you're missing out. You can be sure that plenty of others are, and they're probably doing a great job of it too.

Social media is not only an integral part of modern life; it's a vital tool in your practice communications – a fast and free

---

BOX 2.1 USE OF SOCIAL MEDIA IN EVERYDAY LIFE

- About 83% of adults are online.
- Nearly all 16–24s and 25–34s are now online (98%), and there has been an increase in those ages 65+ going online (42% vs. 33% in 2012).
- The number of adults using tablets has almost doubled, from 16% in 2012 to 30% in 2013.
- Six in ten UK adults (62%) now use a smartphone, an increase from 54% in 2012. This increase is driven by 25–34s and 45–54s, although those ages 65–74 are almost twice as likely to use a smartphone now compared to 2012.
- Two-thirds of online adults say they have a current social networking site profile, unchanged since 2012.
- About 96% have a current profile on Facebook, while 3 in 10 have a Twitter profile and 1 in 5 have a YouTube (22%) or WhatsApp profile (20%).
- About 60% of social media users visit sites more than once a day, an increase from 50% in 2012, and with 83% of 16–24s doing so (69% in 2012).
- On average, Twitter users say they follow 146 people or organisations and have 97 followers.

Ofcom Adults' Media Use and Attitudes Report 2014.

---

way to engage with clients. Box 2.1 shows just how engrained in our lives social media and online activity have become.

Social media is exactly that, it's social – friendly, involving, personal, fun and interactive. It enables practices to talk *with* clients, rather than *at* clients. It may seem a subtle difference, but it's massively important in influencing the 'feel' of your practice. It makes good business sense too – according to Facebook, people who 'like' your page spend twice as much as customers who are not connected to you in this way. Aside from driving turnover, creating an active Facebook community is probably the single best thing you can do to enhance the customer experience at your practice. The two key words in that sentence, though, are 'active' and 'community'; here's why.

Lots of practices have Facebook pages; unfortunately many of them are very sparsely populated with news and photos. There may be a few 'likes' but there is no obvious activity or client involvement. This is *antisocial* media. It does not tell potential clients that your practice is a caring, fun, friendly and helpful place – rather it sulkily shrugs your indifference. The obvious conclusion is that your service will be equally half-hearted.

If you're going to 'do' Facebook, do it properly. Taking responsibility for ensuring that the practice Facebook page works is a really important and fun role for the proactive veterinary nurse, and a great way to demonstrate your team spirit and enthusiasm (always useful at appraisal time).

The following tips will help you manage your Facebook duties more effectively:

- Get a practice smartphone. Updating statuses and adding photos becomes quick and simple if you don't have to log on to a computer at the main desk every time.
- Check the page three or four times a day – if there are any questions that need answering, or messages to pick up, it's much more professional to reply quickly. Similarly, if anyone has left any inappropriate content, you can respond to it swiftly.

- If negative comments are posted, don't delete them, deal with them. If there is a genuine issue, detail what you are doing to rectify the situation. If it's just griping, ask the poster to come and have a chat with you – the practice always wants to deliver the very best service it can, and if someone feels you have fallen short, you want to be able to put things right and learn from it. You'll probably find that other clients will leap to your defence with words of praise and love too.
- Don't tolerate bad language or spiteful comments. You can delete persistent offenders' posts after you've warned them you will do so. Always report trolls or truly nasty comments directly to Facebook.
- Put plenty of photos and videos up. The fact is that people love to look at pictures of funny or cute animals. YouTube is full of videos of animals doing hilarious things, and fortunately you spend your working day meeting these cute and hilarious pets – so while other companies have to spend hundreds of pounds sourcing photos from image banks, you've got a free and endless supply on tap.
- Make sure you get written permission to use photos and videos from your clients. You can easily add some standard words to all your practice literature saying 'I am happy for images of my pet to be used for practice marketing, which will include social media: YES or NO', and the vast majority will be more than happy to oblige.
- Create a library of 'how to' videos and post them to your page. How to … worm a cat, de-flea a dog etc. All done with warmth and humour as appropriate – this shows that your practice understands the realities of managing the routine stuff, and it demonstrates that you get what it's like to own a pet, and all the house-plant-attacking, fox-poo-rolling joy that these day-to-day realities bring.
- If you're really serious about driving word of mouth recommendations and boosting client numbers, then advertise. With Facebook advertising you can specify the location, age and gender of your target audience, so you can be sure that your message will be delivered to people in your area who are ready and willing to spend money with you (Fig. 2.6).

Ideas for Facebook content

Regular updates are key to driving repeat visits to your page and encouraging client interactions. The following is meant as a guide only but gives some ideas for what and when to post over the course of a month. Do try to post over the weekend too – this is when most of your clients may be checking Facebook. Posts can be scheduled for prespecified dates and times so you can set them up during the week (Fig. 2.7).

- **Welcome.** Welcome any new likers and promote your page. Give a brief synopsis of what they can expect to see on your page.
- **Case study.** Document a case study; it could be a routine castration or a fracture repair case. Take lots of pictures from admission to discharge and post with brief description and update. Remember to get permission from the owner.
- **Advice.** Give snippets of free advice such as worming or flea treatment. Invite friends in for a free nurse consultation. Perhaps post a symptom guide.

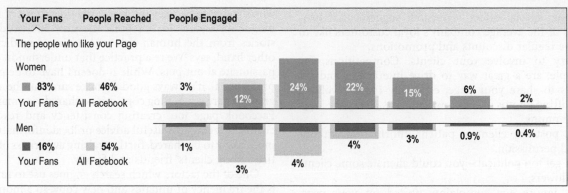

Fig. 2.6 Facebook statistics from a typical practice

	MONDAY	TUESDAY	WEDNESDAY	THURSDAY	FRIDAY	SATURDAY	SUNDAY
	Welcome new followers Case study – continue through week	Veterinary advice Article or link	Cute / funny picture of inpatient	Species / breed information and statistics	Directions / opening times / emergency hours Friday funny	Product offers / discounts	Species / breed information and statistics
	Welcome Case study	Pictures – A day in the life of …	Question / poll / survey	Veterinary advice Article or link	Facilities / equipment	Cute / funny picture of inpatient	Lost and found
	Welcome Case study	Veterinary advice Article or link	Weight-loss success story	Species / breed information and statistics	Meet the team	Charity suggestion	Sunday funny – quote or picture
	Welcome Case study	Species / breed information and statistics	Lost and found Event announcement	Veterinary advice Article or link	Team member profile	Video blog	Link to related community groups (dog shows, training classes etc)

Fig. 2.7 Daily Facebook suggestions

- **Article/link.** Articles can either be written by members of the team or posted via a link to a third-party website – e.g. microchip laws, how to get a pet passport, any outbreaks of disease.
- **Species/breed information and statistics.** Choose a species or breed and give some interesting facts; or help clients decide which pet is best suited to their lifestyle.
- **Pictures.** Post pictures of cute or unusual inpatients. Create a picture gallery of the animal's journey when visiting the practice.
- **Question/survey/poll.** Ask your clients for feedback and suggestions for the practice – what do they like and dislike? Post positive acknowledgements and responses. Or simply ask them about their pets and horses.
- **Weight loss success stories.** Take pictures and give regular updates with weigh-ins.
- **Lost and found.** Post information regarding any strays that have been brought in, or help clients find their lost pets by posting pictures and descriptions.
- **Events.** Post information about open days, charity events, local dog or cat shows, etc.
- **Practice information.** Give details of opening hours, emergency cover and directions to your practice.

- **Facilities/equipment.** Write a brief profile about a piece of veterinary equipment such as the radiography machine or scintigraphy equipment.
- **Friday funny.** Post a funny animal picture or quote.
- **Meet the team.** Team pictures and information on hobbies, pets, horses, etc. add a personal feel.
- **Team member profile.** Write a short profile about one of your team members. Document a 'day in the life' of a veterinary nurse.
- **Video micro blog.** This should be a short video clip of no longer than 2 minutes. It could show you giving advice on keeping your pet cool in hot weather or avoiding fly strike, for example; or it could be about you, where you trained, etc.

Facebook etiquette – do's and don'ts:
- Do vary the subjects of your posts.
- Do carry a case study through to the end.
- Do enrich posts with pictures and videos.
- Do ask questions; your reach will be wider when people comment, share and engage.
- Do ask for testimonials.
- Do direct visitors to your website occasionally.

- Do post special offers – research suggests that two-thirds of the average company's loyal customers like to receive regular discounts and promotions.
- Do try to involve your clients. Competitions, for example, are a great way to drive interaction and get clients to share your page, especially those involving submitting photos of their own animals. Everyone loves a cute puppy.
- Don't post any client or patient information without signed permission.
- Don't get too political – you could alienate some clients or followers.
- Don't ignore any complaints posted on your page. Acknowledge the issue, apologise for the way they feel and offer to chat things through with them privately.
- Don't post more than two or three times a day (but no less than three times a week).
- Don't be too serious all the time.

Beyond Facebook – Twitter and blogs

Facebook is undoubtedly the best place for your practice to start with social media. Once you've established a vibrant page with an engaged community of visitors, then Twitter is probably a good second step. The good thing about Twitter is that it's quick and instant – with only 140 characters it's great for short messages and reminders. Facebook users will generally check in a couple of times a day, whereas Twitter fans are hardwired to their phones for instant updates. So it's very useful for real-time things – drop-in clinic starting now (posted at the end of the working day to remind owners they can call in after work), reduced price flea treatments for the first 10 replies, etc. It's also extremely useful for following veterinary bodies, local pet and horse care businesses, pet stories and local media, giving you immediate notification of news and relevant issues.

Many practices feature blogs on their websites, but this is one example of where it's better not to do anything if you can't commit to doing it properly. Nothing says 'average practice who's trying to be relevant, but really doesn't get it' like a single blog that's a year old. A regular monthly 500-word piece with stories from the human side of veterinary medicine, on the other hand, says 'We're a practice that understands, cares and is passionate about pets'. While it doesn't have to be penned by a professional, it's always good to make sure that the spelling and grammar are good. Blog copy can be shared via emails and your Facebook page too, creating consistency and reaching more clients. If it contains useful advice or local information then it's more likely to be shared, further raising awareness of your practice among clients' friends and family.

One of the factors which search engines use to rank websites is the frequency of updates and new copy, so a monthly blog is also a great way to move your practice website up the rankings and onto the first page without paying for Search Engine Optimisation.

Common sense and consistency

So there you have it – pretty much everything you need to know about communication and the customer experience, and if you only put two things into action after reading this chapter, make it these:

- Use your common sense. Look at your practice, and your own habits and behaviours, through the eyes of a client. Ask yourself, 'How would I like to be treated?' and then make it happen.
- Be consistent. Clients are just as entitled to amazing customer care late on a Friday evening as they are on a Monday morning. It shouldn't depend who you're speaking to, what else is going on in your life, or what time it is – use the five steps when you take phone calls and the seven steps in the consultation room and every client will be delighted with their customer experience.

Because, in the oft-quoted words of Damon Richards, 'Your customer doesn't care how much you know until they know how much you care.'

REFERENCE

Ofcom, 2014. Adults' Media Use and Attitudes Report 2014. Available at: <http://stakeholders.ofcom.org.uk/market-data-research/other/research-publications/adults/adults-media-lit-14/>.

The Institute of Customer Service, 2014. UK Consumer Satisfaction Index, January 2014, Annual Report. The Institute of Customer Service. <https://www.instituteofcustomerservice.com/research-insight/research-library/july-2015-uk-customer-satisfaction-index-the-state-of-customer-satisfaction-in-the-uk>.

Mintel.com report, August 2015. 'Britain's Pet Owners'.

RECOMMENDED READING

Reichheld, F., Markey, R., 2011. The Ultimate Question 2.0 (Revised and Expanded Edition): How Net Promoter Companies Thrive in a Customer-Driven World. Harvard Business Review Press, Harvard.

Buckingham, M., Coffman, C., 2005. First, Break All The Rules. Simon & Schuster, London.

Hsieh, T., 2010. Delivering Happiness: A Path to Profits, Passion and Purpose. Business Plus, New York.

Gladwell, M., 2002. The Tipping Point: How Little Things Can Make a Big Difference. Abacus, London.

Thaler, R., Sunstein, C., 2009. Nudge: Improving Decisions about Health, Wealth and Happiness. Penguin Books, New York.

Silverman, J., Kurst, S., 2013. Skills for Communicating with Patients, third ed. CRC Press, London.

Consulting Skills and Clinics

NICOLA ACKERMAN

KEY POINTS

- Consultation skills are an important aspect of any job that involves communication with clients, whether in specific clinics, during nursing consultation or in surgical admissions and discharges.

- Nursing clinics can aid in animal health and welfare, but also build client bonding and loyalty to the practice.

- The structure of nursing clinics is generic regardless of practice; they just need to be adapted to be workable in each individual situation.

- Additional qualifications can be achieved in order to aid in nursing clinics, but are not mandatory.

Introduction

The role of the RVN has evolved greatly, standing now as a fee-earning regulated professional. Nurses have a vital role to play in the veterinary practice as consulting nurses, not limited just to the offering of advice to clients, but including performing the groundwork in collecting data parameters (blood tests, urine sampling, radiography, complex diet and behavioural histories) in order for the veterinary surgeon to then interpret the collected data and make a diagnosis, the undertaking of preventative health care for animals, postoperative appointments and wound management (see Chapter 4).

For nurses with a keen interest in consulting there is an ideal opportunity in which they can pursue the specialism that interests them while still being of use to the veterinary practice. Veterinary practices are businesses, and nurses that consult need to perform sufficient work not only to cover their costs and overheads, but also to make a profit. This is not necessarily through the charging for nurse clinics, but through the products that are sold, increasing the footfall through the practice and helping with client loyalty and, most importantly, compliance. The aim of this chapter is to provide an introduction to the consultation model around which the consultation process is formed, provide a format for many nursing clinics and give ideas on how to run these clinics.

The changing role of the RVN

RVNs that fully utilise skills learnt during training are more likely to remain with the profession and to feel a more valued member of the practice (LANTRA 2004). Consulting RVNs should not be viewed as 'mini-vets'; they perform a completely different role than veterinary surgeons, though many veterinary surgeons do undertake many roles that should be undertaken by nurses (e.g. blood sampling). These types of appointments need to be scheduled with a RVN, which will 'free up' the veterinary surgeon's time in order for them to undertake tasks that only they can undertake. From a business aspect this is making a much better use of time for the entire workforce. This is also the same argument for the use of animal nursing assistants and dedicated receptionists/telephonists.

Compliance

One of the roles of the RVN is to ensure that the client has good compliance with the recommendations given by the veterinary surgeon. In some cases this can refer to medications, and the nurse can discuss with the owner to determine that the owner is able to administer the prescribed medications. In some cases a different form of medication, liquid instead of tablets, can be of use. In these cases referral back to the veterinary surgeon is required as the client will require a different medication to be prescribed. Many owners do appreciate guidance on the administrations of medications, whether this is verbally or with leaflets. In regards to nursing clinics they are best utilised when the veterinary surgeon offers all newly diagnosed patients an appointment with the nurse in order to discuss all aspects of care for that patient. What this involves in the clinic will vary widely depending on the diagnosis. Items that may be discussed in the clinic can include diet (weight gain or loss, veterinary diets and lifestage diets, assisted feeding), administration of medications, exercise regimens, palliative care, increasing water intake, how to monitor their pets (checking capillary refill time, heart rate, urine output, blood glucose) and why compliance is so important. Discussion of all of these factors will mean that owners are more likely to comply with the veterinary surgeon's recommendations, and therefore bring in more income for the practice and improve the welfare of the pet. The CRAFT model (Box 3.1), developed in 2009, shows that for compliance to occur the *follow-through* aspect of the equation is required. The use of the nursing clinic to provide the follow-through to ensure acceptance from the client is vital.

Setting up nurse clinics

To succeed as professionals conducting their own nurse consultations, nurses need to be able to portray themselves as professionals. This includes how and where the nursing consultations are performed. The consultation room, as with a veterinary surgeon's consultation room, needs to be clean, tidy and fit for purpose. When setting up nurse clinics it is important to ensure that all the resources required are in place in order to make the venture a success. This can range from physical items (such as literature and weighing scales) to personnel training.

BOX 3.1   CRAFT COMPLIANCE

C = R + A + FT

Compliance = Recommendation + Acceptance + Follow-Through

A good, clear recommendation is required, along with acceptance from the client that the recommendation that was made is necessary. Follow-through is needed as many clients will accept the recommendation, but compliance is poor due to many factors (e.g. forgetting, money, time or the recommendation not being clearly made).

American Animal Hospital Association (AAHA), 2009. American Animal Hospital Association Compliance Study Executive Summary. Available from: <https://www.aahanet.org/PublicDocuments/ComplianceExecutiveSummary0309.pdf>.

BOX 3.2   EFFECTIVE LISTENING

GOOD LISTENING SKILLS ARE AN ESSENTIAL PART OF COMMUNICATION

- Seek clarification.
- Take notes.
- Avoid distractions.
- Use pauses and silences.
- Restate and summarise.

The literature that you decide to use within your consultations with clients needs to be of a high standard. The majority of clients will find it difficult to remember everything that is said within a consultation. It is helpful to give clients handouts on what has been discussed, and in some cases it can prove useful to provide written instructions. When clients walk out of the consultation room with information in hand, there is a perception that they have received better value for their money than just walking out empty-handed. Clients that have received written instructions, whether this is a hand-out or specific written instructions, are more likely to comply with the instructions given to them. If your handwriting is poor it can be useful to type instructions or bullet points for the client. This can be printed out or emailed to the client. It can prove useful to be able to direct clients to more information resources, and having more details available on your practice's website can be useful rather than them seeking out websites on their own. All of this needs to be in place before initiating the nurse clinic.

Good, effective communication is one of the most important skills to learn in veterinary practice (Box 3.2). Different forms of communication need to be utilised for the diverse demographics of pet owners that we see. Social media is the communication method of choice for one generation, but would not be for another. Adapting how you convey your message is important.

Consultation training

Several frameworks for consulting have been developed for medical education. However, none have been developed specifically for veterinary use. The Cambridge-Calgary consulting model was adapted by the National Unit for the Advancement of Veterinary Communication Skills (NUVACS) and therefore is the most relevant to all veterinary professionals undertaking consultations (Fig. 3.1). Learning how to conduct consultations is important and leads to more successful outcomes in compliance and understanding from the pet owner. The training of personnel is an important aspect of the overall success of nurse clinics. There are many sources of training for nurse clinics, including webinars, readings and day lectures. There are specific courses for nurses (and veterinary surgeons) who want to learn consulting skills. Theoretical learning of a practical task can be difficult, and the utilisation of practical sessions, workshops and observations can help adapt the theoretical learning into these practical skills. Watching other people consult can be helpful. Everyone conducts their consultations in a different manner, and observing other nurses and veterinary surgeons within practice can give ideas that can be incorporated into the learners' consultations. These methods of coaching can be extended to include video coaching and simulations (Grosdidier 2014).

The success of nurse clinics is directly related to the support from others within the veterinary practice. Clients need to be aware that clinics are being conducted. Marketing of clinics is a key point and needs to be performed in a way that all the practice members are 'on board' for the initiative. Recommendations from colleagues are invaluable, and having one of the veterinary surgeons referring clients is the best way to increase client numbers attending nurse clinics.

As mentioned, the Cambridge-Calgary consulting model (see Fig. 3.1) has been adapted by the National Unit for the Advancement of Veterinary Communication Skills (NUVACS) as the most relevant framework for the veterinary profession. The consultation process is broken down into seven separate sections, which, if followed, help to bring structure and flow to the process.

1.   PREPARATION

As with everything, preparation is key; any equipment required for the consultation should be prepared, the consulting room needs to be clean and the nurse should be familiar with the clinical history of the patient, in particular any relevant details. Make a note of the animal's name, sex and age, and use these when talking about the patient. Your appearance is also highly important as it governs the client's perception of you.

2.   INITIATING THE CONSULTATION

The consultation should be started by confirming the name of the client when calling the client through from the waiting area. Always introduce yourself, and confirm the nature of the appointment at the outset. Clients sometimes make an appointment for one cat, and then bring the other one instead as they could not locate or catch the initial one. If there is a delay, keep the waiting clients updated; not acknowledging increased waiting times will lead to frustration on the client's part.

Spend a few minutes getting acquainted with the patient. Dogs should be patted and spoken to and cats interacted with before removal from their basket; use of the pet's name is vital. If cats are unwilling to leave their baskets, remove the top half of the basket if possible and then either examine them in the bottom half of the basket or lift them out on their blanket onto the consulting table.

This stage is very important for creating rapport with both the client and his or her pet. Remember to use the client's name too, and consider whether it is appropriate to shake hands with

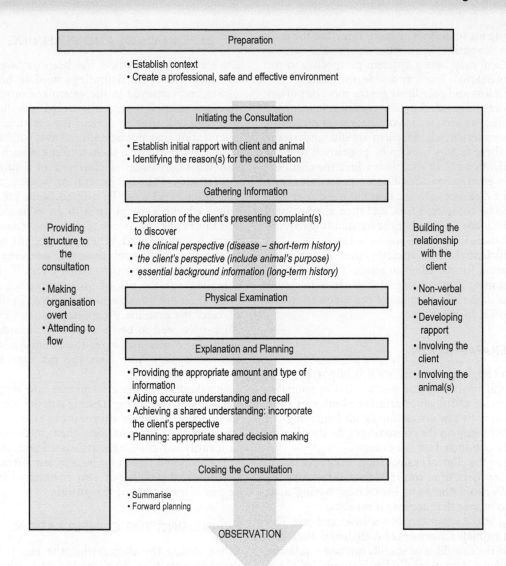

Fig. 3.1 Adapted Cambridge-Calgary model of veterinary consultation skills. (The Consulting RVN, *First Edition. Nicola Ackerman.* © *2012 John Wiley & Sons, Ltd. Published 2012 by John Wiley & Sons, Ltd.*)

the client. Most importantly, involve the pet. To create good rapport, nurses should empathise with the owners; indeed, empathy is an essential trait for all the practice team. In the majority of cases the pet is an integral family member, and this special bond needs to be respected. When children are brought into the consulting room, involving them can prove to be useful. Getting the children to weigh the pet or to read off the weight is a good example of this, especially in weight loss clinics as it helps compliance with the children feeding the pet. Having colouring books and pencils is useful to distract children – just remember to put their pictures on the wall in your consulting room. Whether or not the consultation is regarding the previous clinical history of the animal, if you mention or ask how the pet has been since the incident, the client feels that you care about his or her pet.

3. INFORMATION GATHERING

Background information can be gained from the clinical history, but additional information can be obtained through carefully focused questioning. Many clients are more than happy to offer information, whether it is relevant or not; some need specific questioning in order to retrieve the required information. Both open and closed questions should be utilised, as different types of answers can be gained. Questioning also helps provide information regarding the client's expectations and specific concerns. If conducted appropriately, this part of the process allows you to demonstrate your professionalism and knowledge while helping to build rapport with the client. Questions also help to give you time to think and time to focus. Use communication cues such as nodding your head to demonstrate interest in what the client is saying; listen to what the client is saying, and in some cases repeating back to the client what he or she has said can be helpful to confirm details.

This is a very important stage of the consultation, and one that is often overlooked or not completed to the full. In many situations when the consultation has finished the client often adds, 'And another thing…'. This can be pre-empted by focused questioning of the client at the outset. In some cases the client may have a very long list of queries or tasks. Prioritise the most important ones for the patient by negotiation with the client, if necessary, as the client may have a different perspective to you as a veterinary professional. You may decide, for example, that the dramatic weight loss and polydipsia are the most important factors to be considered whereas the client may be more worried about overlong nails or an increase in vocalisation for no reason. If this situation is experienced, the client should understand why you feel that these factors need to be prioritised over the clipping of the patient's nails. In situations where the client has a long list of non-emergency questions or procedures, it is important to hold a dialogue with the client at the outset as to which things are to be completed first, and then a subsequent appointment can be made to complete the outstanding requirements. Reasons for more than one appointment being necessary may include insufficient time to correctly cover all the items, too much information for the client to retain in one appointment, the pet becoming stressed (e.g. if its coat is matted it would be unfair to undertake removal of the matts all in one consultation) or to aid in compliance.

4. PHYSICAL EXAMINATION

When initiating the physical examination it is important to be aware of the clinical history of the animal. If the animal is known to have a tender abdomen or arthritic joints, care must be taken not to exacerbate any discomfort. With larger dogs, or those that do not like being on the consulting table, the physical examination can be conducted on the floor.

While performing the clinical examination it is important to talk through with the client what you are doing and looking for. Work systematically from the head backwards; having a set routine will help to ensure that nothing is missed.

Start by looking at the symmetry of the head and jaw. This is important when animals are presented with dental disease, as lumps or bumps on the mandible or maxilla can be an indicator of tooth root problems. Any nasal discharge should be noted, along with its colour and whether it is lateral or bilateral. When examining the eyes, the size of the pupils and their symmetry should be noted. The conjunctiva surrounding the eye should be examined to check for infection, and any discharge should be noted. Ears should be checked for discharge, wax, dirt and smell. Examination of the mouth will depend on the cooperation of the animal being examined. If the animal is known to be difficult to handle, in some circumstances asking the owner to lift the animal's lip up so that you can look at the teeth can be appropriate, provided that you are confident that this will not put the owner at risk of being bitten.

When palpating the animal's neck and shoulders, the lymph nodes should be checked, and if palpable this needs to be noted and referred to the veterinary surgeon. The condition of the coat and skin need to be assessed and checked for parasites. Limbs should be checked for range of movement. Cat owners should be questioned carefully about mobility, as most behavioural changes are put down to old age rather than reduced mobility. Examination should also include measuring and assessing heart rate and respiratory rate.

Finally, the overall condition of the animal should be noted, including body condition score (BCS), muscle condition score (MCS), and weight. Even if these parameters are the same as a previous recording, they should be recorded again in order to show stability of the animal's weight.

5. EXPLANATION AND PLANNING

Once all the information has been gathered and the animal examined, your initial findings need to be explained to the owner, and conveyed to the veterinary surgeon if necessary. If your consultation is primarily aimed at dealing with issues such as weight reduction or care of the geriatric patient, veterinary intervention may not be required as it will be your responsibility to explain and plan the next steps in such a way as to ensure that the information is conveyed in a form that the owner understands. This can be oral or written, and in some cases educational DVDs can be utilised. Some points will need to be reiterated, and a useful tip is to do so in a different format as this can enable the owner to fully understand the information that is being conveyed. When planning the next step the owner must agree with the decisions that are being made and be able to comply with the instructions given. If these steps are not complied with the risk of non-compliance increases dramatically. There are three elements involved in the implementation of care: the veterinary professional, the client and the pet. All parties need to be in agreement in order to make a plan work. The owner may agree to administration of oral medication on a daily basis, but the pet may resist, resulting in non-compliance.

Breaking down the information into 'digestible' chunks can be helpful for the owner. During lengthy consultations it can be useful to ask owners if they want to take notes; have a pen and paper ready in order to allow them to do so. Asking the client to identify any challenges associated with the implementation of the proposed plan at home is important as it not only identifies potential pitfalls but also encourages the client to feel a degree of ownership of the process.

6. CLOSING THE CONSULTATION

When closing the consultation the aim is to summarise the decisions that have been made and arrange future appointments as necessary. It is important to confirm that the owner is happy with any agreed-upon protocols such as medications that have been dispensed or diets recommended. Also ensure that the client is provided with contact details, which may be either phone or email; ideally, both are recommended. Reinforce your name by either writing it on any documentation provided or giving a card with your details. While primarily considered the tool of the business person, 'business' cards can be produced very cheaply for all clinical staff and are appreciated by clients.

Professional accountability

The Code of Professional Conduct for RVNs (Royal College of Veterinary Surgeons, 2014) states that RVNs seek to ensure the health and welfare of animals committed to their care and to fulfil their professional responsibilities, by maintaining five principles of practice:
- Professional competence
- Honesty and integrity
- Independence and impartiality
- Client confidentiality and trust
- Professional accountability.

When undertaking nursing clinics these principles need to be adhered to. The RVN is still working under the direction of the veterinary surgeon, and the use of written protocols can help staff. High-quality training is required in order to ensure that RVNs are competent in the process of consultations. There are always situations where the RVN will need guidance from the veterinary surgeon, and protocols can be utilised in these situations.

Life-stage clinics

PUPPY AND KITTEN CLINICS

Puppy and kitten clinics should be held monthly from time of vaccinations through to at least 6 months of age. There are many advantages of these clinics, including the opportunity to bond the client to the practice, as well as for preventative health care. Topics to cover in the clinics include:

- Clinical examination of the pet, to include showing how to perform a BCS
- Handling and grooming techniques, nail clipping, ear cleaning, etc.
- Dental health care, including tooth brushing
- Neutering
- Microchipping, compulsory in dogs in the UK from April 2016
- Nutrition
- Behaviour and training issues
- Parasite control and prevention.

The nurse may also be required to administer additional vaccines depending on the practice policy. These can include Kennel Cough vaccines, the second part of the primary vaccine course, and a 16-week parvovirus vaccination.

Checklists can be used to ensure that all subjects are covered, and are of use when more than one nurse is conducting the clients; this way all subjects are covered and any important points are noted.

SOCIALISATION CLASSES

The role of the RVN in educating clients in the importance of puppy socialisation is paramount. Veterinary practices should openly promote puppy clinics, puppy parties and socialisation groups. Nurses need to understand how puppies assimilate these learning processes in order to fully convey to owners why their puppies display certain behaviours.

The socialisation period begins at 3 weeks of age and is a period of rapid brain development, and coincides with the maturation and myelination of the spinal cord (Shepherd 2002). At this age the puppy becomes fully aware of, and able to respond to, its environment. Many features of socialisation occur in the main socialisation period (4 to 14 weeks), but the features of the most long-term behavioural significance are:

- Development of anticipatory responses as a result of an increased ability to attend to the environment
- Emergence of social behaviour, including determination of relative rank
- Ability to form primary social relationships with conspecifics and with other animals (including people).

In puppies there is a rapid increase in tendency to approach unfamiliar people up to the age of 5 weeks. After 5 weeks puppies can become increasingly cautious of unfamiliar individuals or situations, but social motivation to approach and interact outweighs fear up to the age of 8 weeks. From the age of 12–14 weeks puppies can become easily frightened, and it has been concluded that after 12–14 weeks the growing tendency to react fearfully to novelty puts an end to effective socialisation (Shepherd 2002). During the juvenile period (14 weeks to sexual maturity) gradual improvement of the motor skills occurs and refinement of behaviour patterns in both relevance and context are seen. During this period there is an increased tendency to explore the environment. At about 4 months of age the speed of formation of conditioned reflexes begins to slow down, as associations made previously probably interfere with new learning. There is evidence for a second period of heightened sensitivity to fear-provoking stimuli just before puberty at around 4 to 6 months (Dehasse 1994).

The nurse's role in aiding clients with socialisation of puppies must start from a very early age. Greater results can be achieved if socialisation can be started while still with the bitch. This can only be achieved if breeders are welcome to ideas and take on the responsibility of socialisation of the puppies. Feeding behaviour when with littermates can greatly influence feeding behaviour in adulthood. Puppies, when with littermates, should have their own food bowl; puppies that have to share are more likely to bolt food down (this can result in vomiting if food is eaten too quickly) and to display food guarding and thus aggression towards food.

When puppies are presented to the veterinary practice they are already at roughly 8 weeks of age, a period where socialisation is exceptionally important. Nurse clinics are an ideal opportunity to educate owners on why socialisation is required and how to achieve it. Monthly nurse clinics that are tied in with worming regimens are an ideal opportunity to monitor how clients are doing with socialisation, but this can be too late in many cases. Veterinary surgeons are vital in their role during the primary vaccination course to highlight to clients the importance of socialisation and of attending puppy socialisation parties. It is also important to remember that this visit to the practice is usually the puppy's first visit, and therefore needs to be as atraumatic as possible and positively pleasant for the puppy. These are mainly run by RVNs and are vital in the education of owners in how they are to go about socialising their puppy. Many books have socialisation charts that can be followed by owners and that give them a good indication of the things that they should be looking at achieving with their puppy. It is important to instil in owners that puppies should be socialised in a wide variety of different ways. People's circumstances can change, and therefore puppies should be socialised in everything that they may possibly encounter in their lives. People that live in rural areas should take their puppies into the city, and vice versa, for socialisation. Owners that do not have children still need to socialise their puppy with children. A new baby may come into the house later on in the dog's life, and it is impossible to predict the dog's reactions if it has not been properly socialised as a puppy; this should be strongly emphasised to owners.

ADOLESCENCE HEALTH CHECK

These checks normally occur at 6 months of age. At this stage many owners are considering neutering, though many practices and charities now neuter at much younger ages. Animals need to be checked for whether testicles have descended and for the presence of deciduous teeth. In cases where practices neuter

TABLE 3.1	Differences between male and female cats, and the consequences of neutering			
Parameter	Male	Female	Consequence of neutering	
Body fat (as % of total body weight)	23.8 ± 1	30.1 ± 1.7	Increase M: 32.9 ± 1.7 F: 35.5 ± 1.8	
Energy expenditure (kcal/kg)	57 ± 2	57 ± 2	Decrease M: 50 ± 3 F: 51 ± 2	
Non-esterified fatty acids		Higher in the female	Greater differences between males and females	
Caloric requirements			Requirements reduced in both sexes	
Serum leptin	Regulation of leptin secretion by testosterone	No demonstrated oestrogenic control in cats	M: Increase in the male F: Less noticeable change	
Glucose intolerance		Absent	Unchanged in both sexes	
Insulin	More marked		Continuance of high insulin resistance in the male; in the female, appearance of insulin resistance	

Dethioux et al., 2005.

earlier, these checks should be performed throughout the puppy and kitten monthly checks. Six months can be appropriate time to discuss life-stage diet changes. Once cats have been neutered they need to change to a life-stage diet aimed at young adult neutered cats. Dogs will greatly differ depending on breed size, neuter status and the diet that the owner is feeding. Some diets will have junior stage before changing to adult rather than having a large-breed puppy diet. It is impossible to have detailed knowledge about all of the diets that are available on the market. Having Internet access in the consulting room can prove to be useful to access relevant information.

POST-NEUTERING CLINICS

After neutering there is a gap of usually up to 8 months until the animal is next seen at its first annual booster (at 14 or 15 months of age). There is traditionally a fall of the number of animals that are seen at their first booster vaccination, and an interim visit between neutering and the vaccine can help prevent this. A clinic aimed at roughly 9 months of age can fill this gap. Attaching a reminder to all neutering procedures for a post-neutering clinic 3 months after surgery will ensure that clients receive a reminder for these clinics. Most animals will require some form of worming control at roughly 9 months of age, as most are wormed monthly until 6 months of age and then every 3 months after this. It is also important to weigh the animal and measure its BCS to check that there has not been a large increase in body weight. It is also important to remember that in large breeds of dogs these animals are still growing and therefore monitoring growth rate until adulthood is beneficial.

Advice can be given on dietary matters at this clinic. Some animals have reached maturity by 9 months and therefore can transition to adult diets, whereas some need to remain on a puppy diet for longer.

Many diets have now been introduced to the market specifically designed for neutered cats. As previously discussed, in the immediate post-neutering period the animal's metabolism decreases. In entire cats energy expenditure in both female and male animals is 57 ± 2 kcal/kg. Once neutered, this value decreases to 50 ± 3 kcal/kg in males and 51 ± kcal/kg in females.

There are, however, marked differences in other factors, as demonstrated in Table 3.1. Changes in insulin resistance can suggest predisposition of neutered cats to diabetes mellitus.

PUPPY AND KITTEN PARTIES

Puppy parties are now, fortunately, an almost expected service from new puppy owners and can be a deciding factor on why new puppy owners choose a specific veterinary practice. Parties need to be orderly and well run so as not to cause more problems than they prevent.

Deciding on a format for puppy parties

No matter what format you decide on running your puppy party, it is important that you first do all of your background reading and gain all of the necessary knowledge that is required to successfully run a good-quality puppy party. Puppy parties can be an ideal opportunity to bond clients to the practice, but more importantly enable new puppy owners to achieve a well-rounded puppy that can be fully integrated into the family and environmental setting.

Puppy parties can be singular, a one-off session for the opportunity for puppies to socialise, or a series of parties. Singular parties can be useful and informative for people with limited time to commit to a series of parties, giving a good basis for owners in how to successfully socialise and habitualise their puppies. A series of parties can be in a roll-on roll-off format; that way it is not necessary for a new course to start before being able to attend, and therefore missing out on valuable socialising time. A series of parties is ideal for puppies that are a little hesitant to start with when mixing with the other puppies for the first time. A series gives you a better opportunity to bond clients, as more contact time is achievable.

If you decide on a course of puppy parties, a different subject matter can be covered in each week. Subject matters that clients like to have covered include first aid, training issues (including house training, recalls, play biting), socialisation and behaviour. As these topics are covered in depth it is important that you are giving good, knowledgeable and correct information to clients. With new puppies starting each week, you will get the same questions each week that need answering, but this does give an opportunity to reinforce habitualisation techniques. Also see Chapter 12.

Marketing

When deciding to start running puppy parties, everyone in your practice needs to be on board with promoting the benefits of puppy parties. On initial vaccination of the puppy the veterinary surgeon needs to discuss socialising, and the importance of socialising, and also should discuss the importance that puppy parties play in establishing the groundwork in socialising the puppy with other puppies, the veterinary practice and its staff.

The puppy parties should be advertised on the practice's website, in any newsletters, in puppy packs that are given out to clients, in waiting room displays – anywhere that be seen by the puppy's owner. Prospective clients may call your veterinary practice to check vaccination costs, and promoting the parties at this initial phone call can make a difference to whether that client chooses your practice or not.

Certain parameters need to be set up before starting to promote your parties, and all staff needs to be aware of these so that the correct information is given out. You need to establish an upper age limit on the puppies that can attend the party, and whether they need to have completed their vaccination course or just the first vaccination. Most practices tend to allow only puppies that have had their second vaccination. If you wanted to include puppies that have not received their full vaccination course, you could always hold a second one-off puppy party for those that have received just the first part of their vaccination course. If you decide to run a course of parties and the puppy will reach the upper age limit before completing the course, then this is fine. The puppy will still benefit from attending some of the classes, and some are better than none. It is wise to have a maximum number of puppies that can attend the party; if you find that you are oversubscribed, consider providing another course at a different time.

Running the puppy party

A safe, controlled environment is essential when conducting a puppy party. If you decide to use the practice waiting room, it is important that the floor has been cleaned with a virucidal disinfectant, due to the puppy's immature immunological status.

A natural format is to provide seating in a circle; do not be afraid to move people and their puppies around depending on the nature of the puppy. A very boisterous puppy next to a timid puppy needs to be avoided.

All information that is given out during the puppy party needs to be accurate, clear and concise. Attending seminars, reading around the subject areas and distance learning are essential, and talking to other nurses that have experience running puppy parties is a valuable resource.

Puppies should be kept on their leads, and only two should have off-lead time at any one time. The party should never become a complete free-for-all. Off-lead time should be structured with puppies matched with puppies of a similar character.

Advice to give to owners when things go astray

Not all socialisation experiences will be positive ones. Most bad situations cannot be avoided, and therefore clients that are forewarned are forearmed. Running through a situation where the puppy is spooked by a strange object (a bus, a flapping tarpaulin etc.) and how the owner should react is ideal. Owners should be made aware that the puppy's lead is a means of communication between the handler and the puppy. A nice relaxed lead will help to make the puppy feel relaxed; a tense lead could result in the puppy becoming tense.

Owners should be aware of what to do if the puppy becomes scared. All positive behaviour needs to be rewarded; all negative behaviour should be ignored. If the puppy becomes scared of a bus driving past too closely, this behaviour should be ignored. When the puppy then starts to act "normal" again, walking relaxed on the lead, this needs to be rewarded with attention, a toy or a treat. Lots of positive experiences will outweigh one negative experience.

What to do if things go wrong during a puppy party

If things do start to get out of hand between two or more puppies during a puppy party, it is important to intervene quickly. The puppies should be placed back onto their leads and allowed to calm down. The important fact is to ensure that potentially negative experiences do not occur, and constant monitoring of the puppies interacting is required. This is a prime example of not having too many puppies in the party without having extra help to monitor them interacting. It can be difficult to monitor the puppies while answering the owner's questions, and having an additional pair of eyes can be beneficial.

Quiet puppies

There will always be a collection of puppies that are very quiet, cautious or hesitant about interacting with other puppies when attending puppy parties. If more than one puppy in the group are like this, it is best to sit them next to each other away from the more boisterous ones. If there are no suitable puppies to interact with then it can be beneficial for the puppy just to observe for the first session. In order for the puppy not to become too dependent on its owner, the puppy can just observe from your own lap. In most cases by the end of the session the puppy might be starting to come out a little and might be able to walk around the other puppies (with the others being on their leads).

SENIOR HEALTH-CARE CLINICS

Senior pet clinics are notoriously difficult to set up, whether this is due to a general apathy in pet owners when their pet is older, or more due to people not wanting to take an older and apparently healthy pet to the veterinary practice for professionals to find something wrong. Senior pet clinics should be marketed more as an aid towards preventative health care and improving quality and longevity of life in older pets. Senior clinics can be either nurse led or vet led, and either priced to cover all costs or performed as a loss leader. Those clinics which are nurse led and performed as a loss leader tend to be more successful.

Senior clinics traditionally cover a full clinical history, clinical examination, blood testing, urine testing, and, in cats, blood pressure monitoring. For those clinics that cost these diagnostics out, senior clinics can potentially be very expensive. In clinics performed as a loss leader, the initial consultation and examination is performed at a discounted rate, or free of charge. The reasoning is that the initial consultation will bring in additional work, e.g. dental procedures, blood testing, urine testing and blood pressure monitoring. Several studies have noted that the prevalence of dental disease and arthritis (especially in cats) is approximated at 80% of all animals over 8 years of age, and therefore the likelihood of 'finding' something is fairly high. Even with completely healthy animals advice on senior diets, preventative dental care and making owners aware of which clinical symptoms to be looking out for in their pet is important.

A detailed clinical history needs to be taken from each owner, and this includes behavioural questioning alongside questions relating to feeding patterns, etc. Nurses are in an ideal position to question owners about their pets as they may speak more freely with nurses than with the veterinary surgeon.

Wellness clinics

An ideal clinic for nurses to conduct is the 6-month wellness check. These clinics fall halfway between the annual vaccinations and are an opportunity to ensure that all aspects that may have been raised in the annual health check have been followed. Many animals will require additional parasite control as many formulations are supplied in six-dose boxes.

In older animals there is a recommendation to perform urinalysis and blood pressure every 6 months, and this can be actively promoted in these clinics. Many practices provide these free of charge, at a reduced cost or as part of a monthly budgeting plan. It is much easier to pick up on any weight gain or loss if the animal is seen every 6 months rather than annually.

Medical clinics

Nurse consultations that involve medical conditions are normally to discuss diet and medications, but further information regarding the condition may be required. The client may require further information of the specific condition, or advice on the environmental changes and other factors that can help to increase the animal's quality of life, and compliance from the owner.

This section will discuss individual medical conditions and their requirements in nurse consultations of this type. Additional information regarding clinical nutrition is provided in Chapter 10.

Arthritis (mobility) clinics

The nurse clinic is an important part of helping the owner to improve the quality of life for the pet with osteoarthritis (OA). There are several aspects that owners may need guidance on, along with compliance with any pharmaceuticals that the veterinary surgeon may have prescribed. With the multiplicity of drugs and alternative treatments utilised for chronic pain, management of these patients can be difficult and complex. It is important to emphasise to the owners of these pets that multiple trials may be required to find the right combination of analgesics, supplements and diets, and that not all patients can be effectively managed. For more information on pain management (analgesia) see Chapter 27.

The aims of the nursing clinic are to:
- Perform pain scores in order to assess any improvements or deteriorations in arthritic pain

- Aid the client in compliance with pharmaceutical administration
- Advise on a healthy, balanced diet, with correction of any dietary imbalances, including obesity
- Advise on exercise levels and activities
- Give the client guidance on alternative therapies in order to help mobility in the pet.

MONITORING OF ARTHRITIC PATIENTS

Animals with chronic pain should be rechecked frequently to assess response to therapy and monitor for side effects, and the owners should be consulted with closely as to the effectiveness of treatment. All patients that are going to start on a course of analgesics should undertake blood sampling in order to ascertain renal and liver function. Medications such as non-steroidal anti-inflammatory drugs (NSAIDs) can affect hepatic and renal function. Routine blood screening should occur every 6 months while the animal is receiving the medications. Monitoring of urine specific gravity can prove valuable in the early identification of renal insufficiency. All of these diagnostics can be undertaken by the RVN in clinic, with the veterinary surgeon interpreting the results and guiding to outcomes.

For those animals that have been identified as being arthritic, but have not yet started on any form of treatment, pain scoring should be performed. A scoring system should be utilised that removes any subjectivity. If performed both before and after treatment, the scoring system will give a good indication on whether the treatment has worked and to what degree.

Obesity is a major risk factor of OA. Weight loss must be initiated as soon as possible. Exercising and consequently weight loss can be difficult due to restrictions in mobility. When deciding on a diet for an animal with OA, it needs to meet the requirements for the animal's life stage and BCS. There are many diets designed to aid dogs and cats with OA, and nutritional assessment of these patients will help guide the RVN into the direction of the most appropriate diet for the animal.

It has been long assumed that cats, unlike other species, seldom suffer from arthritis. Studies have been conducted proving that cats do suffer from arthritis. Arthritis is a painful degenerative condition, but the signs exhibited can be very subtle in cats. It has been reported that 90% of cats over 12 years old have been shown to have changes in their bones suggesting arthritis when X-rayed. Being able to recognise whether a cat is suffering from arthritic changes is important, and educating clients on these signs is essential. 'Slowing down' is not an inevitable fact of old age, but rather a possible sign of arthritis, which is a treatable condition. As mentioned the clinical signs are very subtle, as cats are very good at hiding their pain. In order to ascertain whether the cat is suffering from arthritis, there are many signs that the owner can look for. The following questions can be presented in the form of a questionnaire that clients can read through before the consultation so that they are already in the mind frame regarding arthritis:
- Does your cat appear stiff or lame?
- Have there been any weight changes, either gain (as not getting enough exercise) or loss (loss of appetite due to pain)?
- Have you noticed any change in temperament? Some cats can become very clingy and demand attention, some can become reclusive (due to chronic pain) and some can become aggressive.

- Have you noticed any changes in sleep pattern, both increases and decreases? This can be due to not being able to settle (fidgeting) due to pain, or increases due to the exhaustion of pain.
- Has the cat changed where it sleeps? This can indicate pain, as trying to get comfortable by sleeping on softer areas. The cat may not be able to reach up to usual sleeping areas.
- Has the cat shown a reduced ability to jump up or down from surfaces, chairs, steps etc.?
- Have you noticed any changes in toileting behaviour? This can be due to pain and reduced mobility, making climbing into the litter tray uncomfortable/difficult. Some cats can have difficulty getting through the cat flap in order to reach the toileting area outside.
- Have you noticed a reduction in coat condition, due to reduced grooming activities?
- Have you noticed a frequent licking of joints, due to pain in the joints?
- Has there been a reduction in hunting activities?
- Does the cat have longer claws, due to reduction in scratching (either on a scratching post or on surfaces outside)?

If the owner notices any of these signs in the cat, it should be examined by the veterinary surgeon.

Dentistry clinics

Dental disease is the most common problem suffered by adult dogs and cats. Incidence rates show that 85% of dogs and 70% of cats over the age of 3 years suffer from some form of dental disease. The development of periodontal disease is dependent on the host's immunity and inflammatory responses to plaque on the tooth's surface.

The nurse's role in preventative health care is easily demonstrated with dental care. Puppies and kittens that are habitualised into having their mouths handled and their teeth brushed are at an advantage with their dental hygiene. All puppy and kitten owners should have instruction on how to perform these tasks.

The aims of nursing dentistry clinics include (also see Chapter 26):

- Encouraging chewing, which can be achieved by using kibbles of different sizes
- Limiting the components of plaque and the mineralisation of plaque to tartar
- Increasing antimicrobial action with the use of chlorhexidine and xylitol products
- Encouraging the owner to habitualise the animal to having its mouth handled and teeth examined
- Teaching the owner how to achieve effective tooth brushing
- Identifying when other methods such as ultrasonic descaling are required, and referral to the veterinary surgeon in cases where disease or trauma to teeth is evident.

As previously mentioned, owners of all puppies and kittens should have tooth brushing demonstrated and actively encouraged during puppy and kitten clinics. Owners of older animals should also be encouraged through nurse clinics to brush their animals' teeth. An ideal time for referral is annual vaccinations. All animals that have had some form of dental procedure should be referred to nurse clinics. Those that have only received dental hygiene treatment should see the RVN about 3 days after the procedure for guidance in ongoing home care. Those that have extractions or have severe gingivitis should see a veterinary surgeon initially after the procedure; once the veterinary surgeon is happy, the client should be referred to the RVN for home-care advice. All post-procedure protocols depend on the practice's protocols and each individual patient. Owners of all animals that have received dental treatment should be encouraged to use a chlorhexidine-based product, rather than an enzymatic paste.

Follow-up appointments should be as required, with a minimum of 3 months between check-ups with the clinic. Disclosing swabs can be very helpful in identifying areas of the teeth that the owner needs to concentrate on and the effectiveness of the overall home care being used. Many insurance companies now require routine dental hygiene checks, at least two or three a year, before the companies will cover dental procedures.

TOOTH BRUSHING

Tooth brushing is the gold standard in oral hygiene care. Young animals should be habitualised to having their heads, and then mouths, handled. The use of flavoured tooth pastes can facilitate this process. Many clients have difficulty with the pet trying to consume the paste. In these cases pushing the gel or paste into the bristles of the brush can prevent the pet from eating the paste before it reaches the animal's teeth. Enzymatic toothpastes are ideal in healthy mouths of breeds of dogs not predisposed to dental disease. As periodontal disease can start in predisposed breeds from an exceptionally young age, it is recommended that a chlorhexidine-based paste or gel be used in these animals from an early age, i.e. puppy. The staining that can be caused by this product can be easily removed with brushing, and cosmetically it is not a problem in animals as with people.

Instructing clients on how to start tooth brushing with their pet is important. The length of time it takes to reach full brushing will depend on the pet and the proficiency of the owner. The length of each step depends on many factors, and as the person giving guidance you should use common sense on how quickly the owner progresses through:

1. Handling of the pet's head and mouth
2. Habitualising the pet to having a gel or paste applied around its gums
3. Moving up to gently brushing the teeth with a small-headed toothbrush.

The actual brushing of the teeth and gums should be performed with a medium-grade brush. Small-headed brushes are ideal for starting owners off with brushing. Finger brushes tend to be too bulky in the mouth with the rubber 'bristles' too big to perform adequate subgingival brushing. The mouth should always be kept closed when brushing as the lingual aspect of the teeth rarely requires brushing. The front of the mouth is the most sensitive part of the mouth as this is the the area that would 'feel' what the animal is eating, shearing off pieces of food. The rear of the mouth is less sensitive, as it concentrates on the chewing of the food, and thus it can be more difficult to brush the front of the mouth than the rear.

Some gingival bleeding is to be expected when initiating tooth brushing as the gums are not accustomed to the abrasive nature of brushing. This should pass in a few days; however, if it does continue this can indicate gingivitis, and guidance from a veterinary surgeon should be sought.

If advocating the use of finger brushes and other materials such as flannels or swabs to apply gels and pastes, it should be remembered that these animals are not totally comfortable with tooth brushing and there is a potential that the animal can bite. As the owner's fingers are in the animal's mouth, the owner should be warned about the potential for biting. If at any point you feel that the animal could have the potential to bite the owner, whether with intent or not, different forms of dental hygiene should be advocated, e.g. dental diets, oral rinses and drinking water additives.

Cardiac clinics

The nutritional status of the cardiac patient is exceptionally important to ascertain as this can have several effects on the animal. This can include the choice and dose rate of the drugs used in the medical treatment, interpretation of any laboratory results, interpretation of electrocardiogram (ECG) data, prognosis of both surgical and medical intervention and the choice of diet for the patient. As part of the initial clinical assessment a full history of the animal's diet should be taken. Nutrition can be a causative factor in cardiac disease. If the animal receives unusual supplements or is not fed a complete diet, if more than one animal in the household is affected or if it is being fed a homemade or fad diet, cardiac disease can be induced. Micronutrient and macronutrient deficiencies (calcium, potassium) can cause cardiac problems and thus a complete blood workup needs to be performed.

Assessment of body condition and muscle scores of each individual animal is important with cardiac patients. A reduction in skeletal muscle mass might indicate energy malnutrition and possibly a negative nitrogen balance. Animals with catabolic disease such as hyperthyroidism in cats and cardiac failure lose body mass very rapidly, as with anorexic cats. The progression of cardiac disease can be exacerbated in obese animals. This can result in cardiomegaly, circulatory congestion, oedema, ascites and hypocalcaemia. An overweight animal must be subjectively assessed; obesity must be differentiated from abdominal distension due to hepatomegaly or ascites. Obesity can also mask an underlying lean muscle body mass. Obese animals need to lose weight in a controlled and monitored way, the same as in a normal healthy animal. Obesity not only produces clinical signs that mimic those of early heart failure, but can also cause cardiovascular changes that can exacerbate any underlying cardiovascular disease.

The aims of nursing clinics are to:
- Help control signs associated with sodium and fluid retention by avoiding nutritional deficiencies and excesses
- Support patients receiving diuretics or angiotensin-converting enzyme (ACE) inhibitors, aiding the client with compliance in administration of medications
- Maintain optimal weight and body condition score, to aid in preventing cardiac cachexia
- Monitor blood pressure and other diagnostic methods
- Provide support to the owner, as and when required.

CARDIAC CACHEXIA

From 34–75% of dogs suffering with heart disease suffer from anorexia, one of the multifactorial processes associated with the loss of lean body mass in cardiac cachexia. Other factors include increased energy requirements and metabolic alterations. Cardiac cachexia is more commonly seen in dogs than cats and in dilated cardiomyopathy (DCM) or right-sided heart failure. The primary energy source for animals with acute or chronic disease is amino acids from muscle, thus causing a reduction in lean body mass. Cachexia is a slow, progressive process of the loss of lean body mass/muscle. Careful examinations of obese animals should occur, as this lean body mass reduction can occur, creating overcoat syndrome, and be easily missed. Clinical nutrition of these animals includes management of any anorexia.

Obesity clinics

The nature of the veterinary profession is moving towards preventative care rather than 'fire engine medicine'. Obesity has to be viewed as one of the many diseases that can be prevented. Dental disease is a preventable disease, and many clinics are devoted to educating clients in how to prevent dental disease with tooth brushing, diet etc. Obesity should also be viewed along the same lines, rather than at the treatment stage. Obesity is a chronic medical disease that needs to be managed throughout the life of the pet.

The aims of nursing clinics and nutritional management diets to promote weight loss include:
- Monitoring weight loss, alongside BCS and MCS
- Recommending a diet that supplies adequate nutrients, within a reduced-calorie diet
- Promoting smooth weight loss while maintaining a lean body mass as much as possible
- Increasing conversion of stored fat to energy, through exercise programmes
- Motivating the client with the continuation of the weight loss programme
- Educating the client in potential behavioural traits that need to be altered in both the pet and the owner.

Prevention is obviously better than cure, and the ideal place to start is in puppy clinics, first vaccinations and puppy parties. It has been clearly demonstrated that animals that remain at or marginally below their ideal weight throughout their growth phase are less likely to become obese in later life. Following up animals during the post-neutering phase is vital as this is when most fat gain occurs. With a decrease in metabolism and change in diet many animals tend to increase their weight and BCS at this stage in life, and subsequently battle with it into adulthood. The RVN is the ideal person to discuss postoperative changes in diet and feeding amounts. Encourage all owners to bring their animals to see a RVN at 9 months of age for a weight check (most animals will also require worming at this stage) and to discuss diet/feeding. Many animals are about to transition to a junior or adult light/neutered diet at this stage.

OWNER EDUCATION

Owners' perception of their animal's weight can vary, as it does with their own weight. Owners need to be advised/educated as to what is deemed to be obese or overweight. Management systems/protocols need to be in place in veterinary practices in order to aid in obesity prevention. Every animal should be weighed and BCS should be determined at each visit and recorded on the clinical history. The animal's weight can then be tracked throughout its life. It is also easier to estimate an ideal lean body weight for the animal if you know its weight and BCS history. It is also useful to state to an owner when you see a pet at its ideal body weight, 'This is your pet's ideal weight'. Ensure that you log this onto the clinical history. If the animal does subsequently gain weight, you can check the clinical history and ask the owner, 'Do you remember when your pet was this weight? How active was your pet then'?

Obesity is the most prevalent form of malnutrition in pets presented to veterinary practices. *Obesity* is defined as body fat exceeding 15–20% of body weight. Excessive weight is an associative cause or exacerbating factor for specific orthopaedic, endocrine, cardiovascular and neoplastic diseases. Obesity will also make the animal less tolerant or resilient to metabolic stress. The weight and volume of fat in the abdomen of an obese animal can exert enough pressure on the bladder to induce leakage of urine, but also, conversely, to reduce the diameter of the urethra and cause reduced flow of urine. The animal ultimately needs to change from a positive energy balance to a negative energy balance in order to lose fat and then maintain an ideal body weight.

Weight loss is an exceptionally difficult thing to achieve, and not just nutritional advice is required in order to achieve this goal. Behavioural modifications of both the owner and pet are required, alongside advice on exercise; this can be difficult if the animal or owner has a mobility problem. In many cases owners are not receptive to comments that their pets are overweight, and therefore it can be difficult to motivate owners to initiate a weight loss programme. Some owners feel that being overweight by a few kilograms does not make any significant difference to the animal. The effect of being overweight can be easily demonstrated to an owner by asking the owner to put on the practice's lead radiography apron (it weighs about 5 kg, and when you take off the apron you really notice the difference). Illustrate to the client that only a small amount of weight gain can be a significant percentage gain to the animal, depending on the animal's size; for example, a 1-kg weight gain in a 4-kg cat is the same as a woman gaining 2–3 stone.

Satiation (feeling full) is related to the rate of food consumption (animals can overeat before realising that they are satiated), food constituents (protein is more satiating than carbohydrates) and the animal's ability to sense fullness. These three factors should be used in the construction of a dietary plan in obesity control. Nutritional management is only part of a weight loss programme; the animal's exercise levels and lifestyle also need to be considered. Nutrigenomics can play an important part in dietary management (see Chapter 10).

Renal clinics

In all animals, clinical symptoms of renal dysfunction are not evident until 65–75% of renal tissue has been destroyed, and many veterinary practices initiate renal screening for older patients and before the start of pharmaceutical regimens. Nutritional management can affect many consequences of renal failure and is the cornerstone of management. Chronic renal failure (CRF) has many physiological effects, including the decreased ability to excrete nitrogenous waste (and thus build-up of azotaemia), sodium and phosphorus, and an increased loss of potassium. Other clinical symptoms include systemic hypertension, secondary hyperparathyroidism and non-regenerative anaemia, and should be monitored as part of the nursing clinic.

Nurse clinics for animals that have been newly diagnosed with or suspected of renal disease should be initiated as soon as possible. All owners should be referred to the nurse in order to discuss diet, medications (if required), compliance and any future requirements for diagnostics and reviews of the patient. The nurse is also well placed to answer any questions that the owner may have.

The aim for nursing clinics is to:
- Reduce accumulation of nitrogenous waste in the animal's bloodstream (azotaemia) by minimising protein precursors for urea and creatinine and control of blood phosphate levels
- Educate the owner in monitoring hydration status of the animal
- Ensure that the animal gets adequate calories to prevent further catabolism or malnutrition, helping to maintain an ideal BCS
- Ensure compliance of the owner with medications, if any, and repeat diagnostic monitoring methods
- Ensure that the animal's blood pressure is controlled, by routine monitoring and referral back to the veterinary surgeon as required
- Provide support to the client during the later stages of the animal's life.

DIAGNOSTIC MONITORING

The International Renal Interest Society (IRIS) has developed a renal scoring index that helps to identify the progression of the disease in order to facilitate appropriate treatment and monitoring of the patient. The initial staging is based on a fasted plasma creatinine level, and then substaged dependent on proteinuria levels and arterial blood pressure. Fasted blood samples must always be used as even a moderately high protein meal prior to sampling can elevate blood plasma creatinine levels. Repeat blood sampling should occur, as required, but should be performed more regularly if urinalysis shows changes in proteinuria levels.

Owners may need guidance on how to obtain urine samples, as these are the most useful diagnostic tools in the progression of renal failure. Urine concentration should be routinely measured through refractometer, and the urine protein/creatinine (UP/C) ratio should be routinely performed. Medications such as ACE inhibitors should only be administered when proteinuria is present. It should be noted that proteinuria can present at any stage of the renal failure and is not directly linked to the level of azotaemia.

All newly diagnosed renal patients should have their blood pressure monitored. Renal function is directly affected by an increase in blood pressure, and as the kidneys play a role in blood pressure secondary hypertension can result. Hypertension should be treated, as the effects of hypertension are ultimately negative.

PHARMACEUTICALS

The most commonly used pharmaceutical in animals with CRF is benazepril (POM-V), an ACE inhibitor. Inhibition of ACE leads to reduced conversion of inactive angiotensin I into active angiotensin II, therefore reducing the effects mediated by angiotensin II, including vasoconstriction of both arteries and veins, retention of sodium and water by the kidney and modelling changes (including pathological cardiac hypertrophy and degenerative renal changes). In cats with chronic renal insufficiency, benazepril reduces the protein loss in urine and reduces systemic and intraglomerular blood pressure. Benazepril also helps to increase the appetite, quality of life and survival time of cats, particularly in advanced disease. Benazepril is therefore indicated when proteinuria is present, so proteinuria testing is necessary. As ACE inhibitors decrease the intraglomerular blood pressure there will be a refractory increase in nitrogenous waste products.

In some cases additional hypertensive medications may be required in order to return the patient to a normotensive state. In these cases amlodipine (POM) may be added to the regimen. Once initiated, blood pressure monitoring is required in order to taper the dose according to the patient's readings, under veterinary direction.

If medications are prescribed for patients with CRF, it is important that the RVN discusses with clients whether they are able to medicate their pet. Owners may need guidance on the administration of medications.

Feline urinary clinics

Urine is a composite of a complex solution of both organic and inorganic ions. Crystals can grow and form when an imbalance occurs in this complex solution. There are several causes for these imbalances. Diet, decreased water consumption, urine pH alterations or relative lack of inhibitors of crystallisation can cause the solubility of a particular crystal to be exceeded. The result is crystal aggregation and growth. Clinical signs of feline idiopathic cystitis (FIC) include haematuria, proteinuria, dysuria, pollakiuria and/or urethral obstruction. A full diagnostic workup is recommended in all cases, including blood work and imaging. A home-care plan needs to be designed in conjunction with the veterinary surgeon, in order to convey these recommendations to the pet owner.

It is recommended that all cases are given advice on all aspects of husbandry. Dietary manipulation can aid in reducing the risk factors of uroliths, but many other factors need to be taken in to consideration and addressed. Nurse clinics are an ideal place to convey all this information.

The aims of the nurse clinic are to:
- Include a full history of the environmental factors affecting the cat, including other pets in the household or any changes at home (e.g. builders, new baby), and give advice regarding these factors
- Discuss strategies to reduce any stressors for the cat
- Provide instruction regarding dietary manipulation
- Aid the animal to obtain an ideal BCS if required.

Recommendations should be given to clients about preventative measures in all cases. There are clear risk factors associated with FIC; some cannot be helped, such as age, breed and gender, but others, such as lifestyle and obesity, can. Neutering has a significant impact on the risk of bladder stones, the risk of oxalate increasing 7-fold, struvite 3.5-fold. Educating the owner to ensure an adequate water intake and limiting weight gain after neutering is vital.

Struvite crystals ($MgNH_4PO_4.6H_2O$) are commonly seen in cats suffering from FIC. Dietary recommendations for these cats include avoiding excessive dietary protein, avoiding excessive levels of the minerals that are used within the crystals (magnesium and phosphorous) and increasing water consumption.

Urinary pH needs to be within the recommended urinary pH range, as the crystals form in an alkaline environment. A range of 5.9–6.1 is ideal for dissolution, whereas 6.2–6.4 is recommended for prevention. The average urinary pH of domestic cat consuming a natural diet (small rodents) is pH 6.3. Acidifiers are used to prevent struvite uroliths. Cats receiving long-term dietary acidifiers can suffer from a transient negative potassium balance, with phosphoric acid and ammonium chloride acidifiers. Long-term potassium depletion will stimulate ammonia synthesis at the same site as chronic metabolic acidosis. Acidifying therapeutic veterinary diets need to have potassium levels in excess of the National Research Council (NRC) minimum allowance of 0.6% dry matter base (DMB). The use of urinary acidifiers alongside an acidifying food is not recommended, as it can lead to metabolic acidosis. The alterations in pH may increase the solubility of some of the solutes within the urine, and in some cases decrease the solubility of others. This complex and competing interplay between nutritional requirements of the management of oxalate and struvite urolithiasis requires a careful selection in the long-term dietary control of FIC.

Excessive levels of protein need to be avoided in cases where struvite crystals and alkaline urine is present. High protein levels can influence pH; a prime example of this is the difference in urine pH between cats and dogs. Cats have higher protein consumption than dogs, and therefore an increased urinary pH. Increasing the protein level in the diet also increases urinary calcium excretion, uric acid and oxalate excretion. Excess dietary protein should be avoided by feeding a food that contains 30–45% dry matter (DM) protein.

Diets that promote urinary tract health do tend to have a higher fat content. This is due to the increased energy density with overall reduced mineral intake. When metabolised, fat produces the highest metabolic water contribution, which also benefits the animal. Due to the increased fat content some veterinary therapeutic diets are not available in a dry form. Obesity is a major risk factor of FIC, and a diet with a higher fat content may not be the indicated diet in this circumstance.

Cats that suffer from FIC and are overweight need to be placed on an obesity diet. Many of these diets have higher fibre content. The quantity of calcium being absorbed from the digestive system can be reduced by certain sources of dietary fibre. This can be beneficial with cats suffering from recurrent calcium oxalate urolithiasis.

Struvite precipitates form when the urine becomes supersaturated with magnesium, anionic phosphate and ammonium. Therapeutic diets avoid excess dietary magnesium, but low urinary magnesium concentrations have the potential to increase the risk of the formation of calcium-containing uroliths. Highlighting the importance of regular urinalysis is essential when on a therapeutic urinary diet. The intake of magnesium and calcium also influences urinary phosphate concentrations.

The addition of sodium into the diet is occasionally utilised in order to aid in increased water intake. Increasing the salt content of the diet can aid in diuresis and lowers the urine specific gravity.

WATER

Water intake is a vital factor in cats with FIC or a predisposition to FIC. The solute load of the diet influences total water intake by a large factor. Use of a moist diet is preferred, and additional water can also be mixed in if required; however, changing a cat that only eats dry food to a moist diet can cause stress, and therefore the dry diet is less problematic. Encouragement to increase the consumption of water can also be achieved by increasing access, e.g. by placing more bowls of water around the cat's environment. A choice over type and size of water bowls used needs to be considered. Cats can be deterred by the use of fresh tap water due to the chlorine content. Use of bottled, preboiled water or water that has been left to stand will have little or no chlorine that can be detected by the cat.

Increases in water consumption will increase the total volume of urine produced. Crystals precipitate out into the urine when supersaturation occurs. Urine becomes saturated when the salt content completely dissolved within the fluid. Any additional salt or decrease in the relative fluid volume will result in precipitation of the salts, hence the requirement for large volumes of more dilute urine. Owners are advised that the animal's urine should remain dilute and have no strong smell; however, most owners will have difficulty with this as most cats will urinate outside.

Urinalysis should be performed on a regular basis, at least every 3–6 months. Sediment analysis along with pH and specific gravity are good indicators of overall health. FIC can result in haematuria and proteinuria. Fresh urine samples should be used when performing urinalysis. Samples obtained via cystocentesis should be used when obtaining samples for bacterial culture and sensitivity. Voided samples and those not examined immediately can have false positives for bacteria and crystalluria. Many owners will need guidance on how to obtain urine samples from their cats.

FEEDING A CAT WITH FIC

The choice of diet depends on two factors: the body condition of the animal and results of the urinalysis. Correct identification of the type of crystals present (if any) and the pH of the urine is necessary. Use of a diet that promotes urinary health tends to be aimed at preventing struvite formation. Use of these diets in cats with a predisposition to calcium oxalate uroliths may increase the risk of urolith formation. A full dietary history of the cat is required, including any treats, supplements (especially if containing calcium) and whether or not the owner gives the cat milk. Both treats and processed human food (processed meats) are high in mineral levels, such as phosphorous, and should be avoided.

Use of a moist diet is preferable, as is free choice (*ad libitum*) feeding. This might not be possible with this feeding scenario if the cat is overweight. When any animal consumes food, gastric acid is secreted and creates a temporary net acid loss from the body and alkalisation of the urine. This is referred to as the postprandial alkaline tide. The alkaline tide is caused by secretion of bicarbonate into the blood by parietal cells of the stomach. A transient bicarbonisation is produced and increases urinary pH. Acidifiers in the diet will offset this increase in pH. If the diet is offered *ad libitum*, the cat will eat little and often. These feeding habits result in a smaller but more prolonged alkaline tide. This can reduce the likelihood of struvite precipitate formation.

Reducing stress in cats

The influences of behavioural responses in the cat have been widely linked to the occurrence of FIC in cats. Clients need to be made aware of this link and given appropriate advice in order to help their cat. Many cats are presented to the veterinary

practice for behavioural problems with inappropriate urination, but medical issues need to be ruled out before initiation of behavioural treatments. Any of the following behavioural traits can be indicators of stress:
- Food intake disorders (anorexia or overfeeding)
- Overgrooming (bald areas) or undergrooming (matted or soiled fur)
- House soiling, inappropriate urination or defecation
- Decreasing levels of activity, increased resting or feigned sleep
- Appearing withdrawn (reduced desire to play or interact), hiding
- Extreme vigilance and heightened startle response
- Defensive aggression towards people and other cats in the household, e.g. hissing
- Increased dependency or social withdrawal (dependent on personality type)
- Changes in patterns of behaviour, e.g. spending significantly more time indoors, irrespective of normal seasonal changes
- Urine spraying.

Helping the client to understand these sometimes subtle signs can be difficult. In multiple-cat households the presence of other cats can be the main cause, and removal of the cause is impossible. Owners need to be supported in order to make changes to the household to help the stressed family member. There must be sufficient resources in the household to reduce competition for them. This means that more litter trays, food bowls and water bowls are required than cats within the household. All of these resources need to be separate from one another, as cats do not like to eat, drink or eliminate in the same area. Also take into consideration the type of cat litter that is utilised, as cats do have preferences. Multimodal environmental modifications (MEMO therapy) was found to be exceptionally useful in cases of FIC. MEMO involves gaining a thorough environmental history. A detailed client history form, along with additional client and veterinary resources, can be found online at https://indoorpet.osu.edu/veterinarians/environmental-enrichment-resources-and-references.

STRESS AND ANXIETY MODIFICATION SUPPLEMENTS

There are several commercially available nutritional supplements and diets that contain specific nutrients and dietary ingredients that can aid in reducing stress and anxiety. These include L-tryptophan and milk protein hydrolysate (MPH). Tryptophan is an essential amino acid that is a precursor of serotonin in the brain. Tryptophan has been shown to decrease anxiety, stress-related behaviours and house-soiling when placed in the diet after 8 weeks. MPH is a source of peptide which exhibits many biological effects, including a positive effect on the management of anxious disorders in cats, and acts as an antidepressant in dogs.

Postsurgical clinics

The same consultation process should be followed as with life-stage and medical clinics. Read through the clinical history and see what procedure was undertaken; were there any issues with the surgery? Check whether there were any diagnostic results that need following up (histology, etc.).

The aims of the nursing clinic are to ensure that:
- There have been no postoperative complications and that the owner and the animal are happy
- There is no surgical site infection and that surgical wounds are healing with the progress that is expected for the procedure undertaken
- The owner is compliant with medications that may be required, and any follow-up appointments
- Any dressings or bandages (if any) are changed, checked or removed.

It can be useful in clinics to utilise methods such as taking measurements with a ruler and digital photography in order to monitor wound healing. Where different personnel are performing wound checks and/or dressing changes, it can be difficult to assess whether the wound is progressing if not seen before; therefore taking measurements, or taking a photograph that can be attached to the clinical history, can be beneficial. For more information on wound healing and dressing changes, see Chapter 23.

Diagnostic clinics

The RVN's role is ideal in the provision of aiding the veterinary surgeon in the procedure of collection of samples for diagnostics. The RVN should be utilised in the procedure of blood sampling, blood pressure monitoring, Schirmer tear testing, skin sampling and urinalysis. Nurses are not permitted to make a diagnosis, but they are adequately trained in the preparation of the animal and the collection of samples in order for the veterinary surgeon to make a diagnosis. Evidence gathering to aid the veterinary surgeon means that there is better utilisation of the veterinary surgeon's time (see Chapter 4).

BLOOD SAMPLING

Routine sampling for many conditions can be performed by the RVN within the nursing consultation. These can include repeat sampling for fructosamine levels in diabetic patients, haematology for chemotherapy patients and biochemistry parameters for renal patients. When taking samples, you need to make the decision whether or not to have the owners present during the procedure. Many owners expect to remain while you take the sample, but some will not want to be present; however, they do need to be aware of the option. You should also inform owners that it is essential to clip any hair away from the site of sampling in order to prevent infections, as aseptic preparation of the site is required. If the animal requires more than one site to be clipped, it is important to inform the owner of the reasons for this. In all nursing clinics and consultations communication is exceptionally important, and owners like to be aware at all times of things that affect their pet.

Before taking the sample it is important to confirm that the owner understands why the sample is being taken. If it is for a repeat sampling the owner may be fully aware, but if not, the owner may require clarification. Facts concerning when the animal received medication, or if and when fed, need to be gained. It is also a good opportunity to weigh the animal and obtain its BCS. It some cases this appointment may be their only point of contact with a veterinary professional for the few months in between prescription or other veterinary checks. If the animal is suffering from a particular condition, it is also a good opportunity to question the owner on the animal's overall condition, water intake, urine output, food intake, exercise tolerance and general demeanour.

Ensure that all materials required for blood sampling are prepared prior to bringing the client into the consulting room. All blood tubes should be labelled, and slides (if required) identified. When taking bloods for any haematological analysis blood films should always be produced. If performing the sampling in the consulting room with the client present, a competent assistant will be required in order to restrain the animal. Always remember to introduce your colleague to the client.

It is important to note onto the animal's clinic history where you took the sample from and whether or not it was a stressed sampling. Blood samples taken from stressed cats will cause a stress hyperglycaemia and leucogram. If the veterinary surgeon is not present when the sample is taken he or she will not be aware of this, and interpretation of the results can be altered. Always ensure that the correct blood sampling tubes have been used for the types of tests that are to be performed and the laboratory that the samples are to be sent to.

BLOOD PRESSURE MONITORING

Routine blood pressure monitoring should occur in all patients suffering from renal, cardiac disease and diabetes, as well as all patients in the senior (mature) age category. Blood pressure monitoring should ideally be performed in the presence of the owner. Animals, especially cats, tend to be calmer when their owner is present. Cat owners should be encouraged to bring a blanket that the cat normally sits on at home, as this will help the cat to relax. It is important to allow the cat to come out of the basket without dragging it out or by removing the top of the travel box, and for dogs to freely roam around the consulting room prior to monitoring the blood pressure.

All equipment required should be prepared beforehand; the cuff required to be used should be premeasured and the size recorded on the clinical history. If different cuff sizes are used then different readings will be obtained. The secret here is to use the same cuff and site if you wish to monitor a patient long term. The cuff size is determined by the circumference of the limb on which it will be placed. For cats and dogs, the ratio of cuff width to limb circumference should be about 40%. If in between cuff sizes, round up. After placement, the cuff should not be so loose that it can be rotated over the site or so tight that it obstructs venous return. If it does not stay connected when inflated, select the next larger size cuff.

The use of clippers to remove hair from distal to the carpal stopper pad should be avoided as this can inadvertently increase the blood pressure as a stress response in cats. Instead, wiping the area with surgical spirit and then rubbing ultrasound gel well into the hair works just as effectively. To remove any stress response to the noise created by the Doppler probe, headphones can be used. If none are available for use, the volume should be turned off, the probe positioned, and then the volume slowly increased until the pulse is audible.

All animals will react to the increasing pressure exerted by the cuff, and therefore the first reading should always be discarded, as it will be artificially elevated. Different texts state different methods of finding a final measurement. Some recommend taking five readings and taking an average of the five; some state to take the third reading. I repeat the process until three readings that are similar (within 5 mm Hg) are recorded. All excess gel should be wiped from the animal, and it should be noted to the owner that if the animal licks any of it off it is not harmful. The result, the cuff size used and the location where the cuff was placed should all be recorded on the pet's clinical records.

Blood pressure monitoring is a useful diagnostic tool that should be utilised in many areas in veterinary practice. Blood pressure monitoring is a good prognostic indicator for critical animals. The Doppler probes are also very useful for monitoring heart rate in small patients, e.g. rabbits, hamsters, birds, during general anaesthesia.

URINALYSIS

The analysis of urine is a simple task that can provide an excellent insight into the health of the patient. Specific gravity should be conducted on every sample with use of a refractometer, and when conducting microscopy it is important not just to note whether there were crystals present but also the evidence of casts, cells and microorganisms.

Sample collection

The easiest and most commonly used method of collecting a sample is a free flow or voided sample. Collecting a mid-stream overnight sample is the best for routine urinalysis, as it contains the best indicator of the true composition of urine. The specific conditions being investigated will dictate what part of the sample is required. When collecting a sample for urethral plugs, uroliths and bacteria, then the first part of the stream is the best. The end stream is the most appropriate to collect for examination for prostatic disease, haemorrhage or sediment analysis. This is due to the sediment or haemorrhage collecting on the floor of the bladder. Nearly all voided samples in cats are collected in a litter tray with nonabsorbent litter, and these can prove to be invaluable in the treatment of urinary system problems. Many clients will require some guidance in how to collect the urine sample and the importance of compliance in bringing in collected samples.

SCHIRMER TEAR TESTING

Schirmer tear testing (STT) should be used both as a diagnostic tool and for screening programmes. RVNs are in an ideal position to aid in the initiation of screening programmes; predisposed breeds can be targeted for screening. These include Cocker spaniels, Bulldogs, West Highland white terriers, Lhaso apsos, Shih tzus, Pugs and Pekingese. As a diagnostic tool, indications for STT include:

1. Assessment of normal tear production
2. Chronic mucoid epiphora
3. Chronic pigmentary keratitis
4. Epiphora.

The prepackaged, sterile strips are removed and the notched end is placed in the lower conjunctival fornix; the strip should be in direct contact with the cornea. It is important not to touch the notched end as lipids from your skin can affect the movement of the dye. The eye is held closed and the strip allowed to remain in place for exactly 1 minute. If convenient, both eyes may be tested at the same time. The strip is then removed, and, using the standard measurement on the package, the tear production is measured and recorded. Normal dogs should secrete 15 mm or greater in 1 minute. Topical anaesthetic is not used for this test as we are measuring the response of the eye to an irritant. There are three layers to the tear film, and Schirmer only measures the middle layer or aqueous layer; deficiency of the mucin layer (inner) or the lipid layer (outer) may also cause corneal irritation and opacity.

RVN clinics provide a vital role in the provision of services for clients and their pets. There is huge financial sense in providing clinics as they free up veterinary surgeon time, in order for them to perform more profitable services that only they can undertake.

BIBLIOGRAPHY

Ackerman, N., 2012. The Consulting Veterinary Nurse. Wiley Blackwell, Oxford, UK.

American Animal Hospital Association (AAHA), 2009. American Animal Hospital Association Compliance Study Executive Summary. Available from: <https://www.aahanet.org/PublicDocuments/ComplianceExecutiveSummary0309.pdf>.

Dehasse, J., 1994. Sensory, emotional and social development of the young dog. Bull. Vet. Clin. Ethol. 2 (1–2), 6–29.

Dethioux, F., Marniquet, P., Petit, P., Weber, M., 2005. How can we prevent the metabolic consequences of neutering? Focus Special Edition: Preventative nutrition for major health risks in cats. 9–18.

Grosdidier, S., 2014. Video coaching in practice. In Practice. 36 (2), 99–101.

LANTRA, 2004. LANTRA manpower survey: survey into recruitment, retention, education and training issues relating to veterinary nursing. Available from: <http://www.lantra.co.uk/getattachment/17a7efb3-dbb4-427f-b80e-af4cf36dd0b4/Veterinary-Nursing-Man-Power-Report-%28April-2004%29.aspx>.

Royal College of Veterinary Surgeons (RCVS), 2014. Royal College of Veterinary Surgeons Code of Professional Conduct for Veterinary Nurses. Available from <http://www.rcvs.org.uk/advice-and-guidance/code-of-professional-conduct-for-veterinary-nurses/>.

Shepherd, K., 2002. Development of behaviour, social behaviour and communication in dogs. In: Horwitz, D., Mill, D., Heath, S. (Eds.), BSAVA Manual of Canine and Feline Behavioural Medicine. BSAVA Publications, Gloucester UK, pp. 8–20.

Practice and Staff Management

KRISTIE FAULKNER

KEY POINTS

- Regular measurement of Key Performance Indicators of business health plays a vital role in effective practice management. The Balanced Scorecard approach adds vigour and accuracy to this process.

- The customer experience provided by your practice begins long before the client sets foot in the door and continues long after she has left.

- Every successful business must continually attract new customers as well as retain existing ones; a fantastic customer experience is central to both. This customer experience can be quantified through data collection, using industry-standard tools and models.

- Recommendation brings in a huge proportion of your new clients, and recommendation is driven by your existing clients' experience of your practice.

- It is essential that your team are fully engaged with the practice values and ethos; an engaged team is motivated to deliver consistently excellent customer care to your clients.

- Optimising the deployment of facilities, skills and roles will ensure that your business runs effectively, while delivering the best care for patients and their owners. Best practice is best for everyone.

Business health – diagnosis and prognosis

Assessing your business performance is much like the daily diagnosis and treatment we undertake for our patients. Blood results give us present values to compare with 'normal' ranges from which we diagnose and devise a treatment plan to deal with the problem.

The same analytical approach can be used to manage the health of veterinary business, informing a simple model that distils success into five steps:

1. Make the phone ring.
2. Convert the call into an appointment.
3. Convert the consultation into relevant diagnostic and treatment plans.
4. Charge correctly for the work done.
5. Get recommended.

Managers around the world use a process known as the Balanced Scorecard (first proposed by Kaplan and Norton in 1992) to measure and improve the health of their business, and

we will use this model to assess performance in each of four key areas:

- Customer
- Staff
- Finance
- Operational effectiveness.

Often, the very process of collecting, analysing and measuring highlights gaps and areas of weakness which can be overlooked in day-to-day practice management. An assessment of the business based on numbers and hard facts will identify key focus areas and determine a priority order for required actions.

Rolling annual national industry data shows that the growth in new clients at the 'average' practice is −6.48%, i.e. a year-on-year decrease. Not a great picture. Many successful practices, however, are achieving double-digit growth with focus and hard work, demonstrating just how crucial diagnosing and treating business problems in the four areas of the Balanced Scorecard is.

So let us look at each quadrant of the scorecard in more detail. Each section ends with a consideration of the Key Performance Indicators (KPIs) needed to measure its success and improve the customer experience.

Customer

Competition is rife in every profession, and ours is no different; where consumers have a choice, they will place their business with people who they like and trust, and who offer good value. The phrase 'good value' is significant here; note that it is not 'low prices' or 'cheap' – most of us are savvy enough to know that you get what you pay for, and if something seems too good to be true then it probably is.

Pet and horse owners are no different. Nor are you. Where do you choose to service or mend your car? The local garage, where the staff know you and you can drop the car off at your convenience? Sure, it's bit more expensive, but you trust that they won't sell you things you don't need. Or the dealership in town – guaranteed parts and use of a courtesy car are great, but there's always an unexpected 'extra' on the bill. Both have their advantages and disadvantages, so what swings it for you is how you feel about the whole experience.

A practice may think that it has completed its customer service duties by providing free parking outside, but if the marked bays are tiny, the road surface is pot-holed and full of weeds and there is litter blowing around, the customer's experience will be poor. She will feel that if the practice does not pay attention to these external details, how can she trust it to get her bill right, or to recommend the best care for her pet?

Unlike customer service, the customer experience extends way beyond the physical interaction with a practice. If a practice has a reputation for being expensive, if a friend has shared stories of administrative incompetence or rude staff, if the practice sign is misspelled or the website is 'currently under construction', then the potential client's experience of it will be negative. It won't matter if the customer service provided by the team is the brightest, shiniest and loveliest in the area, because this potential client won't set foot in the door. Service is just one thing – the customer experience is everything.

And there is more competition for practices than ever. Whereas in the year 2000 there were 2200 veterinary sites in the UK, in 2015 there are currently 4723. There are more practices offering vaccination, neutering, preventative health-care products and diagnostic services, so it is crucial to understand what your differentiator for the new client is. And are you doing enough to keep your existing clients from having their heads turned?

TOUCH POINTS ON THE CUSTOMER JOURNEY

Every business needs to attract new customers *and* retain them. In order to be successful here, it is important to understand where the touch points with customers occur and ensure that they are aligned with the five-step veterinary business model mentioned earlier.

1. Awareness, or *Marketing:* **Make the phone ring.**

   Marketing conveys what your practice is about, raising local awareness. Depending on your local demographic, a mix of the traditional methods can be used, for example:
   - Local paper advertising
   - Radio
   - Mail drops
   - Signage
   - Community activity at local shows or talks at primary schools.

   In addition to these traditional approaches, there are more powerful ways to raise awareness:
   - Word of mouth: A recommendation from a friend or family member is worth more than any marketing can ever hope to achieve. If someone has taken the time to personally recommend the care and experience received at your practice to a potential client, that potential client will almost certainly be making a call to you.
   - 'Key Opinion Leaders': Take the time to engage with other pet professionals in the local area – visit them with a gift, such as brand-coloured cupcakes to say hello; start a Key Opinion Leader educational programme, holding quarterly meetings at the practice to share education on common topics and introduce them to your practice. More importantly, don't underestimate how many clients and potential clients approach these people for advice before they come to you:
     - Groomers
     - Kennel/cattery owners
     - Pet shops
     - Dog walkers
     - Pet sitters.

   Word of mouth is the most popular reason for clients to choose a new practice, second only to location. It is important for all new clients to be asked how they heard about you, and the answer recorded in a pre-populated section on the practice management system when recording new client details. This is non-negotiable – it allows the practice to see which marketing activity brings the most clients in and therefore helps determine future spending and activity to focus in the most effective areas.

   Clients who encounter your practice marketing will have a perception of you – but does it match what you think of yourself?
   - Brand and materials: Does your branding (logo/colours) stand out? Are the marketing materials you use eye-catching and do they convey your message effectively?
   - Online presence: If potential clients are to Google 'vets in AnyTown' you would hope to be one of the first listed. If potential clients take the time to look at your website, they should find a mirror image of your physical practice. If your website is out of date, unloved and doesn't match how the practice really is, then customers will undoubtedly be put off before they ever got to the point of calling to enquire.

2. Making the call: **Convert the call into an appointment.**
   - If a potential client has received a recommendation, or has found your website warm, informative and engaging, then the next step is for them to actually make an enquiry – generally by phone.
   - The person who answers the phone plays a vital role in determining whether that potential customer chooses your practice, or one of your competitors, to deliver the product or service needed. Does the person simply treat the enquiry as 'just another price checker' and give a price only? Or do they show interest in the caller's pet, creating a sense of value before describing everything that's included in the price? Do they direct the caller to the practice website for more information about the spay procedure, or discuss the fantastic health plan? Is an appointment offered? Imagine a typical puppy vaccine price query over the phone – 'two vaccinations, 2–4 weeks apart and it will cost £xx'. Now imagine that instead of calling, the owner brings this puppy in and asks the same question. The name of the puppy is asked, how pup has been settling in, lots of compliments are given and more often than not the team member will take the pup 'through the back' reluctantly returning only to tell the customer how many of the staff want to take him or her home with them. The client is made to *feel* special, and this is the experience the client will remember. This feeling needs to be transferred to the initial phone call, so that from the very first direct contact with the practice clients feel respected and valued.

   Arrival and waiting:
   - What does the exterior of your practice look like? Clean and tidy with fresh visible signage? Or tired and overrun with rubbish or weeds?
   - Are customers greeted warmly, or at least acknowledged as soon as they get to the reception desk if the customer care team are on the phone? Think about the times you have stood for a few minutes while a receptionist finishes typing/speaking on the phone or, worse, takes an age to realise that you are there. How does it

make you feel? Irritated from the off? This is not what we want for the first impression.

- Is the waiting room clean, with up-to-date notice boards and relevant practice information on show? Hopefully your clients will not be kept waiting for their pre-booked appointment, but while they do sit and wait for a very short time, they will be taking notice of everything they can see.
- If a paying customer books a specific appointment slot then they rightly will expect to be seen on time – don't keep them waiting.

3. The consultation. **Convert the consultation into relevant diagnostic and treatment plans.**
   - The consulting room is the heartbeat of the practice. It is the main area which the customer will see apart from the waiting room, so what happens here really matters. Whether it is a veterinary nurse consultation for second vaccination or a vet consultation for a sick pet, the client must understand what is happening and why. This means creating great rapport from the outset; using open questions to set the agenda, connecting customers to what has been found, and making a clear recommendation as to what the treatment plan or nutritional programme will be, along with how much it will cost. Re-examine appointments are routinely booked with dentists and hairdressers, so there is no reason why our customers wouldn't book in at the time for the re-weigh/second vaccine or follow-up. People are more likely to attend a pre-booked appointment than remember to book one at a later date.
   - The recommendation of blood tests, surgery or flea and worm treatment must be clear and informed. An ambiguous 'you should probably think about having the teeth cleaned' does not say to the client that a dental scale and polish is necessary, and more than likely another year will pass until the next booster appointment, where the same ambiguous recommendation may be made, and ignored, again.

4. The money part. **Charge correctly for the work done.**
   - Once a clear recommendation has been made, all associated costs must be clearly communicated. For in-patients and surgeries, correct charging is imperative. How many times do you visit the local supermarket and get a discount because you are old, shop there frequently or look as though you have no money? The truth is, health care costs money, and undercharging devalues your service, setting a precedent that does no favours for the health of the business and its ability to afford new equipment, continued professional development (CPD) budgets, pay rises for the team or the profession. Miscommunication regarding costs is a common complaint among customers, and it is one reason why they may seek an alternative practice – avoid it at all costs.

5. Lasting impression: **Get recommended.**
   - Once customers have left the consulting room or have collected their pet after surgery or hospitalisation, their lasting impression must be as positive as the first. Running through the invoice clearly, showing an interest in how the consultation went, how pleased the customer must be that the pet has recovered well, or just sharing a smile and the sentiment that you look forward

to seeing the owner and her pet again soon is a warm and caring way to end the in-house experience. From start to finish, the experience must be so great that customers tell their friends and family how good you are.

- 'Friend get friend' recommendation: Vouchers giving £10 off for both recommended clients and the original client are a great way of encouraging recommendation.
- Keep in touch: In Generation Millennial, keeping in touch is easier and more cost effective than ever. Text reminders, progress emails, newsletters and interaction on social media are all musts to ensure a move from once-per-year boosters to more frequent contact between visits. Another non-negotiable must-do: get up-to-date mobile numbers and email addresses. It is the norm for businesses to request this information, and ours is no different; we need this information to keep in touch and to cost-effectively send reminders for pet treatment items.
- Social media: An interactive, informative and frequently updated Facebook page is a great way to show off the practice personality, give insight into practice personnel and inform customers quickly and efficiently regarding practice news or local disease outbreaks. For it to work, however, clients must first 'like' the page. All team members should encourage as many people as possible to like the practice page, and in turn their friends will also see the interaction and become aware that the practice exists.

Customer Balanced Scorecard Key Performance Indicators

ACTIVE CLIENTS PER FULL-TIME-EQUIVALENT VET

The average small animal practice needs around 1000 active clients per full-time-equivalent vet. Active clients are defined as those who have transacted with the practice within a 14- or 16-month window.

NEW CLIENTS PER MONTH: 20 PER FULL-TIME-EQUIVALENT VET PER MONTH

The active client database can decrease by up to 25% each year due to clients moving, pets dying or a competitor practice turning heads. Your practice therefore needs to continue to attract, win and retain clients on an ongoing basis just to survive, never mind grow.

INDEX SCORE: TARGET 85%+ PER MONTH

The Index score measures the experience team members create when a potential new client contacts the practice for the first time. Mystery shopping assesses what is said, the type of language used, levels of engagement and tone used throughout a typical call. Reporting on and recording the calls allows for discussion with the team around ways to improve, and highlights why new client registrations may not be quite where you want them to be.

NET PROMOTER SCORE: TARGET >80%

Fred Reichheld (2003) developed the Net Promoter Score (NPS) as a way of gauging how likely customers are to recommend a business to friends and family. Respondents allocate a score of between 0 (very unlikely) and 10 (very likely), with promoters giving a score of 9 or 10 and considered to be loyal enthusiasts, while detractors respond with a score of 0 to 6 – unhappy customers. Scores of 7 and 8 are passives. The NPS is calculated by subtracting the percentage of customers who are detractors from the percentage of customers who are promoters. In any client survey it is recommended that you also include freehand textboxes so that customers may elaborate further on your service, then share the findings with your clients. Taking visible actions to address any highlighted concerns or requests will improve the customer experience, which is always good for business.

Staff

Human resources (HR) is both the most costly and valuable asset of a business. It can also be the greatest cause of problems. If the practice invested heavily in an expensive piece of equipment, you would expect that it would do its job effectively; it is only sensible therefore to view investment in staff the same way.

For the team to be as productive as possible, each member needs to know what the common goal is – what is your practice vision statement?

The vision statement articulates what a company aspires to be as well as the future it wants to create. It must therefore underpin all business strategy (Mcginnis 1981 cited in David 1989; Thornberry 1997); for example, your vision may be:

'To provide the very best community-based veterinary care in AnyTown, where owners and their pets come first.'

If this vision is to be realised, every single member of staff must be aware of this end goal and understand how their role contributes to reaching it.

Beyond this, your mission statement can be as simple as who the company is and what it does (Falsey 1989 cited in Stallworth Williams 2008). Practices can elaborate further, addressing clients, pets, location and technology, providing areas of focus and building blocks allowing the practice to reach the vision. For example:

'We are a highly trained veterinary team, committed to providing outstanding value and care for your pets for life. Our modern, well-equipped practices are located around the AnyTown area and offer a wide range of services tailored to your pet's individual needs. We endeavour to do our very best for your pet and demonstrate this through excellent customer service.'

This example includes the pet, which is the main concern for both customer and practice (David 1989). It also uses 'we' throughout, joining the practice and owner together and building trust by coming across as 'one of them' (Stallworth Williams 2008). This satisfies the main need of the customer – to care for and look after their pet as an individual – and is something which every team member should be able to deliver in practice.

Veterinary practice is made up of different teams – management, reception, nursing, administration, veterinary – and each team is made up of different individuals.

Let's consider the dictionary definition of team:
1. *A number of persons forming one of the sides in a game or contest: a football team*
2. *A number of persons associated in some joint action: a team of advisers*
3. *Two or more horses, oxen, or other animals harnessed together to draw a vehicle, plough, or the like*
4. *A family of young animals, especially ducks or pigs.*

Two to pay particular notice to are numbers 1 and 3:
1. A football team cannot effectively score goals if only half the team is playing the game, and all players need to know what role they play in that team to result in goals being scored.
3. If animals are harnessed together, they can draw the vehicle, but only if all animals are pulling in the same direction.

It is exactly the same for our practice teams. All team members must be aware of the common goal, or practice vision. Each individual within each team must then understand the impact that his or her role has on reaching this goal, and each team must understand how to work together to achieve the vision.

Another useful description of a team comes from Katzenbach and Smith (1993) who state that 'a team is a small number of people with complementary skills who are committed to a common purpose, performance goals, and approach for which they hold themselves mutually accountable'.

If this does not describe your own practice, then frequent problems are inevitable. Friction between team members and inefficiencies within the practice from day to day will ultimately prevent progression for the business.

Leadership

Back to the football team analogy. What impact does the manager of the team have in the level of success enjoyed? Some would argue not a lot, others would say that a good manager is vital to achieve greatness. So what's the difference between management and leadership?

- *Management: The process of dealing with or controlling things or people.*
- *Leadership: The action of leading a group of people or an organisation, or the ability to do this.*

Notice that even by looking at these definitions, one seems to be more of a dictatorial role; the other involves people following by choice. There is certainly room for, and reason to find, a balance between management and leadership – rotas, admin, paperwork and so on all need to be managed; but when it comes to the people you have working alongside you, wouldn't it be brilliant if they came along with you instead of being dragged?

Bennis (1989) composed a list of the differences between leaders and managers:
- The manager is a copy; the leader is an original.
- The manager maintains; the leader develops.
- The manager focuses on systems and structure; the leader focuses on people.
- The manager relies on control; the leader inspires trust.
- The manager has a short-term view; the leader has long-range perspective.

- The manager asks how and when; the leader asks what and why.
- The manager accepts the status quo; the leader challenges it.

This list shows us how the balance of management and leadership may be achieved, and suggests that the practice may well be held back if the team are managed without also being led.

Leadership allows the practice vision to come alive for the teams; it helps us look beyond what has simply always happened and enables changes that benefit staff, the business, our customers and their pets.

Painting a picture of what practice life could look like is one thing, but direction as to how the teams and individuals can facilitate meeting this vision is another; so we now need to look at who you have on your team, who you may have in the future, and how you can ensure that everyone is pulling in the same direction.

THE CURRENT TEAM

You may have a great team who work really well together and get the job done. Or you may have certain teams who work well and get the job done, or you may have certain individuals who get the job done. Team members firstly need to know where it is you need to get to (vision) and what it is they need to do to get you there.

The culture of your practice may help or hinder you on the journey. Is there a culture of fairness and wanting to be the best that you can be, or one of 'it's not my job' or worse still 'I just want to get paid and go home'? A leader can create a great culture by inspiring people to be the best that they can be. So let's look at a few necessary building blocks:

JOB DESCRIPTIONS

Job descriptions define roles (Box 4.1); they provide boundaries, direction and connection as to how each role assists in reaching the vision while providing accountability. They sit firmly in the 'management' pot, but give a reference point and help towards being able to deliver a meaningful performance appraisal.

All items on the list have to be explained and understood by the team member. If there are areas that the employee feels uncertain about, training needs to be undertaken to enable the task to be completed effectively.

Job descriptions should be reviewed and updated regularly to maintain usability – and must include elements around delivering a great customer experience. Remember, pets don't bring themselves in or pay their own bills.

Performance management

So now that the job outline and duties associated with the role are clear and understood, how do we make sure that said duties are done, and done well? Performance management is more than just an appraisal; it is about ensuring that roles and responsibilities are aligned with supporting the practice vision, and that staff members are in a position to fulfil these roles.

Performance appraisals are not to be ignored, dreaded or done half-heartedly. Nor are they the place for wholly negative feedback, a place to have a good moan or ask for a pay rise. The appraisal process should be viewed as a regular, useful

---

BOX 4.1 EXAMPLE OF A VETERINARY NURSE JOB DESCRIPTION

Job description: Veterinary nurse
Job purpose: To provide high-quality medical care to all patients. To provide outstanding customer service and help to create and maintain an efficient hospital
General responsibilities:
- To be proactive in moving the practice forward
- To provide an excellent customer experience
- To provide veterinary nurse clinics
- To help drive pet health plan sales
- To use 'friend get friend' vouchers
- To ensure own job list is completed

General nursing responsibilities:
- To care for all patients as if they were your own
- To call clients regarding inpatients in a thorough and caring manner
- To admit day patients for surgery correctly
- To prepare patients for surgery in good time, weighing, bleeding and sedating
- To consult alongside vet offering information on all preventative care and pet heath plans
- To assist and monitor anaesthesia correctly with recording sheet
- To perform all duties listed on daily scheduling sheets depending on shift
- To clean and sterilise all theatre equipment after use, ready for next day
- To monitor recovery from anaesthesia and until the patient is discharged
- To discharge day and theatre patients
- To provide excellent customer service should cover or assistance be requested on reception
- To follow up and complete any messages/duties you should encounter
- To price theatre accounts correctly and ensure medical notes are written up at all times
- To quote for surgeries where necessary
- To keep maintenance duties up to date on practice equipment
- To complete all individual duties allocated
- To ensure practice is clean and tidy, ready for the next day's work
- To perform weekly theatre/consult/prep cleans

Administrative duties:
- To complete insurance claim forms
- To input/scan laboratory results/previous histories onto system and file accordingly when vets have seen

---

discussion about employee strengths and weaknesses, clarifying how you as a line manager will enable the individual to make the most of her or his strengths and improve on weaknesses. How well the individual performs, both alone and as part of a team, should be discussed, as should any development and training which may be needed or requested, along with an exploration of how these areas will assist in meeting personal and practice business objectives.

Successful appraisals will increase individual productivity, improve morale and drive motivation and commitment, but only if they are successful. Negative and unproductive annual reviews can actually demotivate staff and make a mockery of the whole process. Performance review should be continuous. An annual performance review is fine, as long as there is a bi-annual 'mini-appraisal' to ensure that the items agreed on such as further training, CPD or additional duties are being carried out and that both parties are 'on the right track'. A year

TABLE 4.1	Example of simple appraisal content

JOB TASK PERFORMANCE TABLE

To be completed by appraiser in conjunction with performance appraisal form

Name: _____ Department: _____

Job task (brief description)	Appraisal rating (tick box)				
	A	B	C	D	E

A Consistently outstanding performance in all aspects of task.
B Has consistently performed more than effectively in most aspects of task.
C Has consistently performed all aspects of task effectively.
D Has generally performed effectively but some aspects of task require improvement.
E Has consistently performed less than effectively in most aspects of task.

1. Which areas of the job have you performed best? How did you go about achieving this?
2. Which areas of the job have you performed less well? Were there any circumstances which prevented performance?
3. What could be done by you, your manager or the practice to help improve your performance in any way?

TABLE 4.2	Job task performance table

OVERALL GRADING OF PERFORMANCE

From your evaluation against the main tasks of the job description and the markings on the Job Task Performance Table, indicate the overall performance achieved by the job holder. Bear in mind particularly the definitions of the ratings. The assessment should reflect the performance actually achieved in the circumstances which prevailed. Any unusual/special factors governing the year's performance should be stated below the assessment.

Tick the appropriate box:

□	□	□	□	□	□
A	B	C	D	E	X

Key:
A: Constantly outstanding performance in most areas of job
B: Constantly more than effective performance in most areas of job
C: Effective performance
D: Some effective performance but some improvement required in many areas of job (review in 6 months)
E: Constantly underachieving and less than effective in most areas of job (review in 3 and 6 months)
X: Too early to assess (review in 6 months)

ALL APPRAISERS SHOULD NOW COMPLETE THE AGREED ACTION PLAN LETTER.

4. The following training and other action will be taken:

5. Employee's comments:

down the line is a little late in the day to find out that the training has not been done, or the steps agreed to improve a particular weakness have not been taken, and in effect there has been zero progress in a 12-month period. It is important to point out that appraisals are two-way as far as commitment and responsibility go; the employee and employer *must* put the same amount of effort into action plans and development to ensure that both the business and the individuals grow.

Appraisal forms should be easy to fill in and to the point, with action plans easy to refer back to at the mini-review or any other time where a meeting with a team member arises. Both line appraiser and appraisee should fill in an appraisal form based on the job outline and duties noted in the job description 2–4 weeks before the appraisal date. It is recommended that you keep a file of areas where the employee has completed tasks effectively, gone above and beyond or has not been able to fulfil elements of the job description to enable specific examples to be given. An example of simple appraisal content is in Table 4.1.

Items detailed on the job descriptions can be appraised in quality and ability, using a job task performance table such as that shown in Table 4.2, which will allow for focus in areas which need assistance.

When it goes wrong

The standards of the practice must be maintained, and if there are members of staff who frequently cause disruption and fail to meet performance criteria, *despite* having been given relevant training and direction, disciplinary action may be necessary. It is worth pointing out, however, that with a clear and communicated practice vision, up-to-date job descriptions and frequent performance review, disciplinary action can be avoided in most cases. Every business needs its own disciplinary policy

detailed in the practice employee handbook, which must be readily available to all staff members. The main areas of disciplinary action usually concern attendance, health and safety, behaviour and job capabilities.

POSITIVE DISCIPLINE

The fact that we work alongside adults would suggest that we should treat them as such. Positive discipline involves putting the responsibility on the employee to change any behaviour that is unacceptable, rather than change being forced upon them. Effective communication is key here – rather than using reactive punishment outright, the option to change should first be given to the team member. By working together based on this decision to change, negative behaviour can be eliminated. Reasons for the behaviour should be sought so that both employee and employer can explore solutions.

If positive discipline fails, it is important to follow a clear and standardised process with regards to issuing warnings, for example:

1. Oral (verbal) warning. Appropriate in cases where unacceptable standards are present
2. Written warning. For a more serious offence, or continued use of the same unacceptable standards that triggered the initial oral warning
3. Final written warning. Continued failure to improve after the written warning, or for serious misconduct such as being rude to a client

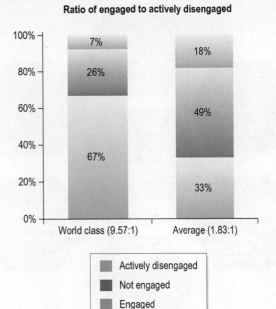

Fig. 4.1 Ratio of engaged to actively disengaged, in an average practice and a 'world class' practice

TABLE 4.3	Twelve core elements represented by 12 questions

KEY

Number	Question
1	Do I know what is expected of me at work?
2	Do I have the materials and equipment I need to do my work right?
3	At work, do I have the opportunity to do what I do best every day?
4	In the last 7 days, have I received recognition or praise for doing good work?
5	Does my supervisor, or someone at work, seem to care about me as a person?
6	Is there someone at work who encourages my development?
7	At work, do my opinions seem to count?
8	Does the mission/purpose of my company make me feel my job is important?
9	Are my co-workers committed to doing quality work?
10	In the last 6 months, has someone at work talked to me about my progress?
11	This last year, have I had opportunities at work to learn and grow?
12	Do I have a best friend at work?

4. Dismissal. Following a further failure to improve after the final written warning, or for gross misconduct such as theft, assault, use of drugs or alcohol on the premises, fraud or falsification of records.

Disciplinary proceedings are essential to undertake professionally and with full regard to employment law – for this reason, outsourcing HR in order to ensure up-to-date, accurate guidance on all employment legislation and misconduct policies is highly recommended.

STAFF SURVEYS

It is important to keep on top of the current mood within the practice team, and bi-annual staff surveys are a great way for team members to safely answer specific, measurable questions while having the opportunity to leave anonymous comments. As much as you would like teams to be able to come to you and voice anything, anytime, this is often not the case.

Employee engagement is crucial to team performance. The following analysis of its importance is provided by the Gallup organisation, and the chart demonstrates how the best-performing businesses have far fewer disengaged employees (Fig. 4.1).

The simple fact is that when employees are engaged with a practice's ethos and vision, they perform better. The 'Gallup 12' is a robust questionnaire developed by the Gallup Organisation identifying 12 core elements that link powerfully to key business outcomes (Table 4.3).

This Gallup survey is used by countless organisations in every area of business around the world, and is the definitive measure of employee engagement. The 12 questions capture the most important information about a workplace – measuring the key elements needed to attract, focus and retain great employees. Analysing the data identifies areas where the team need more support and direction, and ultimately thus builds a stronger team.

WANTS AND OFFERS

This is a great exercise for aligning the wants and needs of employer and employees, highlighting the mutual expectation present in practice.

The manager creates two flip chart lists:
1. **What I will offer** you as a team
2. **What I want** from you as a team

The team are then asked to create two further flip chart lists:
1. **What we want** from you (the manager)
2. **What we will offer** you (the manager)

Each list should match – if not, a discussion will explore where changes are required and keeps everyone focused on that common goal.

PERSONALITIES

We find a vast array of personality types in practice, and understanding each will allow for greater communication, understanding and enhanced productivity and engagement. A useful tool here is DISC profiling, giving insight into the different personality types in the team, providing guidance as to how each personality type is best communicated with and assessing predicted behaviour in certain environments and situations. There are four core personality types, and everyone has a mix of each in different degrees (Fig. 4.2):

- Dominance: driven, direct communicators
- Influential: thrive on praise and recognition
- Steadiness: like clarity, routine and security
- Compliance: perfectionist, information gatherers

Profiling uncovers the things that motivate individuals, as well as informing how best to communicate with each personality type. DISC profiling thus allows the team to understand each other better and can also be used to identify strong candidates to join the team in the future.

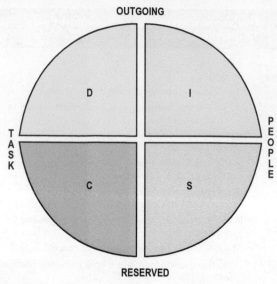

Fig. 4.2 DISC profiling

TRAINING

It is vital that every member of the team is trained to enhance current, or obtain new, skills. Medicines and surgical techniques change so rapidly that we are no strangers to CPD, but how many of these training events are shared or documented as part of a development plan, and how many of these CPD events are non-clinical? Going back to the customer quadrant of the Balanced Scorecard, customer service training for front-of-house teams, telephone skill training and communication training in the consulting room are all vital areas for investment. Unfortunately, unless the pet is killed or cured, customers rarely measure practices based on clinical skills as competence is more often than not assumed. The experience that they have and how they feel is much more likely to drive recommendation than the type of antibiotic prescribed or the size of wound post-surgery.

THE FUTURE TEAM: RECRUITMENT

You may have team members who can be difficult, resist changes and generally create a negative atmosphere. These qualities are to be avoided in future recruitment.

Consider what it is that you look for in a new employee, regardless of position to be filled. It should be much more than simply a pair of hands, tempting as that might be when facing a dearth of applicants.

- Qualifications
- Experience
- In what field
- Confidence
- What else?
- Add something new ... communication and awareness of the client experience.

It is also worth considering the question, What do new staff members look for in you? It is important that both the employer and employee are satisfied, but also that the 'wants' for both drive toward practice vision (Fig. 4.3).

Your job advert must be attractive and eye-catching, with all relevant information included:

- Not too wordy
- Essential information:

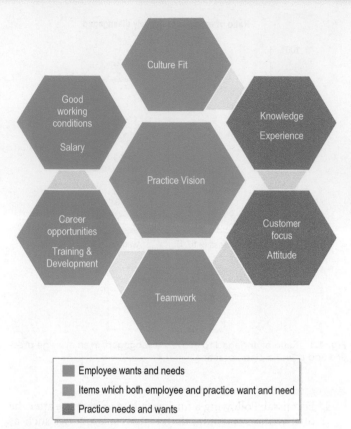

Employee wants and needs
Items which both employee and practice want and need
Practice needs and wants

Fig. 4.3 The practice vision

- Practice logo and name
- Job title
- About us
- About you
- About the job
- Starting salary/benefits
- Application form
- Contact details.

It is recommended that you have an application form for candidates to fill in and return along with their CV – it will weed out those who won't even put in the effort to fill out a form.

Now you have your applicants. Which ones should you interview? Start with those who stand out. Do they have a cover letter for starters? Place all applications into 'yes', 'no' or 'maybe' piles. 'Yes' are those who fit with the job ad and job description specifications. 'No' are those who do not, so don't be tempted to go back to that pile. 'Maybe' applicants can be reviewed if necessary once 'yes' applicants have been contacted. Phone screening is very useful and can save time in the face-to-face interviews.

Once phone screening is complete and you have interviews booked, make sure that you:

- Ensure that the interview is held somewhere where there will be no interruptions
- Interview a realistic number over a few days – each candidate needs the opportunity to stand out individually and not become jumbled into one another
- Prepare questions to establish:
  - Experience and skills
  - Customer service
  - Personality and culture fit
  - Why this practice?

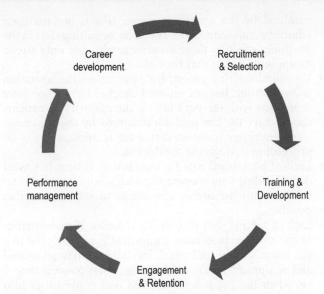

Fig. 4.4 Recruitment and development cycle

Once a candidate has been offered the position and accepted, all the staff considerations we have covered previously need to be adhered to, enabling retention and development of a strong team member, as shown in Figure 4.4.

REGULAR TEAM MEETINGS

Getting everyone together may seem like an impossible task, but it is a necessary one. Whole practice meetings do not have to happen on a regular basis, but team meetings – i.e. veterinary nurse team, reception team, management team and veterinary teams – do. Each team should meet regularly to discuss day-to-day issues, and then the heads of teams should also meet to bring team ideas and solutions to the table, which will reduce negative impact on all teams involved. Whole practice meetings can be timed along with a bi-annual activity such as summer BBQ or Christmas event if they are extremely difficult to coordinate.

Operational effectiveness

Imagine that the practice is a manufacturing warehouse. Managers look to have every square inch of the building as operationally effective as possible at all times, as the costs associated with owning or leasing the warehouse do not pause or get refunded if the plant is not busy enough. This means that the machinery or teams employed within the warehouse must be efficient to ensure that productivity remains high.

Applying this to the veterinary business means looking at where we may be underutilising resources – resulting in higher costs, higher stress levels and reduction in practice potential (Box 4.2). Key touch points where issues can occur are:

ON INITIAL ENQUIRY

If customers do not recommend you, and in turn you do not have enough new clients joining the practice, the pets that we are qualified to treat do not arrive in our surgeries. New customers make enquiries via the phone in most cases, so if your clinic has just one or two inbound lines, and just one member

of staff on reception at any one time, the chances are that your phone will be frequently engaged or simply go unanswered. Putting ourselves in the client's shoes, what happens if you have a choice of company to make an enquiry with, and the first one you call is engaged? You go on to try the next number, and if they pick up, then give a great initial experience, you won't be calling the first number back.

Call data is important here – it shows when the peak call volume times are, what the pattern looks like by hour and by day, when you need to increase staff numbers at reception and what the percentage of calls engaged is, indicating whether there is a need for further phone lines. Analysing inbound call volume will also enable you to work out how effective your phone teams are at converting enquiries into appointments – look at how the total number of inbound calls compares to the number of all first consultation appointments in any one month (include puppy/kitten vaccines and boosters) to calculate the conversion rate. The team should aim to convert half of initial calls into paid consultations.

Answering phones away from reception is a great way to ensure that the face-to-face experience is positive without the interruption of the phone, and also that the phone experience is positive without the distraction of your team member dealing with someone at reception.

THE CONSULTATION DIARY

The consulting room is the heart of the practice. How many consulting rooms are available, who is using them and what happens in them are therefore vital areas to look at when considering operational effectiveness.

Utilise space available

Take a look at how many consulting rooms your practice has. How many of the 24 hours in every day are these rooms available for use? If your consulting hours resemble 9.00am – 11am, a break for surgery, back to consulting around 2pm until 6.20pm, then the rooms are being used only 25% of the time. If you offer extended opening hours, then this percentage will increase, but the focus should be on how to open up consulting time further still. Early consultations, late consultations, weekend opening and shift work allowing consultations to run throughout the day will all increase available consulting time, but the clients have to be there to fill those slots. Which brings us neatly back to the importance of getting recommended and creating local awareness via effective marketing.

Who is using the consulting rooms? Another way of utilising space is to look at who is using the consulting rooms, and what for. If you only have vets consulting at your practice, then almost certainly rooms are being used by vets for things that veterinary nurses are perfectly capable of doing. Each of the examples in the list below can be undertaken by veterinary nurses, thus freeing up vet appointments for those cases that only vets can see and increasing the productivity of the consulting space:

- Pre-vaccine puppy and kitten information appointments
- Second vaccines
- Triage appointments
- Post-op checks
- Admissions
- Discharges
- Bandage changes
- Nail trims/anal gland expressing/ear cleaning
- Medical clinics (including weight, renal, diabetes)
- Pain management clinics
- Diagnostic clinics (blood pressure monitoring, blood sampling)
- Adolescent checks
- Pet health plan checks
- Senior clinics.

Consultation effectiveness. The initial consultation (consultation 1)–to–consultation 2 (re-examination) ratio is important to address. Many practices have consultation 1, 2, 3 and even 4 options on the practice management system. Commonly, the numbers of consultations 1 and 3 are high, but consultations 2 are low. This is usually because there is a feeling of guilt when the pet comes back in for a re-examination, and the cheaper consultation 3 is charged. There are few reasons why a presenting patient with an illness should not need to come back in to get the all clear from a veterinary surgeon, i.e. the person who is qualified to sign the problem off as resolved. An easy way to prevent this from occurring is to remove the consultation 3 option from the system.

The consultations–to–diagnostics/surgery ratio is another area to monitor. We have discussed the importance of a clear recommendation stage, enabling the client to fully understand the diagnosis and why the recommendation is necessary. If the conversion from consultation to any kind of necessary workup, diagnostics or surgery is low, it may be that there is an issue with the consultation process for one or more vets – either an ambiguous recommendation or lack of clarity around value and pricing.

Consultation capacity. Take a look at how many actual appointment slots are on offer throughout your available consulting hours for both vets and veterinary nurses, then at how many of those slots were taken during the last full month. Drilling down further, how many of the vet appointments were for things that a nurse would have been able to do? Quite often, capacity is underutilised and until investigated, it goes unnoticed. Box 4.2 shows figures associated with staff balance.

'Through the back'. Each day in veterinary practice varies hugely in what comes through the door and what type of day everyone has. On average, however, ineffectiveness affecting theatre capacity and day-to-day running can be found in many clinics. Common reasons for operational ineffectiveness are as follows:

- Vets aspinall admitting operations: Unless there is a particularly complicated case, the majority of operations should be admitted by the veterinary nurse. If vets are routinely admitting, this reduces the available consulting slots in the morning, affecting those customers who can only attend an appointment at that time of day.
- Vets administering pre-med: Again, unless the operation is non-routine, has not yet been checked by a vet or there is an issue with the pet's health, the majority of patients should have the pre-med administered by the theatre or ward veterinary nurse so that there is minimal delay on proceeding through the theatre list.
- Lack of established rota for operations: If time is wasted daily deciding who is operating with whom, a rota should be drawn up to enable operations to start as soon as possible.
- Lack of specific shift or individual duties: If maintenance of the X-ray or laboratory equipment is not assigned to a particular shift or individual, inevitably things get missed and equipment breaks down at the worst possible time – i.e. when the pet is anaesthetised and ready to go into X-ray. Shift duties enable daily ownership of areas such as ward/theatre and general cleaning and preparation of the practice.

Veterinary nurses, as with the consultation scenario, should be doing everything which does not specifically need to be done by a vet to enhance productivity of the teams and practice, e.g. in addition to the above:

- Taking and running blood tests
- Placing IV catheters
- Prep for surgery
- Certain X-rays.

INVENTORY CONTROL

This area may seem best suited to the finance section of the chapter, but inefficient stock control can lead to large amounts of cash being tied up on the shelf and an accumulation of out-of-date (OOD) stock items, which have to be discarded. Allocate one team member to be responsible for placing orders, as different orders placed by different people can lead to duplication of products. Frequent stock rotation is key to reduce OOD items, and introducing minimum/maximum order levels can bring structure and standardisation to stock control.

There are useful processes to aid reduction in ineffectiveness and provide structure and guidance in day-to-day running of the practice. **Six Sigma** is described by Henk et al. (2006) in a rather fitting way:

'Six Sigma's approach is similar to that of good medical practice used since the time of Hippocrates – relevant information is assembled followed by careful diagnosis. After a thorough diagnosis is completed, a treatment is proposed and implemented. Finally, checks are applied to see if the treatment was effective.'

Lean management also offers a number of standard solutions to common organisational issues (Henk et al. 2006; Kim et al. 2009). A combination of lean and Six Sigma management is therefore highly effective in everyday practice, and specific concepts that are of use here are:

- **Just-in-time inventory control.** This traditionally means supplying a product or service one at a time just as it is needed by a customer (Novis and Konstantakos 2006). While this would not fit with the ordering of surgical supplies due to unpredictability on a day-to-day basis, it does fit with:

- Minimum/maximum stock re-ordering levels
- Repeat long-term medications with clients 'trained' to order in advance
- Repeat food orders, again 'training' clients to order as they are almost ready to collect
- Preventative products and seasonal promotions.

Using this approach will reduce stock on the shelf along with the costs associated with holding this stock.

- **First in, first out:** This ensures that stock first ordered in is the first used – placing newly ordered stock to the back of the shelf and moving old stock forward is key (Richardson and Osborne 2006).
- Reduce task time and waste by establishing standardised work procedures such as **5S visual management**. 5S stands for *sort, straighten, shine, standardise, and sustain.* 5S uses visual aids to facilitate easy-to-understand instructions, e.g.:
  - Using labels for min/max order levels in the pharmacy
  - Visual document for correct scrub technique
  - Labelling surgical pack contents to reduce time wasted looking for missing instruments
  - In-house laboratory instructions for equipment usage and maintenance
  - Paper identification collars for day and hospitalised patients
  - Colour-coded equipment per consultation room such as nail clippers, flea combs and otoscope to save consulting time looking for these items elsewhere in the building
  - Daily theatre and inpatient boards.
- **DMAIC** – whereby an issue is **D**efined, **M**easured, **A**nalysed, **I**mproved and **C**ontrolled – is useful for cases such as late operating start times and late consultation times. The problem is identified, data is collected and analysed (e.g. frequency of late-running consultation times and average waiting times), improvements are made based on the diagnosis and then efforts to improve are controlled and monitored going forward. This means that common problems are addressed and not just left as a source of frustration for staff and customers alike.

Installing these systems, however, needs more than just protocol – to reap the benefits of increased efficiency resulting in higher productivity and reduced stress, the teams must be committed to finding more efficient ways to work on a day-to-day basis (Novis and Konstantakos 2006). Box 4.3 shows the figures that practices should be aiming to achieve in operational effectiveness.

Finance

While we may not join the veterinary industry to make millions, and finance may not be something which we regularly think about, the reality is that of any other business – customers must be aware that the business exists, choose your practice over the competition, pay for products and services and recommend you to friends and family. By making small, but key, changes to the way you approach and manage practice finances, you can see big results. Box 4.4 shows the finance balance figures which a practice should be aiming for.

Most of us recoil from the word 'sell'. So we will change that word to 'educate'. If we educate our clients on the things which are 'best for pet', then they are best placed to make an informed decision on whether or not to purchase it.

Each and every team member can affect how well clients and potential clients are educated.

RECEPTION TEAM

The reception team takes regular phone enquiries regarding vaccinations, neutering, fleas and general advice. What do the team educate clients in?

- Why vaccination is recommended, vaccination protocol and which diseases they protect against
- Why regular flea and worm treatment is recommended, which products are held in practice and why they are more effective than some pet shop products
- Neutering procedure and why it is recommended
- General advice; why an appointment is recommended.

NURSING TEAM

The nursing team takes phone enquiries as above for reception teams, with additional focus on areas such as general advice, surgical procedures and preventative healthcare recommendations. What do they educate clients in?

- Why vaccination is recommended, vaccination protocol and which diseases they protect against
- Why regular flea and worm treatment is recommended, which products are held in practice and why they are more effective than some pet shop products
- Neutering procedure and why it is recommended
- General advice; why an appointment is recommended
- Nutrition
- Blood profiling
- Pre- and post-op instruction
- Behaviour
- Socialisation
- Administering medication

BOX 4.3 OPERATIONAL EFFECTIVENESS BALANCED SCORECARD FOR KPIS

These are the figures that practices are aiming to achieve:
Consultation 1–to–consultation 2 ratio: >50%
Consults admitted for workup, diagnostics or surgery: >25%
Number of inbound calls per FTE vet per month: >1000
Calls lost or engaged: <5%

BOX 4.4 FINANCE BALANCED SCORECARD FOR KPIS

These are the figures that practices should be aiming/achieving:
Turnover per FTE vet: >£230 000
Gross profit (as % of turnover): 73%
Average transaction value (excluding VAT): >£50. This figure can be calculated simply by dividing the 'cash in the till' by the number of transactions per month
Staff costs: <40% (20% non-vet, 20% vet)
Wholesale spend: <20%

- Explanation of the veterinary surgeon's diagnosis, if the owner wants more information
- Explanation of the treatment plan, to aid in compliance.

VETERINARY TEAM

All consultations undertaken:
- Why vaccination is recommended, vaccination protocol and which diseases are protected against
- Why regular flea and worm treatment is recommended, which products are held in practice and why they are more effective than some pet shop products
- Neutering procedure and why it is recommended
- Explanation of diagnosis
- Explanation of treatment plan.

You will notice that educational themes are duplicated throughout each of the teams, because it is the responsibility of all veterinary team members to know what we recommend and why we recommend it. There must be a consistent recommendation across all staff members.

If we do not educate our clients effectively, then pets may not be treated with an effective veterinary parasitic product, may not be on a correct diet for their breed or life stage, are not brought in soon enough when they show signs of illness and do not receive the necessary diagnostic tests to ensure effective treatment plans. Educating customers in what is best for their pet results in the correct products and services being purchased from your practice, rather than from the Internet, a pet shop or not at all. Purchased products/diagnostics or surgeries then need to be charged for correctly, and paid for.

Profit and loss

Financial accounts are studied with varying vigour from practice to practice, and the two key financial statements are the profit-and-loss account and the balance sheet. We are going to focus on the profit-and-loss account.

Let's look at an example profit-and-loss account, so that we may understand how important it is that we ensure our customers understand recommendations, purchase from the practice and pay for those products and services. The formatting of a profit-and-loss report will vary depending on whether the practice is a limited company, sole trader or partnership, but the overall principles are the same. We can then assess how the sections covered thus far can affect key figures and what can be done to improve these parameters.

The profit-and-loss report shows turnover, or the amount of income (excluding VAT) generated by the practice, less the costs directly linked with producing that turnover, leaving your gross profit figure. Next, all other expenses associated with running a business are deducted, leaving a net profit figure, or 'bottom line'. A simplified trading and profit-and-loss account example based on a four-vet small animal practice is shown in Table 4.4.

From a turnover of £1 million, £132000 net profit can seem a little surprising. So let's look at key profit-and-loss items and how we can influence them on a day-to-day basis.

TURNOVER

This figure is the actual amount of chargeable work done in a given period. It does not, however, bear any relation to the amount of cash the practice has in the bank, as banked

TABLE 4.4	Veterinary practice A: year ended 31 December 2014	
Turnover	£1 million
Less cost of sales	£250 000
Gross profit	£750 000
Staff costs	£400 000 (includes imputed market rate salaries for the owners)
Rent	£50 000
Marketing	£10 000
Bad debts	£5000
Motor/travel	£3000
Other overheads	£150 000
Profit before tax; net profit	£132 000

With thanks to Hazlewoods Accountants for providing example figures.

money includes VAT, whereas the turnover does not, and the money paid into the account is simply the amount paid to the practice and not a reflection of the actual work done. Drug company rebates are not part of practice turnover, but are included in money paid into the bank account (Shilcock and Stutchfield 2008).

Positively influencing turnover

Looking back over previous sections of the chapter, key areas where focus will improve turnover are:
- More clients = more work generated
  - Marketing and word-of-mouth activity results in more enquiries
  - Excellent customer experience on first contact via the phone results in higher caller conversion
  - Increasing numbers of veterinary nurse appointments will free up vet consultations, therefore increasing capacity to see more customers
- Clear explanation and recommendation = improved consultation conversion
  - Clients who understand the need for diagnostics/preventative products and surgery and receive clear recommendations are more likely to agree to said products and services, generating more work
- Correct charging
  - Work done *must* be charged for. No 'X-raying customers' pockets', no reducing fees based on who the consulting vet may be, and no charging lower fees for consultations and surgery times as an example. All work done incurs costs to the practice, which must be paid for.

Cost of sales
- Inventory control
  - Minimising OOD stock wastage (first in, first out)
  - Just-in-time ordering where possible to reduce cash held tied up in stock on the shelf; especially useful for repeat food and prescription medications
  - Reducing duplicate products, i.e. multiple flea products kept in stock
  - Min/max stock levels to aid effective ordering
  - One person in charge of stock control
- Laboratory and cremation fees

- Must be charged at the time of usage. The practice needs to pay for these tests and cremations whether the client pays or not, so prompt billing of items and payment is necessary.

Staff costs

Wages are a huge cost to the business. This means that the team have to have clear direction, boundaries and alignment with the practice vision to ensure that they are as productive and efficient as possible. Good practice suggests:

- Keeping locum costs to a minimum where possible.
- Keeping overtime to a minimum. Effective teams should not need to be claiming overtime on a regular basis. If the teams are efficient, and the overtime bill is still high, then this may indicate that the workload is too high and another team member may be needed. Care should be taken to consider seasonal peaks before adding permanently to the head count.
- Using veterinary surgeons for things that only they can do. Using veterinary nurses in clinics, for admissions, administering pre-meds and imaging where possible will match skill set to task and prevent the practice paying vets to perform tasks that others on a lower pay scale are capable of performing.

Other overheads

Care should be taken by all to ensure that these costs are controlled where possible. For example, taking the initiative to turn off lights and not hoard stationery are areas where all team members can help.

Another way to look at key figures is to have them as a percentage of turnover, for example:

- Percentage of turnover spent with wholesaler(s): 20%
- Percentage of turnover spent on non-vet staff salaries: 20%
- Percentage of turnover spent on veterinary staff salaries: 20%.

Reflecting its importance to the health of every veterinary practice, further reading is recommended on the key elements of financial management, and contracting the services of an accountant experienced in the veterinary sector is always recommended.

In conclusion

We have seen that by approaching our business as we would a patient, using rigour and established processes and protocols, a diagnosis of its general health is easy to obtain. The Balanced Scorecard approach identifies four key areas to focus on here:

- Customer
- Staff
- Finance
- Operational effectiveness.

We have also explored useful tools to help measure and manage performance in each of these four areas. Management and business acumen do not come easy to many of us – after all, we didn't go into veterinary practice because we love numbers. And yet without paying attention to these key aspects of business and applying a healthy dose of commercial common sense, in the light of increasing competition and rising client expectations, before long we might not have a viable practice left. Ultimately, if you adhere to the five-step veterinary business model, everything else will follow:

1. Make the phone ring.
2. Convert the call into an appointment.
3. Convert the consultation into relevant diagnostic and treatment plans.
4. Charge correctly for the work done.
5. Get recommended.

BIBLIOGRAPHY

Bennis, W., 1989. On Becoming a Leader. Hutchinson Business, London.

David, F.R., 1989. How companies define their mission. Long Range Plann. 22 (1), 90–97.

Henk de Koning, J.P.S., Verver, J.H., Soren Bisgaard, R.J.M.M., 2006. Lean Six Sigma in healthcare. J. Healthc. Qual. 28 (2), 4–11.

Kaplan, R.S., Norton, D.P., 1992. The Balanced Scorecard – measures that drive performance. Harv. Bus. Rev. 70 (1), 71–79.

Katzenbach, J.R., Smith, D.K., 1993. The Wisdom of Teams: Creating the High-Performance Organization. Harvard Business School Press.

Kim, C.S., Spahlinger, D.A., Billi, J.E., 2009. Creating value in health care: The case for lean thinking. JCOM. 16 (12), 557–562.

Novis, D.A., Konstantakos, G., 2006. Reducing errors in the practices of pathology and laboratory medicine. Am. J. Clin. Pathol. 126 (S1), S30–S35.

Reichheld, F., 2003. The one number you need to grow. Harv. Bus. Rev. 81, 45–54.

Richardson, F., Osborne, D., 2006. Managing inventory costs. Can. Vet. J. 47 (3), 277–278, 280, 282.

Shilcock, M., Stutchfield, M., 2008. Understanding financial accounts. In: Veterinary Practice Management: A Practical Guide. second ed. Saunders, New York.

Stallworth Williams, L., 2008. The mission statement: A corporate reading tool with a past, present and future. J. Bus. Com. 45 (2), 94–119.

Thornberry, N., 1997. A view about vision. Eur. Manage. J. 15 (1), 23–34.

Legislation and the Veterinary Nurse

SUZANNE MAY

An introduction to legislation

Legislation in the UK refers to both Acts of Parliament and regulations.

Parliament is responsible for approving new laws (legislation). The government introduces most plans for new laws, or changes to existing laws, but they can originate from an MP, a Lord or even a member of the public or a private group. Before they can become law, both the House of Commons and House of Lords must debate and vote on the proposals. It then goes before a parliamentary committee before finally obtaining the Queen's signature to make it law. It is then placed in the Statute Book as an Act of Parliament.

Regulations detail the implications of laws. Further regulations can be added to laws as necessary with the approval of Parliament.

Where animal welfare is concerned, welfare codes are also required to have parliamentary approval. If the provisions of the code are not complied with, it is not an offence. However, this could be used in evidence if prosecution followed.

The Royal Charter

The Royal College of Veterinary Surgeons (RCVS) was created by and still exists by virtue of a Royal Charter of 1844. Most of this original charter has been superseded by the Supplemental Charter of 1967. This revoked the Charter of 1844 except so far as its provisions 'incorporate the College, recognise the veterinary art as a profession, authorise the College to have a Common Seal, to hold property, and to sue and be sued'. The 1967 Charter lays down rules for the transaction of College business and gives powers under which the RCVS awards Fellowships, Diplomas and Certificates.

The Royal Charter came into force in 2014 and recognises Registered Veterinary Nurses (RVNs) as members of a regulated profession who are answerable for their professional conduct. RVNs have the formal status of associates of the College and continue to use the postnominals RVN. The Charter also recognises the Veterinary Nurses' Council as the body which sets standards for the training, education and conduct of RVNs.

Veterinary Surgeons Act 1966

This Act of Parliament controls the work of both veterinary surgeons and veterinary nurses.

Definition of veterinary surgery: the Act defines this as 'the art and science of veterinary surgery and medicine, and without prejudice to the generality of the foregoing, shall be taken to include:
- The diagnosis of diseases in, and injuries to animals including tests performed on animals for diagnostic purposes
- The giving of advice based upon such diagnosis
- The medical or surgical treatment of animals
- The performance of surgical operations on animals.'

The Act prohibits anyone other than a veterinary surgeon who is a Member of the Royal College of Veterinary Surgeons (MRCVS) from practising veterinary surgery. There are, however, a number of exceptions to this rule, some concerning lay persons and two concerning veterinary nurses:
- Schedule 3 of the Act allows anyone to give first aid in an emergency for the purpose of preserving life and relieving suffering. The owner of an animal or a member of the owner's household or employee of the owner may also give it minor medical treatment. There are several exceptions to this general rule, mainly relating to farm animals.

Veterinary nurses, like anyone else, may give first aid and look after animals in a way that does not involve acts of veterinary surgery. However, there are further provisions for qualified listed veterinary nurses under Schedule 3 of the Act.
- Schedule 3 of the Veterinary Surgeons Act 1966 details that RVNs can administer medical treatment and perform

minor surgery (not involving entry into a body cavity) under the direction of the veterinary surgeon that is providing care for that animal (cat, dog or exotic species but NOT equine species, unless a certificate in equine nursing is also held). The veterinary surgeon must be satisfied that the nurse is competent to carry out their instructions as he or she is ultimately responsible and accountable for their actions.

Amendment to paragraphs 6 & 7 of Schedule 3 to the Veterinary Surgeons Act 1966, as amended by the Veterinary Surgeons Act 1966 (Schedule 3 Amendment) Order 2002 clarifies the term 'veterinary nurse' within the Act as one whose name is entered on to the register of veterinary nurses maintained by the RCVS. It also makes provisions for the training of student veterinary nurses, allowing them to perform Schedule 3 procedures as detailed earlier, but only with direct, continuous and personal supervision from a registered veterinary surgeon, or veterinary nurse under veterinary instruction where surgery is concerned. The definition of a student veterinary nurse is one who 'has been enrolled under the RCVS bylaws for the purposes of training as a veterinary nurse and who is employed at an approved training practice'.

Occupational health

WHAT IS HEALTH AND SAFETY ALL ABOUT?

Health and safety laws exist to assist in the provision of a satisfactory, safe working environment, preventing people from being injured or harmed at work by taking the right precautions and knowing what action to take when things go wrong.

The Health and Safety Commission (HSC) is the body which oversees and monitors health and safety, producing reports and advising the government on health and safety matters. The Health and Safety Executive (HSE) is the enforcement body of the HSC, and at present veterinary practices come under the jurisdiction of HSE inspectors, whereas shops, offices, hotels, etc. are the responsibility of local authority environmental health officers.

HSE inspectors can visit any practice at any time to ensure that all relevant legislation is being complied with. Their job is to advise and enforce accordingly. Where they find a breach in health and safety law, there are a number of actions they can take based on how severe the problem is:

- If the breach is minor, an inspector will usually informally tell the employer what the problem is and how to correct it.
- If the breach is more serious, an **improvement notice** may be issued which identifies the situation that needs to be corrected and sets a specific date by when this should be done.
- Where an inspector believes that a breach could cause serious personal injury, a **prohibition notice** can be used to halt an activity immediately, i.e. this notice takes effect as soon as it is issued.

Failure to comply with either an improvement notice or a prohibition notice can result in fines of up to £20 000. Both types of notice can be appealed against through the Employment Tribunal.

The main Acts of Parliament affecting occupational health within veterinary practices are as follows.

Health and Safety at Work Act 1974

This applies to all businesses, however big or small, and to those who are self-employed. It generally places the responsibility for minimising health and safety risks onto those who create them, usually the employer.

Employer responsibilities include:
- Appointing a competent person to oversee health and safety
- Carrying out risk assessments
- Supplying health and safety information to employees and visitors
- Providing health and safety training for employees.

Employee responsibilities include:
- Taking reasonable care of their own health and safety, and that of others
- Cooperating with the employer over health and safety matters
- Using equipment and substances in accordance with health and safety training
- Informing the employer of any health and safety risks or lack of protection.

A health and safety policy is required by any business that employs five or more people. This written policy contains information as to how employers will maintain the health and safety of their employees, and usually includes the following information:
- Responsibilities for health and safety, i.e. who has overall responsibility and to whom specific responsibilities have been delegated
- The risk assessments that will be undertaken
- How the practice will organise consultation with its employees
- How the safety of equipment will be maintained and who is responsible for this
- Implementation of COSHH
- Arrangements for the provision of health and safety training
- Accident and first-aid arrangements
- Fire and emergency evacuation procedures
- How reviews of health and safety will be undertaken.

Management of Health and Safety at Work Regulations 1999

These regulations follow on from the Health and Safety at Work Act 1974, redefining and reinforcing the requirements of the Act to include the following activities:
- Planning
- Organisation
- Control
- Monitoring
- Review.

Health and Safety at Work Regulations 1992

The 1992 Health and Safety at Work Regulations state that 'it shall be the duty of every employer to ensure so far as is reasonably practicable the health, safety and welfare of all their employees.' With this legislation came the requirement for

TABLE 5.1	Example of a risk assessment	
Activity	Radiography	
Location	Radiography room	
Potential hazards (the actual things that are likely to cause harm)	Primary beam Secondary radiation (scatter) Animal (if conscious)	
Risk (the likelihood of the potential hazard causing harm)	Consider: Protective clothing Protective screening Persons inside the controlled area Any manual restraint of animal Any protective restraint of animal, e.g. muzzle Possibility of machine malfunction – continuous emission of X-rays	
Who is at risk? Is anyone more at risk than others?	Any persons remaining within the controlled area are most at risk. Those more at risk but who should not be participating anyway are those who are pregnant, under 18 or who have been advised not to undertake radiography by their GPs	
Control measures	Authorised personnel only Personal dosimeters Protective clothing/screens Extension enabling radiographer to stand out of the controlled area when exposure is taken	
Training required	Health and safety training on radiography. Those involved must have read and understood the local rules and systems of work	
Emergency action	Shut off power to X-ray machine from fuse box Inform RPS and RPA and arrange for immediate service of the machine	

employers to carry out risk assessments, and later that year the first six regulations requiring risk assessments were published:

- Manual Handling Operations Regulations
- Workplace (Health and Safety at Work)
- Personal Protective Equipment Regulations
- Provision and Use of Work Equipment Regulations
- Health and Safety (Display Screen Equipment) Regulations
- Management of Health and Safety at Work Regulations.

Leading from these, other areas have since been identified as also requiring risk assessment including:

- Fire
- First aid
- Electrical safety
- Ionizing radiation
- Young people at work
- Lone workers
- Noise
- New and expectant mothers
- Working time
- Work-related stress
- COSHH.

In 2013 new regulations came into force. These regulations are implemented by the EU law (the 'sharps directive') European Council Directive 2010/32/EU, and extend from existing UK health and safety law. It is required that employers consider engineering-specific controls to reduce employee exposure to blood-borne pathogens through the use of 'safer medical devices'. Exposure control plans must be developed and reviewed annually, with updates based on changes in technology. Needleless systems and related protective devices are not mandated but their annual consideration is. Employers are required to maintain a sharps injury log containing information about the type and brand of device involved, the area in which the exposure occurred and an explanation of how the injury happened.

RISK ASSESSMENTS

A risk assessment involves looking at the workplace and the type of work undertaken, and identifying anything that could cause harm to people. The assessment involves identifying **hazards,** and then determining the level of **risk** each hazard is likely to have to employees.

- A *hazard* is anything that can cause harm.
- A *risk* is the likelihood that someone will be harmed by the hazard.

The HSE recommends the following three actions with regards to hazards:

1. Eliminate the source of the hazard wherever possible.
2. Substitute the source of the hazard if it cannot be eliminated.
3. Control the source of the hazard if it cannot be substituted.

The following steps should be considered when undertaking risk assessment:

- Careful consideration of the task/situation
- Identification of the hazards
- Identification of those people who carry out the task or are exposed to the hazard
- Assess the level of risk involved
- Consider what control measures are already in place
- Identify any other control measures needed
- Record all of the findings of the assessment
- Implement control measures that have been identified as being required
- Inform all relevant staff of the risk assessment and its outcomes – development of a standard operating procedure (SOP) may be required if not already in place
- Train staff if required
- Monitor and review on a regular basis.

An example risk assessment can be seen in Table 5.1.

Fig. 5.1   Some common hazard warning signs

STANDARD OPERATING PROCEDURES (SOPS)

These are written documents designed to cover the full range of work performed within the practice. They provide clear and concise information in line with the individual protocols of the practice.

Control of Substances Hazardous to Health Regulations 2002

The Control of Substances Hazardous to Health Regulations 2002 (COSHH) were introduced specifically to cover the management of risks associated with hazardous substances. This includes all pharmaceutical products and chemicals used in veterinary practice.

Risk assessments should be in place for all such substances. In assessing the level of risk involved, the following should be considered:

- Who uses it?
- How is it used?
- How long are people exposed?
- By which route would the substance enter the body?
- Are there any particular people at risk (e.g. asthmatics, expectant mothers)?

Employees should be familiar with the common hazard warning symbols illustrated in Figure 5.1 when dealing with a substance and what personal protective equipment is needed.

In addition the particular hazards of a substance can be identified by using a numerical code system introduced in 1996 as a result of the Chemicals (Hazard Information and Packaging for Supply) Amendment Regulations 2002 (CHIP 96). Manufacturers should also supply COSHH data sheets to help the practice produce its risk assessments. The practice should have easy access to these data sheets in case of an accident.

Standard operating procedures should be in place for substances which present a hazard and for how to deal with spillages, i.e. the cleaning-up procedure and whether any protective equipment is required (Box 5.1).

It should be noted that clinical waste also comes under COSHH regulations in terms of risk assessment, but there are also different legal requirements as to its disposal.

Hazardous Waste (England and Wales) Regulations (HWR) 2005

DISPOSAL OF WASTE FROM THE PRACTICE

The legal definition of clinical waste is given in the Controlled Waste Regulations 1992 as 'any waste which consists wholly or partly of human or animal tissue, blood or other bodily fluids, excretions, drugs or other pharmaceutical products, swabs or

BOX 5.1   RULES FOR WORKING WITH CHEMICALS

- Never eat, drink or smoke when working with chemicals.
- Ensure area is adequately ventilated.
- Use the appropriate protective clothing.
- Ensure the chemical is correct for use in this situation.
- Keep the chemicals in their original containers with the label intact and legible.
- Use the correct concentration.
- Read the label and the product COSHH sheet.
- Store appropriately according to manufacturer's instructions – out of direct sunlight, away from animals and children – in a locked cupboard if necessary.
- Do not mix unless recommended by the manufacturer.
- Dispose of chemical according to manufacturers' guidelines.
- Wash hands after use.
- Deal with accidental spillage immediately and report as necessary.

TABLE 5.2   Colour coding for waste containers

Container colour	Contents
• Yellow	Infectious waste which requires disposal by incineration
• Orange	Infectious waste which requires treating to render it safe or it is incinerated
• Purple	Cytotoxic and cytostatic waste
• Yellow and black	Offensive or hygiene waste
• Black	Domestic waste which cannot be recycled

dressings, or syringes, needles or other sharp instruments, being waste which unless rendered safe may prove hazardous to any person coming into contact with it'. This includes waste from medical, nursing, dental, pharmaceutical, teaching, research and veterinary practices.

The Environmental Protection Act 1990 states that 'all establishments are responsible for their own waste' but this was amended in 1992 to include 'a duty of care for controlled waste'. This means that the responsibility for disposing of waste created by a business lies with the employer or self-employed person, which includes ensuring that waste disposed of by an outside company, e.g. collectors of clinical waste from a veterinary practice, is disposed of legally and safely. Should the outside company be found to be negligent according to law then the people who employ that company are also liable for prosecution.

Within the veterinary practice there must be a waste storage area separate from any other area, which must be secure (locked) against both humans and vermin, with access only to authorised personnel. Within the area the waste is stored in appropriate receptacles ready for disposal and collection by the designated company.

There are many different types of waste, which must be disposed of correctly. They can be classed as:

- Hazardous waste – the premises must keep a waste register, use consignment notes and keep these records for 3 years.
- Non-hazardous waste.

All waste has an EWC classification number for identification. There is also a colour-code system of containers for the disposal of waste (see Table 5.2).

HAZARDOUS WASTE

In 2005, the Hazardous Waste Regulations replaced the Special Waste Regulations and introduced new definitions of hazardousness for infectious and pharmaceutical wastes.

This group is divided into:

1. Cytotoxic and cytostatic pharmaceuticals – includes medicinal products which are toxic, carcinogenic and/or mutagenic. Following identification, these may include glass containers, syringes and sharps, animal bedding and clinical items such as swabs and gloves. They must be disposed of by segregating into purple or yellow containers for high-temperature incineration.
2. Contaminated sharps – includes all sharps contaminated with blood or pharmaceuticals (other than cytotoxic or cytostatic as above). They must be disposed of by segregating into yellow sharps containers for high-temperature incineration. Non-contaminated sharps can be disposed of in orange-lidded containers for treatment such as autoclaving.
3. Infectious waste – includes waste containing microorganisms or their toxins which are believed to have caused disease in another living organism. Following identification, these may include clinical items such as swabs and gloves and animal bedding from an infectious case, disposed of into orange waste bags. Body parts need to be disposed of in anatomical waste bins (red-lidded bins).
4. Photographic chemicals – includes waste fixer and developer solutions. They must be disposed of by segregating into separate containers and treated at a permitted facility which can be arranged via the practice waste contractor. There is no standard packaging.

NON-HAZARDOUS WASTE

This group is divided into:

1. Pharmaceuticals – does not include cytotoxic or cytostatic pharmaceuticals but it does include controlled drugs, prescription-only medicines, out-of-date drugs and contaminated bottles, syringes and packaging. It can be further divided into:
   - Disposal of controlled drugs – all controlled drugs should be denatured before disposal with other pharmaceuticals above. Schedule 2 drugs required denaturing in the presence of a person authorised by the Secretary of State, e.g. a police officer.
   - Disposal of other pharmaceuticals – should be segregated into leak-proof containers and done without mixing them together. There is no standard packaging. They should be incinerated at a permitted facility which can be arranged via the practice waste contractor.
2. Offensive waste – this is soft waste, e.g. swabs, gloves and animal bedding that is not infectious but is unpleasant to the senses. It should not present risk of infection or hazard to another living organism. Material containing bodily fluids should not be placed in this waste unless the veterinary surgeon can demonstrate that procedures that ensure the waste does not pose a threat of infection to another living organism have been implemented. The waste should be segregated into yellow and black containers for disposal into landfill.

3. Non-infectious cadaver – any pet cadavers that are not infectious can be buried at home, buried in a pet cemetery or cremated. There is no standard packaging and disposal can be arranged via the waste contractor for the practice.
4. Domestic waste – includes domestic waste such as unsoiled newspaper, food waste and other household waste not fit for recycling. This waste goes to landfill.

Further information on the disposal of waste can be found on the BVA website at <http://www.bva.co.uk> or in the BVA Good Practice Guide to Handling Veterinary Waste (Fig. 5.2).

Manual Handling Regulations 1992

This Act expands on the general provisions of the Health and Safety at Work Act 1974. The requirements and applications of these regulations are clearly outlined in the booklet *Manual Handling, Guidance on Regulations*.

General provisions outlined include:
- Avoid hazardous manual handling operations so far as is reasonably practicable
- Assess any hazardous manual handling operations that cannot be avoided
- Reduce the risk of injury so far as is reasonably practicable.

The regulations do not set out any guidelines for weight limits, etc. It is expected that each individual task will be assessed according to:
- The task
- The load (an animal being carried may suddenly move, which makes it different from carrying a box)
- The working environment (moving around objects, slippery floors, etc.)
- The individual's capabilities (these vary with age, pregnancy, etc.).

The Health and Safety Executive (HSE) guidance for manual lifting and the main elements of a good lifting technique can be found in Figures 5.3 and 5.4, respectively.

The Health and Safety (First Aid) Regulations 1981

This requires employers to provide adequate and appropriate equipment, facilities and personnel to enable first aid to be given to employees if they are injured or become ill at work. The minimum first-aid provision in any workplace is:
- A suitably stocked first-aid box
- An appointed person to take charge of first-aid arrangements.

Requirements increase with the size of the workforce and the type of work being done. A veterinary practice is considered as a medium-risk environment, and as such must appoint a person responsible for first aid if there are fewer than 20 employees. If there are between 20 and 50 employees, a trained first aider must be appointed.

WHAT IS THE DIFFERENCE BETWEEN AN APPOINTED PERSON AND A FIRST AIDER?

An *appointed person* is someone who is appointed by management to take charge when someone is injured or ill. This includes calling an ambulance if required. Appointed persons are also

	Details	Disposal	Colour Coding
HAZARDOUS WASTE			
Cytotoxic and Cytostatic Pharmaceuticals	Waste contaminated with cytotoxic / cytostatic products: • Glass vials and bottles • Clinical consumables • Syringes and sharps • Animal bedding	High temperature incineration. EWC 18 02 07	Purple and yellow containers, sharps into purple-lidded sharps bins
Photographic Chemicals	Waste fixer and developer	Leak proof approved container EWC 09 01 01 (developer) EWC 09 01 04 (fixer)	No standardised packaging, specific requirements should be discussed with the waste contractor
Infectious Waste	Any waste containing viable micro-organisms (or their toxins) which are known to be zoonotic to people or other animals • Clinical consumables • Animal bedding • Blood, body parts and cadavers	High temperature incineration only EWC 18 02 02 Highly infectious waste can be segregated into orange containers for suitable alternative treatment (e.g. autoclaving) EWC 18 02 02	Yellow containers, or orange bags
Contaminated Sharps	All sharps that have been contaminated with animal blood or pharmaceuticals (other than cytotoxic/cytostatic) • Hypodermic needles • Scalpel blades • Other sharp instruments	High temperature incineration only EWC 18 02 02	Yellow lidded sharps bins
NON-HAZARDOUS WASTE			
Pharmaceuticals (non-cytotoxic or cytostatic)	Waste contaminated with pharmaceuticals (not cytotoxic or cytostatic) • Prescription-only medicines • Out-of-date drugs • Un-required (returned) drugs • Contaminated bottles, syringes and packaging	Incineration at approved facility EWC 18 02 08	Leak proof container, there is no standardised requirement
Pharmaceuticals (controlled drugs)	All controlled drugs should be denatured or made not readily recoverable and then disposed of with other pharmaceutical waste. Sch2 drugs need to be denatured in the presence of a person authorised by the Secretary of State (e.g. a Police Officer).	EWC 18 02 08	Leak proof container, there is no standardised requirement
Domestic Waste	Waste that only includes domestic waste • Unsoiled newspaper/magazines • Food cans	Landfill or recycling if possible EWC 20 03 01	Black household rubbish bags
Offensive Waste	Veterinary waste that doesn't demonstrate a risk of infection or other potential hazard to any animal or person that may come in contact with it, even if mismanaged • Clinical consumables • Animal bedding • Materials contaminated with body fluids, providing the veterinary surgeon is able to demonstrate that there is no risk of infection	Landfill or other suitable permitted facility EWC 18 02 03	Yellow bags with a black strip, sometimes referred to as 'Tiger' bags
Non-Infectious Cadavers	Any pet carcasses that are not considered to be infectious	Burial at home Burial in a pet cemetery Cremation EWC 18 02 03	There is no standardised packaging requirements

EWC = European Waste Catalogue

Fig. 5.2 *Good Practice Guide to Handling Veterinary Waste (From BVA)*

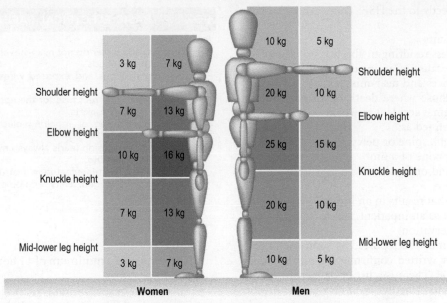

Fig. 5.3 Health and Safety Executive guidance for manual lifting *(Crown copyright material, with permission of the Controller of HMSO and the Queen's Printer for Scotland)*

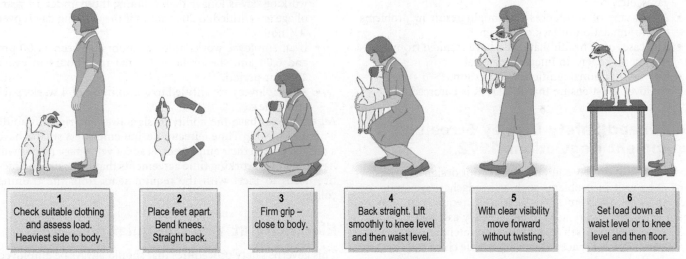

| 1 Check suitable clothing and assess load. Heaviest side to body. | 2 Place feet apart. Bend knees. Straight back. | 3 Firm grip – close to body. | 4 Back straight. Lift smoothly to knee level and then waist level. | 5 With clear visibility move forward without twisting. | 6 Set load down at waist level or to knee level and then floor. |

Fig. 5.4 The main elements of a good lifting technique

responsible for keeping the first-aid box stocked and recording any treatments given.

A *first aider* is someone who has undergone an HSE-approved training course in First Aid at Work and holds a certificate to prove this. Training should be repeated every 3 years to ensure that the certificate is kept up to date.

The *First Aid at Work: Approved Code of Practice and Guidelines* 1997 states that staff must know who the first-aid officer is and where the first-aid box is kept. First-aid boxes should be clearly marked with a white cross on a green background. There is no 'standard' list of items that should be kept in the first aid box; it depends on what the practice assess the needs to be. The HSE offers further guidance on this.

All accidents that occur within the workplace must be recorded in an Accident Book approved by the HSE (form B1 510). Details of what should be recorded in the Accident Book include:

- Full name, address and occupation of individual who had the accident

- The signature of the person who is filling in the Accident Book and the date of the occurrence
- When and where the accident took place
- Details of occurrence and record of injuries.

Indicate whether the incident needs to be reported to the HSE under RIDDOR (see below).

Any injury that involves an adverse reaction to a veterinary medicine or a needle-stick injury also needs to be reported to the Veterinary Medicine Directorate (VMD) as a pharmacovigilance report.

Reporting of Injuries, Diseases and Dangerous Occurrence Regulations 1995 (RIDDOR)

The Reporting of Injuries, Diseases and Dangerous Occurrence Regulations 1995 (RIDDOR) legislate for the reporting of certain serious events directly to the HSE. These can be broadly divided into:

- Major or fatal accidents
- Any accident or illness resulting in absence from work for more than 3 days because of an incident at work
- Dangerous occurrences and near-misses.

Fatal accidents include those where death occurred within 1 year as a result of an original accident at work.

Major accidents are defined as:

- A fracture of the skull, spine or pelvis
- A fracture of a long bone of a limb
- Amputation of a hand or foot
- Loss of sight of an eye
- Any other accident that results in an injured person being admitted to hospital as an inpatient, unless he or she was only kept in for observation.

Major or fatal accidents must be reported as soon as possible by telephone, followed by written confirmation within 7 days using the HSE form F2508. There is a list of dangerous occurrences that must be reported whether an injury occurs or not. These include:

- Explosion from a gas cylinder or steriliser
- Uncontrolled release of substance (including X-radiation, gases, etc.)
- Any escape of substances that might result in problems due to inhalation or lack of oxygen
- Any cases of ill health that could have resulted from exposure to pathogens in infected material
- Any unintentional ignition or explosion.

The employer must ensure that RIDDOR is enforced.

Health and Safety Display Screen Equipment Regulations 1992

Incorrect use of display equipment and poor design of workstations can result in problems such as headaches, eye strain, or neck and back problems. This legislation requires the way in which workstations are used to be regularly assessed.

The workstation itself should be adequately lit with appropriate room and leg space with an adjustable chair and foot rest if required.

Equipment should be of a low-radiation type, have no glare and have good contrast with a stable image. Monitors should be adjustable and keyboards should be legible with a wrist rest provided if needed.

Noise at Work Regulations 1989

These regulations state that the employer must assess the level of noise to which employees are exposed and take any necessary action to eliminate, control or reduce exposure. If noise levels are found to be above the 'first action noise level' of 85 decibels for continuous periods, e.g. due to barking dogs, then hearing protection **must be provided**.

The Working Time Regulations 1998

These set out entitlement for rest periods, night work and annual leave in line with the hours worked. They state that:

- The average working time is limited to 48 hours during each 7-day period.

- There must be a minimum of 11 hours rest in any 24-hour period.
- There must be a minimum rest period of 24 hours in each 7-day period. This increases to 48 hours for persons under 18 years of age.
- There must be a minimum rest break of 20 minutes if the working day is longer than 6 hours; those under 18 years of age are entitled to 30 minutes if the working day is over $4\frac{1}{2}$ hours.
- If an employee works at least 3 hours between 11.00 pm and 6.00 am, she or he is limited to 8 hours in every 24-hour period.
- All employees are entitled to a minimum of 4 weeks paid annual leave.

All employees have the ability to sign away the right to abide with the Working Time Directorate, but employers still do have a duty of care to their employees. Student veterinary nurses will have their own working time agreements that the training practice needs to meet with the requirements from the training college.

Electricity at Work Regulations 1989

This governs safety procedures that should always be employed when dealing with electrical equipment (Box 5.2).

PORTABLE APPLIANCE TESTING

Portable appliance testing (PAT) comes under these regulations. Appliances that have been tested will often have a label attached to the cable detailing the date and who tested it. The frequency of testing is dependent on the type of equipment and is usually somewhere between every 6 months and every 2 years.

ELECTRICAL CIRCUITS AND CIRCUIT BREAKERS

Every electrical circuit should have a fuse in it, which is a simple safety device. A fuse is simply a thin wire through which the current of electricity flows. If a fault occurs in the circuit it usually causes an increase in the electrical current. This results in the wire melting, which breaks the circuit. It is very important to use the correct fuse within a circuit (Fig. 5.5). If a fuse that is used in a circuit has too low a value, the fuse will constantly 'blow'. However, if a fuse is used with too high a value, a fault may result in the risk of fire or electrocution.

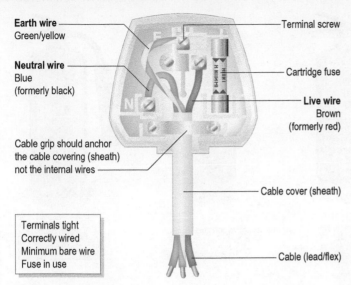

Earth wire
Green/yellow

Neutral wire
Blue
(formerly black)

Terminal screw

Cartridge fuse

Live wire
Brown
(formerly red)

Cable grip should anchor
the cable covering (sheath)
not the internal wires

Cable cover (sheath)

Terminals tight
Correctly wired
Minimum bare wire
Fuse in use

Cable (lead/flex)

Fig. 5.5 How to wire a plug

A circuit breaker is a device used to protect against short-circuits and is found on the main fuse board. These electromagnetic devices switch off the current if a fault occurs. A trip switch or RCD (residual current device) can be plugged into a socket to give added protection for a portable appliance. Circuit breakers are reset by either pressing a button or by switching them back on.

The Regulatory Reform (Fire Safety) Order 2005

This legislation came into force in October 2006 and replaces most of the previous fire legislation. It requires the following to be undertaken:

- Risk assessment with reference not only to employees but also to clients and other visitors who may be in the practice
- Implementation of fire precautions such as fire detection systems, firefighting equipment and suitable escape routes.

On discovering a fire, the alarm should be raised and the fire brigade alerted immediately. A specified member of staff should be appointed as Fire Officer and it is this person's responsibility to ensure that the building is evacuated, that all occupants are accounted for and that no-one re-enters the building until the all-clear is given by the Fire Department. Local fire rules describing what to do in the event of a fire should be displayed within different areas within the building. Fire exits should be well labelled and well lit and not blocked with rubbish, etc., as should fire assembly points. There should be adequate firefighting equipment, and staff must know the location of the equipment. Fire doors should be kept shut at all times. Care should be taken with the handling and storage of flammable and explosive materials.

FIRE EXTINGUISHERS

These are now all red, with a coloured strip indicating the contents and usage. There should also be a label mounted on the wall above the extinguisher, showing in green the fires that can safely be extinguished with that particular fire extinguisher and in red those that cannot (Fig. 5.6). **The requirement is that they should be installed and commissioned by a competent person, then serviced at least annually thereafter.**

Ionizing Radiation Regulations 1999

Damage from radiation is cumulative, i.e. exposure to tiny amounts of radiation over a period of time can be just as serious as one exposure for a length of time. In addition to damaging cell structure, genes of reproductive cells (sperm and ova) can also be harmed, causing gene mutation. The effects of this may not be immediately obvious and may take a long while to emerge.

Harmful effects of radiation:
- Inflammation
- Blood disorders
- Death of tissue
- Death or mutation of developing foetus
- Damage to gonads
- Infertility
- The production of tumours.

The main beam that is produced when making an exposure is called the primary beam. This represents the biggest hazard to personnel. No part of the operator's body should ever be placed in the primary beam.

Secondary radiation or scatter is produced when particles of energy from the primary beam hit a surface (such as tissue or inanimate objects) and cause the production of lower-energy particles. These lower-energy particles 'bounce' off the surface at random and, like X-rays, travel in straight lines (Fig. 5.7).

Everyone who is involved with radiography must be protected from its dangers.

All practices should have written local radiation rules and a system of work, a copy of which should be displayed in the designated X-ray room. This should include a list of all personnel within the practice who are authorised to undertake radiography.

The main principles associated with radiation protection are:
- Radiography should only be undertaken if there is a definite clinical justification for the use of the procedure.
- Exposure of personnel should be kept to a minimum.
- There must be personal monitoring of staff involved with radiation to ensure that dose limits are not exceeded.

Under the legislation, practices must appoint:

A **Radiation Protection Supervisor (RPS)** – A listed veterinary nurse or veterinary surgeon employed in the practice whose responsibility it is to ensure that radiography is carried out safely and in accordance with local rules and the associated system of work

A **Radiation Protection Advisor (RPA)** – A suitably qualified person not employed by the practice who is responsible for periodically visiting the practice and inspecting/giving advice regarding aspects of radiation protection. The RPA is responsible for writing the local rules. They must either:
- Hold a Diploma in Veterinary Radiography (DVR) or
- Be qualified in appropriate radiation physics with an interest in veterinary radiography.

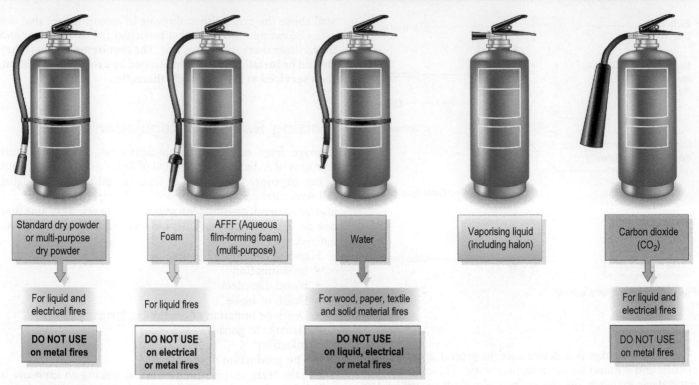

Standard dry powder or multi-purpose dry powder	Foam	AFFF (Aqueous film-forming foam) (multi-purpose)	Water	Vaporising liquid (including halon)	Carbon dioxide (CO$_2$)
For liquid and electrical fires	For liquid fires		For wood, paper, textile and solid material fires		For liquid and electrical fires
DO NOT USE on metal fires	**DO NOT USE** on electrical or metal fires		**DO NOT USE** on liquid, electrical or metal fires		**DO NOT USE** on metal fires

Fig. 5.6 Use of fire extinguishers (redrawn with permission from Health and Safety Executive 2004 Fire Safety: An Employer's Guide. Stationery Office, London)

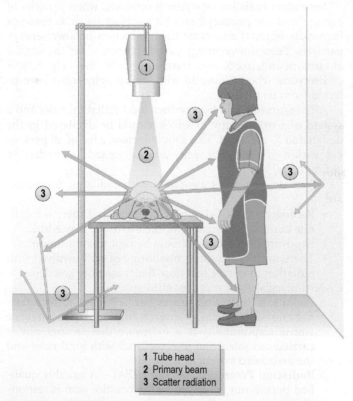

1 Tube head
2 Primary beam
3 Scatter radiation

Fig. 5.7 The hazards of radiation (redrawn from Lane and Cooper 2003 Veterinary Nursing, third ed. Butterworth-Heinemann, Oxford)

CONTROLLED AREA

A specified room should be identified for small-animal radiography. It should have sufficiently thick walls and no part of the controlled area should extend beyond it (brick walls are adequate; thin walls may be reinforced with barium plaster or lead ply).

The room should be large enough to allow any people that have to remain in it during exposure to stand at least 2 metres from the primary beam. If this is not possible, a protective lead screen must be provided. Unshielded doors and windows may be acceptable if the workload is low and the room is large enough. Special recommendations are made for flooring in rare cases where there is an occupied area below the radiography room.

Technically, the controlled area is the area around the primary beam within which the average dose rate of exposure exceeds a given limit. This is usually within a radius of 2 metres (6 metres for large animal work) as specified in the regulations. The controlled area must be clearly labelled and a red warning light should be displayed (usually by the entrance to the controlled area) when radiography is taking place, warning others not to enter.

In addition, all X-ray machines should have lights visible from the control panel indicating:

- When the machine is switched on and being supplied by electricity
- When exposure is taking place.

Once radiographic examination has been completed the machine should be disconnected from the electricity supply. All staff should be aware of what to do in an emergency, i.e. if the machine jams while emitting X-rays. This usually involves knowing where to shut down power without having to re-enter the controlled area. Any fault must be reported to the RPA.

Date	Owner Details	Animal Name	Breed	Wt (kg)	Consc Or GA	View	Plate	Grid Y/N	Exposure	Comments	Initials
1.6.01	Jones	Sam	GSD	37	GA	VD Hips	Large	Y	85 x 5	V. good	DM SKM

Fig. 5.8 Example of records kept in a radiography book

STAFF INVOLVED WITH RADIOGRAPHY

Persons 16–18 years of age have restrictions on radiography work. There is a smaller dose limit for them, although if possible they should not be allowed in the controlled area as their bodies are still developing and are at a slightly greater risk.

MAXIMUM PERMISSIBLE DOSE

The maximum permissible dose (MPD) is the amount of radiation that can be received by the body or a specific part of it without causing harm.

PERSONAL MONITORING

Designated persons (a list of whom will be displayed in the local rules) should all have a doiemeter that they wear while at work. The doiemeter should only be worn by its designated wearer. There should be no swapping and sharing. Dosimeters should be worn on the trunk beneath any lead apron.

Different types of dosimeter are available. Commonly used types include:
- Film badge (blue holder)
- Thermolucent crystal badge (bright orange holder).

They should not leave the building, nor be placed in direct sunlight or next to any other sources of radiation, e.g. a computer. Dosimeters are supplied by the National Radiation Protection Board (NRPB) and are periodically exchanged, when the old dosimeters are sent back for reading. A printout of all readings is sent to the practice so staff can see if they have registered any exposure. Records of these printouts must be kept in the practice for at least 2 years.

Persons who should not take part in radiography:
- Persons under 16 years of age
- Pregnant women
- Those advised not to by their GP.

PROTECTIVE CLOTHING

It is important to realise that any protective clothing protects against scatter and not the primary beam. Clothing available may include:
- Aprons
- Gloves
- Sleeves
- Thyroid guards.

They are made of plastic or rubber that is impregnated with lead and known as 'lead rubber'. Aprons may be single- or double-sided (double-sided giving better protection). They should be long enough to reach mid-thigh level. The aprons should be worn by any persons remaining in the controlled area while an exposure is taken, even if standing behind a lead screen. Gloves and sleeves are worn when manual restraint of an animal is necessary. Even when wearing these, the hands should not be placed in the primary beam.

Protective clothing must be checked regularly for signs of wear and tear. Visual inspection is usually enough but, where further investigation is needed, X-raying the clothing may be necessary. Aprons should never be folded; they should be hung up to prevent cracking of the lead.

X-RAY RECORDS BOOK

Every practice should have a record of exposures taken. Columns may be detailed, as shown in Figure 5.8. This is used to keep an accurate record of exposures and also enables staff to see which exposures have produced diagnostic radiographs, thus helping to reduce the number of unnecessary radiographs.

MANUAL RESTRAINT

Manual restraint while taking radiographs:
- Should only be done when there is just cause, e.g. if the patient is a severe anaesthetic or sedation risk
- Details of any persons manually restraining during X-rays should be recorded in the X-ray book so their exposure can be monitored.

PROCESSING CHEMICALS

Processing chemicals for use in automatic or wet processors may be supplied as powders, liquid concentrates or ready-to-use liquids. All chemicals should be handled with care in a well-ventilated room. Gloves, goggles and face mask should be worn.

When spent, waste chemicals should be placed in the original container and collected by an authorised person. Local hospitals and laboratories may provide this service. As with all potentially hazardous substances, a risk assessment and standard operating procedure should be in place for use and disposal of these chemicals.

A summary of other legislation designed to protect the public is included in Table 5.3.

TABLE 5.3	Summary of laws that protect the public
Animal Health Act 1981 and Quarantine regulations	This Act gives government ministers powers to make orders to prevent and control the introduction and spread of zoonotic disease and assist in the eradication of diseases carried by animals in the UK. The orders and regulations covered include the following: • The Rabies (Control) Order 1974, now incorporated into the Animal Health Act • Quarantine for imports and exports • Points of entry into Britain • Transport method and conditions • Seizure of animals and their disposal (dogs and wildlife) • Disinfection of places and vehicles.
The Pet Travel Scheme (PETS)	PETS, introduced in 2001, allows dogs and cats coming from EU countries, certain other European countries and rabies-free islands to enter the UK without having to undergo quarantine provided they can be shown to meet the necessary criteria regarding vaccination and identification. Requirements: • Microchipped with electronic chip • Vaccinated against rabies using an inactivated vaccine • Treated for exotic diseases not present in the UK • Blood-tested at an approved laboratory to prove efficacy of vaccine • Has an official health certificate • 24–48 h before re-entry into UK the dog or cat must be treated against ticks and tapeworm • Pre-entry checks carried out by train operators, ferry companies and airlines • Random spot checks on animals arriving in the UK by the Department of the Environment, Farming and Rural Affairs (DEFRA) and official carriers.
Dangerous Dogs Act 1991, 1997	Applies to the following breeds of dog: • American pit bull terrier • Japanese tosa • Dogo argentino • Fila braziliera. The Act states that the rules for ownership of a dangerous named breed of dog are as follows: • Notifying the police of ownership • Obtaining a certificate of exemption from the police, which is issued when the dog has been neutered and identified with a microchip or other permanent method • The dog is covered by third-party liability insurance • In public places, the dog is always muzzled and on a lead • The dog is always in the company of a person over 16 years of age • It is an offence to sell, exchange or abandon the dog • It is an offence to breed from these dogs. Any dog dangerously out of control and a risk to the general public comes under the remit of this Act. Where such a dog has caused injury, the owner may be subject to prosecution and an unlimited fine
Guard Dogs Act 1975	Governs the safe use and control of dogs that guard property or sites. This must be done in a way that does not put the general public at risk. A notice must be displayed to inform the public that a dog is in use and the dog must only be off the lead if accompanied by a handler
Animals Act 1971	This Act covers liability for damage that has been caused by animals, including damage, death and injury caused to people, property and livestock. The owner of a dangerous animal must take precautions to ensure that it has no opportunity to inflict damage as defined by this law. If a dog kills or harms farm animals, farmers are entitled to protect the stock in their care. If, for example, a dog is found injuring sheep, the farmer may kill the dog but must report the incident to the police
Dog Fouling of Land Act 1996	Local authorities and councils use this Act to prevent dogs fouling where there is public access to property or pavements, but allowing the exemption of guide dogs for the blind.
The Microchipping of Dogs Regulations 2014	All dogs will be required to be microchipped, and owner details must be current on the database. It will be enforced by local authorities, police constables, community support officers and any other person which the Secretary of State may authorise to act as an enforcer of the regulations.

Animal Welfare Act 2006

The Animal Welfare Act 2006 defines an 'animal' as being any living vertebrate animal.

It imposes a 'duty of care' (a legal phrase which means that someone is obligated to do something) on those persons responsible for animals. This includes if he or she is:
• The owner of the animal
• In charge of the animal, e.g. the owner of a cattery, or looking after a neighbour's dog while the owners are on holiday
• A parent or guardian of a person under 16 years of age who is responsible for an animal.

Before the Animal Welfare Act was introduced, people only had a duty to ensure that their animal did not suffer unnecessarily.

This new Act builds on this, making owners and keepers responsible for ensuring that the welfare needs of their animals are met, including the need for:
• A suitable environment
• A suitable diet
• The ability to exhibit normal behaviour
• Any need the animal has to be housed with; or apart from other animals
• Protection from pain, suffering, injury and disease.

Collectively, the above are known as the 'Five Freedoms' (see also Chapter 1).

Under the Act, two different types of action can be taken in the event of someone breaking the law:
• An improvement notice can be issued. This explains why someone is failing to meet the welfare needs of the

animal, what they need to do to rectify the situation, the time in which they must comply with the notice and the action that will be taken if they fail to do so. It is not a criminal penalty, but can lead to a criminal record if there is failure to meet the welfare requirements of the notice.

- Criminal prosecution can be pursued; if found guilty a person can be fined up to £20 000, imprisoned, have the animals taken away or be banned from keeping animals in the future.

A summary of other animal welfare legislation is included in Table 5.4.

TABLE 5.4	Current animal welfare legislation
Animal Boarding Establishments Act 1963	Boarding kennels or catteries must be licenced by their local authority in order to trade. The following conditions apply: • Records kept of animal arrivals and departures and details of owners • Provision of suitable accommodation • Adequate and appropriate supplies of food and water • Exercise facilities available • Animals protected from disease and risk of fire. In order to ensure that the conditions of the licence are met, the local authority can at any time instruct inspection by an authorised officer or veterinary surgeon. Licences are renewed annually.
Breeding of Dogs Act 1973	The law was altered in 1991, allowing authorised officers or veterinary surgeons to enter premises with a warrant if they suspect an offence under the 1973 Act has been committed. The term 'breeding establishment' refers to any premises where more than two bitches are kept for the purpose of breeding animals for selling. The 1973 Act prohibits: • Obstruction of inspection by authorised personnel • Breeding dogs for sale without a licence from the local authority • If disqualified under other Acts of Parliament, holding a licence for the breeding of dogs.
Pet Animals Act 1951, 1983	Prohibits the keeping of a pet shop without a licence. A licence is granted after inspection of the premises by an approved veterinary surgeon authorised by the local authority. An amendment in 1983 now makes it illegal to sell pets in public places. A licence is granted if the following conditions are met: • Proper care • Suitable accommodation • Housed in the correct conditions with reference to heating, lighting, etc. • Provided with appropriate food • Observed and checked at suitable intervals during the day • Sold only after weaning and after a suitable age has been reached • Prevention of spread of disease • Emergency and fire precautions for the premises are in place and operational.
Protection of Animals Acts 1911, 1988	This series of Acts forms the main statutory control on cruelty to animals by humans. These Acts are used when bringing prosecutions related to animal welfare cases. The Act makes it an offence to cause unnecessary suffering to any domestic or captive animal either deliberately or by omission (neglect). The Act lists offences such as: • Inflicting physical cruelty by beating, kicking, etc. • Inflicting mental cruelty by teasing or terrifying • Causing unnecessary suffering during transportation by failing to provide food or water at appropriate intervals • Performing surgery or operations without anaesthetic • Poisoning without reason.
Protection of Animals (Anaesthetics) Acts 1954, 1982	It is illegal for any operation to be conducted on an animal that will cause pain unless under anaesthetic (local or general). There are, however, several exceptions to this Act. • Does not apply to birds, fish or reptiles • In emergency first-aid situations • Under permitted Home-Office-licenced procedures • Minor painless operations carried out by a veterinary surgeon or a listed veterinary nurse.
Welfare of Animals during Transport 1973, 1994 (Amendment) Order 1995	This order is designed to protect all animals during transport by road, rail, sea and air. From 1997, a standard set of regulations covering EU countries on journey times, hauliers' journey plans and routes amended the original order. The regulations cover: • Loading and unloading of animals • Housing and containers for transit • Access to food and water • Specified number of animals contained together for transit.
Abandonment of Animals Act 1960 Dangerous Wild Animals Act 1976	This Act applies to the abandonment of an animal in circumstances likely to cause it unnecessary suffering, whether temporarily or permanently. This Act was introduced following a rise in the 1960s and 1970s in the numbers of members of the public keeping animals more associated with zoos and wildlife parks. There was cause for concern over their standard of living and also about the danger posed to the general public. The legislation involves strict control and inspection by authorised veterinary surgeons, who may inspect premises in which these animals are kept. If the inspection is approved, a licence may be issued by the local authority. The Secretary of State has the power to change the list of animals at any time and any animal on the list is classified as a 'dangerous wild animal'. The Act states that anyone keeping these listed animals must: • Pay a fee to the local authority for the issue of the licence • Take out liability insurance • Provide suitable accommodation • Be over 18 years of age.

Continued

TABLE 5.4	Current animal welfare legislation—cont'd
Performing Animals (Regulation) Act 1925	This Act was introduced following public concern over the treatment of animals in circuses. As a result, the local authority must be informed of anyone who trains animals for exhibition to the public or exhibits a performing animal to the public, even if it is free of charge, and any such person must be registered to that effect. The exceptions to this rule are when animals are trained for sporting purposes, military or police work and display.
Zoo Licensing Act 1981	The term 'zoo' refers to the exhibiting of wild animals to the public for educational purposes. It applies to animal collections that are open to the public for 7 days or more in any year. This Act was passed after the dramatic increase of zoos and wildlife/safari parks in the 1960s. It is intended to protect the zoo animals and the general public by ensuring that measures to safeguard standards of care, the welfare of the animals and the safety of the public are in place. The zoo must obtain a licence from the local authority, which is renewed initially after 4 years and then every 6 years.
The Wildlife and Countryside Acts 1981, 1985	These Acts replace several existing laws and regulations and cover the protection and conservation of wild animals and their habitats. Land, sea and airborne species of wild animals are protected. The minister can add or remove species on this list, which may not legally be injured, killed or taken from the wild. The Act protects habitat from humans and species in captivity which, if released into the wild, would seriously affect many other species. Within the Act, licences can be granted which exempt the holder from the above provisions: • Relating to the protection of farming or forestry interests • Relating to the conservation, reintroduction, photographing and identification of wildlife.
Convention of International Trade in Endangered Species of Wild Flora and Fauna (CITES) 1973	This is an international agreement in place to protect the world's endangered species. This is done through control of their export and import on a worldwide scale. Animals within this agreement fall into one of two categories: • Those that are threatened with extinction • Those likely to become so threatened.

BIBLIOGRAPHY

Cooper, B., Mullineaux, E., Turner, L. (Eds.), 2012. BSAVA Textbook of Veterinary Nursing, fifth ed. British Small Animal Veterinary Association, Gloucester.

Dallas, S., 2002. Animal Biology and Care. Blackwell Science, Oxford.

Hotston-Moore, A., Rudd, S. (Eds.), 2008. Manual of Advanced Veterinary Nursing, second ed. British Small Animal Veterinary Association, Gloucester.

Hughes, P., Ferrett, E., 2003. Introduction to Health and Safety at Work. Butterworth-Heinemann, Oxford.

Mullineaux, E., Jones, M. (Eds.), 2007. Manual of Practical Veterinary Nursing. British Small Animal Veterinary Association, Gloucester.

Shilcock, S., Stutchfield, G., 2003. Veterinary Practice Management; A Practical Guide, second ed. Saunders Elsevier, Oxford.

USEFUL WEBSITES

British Veterinary Association: <http://www.bva.co.uk>

DEFRA: <www.gov.uk/government/organisations/department-for-environment-food-rural-affairs>

Health and Safety Executive (HSE): <http://www.hse.gov.uk>

Royal College of Veterinary Surgeons: <http://www.rcvs.org.uk>

RECOMMENDED READING

Cooper, B., Mullineaux, E., Turner, L. (Eds.), 2012. BSAVA Textbook of Veterinary Nursing, fifth ed. British Small Animal Veterinary Association, Gloucester.

Hotston-Moore, A., Rudd, S. (Eds.), 2008. Manual of Advanced Veterinary Nursing, second ed. British Small Animal Veterinary Association, Gloucester.

A detailed discussion about the legal responsibilities of a veterinary nurse within a practice.

Mullineaux, E., Jones, M. (Eds.), 2007. Manual of Practical Veterinary Nursing. British Small Animal Veterinary Association, Gloucester.

Both manuals provide added information about animal welfare law and the responsibilities of a veterinary nurse.

6

Canine and Feline Anatomy and Physiology

SUE DALLAS | NICOLA ACKERMAN

KEY POINTS

- The cell is the basic unit of the body. All cells contain a nucleus, a cell membrane and cytoplasm. They also possess other features that are specific to their type and function.
- Cells form the four basic tissues (muscular, epithelial, connective and nervous), which are arranged into organs, which form the body systems.
- The systems of the body comprise a set of organs, each of which has a function that contributes to the overall function of the system.
- Anatomy is the study of the structure of the organs; physiology is the study of how the organs function.

Introduction

Knowledge of the anatomy and physiology of the dog and cat is essential as a foundation to many aspects of veterinary nursing and care. From this knowledge evolves an appreciation of how disease and injury affect normal function and how treatment can be designed to alleviate the symptoms. This chapter is not an all-inclusive description of anatomy and physiology; a recommended reading list for more in-depth coverage is included at the end of the chapter.

Cells and basic tissues

The cell is the functional unit of all tissues and each cell has the ability to perform all the essential life functions (reproduction, respiration, metabolism, synthesis, growth, excretion, transport and homeostasis). Within the various tissues of the body, the constituent cells show a wide range of adaptations to perform a particular functional specialisation. All cells conform to a basic structure (Box 6.1).

THE DIVERSITY OF CELLS

Cells are not identical and their shape and contents show variation according to their function, but wherever they are found in the body they have the same basic features. Some examples of different cells are:

- **Epithelial cells** – found lining the surface of the body, the body cavities and the organs within it.
- **Glandular cells** – responsible for producing some kind of secretion, e.g. mucus to lubricate the tissues.
- **Osteoblasts** – produce bone tissue.

- **Erythrocytes (red blood cells)** – their biconcave shape is designed increase the surface area of the cell that contains the red pigment haemoglobin. They are one of a few type of cells in the body that has no nucleus in the mature form.
- **Nerve cells, or neurons** – have slender arm-like processes that transmit electrical impulses through the nervous system to reach the whole body.
- **Muscle** – capable of contracting to bring about body movement.

CELLS

All animal cells have the following features in common:

- **Cell membrane** – encloses the cytoplasm and controls the internal environment of the cell
- **Cytoplasm** – a jelly-like material that contains all the structures (organelles) and chemicals that make the cell function
- **Nucleus** – to control all the functions of the cell and to hold the inheritable material in the form of chromosomes. (See also Chapter 15.)

Cell membrane

The cell membrane is 0.00001 mm thick and forms the outer boundary of the cell. It is here that all exchanges take place between the cell and its surrounding environment. The cell membrane allows certain chemicals to pass in and out of the cell but prevents the passage of others – the cell membrane is said to be selectively permeable.

Cytoplasm

The term cytoplasm refers to all the living parts of a cell except the nucleus and is a jelly-like material containing a large number of important structures and substances, many of which are concerned with metabolism (Fig. 6.1). It contains:

- Organelles – the free-living structures within the cell other than the nucleus
- Mitochondria – some of the most important organelles in which the chemical reactions involved in cellular respiration take place; energy is released for cellular function
- Rough endoplasmic reticulum – lined by ribosomes produced in the nucleus; protein is synthesised here and the cell may transport it for use in the manufacture of digestive enzymes and hormones
- Smooth endoplasmic reticulum – not lined by ribosomes but is concerned with the synthesis and transport of lipids (fats) and steroids of body origin
- Ribosomes – these granules, rich in ribonucleic acid, are sites of protein synthesis

- Centrosome – lies near the nucleus and is made up of two centrioles; it is important during cell division and the formation of the cilia and flagella, which are slender projecting hairs needed by some cells
- Lysosomes – dark, round bodies containing enzymes (lysozymes) responsible for splitting complex chemical compounds into simpler ones. They also destroy worn-out organelles within the cell
- Golgi body or complex – a system of flattened tubes in which lysozymes are stored.

Nucleus

A nucleus is found in the living cells of all organisms. The nucleus of a cell contains rod-shaped objects called chromosomes. These are only visible when a cell is about to divide into two during mitosis and meiosis. Chromosomes contain a complex chemical called deoxyribonucleic acid (DNA). DNA controls the development of the features that an organism inherits from its parents. In other words, it contains the chemical 'blueprints' for making an organism.

BOX 6.1   STRUCTURE OF THE BODY

The body is made up of:
- *Cells*, which make up
- *Tissues*, which make up
- *Organs*, which make up
- *Systems*, which have a specific function to perform in the living body.

BASIC TISSUE TYPES

Muscular tissue

Brings about movement.
- Skeletal (voluntary, striated) – causes movement of the skeleton, e.g. locomotion
- Smooth (involuntary, non-striated) – concerned with movement within organs and blood vessels, e.g. vaso-constriction, peristalsis
- Cardiac – concerned with the beating of the heart.

Epithelial tissue

Forms a protective layer both inside and on the surface of the body, e.g. skin, glands and linings of the various body systems. Its function is to protect and, depending on its location and density, to allow absorption. Epithelial tissue may be simple or compound (Fig. 6.2). The many and varied functions of epithelium mean that it takes many different forms.

a. **Simple.** The layer of cells is one cell thick:
- Squamous – cells are flat and plate-like. Found where absorption is required, e.g. blood vessel walls and lining the renal nephrons
- Cuboidal – cells are cube-shaped with a central spherical nucleus. Found in glands and ducts
- Columnar – tall and rectangular; the layer of cells may contain mucus-secreting goblet cells or may be ciliated, i.e. covered in a fine covering of hairs. Found in the respiratory tract (ciliated), lining the gut with a covering of microvilli, and in secretory glands of the digestive and endocrine systems.

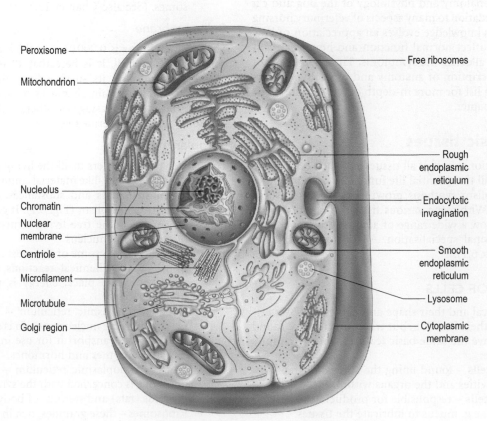

Peroxisome
Mitochondrion
Free ribosomes
Rough endoplasmic reticulum
Endocytotic invagination
Nucleolus
Chromatin
Nuclear membrane
Centriole
Smooth endoplasmic reticulum
Microfilament
Microtubule
Lysosome
Golgi region
Cytoplasmic membrane

Fig. 6.1   Ultrastructure of a generalised cell

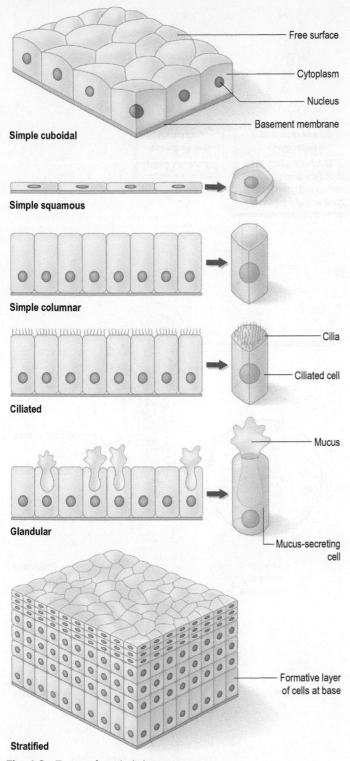

Simple cuboidal
- Free surface
- Cytoplasm
- Nucleus
- Basement membrane

Simple squamous

Simple columnar

Ciliated
- Cilia
- Ciliated cell

Glandular
- Mucus
- Mucus-secreting cell

Stratified
- Formative layer of cells at base

Fig. 6.2 Types of epithelial tissue

b. Compound. More than one layer of cells.
- Stratified – the first layers of cell are cuboidal, becoming flatter as they are moved towards the surface of the tissue by new cells forming beneath them, e.g. in skin
- Transitional – modified, stratified, containing a combination of shapes; found where ability to stretch is required, e.g. urinary bladder.

- Glandular – consisting of either individual goblet cells with a single unbranched duct or a mass of secretory cells with a branched duct system forming a gland; there are two types:
  a. Endocrine – surrounded by an extensive capillary network and are ductless, secreting hormones directly into the blood stream, e.g. thyroid gland (Fig. 6.3)
  b. Exocrine – defined as simple or compound, have ducts and secrete on to an epithelial surface, e.g. sweat glands.

Connective tissue

Connective tissue is a kind of animal tissue that supports, connects, or separates different types of tissues and organs of the body. These tissues also act as a transport system to move essential materials, e.g. nutrients around the body. Examples of this tissue are:

- Loose connective tissue (also called areolar tissue) – this consists of a loose network of collagen fibres and surrounds organs providing support and flexibility, e.g. under skin, around blood vessels. Adipose tissue is similar to areolar tissue but has an increased proportion of fat cells, which provide an energy reserve, insulation and protection.
- Dense connective tissue – has a large proportion of collagen fibres, which provide great strength, e.g. tendons, which connect muscle to bone, and ligaments, which connect bone to bone.
- Blood – transports essential nutrients, gases, waste products, hormones and enzymes to and from all body cells. Consists of many cell types, e.g. erythrocytes, leucocytes and thrombocytes, suspended in a liquid matrix called plasma.
- Cartilage – a mixture of collagen and elastic fibres provides shape, provides protection for organs and allows movement. It is a dense, clear, blue/white material that is tough and can be elastic or rigid. Found mainly in joints, it has no blood vessels but is covered by a membrane called the perichondrium from which it receives its blood supply. The cells of cartilage are called chondrocytes.
- There are three types of cartilage:
  a. Hyaline – chondrocytes lie within a hyaline matrix with collagen fibres running through, e.g. forming the articular surfaces of the joint; C-shaped rings that keep the trachea open for air passage into the lungs
  b. Fibrocartilage – stronger than hyaline cartilage and the matrix contains more fibrous collagen fibres, e.g. surrounds the articular surface of some bones, e.g. in the hip joint and the shoulder joint; also found in the stifle as pads of cartilage called menisci; intervertebral discs within the vertebral column
  c. Elastic – has a hyaline matrix and many elastic fibres that gives it elastic properties, e.g. in the ear pinna; in the epiglottis.
- Bone – provides support for the body and a means of attachment for skeletal muscles. It consists of cells embedded in a comparatively hard matrix or ground substance. The cells are arranged as cylinders in layers known as Haversian systems, which give bone its strength (Fig. 6.4). Bone is made of three types of cell:
  a. Osteoblasts – responsible for the secretion of material which, when mineralised or calcified, will become bone

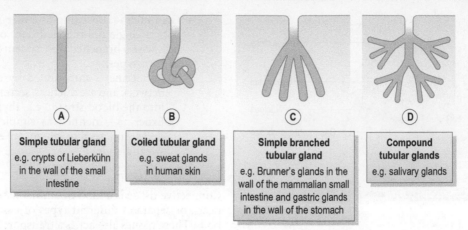

Fig. 6.3 Examples of endocrine glands

b. Osteoblasts – become trapped in the forming bone and are then called osteocytes
c. Osteoclasts – responsible for reabsorbing materials and for the remodelling of bone, e.g. after a fracture.

Long bones, e.g. femur, humerus (Fig. 6.4), are made up of two types of bone tissue:

- Compact bone – forming the dense walls of the bone shaft
- Cancellous or spongy bone – forming the central medullary cavity and providing support for haemopoietic tissue.

The medullary cavity of most bones contains red marrow, which is responsible for the production of platelets or thrombocytes and red and white blood cells. The yellow, rather fatty-looking material sometimes found in the medullary cavities is inactive bone marrow. The outer surface of bone is covered with a layer of dense fibrous connective tissue called the periosteum into which are inserted tendons and ligaments for the attachment of muscles. The inner surface of bone is covered by a delicate connective tissue layer called the endosteum. Both the periosteum and endosteum contain osteoclasts, which assist in the remodelling and repair of bone if it becomes damaged.

- Haemopoietic tissue – responsible for the formation of all blood cells from haemopoietic stem cells which are found in the spleen, liver, lymphoid tissue and in bone marrow. As the animal reaches maturity the bone marrow is the main site of haemopoiesis.

Nervous tissue

Conducts electrical or nerve impulses to and from the central nervous system by means of neurons. Each neuron consists of a cell body, many dendrons, which conduct impulses towards the cell body, and a single axon, which conducts impulses away from the cell body. Neurons are supported by neuroglial cells, which are a form of connective tissue (see Nervous system section).

BODY FLUIDS

The body consists of approximately 60% fluid, which is often referred to as body water and is distributed into 'compartments'

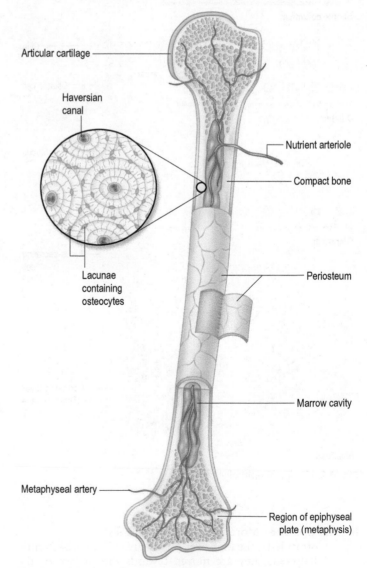

Fig. 6.4 Structure of compact bone

(Fig. 6.5), which are delicately balanced. The total volume of body fluids is affected by:

- Input, i.e. by drinking and eating
- Output, i.e. major losses include:
  Respiration – within exhaled gases
  Skin – sweating
  Gastrointestinal – faeces
  Kidneys – urine.

The proportion of body fluids varies between individuals:

- Fat animals – lower percentage of fluid, as fat displaces water within the cells
- Very young animals – higher percentage of fluid, as the solid elements of the body are underdeveloped. Neonates have a very low proportion of fat, and this in turn effects fluid percentage.

The daily fluid loss in terms of body weight is calculated as:

- 20 ml/kg body weight/day – respiration and sweating
- 10–20 ml/kg body weight/day – faeces
- 1–2 ml/kg body weight/hour – urine.

The total loss of fluid from the body is estimated to be 50–60 ml/kg body weight/day.

The losses from the respiratory tract and the skin cannot be regulated and are described as insensible or inevitable water loss. Losses from the kidney are linked to thirst and osmoregulatory mechanisms involved in the maintenance of extracellular fluid volume (Fig. 6.6).

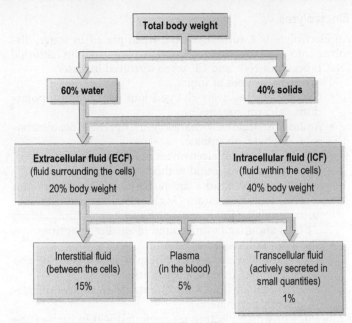

Fig. 6.5 Distribution of body fluids into compartments

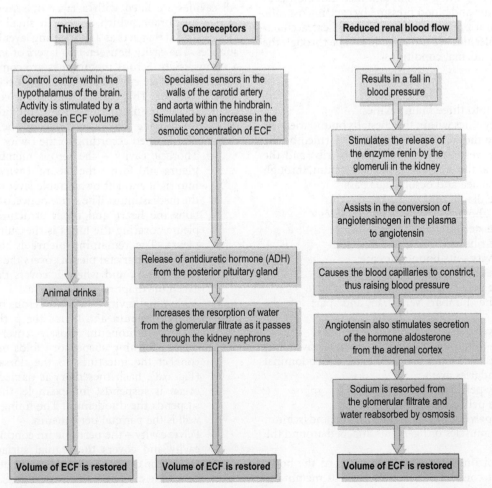

Fig. 6.6 Physiological reactions that regulate the volume of extracellular fluid (ECF)

Electrolytes

An electrolyte is a substance that, when placed in water, dissolves into ions or charged particles, e.g. sodium chloride (NaCl) becomes Na^+ and Cl^- when dissolved in water.

There are two types of ion:

- Cations are positively charged ions, e.g. sodium, potassium, calcium, magnesium.
- Anions are negatively charged ions, e.g. chloride, bicarbonate, sulphate, phosphate.

The body fluids contain electrolytes as follows:

- The main **cations** found within:
  a. Intracellular fluid – are potassium (K), with sodium (Na) and magnesium (Mg) in smaller quantities
  b. Extracellular fluid – are sodium, with potassium, calcium (Ca) and magnesium found in smaller quantities.
- The main **anions** found within:
  a. Intracellular fluid – are phosphate with chloride and bicarbonate in smaller quantities
  b. Extracellular fluid – are chloride with smaller quantities of phosphate.

Knowledge of which electrolytes are found within each of the fluid compartments enables the veterinary surgeon to decide which type of fluid replacement therapy is appropriate in different disease conditions (see Chapter 25).

Plasma proteins

Plasma contains plasma proteins – the main ones are albumin, prothrombin, fibrinogen and globulin and their function is to maintain blood volume and blood pressure by exerting osmotic pressure. These are not present in other forms of extracellular fluid because the molecules are too large to escape through the capillary walls under normal conditions.

BODY CAVITIES

The body is divided into three main cavities:

1. **Thoracic cavity** – lies within the chest. Its boundaries are:
   - Cranial – the thoracic inlet or aperture formed by the first thoracic vertebrae, the first pair of ribs and the manubrium at the cranial end of the sternum, through which the trachea and oesophagus pass
   - Caudal – the diaphragm
   - Dorsal – the thoracic vertebrae and muscles
   - Ventral – the sternum
   - Lateral – the ribs and intercostal muscles.
2. **Abdominal cavity** – its boundaries are:
   - Cranial – the diaphragm
   - Caudal – the pelvic opening
   - Dorsal – the lumbar vertebrae and part of the diaphragm
   - Lateral and ventral – the abdominal muscles.
3. **Pelvic cavity** – often described as a separate cavity but there is no physical barrier between it and the abdominal cavity. Its boundaries are:
   - Cranial – the pelvic inlet
   - Caudal – the pelvic outlet
   - Dorsal – the pelvic girdle – the pubis, ileum and ischium
   - Lateral – the muscles or ligaments attached around the pelvic girdle.

The pericardium, not one of the major cavities of the body, contains the heart. It consists of a double layer of membrane and lies within the mediastinum in the thoracic cavity.

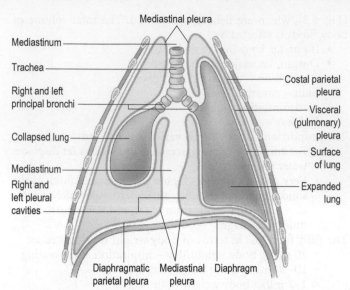

Fig. 6.7 Longitudinal section through the thorax showing the arrangement of the pleura

Other cavities include the cranial cavity, formed by the bones of the cranium and containing the brain, and the oral cavity.

Body cavity linings

All cavities are lined with a layer of serous endothelium or serous membrane, which secretes a small amount of serous (watery) fluid that acts as a lubricating layer between two tissue surfaces. The cavity between two layers of serous membrane is a serous cavity. Serous membranes are composed of a simple squamous surface epithelium and a connective tissue groundwork or stroma. This connective tissue is composed of yellow elastic and white fibrous tissue and provides support to the delicate membrane. The layer covers all the organs within the cavity and is named according to the cavity.

- Thoracic cavity – the serous membrane is called the **pleura** and forms the pleural cavity, which is divided into right and left by a double layer of pleura known as the mediastinum. The space between the two layers contains the heart and other structures (Fig. 6.7). The pleura covering the lungs is the pulmonary or visceral pleura. The remaining pleura is the parietal pleura. Where the parietal pleura covers the ribs it is called the costal pleura and where it covers the diaphragm it is called the diaphragmatic pleura.
- Abdominal cavity – here the serous membrane is called the **peritoneum** and forms the peritoneal cavity. The visceral peritoneum closely covers the abdominal organs, forming suspensory folds or mesenteries that connect the intestines to the dorsal abdominal wall (Fig. 6.8). Each mesentery is named according to the organ it suspends; for example, the mesoduodenum suspends the duodenum. The lining of the abdominal wall is the parietal peritoneum.
- Pelvic cavity – the peritoneum continues into the pelvic cavity and covers the cranial surfaces of the organs within the cavity, e.g. bladder and uterus. The remainder of the cavity is filled with organs, muscles and connective tissue and is not lined by a serous membrane.

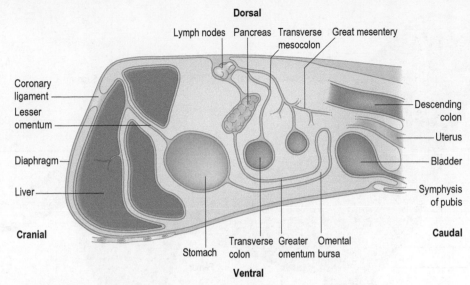

Fig. 6.8   Sagittal section through the abdominal cavity to show the arrangement of the peritoneum

Locomotor system

The function of the locomotor system is to bring about movement of the animal. It consists of two major systems:
- The skeletal system – made up of the skeleton and the joints
- The muscular system – made of the muscles attached to the skeleton.

THE SKELETAL SYSTEM

The skeleton is divided into three parts:
- Axial skeleton – the skull, vertebral column, ribs and sternum
- Appendicular skeleton – the fore and hind limbs
- Splanchnic skeleton – bones that develop in soft tissues, e.g. the os penis.

The skeletal system consists of bone and cartilage whose function is to provide support for the body and a rigid but all-moving framework (see Basic tissues types).

Bone growth or ossification

Bone develops within the embryo in two ways:
- Intramembranous – bone formed directly from fibrous tissue, e.g. flat bones of the skull
- Endochondral – bone formed within a preformed cartilaginous model.

The **functions** of the skeletal system are:
- To support the body
- Movement by providing leverage for muscle contraction
- Protection of the organs, e.g. heart, lungs, brain
- Mineral balance, maintaining calcium and phosphorus levels in the body
- Red blood cell production, within the bone marrow
- Endocrine regulation.

There are over 200 bones in the skeleton, many of which are shown in Figure 6.9. For more detailed descriptions of the skeleton you are advised to look at a more specialised anatomy book (see Recommended reading).

Joints

Joints are places where two or more bones meet. There are several methods of joint classification:

Degree of movement

- Synarthrosis – joint that is immovable, e.g. joints of the skull, known as sutures
- Diarthrosis – joint in which there is a great deal of movement; these are usually related to the limbs, e.g. synovial joints (Fig. 6.10)
- Amphiarthrosis – joint that shares some of the characteristics of the synarthroses and diarthroses and has limited movement, e.g. between the vertebrae of the spine
- Syntosis – joint that becomes fused with bone as the animal ages, e.g. pubic symphysis, sutures of the skull.

Structure

- Fibrous – connected by dense fibrous connective tissue that allows very little movement, e.g. sutures of the skull
- Cartilaginous – connected by cartilage and found where the right and left sides of the body join, e.g. mandibular symphysis and pubic symphysis
- Synovial – allow plenty of movement (see Fig. 6.10). Synovial joints have several anatomical features:
  - Hyaline cartilage covers the bone ends to form the articular surfaces.
  - The surfaces of the joint are linked by a dense, fibrous, connective-tissue joint capsule.
  - The capsule is lined by a synovial membrane which secretes synovial fluid.
  - The joint cavity is filled with synovial fluid, which acts as a lubricant and a 'shock absorber'.

Synovial joints may be called simple joints if they contain two articular surfaces, e.g. the shoulder joint formed by the glenoid cavity of the scapula and the head of the humerus. Compound joints have more than two articular surfaces, e.g. the elbow formed by the distal end of the humerus, the proximal ends of the ulna and radius.

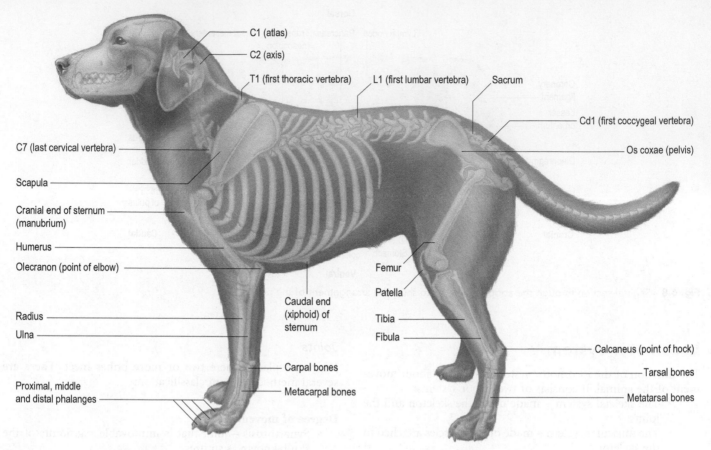

Fig. 6.9 The skeleton of the dog

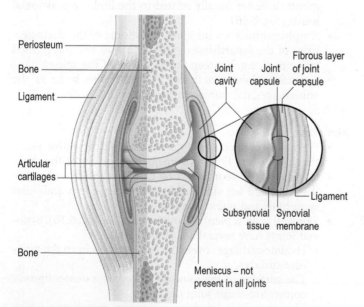

Fig. 6.10 Structure of a synovial joint

Type of movement

- Pivot (radius/ulna or atlas/axis)
- Ball and socket (femur/acetabulum)
- Hinge (humerus/radius and ulna)
- Plane or gliding (between carpals/tarsals)
- Saddle (between phalanges)
- Condylar (stifle).

During locomotion joints undergo a great deal of stress and strain and their stability is improved by:

- Surrounding muscle and tendons
- Ligaments, which link one bone to another
- Correct bone conformation, particularly at the articular surfaces, which ensures that the weight is supported by the correct part of the bone – poor conformation leads to lameness and arthritis.

THE MUSCULAR SYSTEM

The main tissue of the muscular system is striated or skeletal muscle, i.e. that which is attached to the bones of the skeleton via tendons. Its contraction is controlled voluntarily.

Skeletal muscle structure

Muscle tissue consists of cells that are long, thin and thread-like and are referred to as muscle fibres. They vary in size from about 1 mm to 5 cm in length. Under the microscope the fibres of striated muscle appear striped, which gives them their name. This is due to the microscopic appearance of the two contractile proteins actin and myosin.

Skeletal muscles attached to a bone are formed from parallel muscle fibres held together in small bundles or fascicles by connective tissue. These are collected into larger groups, also enclosed in connective tissue, and ultimately form the muscle, which is surrounded by yet more connective tissue, commonly called the muscle sheath (Fig. 6.11). When muscles lie close to one another, the sheaths may thicken to form what is called an intermuscular septum. During muscle contraction the

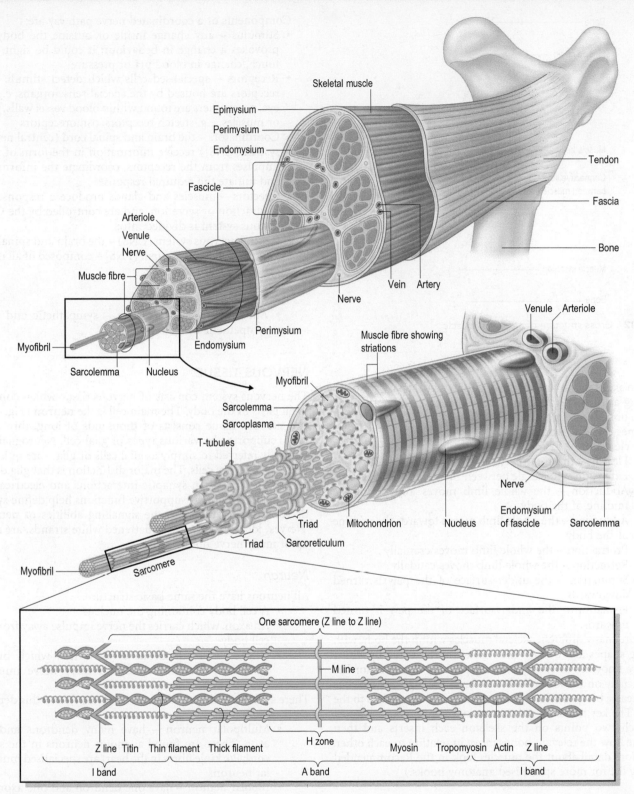

Fig. 6.11 Microscopic structure of skeletal muscle

arrangement of the myofilaments, both thick and thin, remain constant in length regardless of the muscle contractions. Thick filaments remain parallel, whereas thin filaments are united in a disc-like formation; this allows the thick and thin filaments to slide over each other, altering the length of the sarcomere (see Fig. 6.11).

All the connective tissue within and around the muscle merges into the connective tissue of the periosteum of the bone to which the muscle is attached, forming a tendon (Fig. 6.12) or a fibrous sheet called an aponeurosis. Aponeuroses are seen attached to the abdominal muscles and within the diaphragm.

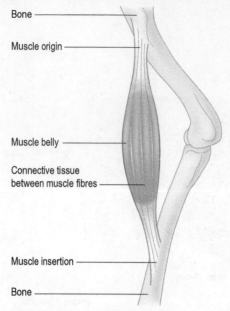

Bone

Muscle origin

Muscle belly

Connective tissue
between muscle fibres

Muscle insertion

Bone

Fig. 6.12   Gross structure of a skeletal muscle

Each skeletal muscle consists of a thick central part, the belly, tapering at each end to form a head that inserts via a tendon on to a bone (see Fig. 6.12). When the muscle contracts it pulls the bones closer together.

Muscle action is defined in the following terms:

- Flexion – the angle between the bones is reduced
- Extension – the angle between the bones is increased
- Abduction – the whole limb moves away from the midline of the body
- Adduction – the whole limb moves towards the midline of the body
- Protraction – the whole limb moves cranially
- Retraction – the whole limb moves caudally
- Supination – the under-surface of the paw is turned downwards
- Pronation – the under-surface of the paw is turned upwards.

There are many different skeletal muscles within the body, with varying shapes and actions that influence the name by which they are known. For example, the superficial digital flexor lies superficially on the lower limb and flexes the digits; triceps has three heads; biceps femoris has two heads and is attached to the femur. The key to learning the action of each muscle is to know at which two points on the skeleton each inserts and then imagine how the relevant bones move in relation to each other. (For more detail about the muscles look in the Recommended reading list for more specialised anatomy books.)

Nervous system

The nervous system provides a rapid means of communication and coordination for all body systems and enables the body to respond to events within its environment and thus survive.

The functions of the nervous system are to receive information from both the internal and external environment, to integrate and analyse this information and to bring about the appropriate response.

Components of a coordinated nerve pathway are:

- Stimulus – any change inside or outside the body that provokes a change in behaviour; it could be sight, pain, touch, change in blood pH or pressure
- Receptors – specialised cells which detect stimuli: some receptors are housed by the special sense organs, e.g. ear, eye, nose; others are found within blood vessel walls, joints or muscles, e.g. stretch receptors, osmoreceptors
- Coordinators – the brain and spinal cord (central nervous system [CNS]) receive information in the form of nerve impulses from the receptors, coordinate the information and initiate the required response
- Effectors – muscles and glands produce a response, e.g. contraction or secretion, and are controlled by the CNS.

The nervous system is divided into:

- Central nervous system (CNS) – the brain and spinal cord
- Peripheral nervous system (PNS) – composed of all nerves extending from the CNS:
  - Cranial nerves
  - Spinal nerves
  - Autonomic nervous system – sympathetic and parasympathetic branches.

NERVOUS TISSUE

The nervous system consists of nervous tissue which connects to all parts of the body. The main cell is the **neuron** (Fig. 6.13), and nervous tissue consists of thousands of long, thin nerve fibres supported by various types of glial cell. Neuroglial cells – usually referred to simply as glial cells or glia – are quite different from nerve cells. The major distinction is that glia do not participate directly in synaptic interactions and electrical signalling, although their supportive functions help define synaptic contacts and maintain the signalling abilities of neurons. 'Nerves', identified grossly as flattened white strands, are made up of many nerve fibres.

Neuron

All neurons have the same basic structure:

- A cell body containing the nucleus
- An axon, which carries the nerve impulse away from the cell body
- One or more dendrons or dendrites, which branch extensively like tiny trees and carry nerve impulses towards the cell body.

There are several shapes of neuron (Fig. 6.14), and this depends on their function:

- Multipolar neuron – have many dendrons and one axon. These are found as motor neurons in the spinal cord; Purkinje fibres in the heart are specialised multipolar neurons
- Bipolar neuron – have one dendron and one axon and are found in the retina of the eye and in the nasal mucosa
- Pseudo-unipolar neuron – appear to have only one fibre leaving the cell body (see Fig. 6.14), but in fact they have one dendron and one axon which are wound around each other giving this appearance. They are found as sensory nerves.

The majority of the axons leaving the neurons are enveloped by specialised Schwann cells, which provide both structural and

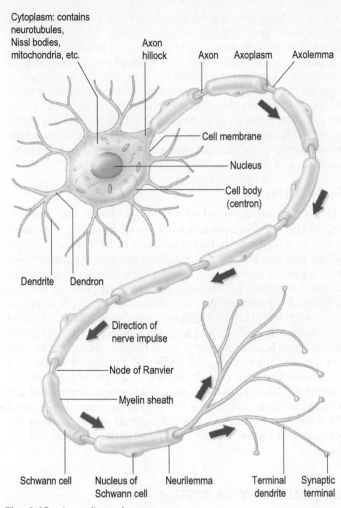

Fig. 6.13 A myelinated neuron

metabolic support and secrete a lipoprotein material known as myelin (see Fig. 6.13). Large-diameter fibres are wrapped by a variable number of concentric layers of the Schwann cell plasma membrane forming the so-called myelin sheath. These nerve fibres are said to be myelinated. Non-myelinated fibres are found within the cornea of the eye and within the grey matter of the CNS. The myelin sheath increases the rate and efficiency of electrical conduction along the axon by allowing the impulse to jump between gaps within the myelin (between the Schwann cells), called the nodes of Ranvier. At this point the axon is exposed to the external environment. The jumping from node to node is known as saltatory conduction and greatly enhances the conduction speed of axons.

Nerve impulses pass along nerve fibres in one direction only and are named accordingly:

- Sensory neurons – conduct impulses from receptors such as those in the eyes, ears and stretch receptors in the muscles and carry them *towards* the CNS
- Motor neurons – conduct impulses *away* from the CNS towards effector organs, e.g. muscles and glands.

Nerves that supply the visceral organs, i.e. those of the respiratory, digestive, urinary and reproductive systems and the heart, are known as visceral nerves. They may be visceral sensory or visceral motor nerves.

Nerves that supply all other organs, e.g. skin, joints, skeletal muscles, are known as somatic nerves. They may be somatic sensory or somatic motor nerves.

Neuroglial tissue

Neuroglial tissue provides support for the neurons and their processes and there are four types:

- Astrocytes – numerous star-shaped cells thought to provide mechanical and metabolic support for neurons. They cover the capillaries in the brain and help to form the blood–brain barrier.
- Oligodendrocytes – similar to the Schwann cell of peripheral nervous tissue and are responsible for myelination and holding nerve fibres together.

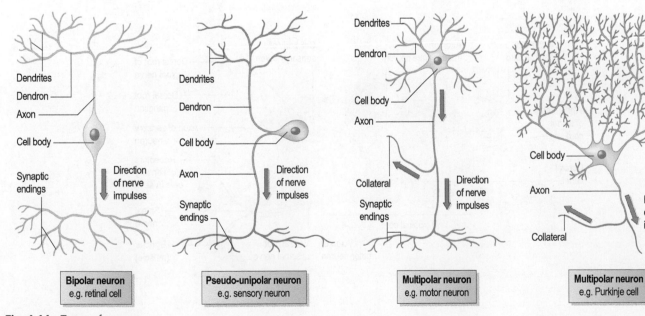

Fig. 6.14 Types of neuron

- Microglia – small phagocytic cells that are thought to be the CNS representatives of the macrophage/monocyte defence system.
- Ependymal – a simple epithelium that lines the cerebral ventricles of the brain and central canal of the spinal cord.

Nerve impulses

Nerve impulses can be considered to be a form of electrical impulse resulting from a chain reaction in the form of a wave of rearrangements of sodium and potassium ions across the cell membrane. The nerve fibre must recover before it can conduct another impulse. This recovery period, known as the refractory period, lasts for only a few thousandths of a second.

Impulses passing along a nerve fibre eventually reach the end of it, where they encounter a microscopic gap called a synapse (Fig. 6.15) lying between the tip of one fibre and the beginning of the next. Transmission of the impulse across the gap is dependent upon the presence of chemical or neurotransmitters, e.g. acetylcholine (most common), epinephrine (adrenaline) or serotonin (5-hydroxytryptamine). The neurotransmitter is released from vesicles in the axon terminal to activate (excite or inhibit) other impulses in the dendrites of the connecting neuron. The neurotransmitters facilitate their effects by interacting with specific receptors in the opposing plasma membrane. Nerve fibres that terminate on muscle fibres at a motor endplate or a neuromuscular junction.

Reflex action

The simplest arrangement of neurons is seen in the reflex arc (Fig. 6.16). A reflex action is a behaviour in which a stimulus results in a response that does not have to be learned and that occurs very quickly without conscious thought, e.g. withdrawal from a painful stimulus is an involuntary reaction. Stimulation of pain receptors in the skin fires off impulses in sensory neurons that pass through the spinal cord along spinal nerves. They enter the spinal cord via a separate dorsal root (containing the sensory nerve fibres) and leave via a ventral root (containing motor nerve fibres) (see Fig. 6.16). The grey matter of the cord contains the nerve cells and bodies of the motor nerve cells whose axons run out into the ventral roots. Nerve impulses are conveyed to the appropriate muscle by motor nerves and the muscle contracts and moves the limb away from the cause of the pain. The stimulus is also transmitted up the CNS to the brain, so that the animal can acknowledge the stimulus and feel the pain.

CENTRAL NERVOUS SYSTEM

The CNS is the control area of the nervous system comprising the brain, located in the cranium, and the spinal cord, lying within the spinal cavity of the vertebral column. Both are protected by the skeletal system. It is composed entirely of neurons and neuroglia arranged as white matter and grey matter.

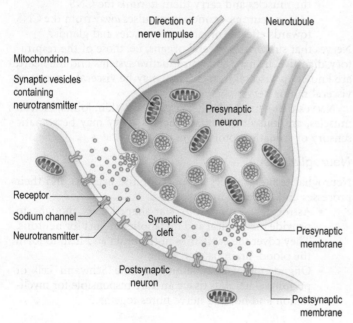

Fig. 6.15   A synapse

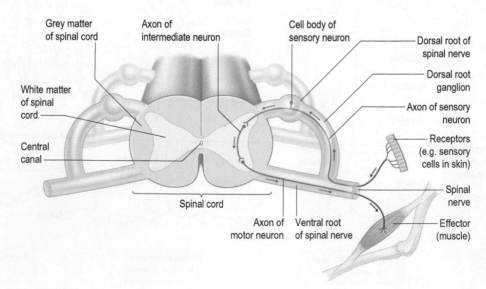

Fig. 6.16   Components of a reflex arc

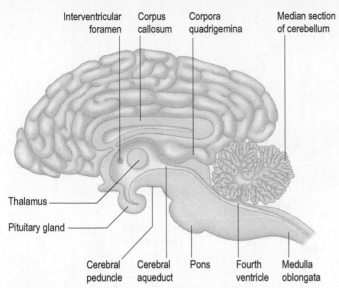

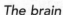

Fig. 6.17 Median section through the canine brain

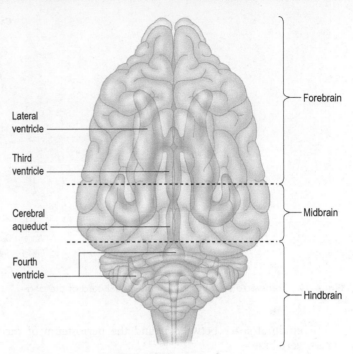

Fig. 6.18 Ventricular system of the brain

The brain

The brain is subdivided into three regions

Forebrain – telencephalon and diencephalon. This consists of the right and left cerebral hemispheres connected in the midline by a band of tissue known as the corpus callosum (Fig. 6.17). The cerebral hemispheres are concerned with conscious thought. The outer layer of grey matter is known as the cerebral cortex and is divided into lobes whose names correspond to the skull bone nearest to the lobe:

- Frontal lobe – the most anterior of all the lobes, is the centre of voluntary movement. It is often referred to as the motor area, containing areas for control of gross, fine and complicated muscle movements.
- Parietal lobe – collects, recognises and organises sensations of pain, temperature, touch, position and movement.
- Temporal lobe – contains the centres for awareness and correlation of auditory stimuli.
- Occipital lobe – forms the posterior extremity of each cerebral hemisphere. It involves visual perception and visual memory with a role in eye movements.

On the ventral surface of the forebrain is the optic chiasma, which is a cross-shaped arrangement of nerve fibres associated with the eye and the pituitary gland, part of the endocrine system. Dorsal to the pituitary gland and lying within the brain tissue is the hypothalamus, which is the coordinating centre of the endocrine system. At the anterior point of the cerebral hemispheres are the olfactory bulbs. These paired structures lie close to the nasal chambers and are concerned with the sense of smell. The thalamus at the base of the cerebral hemispheres acts as a relay station for sensory impulses. The epithalamus holds the pineal body, which is involved in the regulation of gonad hormones. Cranial nerves I (olfactory nerve) and II (optic nerve) are attached to the forebrain. Running through the centre of the forebrain are the lateral ventricles – part of the ventricular system, which contains cerebrospinal fluid (CSF). Damage to tissue in the forebrain can cause personality change.

Midbrain – mesencephalon. Consists of a tube through which runs part of the ventricular system known as the cerebral aqueduct, carrying the CSF. It contains centres for control of muscle, sight and hearing and is involved in the positioning of the body to maintain balance. Cranial nerves III (oculomotor nerve) and IV (trochlear nerve) are attached to the midbrain. Damage to tissue in the midbrain results in coma.

Hindbrain – metencephalon and myelencephalon. Consists of the cerebellum, which has a ridged surface resembling a small cauliflower and is composed of two hemispheres joined in the midline (Fig. 6.18). Each hemisphere controls and coordinates balance and movement. Ventral to the cerebellum is the medulla oblongata, which passes through the foramen magnum of the skull and becomes the spinal cord. It contains centres that control respiration, heart rate and blood pressure. Linking the cerebrum, cerebellum and the medulla oblongata is the pons, which forms a crossover tract of white matter involved in the control of respiration. Within the hindbrain is the fourth ventricle, which is continuous with the cerebral aqueduct and the central canal within the spinal cord. Cranial nerves V (trigeminal nerve), VI (abducens nerve) and XII (hypoglossal nerve) are located on the ventral surface. Damage to the hindbrain results in rapid death.

Protection of the central nervous system

If an animal is to survive, the CNS must be protected from mechanical and chemical damage.

- Cranium – the bones of the skull form a hard outer covering to the brain
- Vertebral column – protects the spinal cord
- Meninges – three layers of membrane composed of white, fibrous connective tissue envelope the entire CNS providing support and protection:
  - **Dura mater** – the outermost layer is tough, fibrous and lines the cranium. In the vertebral canal there is an

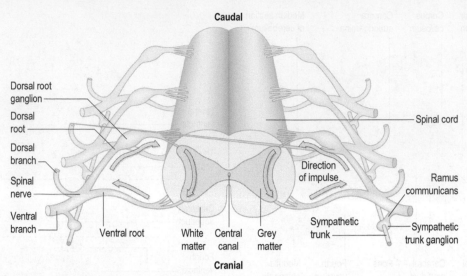

Caudal

Dorsal root
ganglion

Dorsal
root

Dorsal
branch

Spinal
nerve

Ventral
branch

Ventral root

White
matter

Central
canal

Grey
matter

Direction
of impulse

Spinal cord

Ramus
communicans

Sympathetic
trunk

Sympathetic
trunk ganglion

Cranial

Fig. 6.19   Transverse section through the spinal cord of the dog

epidural space between it and the periosteum of the vertebrae

- **Arachnoid mater** – named for its web-like appearance. More delicate and cushions the CNS and facilitates diffusion of oxygen and nutrients into the nervous tissue beneath. CSF runs in the subarachnoid space below this layer.
- **Pia mater** – the innermost layer; delicate, very vascular supplying blood to the CNS tissues and closely follows the contours of the brain surface.

Cerebrospinal fluid (CSF) consists of a watery, transparent fluid, similar to plasma with less protein, which flows within the ventricular system of the brain, the central canal of the spinal cord and subarachnoid spaces (Fig. 6.19). It is secreted by networks of capillaries referred to as choroid plexuses located within each ventricle. The function of CSF is to act as a shock absorber during movement, provide an antibacterial effect and transport nutrients and waste materials from the nervous tissue.

The spinal cord

The spinal cord runs from medulla oblongata to the lumbar region terminating at the sixth or seventh lumbar vertebrae as the cauda equina or 'horse's tail'. Pairs of spinal nerves leave the cord throughout its length via intervertebral spaces, linking the brain to all the organs of the body.

The spinal cord is composed of nerve fibres running in organised tracts. Its structure is similar over its entire length and the tissue is divided into outer white matter surrounding the central grey matter. It is covered by the meninges and bathed in CSF, which also flows in the central canal (see Fig. 6.19).

In transverse section (see Fig. 6.19) the grey matter has a characteristic butterfly shape. The ventral horns are more prominent and contain the cell bodies of the large motor neurons. The dorsal horns contain the cell bodies of smaller sensory neurons. Sensory information, particularly concerning pain and temperature, is relayed to the brain via afferent neurons. Smaller lateral horns, containing the cell bodies of preganglia and sympathetic efferent neurons, are located in the upper lumbar and thoracic regions. This corresponds to the level of sympathetic outflow from the cord. More grey matter is required in the cervical and lumbar regions because of the greater activity of both

sensory and motor innervation of the limbs. This in turn increases the diameter of the spinal cord in these areas.

The white matter contains a greater proportion of myelin and consists of ascending tracts of sensory fibres and descending motor tracts that increase in volume, especially in the sacral to cervical regions, as more and more fibres pass up towards the brain.

PERIPHERAL NERVOUS SYSTEM

The peripheral nervous system is made up of the nerves which leave the central nervous system. It links the CNS to all the organs of the body.

Cranial nerves

Cranial nerves are given off by the brain and leave the cranium via foramina in the bones (Fig. 6.20). Most supply structures on the head and are relatively short. They may carry sensory or motor nerve fibres or a mixture of the two. These nerves have specific names and are always referred to by Roman numerals (Table 6.1); there are many acronyms to remember these.

Spinal nerves

Spinal nerves are given off by the spinal cord. They contain both sensory and motor fibres and are, therefore, mixed nerves. They supply all the musculoskeletal system and are numbered according to the number of the vertebra in front of their point of exit from the cord. The exception is in the cervical region, where the first nerve leaves the cord *before* the first vertebra – there are eight cervical nerves in total.

The spinal nerves on each side of the cord are divided into two roots:

- The dorsal root carries sensory fibres into the cord and the cell bodies of the nerves are contained in the dorsal root ganglion (see Fig. 6.19).
- The ventral root carries motor fibres away from the cord and their cell bodies are within the grey matter of the cord. The nerve supply to the limbs is:
  - Fore limb – spinal nerves Cervical 6 (C6) to Thoracic 2 (T2; forms the radial nerve). Together these form the brachial plexus

TABLE 6.1	Cranial nerves		
Cranial nerve number	Name	Nerve type	Function
I	Olfactory	Sensory	Smell
II	Optic	Sensory	Vision, pupil light response
III	Oculomotor	Motor + parasympathetic	Eye movement, pupil constriction, focus
IV	Trochlear	Motor	Eye movement
V	Trigeminal	Mixed	Muscle for mastication, upper and lower jaws, face
VI	Abducens	Motor	Eye movement
VII	Facial	Mixed (motor) + parasympathetic	Salivation, facial expression, taste, ears, head
VIII	Auditory/vestibulocochlear	Sensory	Hearing, balance
IX	Glossopharyngeal	Mixed + parasympathetic	Taste, laryngeal muscles, swallowing, salivation
X	Vagus	Mixed (motor) + parasympathetic	Vocalisation, swallowing, gastrointestinal tract, thoracic organs, abdominal organs
XI	Accessory	Motor	Head and shoulder movement, vocalisation, swallowing
XII	Hypoglossal	Motor	Tongue movement, swallowing, vocalisation

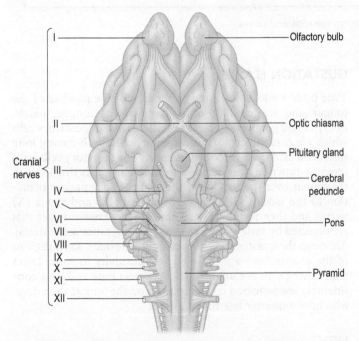

Fig. 6.20 Ventral view of brain showing cranial nerves

- Hind limb – spinal nerves Lumbar 4 (L6) to Sacral 2 (S2; forms the sciatic nerve). Together these form the lumbo-sacral plexus.

Autonomic nervous system

The autonomic nervous system (ANS) consists of spinal nerves that supply motor fibres to the viscera and may be described as the visceral motor system. It is considered to be self-governing, i.e. it is not under conscious control but will assist in the regulation of the internal body organs by means of both sympathetic and parasympathetic innervation.

Sympathetic system. The nerves for this system are located in the thoracolumbar areas of the spinal cord, i.e. T1 to L4

TABLE 6.2	Comparison between the functions of the sympathetic and parasympathetic systems
Sympathetic system	**Parasympathetic system**
Neurotransmitter chemical – norepinephrine (noradrenaline)	Neurotransmitter – acetylcholine
Prepares body for fight, flight or frolic, e.g. dilates the pupils	Assists in the day-to-day functions of the body
Inhibits salivation and slows gut movement	Stimulates gut movement and salivation
Increases heart rate	Returns heart rate to normal
Increases respiratory rate	Decreases respiratory rate
Dilates the bronchi and bronchioles	Lacrimal secretions increase

or L5. Short preganglionic fibres synapse within a series of ganglia on each side of the vertebral column forming a nodular cord (looking like a string of beads) known as the sympathetic chain. Long postganglionic fibres then travel to their intended organs using the routes of blood vessels. The function of the sympathetic system is to prepare the body for stressful or hazardous situations (the fight, flight or frolic reflex) and relies on noradrenaline (norepinephrine) as a transmitter at the synapses within the system (Table 6.2 and Fig. 6.15).

Parasympathetic system. This originates in the brain stem, sending impulses via the oculomotor (III), facial (VII), glossopharyngeal (IX) and vagus (X) cranial nerves and via the sacral nerves S1 and S2. The ganglia are embedded in the wall of the effector organ, thus requiring long preganglionic and short postganglionic nerve fibres. The function of the system is the opposite of the sympathetic system and relies on the use of acetylcholine at all the synapses (see Table 6.2).

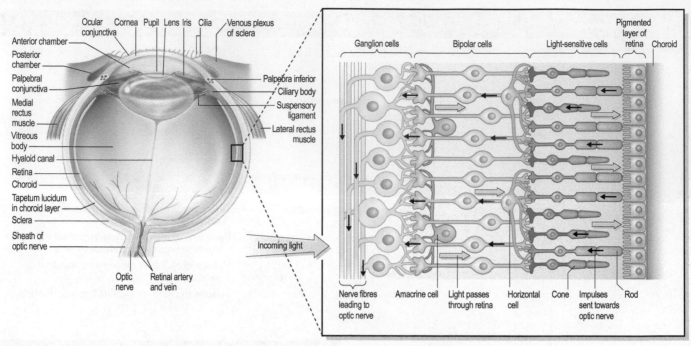

Fig. 6.21 Cross-section through the eye. Section through the retina showing the rods and cones

Special senses

The special senses, i.e. sight, hearing and balance, smell and taste, are detected by sophisticated sensory receptors that respond to a stimulus or change in the environment. These specific neural receptors are housed within the special sense organs, e.g. eye or ear, which enhance and refine the reception of incoming stimuli before it is passed on the CNS.

Sensory receptors are found all over the body and can be divided into:

- Proprioceptors – lie within muscle and joints and are used to detect the body's spatial position in the environment; also linked to the ear for balance
- Exteroceptors – involved in the response to external stimuli collected by the special sense organs
- Interoceptors – respond to changes in the internal environment of the body, e.g. blood pH or blood pressure, and stimulate homeostatic mechanisms, e.g. respiration, vasodilation.

OLFACTION (SMELL)

The chemoreceptors for the sense of smell are located in the nasal mucosa covering the turbinate bones in the nasal cavity. In the dog and cat the olfactory tissue is extensive and is an essential function for survival in the wild. The olfactory receptor cells are true bipolar neurons containing a single dendritic process extending from the cell body to the tissue surface and terminating as a small swelling giving rise to a number of long, modified cilia. The cilia receive information from smell chemicals dissolved in the mucus over the epithelium, passing it to receptor cells. Nerve impulses travel along the olfactory nerve (cranial nerve I) and reach the olfactory bulbs in the forebrain. The sense of smell and taste are linked, with smell being by far the more sensitive of the two.

GUSTATION (TASTE)

Taste buds are located in the epithelium of the papillae of the tongue and scattered in other parts of the tongue, palate, pharynx and epiglottis. The taste bud consists of gustatory cells which are chemoreceptors and support cells, both having long microvilli extending into the taste pore. The gustatory cells have receptor function and respond to taste chemicals dissolved in the mucus over the surface of the tongue. They pass information to the facial (VII), glossopharyngeal (IX) and vagus (X) nerves and then to the brain. There are five known tastes that are detected by taste buds: sweet, salty, sour, bitter and umami. Although these tastes are detected by all taste buds, some regions of the tongue have a slightly higher sensitivity to some tastes than others. Cats are unable to detect sweet taste and have considerably less taste bud concentrations on the tongue than dogs, who have a quarter less than humans.

SIGHT

The eye is a highly specialised organ of photoreception that involves the conversion of different wavelengths of light into nerve impulses.

The eye

Perception of an image. Light radiating from an image is received by photoreceptor cells which are located in the inner layer of the eye, the retina. These cells are modified dendrites of two types of nerve cell (Fig. 6.21):

- Rods – receptive to light of differing intensity seen in black and white images and used in night vision; located outside the fovea in the more peripheral parts of the retina
- Cones – receptive to different colours, enabling a coloured image to be perceived in daylight levels; located in the fovea to give high levels of visual accuracy.

The tapetum lucidum lies over the retina of the dog and cat, within the uvea. It is a reflective layer, enhancing light entering the eye and improving vision when there are low light levels by reflecting it back to the retina. The retina contains many sensory and connector neurons and processes. At an area in the back of the retina, there is an optic disc where the nerve fibres from the eye meet to form the optic nerve (II). The optic nerve is joined by an artery and vein from the choroid, which together form a blind spot in which there are no rods and cones.

Light passes through the overlying retinal layers to the photoreceptor cells where an inverted image is produced. The light that misses the receptor cells on its way through the retina is reflected back to the retinal layers by the tapetum lucidum. The bipolar receptor cells then transmit the image through the optic nerve to the cerebral cortex of the brain.

Structure of the eye. The remaining structures of the eye (see Fig. 6.21) support the retina and assist in the focusing of light rays on to the retina.

The eyeball comprises three layers:
- Sclera – the tough outermost layer of dense connective tissue, divided into the cornea and the sclera
- Uvea – the vascular pigmented layer, divided into the choroid, tapetum lucidum, suspensory ligament, ciliary body and iris
- Retina – the innermost layer, which contains the photoreceptor cells.

The eye is situated within the orbit of the skull and is cushioned in fat and connective tissue. Attached to the eyeball are the optic nerve (II), ocular musculature, other nerves and its blood supply. The eye is protected by the eyelids, covered by a thin, highly folded skin externally and by smooth conjunctival epithelium on the inner surface. The upper and lower eyelids are hairy and meet at the medial canthus close to the nose and the lateral canthus nearer to the ear. The third eyelid or nictitating membrane comes from the medial canthus and is hairless. In the dog and cat this eyelid is stiffened with a T-shaped piece of cartilage. The conjunctiva lines the inner eyelids and lines the surface of the sclera. The fold in the conjunctiva between the layer lining the eyelids and the layer lining the sclera is the fornix. The conjunctival mucous secretions contribute to the protection of the exposed surface of the eye.

Lachrymal glands are responsible for the secretion of tears. The tears are evenly distributed over the eye surface by the eyelids, collecting near the medial canthus to drain via the nasolacrimal duct into the nasal cavity. The Meibomian glands lie under the lashes of the upper and lower eyelids. They are a specialised sebaceous gland attached to the hair follicle of each eyelash and open directly on to the edge of the eyelid, producing oily tears. These tears float on the surface of the watery tear film and help prevent evaporation.

The front of the eye is protected by a thick, transparent cornea behind which lies the iris, which is continuous with the ciliary body and contains circular and radial muscles. Contraction of these muscles alters the size of the aperture or pupil and controls the amount of light falling on to the retina. The transparent biconvex lens is located directly behind the iris of the eye, supported by the suspensory ligament and attached to the ciliary body, which encircles the lens. The lens focuses light rays on to the retina.

The fundus of the eye comprises the anterior and posterior chambers formed by the iris extending in front of the lens from the ciliary body (see Fig. 6.21). Both the chambers contain a watery fluid, the aqueous humour, secreted into the posterior chamber by the ciliary body and circulated through the pupil to drain into the canal of Schlemm in the anterior chamber. The aqueous humour is a source of nutrients for the lens and the cornea, which are non-vascular. It also acts as a non-refractive optical medium, maintaining the shape of the cornea by the resulting intraocular pressure. The vitreous chamber at the back of the eye, behind the lens, contains a gelatinous mass called the vitreous body or humour, which also provides a non-refractive optical medium and supports the lens and retina.

HEARING AND BALANCE

Hearing is the detection of sound waves or vibrations in the air. These sound waves have differing frequencies and are detected by the ear and interpreted by the brain as differences in pitch. Balance is perceived by the semicircular canals within the inner ear.

The ear

The ear (Fig. 6.22) can be divided into the:
- External ear – concerned with reception of sound
- Middle ear – involved with transmission and amplification of incoming sound waves
- Internal (inner) ear – containing specific sensory receptors for both movement and sound.

The external ear. Receives and conducts sound waves to the ear drum or tympanic membrane. The external auditory meatus or ear canal (see Fig. 6.22) is lined by hairy skin containing sebaceous glands and modified apocrine sweat glands that secrete a waxy material called cerumen. The shape of the ear canal and the pinna or ear flap are maintained by elastic cartilage. The ear canal consists of a vertical and then a horizontal section.

The middle ear. The middle ear is an air-filled cavity located within the tympanic bulla of the temporal bone and separated from the external ear by the tympanic membrane. The Eustachian or auditory tube links it to the pharynx and equalises the air pressure on either sides of the tympanic membrane. Sound waves reaching the tympanic membrane are converted into mechanical vibrations, which are then amplified by a system of levers made up of three small bones called ossicles. These are the malleus, nearest to the tympanic membrane, the incus and the stapes, next to the oval window below which is a membrane called the round window (see Fig. 6.22). The ossicles articulate with each other via synovial joints and ligaments. The muscle linking the tympanic membrane and stapes reduces excessive sound vibrations that might otherwise damage the middle and inner ear. The oval window is covered by the base of the stapes to assist transmitted vibrations. The round window permits vibrations passed to the sensory receptors for sound to be dispersed.

The inner ear. The inner ear consists of an interconnected fluid-filled membranous labyrinth located within a bony labyrinth within the temporal bone. This is shaped specifically to house the membranous labyrinth.

The two are separated by fluid known as perilymph and the membranous labyrinth is filled with endolymph (see Fig. 6.22).

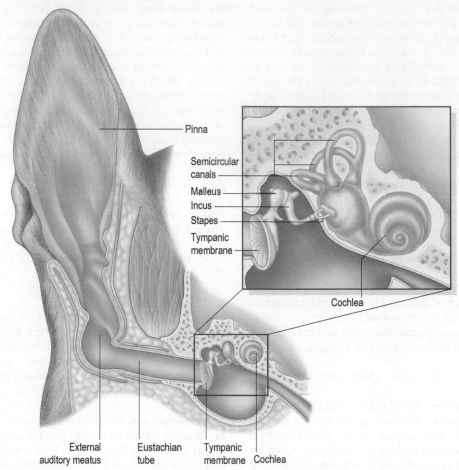

Pinna

Semicircular canals

Malleus

Incus

Stapes

Tympanic membrane

Cochlea

External auditory meatus

Eustachian tube

Tympanic membrane

Cochlea

Fig. 6.22 The structure of the ear

The membranous labyrinth consists of the:
1. Vestibular apparatus
2. Cochlea.
1. Vestibular apparatus – the vestibule gives rise to three semi-circular canals which lie in vertical, horizontal and transverse directions perpendicular to each other. They are concerned with balance and the detection of movement. The vestibule also contains the utricle and the saccule, whose walls contain a specialised area of sensory receptor cells known as a macula. Axon fibres pass from the macula into the vestibulocochlear or auditory nerve (VIII), serving as part of the sensory input for balance.

Close to one end of each semicircular canal is a dilated area called the ampulla. In each ampulla there is a ridge called a sensory crista containing sensory receptors (hair cells) which move back and forth influenced by the movement of the head and thus the endolymph in the canals. The hair cells send nerve impulses along the vestibulocochlear nerve to the brain to record movement of the head in all directions.

2. Cochlea – this takes a spiral form similar to a snail shell with a canal divided into channels within which is the organ of Corti. This contains receptor hair cells, which respond to movement of the endolymph caused by the vibrations of the sound waves and convert it into sensory receptor information. The resulting nerve impulses are carried by the vestibulocochlear nerve to the brain where they are interpreted as sound.

Endocrine system

The endocrine glands are the sites of synthesis and secretion of proteins called hormones. The hormones are disseminated throughout the body by the blood and act on specific target organs. Hormones coordinate and integrate the functions of all the body systems in conjunction with the nervous system. Both systems provide a means of communication within the body and both involve the transmission of a message, triggered by a stimulus to produce a response. The difference between the two systems concerns the nature of the message – in the endocrine system the message takes the form of a chemical substance conveyed through the blood system while in the nervous system it is a rapid nerve impulse.

Endocrine glands are ductless and are composed of secretory cells of epithelial origin supported by connective tissue that is rich in blood and lymphatic capillaries. The secretory cells discharge hormones into the interstitial spaces from which they are rapidly absorbed into the circulatory system.

Some endocrine glands form organs, e.g. pituitary, thyroid, parathyroid, adrenal, while others are associated with exocrine glands, e.g. pancreas. Some form a part of complex organs, e.g. kidney, testis and ovary.

For the full list of endocrine glands see Table 6.3, but some of the more significant endocrine glands are as follows.

TABLE 6.3	The endocrine glands and their hormones	
Gland	**Hormone**	**Action**
THYROID	Thyroxine	Increases metabolic rate
	Calcitonin	Regulates calcium levels
PARATHYROID	Parathormone (parathyroid hormone)	Regulates calcium and phosphorus levels
ADRENAL CORTEX	Glucocorticoids	Protein and carbohydrate metabolism and anti-inflammatory
	Mineralocorticoids	Stress resistance, potassium and sodium levels
	Gonadocorticoids	Male/female sex hormones
ADRENAL MEDULLA	Epinephrine (adrenaline)	Sympathetic nervous system
	Norepinephrine (noradrenaline)	Sympathetic nervous system
ANTERIOR PITUITARY	Growth hormone	Stimulates growth
POSTERIOR PITUITARY	Thyroid-stimulating hormone (TSH)	Stimulates thyroid gland activity
	Adrenocorticotrophic hormone (ACTH)	Stimulates adrenal cortex
	Follicle-stimulating hormone (FSH)	Stimulates growth of ovarian follicle
	Luteinizing hormone (LH)	Ovulation and development of the corpus luteum
	Interstitial cell-stimulating hormone (ICSH)	Stimulates interstitial cells of the testis
	Prolactin	Stimulates formation of milk
	Oxytocin	Milk 'let down'; uterine contraction in parturition
	Antidiuretic hormone (ADH)	Reabsorption of water from renal collecting ducts
PANCREAS	Insulin	Decreases blood glucose
	Glucagon	Increases blood glucose
	Somatostatin	Smoothes out blood glucose fluctuations
OVARY	Oestrogen	Female sex characteristics and oestrus behaviour
	Progesterone	Prepares uterus and uterine horns; maintains the pregnancy
TESTIS	Testosterone	Male sex characteristics; spermatogenesis
PINEAL	Melatonin	Coordinating circadian and diurnal rhythms

ADRENAL GLAND

This can be considered to be two separate glands wrapped around each other:

- The **medulla** – produces the hormones norepinephrine (noradrenalin) and epinephrine (adrenalin). Their effects on body organs are identical to those produced by the stimulation of the sympathetic nervous system, i.e. they raise heart rate and systolic blood pressure and cause peripheral vasoconstriction in preparation for the 'fear, flight or fight' response. Norepinephrine is the more potent hypertensive agent.

Adrenaline also decreases gut motility and increases:

- Cardiac output
- Glycogen breakdown in liver and muscle
- Fatty acid release
- Skeletal muscle tone.

The action of epinephrine and norepinephrine is short-lived as they are rapidly inactivated. Both are regarded as 'emergency hormones' and the adrenal medulla is not essential to life.

- The **cortex** – surrounds the medulla and consists of three concentric layers each of which secretes a different group of steroid hormones belonging to two groups:
  1) **Corticosteroids** – these are essential for life. Individual corticosteroids vary in their ability to produce the full glucocorticoid or mineralocorticoid effects (see Table 6.3). In the dog and the cat the two most important corticosteroids are cortisol, which has mainly glucocorticoid effects, and aldosterone, which has primarily mineralocorticoid effects.
  2) **Adrenal sex hormones**, i.e. androgens, oestrogens and probably progestagens. These are produced in small quantities and may be called gonadocorticoids.

Adrenocorticotrophic hormone (ACTH), secreted by the anterior pituitary gland, controls the formation of cortisol and androgens but has little effect on the formation of aldosterone, which is controlled by the renin–angiotensin pathway in the kidney.

THYROID GLAND

This lies as paired bilateral glands below the larynx near to the upper trachea. It produces:

- **Tri-iodothyronine (T_3) and thyroxine (T_4)**, together known as thyroid hormone and based on iodine. They are vital for growth and the regulation of the metabolism. Secretion of these hormones is regulated by thyroid-stimulating hormone (TSH), secreted by the anterior pituitary (see Table 6.3).
- **Thyrocalcitonin or calcitonin** regulates blood calcium levels in conjunction with parathormone. Calcitonin lowers blood calcium levels by inhibiting the rate of decalcification of bone by osteoclasts and by stimulating bone growth or osteoblast activity.

PANCREAS

This is a mixed gland lying within the loop of the duodenum (see Digestive system and Fig. 6.31). Hormones are secreted by discrete areas of endocrine tissue known as the islets of Langerhans lying within the exocrine tissue. The islets consist of three types of cell, each secreting a different hormone:

- α cells secrete glucagon, which increases blood glucose levels by breaking down stores of glycogen in the liver by a process of glycogenolysis.

- β cells secrete insulin, which reduces blood glucose levels by enabling glucose to pass into the cells where it is used as a vital source of energy, in the presence of adequate potassium levels. Excess glucose is stored as glycogen in the liver by a process of glycogenesis.
- δ cells secrete somatostatin, which smoothes out the daily fluctuations in blood glucose levels.

Cardiovascular system

The cardiovascular system consists of four separate components:
- Blood
- The heart
- The circulatory system
- The lymphatic system.

BLOOD

Blood is a highly specialised connective tissue consisting of several types of cell suspended in a fluid medium called plasma. Blood performs a wide range of functions:

1. **Transportation** – blood is responsible for carrying the following vital components around the body:
   - Oxygen – carried by haemoglobin in the red blood cells
   - Carbon dioxide – formed by the tissues and carried in solution in the plasma to the lungs
   - Nutrients – products of digestion carried from the small intestine to the liver and other tissues
   - Waste products – resulting from metabolism and transported to the point of excretion, e.g. kidney and liver
   - Hormones and enzymes – carried to their target organs.
2. **Homoeostasis** – regulation of the systems responsible for maintaining the internal equilibrium of the body:
   - Defence against disease – white blood cells and immunoglobulins protect against invasion by antigens
   - Body temperature – blood conducts heat around the body to where it is needed
   - Acid–base balance – presence of buffers in the blood maintain pH at approximately 7.4
   - Osmotic concentration and volume of body fluids – presence of plasma proteins and electrolytes controls fluid flow between compartments and maintains blood volume and pressure
   - Blood clotting – cascade mechanism controls blood loss from injuries and prevents entry of infection.

Composition of blood

Blood is a connective tissue that circulates around the body in a continuous system of blood vessels. It makes up about 7% of the body weight and has a pH of 7.35–7.45. Plasma makes up about 60% of the volume and the cells and other materials in transit make up the remaining 40%.

Plasma. Plasma is an aqueous solution containing a variety of dissolved substances, e.g. oxygen, hormones and nutrients, which are transported from one part of the body to another and constantly exchanged with the interstitial fluid of the tissues.
Plasma consists of:
- Water
- Electrolytes, e.g. sodium, chloride, potassium
- Plasma proteins, e.g. albumin, globulin, fibrinogen, prothrombin

- Nutrients, e.g. amino acids, fatty acids, glucose
- Gases, e.g. oxygen, carbon dioxide
- Waste products, e.g. urea, creatinine
- Hormones, e.g. adrenaline, insulin, thyroxine, oestrogens
- Enzymes, e.g. alanine aminotransferase (ALT), amylase, lipase
- Antibodies.

Plasma proteins. Plasma proteins are large molecules in the blood, which exert a colloidal osmotic pressure within the circulation to help regulate the exchange of fluid between the plasma and the extracellular fluid. The main plasma proteins are:
- Albumin – binds with plasma calcium, which is required for clotting, bone formation and restructuring. It maintains blood pressure by keeping fluid within the plasma by osmosis (the colloid osmotic pressure [COP]) – its large molecular size means that under normal circumstances it cannot pass between the endothelial cells of the blood capillaries into the extracellular fluid. Albumin can also become glycosylated when blood glucose levels are high – this molecule is called fructosamine
- Globulin – binds with thyroxine and bilirubin, iron, cholesterol and vitamins A, D and K, and is involved in defence against infection. They also maintain blood pressure
- Fibrinogen and prothrombin – are both involved in the clotting mechanism. Fibrinogen is converted to fibrin and used in the formation of a clot. The remaining fluid seen at the site of an injury is serum. Serum is thus plasma without fibrinogen/fibrin.

Blood cells. Haemopoiesis is the process by which mature blood cells develop from precursor or stem cells. Production takes place in the liver and spleen of the embryo and the bone marrow, mainly of the pelvis, ribs, long bones and lymph nodes in the neonate and adult animal. The exception is the lymphocyte, which is formed in lymphoid tissues in the lymph nodes and the spleen. Erythrocytes and platelets function entirely within blood vessels, while the leucocytes are able to function outside the blood vessels in the interstitial tissue spaces. They are found in circulating blood only in transit between their various sites of activity.

Red blood cells – erythrocytes – are produced in the red or active bone marrow. They are non-nucleated biconcave discs filled with the protein haemoglobin and are about 7 μm in diameter once mature – those of the cat are slightly smaller than those of the dog (Fig. 6.23). Their main function is to carry oxygen, as oxyhaemoglobin, from the lungs to the tissues.

Erythropoiesis – the production of erythrocytes – takes about 1 week and is controlled by the hormone erythropoietin, secreted by the kidney and regulated by the amount of oxygen reaching the tissues. Haemoglobin is synthesised from iron, folic acid and vitamin B_{12}. Immature erythrocytes are known as reticulocytes and their presence in the blood is an indication of red cell regeneration – a significant factor in some types of anaemia. Cat erythrocytes live for 58–68 days while those of the dog live for 107–120 days.

White blood cells – leucocytes – are fewer in number and can be divided into two groups:

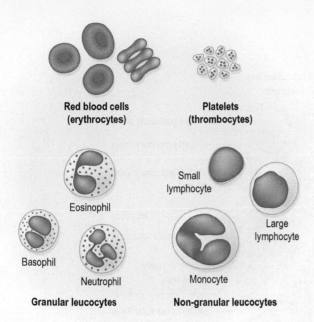

Red blood cells (erythrocytes)

Platelets (thrombocytes)

Small lymphocyte

Eosinophil

Large lymphocyte

Basophil

Neutrophil

Monocyte

Granular leucocytes

Non-granular leucocytes

White blood cells (leucocytes)

Fig. 6.23   Blood cells

1. Granulocytes – have granular cytoplasm and a multilobed nucleus. Also known as polymorphonuclear leucocytes (see Fig. 6.23). They are:
   - Neutrophils – phagocytic cells which increase rapidly as juvenile or band cells in acute infections described as a neutrophilia. The granules stain purple.
   - Eosinophils – involved in the inflammatory reaction to tissue damage and in allergies. Also seen where there is a large parasite burden. The granules which are released from the cytoplasm, deactivating histamine and heparin, take up acid dye and stain red.
   - Basophils – granules produce heparin and histamine, take up alkaline dyes and stain blue.
2. Agranulocytes – have a clear cytoplasm:
   - Lymphocytes – round nucleus that almost fills the cells (see Fig. 6.23). They support the immune system and are classified as B lymphocytes and T lymphocytes depending on their origin.
   - Monocytes – are the largest of the white cells and their function is phagocytosis. They have a horseshoe-shaped nucleus and are highly motile cells, migrating into connective tissues, where they are termed histiocytes or macrophages. Macrophages play an important role in the immune defence system. Monocytes appear to have little function in circulating blood and are seen in chronic conditions, assisting in the removal of debris arising from normal turnover of cells within the tissues.

Thrombocytes or platelets – small, non-nucleated cells formed in the bone marrow by break-up of huge megakaryocyte cells. They participate in blood clotting in two main ways:
   - They clump together to plug small defects in the walls of small blood vessels.
   - In the presence of damaged vessels they release a substance called serotonin that reduces blood flow by constriction of the area.

THE HEART

The heart is a muscular pump located in the thorax and held within the mediastinum, slightly to the left of the midline and covered in a double layer of serous membrane known as the pericardium. Between the two layers is the small pericardial cavity.

The heart, whose sole function is to pump blood around the circulatory system, is a hollow, muscular, cone-shaped organ divided into four chambers – the right and left atria and the right and left ventricles (Fig. 6.24). Its size varies depending on the size of animal, and it lies between the third and sixth rib. The right side of the heart receives deoxygenated blood from the systemic veins, and the left side of the heart receives oxygenated blood from the lungs via the pulmonary circulation.

The heart wall consists of three layers:
- Endocardium – a smooth inner layer of epithelium involved in the formation of valves and continuous with the endothelium of the blood vessels
- Myocardium – the cardiac muscle layer; the left ventricle muscle is three times thicker than the right. Blood supply to this muscle is through the coronary vessels
- Epicardium or serous pericardium – the outer layer of the heart covering the muscle wall. It produces serous fluid, which lies within the pericardial cavity and lubricates the movements of the heart.

Heart valves

These ensure that the flow of blood through the heart goes in one direction only (see Fig. 6.24). There are two sets of valves:
1. Left side
   - Left atrioventricular valve, also known as the bicuspid or mitral valve, lying between the left atrium and ventricle. It has two cusps or flaps.
   - Aortic valve, which lies at the base of the aorta. This is described as being a semilunar valve because of the shape of its three cusps.
2. Right side
   - Right atrioventricular valve also known as the tricuspid valve, lying between the right atrium and ventricle. It has three cusps.
   - Pulmonary valve lies at the base of the pulmonary artery. This is also a semilunar valve and has three cusps.

Each cusp of the right and left atrioventricular valves has several tendinous attachments or chordae tendinae running from their margin to the papillary muscles on the ventricular surface of the heart. They prevent the valves everting as blood is forced out during the strong ventricular contractions.

Nervous control of the heart

Cardiac muscle has an inherent ability to contract at a set rate and contraction is coordinated by a conduction system (Fig. 6.25), which consists of:
- Sinoatrial node (SA node) – situated in the wall of the right atrium. This initiates each heartbeat and is known as the pacemaker.
- Atrioventricular node (AV node) – lies at the top of the interventricular septum between the right and left sides of the heart.

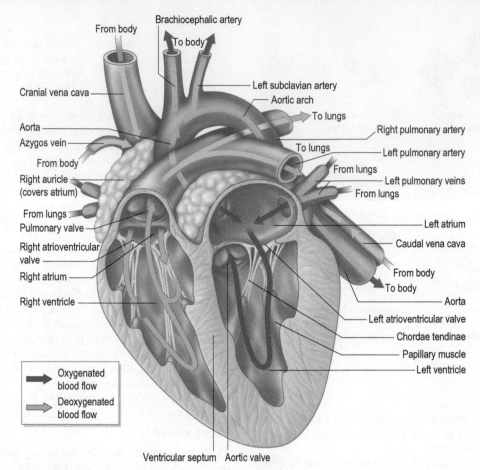

Fig. 6.24   Structure of the heart

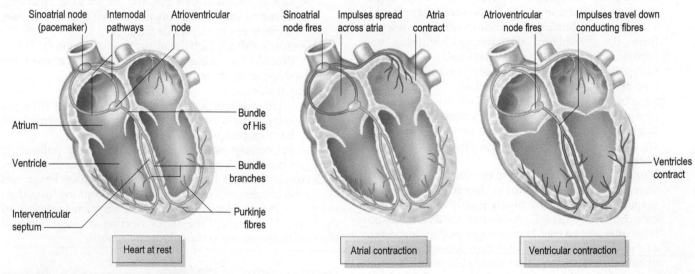

Fig. 6.25   Conduction system of the heart

- Bundle of His – specialised cells within the interventricular septum.
- Purkinje fibres – specialised nerve cells within the walls of the ventricles.

Nerve impulses, initiated by the SA node, travel across the atrial walls and stimulate the AV node. They then continue down the bundle of His to the Purkinje fibres at the apex of the ventricles. As a result of this electrical wave, the atria contract (atrial systole), forcing blood into the ventricles. The atria relax (atrial diastole) and the ventricles then contract (ventricular systole) and blood is forced upwards, closing the AV valves but opening the aortic and pulmonary valves and moving blood from the ventricles into the systemic and pulmonary circulations. The ventricles then relax (ventricular diastole) and the semilunar valves close.

In order to meet the changing demands of the body, the heart rate must be able to alter. This is done by nerves of the autonomic nervous system, which act on the SA node – the sympathetic branch of the autonomic nervous system increases the heart rate, while the parasympathetic branch (the vagus nerve) slows the heart rate.

Pulse rate – the number of heartbeats per minute

The pulse is produced by the heart pumping blood into the aorta, increasing and decreasing the expansion of the arterial vessel wall with each heartbeat. The pulse is measured by palpation of a superficial vessel as it passes over a bone. The pulse quality, i.e. its rate, rhythm and character, is a reflection of the function of the heart. Normal sites for measuring the peripheral pulse in the dog and cat are the femoral, brachial, lingual and coccygeal arteries.

CIRCULATORY SYSTEM

This consists of a continuous series of blood vessels that transport the blood pumped by the heart around the body. Figure 6.26 shows the route taken by the blood around the body.

Blood vessels

Table 6.4 compares the characteristics of the different types of blood vessels:

- Arteries – carry blood *away* from the heart, except for the pulmonary artery, which carries blood towards the heart. Arteries carry oxygenated blood.
- Veins – carry blood *towards* the heart, except for the pulmonary vein, which carries blood away from the heart. Veins carry deoxygenated blood.
- Capillaries – thin-walled vessels that link arteries to veins and are the site of gaseous and nutrient exchange within the tissues.

Lymphatic system

The lymphatic system is closely linked to the circulation and is a means of returning lymph or excess interstitial tissue fluid back to the circulation via a system of lymphatic vessels and ducts.

The functions of the lymphatic system are:

- To return excess tissue fluid or lymph to the circulation
- To produce lymphocytes to fight infection
- To transport fatty acid molecules, produced during digestion, as chyle, which is collected by the lacteals; these are a form of lymphatic capillary found within the finger-like villi of the small intestine and they drain the chyle into the cisterna chyli in the dorsal abdomen
- To act as a filter for lymph.

Formation of lymph takes place at the arterial end of blood capillaries, where the hydrostatic pressure exceeds the colloidal osmotic pressure exerted by plasma proteins. Fluids and electrolytes pass out of the blood capillaries into the extracellular spaces with some plasma proteins, which leak through the endothelial wall. At the venous end of the blood capillaries the pressure relationships are reversed and fluid is drawn back into the blood vascular system. In this way about 2% of plasma passing through the capillary bed is exchanged with the extracellular tissue fluid. The rate of tissue fluid formation

at the arterial end of capillaries generally exceeds the reuptake of fluid at the venous end, leaving quantities in the interstitial spaces. The excess fluid becomes known as lymph once it drains into the system of lymphatic capillaries, which converge to form progressively larger-diameter lymphatic veins or vessels. Movement of lymph along the vessels relies on the surrounding tissues, particularly skeletal muscles, squeezing the fluid past non-return valves in the walls.

Lymph re-enters the venous circulation via the right atrium of the heart via a single duct on each side of the body:

- The right lymphatic duct and the right and left tracheal ducts drain lymph from the right forelimb and from the head and neck.
- The thoracic duct drains lymph from the whole of the rest of the body. The contents of the cisterna chyli in the abdominal cavity also empty into the thoracic duct.

Lymph nodes. Along the route of the regional lymphatic vessels are lymph nodes from which lymphocytes and antibodies enter the general circulation. Lymph nodes are small kidney-bean-shaped organs whose function is to filter lymph or bacteria or other particulate matter by the phagocytic activity of macrophages and to produce and store the T and B lymphocytes. Lymph passes through one or more nodes before re-entering the circulation.

A lymph node is an encapsulated mass of lymphoid tissue supported by dense connective tissue trabeculae between which are channels containing the flowing lymph (Fig. 6.27). Each node is supplied by many afferent lymphatic vessels and drained by a single efferent vessel, which leaves at the hilus of the node. As lymph nodes are responsible for draining lymph from specific regions of the body, they monitor the health status of that area. All areas of the body have their own nodes, e.g. bronchial or mesenteric lymph nodes, but some nodes are quite superficial and can be palpated, particularly if they become enlarged or diseased (Fig. 6.28).

Lymphoid tissue is also found in other sites:

- Spleen – located in the left cranial abdomen, it is highly vascular and acts both as a lymph node and a blood reservoir
- Tonsils – three pairs located within the pharyngeal area and referred to as the palatine, lingual and pharyngeal tonsils
- Thymus – located in the anterior part of the thoracic cavity, its role is vital to the developing immune system in young animals.

Respiratory system

Respiration describes two interrelated processes:

- Cellular respiration – the process in which cells derive energy from the breakdown of organic molecules in the presence of oxygen
- Mechanical respiration – the process by which oxygen required for cellular respiration is absorbed from the atmosphere into the blood and the process by which carbon dioxide produced by the cells during metabolism is excreted into the atmosphere.

It is mechanical respiration that occurs in the respiratory system.

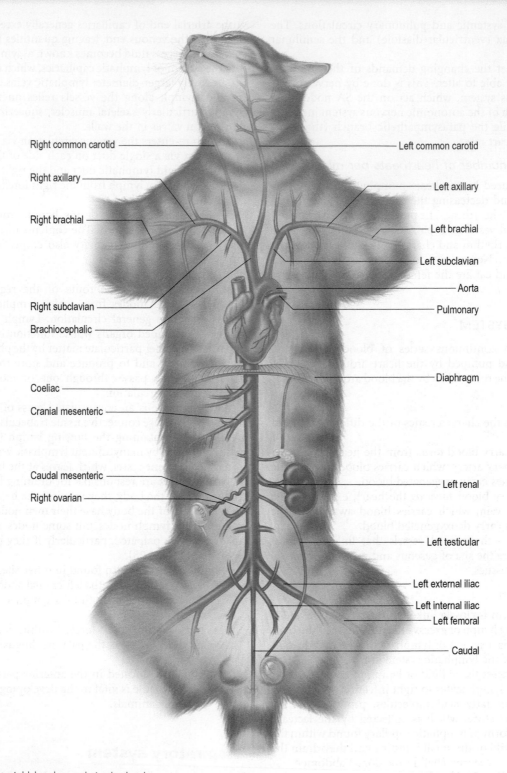

Fig. 6.26 Major arterial blood vessels in the body

The respiratory system has two functional components:

- A conducting system or the respiratory tract, for the transport of inspired and expired gases between the atmosphere and the circulatory system
- An interface for the passive exchange of gases between the atmosphere and the blood – the pulmonary membrane.

NASAL CAVITY

The entrance to the cavity is via the nostrils or external nares and the exit is via the internal nares or the opening to the pharynx. The nasal cavity is divided into left and right chambers separated by a septum and filled by coiled turbinate bones. These are covered with ciliated mucous membrane to filter out

TABLE 6.4	Characteristics of the different types of blood vessels		
Artery	**Capillary**		**Vein**
Transport blood away from the heart	Link arteries to veins. Site of exchange of materials between blood and tissues		Transport blood towards the heart
Tunica media thick and composed of elastic, muscular tissue	No tunica media. Only tissue present is squamous endothelium. No elastic fibres		Tunica media relatively thin and only slightly muscular. Few elastic fibres
No semi-lunar valves	No semi-lunar valves		Semi-lunar valves at intervals along the length to prevent backflow of blood
Pressure of blood is high and pulsatile	Pressure of blood falling and non-pulsatile		Pressure of blood low and non-pulsatile
Blood flow rapid	Blood flow slowing		Blood flow slow
Low blood volume	High blood volume		Increasing blood volume
Blood oxygenated except in pulmonary artery	Mixed oxygenated and deoxygenated blood		Blood deoxygenated except in pulmonary vein

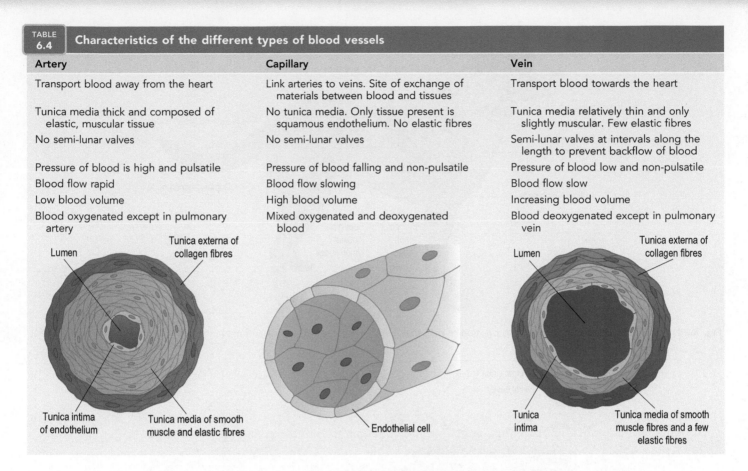

PHARYNX

The pharynx is divided by the soft palate into the nasopharynx and the oropharynx. It has six openings into it: i.e. from the nasal chambers, the mouth, the Eustachian tube from the middle ear on each side, the oesophagus and the larynx. It acts as a crossover point between the digestive and respiratory tracts (Fig. 6.29).

LARYNX

A hollow box-like structure consisting of cartilage, muscle, fibrous tissue and ciliated mucous membranes, its function is to:

- Provide the means of vocalisation
- Control the flow of inspired gases during breathing
- Prevent the entry of solid particles into the trachea.

The larynx consists of a collection of cartilages, the most cranial of which is the epiglottis, which closes the glottis or the opening of the larynx. Inside the larynx, paired vocal folds form a narrow passageway for air flow. Movement of the cartilages controls the size of the glottis and regulates the flow of air through it. During normal breathing the larynx lies in its resting position with the epiglottis lying above the soft palate, making a continuous opening for the air to pass through and the glottis is open (see Fig. 6.33). During swallowing the epiglottis lies over the glottis, closing it and preventing the passage of food down the trachea.

TRACHEA

The trachea is a non-collapsible tube extending from the larynx through the thoracic inlet to the bifurcation or point of division

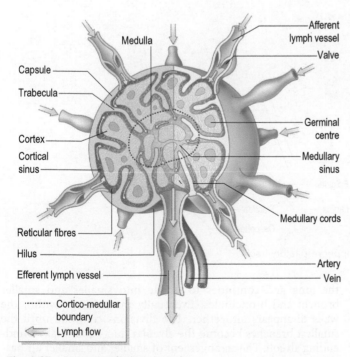

Fig. 6.27 Structure of a lymph node

dust and other foreign matter and it also enables the air to be moistened and warmed prior to entry into the lower tract. Leading from each chamber are the air-filled frontal and maxillary sinuses which assist in this function and reduce the weight of the skull.

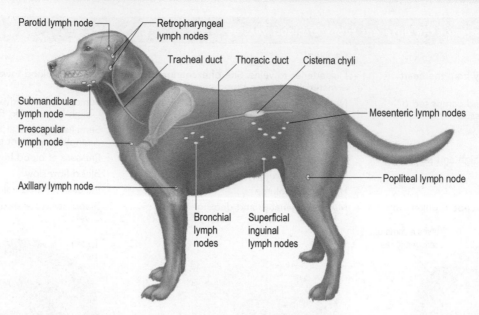

Fig. 6.28 Lateral view of a dog showing the position of palpable lymph nodes. NB. Bronchial and mesenteric lymph nodes are not palpable.

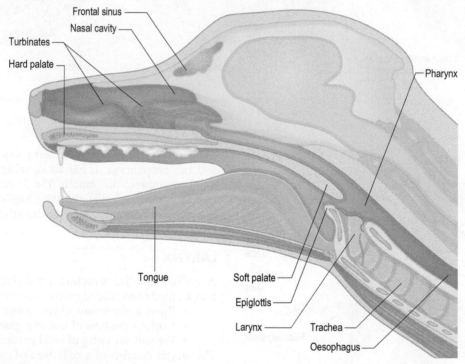

Fig. 6.29 Longitudinal section through the head of a dog to show the upper respiratory tract

into the left and right bronchi. It is made up of a series of incomplete C-shaped rings of hyaline cartilage separated by fibrous connective tissue and smooth muscle and lined with ciliated epithelium. The open area of each ring is on the dorsal aspect, which enables the oesophagus, lying close to it, to expand without hindrance when a bolus of food passes through.

BRONCHI, BRONCHIOLES AND ALVEOLAR DUCTS

The bronchi are similar in structure but the cartilage rings are complete. Each bronchus enters the lung tissue at the root of

the lung and continues to divide into smaller and smaller bronchi and bronchioles. Eventually the cartilage within the walls disappears altogether. The divisions continue until the smallest branches become the alveolar ducts and finally blind-ending alveoli. The arrangement of smaller and smaller air passages is referred to as the bronchial tree.

The lining epithelium of the tract is a ciliated mucous membrane. The cilia and the mucus trap particles and pass them up to the pharynx where they are either coughed out or swallowed. Deeper into the bronchial tree the alveolar ducts and alveoli are lined by a thin simple squamous epithelium known as the pulmonary membrane – it is across this that gaseous exchange takes place.

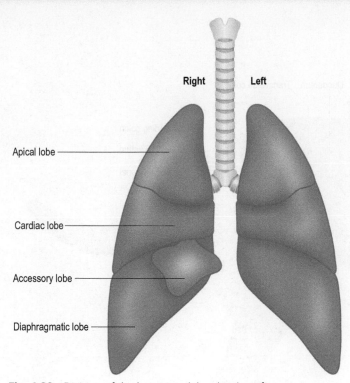

Right · Left

Apical lobe

Cardiac lobe

Accessory lobe

Diaphragmatic lobe

Fig. 6.30 Division of the lungs into lobes by deep fissures

LUNGS

The right and left lungs are essentially spongy organs that lie in the thorax on either side of the mediastinum (Fig. 6.30). They are divided into lobes – the right side is larger than the left. The lung tissue is covered by the pulmonary pleura and enclosed within the pleural cavity, in which there is nothing but a vacuum and a little serous fluid. These are essential to provide smooth movement between the lungs and thoracic wall during breathing and to bring about inflation of the lungs.

THE MECHANICS OF BREATHING

Lung tissue contains no muscle, so it cannot expand on its own. It is, however, very elastic and will return to its collapsed state when there is nothing to expand it. Breathing occurs in two phases:

- **Inspiration** – the cavity volume increases by the flattening of the diaphragm (a dome-shaped muscular partition separating the thoracic and abdominal cavities) and the lifting of the ribs by contraction of the external intercostal muscles. The lungs increase in size as they are sucked outwards by the vacuum in the pleural cavity. The pressure in the lungs reduces and air passes from the outside down into the lungs, which fill the pleural cavity.
- **Expiration** – the diaphragm relaxes and returns to its domed position and the ribs return to their natural position, decreasing the volume of the cavity and increasing the pressure of the air in the lungs. Air is forced up the trachea and out of the body.

Control of respiration

Respiratory centres in the pons and medulla oblongata of the hindbrain control:

- Inspiration via the inspiratory centre
- Expiration via the pneumotaxic and apneustic centres
- Hering–Breuer reflex – prevention of overinflation of the lungs by stretch receptors in the bronchiole walls. When stretched by air in the bronchioles, these receptors provide information to the hindbrain and stimulate expiration
- Blood pH – chemoreceptors in the aortic and carotid artery walls and within the medulla oblongata receive information on the changing levels of carbon dioxide and oxygen in the blood which affect the pH. They stimulate respiration to restore the correct pH by expelling the carbon dioxide.

Respiratory terminology

- External respiration – transfer of gases between the external environment and the circulation
- Internal or tissue respiration – transfer of oxygen from the blood to the tissues and carbon dioxide from the tissues to the blood
- Tidal volume – the amount of air breathed in and out in one respiration
- Residual volume – the air left in the lungs following a forced exhalation
- Functional residual volume or capacity – the amount of air left in the lungs after normal exhalation
- Total lung capacity – the total amount of air in the lungs
- Vital capacity – the greatest volume of air that can be made to pass out of lungs following forced exhalation
- Anatomical dead space – the volume of air in the trachea, bronchi and bronchioles that never reaches the alveoli.

Digestive system

The digestive or gastrointestinal tract is a muscular tube lined by a mucous membrane which runs from the mouth to the anus. It comprises a variety of structures, reflecting the many functions of the system that work together to bring about the digestion of food in order to provide a source of energy to the body tissues (Fig. 6.31).

ORAL CAVITY

Forms the beginning of the tract and consists of the tongue, teeth, cheeks and lips. Its boundaries are (Fig. 6.32):

- Laterally, the cheeks and teeth. Each cheek holds a pad of fat, the buccal pad, which during eating prevent the cheeks from being bitten
- Dorsally, the palate, which is divided into the hard and soft palates – the hard palate is a bony structure covered with mucous membrane, parts of which are set out in thickened ridges on its surface. The soft palate is a flap of tissue dividing the pharynx into the nasopharynx and oropahrynx
- Ventrally, the tongue and sublingual muscles, which anchor the tongue, enabling it to assist with prehension, swallowing of food and water, grooming and licking
- Cranially, the lips and teeth.

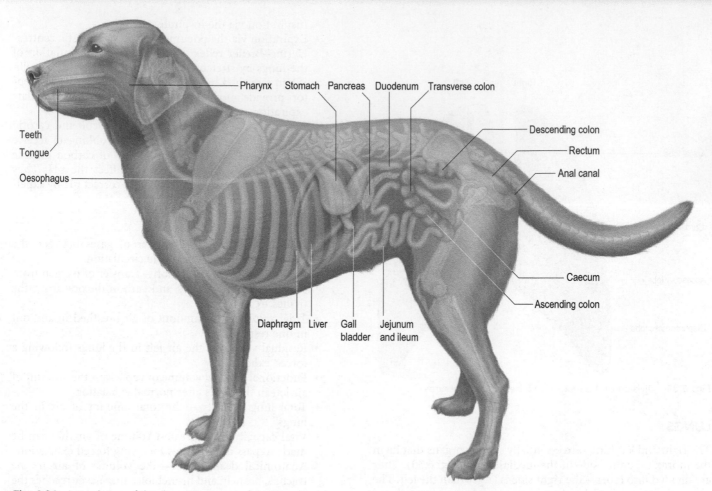

Fig. 6.31   Lateral view of the digestive system of the dog

SALIVARY GLANDS

Paired primary salivary glands include:
- Zygomatic or dorsal buccal
- Sublingual
- Mandibular.

Minor glands also secrete saliva and include the labial, lingual and palatine glands. These glands all have ducts which pass saliva directly into the mouth when stimulated by the smell, sight or thought of food. Saliva is used for moistening food in the mouth and for the formation of a bolus which is swallowed and passed down the oesophagus. In some species, enzymatic digestion of food occurs during mastication as amylase (an enzyme that breaks down starches) is contained within the saliva.

PHARYNX

The pharynx is a short muscular tube that acts as a crossover between the digestive and respiratory tracts and serves as a common passageway for air and for food. When food enters the pharynx, all other openings, including the larynx, are blocked in order to direct the food to the oesophagus (Fig. 6.33). The tongue presses against the hard palate to close the oral cavity and the food bolus passes through the pharynx. The larynx, attached to the hyoid apparatus, then moves backwards, and the epiglottis falls forward, leaving the larynx open again when swallowing or deglutition is complete. The bolus of food

enters the oesophagus and moves downwards by peristalsis into the stomach.

OESOPHAGUS

A hollow muscular tube which is capable of considerable distension during the passage of a food bolus. It has a good supply of nerves, blood vessels and mucous glands that lubricate the inner lining during the passage of food material by peristalsis. It extends from the pharynx through the thorax and diaphragm via the oesophageal hiatus (a hole in the diaphragm through which the oesophagus and the vagus nerve pass) to the stomach.

STOMACH

Lies within the abdomen on the left side of the cavity. It is divided into sections:
- Cardia – area adjacent to the cardiac sphincter, a poorly defined ring of muscle at the junction with the oesophagus which controls the passage of food into the stomach
- Fundus – major area of digestive glands, which secrete gastric juices and some protective mucus
- Body – or corpus, which is a continuation of the fundus
- Pylorus – a narrowing of the body in which mucus and the hormone gastrin are secreted. It joins the duodenum at its narrowest point as the pyloric sphincter and

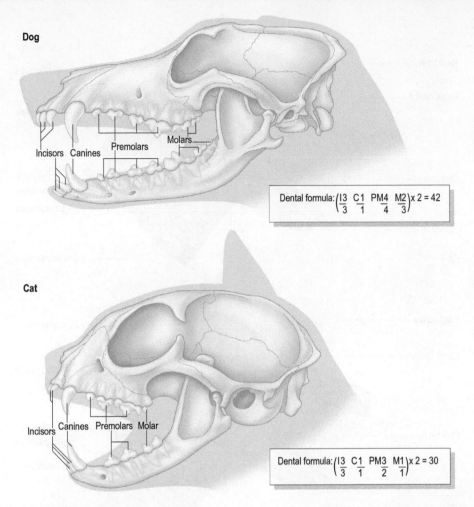

Dog

Incisors Canines Premolars Molars

Dental formula: $\left(\dfrac{I3}{3}\ \dfrac{C1}{1}\ \dfrac{PM4}{4}\ \dfrac{M2}{3}\right) \times 2 = 42$

Cat

Incisors Canines Premolars Molar

Dental formula: $\left(\dfrac{I3}{3}\ \dfrac{C1}{1}\ \dfrac{PM3}{2}\ \dfrac{M1}{1}\right) \times 2 = 30$

Fig. 6.32 Skull of dog and cat to show the dentition

controls the passage of liquid, partially digested food or chyme, which is squirted into the duodenum.

The stomach is composed of an inner mucous membrane supported on a submucosal layer and known as the gastric mucosa. It is arranged in numerous folds or rugae, which become flattened when the stomach is distended with food. Gastric pits or glands within the gastric mucosa produce hydrochloric acid, mucus and the enzyme pepsin. The lining of the stomach is protected from autodigestion by a thick surface covering of mucus. The middle layers of the stomach consist of smooth muscle, which is responsible for the mixing of food. The outermost layer is a layer of mesentery or visceral peritoneum forming the omentum, which suspends the stomach from the dorsal body wall.

The function of the stomach is to store and mix food with the gastric digestive enzymes. The process of digestion in the stomach varies in time, dependent on the nutrient constituents of the diet. Digestion requires the muscular contractions of the stomach wall and results in the formation of chyme, which passes into the duodenum.

Within the lining of the stomach wall are gastric pits that secrete gastric juices in response to the hormone gastrin, which is secreted in response to the presence of food passing through the cardiac sphincter. The gastric pits are made up of:

- Goblet cells in the fundus and body of the stomach which secrete mucus which lubricates the passage of food and protects against autodigestion

- Parietal or oxyntic cells distributed in the gastric pits of the fundus and secrete hydrochloric acid. This protects the gastrointestinal tract from harmful bacteria by creating an environment in which they cannot survive and it also denatures protein prior to its digestion
- Chief cells secrete pepsinogen and are clustered at the base of the gastric pits. Pepsinogen is converted into the active enzyme pepsin in the presence of hydrochloric acid and it digests protein.

SMALL INTESTINE

Acidic chyme is received from the stomach (see Fig. 6.31) via the pyloric sphincter, and the addition of bicarbonate ions from the pancreas neutralise the acidity. Here the process of digestion is completed and the digested food products are absorbed. Effective absorption depends on a large surface area and this is achieved by the development of finger-like villi within the intestinal mucosa. These are covered by a layer of epithelium within which lie the digestive glands (Fig. 6.34). The small intestine is divided into three parts:

- Duodenum – lies on the right side of the abdomen, and within its U-shaped loop lies the pancreas. It is held in position by part of the visceral peritoneum known as the mesoduodenum. The duodenal mucosa has characteristic villi and Brunner's glands, which open between

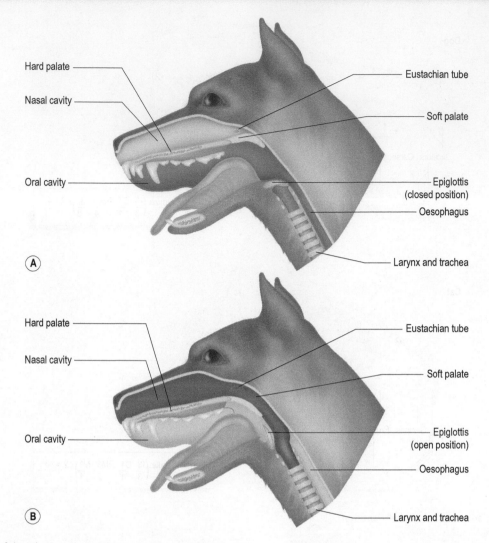

Fig. 6.33 Function of the pharynx during (A) swallowing and (B) breathing

the villi. The presence of chyme in the duodenum stimulates the Brunner's glands to secrete a mixture of enzymes known as succus entericus. There are ducts opening into the duodenum from the pancreas and the bile duct.

- Jejunum and ileum – it is difficult to distinguish between these two parts, which form a long mobile tube with no fixed position within the abdominal cavity. It is suspended by the mesojejunum and the mesoileum. The lining epithelium contains villi at the base of which are digestive glands known as the crypts of Lieberkühn. The ileum terminates at the ileocaecal junction.

PANCREAS

Lies within the U of the duodenum and is a mixed gland, i.e. has exocrine and endocrine parts. It is an elongated gland, highly lobulated and covered by a loose connective tissue capsule.

- Endocrine tissue – consists of the islets of Langerhans, which secrete several hormones including insulin (see Endocrine system)
- Exocrine tissue – consists of closely packed secretory cells forming the major part of the gland. Pancreatic

juices drain into a highly branched duct system and then into the main pancreatic duct which joins the common bile duct to drain into the duodenum. The secretions are alkaline because of a high content of bicarbonate ions, which helps to neutralise the acidic chyme. They are also rich in enzymes which digest proteins, carbohydrates and fats. Many are in an inactive form, preventing autodigestion of the pancreas, and must be activated by other enzymes before they can function.

The secretion of pancreatic juices occurs in response to the sight, smell and taste of food. In addition, food entering the duodenum as chyme stimulates secretion via the gastrointestinal hormones cholecystokinin and secretin from the duodenal mucosa.

GALL BLADDER

Lies within the lobes of the liver and stores bile produced by the liver. Bile containing bile salts is required for the emulsification of fat prior to its digestion and is added to the ingesta via the common bile duct in the duodenum.

DIGESTION

Food eaten by an animal consists of a mixture of protein, carbohydrate and fat. These food materials are too large to be

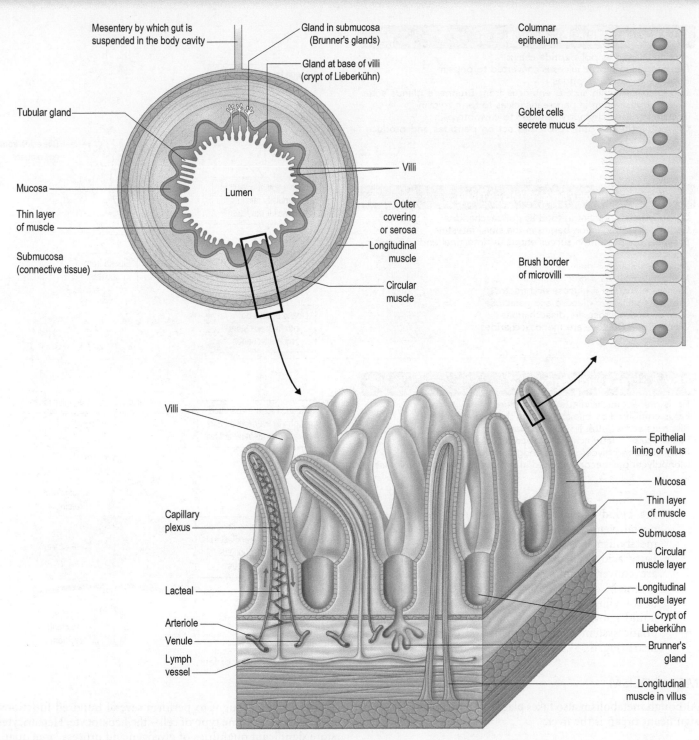

Fig. 6.34 Cross-section through the small intestine showing its structure

absorbed into the blood stream and must undergo the process of enzymic digestion (Boxes 6.2–6.4). A cocktail of digestive enzymes are secreted by the gastric pits, Brunner's glands within the duodenum, the crypts of Lieberkühn in the jejunum and ileum, the pancreas and the gall bladder. Enzymes are proteins that act as catalysts to increase the speed of a chemical reaction. Each enzyme is specifically adapted to act on a particular substrate: e.g. lipases act on lipids; proteases act on proteins. The result of the digestive process is the production of small molecules that can be absorbed into the blood stream and carried

to the tissues and the liver where they are used for the metabolism of the body.

ABSORPTION

The main site for absorption into the blood stream is within the small intestine.

- Amino acids resulting from protein digestion and monosaccharides and disaccharides from carbohydrate digestion pass through the walls of the villi into

BOX 6.2   PROTEIN DIGESTION

Protein in food as polypeptide chains
Pepsinogen in gastric juices is converted to pepsin
Pepsin + protein = peptides
Enterokinase within succus entericus from Brunner's glands activates trypsinogen in pancreatic juices to form trypsin
Trypsin converts chymotrypsinogen to chymotrypsin
Chymotrypsin and other proteases act on peptides and produce amino acids

BOX 6.3   CARBOHYDRATE DIGESTION

Carbohydrates present in food as polysaccharides
Carbohydrate digestion begins in the small intestine
Enzymes are present in succus entericus, intestinal and pancreatic juices
Amylase + starch = maltose
Maltase + maltase = glucose
Sucrose + sucrase = glucose and fructose
Lactose + lactase = glucose and galactose
Sucrose and maltose are disaccharides
Glucose and fructose are monosaccharides

BOX 6.4   FAT DIGESTION

Fat is present in the diet as triglycerides
Fat is emulsified by bile salts within the duodenum
Bile salts activate the lipase enzymes
Fats + lipase = fatty acids and glycerol
Fatty acids and glycerol are monoglycerides
Monoglycerides become coated in protein to form chylomicrons

the blood capillaries and are carried by the hepatic portal vein to the liver, where they are used for metabolism.

- Fatty acids and glycerol resulting from fat digestion are converted into chylomicrons by the addition of a protein coat. These are absorbed through the walls of the villi into the lacteals and are carried as a milky liquid known as chyle to the cisterna chyli (see Lymphatic system) before entering the circulation via the heart (Fig. 6.35).

METABOLISM

Although metabolism also takes place in many tissues, the most significant organ is the liver.

Liver

The liver is the largest organ in the body, occupying approximately 3–4% of total body weight in an average dog or cat. It lies just behind the diaphragm, cranial to the duodenum and the right kidney, resting against the stomach. It is attached to the abdomen wall by a fold of fibrous tissue and fat called the falciform ligament, which is the remains of the umbilical blood vessels in the foetus. Approximately 75% of the liver's blood supply comes from the hepatic portal system, which delivers blood from the small intestine carrying the products of digestion. The remaining 25% of the blood supply comes from the hepatic artery, which delivers oxygenated blood. The hepatic vein carries waste materials, including carbon dioxide, away.

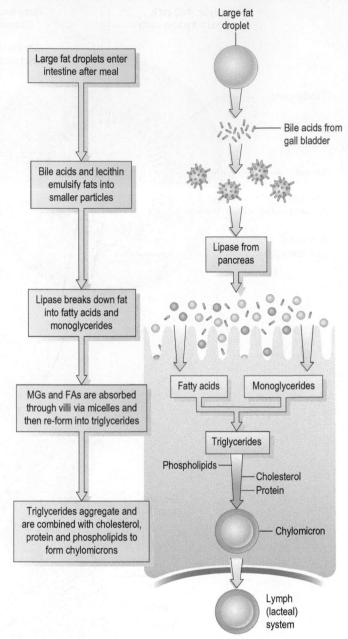

Fig. 6.35   Digestion of fats

The liver is thought to perform several hundred functions, all carried out by one type of cell – the hepatocyte. Hepatocytes store significant quantities of glycogen and process large quantities of lipid. The hepatocytes are arranged in hexagonal lobules with the cells arranged in rows radiating from the centre of each lobule towards the periphery. Running alongside each lobule are branches of the hepatic artery, hepatic portal vein and bile duct (Fig. 6.36).

The hepatic artery and hepatic portal vein may be referred to as the interlobular blood vessels since they are located between adjacent lobules. In the centre of each lobule is a branch of the hepatic vein, referred to as the central or intralobular vein. The vessels are connected with the central vein by a system of capillary-like sinusoids that run parallel to, and come into close contact with, the chains of lower cells. The sinusoids are surrounded by fine channels called canaliculi.

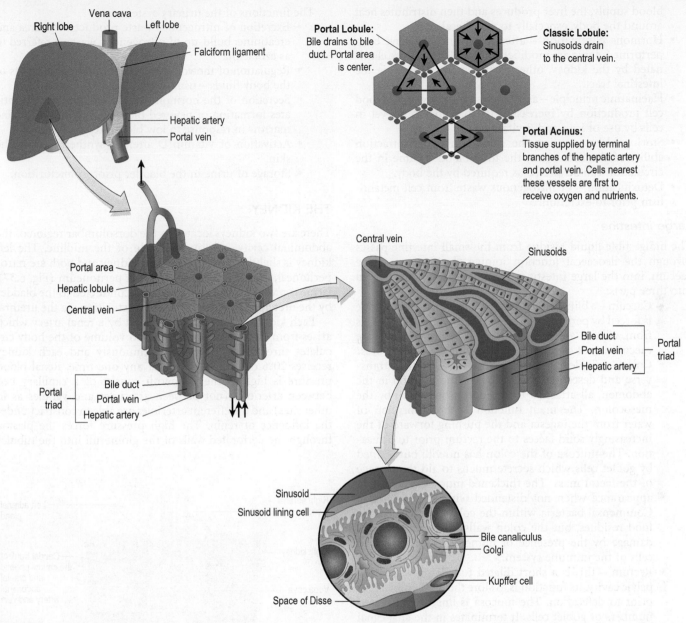

Portal Lobule: Bile drains to bile duct. Portal area is center.

Classic Lobule: Sinusoids drain to the central vein.

Portal Acinus: Tissue supplied by terminal branches of the hepatic artery and portal vein. Cells nearest these vessels are first to receive oxygen and nutrients.

Fig. 6.36 Liver cells

These connect up with the bile ducts at the edge of the lobule. The hepatocytes are located close to both sinusoids and canaliculi.

Blood reaches each lobule via the interlobular vessels, flowing along the sinusoids towards the central vein. The liver cells take up from the blood what they require and shed products into it. The only exception is bile, which is secreted not into the sinusoids but into the canaliculi to flow into the gall bladder where it is stored until it is needed.

Functions of the liver include:

- Bile production – synthesised by liver hepatocytes. Contains bile salts and the pigment bilirubin, reduced from the green pigment biliverdin, which results from erythrocyte breakdown. Stored in the gall bladder until food enters the stomach and duodenum. This stimulates contraction of the gall bladder and the bile is squirted along the common bile duct into the duodenum.

- Carbohydrate metabolism – occurs when glucose molecules arrive in the liver via the hepatic portal vein. They are polymerised to become glycogen and are stored in the liver. When energy is required by the body, glycogen is broken down to release glucose by a process known as glycogenolysis.
- Fat metabolism – lipids are synthesised to produce cholesterol and fatty acids used to produce energy or stored around the body in adipose tissue.
- Protein metabolism – needed for the following purposes:
  - Use in cells
  - Polymerised to make plasma proteins, e.g. albumin, globulin, fibrinogen and prothrombin
  - As an energy source
  - Deaminated to form urea and eliminated by the kidney.
- Heat production – from synthesis, deamination and transporting of products through the liver combined with its

blood supply, the liver produces and then distributes heat around the body, especially to peripheral sites.

- Hormone elimination – after their functions have been performed, some are modified chemically, some are eliminated by the kidney, others expelled in the bile via the intestinal tract.
- Haematinic principle – assisting in the quality of the blood cell production by increasing the haemoglobin level in cells by use of iron and B vitamins.
- Storing blood – using the expansion and contraction ability of the liver veins, the total blood volume in the circulation can be altered as required by the body.
- Detoxification – of nitrogenous waste from cell metabolism prior to excretion.

Large intestine

The indigestible liquid residue from the small intestine passes through the ileocaecal junction joining the ileum and the caecum, into the large intestine. The large intestine is divided into three parts:

- Caecum – a blind-ended sac through which food residue is forced by peristalsis (see Fig. 6.31). The lining changes from villi to a glandular form. The function of the caecum is not significant in carnivores and omnivores.
- Colon – divided into three sections, ascending, transverse and descending according to the position in the abdomen, all attached to the dorsal body wall by the mesocolon. The main function is the absorption of water from the ingesta and the pushing forward of the increasingly solid faeces to the rectum prior to defecation. The mucosa of the colon has no villi but is lined by goblet cells which secrete mucus to aid the passage of the faecal mass. The thickened mucosa is folded in appearance when not distended with faecal material. Commensal bacteria within the colon further degrade food residues, but the colon walls are protected from damage by the presence of numerous leucocytes and cells of the immune system.
- Rectum – this is a short dilated tube lying within the pelvic cavity. Its function is to store the semi-solid faeces prior to defecation. The mucosa is lined by increased numbers of goblet cells. It terminates in the anal canal and internal and external anal sphincters which control the passage of faeces to the outside. Lying within the anal sphincters are a pair of modified cutaneous glands – the anal sacs – which produce a smelly secretion used to coat the faeces as a form of territorial marking.

The gastrointestinal biome

The gastrointestinal biome refers to the commensal bacteria that are present in large numbers, especially within the large intestine. Their functions are vast, ranging from immunity of the digestive system to fermentation of certain types of carbohydrates and starches.

Urinary system

The urinary system is primarily responsible for maintaining the balance of water and electrolytes within the body fluids, i.e. homeostasis. The kidney provides the route by which excess water and electrolytes are eliminated as urine, which is then stored within the bladder before being excreted.

The functions of the urinary system are:

- Excretion of nitrogenous waste products, e.g. urea and creatinine; build-up of nitrogenous waste is referred to as azotaemia
- Regulation of the volume and chemical constituents of the body fluids – osmoregulation
- Secretion of the hormone erythropoietin, which initiates formation of new red blood cells within the bone marrow in response to low blood oxygen levels
- Activation of vitamin D after its synthesis within the skin
- Storage of urine in the bladder prior to micturition.

THE KIDNEY

There are two kidneys located in the dorsolumbar region of the abdominal cavity, one on each side of the midline. The left kidney is slightly caudal to the right kidney and both are retroperitoneal, i.e. lie beneath the parietal peritoneum (Fig. 6.37). Urine is produced by the kidneys and conducted to the bladder by the ureters to be stored, prior to micturition via the urethra.

Each kidney is supplied with blood by a renal artery which arises from the aorta. The total blood volume of the body circulates through the kidneys continuously and each kidney receives 20% of cardiac output at any one time. Renal blood pressure is high as the glomeruli consist of a capillary bed between arterioles (not between arterioles and venules as in other sites) and the efferent arterioles are able to constrict under the influence of renin. The high pressure forces the plasma through the perforated walls of the glomeruli into the tubules

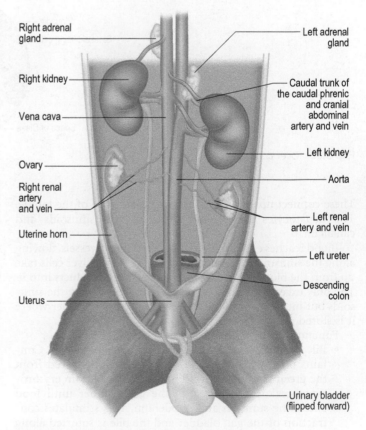

Fig. 6.37 Ventrodorsal view of the urinary tract

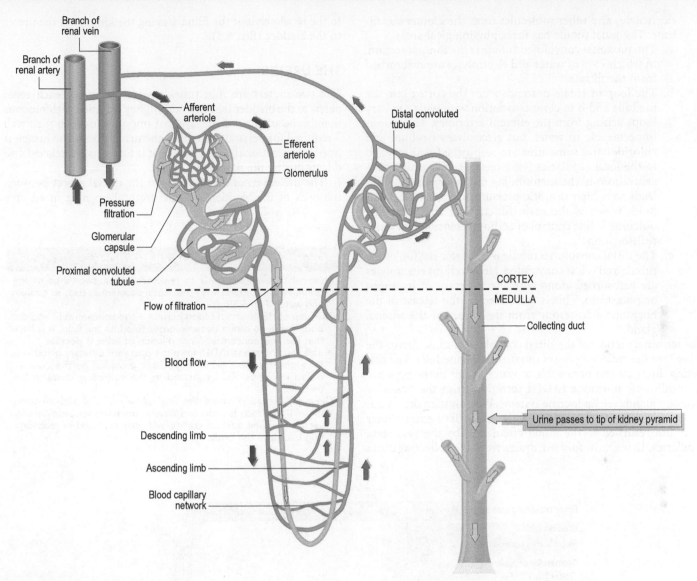

Branch of
renal vein

Branch of
renal artery

Afferent
arteriole

Efferent
arteriole

Glomerulus

Distal convoluted
tubule

Pressure
filtration

Glomerular
capsule

Proximal convoluted
tubule

Flow of filtration

CORTEX

MEDULLA

Collecting duct

Blood flow

Descending limb

Ascending limb

Blood capillary
network

Urine passes to tip of kidney pyramid

Fig. 6.38   A renal nephron

for modification. Blood is then returned via the renal vein directly to the caudal vena cava. Both the renal artery and vein are positioned in a depression on the medial side of the kidney called the hilus.

The substance of the kidney is contained within a tough, fibrous capsule and is divided into two layers:

- Cortex – outer layer containing the major part of each kidney nephron, including the glomeruli
- Medulla – the inner area arranged in pyramid-shaped units separated by extensions of cortical tissue. Each pyramid is formed by several collecting ducts which discharge urine into the renal papillae. The calyx, into which the papillae link, forms the larger renal pelvis to conduct urine to the bladder via the ureter.

Nephron structure

The functional unit of the kidney is called a nephron (Fig. 6.38) and each healthy kidney will contain about one million nephrons. Each nephron consists of:

- The **glomerular or Bowman's capsule** – consists of a double layer of flattened cells connecting with a perforated

basement membrane forming a hollow, distended, cup-shaped structure.

- The **glomerulus** – a tightly coiled network of capillaries that is closely applied to the basement membrane of the glomerular capsule. A glomerulus sitting within its glomerular capsule is known as a renal corpuscle. It is here that a process of ultrafiltration, in which plasma is forced from the glomerular capillaries into the glomerular space, takes place. The filtering action of the glomerulus holds back molecules the size of the plasma proteins or larger. It also retains substances bound to these proteins, e.g. hormones and calcium. Any molecule that is smaller and freely dissolved in plasma will appear in the ultrafiltrate or primitive urine, e.g. sugars, amino acids, small proteins such as myoglobin and haemoglobin, drugs, toxins and electrolytes. The ultrafiltrate then passes into the next section of the renal tubule.
- The highly convoluted renal **tubule** extends from the glomerular capsule to the connection with the collecting duct. The duct is lined by a single layer of epithelial cells. The function of the tubule is to selectively reabsorb water,

electrolytes and other molecules from the glomerular filtrate. The renal tubule has three physiological areas:

a. The proximal convoluted tubule is the longest section, in which 75% of water and electrolytes are reabsorbed from the filtrate.

b. The loop of Henle descends from the cortex into the medulla and is in close association with wide capillary loops arising from the efferent arterioles. The loop is impermeable to water, but electrolytes (sodium and chloride) and some urea are reabsorbed and recycled in the local capillaries (vasa recta), causing high concentrations in the surrounding medullary tissues. This leads to a high osmotic pressure in the extracellular fluid, which is the main function of this area. The outcome is fine control of sodium, chloride and water reabsorption.

c. The distal convoluted tubule is a shorter section of the tubule and is less convoluted. Here sodium electrolytes are reabsorbed along with the secretion of hydrogen or potassium. This is controlled by the release of the hormone aldosterone from the cortex of the adrenal gland.

The terminal section of the distal convoluted tubule drains the urine into the collecting ducts situated in the medulla. The collecting ducts are not permeable to water except in the presence of antidiuretic hormone (ADH) secretion from the posterior pituitary gland (see Endocrine system). Water is then drawn out by the high osmotic pressure of the medullary extracellular fluid and returned to the blood circulation by the vasa recta capillaries. Urine, now formed, drains from the collecting ducts

to the renal pelvis at the hilus, leaving the kidney via the ureter to the bladder (Box 6.5).

THE URETER

The two ureters are thin tubes, one leading from each renal pelvis to the bladder (see Fig. 6.37). They are lined with mucous membrane and have three layers of smooth muscle in their wall – required for peristalsis to move the urine along. The lumen is lined by transitional epithelium that is folded when relaxed and dilates during the passage of urine.

The ureters enter the bladder on the dorsal aspect between the neck of the bladder and the urethral opening in an area

---

BOX 6.5 PHYSIOLOGY OF FILTRATION

Proximal tubule function is to reabsorb about two-thirds of the primitive urine, along with the useful substances such as sodium and water (Fig. 6.39).

The loop of Henle acts if blood plasma is too concentrated and the body needs to retain water in order to dilute the fluid. It is here that the final concentration or dilution of urine is decided.

Antidiuretic hormone (ADH) from the posterior pituitary gland acts in response to the osmotic gradient provided by the concentrated interstitial fluid surrounding the collecting ducts in the medulla.

The distal tubule is where the final urinary loss of sodium takes place. If the body is sodium-deficient, the hormone aldosterone, secreted by the adrenal cortex, will promote sodium reabsorption back into the body.

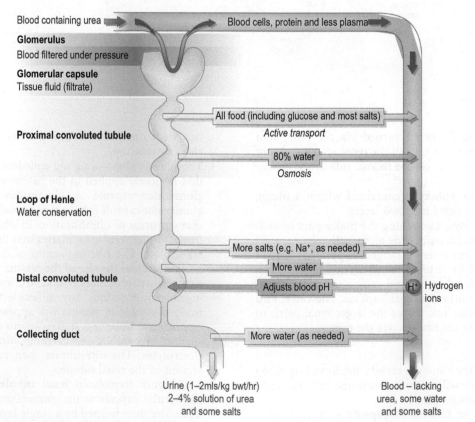

Fig. 6.39 Diagrammatic representation of nephron function

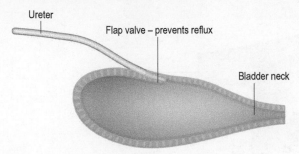

Fig. 6.40 Site of entry of the ureters into the bladder

called the trigone. Urine is prevented from re-entering the ureter if the bladder is full by a flap-valve within each ureter that compresses against the bladder wall (Fig. 6.40).

THE BLADDER

The bladder is a vesicle or sac used for the temporary storage of urine (see Fig. 6.37). It is a pear-shaped sac with three layers of smooth muscle in its walls, which contract during micturition. The lining of transitional epithelium resembles that of the ureters. When empty the bladder lies on the pelvic cavity floor and the lining epithelium is folded; when full it may expand as far forward as the umbilicus within the ventral abdomen.

Micturition or bladder emptying occurs when stretch receptors in the bladder wall monitor the degree of filling and relay the message to the spinal cord via the pelvic nerve. Nerve impulses from the spinal cord are sent to the internal bladder sphincter at the neck of the bladder, which is made of smooth muscle and allows urine to pass down the urethra. Emptying is a reflex action but voluntary control involving the external bladder sphincter, which is made of striated muscle, can be learned using reward training.

THE URETHRA

The urethra carries urine from the bladder to the outside. It is a tubular canal lined with transitional epithelium. There is a difference between the urethra of the male and of the female animal.

1. **Female urethra**
   - Shorter than in the male
   - Serves only the urinary system
   - Exterior opening embedded in the vaginal wall and called the urinary meatus.
2. **Male urethra** (Fig. 6.41)
   - Longer and narrower than in the female
   - Divided into three sections:
     - Prostatic – surrounded by prostate gland, ducts from prostate open into it
     - Membranous or pelvic – narrowest part of the urethra, passing along pelvic floor
     - Cavernous or penile – lies within the body of the penis and opens to the outside
   - Urethral opening is called the urinary meatus
   - Serves both urinary and reproductive systems.

In the tomcat, the urethra is short, the opening lies within the perineum and is directed caudally.

URINE PRODUCTION

Normal urine contains the following:
- 96% water and 4% solids
- Electrolytes
- Urea
- Other metabolic waste:
  - Creatinine
  - Phosphate
  - Sulphate.
- Volume: approximately 1–2 ml/kg body weight/hour.
  - Specific gravity: dog – 1.016–1.060; cat – 1.020–1.040
  - pH: dog – 7.5; cat – 6.5.

The rate of urine production varies with ambient temperature, water intake (including diet) and disease processes. Factors affecting urine composition, other than disease, include:
- Species – variation in specific gravity, which varies with the ability to concentrate urine (compare the volume produced by a cat to that produced by a horse)
- Diet – affects pH values – herbivores produce alkaline urine while carnivores produce a more acidic urine. The moisture content of the diet can directly affect the volume of water consumed by the animal, and thus the concentration of the urine
- Fluid intake – affects specific gravity concentration
- Exercise – influences fluid loss from body by sweating
- Medication – some drugs are excreted unchanged in the urine.

Reproductive system

THE MALE TRACT

Testis

The testes are paired, oval in shape and develop embryonically within the abdomen close to the kidneys (see Fig. 6.41). At later stages of embryonic development they migrate caudally through the abdominal cavity, taking their blood supply with them, and pass out through the inguinal canal to lie in the scrotum. This is complete by the age of 12 weeks – if the testis fails to descend the animal is described as being a cryptorchid. The scrotum consists of thin, pigmented skin supplied with sweat glands and is divided into two cavities surrounded by a double fold of peritoneum, the internal and external tunica vaginalis (Fig. 6.42). In mammals the testes are held outside the body because the normal internal body temperature is too high for sperm development. The blood vessels, nerves and ducts supplying the testes run from abdomen to scrotum in the spermatic cord. The cremaster muscle surrounds the spermatic cord and controls the position of the scrotum in relation to the body.

The testicular tissue is divided into numerous conical compartments, each containing a coiled mass of seminiferous tubules between which lie the interstitial cells or cells of Leydig, which secrete the male hormone testosterone (see Table 6.3). The seminiferous tubules are lined by two types of cell:
- Spermatogenic cells to produce sperm
- Sertoli cells, which provide support, nutrients and protection for the developing sperm. They also secrete small amounts of the hormone oestrogen.

The seminiferous tubules eventually join to form the epididymis, which runs on the dorsolateral border of the testis and leads into the deferent duct or vas deferens. This then passes

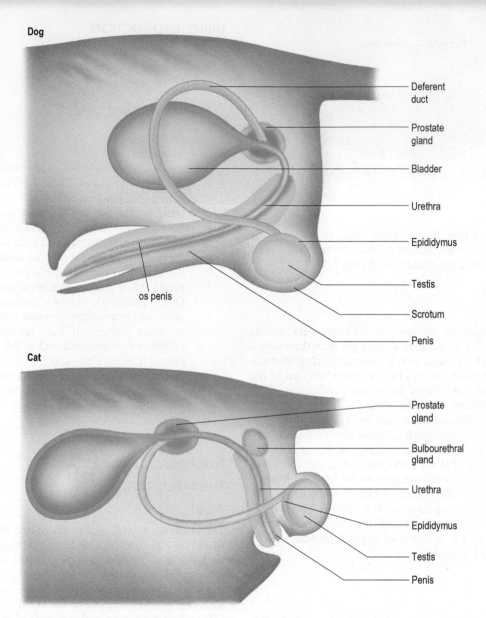

Dog

- Deferent duct
- Prostate gland
- Bladder
- Urethra
- Epididymus
- Testis
- Scrotum
- Penis

os penis

Cat

- Prostate gland
- Bulbourethral gland
- Urethra
- Epididymus
- Testis
- Penis

Fig. 6.41 Male urino-genital system of the dog and cat

through the inguinal canal and joins the urethra in the area of the prostate gland.

Sperm formed in the seminiferous tubules mature during their passage into the epididymis, where they are stored within the cauda epididymis before being propelled along the deferent duct during ejaculation.

The prostate gland surrounds the junction of the deferent ducts with the urethra close to the neck of the bladder and secretes prostatic fluid. This is alkaline, in order to protect the sperm from possible damage by the acidity of urine, and helps to increase the volume of sperm in order to wash it into the female tract. Bulbourethral glands, found only in the cat, contribute to the action of the prostate gland.

Penis

The penis consists of the urethra surrounded by layers of cavernous erectile tissue which becomes engorged with blood during sexual arousal, enabling its entry into the female vagina during coitus. Embedded within the erectile tissue close to the

tip is the os penis. This is a tunnel-shaped bone that in the dog lies dorsal to the urethra and in the tomcat lies ventral to it. Its function is to aid the entry of the penis into the female tract before erection is fully complete.

The tissues of the penis are protected by a covering of hairy skin known as the prepuce, which is well supplied with lubricating glands. In the dog this is suspended from the ventral abdomen and in the tomcat is much shorter, as the opening to the urethra and the scrotum lie in the perineum ventral to the anus. The tip of the tomcat's penis is covered in barbs, which play a part in the induction of ovulation during coitus.

Spermatozoon structure

Spermatozoa or sperm are formed within the seminiferous tubules of the testes by a process of spermatogenesis. This is influenced by the hormone testosterone, secreted by the cells of Leydig. Cell division occurs by meiosis and the nucleus of each sperm contains the haploid number (half the normal number) of chromosomes (see Chapter 15).

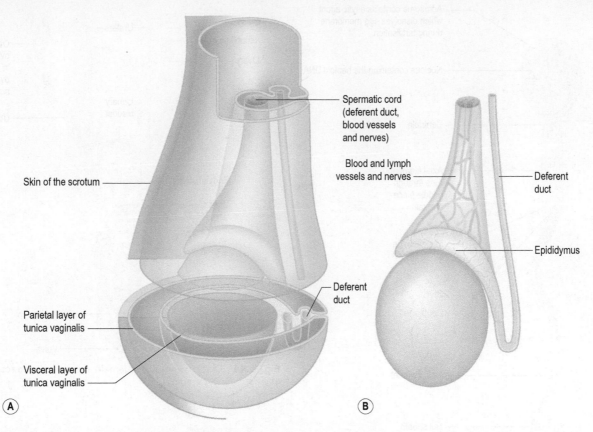

Fig. 6.42 The testis within the scrotum. (**A**) Testis enclosed within the internal and external tunica vaginalis. (**B**) Testicular structure

Each sperm (Fig. 6.43) consists of the following:

- **Head** – this carries the chromosomes (DNA) within a large nucleus and accounts for more than half the dry weight of the head. The nucleus is surmounted by a thin acrosome cap, which contains the enzymes necessary for penetrating the outer membrane of the ovum.
- **Neck and midpiece** – within the midpiece, the axial core is surrounded by densely packed mitochondria rich in respiratory enzymes. This section is concerned with releasing energy for driving the sperm.
- **Tail** – a modified flagellum, which, by lashing from side to side, propels the sperm along the female tract towards the ovum.

THE FEMALE TRACT

Ovary

There are two ovaries found in the dorsal abdomen caudal to the kidneys at the level of the third and fourth lumbar vertebrae (Fig. 6.44 and Fig. 6.37). Each is a small, round structure consisting of a central medulla and an outer cortex of connective tissue surrounded by a layer of epithelial cells continuous with the peritoneum known as the mesovarium. This forms a pouch known as the ovarian bursa, which masks the ovary and contains an opening into the peritoneal cavity.

Within the ovarian connective tissue are many primary follicles, each of which can develop into a mature or Graafian follicle. Each mature follicle contains a small amount of fluid and an ovum. The bitch and the queen are litter-bearing (multiparous) species, so they release several ova at the same time.

During ovulation, the follicle ruptures on the surface of the ovary, releasing the ovum, which passes down the uterine tube. After ovulation there may be some bleeding into the ruptured follicle. This is resorbed and replaced by a corpus luteum, which releases progesterone to maintain the pregnancy. In the bitch the corpus luteum remains even in the non-pregnant animal for several weeks and the resulting high levels of progesterone may cause a false pregnancy.

Uterine tube

The uterine tube, oviduct or Fallopian tube is a narrow tube running from the trumpet-like infundibulum, which encloses the ovary, to the uterine horn. The edges of the infundibulum are fringed with fimbriae, which aid in the capture of the newly released ova. The tube is convoluted, lined with ciliated epithelium and suspended by the mesosalpinx, which is continuous with the mesovarium. Its function is to convey the ova to the uterus. Fertilisation takes place within the uterine tube.

Uterus

The function of the uterus is to contain the embryos/foetuses during pregnancy and provide nourishment for them to develop to full term. The non-pregnant uterus lies in the pelvic and abdominal cavities; when pregnant the weight of the foetuses pulls the uterus down into the abdominal cavity.

The uterus is a Y-shaped, hollow, muscular organ composed of two long uterine horns, which unite, forming the small body or fundus. This is described as being a bicornuate uterus and is characteristic of litter-bearing species. The inner layer of epithelial and glandular tissue is called the endometrium and this

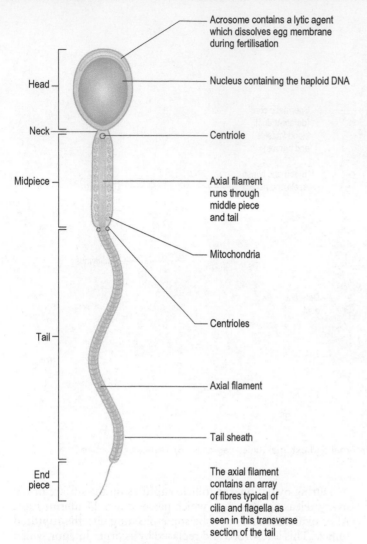

Acrosome contains a lytic agent which dissolves egg membrane during fertilisation

Nucleus containing the haploid DNA

Head

Neck

Centriole

Midpiece

Axial filament runs through middle piece and tail

Mitochondria

Centrioles

Tail

Axial filament

Tail sheath

End piece

The axial filament contains an array of fibres typical of cilia and flagella as seen in this transverse section of the tail

Fig. 6.43 Structure of a spermatozoon

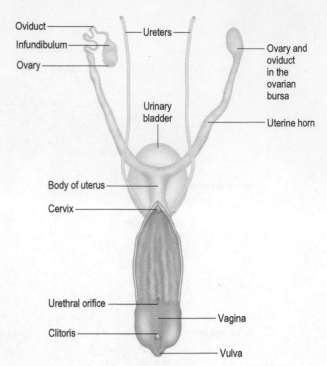

Oviduct

Infundibulum

Ovary

Ureters

Ovary and oviduct in the ovarian bursa

Urinary bladder

Uterine horn

Body of uterus

Cervix

Urethral orifice

Vagina

Clitoris

Vulva

Fig. 6.44 Dorsal view of the female reproductive tract of the dog and cat

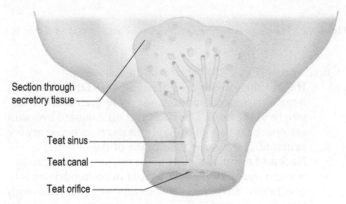

Section through secretory tissue

Teat sinus

Teat canal

Teat orifice

Fig. 6.45 Section through a mammary gland

thickens during pregnancy to receive the placenta. The endometrium is surrounded by layers of smooth muscle that form the myometrium. It is suspended from the abdominal wall by the mesometrium or broad ligament, which forms the outermost layer.

The uterus has a dual blood supply:

- An ovarian artery arises from either side of the aorta just caudal to the kidney to supply each ovary and the uterine horn.
- Each ovarian artery anastomoses with a uterine artery, which runs down the side of the uterine body and cervix, and supplies the more caudal parts of the tract.

Cervix, vagina and vulva

The cervix lies between the uterus and the vagina and is a thick-walled structure through which runs the cervical canal. It acts as a sphincter, only opening in the healthy animal during oestrus, mating and parturition. The vagina is a hollow muscular organ that extends from the cervix to the external genitalia. It is capable of great dilation and is lined by stratified epithelial cells. These cells change throughout the oestrous cycle under the influence of oestrogen and progesterone.

The vagina continues into the vestibule, a short passage that is shared by both reproductive and urinary systems – the urethra enters in the floor of the tract and marks the change from vagina to vestibule. It contains vestibular glands, which lubricate the caudal genital tract. The muscles in the wall of the vestibule constrict around the dog's penis and aid the 'tie' during coitus.

The vulva forms the external opening of the tract guarded by a pair of vertical labia. These contain striated muscle and under normal conditions are held closed to keep the vulva sealed. It is the vulval labia that become visibly engorged with blood when the bitch is in season. Lying ventrally between the labia is a knob of erectile tissue known as the clitoris.

Mammary glands

Mammary glands are highly modified sweat glands. The glandular tissue is surrounded by connective tissue and fat (Fig. 6.45). The secretion – milk – is produced by secretory

TABLE 6.5	Interaction between gonadotrophins and sex hormones		
	Follicle-stimulating hormone (FSH)	**Luteinizing hormone (LH)**	**Luteotrophic factors**
Site of action by hormone	Developing follicle	Mature follicle and corpus luteum	1. Corpus luteum 2. Mammary glands
Effect of hormone	1. Follicular growth 2. Secretion of oestrogen	1. Ovulation and formation of the corpus luteum 2. Secretion of progesterone	1. Progesterone secretion maintained 2. Stimulates mammary gland enlargement
Action/effect on the pituitary gland	Oestrogen secretion exerts negative feedback and prevents further secretion of FSH but positive feedback stimulates secretion of LH	Progesterone exerts negative feedback on the hypothalamus and prevents further release of GRH	

TABLE 6.6	Phases of the oestrous cycles of the bitch and the queen				
The bitch			**The queen**		
Notes: Spontaneous ovulator. Monoestrous. Age at puberty – approx. 6 months but breed-dependent			Notes: Induced ovulator. Seasonally polyoestrous – breeding season is between January and September. Age at puberty – approx. 5 months but depends on month of birth		
Phase	**Length**	**Signs**	**Phase**	**Length**	**Signs**
Pro-oestrus	9 days	Enlarged vulva, blood-stained vaginal discharge. Flirty, excitable behaviour. Will not allow mating	Oestrus	4–10 days	No external signs. Very affectionate, rubs against objects, rolls over, lordosis, loud 'calling'
Oestrus	Approx. 9 days. Ovulation occurs on day 10 of the complete cycle	Vaginal discharge becomes straw-coloured. Vulva even more enlarged. Excitable, flirty, stands to allow mating	Dioestrus	Up to 14 days	Behaviour returns to normal
Metoestrus I	Approx. 20 days	Vulva shrinks, discharge dries up, behaviour returns to normal	Anoestrus	Up to 4 months. Occurs only in the non-breeding season	Normal behaviour
Metoestrus II	Approx. 70 days	Behaviour and appearance is normal			
Anoestrus	Variable – 3–9 months	Behaviour and appearance is normal			

epithelial cells and drains into gland sinuses and then into teat sinuses. These narrow into teat canals and link to the outside via the teat orifices. In the bitch and the queen the mammary glands lie between the musculature of the body wall and the skin, in two parallel rows along the ventral abdomen and thorax. The bitch has five pairs and the queen has four pairs.

Mammary glands enlarge during pregnancy and start to produce milk a few days before parturition. Their development is controlled by the following hormones:

- Oestrogen – causes initial development at puberty
- Progesterone – enlargement during pregnancy
- Prolactin – formation of milk during last third of pregnancy
- Oxytocin – causes contraction of smooth muscle around the glands and squeezes milk out of teats – known as milk 'let down'.

The oestrous cycle

The oestrous cycle is the regular cycle of events that occurs in the ovary and the reproductive tract of the postpubertal non-pregnant female.

Reproductive function is under the control of gonadotrophins produced by the anterior pituitary gland (Table 6.5). Gonadotrophins are hormones that stimulate the gonads, i.e. ovary or testis. The release of gonadotrophins is controlled by gonadotrophin-releasing hormone (GRH), which is produced in the hypothalamus and transported down the pituitary blood portal system. The hypothalamus is sensitive to both internal and environmental stimuli such as heat, light and particularly the day length. It may also be stimulated by pheromones, secreted by other females and by the male animal. The oestrous cycle is controlled by a complex interplay between these stimuli, the hypothalamus and the reproductive tract.

The oestrous cycle occurs in distinct phases during which events take place within the ovary, the reproductive tract and in the female animal's behaviour. (For further details see Chapter 16.) Table 6.6 shows the details of the oestrous cycle of the bitch and the queen.

FERTILISATION

The ova released at ovulation from the ovaries are propelled down the uterine tubes by the ciliated epithelium and the peristaltic action of the muscles lining the tube walls. At the time

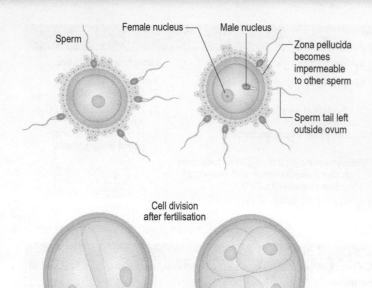

Fig. 6.46 Fertilisation of the ovum

of ovulation the ova contain the haploid number of chromosomes (half the normal number) and are immature and incapable of being fertilised. They are known as primary oocytes and they mature to become secondary oocytes approximately 3 days later.

Mature spermatozoa (sperm) pass from the seminiferous tubules of the testes into the epididymis where they undergo a maturation period within the cauda epididymis. During ejaculation they are propelled up the ductus deferens into the urethra, through the penis and into the female tract. The sperm, containing the haploid number of chromosomes, use their tails to swim from the vagina through the cervix into the uterus. They then enter the uterine tubes where fertilisation takes place. Sperm are able to survive within the female tract for up to 7 days waiting for mature ova to be available. Fertilisation occurs when a single sperm penetrates an ovum and the nuclei coalesce (Fig. 6.46).

Each ovum released from the ovary is protected by a double layer of cells – an inner layer of glycoprotein, the zona pellucida, and the outer layer of cells, the corona radiata. Sperm come into contact with the ova by random movement. When the head of a sperm hits the zona pellucida, the acrosome, the tip of the sperm head, bursts open, releasing an enzyme that softens the connecting tissue membrane of the ovum. The sperm is then able to penetrate into the cytoplasm of the ovum. Further spermatozoa are prevented from entering by a rapid chemical change known as the fertilisation reaction, which causes thickening of the surface of the ovum. After penetrating the ovum, the sperm tail is discarded. The head and midsection are drawn through the cytoplasm toward the nucleus. The nuclear membrane breaks down, forming a spindle along which the chromosomes of the sperm and ovum arrange themselves as in mitosis (see Chapter 15).

Fertilisation of the ovum by the sperm results in a zygote (Box 6.6). The diploid number of chromosomes is restored (haploid + haploid = diploid) and the fertilised ovum or zygote is ready for its first mitotic division (see Fig. 6.46). As further

divisions take place the zygote continues to move down the uterine tube towards the uterine horns.

Pregnancy

After fertilisation the zygote moves down the uterine tube and by the time it reaches the uterine horns it has already divided several times. At the stage in which the cell contains 16–32 cells the structure is called a morula and is a solid mass of cells resembling a blackberry. Following a long journey down the tube during which the ball of cells floats free in the lumen of the tube it develops a fluid-filled cavity and is known as a blastocyst. By about the 19th day the blastocysts space themselves evenly along the uterine horns and implantation begins (Fig. 6.47). In order to create equal numbers within each uterine horn, thus allowing equal space for development, one or more blastocysts may cross the body of the uterus to implant in the opposite horn – this is known as transuterine migration.

During the oestrous cycle the uterus prepares to receive the fertilised ova. In the follicular phase of the cycle there is growth both of the myometrium and endometrium and an increase in the blood supply of the uterus. The endometrium thickens, new blood vessels grow and glandular structures hypertrophy. In the luteal phase of the cycle these changes continue and the endometrium becomes secretory. When the blastocysts reach the uterine horns they are bathed in the uterine secretions, which provide nutrients and create the correct environment for survival.

EMBRYONIC DEVELOPMENT

The cells of the blastocyst become organised to form on one side of the cyst the inner cell mass and on the other side a thinner layer known as the trophoblast. The inner cell mass becomes the embryo and divides into three germ cell layers, each of which has a specific role (Box 6.7). The inner cell mass curves around to become C-shaped, enclosing the endoderm and mesoderm, which form the internal organs. Table 6.7 shows the stages and timing of puppy development. Kittens develop in a similar way but are usually slightly in advance of puppies.

FORMATION OF THE EXTRA-EMBRYONIC MEMBRANES

The trophoblast consists of the peripheral cells of the blastocyst and is eventually responsible for attachment to the uterine wall, i.e. implantation (see Fig. 6.47). It develops small, finger-like

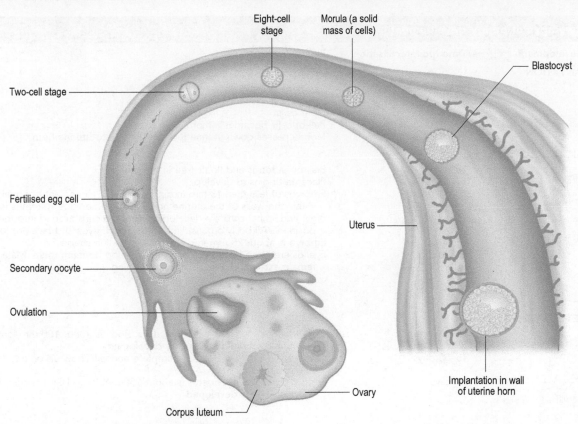

Fig. 6.47 Development and implantation of the embryo

---

outgrowths that project into the surrounding tissue of the uterine wall, contributing to the placenta and the extra-embryonic membranes and enabling absorption of nutrients across the villi.

There are four extra-embryonic membranes that surround the developing embryo. They protect the embryo and provide a means of attachment to the uterine wall (Fig. 6.48).

1. Cells from the endoderm multiply and line the trophoblast, forming the **yolk sac**. This shrinks away sometime before birth.
2. Between the yolk sac and the trophoblast, mesodermal cells divide into two layers forming a cavity – the outer layer lies close to the trophoblast and forms the **chorion**, and the inner layer lies close to the yolk sac.
3. The trophoblast and mesoderm expand and push up around the embryo, forming a fluid-filled cavity – the amniotic cavity. This is entirely separate from the other cavities and it is the surrounding membrane or **amnion** in which the foetus is delivered.
4. Around the outer surface of the amnion creating a double layer is the chorion, which is now in contact with the uterine endometrium. Projections called chorionic villi

grow out from its surface to connect with the maternal tissues as the placenta. Both amnion and chorion consist of ectoderm and mesoderm.

5. From the caudal end of the primitive embryonic gut endodermal cells multiply and form a diverticulum known as the **allantois**, which lies beside the yolk sac. This collects urine from the foetal kidneys via a tube or urachus that connects to the foetal bladder. During development the allantois increases in size, pushing between the amnion and the chorion, eventually surrounding the embryo. The inner layer fuses with the amnion, forming the allantoamnion, which contains lubricant fluids to assist movement towards the birth canal during parturition. The outer layer forms the **chorioallantois** with the chorionic layer and is known as the 'water bag'. This ruptures during parturition as the foetus moves toward the birth canal.

DEVELOPMENT OF THE PLACENTA

The placenta is the organ responsible for providing nourishment to the developing embryo and foetus while aiding in the removal of waste products. Villus structures develop from the chorioallantois and contain capillary loops derived from the umbilical artery (Fig. 6.49). They burrow into the endometrium of the uterus and project into the maternal blood spaces, which receive blood from the uterine artery. Only a thin endothelial layer separates the foetal and maternal systems and here nutrients and oxygen are able to pass into the foetus and waste gases and nitrogenous waste pass from the foetus into the maternal circulation.

TABLE 6.7	The stages of puppy development	
Stage of development	**Time (post-fertilisation)**	**Event**
PRE-IMPLANTATION		
	96 hours	Fertilised ovum divides into two cells
	20 hours	Four cells
	144 hours	Eight cells
	192 hours	Ball of cells becomes a morula
	8–9 days	Morula passes down uterine tube and then into uterine horn
EMBRYONIC DEVELOPMENT		
	15 days	Blastocyst forms and floats free in the uterus
	17–18 days	Placenta begins to develop
	20–21 days	Embryos of less than 13 mm in diameter begin to implant at equal distances within the walls of the uterine horns. Central nervous system is forming
	21–28 days	Brain and spinal cord are developing. Embryo curls around into the 'foetal position'. All body organs, limb buds, head, eyes and face are forming
	28 days	Embryo is about 25 mm in diameter and oval in shape
	29–30 days	Eyelids are closed and eyes begin to develop beneath them. Male and female external characteristics are forming
FOETAL DEVELOPMENT		
	35–44 days	Organogenesis is complete by 35 days. Body is about 100 mm long. Body hair and coloured markings are developing
	45–55 days	Calcification of the skeleton is complete and will show up on a radiograph. Foetus grows rapidly
	57 days	Further rapid growth. Foetus is about 150 mm long. Hair covering is complete; pads developed

The placenta forms a thickened band around the conceptus and is described as being a zonary placenta (Fig. 6.50). At the edges are areas of capillary degeneration and haemorrhage into the uterine endothelium caused during implantation. These are referred to as the marginal haematoma. During parturition the broken-down blood in these haematomata colours the parturient discharges. It is normal to see a green discharge in the bitch and a brown discharge in the queen – any other colour should be a cause for concern.

The placenta produces small amounts of oestrogen and progesterone, which act together to prevent further ovulation and oestrous cycles during pregnancy. Their effects are responsible for more vascular development of the uterine endometrium and glandular secretions. The uterine muscle relaxes and size increase becomes possible during the pregnancy.

CHANGES DURING PREGNANCY

The gestation period may be defined as the time between mating and parturition. The time is always expressed as a range as there is great individual variation and the exact timing of fertilisation is difficult to determine.

- Bitch 59–72 days – average 63 days or 9 weeks. Smaller breeds whelp earlier than larger breeds.
- Queen 61–70 days – average 63 days or 9 weeks. Siamese and Persians will often go to 70 days.

Changes during pregnancy include:

- Enlargement of abdomen
- Mammary gland enlargement
- Enlargement of the teats
- Vulva remains enlarged and elastic throughout pregnancy
- Clear mucoid vaginal discharge may be seen in some animals.

Relaxation and loosening of the ligaments in and around the pelvic girdle area occurs a few days before actual birth, by the hormone relaxin that it produced by the placenta and the ovaries. Alterations in abdominal configuration accompany such ligament relaxation. The abdomen, which earlier shows a uniform bulge, develops a 'hollow' in the flank area. This change is clearly visible both in profile and from above and is frequently referred to as a 'pear-shaped' abdomen, though it may not be obvious in all cases.

Parturition

Parturition occurs in three stages:

- First stage – uterine contractions begin and cervix dilates

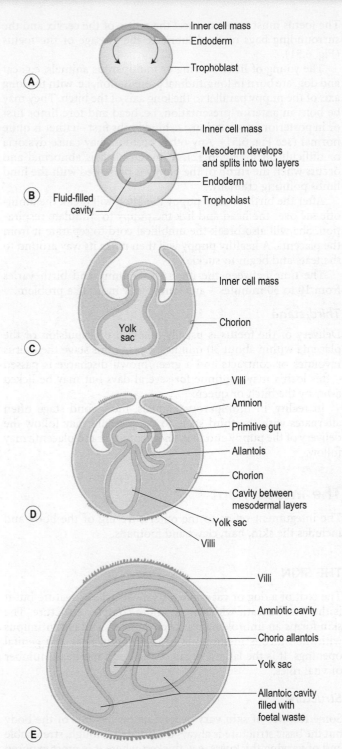

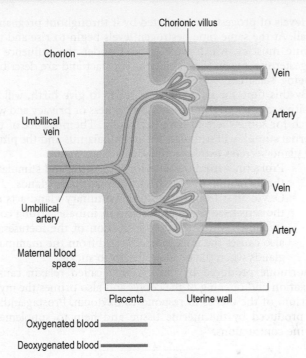

Fig. 6.49 Arrangement of blood capillaries within the placenta

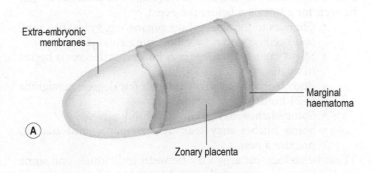

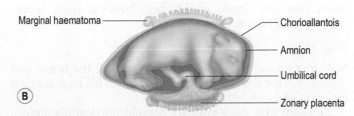

Fig. 6.50 The zonary placenta of the dog and cat. (A) Conceptus, showing zonary placenta. (B) Section through the conceptus

Fig. 6.48 Stages in the development of the extra-embryonic membranes. (A) Cells of the endoderm multiply and line the trophoblast. (B) Mesodermal cells divide into two layers forming a cavity between them. (C) The trophoderm and mesoderm expand and push up around the inner cell mass or embryo. (D) The amniotic cavity is formed; the yolk sac begins to shrink and the allantois develops from the primitive hindgut. (E) The allantois fills with waste products and extends around the embryo. Placental villi form around the outer surface and aid implantation

- Second stage – delivery of the foetuses
- Third stage – expulsion of the membranes and placenta or afterbirth.

It may be referred to as whelping in the bitch and kittening in the queen. Other species also have colloquial names for

parturition, e.g. calving in cows, foaling in horses and lambing in sheep.

HORMONAL CHANGES

Parturition is the expulsion of the foetus and its membranes from the uterus. It involves interaction between the hormonal and nervous system control mechanisms. It is thought to be initiated by the foetuses within the uterus. As they grow larger they outgrow the available space, which results in distress and the secretion of cortisol from the foetal adrenal glands. Cortisol causes the corpus luteum within the ovary to degenerate and the levels of progesterone secreted by it throughout pregnancy to fall. At the same time oestrogen levels begin to rise and the uterine muscles, which were relaxed under the influence of progesterone, regain their ability to contract and are described as being 'sensitised'.

By this time the dam may feel ready to give birth, will be sensitive to external stimuli such as darkness or privacy and will search for somewhere to have her young. The presence of the external stimuli will stimulate the hypothalamus and the pituitary gland secretes two hormones:

- Prolactin – from the anterior pituitary gland stimulates the formation of milk from the mammary glands
- Oxytocin – from the posterior pituitary gland acts on the sensitised uterine muscle and initiates strong contractions, which result in expulsion of the foetuses. It also causes the milk to be released from the mammary glands when the neonates begin to suckle.

A hormone produced by the placenta called relaxin causes relaxation and opening of the cervix and also primes the myometrium of the uterus to respond to oxytocin. Prostaglandins are produced by the uterine tissue and help to supplement uterine contractions.

SIGNS OF IMMINENT PARTURITION

Subtle signs that indicate that parturition will soon occur may be seen for a few days before the event.

- Changes to the external sex organs, e.g. vulval lips swell and become softer; vulval opening enlarges
- Slight vaginal discharge may be seen as the cervix begins to dilate
- Body temperature may drop by a few degrees centigrade 6–24 hours before parturition
- Some bitches may go off their food
- Some bitches may tear up newspaper and start to prepare a nest.

These behaviour patterns vary between individuals and some bitches show no signs at all (see Chapter 16). Most queens will search for somewhere to give birth and this is usually in private where they can remain undisturbed; however, some queens seem to need human company.

First stage

Mild uterine contractions start sweeping over the uterus and gradually bring about dilation of the cervix. This stage may last for up to 48 hours but is very variable.

The dam may show evidence of mild physical discomfort, e.g. restlessness, agitation, panting, licking the vulva. Strings of mucus may hang from the vulva and the first 'water bag' or chorioallantois may rupture within the vagina. Milk may be present in the mammary glands. The foetus becomes active and moves from the curled foetal position to the extended position ready for birth and the immature cardiac and respiratory systems become ready to take over from the placental exchanges that occur in utero. The contractions push the first foetus up against the cervix as it starts to dilate. Once the cervix is fully dilated the second stage begins.

Second stage

Increased uterine contractions propel the foetus through the cervix into the vagina. Once the foetus is in the birth canal abdominal contractions help to increase the propulsive force.

The foetus must rotate to meet the centre of the cervix and the surrounding bags of fluid lubricate the passage of the foetus (Fig. 6.51).

The young of litter-bearing or multiparous animals, e.g. cat and dog, are born in longitudinal presentation, i.e. with the long axis of the puppy parallel to the long axis of the bitch. They may be born in anterior presentation, i.e. head and fore limbs first or in posterior presentation, i.e. hind limbs first – either is quite normal (see Fig. 6.51). Any other position may cause dystocia or difficult birth (Fig. 6.52). A breech birth is abnormal and occurs when the rump of the puppy is presented with the hind limbs pointing cranially.

After the birth of each puppy the bitch will break the amniotic sac over the head and lick the puppy to stimulate respiration. She will also break the umbilical cord to separate it from the placenta. A healthy puppy will then make its way around to the teats and begin to suckle.

The time between the onset of straining and birth varies from 10 to 30 minutes – any longer may indicate a problem.

Third stage

Delivery of the foetus is usually followed by expulsion of the placenta within about 30 minutes. During this stage the uterus involutes or contracts and a green/brown discharge is passed – this lochia may continue for several days but may be licked away by the bitch or queen.

In reality, in multiparous animals, the second stage often alternates with the third stage so the placenta may follow the delivery of the puppy and then another puppy and placenta may follow.

The integument

The integument refers to the outer covering of the body and includes the skin, hair, claws and footpads.

THE SKIN

The coat of a dog or cat is often its most striking feature but it is the skin beneath which is the more complex structure. The skin forms an unbroken layer over the body and is continuous with the mucous membranes of the mouth, nose and genital openings. It is the largest organ of the body and has a number of vital roles.

Structure

Some features of skin vary depending on the area of the body but the basic structure is always the same. It is tough, stretchable and of varying thickness, e.g. thickest where it is most exposed such as the footpads of the dog. It is also thicker over the dorsal and lateral surfaces of the body but at its thinnest over the ear flap, thorax, ventral surface of the abdomen and inner surface of the legs.

The skin (Fig. 6.53) is composed of three main layers:

1. **Epidermis** – layer of non-vascular stratified epithelium of varying thickness. The epidermis is composed of four layers of cells:
   - **Stratum basale** or **germinativum** – lowest layer in which cells divide rapidly by mitosis. Melanocytes (pigment cells) are found in this layer and are responsible for skin colour.

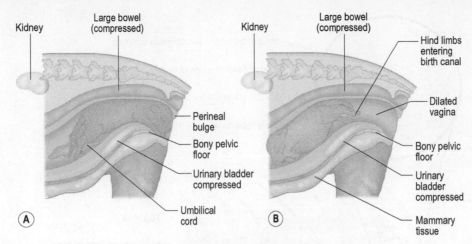

Fig. 6.51 Position of puppy during normal birth. (**A**) Anterior presentation. (**B**) Posterior presentation

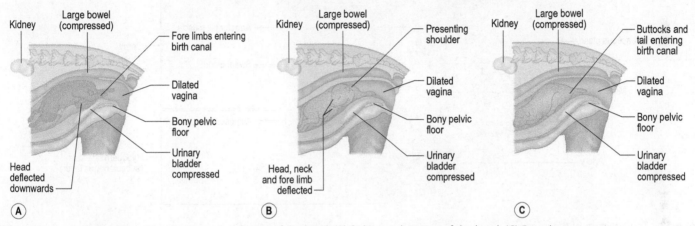

Fig. 6.52 Incorrect presentation. (**A**) Downward flexion of the head. (**B**) Sideways deviation of the head. (**C**) Breech presentation

- **Stratum granulosum** – cells contain granules in the cytoplasm and begin to die as they gradually move to the surface. Keratin, a fibrous protein, develops and gives a hardened texture to the cells.
- **Stratum lucidum** – cells lose their nuclei and develop a clearer appearance. This layer develops in areas of harder wear.
- **Stratum corneum** – flat, cornified cells, overlapping each other as dry scales. If these scales remain intact, this top layer prevents the entry of harmful materials. Keratinisation is completed here and gives the modified epidermal structures, e.g. hooves, beaks and hair, their strength. Dead cells or squames from this layer are continuously sloughed off as dandruff, scurf or dander and replaced by new cells growing up from the base layer.

2. **Dermis or corium** – made up of dense, fibrous, elastic connective tissue, which contains blood vessels and nerves. Bundles of smooth muscle called the arrector pili muscles are attached to hair follicles and when contracted cause hairs to become erect. The effect of this action increases the animal's ability to keep warm in cold weather and, if used in the 'fight or flight' reaction when the animal raises its hackles along the back and neck, increases the animal's apparent size. This layer also contains sebaceous glands, sweat glands, sensory nerves and blood capillaries.

3. **Hypodermis or subcutaneous layer** – contains connective tissue and adipose tissue, allowing the skin to move over deeper structures without tearing or damage.

Function

The many functions of skin include:

1. **Protection**
   - Acts as a barrier between the internal structures and the external environment
   - Prevents entry of microorganisms
   - Protects underlying structures from injury
   - Protects against damage from water loss, mechanical trauma and ultraviolet light
   - Prevents absorption of toxic or harmful substances.

2. **Production**
   - Vitamin D, required for the absorption of calcium from the intestines, is synthesised from dihydrocholesterol in sebum by the action of ultraviolet light
   - Sebum from sebaceous glands forms a water-repellent layer over the skin and helps control bacterial growth
   - Sweat, which assists in the removal of some waste products

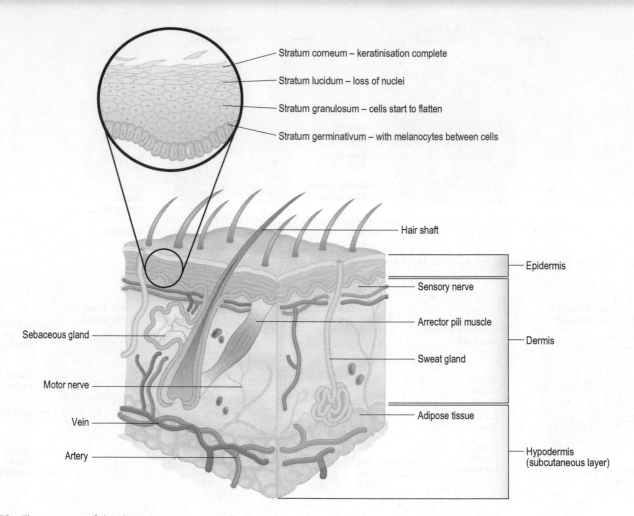

Stratum corneum – keratinisation complete
Stratum lucidum – loss of nuclei
Stratum granulosum – cells start to flatten
Stratum germinativum – with melanocytes between cells

Hair shaft
Epidermis
Sensory nerve
Arrector pili muscle
Dermis
Sebaceous gland
Sweat gland
Motor nerve
Vein
Adipose tissue
Artery
Hypodermis (subcutaneous layer)

Fig. 6.53   The structure of the skin

- Pheromones, produced in special scent glands, are used for communication with other animals for reproductive or territorial purposes
- Milk, released from the mammary glands.

3. **Sensation**
   - Sense organ with receptor nerves throughout the skin's surface needed to perceive touch, temperature, pressure and pain.

4. **Storage**
   - Fat, as adipose tissue, is an energy store and acts as an insulation layer to help maintain the body temperature in cold weather. It also helps to protect some organs such as the kidney.

5. **Thermoregulation**
   - Heat loss – dilation of surface blood vessel walls and sweating from the skin glands assists in the loss of water and salts that evaporate and cool the skin surface
   - Heat gain – constriction of surface blood vessel walls conserves heat in the body
   - Insulation – adipose tissue under the skin insulates the body. Erection of hairs traps a layer of warm air.

6. **Communication**
   - Pheromones – scents produced by special skin glands and used for communication with other animals of the same species. The production of pheromones is used mainly for reproductive purposes

- Visual communication or camouflage involving coat colour or pattern
- Response to threat or attack, the animal will raise its 'hackles' in order to appear larger.

Skin glands

Glands in the skin produce a variety of secretions:
- Sebaceous glands opening into the hair follicles secrete sebum whose function is to form a thin, oily, water-repellent layer over the skin surface. It gives the coat hair a shiny appearance and encourages the growth of bacteria that produce an acid pH. This acidity protects the skin from growth of other bacterial species.
- Sweat glands or sudoriferous glands open on to the skin surface. Sweat evaporates and causes cooling of the body and also contains some waste from the body.
- Anal glands or anal sacs – lie on either side of the anal sphincter. Their secretion has an unpleasant smell and is thought to be used as a pheromone for territorial marking. These sacs are intermittently emptied by the passage of faeces.
- Mammary glands – their function is to produce milk. They are the characteristic feature of mammals and are present in both male and female animals.

MODIFIED EPIDERMAL STRUCTURES

Hair

Individual hairs develop from pegs of epidermal cells which project downwards into the dermis and form a hair follicle. A small area at the base invaginates and fills with a knot of blood capillaries forming the hair papilla. Cells above the follicle divide to produce the keratinised hair shaft, which pushes up through the centre of the follicle and on to the centre. Each follicle develops an arrector pili muscle and a sebaceous gland.

There are three main types of hair:

- **Guard hairs** – longer and coarser than the other hairs; prevent water soaking into the coat and protect against mechanical damage
- **Wool hairs** – softer and wavier than other hairs; lie close to the body surface forming an insulating layer
- **Sinus hairs** (includes the vibrissae or whiskers) – long coarse hairs that protrude beyond the outline of the body. The base of each hair is in contact with a blood-filled sinus with a good nerve supply. Movement of the hair 'tweaks' the nerve fibres and a nerve impulse is sent to the brain, where it is interpreted.

Claws

These are beak-shaped structures forming the protective outer covering of the distal phalanges of each digit. Each claw consists of two sheets of epidermis which form the claw walls. The sole lies between them, facing the ground surface, and is filled with a soft, flaky horn. At the base of the claw, where it attaches to the skin covering the digit, is a fold of skin called the claw fold. In the centre of the claw between the last bone of the toe and the horn of the claw is the dermis, which contains blood capillaries and nerve fibres – often referred to as the 'quick'.

The functions of a claw include:

- Assisting in locomotion by providing grip
- Obtaining food
- Fighting, especially in cats.

Each of the five digits of the foot has a claw. The first digit or dewclaw is small and bears no weight so the claw is not worn down and may cause problems with overgrowth. The claws of the cat are narrower than those of dogs and are usually retracted into the claw fold by ligaments. The claws can be quickly unsheathed by muscular action when required.

Footpads

These are the weight-bearing surface of the animal's foot. The footpad is hairless and covered in specialised epidermis that is thick, roughened and normally pigmented. Sweat glands are present in the dermis and beneath this is the toe or digital cushion, made of fatty or adipose tissue with a good blood supply. The pads are oval or heart-shaped depending on their location in the dog, and are more rounded in the cat. The pads provide protection against wear, provide grip when walking and act as shock absorbers when running or jumping.

BIBLIOGRAPHY

Allen, W.E., 1992. Fertility and Obstetrics in the Dog. Blackwell Scientific Publications, Oxford.

Aspinall, V., O'Reilly, M., 2015. Introduction to Veterinary Anatomy and Physiology, third ed. Butterworth-Heinemann, Oxford.

Cooper, B., Mullineaux, E., Turner, L. (Eds.), 2012. BSAVA Textbook of Veterinary Nursing, fifth ed. British Small Animal Veterinary Association, Gloucester.

McBride, D., 1996. Learning Veterinary Terminology. C V Mosby, St Louis, MO.

Tighe, M., Brown, M., 1998. Mosby's Comprehensive Review for Veterinary Technicians. C V Mosby, St Louis, MO.

RECOMMENDED READING

Aspinall, V., 2005. Essentials of Veterinary Anatomy and Physiology. Butterworth-Heinemann, Oxford.
   Quick reference guide to all the important facts – useful for revision.

Aspinall, V., O'Reilly, M., 2015. Introduction to Veterinary Anatomy and Physiology, third ed. Butterworth-Heinemann, Oxford.
   This book is designed to cover the veterinary nursing syllabus and provides the correct depth of knowledge for student veterinary nurses.

Aspinall, V., Bowden, S., Capello, M., 2009. Introduction to Veterinary Anatomy and Physiology Workbook. Butterworth-Heinemann, Oxford.
   The fun way to revise anatomy and physiology! Provides a series of games and exercises to test your knowledge.

Tartaglia, L., Waugh, A., 2002. Veterinary Physiology and Applied Anatomy. Butterworth-Heinemann, Oxford.
   Provides in-depth coverage of the subject at a more advanced level. Recommended for those who wish to take the subject further.

Comparative Anatomy and Physiology of the Exotic Species

VICTORIA ASPINALL

KEY POINTS

- The rabbit is a warm-blooded mammal that is subjected to constant predation by many carnivorous species. As a prey species, much of its anatomy and physiology is adapted to sensing danger and making a rapid escape.

- Rodents make up 40% of all mammalian species, but only a few species are commonly kept as captive pets.

- The digestive system of the small captive rodent is the most likely to cause clinical problems, due to poor husbandry. These problems are usually linked to the fact that rodent teeth grow constantly and incorrect dietary care can lead to malocclusion.

- The domestic ferret is a true carnivore and shares many anatomical features with the domestic cat.

- The anatomy of the bird is unlike that of any other group of animals, and the metabolic and physical demands of flight are shown in almost every system of the body.

- Reptiles are cold-blooded animals that breed on land. There are approximately 6500 species and they share many anatomical features, but they also exhibit individual species variation that reflects their habitat and lifestyle.

- Fish are vertebrates that show numerous anatomical and physiological adaptations to life in water. The most obvious is the ability to breathe by means of gills.

Introduction

It is no longer rare to be presented in the surgery with an animal that is classed as an exotic species, i.e. one that is neither a cat nor a dog. In order to understand their care within the practice, it is necessary to have some knowledge of their individual anatomy and physiology. This chapter will take the basic plan of the mammal as exemplified by dogs and cats and highlight the differences.

Small mammals

THE RABBIT

Rabbits are warm-blooded mammals and members of the class Lagomorpha, which also includes the hare and a guinea-pig–like creature known as the pika. The feature that distinguishes them from members of the rodent family is that they possess two pairs of upper incisor teeth whereas the class Rodentia has only one pair. In the wild, rabbits are subject to constant predation by carnivorous species. As a prey species, much of the anatomy and physiology of the rabbit is adapted to sensing danger and making a rapid escape.

Morphology

The wild rabbit is covered in brown-ticked fur, which camouflages it. The average rabbit weighs about 2.5 kg but selective breeding has led to the development of at least 50 different breeds, which vary in colour and size. The head is rounded, with protuberant eyes set laterally, providing a wide field of monocular vision that enables the individual to detect predators. The ears are long and black-tipped and can be moved independently to pick up sound. They represent about 12% of the body surface and are extremely vascular, making them a useful means of thermoregulation. The lips are soft and the upper lip is divided by a deep philtrum, which allows the rabbit to nibble grass very short. Food is taken into the rabbit's mouth by the lips.

The skin of the rabbit is well supplied with scent glands, particularly under the chin, around the anus and in the inguinal region. The rabbit is strongly territorial, and the development of these glands, which is affected by the reproductive hormones, reflects the degree of sexual activity. As the female rabbit matures, she develops a large flap of skin or the dewlap under her chin from which fur is pulled to line the nest prior to giving birth.

The fore limbs are relatively short and used for digging while the hind limbs are long and powerful. They provide the main force needed for the hopping motion that is a characteristic of the rabbit. There are no footpads and the undersurface of the foot is covered in coarse fur. There are five toes on each forepaw and four on each hind paw, each of which ends in a sharp claw. The tail is short and fluffy and its white underside 'flashes' as the animal runs, acting as a warning to other members of the group.

Musculoskeletal system

The skeleton represents only 7–8% of the body weight and the bones are thinner and much more fragile than those of the cat, whose skeleton occupies 12–14% of the body weight. Incorrect or clumsy handling of the animal may cause fractured limbs or spine. In addition, older rabbits, those that are overweight or those not given sufficient exercise may develop osteoporosis or thinning of the cortex.

Apart from obvious differences in conformation (Fig. 7.1), the skeleton is largely similar to that of the cat. The number of vertebrae in the vertebral column is C7, T12–13, L7, S4, Cd16.

Digestive system

The rabbit is a herbivore and thrives on coarse plant material with a high fibre content. The oral cavity is long and narrow and the tongue is fleshy. The teeth are all open-rooted, which

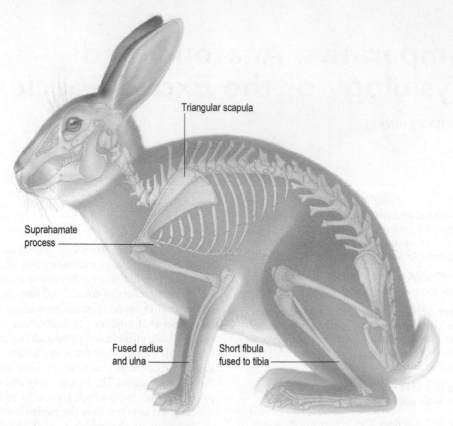

Fig. 7.1 Skeleton of the rabbit

TABLE 7.1	Dental formulae of the commonly kept small mammals	
Species	**Latin name**	**Dental formula**
Rabbit	Oryctolagus cuniculus	[I 2/1 C 0/0 PM 3/2 M 3/3] × 2 = 28
Mouse	Mus musculus	[I 1/1 C 0/0 PM 0/0 M 3/3] × 2 = 16
Rat	Rattus norvegicus	[I 1/1 C 0/0 PM 0/0 M 3/3] × 2 = 16
Syrian or golden hamster	Mesocricetus auratus	[I 1/1 C 0/0 PM 0/0 M 3/3] × 2 = 16
Gerbil	Meriones unguiculatus	[I 1/1 C 0/0 PM 0/0 M 3/3] × 2 = 16
Chipmunk	Tamias sibiricus	[I 1/1 C 0/0 PM 0/0 M 3/3] × 2 = 16
Guinea pig	Cavia porcellus	[I 1/1 C 0/0 PM 1/1 M 3/3] × 2 = 20
Chinchilla	Chinchilla lanigera	[I 1/1 C 0/0 PM 1/1 M 3/3] × 2 = 20
Ferret	Mustela putorius furo	[I 3/3 C 1/1 PM 3/3 M 1/2] × 2 = 34

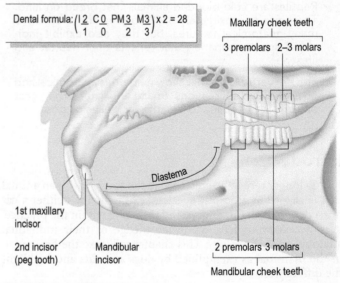

Dental formula: $\left(\dfrac{I\,2\ \ C\,0\ \ PM\,3\ \ M\,3}{1\ \ \ \ 0\ \ \ \ 2\ \ \ \ 3}\right) \times 2 = 28$

Fig. 7.2 Normal dentition of the rabbit

enables them to grow continuously throughout life. Dental problems are the most common reason for visiting the veterinary surgery. The dental formula is shown in Table 7.1. The incisor teeth are chisel-shaped for nibbling food, while the premolars and molars are flatter and ridged for grinding fibrous grass and hay. There are no canine teeth (Fig. 7.2). The gap between the incisors and the premolars is known as the diastema.

The digestive tract is long compared to that of the dog and cat as plant material is relatively difficult to digest. The stomach is simple and thin-walled and acts as a reservoir for food and ingested faeces. Both the cardiac and pyloric sphincters are well developed and rabbits are unable to vomit, making starvation prior to anaesthesia unnecessary, though their mouths should be checked for any food in order to prevent aspiration. The duodenum, jejunum and ileum are long, with a small lumen. The ileum terminates at the caecum in a rounded structure separate the fibrous from the non-fibrous components. The fibrous material travels on down the digestive tract and is passed out as hard pellets within about 4 hours of eating. The remaining softer and more fluid material passes back into the caecum where it undergoes fermentation by colonies of microbes that are able to produce the enzyme cellulase for the breakdown of the cellulose plant cell walls. At intervals the now digested material is squeezed into the colon by peristalsis and leaves the anus as softer pellets or caecotrophs, which are eaten by the rabbit – a process known as coprophagia or caecotrophy. These are produced within 3–8 hours of ingestion of the original food material, often at night, and are covered in mucus, which protects them from the stomach acid. Food ingested by the rabbit passes through the digestive tract twice in 24 hours and in this way nutrients produced by microbial fermentation are made available to the rabbit. Although fibre has very little nutritional value it is an essential component of a rabbit's diet to wear the teeth down and to stimulate peristalsis and digestive function.

Urinary system

The kidneys are unipapillate in contrast to the multipapillate kidneys of the dog and cat. The structure of the kidney varies with the species of rabbit and its associated environment. Desert-living rabbits have large kidneys with an extremely well-developed ability to concentrate urine, and thus conserve water, while those of alpine rabbits are small and produce more dilute urine.

The urine of the rabbit is the main method of calcium excretion and the urine, depending on the intake of calcium in the diet, is often thick and creamy because of its high calcium carbonate content. The colour also varies from white to yellow or even red. These changes are normal and are due to certain pigments excreted by the kidney.

Reproductive system

Male or buck. The almost hairless scrotum contains two testes and lies cranial to the penis. This position is unlike that of any other placental mammal, where the scrotum lies caudal to the penis. The testes descend at about 12 weeks of age and the inguinal canal remains open. There is no os penis. The buck has no nipples.

Female or doe. The bicornuate uterine tract has evolved to produce large litters of young and consists of two long uterine horns, each of which enters the vagina via its own cervix. There is no uterine body. The mesometrium that suspends the tract within the peritoneal cavity contains abundant amounts of fat and is a major fat storage area.

The doe is an induced ovulator and does not have a well-defined oestrous cycle. Periods of sexual receptivity occur in domestic rabbits at 4–6-day intervals. Ovulation takes place within 10 hours of coitus. (For further details of reproduction see Table 7.2.) The doe has four or five pairs of nipples. The young are altricial, i.e. blind, deaf and bald, and entirely dependent on their mother until they are weaned.

SMALL RODENTS

Members of the order Rodentia – the rodents – make up 40% of all mammals, but only a few species are kept as pets. Those that are kept in captivity include mice, rats, gerbils, hamsters, chipmunks, guinea pigs and chinchillas. Their common

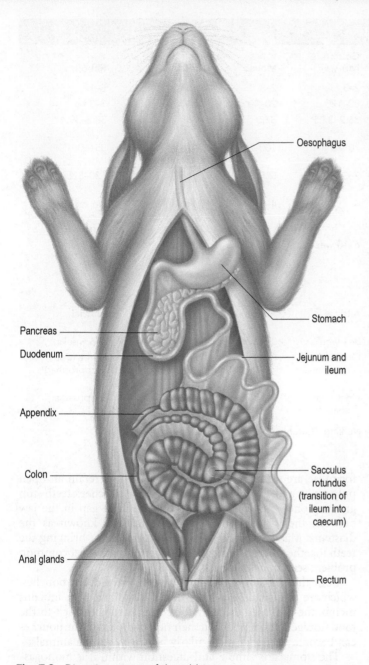

Fig. 7.3 Digestive system of the rabbit

known as the sacculus rotundus or the ileo-caecal tonsil (Fig. 7.3) inside which is a network of lymphoid follicles.

The caecum is the largest organ in the abdominal cavity, occupying most of the right side. It is thin-walled, sacculated and coils in on itself, ending in a vermiform appendix, which also contains lymphoid material. The colon is also sacculated and leads into the rectum.

Digestion

The rabbit is a herbivorous, monogastric hindgut fermenter. Plant material is masticated within the oral cavity with the aid of the flattened surfaces of the molars and premolars. After swallowing, the food undergoes monogastric digestion within the stomach in a similar way to that seen in the dog and cat. The ingesta passes into the small intestine and then into the caecum. When it enters the colon, muscular contractions

TABLE 7.2	Biological data relating to rabbits and small mammals						
	Chinchilla	**Gerbil**	**Guinea pig**	**Golden hamster**	**Mouse**	**Rat**	**Rabbit**
Life span (years)	10–12	3–4	4–8	2–3	2–3	3–4	5–12
Adult weight	400–600 g	50–60 g	750–1000 g	80–120 g	20–40 g	400–800 g	1–8 kg
Body temperature (°C)	38–39	37.4–39	38.6	36.2–37.5	37.5	38.0	38.3–39.4
Respiratory rate (breaths/min)	40–80	90–140	90–150	70–80	100–250	70–150	35–60
Pulse rate (beats/min)	100–150	250–500	130–190	280–412	500–600	260–450	130–325
Oestrus cycle (days)	41; seasonally polyoestrous	4–6	15–17	4	4–5	4–5	No regular cycle; induced ovulator
Age at puberty	8 months	10 weeks	M 8–10 weeks; F 4–5 weeks	6–10 weeks	6–7 weeks	8–10 weeks	4–6 months
Gestation period (days)	111	24–26	63	16	19–21	20–22	28–32
Development of young at birth	Precocial	Altricial	Precocial	Altricial	Altricial	Altricial	Altricial
Weaning age	6–8 weeks	24–27 days	2–3 weeks	3–4 weeks	3–4 weeks	3–4 weeks	4–6 weeks
Type of diet	Herbivorous; coprophagic	Omnivorous; coprophagic	Herbivorous; need vitamin C	Omnivorous; coprophagic	Omnivorous; coprophagic	Omnivorous; coprophagic	Herbivorous; coprophagic
Natural behaviour	Nocturnal; social	Nocturnal; monogamous	Diurnal; social	Nocturnal; solitary	Nocturnal; social	Nocturnal; social	Crepuscular; social

Source: Adapted from Aspinall, V., 2003. Clinical Procedures in Veterinary Nursing. Butterworth-Heinemann, Edinburgh.

characteristic is that they have incisor teeth with a persistent pulp cavity, i.e. the cavity remains open, unlike the pulp cavity of the incisors of the cat and dog, which shrinks once the tooth is fully developed. As a result the teeth continue to grow and the animal must gnaw on hard food, wood or stone to keep the incisors at a normal length.

Rodents can be subdivided into three groups:

1. The myomorphs – the mouse-like rodents. They are all omnivores and include rats, mice, gerbils and hamsters. The young are altricial.
2. The sciuromorphs – the squirrel-like rodents. They are all omnivores and include the chipmunks. The young are altricial.
3. The histricomorphs – relates to their reproductive patterns. They are all herbivores and include guinea pigs and chinchillas. The young are precocial, i.e. born fully furred with their eyes open and capable of eating solid food within the first 24 hours of life.

Rodents are warm-blooded mammals and as such they have many similarities with the dog and cat. The most notable difference is in the anatomy of the digestive system, which has evolved to deal with a range of diets.

Digestive system

Omnivores, e.g. mouse, rat, gerbil, hamster and chipmunk. These species eat a wide variety of different foodstuffs, including leaves, seeds, roots, fruit, insects such as crickets and locusts, cheese, hard-boiled egg and cooked meat. Their dentition consists of one pair of chisel-shaped incisors designed to gnaw and bite the food and flattened premolars and molars or cheek teeth for grinding and breaking up the plant material. Dental

formulae are shown in Table 7.1. The incisors retain an open pulp cavity and grow throughout life, while the cheek teeth stop growing once they have reached full size. The gap in the jaw between the incisors and the cheek teeth is known as the diastema. Malocclusion or difficulty in closing or bringing the teeth together caused by abnormal growth is the most common problem seen in pet rodents.

Both the hamster and the chipmunk have cheek pouches, which are diverticula from the oral cavity lined with mucous membrane and used to carry food long distances back to the food storage chambers within their nest complexes. The pouches can become impacted, particularly in newly weaned animals.

The stomach is simple and digestion within it is monogastric. In the rat, mouse and gerbil the lining epithelium is mostly non-glandular. Lying between the oesophagus and the cardiac region is a ridge that prevents regurgitation and makes vomiting impossible. The intestine is relatively longer than that seen in the carnivorous dog and cat but shorter than that seen in the herbivores. As plant material makes up only part of the diet, there is no organ specifically adapted for microbial fermentation and breakdown of cellulose; however, the hamster has a distinct forestomach which is adapted for this purpose. The rat has no gall bladder but it is present in the other omnivores.

All omnivores show a degree of caecotrophy or coprophagia and the faecal pellets are thought to contain a significant amount of vitamin B produced by the microbial flora living in the colon.

Herbivores, e.g. guinea pig and chinchilla. These species live mainly on the leafy parts of plants, and in the guinea pig in particular it is essential that it receives fresh green food daily.

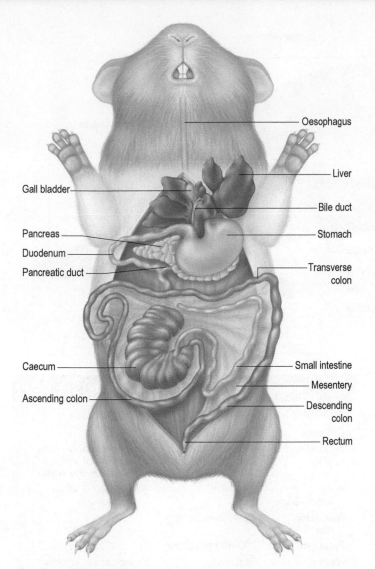

Fig. 7.4 Digestive system of the guinea pig

The liver of the guinea pig is unable to manufacture vitamin C, and if deprived of green food containing the vitamin it will begin to show symptoms and will eventually die.

The dentition consists of chisel-shaped incisor teeth and flattened premolars and molars, all of which retain an open pulp cavity and grow throughout the animal's life. The dental formulae are shown in Table 7.1. As with the other species, malocclusion is a common problem. The stomach is simple and lined with a glandular epithelium, and digestion is monogastric. The small intestine is moderately long and lies mainly on the right of the side of the peritoneal cavity.

The much longer large intestine fills the left and central parts of the cavity. The most significant part of the large intestine is the caecum, which is large and thin-walled and has many lateral pouches created by bands of smooth muscle in the walls (Fig. 7.4). Inside the caecum are large numbers of microorganisms, which are responsible for the fermentation and breakdown of cellulose within the plant cell walls. They also contribute extra nutrients such as vitamin B to the digested food mixture. Both guinea pigs and chinchillas exhibit caecotrophy. Animals deprived of the opportunity to eat their own faeces may suffer from malnutrition.

THE FERRET

The domestic ferret is a member of the family Mustelidae and is therefore related to other members of the family such as the polecat, weasel, stoat and badger. These species are noted for their pungent smell, which comes from sebaceous glands distributed within the skin and also the anal glands. They are carnivorous mammals and as such show many similarities to the cat. Working ferrets are used to kill rats and rabbits but they are also becoming popular as domestic pets.

Morphology

The tubular body is long and very flexible and is designed to go down holes in pursuit of prey. The neck is long and muscular with a similar diameter to that of the rest of the body. The head is small, with small ears set on the crown of the head and eyes that point forwards. These provide binocular three-dimensional vision, which enables the ferret to locate its prey accurately. Their eyesight is poor and is adapted to the low light levels found within tunnels.

The legs of the ferret are short and are used mainly for digging. Ferrets are excellent climbers and if the surface is rough enough to grip they may reach great heights. There are five toes on each foot, each ending in a non-retractable claw. The skin is thick to provide protection from bites and the fur is very dense. The natural colour is cream, with black guard hairs, black feet and tail and a black mask on the face. This is the colour of the closely related polecat and in the ferret is described as 'fitch'. Other colours that may also occur naturally include albino, sandy or cinnamon.

Musculoskeletal system

The pattern of the skeleton is similar to that of the cat (Fig. 7.5). The spine is extremely flexible and allows the ferret to bend at an angle of at least 180°. The arrangement of the vertebral column is C7, T15, L5–6, S3, Cd18. The thoracic inlet is small and may quite easily be blocked by an abnormal mass, which will interfere with breathing and swallowing.

Digestive system

The ferret is a true carnivore and this is reflected in its dentition and the anatomy of the digestive tract. The teeth are extremely sharp and are adapted for killing prey and tearing flesh off the bone. The incisors are prominent; the canines are large and may be visible when the mouth is closed. The premolars and molars are similar to those of the cat. The third upper premolars are the largest of the cheek teeth and are known as the carnassials. The dental formula is shown in Table 7.1.

As in all carnivores the digestive tract is quite short as meat is easily digested and therefore takes less time. The stomach is simple and small but capable of enormous distension with food. The small and large intestines follow a similar pattern to that seen in the cat. There is no caecum or ileocaecal valve. The ferret has a six-lobed liver, a gall bladder and a pancreas that has two parts, which open into the duodenum close to the pylorus.

Reproductive system

Male or hob. The two testes lie externally within the scrotum and once the testes have descended the inguinal ring closes. During the breeding season the testes become noticeably enlarged as spermatogenic activity increases. There is a J-shaped os penis lying within the caudal section of the penis and dorsal

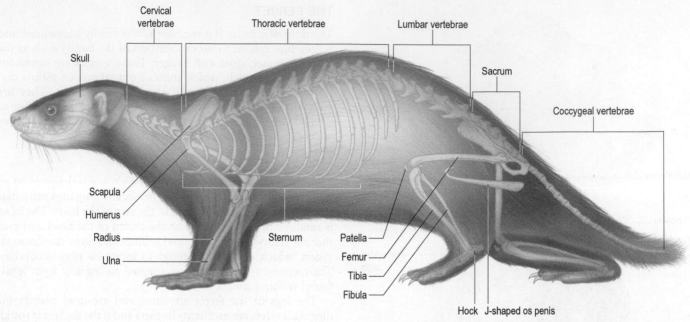

Fig. 7.5   Skeleton of the ferret

to the urethra (Fig. 7.5). The opening of the prepuce is on the ventral abdomen in a similar position to that of the dog. The male ferret has teats. Further reproductive details are shown in Table 7.3.

Female or jill. The bicornuate uterus consists of two long uterine horns with no uterine body. This adaptation is essential to produce the litters of 8–10 young commonly seen in the ferret. The small slit-like vulva lies ventral to the anus and becomes enlarged during the oestrous cycle. The jill is seasonally polyoestrous and an induced ovulator. Coitus may last for 1–3 hours and can be a violent procedure. Ovulation takes place within 30–40 hours of coitus. The young, known as kits, are altricial. (For further details see Table 7.3.)

Birds

Birds are members of the class Aves and as such have an outer covering of feathers. There are about 8500 species of bird, but only a relatively few species are commonly kept as cage and aviary birds; examples of these are shown in Table 7.4. Most species of bird are able to fly although there are some species, e.g. penguin, ostrich, kiwi, which remain land-bound. The ability to fly has contributed to their great ecological success and they are distributed within most habitats in the world. Their anatomy and physiology is very different to that seen in the mammal, and adaptations to the metabolically demanding ability to fly are shown in almost every body system and affect such factors as metabolism, body weight, stability and wind resistance.

THE SKELETON

The skeleton of the bird (Fig. 7.6) is adapted to support both walking and flying and has many specialised features, which result in a strong but light framework. These include:
- A reduction in the total number of bones
- Fusion of some joints to form strengthening plates of bone

TABLE 7.3	Biological data relating to the ferret	
Parameter	**Measurement**	**Comment**
Life span	5–11 years	
Adult weight	Jill: 600–900 g Hob: 1–2 kg	Weight fluctuates with the time of year – heavier in the winter
Body temperature	37.8–40°C	Rises to 40°C when excited
Respiratory rate	30–40 breaths/min	
Pulse rate	200–400 beats/min	
Oestrous cycle	Seasonally polyoestrous Induced ovulator	Season starts in March and continues until September. Female remains in oestrus until mated. Ovulation occurs 30–40 h after mating
Age at puberty	Jill: 7–10 months Hob: 5–14 months	Puberty occurs in the spring after birth, so age varies
Gestation period	38–44 days	Young are altricial. May be eaten by the jill if disturbed
Litter size	2–6	
Weaning age	6–8 weeks	
Diet	Carnivorous	Require 30% protein, 30% fat. Can be fed on tinned or dry cat food

Source: Adapted from Aspinall, V., 2003. Clinical Procedures in Veterinary Nursing. Butterworth-Heinemann, Edinburgh.

- A reduction in the density of bone – many bones have a thin cortex which is strengthened by the addition of a network of bony struts
- Loss of the internal components – many bones are hollow and filled with air sacs.

TABLE 7.4	Commonly kept species of cage and aviary birds		
Order	**Species**	**Common name**	
Psittaciformes – noted for their bright plumage and ability to mimic sounds	Psittacus erithacus	African grey parrot	
	Amazona species	Amazon parrots	
	Ara species	Macaws	
	Eclectus species	Eclectus parrots	
	Nymphicus hollandicus	Cockatiel	
	Melopsittacus undulatus	Budgerigar	
	Trichoglossus species	Lories and lorikeets	
	Cacatua sulphurea	Lesser sulphur crested cockatoo	
Passeriformes – so-called perching birds; contains over half the living species of bird	Serinus canaria	Canary	
	Poephila quattata	Zebra finch	
	Chloebia gouldiae	Gouldian finch	
	Gracula religiosa	Mynah bird	
Columbiformes	Columbia livia	Pigeons and doves	
	Coturnix species	Quail	

Axial skeleton

- The skull shows many adaptations, which contribute to the overall reduction in weight. A lightweight beak covers the mandible and replaces the teeth. The upper beak articulates with the rest of the skull by means of the craniofacial hinge, which increases the mobility of the beak during feeding. The lower beak hinges on the quadrate bone, which enables the beak to open wide and makes dislocation of the beak very unlikely. The large eyes are housed within a pair of thin-walled orbits. Each orbit is surrounded by a ring of bony plates, known as the sclerotic ring, which protects and supports the structure of the eyeball.
- The vertebral column is divided into the different regions as in other animals; however, there are fewer vertebrae in the central regions and more in the cervical and coccygeal regions, which allows greater flexibility. The neck may contain as many as 25 vertebrae, depending on the species. Birds have 12 caudal or coccygeal vertebrae, the first few of which are mobile to enable movement of the tail and the remaining ones are fused to form the pygostyle, which

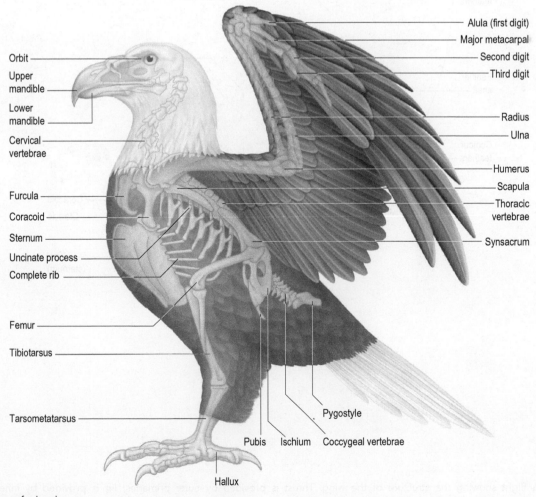

Fig. 7.6 Skeleton of a hawk

carries the tail feathers. The thoracic, lumbar and sacral vertebrae are fused to form a rigid frame to support the rib cage and the legs.

- The sternum is extended into a large concave keel, which provides an increased surface area for the attachment of the flight muscles. Flightless birds do not have a keel.

Appendicular skeleton

- The pectoral girdle is formed from three pairs of bones – the coracoids, scapulae and clavicles. On each side the glenoid cavity is formed by the junction of the coracoid and the scapula and the humerus of the upper wing inserts into this cavity, forming the shoulder joint. The pair of clavicles, often referred to as the wishbone, keep the shoulders separated.
- The wings (Fig. 7.7) attach to the body at the shoulder joint, which allows rotation in several planes. The bones of the wing are reduced to the humerus, a separate radius and ulna, fused carpal and metacarpal bones and two

digits. Digit 3 is fused to the metacarpal bones and is the main digit. It carries the primary feathers. Digit 1 forms the alula or bastard wing and carries a few feathers for controlling takeoff and landing. The shape of the wing, which varies with the species and affects the type and speed of flight, is slightly curved from front to back, forming an aerofoil shape that creates lift as the bird flaps its wings.

- The pelvic girdle is formed by three pairs of bones – the ilium, ischium and pubis – which join to form the joint into which the femur of the leg inserts. The distal ends of the three bones are not fused, leaving the lower part of the pelvis open to allow the passage of eggs out of the body cavity.
- The upper leg is formed by a short, wide femur which ends at the stifle joint. This is directed forward so that the lower leg is under the bird's centre of gravity. The middle of the leg consists of a fused tibia and fibula known as the tibiotarsus, which ends at the hock joint, consisting of a single

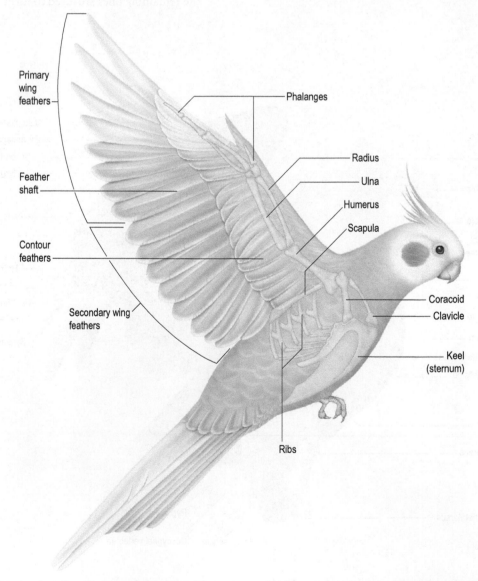

Fig. 7.7 Bird in flight showing the structure of the wing. Thrust is provided by outer primaries; lift is provided by inner primaries and secondaries.

fused tarsometatarsus. Most species of bird possess four toes, with three pointing forwards and one pointing back. However, the members of the parrot family and the woodpeckers have two toes pointing forwards and two pointing backwards. Owls and ospreys have a fourth toe that is opposable and can face backwards or forwards, which enables them to use their feet to pick up their prey.

MUSCULAR SYSTEM

The average bird has between 175 and 200 muscles, many of which are placed on the ventral surface of the body close to the centre of gravity.

Wing muscles

The most prominent are the pectorals, which are large and superficial and responsible for the powerful downbeat of the wing, and the supracoracoids, which lie deep to the pectorals and are responsible for the upbeat of the wing. Both pairs originate on the keel, with the pectoral inserting on the underside of the humerus and the supracoracoid inserting on the upper surface of the humerus. In strong, long-distance fliers these muscles make up about 25% of the body weight and in the pigeon they make up 40% of body weight.

Leg muscles

Most of the muscles lie high up the leg or on the body itself and they control movements by means of long tendons that run down the leg. Extensor tendons run down the front of the tibiotarsus and the tarsometatarsus while the flexor tendons run down the back of the leg. The digital flexor tendon runs in a groove at the top of the tarsometatarsus and supplies each of the digits. As the bird bends its leg to perch, the tendon is pulled taut and the toes flex and tighten the hold on the branch. This is the perching reflex and is the reason why birds can sleep on a branch without falling off.

INTEGUMENT

The integument of the bird consists of skin and its derivatives – the claws, beak and feathers. The structure of the skin and its associated glands is similar to that of the dog and cat and the claws and the beak are made of a tough horn that grows throughout the bird's life. However, it is the feathers that are the distinctive characteristic of the bird family.

Feathers derive from epidermal cells in a similar way to the hairs of mammals. They are made of keratin and have several functions. They:

- Form a waterproof covering that protects the thin skin from physical and chemical damage
- Create a smooth outer covering to the wing that cannot be penetrated by air, enabling the downward force of the wing to bring about lift
- Provide insulation of the body
- Provide camouflage
- Are involved in communication between birds of the same species.

All feathers have a similar structure, consisting of a central shaft or rachis that is filled with blood capillaries during growth but later becomes hollow (Fig. 7.8). The shaft gives off the flattened vane, which consists of barbs and interlocking barbules that hook together to produce a wind-resistant surface. It is

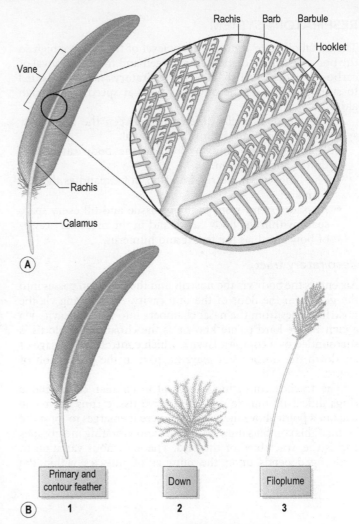

Fig. 7.8 (A) Feather structure and (B) types of feather

essential that the feathers are kept in good condition, and a healthy bird will constantly preen itself and apply sebum obtained from the preen gland at the base of the tail to the feathers. This helps to 'zip up' the barbules and makes the feathers waterproof.

There are four main types of feather (see Fig. 7.8):
- **Flight** – long rigid feathers attached to the wing and tail. The primaries are attached to digit 3 and to the fused metacarpals bones. The major thrust of the downbeat is provided by the outer primaries. The shorter secondaries are attached to the ulna and, in combination with the inner primaries, provide lift during flight.
- **Contour** – cover the rest of the wing and may be known as coverts. They create a smooth cover over the body. They are shorter and more flexible than the flight feathers and the lowest part closest to the body may be fluffier.
- **Down** – lie close to the body underneath the contour feathers, forming an insulating layer.
- **Filoplume** – also lie close to the body. Designed to break up and form feather dust, which absorbs dirt and moisture, helping to keep the bird clean. Both down and filoplume feathers are barbless, so they look fluffy (see Fig. 7.8).

RESPIRATORY SYSTEM

The metabolic rate and the energy level of the bird are high so the body has a high demand for oxygen and for the removal of carbon dioxide. To satisfy this, the respiratory system is adapted to supply oxygen as the bird flies both at speed and at high altitudes.

There are three main differences between the respiratory system of the bird and that of the mammal:

- There is no diaphragm dividing the body cavity into thorax and abdomen.
- The lungs are more rigid and do not expand as they fill with air.
- Air sacs extend from the lung tissue and fill every spare space within the body cavity and in the medullary cavity of bones such as the femur and humerus.

Respiratory tract

Air enters the body via the nostrils and the beak and passes into the glottis on the floor of the oral cavity. Air entering via the nostrils passes from the nasal chambers into the oral cavity via a cleft in the hard palate known as the choana. The glottis is surrounded by a complex larynx, which controls the passage of air down the trachea but plays no part in the production of sound.

The trachea consisting of complete circular cartilaginous rings linked by muscle and connective tissue runs down the neck to a point above the sternum where it enlarges to form the syrinx. This contains muscles, air sacs and vibrating membranes and is the 'voice box' of the bird. The enormous variation in birdsong depends upon the number of muscles within the

syrinx, which is dependent on the species. Just distal to the syrinx the trachea bifurcates into two bronchi, which pass along the ventral side of each lung, ending in the posterior air sacs. Within the lung tissue the bronchi lose their cartilaginous rings and are known as mesobronchi. These give rise to four to six ventrobronchi which further divide to form parabronchi. The parabronchi are connected to air capillaries, which are surrounded by pulmonary blood capillaries, and it is here that gaseous exchange takes place. Gaseous exchange is a similar process to that seen in mammals.

Leading from the various bronchi are thin-walled air sacs. These are covered in minute capillaries and account for 80% of the respiratory volume. Most birds have nine pairs of air sacs (Fig. 7.9), which fill the spaces within the body cavity and penetrate into the insides of many bones. They are not involved in gaseous exchange but act as a reservoir for air and have a bellows-like effect that helps to push the air back through the lungs. They also reduce the weight of the skeleton, so aiding flight and the buoyancy of water birds.

The lungs containing the different bronchi are bright red, vascular and quite rigid and are attached to the thoracic vertebrae and ribs in the dorsal part of the body cavity. The volume of the lungs is only 2% of the total body volume.

Respiration

Air flows through the lungs and air sacs via the following route:

1. The bird inspires by muscular expansion of the body cavity, which reduces the pressure within the respiratory tract and air is drawn in; most of the air is drawn into the posterior air sacs where it is warmed and moistened. The keel bone moves during muscular expansion, and it is

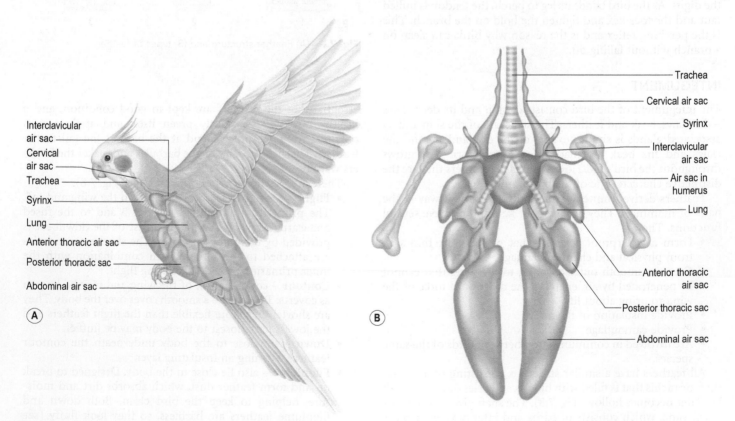

Interclavicular air sac
Cervical air sac
Trachea
Syrinx
Lung
Anterior thoracic air sac
Posterior thoracic sac
Abdominal air sac

(A)

Trachea
Cervical air sac
Syrinx
Interclavicular air sac
Air sac in humerus
Lung
Anterior thoracic air sac
Posterior thoracic sac
Abdominal air sac

(B)

Fig. 7.9 Respiratory system of a bird

important when restraining the bird not to restrict movement of the keel.

2. The bird expires and the air is pushed from the posterior air sacs into the lung tissue where gaseous exchange takes place.
3. The bird inspires again and the air moves out of the lungs into the anterior air sacs.
4. The bird expires again and the air leaves the anterior air sacs and exits the body via the trachea.

In order to make use of one 'unit' of air the bird has two inspirations and two expirations. Fresh air follows a one-way path and does not get mixed with the air containing carbon dioxide. This allows almost all the oxygen within the inspired atmospheric air (21%) to reach the capillaries, and it is thought that the respiratory system of the bird is about 10 times more efficient than that of the mammal.

DIGESTIVE SYSTEM

The digestive system is very efficient and enables the energy in food to be used rapidly to satisfy the high metabolic rate of the bird.

The basic plan of the digestive tract is similar to that in other groups of animal but there are certain modifications.

Oral cavity

A lightweight beak replaces the lips and teeth. Its shape varies with the species and is adapted to the type of diet. In most species the tongue is not very mobile but in members of the parrot family it is large and fleshy and is used to move food around for easy swallowing. Most birds have salivary glands, which secrete saliva consisting of mucus and a starch-digesting enzyme. Those species eating dry food such as seeds have many glands whereas those eating a wetter diet such as fish have very few.

Oesophagus and crop

Food passes down the muscular oesophagus on the right side of the neck into a diverticulum known as the crop. This lies outside the body cavity and is mainly used for food storage. Its size varies according to the species – granivorous birds have large, bilobular crops while species such as the insectivores and the owls have no crop. Some species, particularly members of the pigeon family, secrete 'crop milk' from the lining to feed their young. This is rich in proteins and fat and is stimulated by the hormone prolactin.

Stomach

The stomach is divided into two parts:
- Proventriculus – lined by an epithelium, which secretes mucus, hydrochloric acid and pepsin; here food is stored, mixed with these digestive juices and protein digestion begins.
- Gizzard – the walls are lined with bands of muscle that contract and expand to grind up the harder components of the diet such as seeds, bones and scales; in addition, many birds actively ingest small stones or grit to help with the physical breakdown of food in the gizzard.

Small intestine

Consists of a duodenum, jejunum and ileum that are not clearly delineated. The duodenum is the major site of digestion and absorption. The pancreas is relatively large and lies in the loop of the duodenum, pouring its secretions into the lumen of the duodenum via three ducts. The liver is bilobed; the right lobe is usually larger than the left.

Large intestine

Consists of a pair of blind-ending caeca, which lie at the junction of the small and large intestines. Their function seems to be associated with the bacterial fermentation of cellulose and the reabsorption of water, and their presence varies with the diet of the species. The rest of the large intestine, whose main role is concerned with water and mineral reabsorption, is the relatively short length between the small intestine and the cloaca.

Cloaca

This is the common exit from the body shared by the digestive, urinary and reproductive systems. It is divided into three parts:
- Coprodeum – anterior part, which receives faeces from the intestine
- Urodeum – middle part, which collects the discharge from the kidney and the reproductive system
- Proctodeum – posterior part, which collects and stores the discharges from all three systems. It is closed by a muscular anus, which controls the passage of 'bird droppings' or mutes and, in the case of the hen bird, the passage of eggs out of the body. In the wall of the cloaca is an area of lymphoid tissue known as the bursa of Fabricius.

URINARY SYSTEM

The function of the urinary system, which consists of a pair of kidneys and a pair of ureters but no bladder, is the same as that in the mammal. However, birds excrete nitrogenous waste in the form of uric acid and urates rather than the familiar mammalian urea. The waste materials are suspended in urinary water rather than being dissolved and the resulting semi-solid urine leaves the kidneys via the ureters. It enters the urodeum of the cloaca and then passes by retroperistalsis into the large intestine, where more water is reabsorbed. The resulting mutes consist of white urates, greeny-brown faeces surrounded by clear urine.

Birds, like reptiles, possess a renal portal system. This consists of a valve at the junction of the common iliac vein with the renal portal vein that enters the kidney. The valve consists of a muscular sphincter that opens and closes in response to nervous stimulation – when it is closed blood flows into the kidney and when it is open blood bypasses the kidney and flows into the caudal vena cava. This may be of significance when administering medication by injection to the caudal part of the body – the drug may be excreted by the kidneys without reaching the cranial parts of the body.

REPRODUCTIVE SYSTEM

Male

The two bean-shaped testes lie within the body cavity and are connected to the urodeum of the cloaca by the vas deferens. In many species the left testis is much larger than the right and in the non-breeding season both may be relatively small. The anatomy and physiology of the system is similar to that of mammals except that the seminal fluid needed to wash the sperm along the tract is produced by the testes rather than by accessory glands. At the distal end of each vas deferens is a seminal vesicle, which acts as a storage organ for the sperm prior to their use.

Sperm is transferred into the female vagina either by means of the grooved erectile penis attached to the wall of the cloaca in species such as geese, ducks, storks and flamingos or, as in most other species, by the male and female simply bringing their cloacae close together.

Female

The tract consists of a pair of ovaries and oviducts, which lead to the cloaca. In most species the right side is rudimentary and in the non-breeding season the left ovary may be quite small. The ovum is released by the ovary and begins to pass down the tubular oviduct, which is divided into several different parts:

- Infundibulum – funnel-shaped opening, which engulfs the ovum, preventing it falling into the body cavity; fertilisation takes place here and the first layer of albumen is added.
- Magnum – glandular part, which adds the remaining albumen.
- Isthmus – walls are lined by layers of thick circular muscle; inner and outer shell membranes are added.
- Uterus or shell gland – walls are lined by thick layers of longitudinal muscle lined with goblet cells; the egg spends as much as 15 hours in this part while the shell and any pigmentation is added.
- Vagina – mucus is secreted to aid egg laying and sperm from the male may also be stored for several days.

The female bird lays her eggs in a clutch and then begins incubation. The number within the clutch and the number of clutches per year varies with the species of bird. Many species lay one egg per day while others, such as ducks and geese, lay every other day. During incubation the eggs must be kept warm and damp – the average temperature is 35°C. The bird will also turn the eggs at regular intervals using her feet. This prevents the embryo from sticking to the side of the shell, which may impair the development of the chick. Incubation times vary with the species. Smaller birds have short incubation times: for example, many passerines hatch their eggs within 14–21 days, while larger birds such as hawks have an incubation time of around 30 days. The young may be described as being:

- **Nidicolous**, i.e. they are featherless and blind and dependent on the parent birds until fledged; for example, young pigeons (known as squabs), robins and sparrows
- **Nidifugous**, i.e. they are covered in down feathers, eat adult food and are capable of surviving away from their mother; for example, ducklings, goslings and chicks.

Reptiles

Reptiles are members of the class Reptilia and as such are cold-blooded vertebrates that breed on land. They are dependent on the external environment to raise their internal body temperature and increase their metabolic rate. To do this they alter their behaviour patterns and will seek out warm spots or flatten themselves on the ground in order to increase the surface area exposed to the sun.

There are about 6500 species, which can be classified into four separate orders:

- Rhynchocephalia – includes the tuatara, which is rare and unlikely to be encountered as a captive pet

- Crocodilia – crocodiles and alligators – rarely kept as pets
- Squamata – further divided into suborder Sauria (lizards), suborder Serpentes (snakes) and suborder Amphisbaenia, members of which are not kept in captivity
- Chelonia – shelled reptiles, which includes the tortoises, terrapins and turtles.

All the orders of reptiles have a common evolutionary pathway so they share many anatomical features. For the purposes of this book the common features will be described, followed by the notable characteristics of each group.

GENERAL ANATOMY

Skeletal system

Reptiles are vertebrates and have an internal skeleton that in most cases follows a similar pattern to that of the mammal.

Integument

Reptilian skin is covered in thick, keratinised protective scales. They grow by moulting or shedding this covering of scales in a process known as ecdysis. The underlying new skin is soft and enables the body to expand rapidly until the replacement scales harden. Snakes usually shed their skin in one piece, wriggling backwards out of it, whereas lizards shed their skin in several pieces, many of which may then be eaten. The integument of the chelonians is modified into a tough outer shell.

Cardiovascular system

All reptiles have a heart that comprises two atria and one ventricle. This is functionally divided into three subchambers and receives blood from both atria. Reptiles also possess a renal portal system that is similar to that seen in the bird. Blood from the hind legs and tail may drain directly into the kidneys, so any drug injected into the hind end may be excreted via the kidneys without circulating around the fore end.

Respiratory system

Reptiles use oxygen taken from atmospheric air. They possess lungs but they do not have a diaphragm so the body cavity is not divided into two. Gaseous exchange takes place in the same way that it does in the mammal.

Digestive tract

The anatomy of the digestive tract varies with the species and with the type of diet on which the animal depends. Many species possess a specialised olfactory organ in the roof of the oral cavity that is known as Jacobsen's organ. This is used in conjunction with the tongue, which 'tastes' the environment by flicking in and out of the mouth and is then drawn across the organ. Information is then conveyed to the brain via branches of the olfactory nerve. In all species the tract ends in a cloaca. As in the bird this is divided into the coprodeum to collect faeces, the urodeum to collect urinary waste and the proctodeum, which is the final collecting chamber before elimination of the combined waste.

Urinary system

The paired kidneys do not have loops of Henle, which means that the excreted urine is very dilute. Snakes do not possess a bladder but this is present in lizards and chelonians.

Reproductive system

All reptiles lay eggs, i.e. they are oviparous, and the yolk within the egg provides nourishment for the developing embryo. Some species of reptile are ovoviviparous, which means that they appear to give birth to live young. In fact the egg is retained within the oviduct and hatches to release the young. Nutrition is still supplied to the young via the yolk and not via a placenta, as happens in mammals.

LIZARDS

Most lizards (Fig. 7.10) have four legs, which are attached to the body at right angles and allow the body to be raised off the ground. The tail is well defined, and some species are able to shed their tail as a defence against predators. This process, known as autotomy, means that once the tail has been shed it continues to squirm, diverting the predator's attention while the lizard escapes.

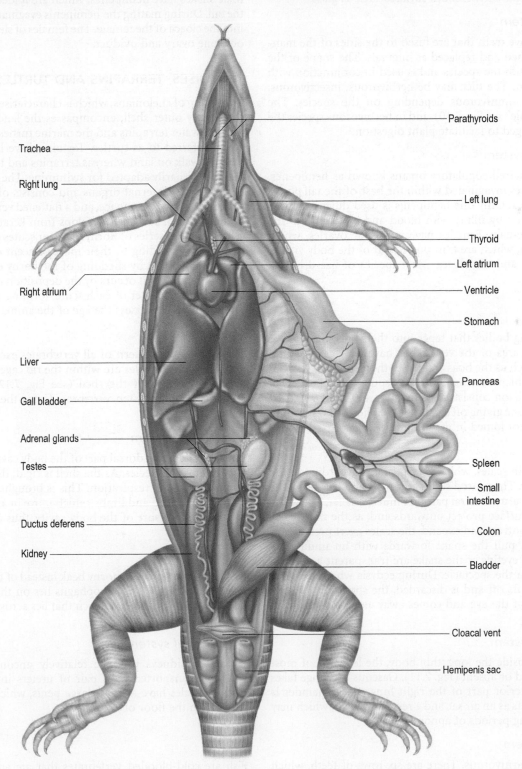

Parathyroids

Trachea

Right lung

Left lung

Thyroid

Left atrium

Right atrium

Ventricle

Stomach

Liver

Pancreas

Gall bladder

Adrenal glands

Testes

Spleen

Small intestine

Ductus deferens

Colon

Kidney

Bladder

Cloacal vent

Hemipenis sac

Fig. 7.10 Internal anatomy of the male lizard

The skin is thick and scaly and its texture varies according to the species. Some lizards, such as the skinks, have scales that fit tightly together, creating a smooth outline, while others are covered in much thicker and more protective scales. Species such as the chameleons have cells known as chromatophores within the skin that are able to alter the colour of the skin and thus camouflage the lizard. The gecko family has layers of overlapping scales on the underside of their feet which enable them to grip on to apparently smooth surfaces such as glass.

Digestive system

Most species have teeth that are fused to the sides of the mandible and are shed and replaced at intervals. The shape of the tongue varies with the species and is used in conjunction with Jacobsen's organ. The diet may be herbivorous, insectivorous, carnivorous or omnivorous depending on the species. The stomach is simple (see Fig. 7.10), and in herbivorous species the caecum is enlarged to facilitate plant digestion.

Urinogenital system

Males possess paired copulatory organs known as hemipenes, each of which lies invaginated within the base of the tail posterior to the cloaca. Only one hemipenis is used during mating, when it is erected by filling with blood and inserted into the cloaca of the female. Females have a pair of ovaries, which produce the ova, which are transported out of the body via the paired oviducts and the cloaca. Most species of lizard have a bladder.

SNAKES

Snakes have long bodies that taper into their tails, the start of which is in the area of the vent. They have no legs, although some species such as the boas and the pythons possess vestigial pelvic limbs, which are manifested as spurs on the external surface. The skeleton consists of as many as 400 similar-shaped vertebrae, each one giving off a pair of ribs. There is no sternum, so the ribs are not joined in the midline.

Integument

This is covered in scales, which vary in shape according to the area of the body. The ventral scales are larger and thicker, while those in the dorsal and lateral parts are much smaller. The scales on the ventral surface project outwards and, as the muscles of the body wall contract and expand, the scales exert pressure on the surface and pull the snake forwards with an undulating movement. The eyelids of the snake are transparent and fused together to form the spectacle. During ecdysis when the outer layer of scales lifts off and is discarded, the spectacle also lifts off the surface of the eye and comes away as part of the shed skin.

Respiratory system

In order to fit inside the long, thin body, the left lung of most snakes is reduced or absent (Fig. 7.11). Gaseous exchange takes place in the anterior part of the right lung; the remainder is avascular and acts as an air sac and a reservoir of air, which may be needed during periods of apnoea.

Digestive system

All snakes are carnivorous. There are six rows of teeth, which are fused to the mandibles and replaced continuously. Some species have modified fangs connected to poison glands above the oral cavity and used to inject venom into the prey. The forked tongue is used to 'taste' the environment and is used in conjunction with Jacobsen's organ. The stomach is elongated and the intestines are relatively short. The organs are arranged in an elongated fashion to fit into the thin body (see Fig. 7.11).

Urinogenital system

Male snakes have hemipenes, which are folded into the base of the tail. During mating the hemipenis evaginates and is inserted into the cloaca of the female. The females of slender species have only one ovary and oviduct.

TORTOISES, TERRAPINS AND TURTLES

This group of chelonians, which is characterised by the presence of a horny outer shell, encompasses the land-living tortoises, the freshwater terrapins and the marine turtles. In the USA they are all referred to as turtles. Tortoises have limbs that enable them to walk on land whereas terrapins and turtles have limbs that are primarily adapted for swimming. The shell forms a box to protect the internal organs and consists of a domed upper part, known as the carapace, and a flattened ventral part, known as the plastron. The shell develops from keratinised epidermal cells, forming a series of horny plates or scutes (Fig. 7.12), which are named according to their most adjacent organ. Growth is not brought about by shedding of the horny epidermis, as it is in other reptiles, but occurs by the deposition of epidermal cells around the perimeter of each scute, forming annual rings that can be counted to assess the age of the animal.

Skeletal system

This follows the pattern of all vertebrates except that the pectoral and pelvic girdles are within the rib cage and are directed vertically to support the shell (see Fig. 7.12). The vertebral column, comprising ten vertebrae, forms the undersurface of the carapace.

Respiratory system

The lungs lie in the dorsal part of the body cavity and aid buoyancy in aquatic species. As the shell is rigid, the body is unable to expand during respiration. This is brought about by movements of the head and limbs, which move in and out, changing the internal pressure of the body cavity, thus drawing air in or pushing it out.

Digestive system

All chelonians possess a horny beak instead of teeth. The tongue is large and fleshy. The oesophagus lies on the left side of the neck, entering a simple stomach that lies across the body cavity (see Fig. 7.12).

Urinogenital system

A pair of kidneys produce relatively unconcentrated urine, which is transported by a pair of ureters into a thin-walled bladder. Males have a single large penis, which is able to protrude from the floor of the cloaca.

Fish

Fish are cold-blooded vertebrates that are adapted to live in water, from which they extract the oxygen needed for their

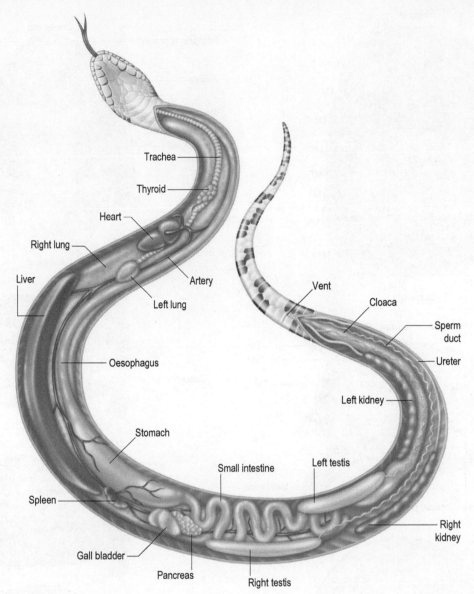

Fig. 7.11   Internal anatomy of the snake

metabolism. There are approximately 30 000 species of fish, which can be divided into two main groups:

- Cartilaginous fish – comprising the rays and sharks
- Bony fish – comprising all other species. These can be further subdivided into:
  - Lower teleosts, e.g. carp and salmon
  - Higher teleosts, e.g. perch and mackerel.

Although these bony fish show an enormous range of external shapes and sizes, they all have a similar basic anatomy.

EXTERNAL ANATOMY

Most species of fish have a typical fusiform shape that enables them to pass through the water with a minimum of energy expenditure. Most fish are covered in flexible, overlapping plates known as scales. Each scale is formed by and is embedded within the dermis, with the free edge covered in a thin layer of epidermis. The scales are covered in a layer of mucus called the glycocalyx, which reduces frictional drag as the fish swims and also has a fungicidal and bactericidal action. The scales contain

pigment cells that give the fish its colour and many species are able to change their colour to blend into the background.

The fish is able to swim, manoeuvre and maintain its balance in the water by the presence of flexible fins, which consist of a web of skin supported by bony or cartilaginous rays. Each fin is attached to muscle, enabling the fin to make rapid precise movements. Most fish have seven fins. These are the:

- Caudal fin or tail – shape indicates the swimming pattern
- Dorsal fin – set vertically along the back
- Anal fin – on the underside close to the tail; in some species this is adapted to form the gonopodium, which assists in internal fertilisation of the female
- A pair of pectoral fins – set on either side just behind the head
- A pair of pelvic fins – set just below and behind the pectoral fins.

Fish have the range of special senses seen in mammals but in addition they have a lateral line system. This is used to detect vibrations in the water caused by the presence of other fish, which might be prey or predators. It consists of a series of

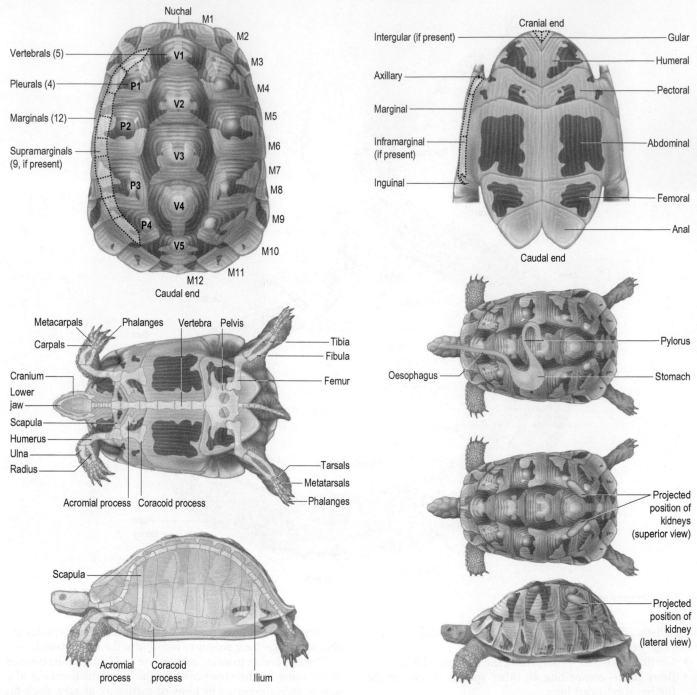

Fig. 7.12 Anatomy of the tortoise

shallow channels running over the surface of the body along the lateral midline. Along the line, arranged at intervals, are groups of hair cells embedded within a cup or cupula. Vibrations cause movement of the hairs, which stimulate nerve impulses, which reach the brain and the appropriate nerve impulse is initiated.

INTERNAL ANATOMY

Musculoskeletal system

Although the skeleton (Fig. 7.13) appears to be completely different from that of the mammal, it has similar components. The pectoral and pelvic girdles comprise the remnants of the

pentadactyl limb (five digits) seen in mammals, birds and reptiles and provide a key to the evolutionary pathway of the fish. The muscles of the body are arranged in blocks or myomeres attached on either side of the axial skeleton. They enable the body to flex laterally, providing the propulsive force to move forward. The number of vertebrae varies with the species. The ribs in the thoracic region articulate with the vertebrae and support the walls of the body cavity.

In order to maintain buoyancy in the water most bony fish possess a swim bladder, which lies just below the vertebral column within the body cavity. The specific gravity of the fish is greater than that of the surrounding water, so it sinks if it

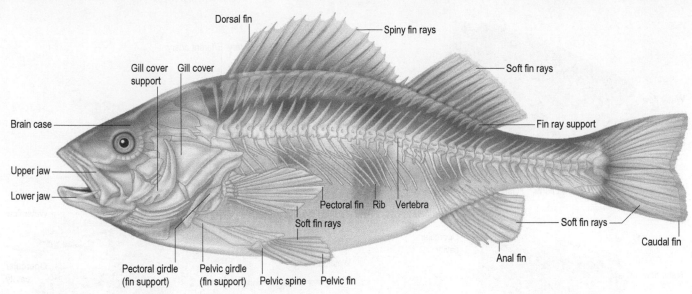

Fig. 7.13 Skeletal structure of a fish

stops swimming. This is overcome by altering the volume of gas within the swim bladder and the fish is able to rise or fall according to its needs. The structure of the swim bladder depends on the species of fish:

- Lower teleosts – the swim bladder is said to be physostomous and is a diverticulum of the foregut linked by a pneumatic duct. The swim bladder is refilled by the fish rising to the surface and taking a mouthful of air and is mainly seen in shallow water species.
- Higher teleosts – the swim bladder is said to be physoclistous. There is no connection between the swim bladder and the foregut and depending on the species it is either filled during larval development, when there may be a temporary connection, or it may be filled by specialised cells forming a gas gland within the sac. The secreted gas is mainly carbon dioxide and it is kept in the bladder by an impermeable lining.

In addition to its function as a buoyancy aid the swim bladder acts as resonator for sound, giving the fish a more acute sense of hearing than is provided by its inner ear.

Cardiovascular system

The heart is a long, folded organ consisting of a single atrium and a single ventricle. The circulation is described as being single because blood passes once through the heart in a complete circuit. This is compared to the double circulation of the mammal. Oxygenated blood leaves the ventricle and is pumped to the tissues, where it gives up its oxygen. The blood picks up carbon dioxide from the tissues and is carried to the gills, where it is excreted into the water. At the same time the blood picks up oxygen and is carried to the atrium of the heart.

Respiratory system

Fish breathe using a system of gills (Fig. 7.14). Each gill consists of a bony gill arch supporting the gill filaments. Projecting from these are delicate secondary filaments or lamellae, which contain the blood vessels through which gaseous exchange occurs. On each side of the pharynx are five lateral gill slits

through which water drawn in through the mouth passes. The entrance to each gill slit is 'guarded' by stiff projections known as gill rakers, which act as a screen to filter out food particles which could damage the delicate gills. On the external surface of the head the gills are covered by cartilaginous protective flaps or opercula (sing. operculum). Water is drawn in through the mouth by constant opening and closing, forced into the pharynx, over the gills and out through the opercula. Because of the difference in concentration between the gases in the blood and the water, oxygen dissolved in the water diffuses into the blood and carbon dioxide in the blood is released into the water.

Digestive system

This varies according to the diet of the species. Predatory species have teeth on the front and the roof of the mouth and they may also have throat teeth just in front of the oesophagus. These are mainly used to hold the prey and position it ready for swallowing head first. Some species have teeth for biting; some have teeth to rasp food from rocks; and some have no teeth at all. Ingested food travels down the oesophagus into a tube-like stomach and then into an intestine of uniform diameter. The length depends on the type of diet, herbivorous species having the longest intestine. Faeces are evacuated from the body via the rectum and anus.

Urinary system

The kidneys lie below the vertebral column and in some species may sit like a saddle over the swim bladder. They have several functions, e.g. haemopoiesis, excretion, osmoregulation and secretion of hormones. Nitrogenous waste is excreted in the form of ammonia, which is extremely toxic and is only excreted by organisms that live in a watery environment where it can flow away. The main site for excretion is the gills, not the kidneys as occurs in mammals.

Reproductive system

Among the huge number of fish species there are examples of a range of reproductive patterns, including parthenogenesis and

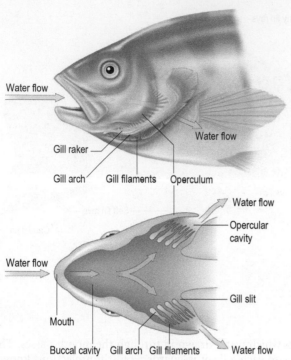

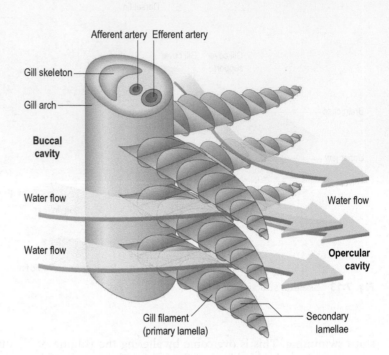

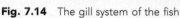

Fig. 7.14 The gill system of the fish

hermaphroditism. However, the majority of teleosts have separate sexes. Fertilisation may be:

- Internal – the male introduces the sperm into the female. She retains the fertilised eggs in her body until they hatch to produce live young.
- External – the female lays her eggs in the water and the male adds his sperm or milt in a process known as

spawning. Many of these eggs and sperm are lost so millions are produced. The eggs may then be scattered or deposited in a nest or in the mud on the river bed. Some species are mouth brooders and incubate the eggs in the mouth. This is often done by the male and once the young are hatched they may continue to use the mouth as a refuge from predators.

BIBLIOGRAPHY

Aspinall, V., O'Reilly, M., 2015. Introduction to Veterinary Anatomy and Physiology, third ed. Butterworth-Heinemann, Oxford.

Bowden, C., Masters, J. (Eds.), 2001. Pre-veterinary Nursing Textbook. Butterworth-Heinemann, Oxford.

Colville, T., Bassett, J.M., 2015. Clinical Anatomy and Physiology for Veterinary Technicians. Mosby, St Louis, MO.

Cooper, B., Mullineaux, E., Turner, L. (Eds.), 2012. BSAVA Textbook of Veterinary Nursing, fifth ed. British Small Animal Veterinary Association, Gloucester.

Cooper, J.E., 2002. Birds of Prey – Health and Disease. Blackwell Scientific Publications, Oxford.

Dyce, K.M., Sack, W.O., Wensing, C.J.G., 1996. Textbook of Veterinary Anatomy, second ed. W B Saunders, Philadelphia.

Girling, S., Raiti, P., 2004. Manual of Reptiles, second ed. British Small Animal Veterinary Association, Cheltenham.

Harcourt, B., Chitty, J. (Eds.), 2005. Manual of Psittacine Birds, second ed. British Small Animal Veterinary Association, Cheltenham.

Harvey Pough, F., Heiser, J.B., McFarland, W.N., 1993. Vertebrate Life, third ed. Macmillan, Basingstoke.

Hillyer, E.V., Quesenberry, K.E., 1997. Ferrets, Rabbits and Rodents – Clinical Medicine and Surgery. W B Saunders, Philadelphia, PA.

King, A.S., McClelland, J., 1984. Birds – Their Structure and Function. Baillière Tindall, London.

Laber-Laird, K., Swindle, M.M., Flecknell, P. (Eds.), 1996. Handbook of Rodent and Rabbit Medicine. Pergamon, Oxford.

McArthur, S., 1996. Veterinary Management of Tortoises and Turtles. Blackwell Science, Oxford.

Mader, D.R., 1996. Reptile Medicine and Surgery. W B Saunders, Philadelphia, PA.

Meredith, A., Johnson-Delaney, C. (Eds.), 2010. Manual of Exotic Pets, fifth ed. British Small Animal Veterinary Association, Quedgeley.

Meredith, A., Lord, B. (Eds.), 2014. Manual of Rabbit Medicine. British Small Animal Veterinary Association, Quedgeley.

Okerman, L., 1994. Diseases of Domestic Rabbits. Blackwell Scientific, Oxford.

Phillips, W.D., Chilton, T.J., 1989. A-level Biology. Oxford University Press, Oxford.

Roberts, R.J. (Ed.), 2001. Fish Pathology, third ed. W B Saunders, Philadelphia, PA.

Sturkie, P.D. (Ed.), 1976. Avian Physiology. Springer Verlag, New York.

Warren Dean, M., 1995. Small Animal Care and Management. Delmar, New York.

Wildgoose, W. (Ed.), 2001. Manual of Ornamental Fish, second ed. British Small Animal Veterinary Association, Gloucester.

RECOMMENDED READING

Aspinall, V., Capello, M., 2015. Introduction to Veterinary Anatomy and Physiology, third ed. Butterworth-Heinemann, Oxford.

This book provides three chapters on comparative exotic animal anatomy and physiology, and in the third edition there is a new chapter on farm animal anatomy.

Bowden, S., 2012. Introduction to Veterinary Anatomy and Physiology – Workbook. Butterworth-Heinemann, Oxford.

Fun way to revise your knowledge of exotic anatomy using a wide variety of games and tests.

Colville, T., Bassert, J.M., 2015. Clinical Anatomy and Physiology for Veterinary Technicians, third ed. Mosby, London.

Very detailed coverage of the anatomy of the bird.

Cooper, B., Mullineaux, E., Turner, L. (Eds.), 2012. BSAVA Textbook of Veterinary Nursing, fifth ed.

British Small Animal Veterinary Association, Gloucester.

New chapter on exotic anatomy.

Hillyer, E.V., Quesenberry, K.E., 2012. Ferrets, Rabbits and Rodents – Clinical Medicine and Surgery, third ed. W B Saunders, Philadelphia, PA.

Each section begins with detailed descriptions of the relevant anatomy and physiology.

8

Equine Anatomy and Physiology

CATHERINE PHILLIPS

KEY POINTS

- All species of horse belong to the class Mammalia and as such they have much in common with other mammals, e.g. respiratory system, urinary system, structure of the integument, etc.

- The horse has evolved the ability to run fast for long distances and this is reflected in the anatomy and physiology of its skeleton and muscular system.

- Horses are adapted to eating relatively poor-quality roughage over long periods of the day and this is reflected in the anatomy and physiology of their digestive tract.

Introduction

In Chapter 6 we looked at the anatomy and physiology of the dog and cat, which, as they are mammals, show many similarities to those of the horse so in this chapter we will only look at the systems in which there are differences.

The horse has evolved from a small multi-toed animal, *Eohippus,* into the creature that we know today with a specialised digestive tract to allow the consumption of grass and grains and a single-digit elongated limb which enables the horse to make a rapid escape from predators. Knowledge and understanding of these complex anatomical and physiological structures are essential to allow us to plan the management and nursing of this species.

The skeletal system

The skeleton (Fig. 8.1) can be divided into two main sections:
- The axial skeleton – made up of the skull, vertebral column, ribcage and pelvis
- The appendicular skeleton – made up of the bones of the limbs.

The skeleton is a framework of hard structures creating strength and rigidity that will support and protect the soft tissues, facilitate movement and allow locomotion. Note that there is no splanchnic skeleton in the horse as there is in the dog and cat.

THE AXIAL SKELETON

The skull

The skull is constructed of a large number of bones joined by fibrous joints or sutures that allow little movement between them (Fig. 8.2). The main function of the skull is to protect the brain, inner ear, parts of the eye and nasal passages.

The major part of this structure comprises the following bones:
- The mandible (the lower jaw)
- The maxilla, incisive and palatine bones (the upper jaw, hard palate and base of the nasal cavity)
- The nasal bone (completing the nasal cavity)
- The frontal bone (forming the rostral section of the cranium)
- The supraorbital process (supporting and protecting the eye)
- The temporal bone (containing and protecting the middle ear)
- The occipital bone (forming the back of the skull)
- The hyoid bones (constitutes the apparatus that supports the guttural pouches, pharynx, larynx and base of the tongue).

The nasal septum divides the nasal cavity into two nasal chambers and a bony, membranous septum divides the maxillary sinus into rostral and caudal compartments. The maxillary sinus communicates with the nasal cavity through an opening into the middle nasal meatus.

Teeth. Dental formula:

Deciduous teeth – (I3/3 PM3/3) × 2 = 24

Permanent teeth – (I3/3 C1/1 PM3/3 or 4/3 M3/3) × 2 = 40 or 42

The roots of premolar teeth 4 and molar 1 extend into the rostral maxillary sinus and the last two cheek teeth, i.e. molars 2 and 3, communicate with the floor of the caudal maxillary sinus. If these teeth suffer injury or infection, then infection of the sinus may also occur.

The horse has hypsodontic teeth, i.e. they do not have a surface covering of enamel and they are all of the same height (Fig. 8.3). This creates an abrasive surface necessary for the grinding up of plant material and includes vast reserve crowns that allow the teeth to continually grow for some years, ensuring a long working life. As the horse chews, the occlusal surfaces are worn down by about 2–3 mm a year. The extent of wear and the appearance of the occlusal surface of the tooth can be used to identify the approximate age of the horse (Fig. 8.4).

Canine teeth may not be present or may be vestigial in the mare. The wolf tooth is a small upper premolar that is often extracted to prevent interference with the bit during training.

The vertebral column

The vertebral column (see Fig. 8.1) is made up of groups of vertebra as seen in the dog and cat. The functions of the vertebra are to house the spinal cord, support the skull and thorax and provide attachment for the pelvis and insertion of many of the muscles.

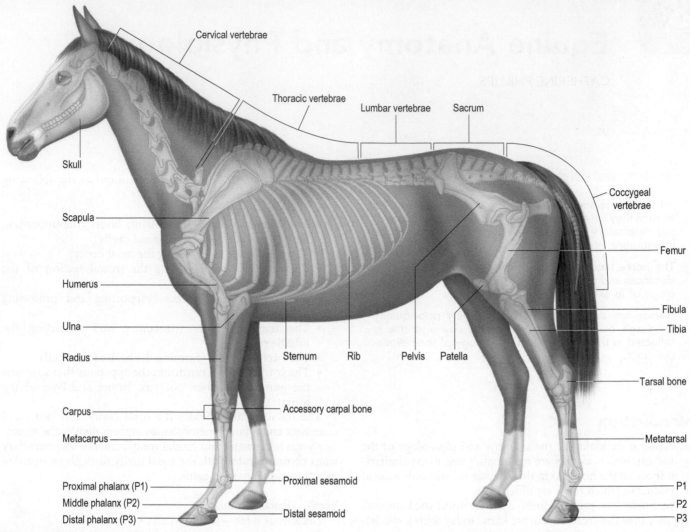

Fig. 8.1   Skeleton of the horse

There are five different types of vertebra (Fig. 8.5), making up the column as follows:

- Cervical vertebrae – 7 bones, the first 2 being the atlas and axis
- Thoracic vertebrae – 18 bones
- Lumbar vertebrae – 6 bones, occasionally 5 or 7 are found in some Arabian horses
- Sacral vertebrae – 5 bones, fused to form a triangular sacrum
- Coccygeal vertebrae – 15–20 (average 18 bones), sometimes called caudal vertebra.

The vertebral formula may be quoted as follows: C7 T18 L6 S5 Cd15–20.

The ribs

The horse has eighteen pairs of ribs – the first eight pairs are described as being true, as they articulate directly with the sternum. The remaining ribs are false or asternal, as they articulate with the rib in front to form the costal arch.

The sternum

The sternum forming the ventral surface of the thorax is composed of seven sternebrae. The first sternebra is called the manubrium and the terminal segment is called the xiphoid process or xiphisternum.

THE APPENDICULAR SKELETON

This comprises the limbs, which have been adapted to allow great leverage for the application of speed, and the bony girdles that attach them to the body.

The fore limb

This is attached to the trunk by means of the scapula (see Fig. 8.1), which in turn is attached by strong muscles.

The fore limb (Fig. 8.6) comprises the following bones running from proximal to distal:

- The scapula (shoulder blade)
- The humerus
- The ulna and radius
- The proximal row of carpal bones (medial to lateral) – radial carpal bone, intermediate carpal bone, ulnar carpal bone, accessory carpal bone (Fig. 8.7)
- The distal row of carpal bones (medial to lateral) – first carpal bone (may be absent), second carpal bone, third carpal bone, fourth carpal bone

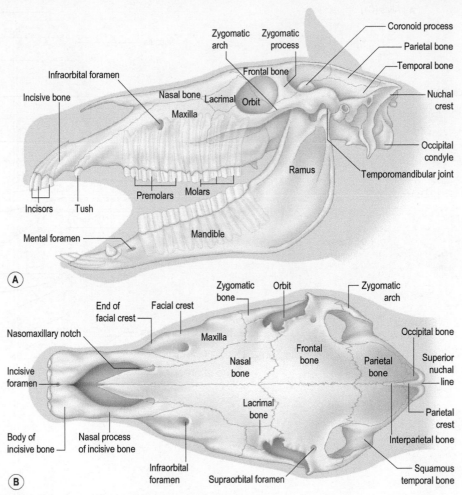

Fig. 8.2 The equine skull. (A) Lateral view. (B) Dorsal view.

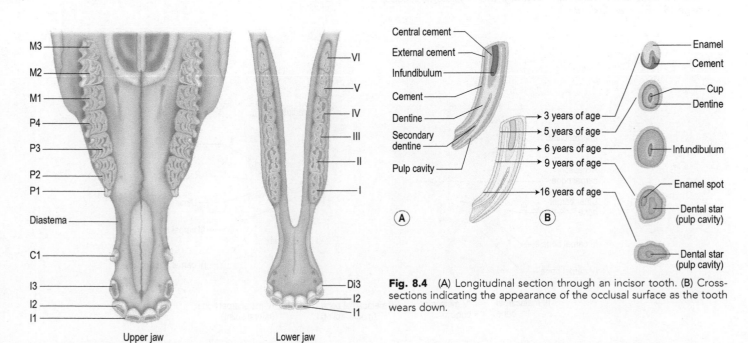

Fig. 8.3 Teeth in the jaw of a 4½-year-old horse

Fig. 8.4 (A) Longitudinal section through an incisor tooth. (B) Cross-sections indicating the appearance of the occlusal surface as the tooth wears down.

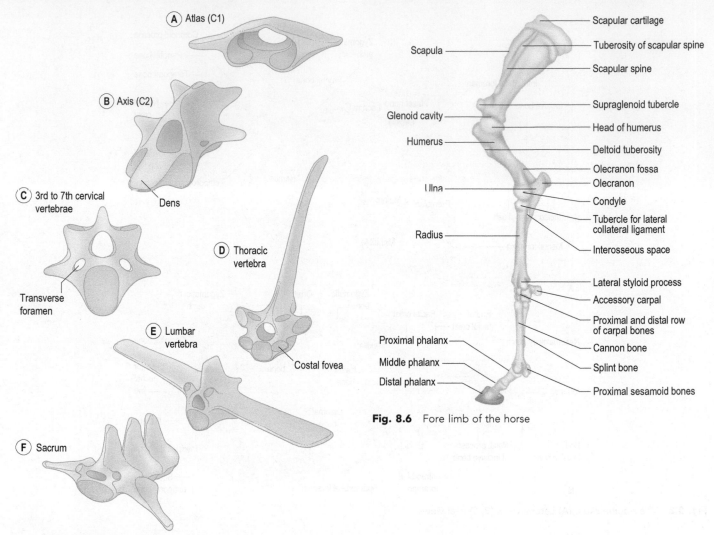

(A) Atlas (C1)

(B) Axis (C2)

Dens

(C) 3rd to 7th cervical vertebrae

Transverse foramen

(D) Thoracic vertebra

(E) Lumbar vertebra

Costal fovea

(F) Sacrum

Fig. 8.5 The shape of each vertebral type – *from Aspinall, V., Capello, M., 2009. Introduction to Veterinary Anatomy and Physiology, second ed., page 192. Elsevier, Oxford.*

Scapular cartilage

Scapula

Tuberosity of scapular spine

Scapular spine

Supraglenoid tubercle

Glenoid cavity

Head of humerus

Humerus

Deltoid tuberosity

Olecranon fossa

Ulna

Olecranon

Condyle

Tubercle for lateral collateral ligament

Radius

Interosseous space

Lateral styloid process

Accessory carpal

Proximal and distal row of carpal bones

Proximal phalanx

Cannon bone

Middle phalanx

Splint bone

Distal phalanx

Proximal sesamoid bones

Fig. 8.6 Fore limb of the horse

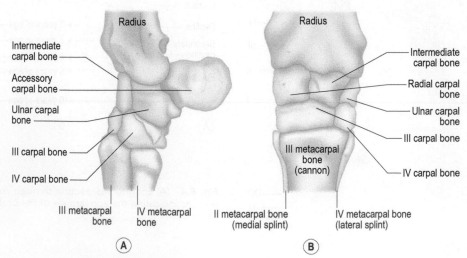

Radius

Radius

Intermediate carpal bone

Intermediate carpal bone

Accessory carpal bone

Radial carpal bone

Ulnar carpal bone

Ulnar carpal bone

III carpal bone

III carpal bone

III metacarpal bone (cannon)

IV carpal bone

IV carpal bone

III metacarpal bone

IV metacarpal bone

II metacarpal bone (medial splint)

IV metacarpal bone (lateral splint)

(A)

(B)

Fig. 8.7 Left carpus of the horse. (A) Lateral view. (B) Dorsal view.

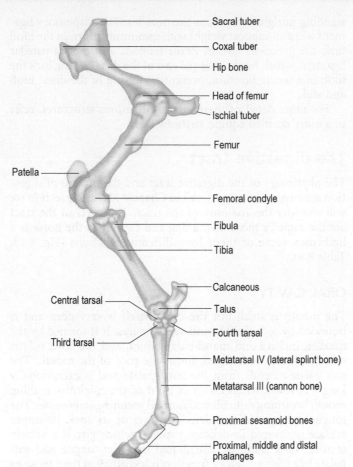

Fig. 8.8 Hind limb of the horse

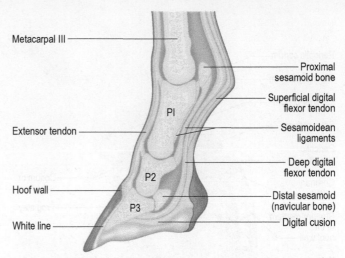

Fig. 8.9 Lateral view of the distal part of the fore limb

- The metacarpal bones (medial to lateral) – second metacarpal bone, third metacarpal bone, fourth metacarpal bone. The second and fourth metacarpal bones are also called medial and lateral splint bones, respectively.
- The medial and lateral proximal sesamoid bones
- Proximal phalanx (P1, long pastern)
- Middle phalanx (P2, short pastern)
- Distal sesamoid bone (navicular bone)
- Distal phalanx (P3, pedal bone).

The hind limb

This is attached to the body by means of the pelvic girdle, which is made up of three fused bones:
- Ilium
- Ischium
- Pubis.

The hind limb (Fig. 8.8) comprises the following bones, running from proximal to distal:
- The femur
- The patella
- The tibia and fibula
- The calcaneus
- The talus
- The central tarsal bone
- The first and second tarsal bones – fused
- The third tarsal bone
- The fourth tarsal bone

- The second metatarsal bone – also known as the medial splint bone
- The third metatarsal bone
- The fourth metatarsal bone – also known as the lateral splint bone
- The medial and lateral proximal sesamoid bones – found on the plantar surface
- Proximal phalanx (P1, long pastern)
- Middle phalanx (P2, short pastern)
- Distal sesamoid bone (navicular bone)
- Distal phalanx (P3, pedal bone).

The foot

The equine foot has a bony base that consists of the distal half of the middle phalanx (short pastern), the complete distal phalanx (pedal bone) and the distal sesamoid (navicular bone) (Fig. 8.9). Several important soft-tissue structures are also housed within the foot, including the digital cushion and the navicular bursa. Covering this is a highly vascular modified dermis called the corium, which is named according to the insensitive structures that it underlies, i.e. perioplic corium, corium of the frog, corium of the sole, etc. (Fig. 8.10). The hoof is the insensitive cornified layer of epidermis that covers the distal end of the digit. The insensitive structures of the hoof include the periople, wall, bars, laminae, sole and frog. These are all produced by the germinative layer of the epidermis, which lies close to the corium of the same name, which is well supplied with blood capillaries and nerve fibres (see Fig. 8.10).

Joints of the fore and hind limbs

The joints of the limbs are extremely important if the horse is going to be able to move fast. Table 8.1 summarises the anatomy of the major joints of both limbs.

The muscular system

The muscular system brings about movement of the horse. Muscles are often found in pairs, working together with opposite actions, e.g. flexion and extension, which creates coordinated movement and balance (Table 8.2).

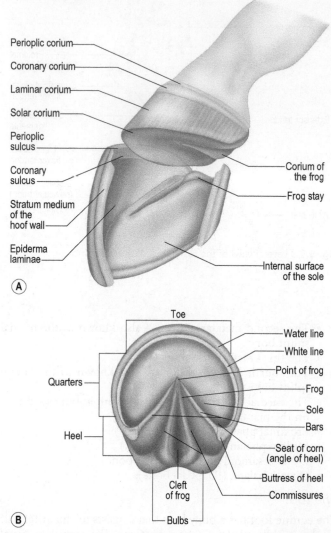

Fig. 8.10 The hoof. **(A)** Dissected view of the relationships of the hoof to the underlying regions of the corium. **(B)** Weight-bearing surface.

THE SUSPENSORY APPARATUS

The suspensory apparatus consists of a collection of ligaments connected with the proximal sesamoid bones in both the fore and hind limb, as follows:

- Suspensory ligament
- Intersesamoidean ligament
- Collateral sesamoidean ligament
- Distal sesamoidean ligaments.

This apparatus acts to suspend and support the fetlock joints and prevent overextension and collapsing of the limb. The suspensory apparatus also forms part of the stay apparatus (Fig. 8.12).

THE STAY APPARATUS

The stay apparatus consists of an arrangement of muscles, tendons and ligaments in both the fore and hind limbs that allows the horse to stand and sleep while using minimum muscular effort (see Fig. 8.12). The apparatus locks the joints in position so that they can bear the weight of the body for long periods. The flexor tendons allow extension to a certain point, in combination with the check ligament to take the work of

standing upright away from the muscles. The suspensory ligament will also support weight with minimum effort. In the hind limb the peroneus tertius, flexor tendons and medial patellar ligament, which hooks over the end of the distal femur, lock the limb in a secure position, preventing flexing of the distal limb and stifle.

For more detail of these vital ligamentous structures, refer to a more detailed equine anatomy text.

The digestive tract

The physiology of the digestive tract and the process of digestion are covered in more detail in Chapter 11. In this section we will consider the anatomy of the tract. The parts of the tract are the same as those of the dog and cat but as the horse is a herbivore, some of them have different functions (Fig. 8.13, Table 8.3).

ORAL CAVITY

The mouth is small but the cavity itself is very deep and is bounded by soft, flexible and sensitive lips. It is formed by the maxilla, incisive and mandibular bones, and the hard palate, which is broad and ridged, forms the roof of the mouth. The soft palate extends from the hard palate and is exceptionally long – at rest it hangs down in front of the epiglottis, making mouth breathing difficult and normal vomiting impossible. The tongue is long and broadens out towards its apex. Its upper surface is covered in delicate papillae, which give it a velvety texture. Taste buds are distributed over the tongue and soft palate but their gustatory function is less efficient than those of the dog and cat. Teeth have been covered within the skeletal system.

PHARYNX

The pharynx lies entirely within the skull. Part of the roof and the lateral walls are enveloped by the guttural pouches, which are found only in the horse. They are large caudo-ventral diverticula of the auditory tube that connect the nasopharynx to the middle ear. Several large and vital blood vessels, e.g. internal carotid artery, and cranial nerves, e.g. glossopharyngeal (IX) and vagus (X), run over their surface. They are lined with mucous membrane and mucus drains from them into the pharynx – the normal downwards position of the head during grazing promotes drainage.

The pharynx is divided into the upper nasopharynx and lower oropharynx by the soft palate. The walls of the oropharynx contain diffuse areas of lymphoid tissue. The function of the pharynx, which acts as a crossover point between the digestive and respiratory systems, is similar to that of the cat and the dog. During swallowing, the back of the tongue raises and pushes the food material against the hard palate while the laryngeal entrance to the respiratory tract is covered with the epiglottis. The movement of these structures creates pressure within the pharynx and the food is forced into the oesophagus. Peristalsis pushes the food material towards the stomach.

OESOPHAGUS

The oesophagus is located close to the trachea on the ventral surface of the neck and slightly to the left of the trachea. The

TABLE 8.1	Joints of the fore and hind limbs of the horse	
	Fore limb	**Hind limb**
Shoulder joint	Consists of the glenoid cavity of the scapula and head of the humerus	
Elbow joint	Consists of the condyles of the humerus, radius and ulna	
Carpal joints (knee)	1. Radiocarpal joint – radius and proximal row of carpal bones 2. Midcarpal joint – proximal and distal row of carpal bones 3. Carpometacarpal joint – distal row carpal bones and metacarpal bones 2–4	
Metacarpophalangeal joint (fetlock) or metatarsophalangeal joint	Metacarpal bone III or metatarsal bone III, proximal phalanx P1, medial and lateral proximal sesamoid bones	
Proximal interphalangeal joint (pastern)	Proximal phalanx P1 and middle phalanx P2	
Distal interphalangeal joint (coffin)	Middle phalanx P2, distal phalanx P3 and distal sesamoid bone (navicular)	
Hip joint		Ilium, pubis, ischium all combine to form the acetabulum, head of femur
Stifle joint		1. Femorotibial joint – femur and the medial and lateral condyles of the tibia 2. Femoropatellar joint – femoral trochlea with the patella
Tarsal joint (hock; Fig. 8.11)		1. Tarsocrural joint – cochlea of tibia with trochlea of talus 2. Proximal intertarsal joint – talus and calcaneus with central and fourth tarsal bones 3. Distal intertarsal joint – central tarsal with I–III tarsals 4. Tarsometatarsal joint – I–IV tarsals with II–IV metatarsals

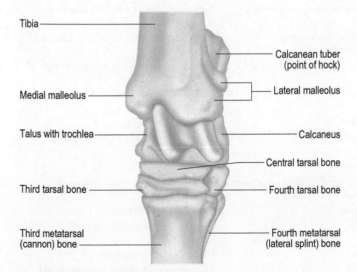

Fig. 8.11 Dorsal view of the left hock

structure passes through the mediastinum and oesophageal hiatus into the stomach.

STOMACH

The stomach is a small, J-shaped organ and food enters from the oesophagus via the cardiac sphincter. The oesophageal region of the stomach is similar to the oesophagus in that it does not contain secretory glands. The cardiac and pyloric gland regions contain digestive and mucus glands to initiate the process of protein digestion. The exit of the stomach is via the pyloric sphincter, which controls the flow of stomach contents into the small intestine.

SMALL INTESTINE

The small intestine (see Fig. 8.13) is a tube which is approximately 22 m in length divided into three regions:
- Duodenum
- Jejunum
- Ileum.

The bile and pancreatic ducts empty into the duodenum close to the pyloric sphincter. The ileum is the terminal section of the small intestine, joining with the caecum of the large intestine at the ileocaecal junction.

LARGE INTESTINE

The horse has the largest and most complex large intestine of all domestic animals (Fig. 8.14). It has an enormous capacity and consists of the:
- Caecum
- Colon
- Rectum.

The walls of the caecum and colon are characteristically sacculated by the presence of bands of muscle and elastic fibres. In

TABLE 8.2	Important muscles, ligaments and tendons of the equine muscular system		
Muscle/ligament/tendon	**Origin**	**Insertion**	**Action**
Rhomboideus	Nuchal ligament	Medial scapula	Lifts head and pulls scapula forward and up
Brachiocephalicus	Cranial cervical vertebra	Shoulder to humerus	Protraction of limb, extends shoulder, bending of head and neck
Sternocephalicus	Sternum	Mandible	Moves the head and neck
Splenius	Base of skull	Beginning of trapezius muscle	Lifts head and bends neck
Trapezius	Occipital bone and vertebra C7–T10	Spine of the scapula	Pulls shoulder forward and backward in addition to upward movement
Latissimus dorsi	Lower thoracic and lumbar vertebrae	Caudal humerus	Flexes the shoulder and retracts the fore limb
Longissimus dorsi	Ilium, sacrum and thoracic spine	Cervical spine 4–7, lumbar and thoracic vertebrae, ribs	Raises and supports head lateroflexion and extension of the back
Nuchal ligament	Skull	Cranial thoracic spine	Aids muscles of the neck to support the head
Deltoid	Scapula	Proximal humerus	Flexes and abducts shoulder
Supraspinatus	Below the trapezius	Point of the shoulder	Maintains shoulder extension
Pectoral	Sternum and ribs 1–4	Humerus and scapula	Protracts, retracts and adducts limb
Triceps brachii	Scapula and humerus	Olecranon	Extends the elbow
Biceps brachii	Distal scapula	Radius	Flexes the elbow
Extensor carpi radialis	Humerus	Metacarpals	Extends carpus and flexes elbow
Flexor carpi radialis	Humerus	Metacarpal III	Flexes carpus and extends elbow
Common digital extensor tendon	Distal humerus	P1–P3	Extension of P1–P3, carpus and flexion of elbow
Lateral digital extensor tendon (fore limb)	Lateral aspect of the elbow	P1	Extension P1–P3 and carpus
Superficial digital flexor tendon (fore limb)	Medial humerus and posterior radius	Distal P1 and proximal P2	Flexion of P1–P3 and carpus, extension of the elbow
Deep digital flexor tendon (fore limb)	Medial humerus and olecranon	Palmar aspect of P3	Flexion of P1–P3 and carpus and extension of the elbow
Long digital extensor tendon	Distal femur	Dorsal proximal aspects of P1–P3	Extension of distal P1–P3 and flexion of hock
Lateral digital extensor tendon (hind limb)	Lateral stifle and proximal tibia	Long extensor tendon mid metacarpal III	Extension of distal limb and flexion of hock
Superficial digital flexor tendon (hind limb)	Distal femur	Tuber calcis, proximal and distal P2	Flexion of distal limb and extension of hock
Deep digital flexor tendon (hind limb)	Proximal tibia	Palmar aspect P3	Flexion of distal limb and extension of hock
Intercostal muscles	Between ribs	Between ribs	Aids breathing
External and internal abdominal oblique	Ribs	Pelvic bones	Supports internal organs and aids breathing
Superficial gluteal	Tuber coxae	Proximal femur	Hip flexion
Biceps femoris	Sacroiliac ligament, and tuber ischii	Distal femur, patella, tibia crest and tuber calcis	Extension of hip, stifle and hock
Semitendinosus	Tuber ischii and tail base	Proximal tibia	Extends hip and hock
Semimembranosus	Tuber ischii and sacrosciatic ligament	Distal femur	Extends hip and adducts limb
Gastrocnemius	Caudal femur	Point of hock	Maintains hip extension
Peroneus tertius	Femur	Metatarsal III	Flexion of hock when stifle in flexion
Achilles tendon	Distal gastrocnemius	Point of the hock	See Gastrocnemius
Radial check ligament	Distal radius	Proximal superficial flexor tendon	See Superficial digital flexor tendon
Carpal check ligament	Distal carpus	Proximal deep digital flexor tendon	See Deep digital flexor tendon
Tarsal check ligament	Distal tarsus	Proximal deep digital flexor tendon	See Deep digital flexor tendon
Suspensory ligament	Proximal palmar metacarpus	Dorsal extensor tendon at the level of distal P2	Suspends and supports fetlock joint

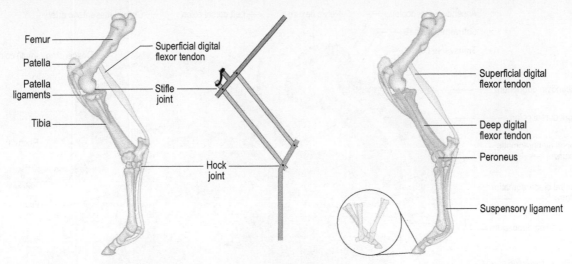

Fig. 8.12 The stay apparatus and the suspensory apparatus of the hind limb. There is a similar mechanism in the fore limb.

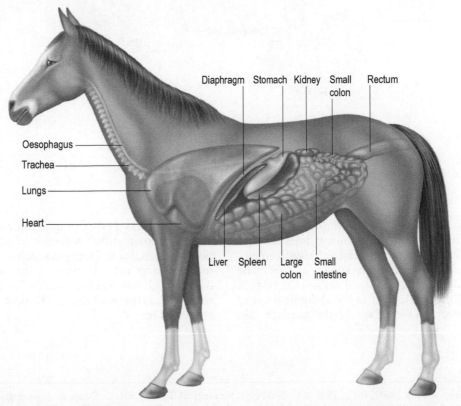

Fig. 8.13 Left lateral view of the equine digestive tract

TABLE 8.3	Size and function of the parts of the equine digestive tract	
Structure	**Approximate length or capacity**	**Function**
Oesophagus	1.5 m	Passage of food from mouth to stomach at approximately 35–40 cm per second
Stomach	18 l	Mixing of food with acids, enzymes and mucus; protein digestion
Small intestine	22 m, 64 l	Absorption of nutrients, breakdown of non-fibrous material and addition of pancreatic juices and bile
Caecum	1 m, 30 l	Microbial fibre breakdown into fatty acids and absorption of water
Large colon	3.5 m	Continuation of microbial breakdown of fibre, absorption of water and nutrients
Small colon	2.5 m	Absorption of water and nutrients
Rectum	0.5 m	Transfer of faeces through anus as excreta

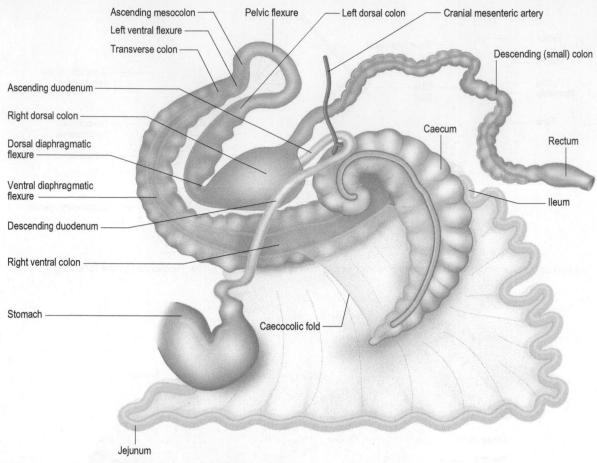

Fig. 8.14 Diagrammatic representation of the equine digestive tract

order that the large intestine can fit into the relatively small abdominal cavity of the horse it is folded many times and this predisposes to various types of obstruction and displacement, which lead to the group of conditions known as colic. The caecum is a blind-ending, comma-shaped organ that extends from the right side of the pelvic inlet to the abdominal cavity floor just behind the xiphoid cartilage of the sternum (see Fig. 8.14). It has a capacity of about 30 litres. It leads into the ascending colon at the caecocolic orifice. The colon is divided into the ascending and transverse colon, which are often referred to as the large colon because of their diameter, and then the descending colon, which is long and arranged in coils and often referred to as the small colon. The descending colon terminates at the rectum.

BIBLIOGRAPHY

Budras, K.-D., Sack, W.O., Röck, S., et al., 2001. The Equine Veterinary Nursing Manual. Blackwell Science, Oxford.

Budras, K.-D., Sack, W.O., Röck, S., et al., 2003. Anatomy of the Horse, fourth ed. Schlütersche, Hanover.

Dyce, K.M., Sack, W.O., Wensing, C.J.G., 2002. Textbook of Veterinary Anatomy and Physiology, third ed. W B Saunders, Philadelphia, PA.

Frandson, R.D., Spurgeon, T.L., 1992. Anatomy and Physiology of Farm Animals, fifth ed. Lea & Febiger, Philadelphia, PA.

Sisson, S., Grossman, J.D., 1969. Anatomy of the Domestic Animals, fourth ed. W B Saunders, Philadelphia, PA.

RECOMMENDED READING

Aspinall, V., Capello, M., 2015. Introduction to Veterinary Anatomy and Physiology, third ed. Elsevier, Oxford.
    This new edition includes a chapter on equine anatomy and physiology.

Aspinall, V., Capello, M., Bowden, S., 2012. Introduction to Veterinary Anatomy and Physiology – Workbook. Elsevier, Oxford.

    This provides a fun way of revising anatomy and physiology.

Dyce, K.M., Sack, W.O., Wensing, C.J.G., 2009. Textbook of Veterinary Anatomy and Physiology, fourth ed. W B Saunders, Philadelphia, PA.
    Provides an excellent detailed section on the horse.

Sisson, S., Grossman, J.D., 1969. Anatomy of the Domestic Animals, fourth ed. W B Saunders, Philadelphia, PA.
    Old-fashioned but very detailed text and photographs.

Canine and Feline Nutrition

ALISON JONES | NICOLA ACKERMAN

KEY POINTS

- Nutrients are divided into six classes – protein, fat, carbohydrates, minerals, vitamins and water – and these essential nutrients must be present in the correct proportions if an animal is to remain healthy.

- Each of the food classes has a specific function within the metabolic processes of the body.

- Animals have a basic energy requirement, which satisfies the energy used in sleep, and a maintenance energy requirement, which satisfies the energy used in moderate activity.

- Pet food for dogs and cats is available as home-made diets and commercial diets, which in turn are available as wet (including canned, trays and pouches), semi-moist and dry foods.

- The nutritional demands of the different life stages of an animal, e.g. puppy/kitten, pregnancy and old age, must be satisfied by specifically designed diets.

Introduction

The correct diet is vital in maintaining health and in the management of disease. Understanding nutrition and its role in both health and disease is an important skill for all qualified veterinary nurses, and your advice will frequently be sought by your clients.

Domesticated dogs have little opportunity to select their own diet, so it is important to realise that they are solely dependent upon their owners to provide all the nourishment they require. Pet cats are less reliant on their owners' dietary selection as they are able, through hunting, to supplement their diet. This chapter will explain the principal components of healthy nutrition to allow you to recommend a balanced diet which avoids both nutritional excess and deficiency. It will look at the practical feeding of dogs and cats of all ages, while giving you an insight into the key nutritional differences between dogs and cats as well as the different types of pet food available commercially.

Before any nutritional recommendation is given, it is important to look at the full diet history and to take a nutritional assessment of the animal (see Chapter 10 for more details).

Essential nutrition

Dogs have a common ancestry with, and are still often classified as, carnivores, although from a nutritional point of view they are actually omnivores. This means that dogs can obtain all the essential nutrients that they need from dietary sources consisting of either animal or plant material. The same is not true for domesticated cats, which are still obligate carnivores.

A nutrient is any food component that helps support life. Any nutrient required by the animal that cannot be synthesised in the body is called an essential nutrient. It must be present in the diet. If any essential nutrient is missing or present in too low a level then the diet as a whole is inadequate.

Nutrients are divided into six basic classes:
- Protein
- Fat
- Carbohydrates
- Minerals
- Vitamins
- Water.

WATER

Water is the most important nutrient of all, and even small losses can cause clinical signs (Table 9.1). Animals can lose almost all their fat and half their protein and still survive. Good-quality clean water should always be available except when an animal is persistently vomiting, when temporarily withholding oral fluid intake may be advised, or if water deprivation tests are being undertaken. Water intake increases with habit, behavioural changes (polydipsia due to pain), increased salt intake and clinical signs that increase water losses – bleeding, diarrhoea, polyuria, lactation or increased body temperature. The amount of water animals should consume per day in millilitres is roughly equivalent to their daily energy intake in kilocalories. Many texts quote 20–70 ml/kg of body weight per day; polydipsia is defined when the cat's or dog's intake is greater than 100 ml/kg/day.

ENERGY

In addition to providing specific nutrients, food also provides energy. The energy content of the diet is derived solely from the fats, proteins and carbohydrates, and the proportion of these energy-producing nutrients in the diet will determine its energy content (also referred to as the energy density).

All living cells require energy, and the more active they are the more energy they use. Individual animals have unique energy needs, which can vary, even between members of the same breed, age, sex and activity level. Breeders will recognise the scenario in which some littermates develop differently, one tending towards obesity, another on the lean side, even when they are fed exactly the same amount of food. If your clients are feeding a commercially prepared food, you should be aware that the feeding guide recommended by the manufacturer is also based on average energy needs, and therefore you may need to increase or decrease the amount you recommend to meet the individual pet's requirements. Some food manufacture companies print the energy density on the packaging or have this information readily available if required.

When considering different foods, it is important to compare the metabolisable energy (ME),which is the amount of energy in the food that is available to a pet; this is normally measured in kcal/100 g of food fed. If requesting energy density of the food, some companies will provide you with figures for the gross energy. Gross energy is not as useful because some of that energy (sometimes a substantial amount) will not be available to the animal due to the digestibility of the food (Fig 9.1).

Water has no energy value, and so a diet with a high moisture content will contain a lower energy density and therefore fewer calories compared to a diet with a lower water percentage

content. It is important that energy intake is carefully controlled to allow the animal to reach and maintain optimum body condition. Excess energy can lead to growth abnormalities during the growth phase and obesity at any point in the life stage. Inadequate energy intake leads to poor growth and weight loss. Both conditions are potentially damaging to health and should be avoided by careful dietary management.

Animals eat to satisfy their energy requirements unless a diet is excessively palatable, when overeating may occur. In a balanced diet when an animal has consumed the amount of diet to meet its energy needs then the requirements for all other nutrients should also have been met. If the energy density of the diet is low, nutrient deficiencies may occur since the animal will stop eating when the gut is full but before all the nutritional requirements have been met. The diet is said to be bulk-limited; examples of bulk-limited diets are:

- Puppies and kittens on a poor-quality diet or an incorrect life-stage diet
- Weight loss in lactating bitches fed on a maintenance or a poor puppy diet
- Some weight-control foods are bulk-limited for the energy-producing nutrients but not for the non-energy-producing nutrients – this is deliberate to achieve weight loss.

Energy requirements vary from individual to individual according to an animal's:

- Age
- Breed
- Sex
- Activity level
- Reproductive status
- Environment
- Health status.

TABLE 9.1	Assessing levels of dehydration in an animal
Percentage of dehydration	**Clinical signs**
<5%	No obvious outward signs Concentrated urine
5–8%	Slightly prolonged CRT Slight tenting of the skin Mucous membranes feel tacky Third eyelid visible
8–10%	Sunken eyes Prolonged CRT Obvious tenting of the skin
10–12%	Oliguria Tented skin remains in place Clinical shock can be experienced
>12%	Progressive shock Coma and death

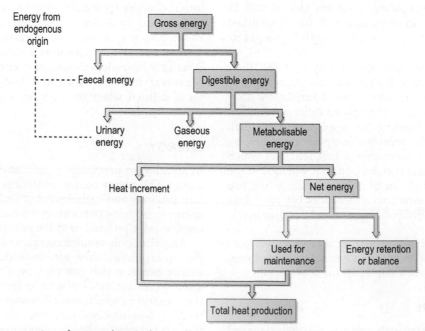

Fig. 9.1 Diagrammatic representation of energy losses during digestion. *Heat increment:* heat produced from the digestion, absorption and metabolism of food. *Digestible energy:* energy remaining after the energy lost in faeces is subtracted from gross energy (GE). *Metabolised energy:* energy available to the animal after energy from faeces, urine and combustible gases has been subtracted from the GE.

TABLE 9.2	Daily maintenance energy requirements
Weight in kg	Energy in kcal/kg
DOGS	
3	110
6	85
10	75
>25	65
CATS	
2.5–5.5	65–70

TABLE 9.3	Daily energy requirements for cats and dogs
One full day's work	1.5 × maintenance energy requirement (MER)
Gestation post 3 weeks	1.3 × MER
Peak lactation	2–4 × MER
Birth to 3 months	2.0 × MER
Sub-freezing temperatures	1.7 × MER
Tropical heat	2.5 × MER
Resting	0.8 × MER
Obesity	0.6 × MER
Geriatric	0.6 × MER

TABLE 9.4	Gross energy content of nutrients
Nutrient	kcal/g
Protein	5.64
Fat	9.40
Carbohydrate	4.15

TABLE 9.5	Metabolisable energy content of nutrients
Nutrient	kcal/g
Protein	3.5
Fat	8.7
Carbohydrate	3.5

This should be borne in mind when advising your clients on the most appropriate diet for the pet and when calculating the daily feeding amount.

Owners may think that protein does not contain calories and is used to provide the building blocks for growth and repair. Excess protein is used as an energy source, and produces the same amount of calories per gram as carbohydrates. It is a relatively poor source of energy because a large amount of the energy theoretically available from it is lost in meal-induced heat. Meal-induced heat is the metabolic heat 'wasted' in the digestion, absorption and utilisation of the protein. Fat and carbohydrates are better sources of energy for performance.

For obese or obesity-prone dogs a low energy intake is indicated, and there are specially prepared diets that have a very low energy density.

Energy requirements

The basal energy requirement (BER) is the amount of energy expended while asleep, 12–18 hours after feeding in a thermoneutral environment.

The maintenance energy requirement (MER) is the amount of energy required by a moderately active animal in its daily search for and utilisation of food (Table 9.2). It does not include the energy required for growth, repair, pregnancy, lactation or work.

- MER in dogs is approximately 2 × BER.
- MER in cats is approximately 1.4 × BER.

Most of the energy used by the body is given off as heat through radiation and convection from the body surface. Energy expenditure is related to body surface area. Small animals have a larger body surface area related to body weight and therefore have greater heat loss, and so a greater BER. Surface area can be determined from conversion tables using the animal's body weight, but this can be complex and time-consuming.

Resting energy requirement (RER). The RER differs from the BER as it includes energy expended for recovery from physical activity and feeding, and is calculated from these equations dependent on the weight of the animal. The RER for dogs and cats can be calculated with these two formulas:

$$RER\,(kcal/day) = 70\,(BW_{kg})^{0.75}$$

(if body weight [BW] is less than 2 kg).

Or, $30\,(BW_{kg}) + 70$ (if BW is between 2 and 45 kg).

It has been calculated that RER may be 1.25 BER, but many texts regard the two as interchangeable values.

In sickness the energy requirement varies considerably. Pets are often less active, sleep more and lie in a warm environment. The BER can sometimes be lower; however, if the animal has suffered from trauma, surgery or sepsis, the BER rises sharply. The precise rise will depend upon the illness factor involved. Illness factors can be used to calculate the daily energy requirements for patients with varying requirements, but these should only be used as a starting calorific guideline and adjusting nutritional assessment accordingly. During pregnancy, lactation, growth and the control of obesity, the energy needs also vary (Table 9.3).

The gross energy of nutrients (Table 9.4) varies but only a proportion of these nutrients are actually digested by the animal. The figures must therefore be adjusted to provide accurate values of the metabolisable energy obtained from the nutrient. The figures shown in Table 9.5 allow for digestibility. If a diet is highly digestible, the energy content (density) is higher; if a diet is poorly digestible because of lower-quality ingredients, the energy density is lower.

- The only way to accurately determine the nutrient content of a diet as shown in Table 9.6 is by laboratory analysis. The carbohydrate content may not be stated on the label but can be calculated by subtracting the total amount of all other nutrients from 100.
- The water content may not be given for all dry diets. Assume a figure of 10% if none is stated.
- This diet therefore contains 333.8 kcal/100 g of food, i.e. 3.338 kcal/g.

TABLE 9.6	Nutrient content of a typical diet		
Nutrient	Amount (%)	kcal/g nutrient	kcal/100 g diet
Protein	22	× 3.5	77.0
Fat	9	× 8.7	78.3
Fibre	3	0	0
Water	10	0	0
Ash	5	0	0
Carbohydrate	51	× 3.5	178.5
Total			333.8

Using the above information, the energy provided by each nutrient can be calculated as a percentage of the total energy:

Percentage protein calories = 77/333.8 × 100 = 21%

Percentage fat calories = 78.3/333.8 × 100 = 21.3%

Percentage carbohydrate calories = 178.5/333.8 × 100 = 48.6%.

PROTEIN

Proteins are complex molecules composed of chains of amino acids. There are only 23 amino acids and all animals need all 23 of them. These 23 amino acids can be arranged in any combination, giving an almost infinite variety of naturally occurring proteins, each with its own characteristic properties, e.g. hair, skin, muscle, hormones, antibodies.

Many amino acids can be synthesised within the animal's body and so do not have to be provided in the diet. There are some, however, that cannot be synthesised and so must be included in the diet; these are termed the 'essential' amino acids. There are 10 amino acids essential in the diets of dogs and 11 amino acids essential in the diets of cats. These are:

- Phenylalanine
- Valine
- Tryptophan
- Threonine
- Isoleucine
- Methionine
- Histidine
- Arginine
- Leucine
- Lysine.

The eleventh amino acid that is essential for cats only is called **taurine**. Inadequate taurine in the diet of cats can cause irreversible blindness and heart problems. Plant proteins do not contain taurine. The only source of taurine is animal protein, providing evidence that the cat is an obligate carnivore. Arginine is a conditionally essential amino acid, meaning that whether or not it is required is conditional on the health status or life cycle of the individual. The biosynthetic pathway, however, does not produce sufficient arginine, and some must still be consumed through diet. Individuals with poor nutrition or certain physical conditions may be advised to increase their intake of foods containing arginine.

Proteins are essential components of all living cells, in which they have several functions including regulation of metabolism, a structural role in cell walls and muscle fibres. They are an important requirement for tissue growth and repair. Proteins may also be used as a source of energy in the diet. Animals cannot synthesise new amino acids so they require a dietary protein source to prevent a loss of body function or an inability to produce new tissue.

The quality of a protein varies with the number and amount of essential amino acids it contains. The quality of a protein is referred to as its **biological value (BV)**. This will depend on how:

- Acceptable (palatable)
- Digestible
- Utilisable

the protein is: e.g. leather is not edible and so has 0% acceptability, and therefore 0% biological value; chicken is edible, is 80% digestible and is 70% utilisable – the biological value is 87% or 0.87. Egg has the highest BV at 100% or 1.

Dietary protein in **excess** of the animal's requirements cannot be laid down as muscle but is broken down in the liver by a process of deamination. The amino part is converted to urea, which is excreted by the kidneys. The acid part of the amino acid is converted to glycogen or fat and is stored. Excess dietary protein can therefore be damaging to animals with liver and kidney problems, and so controlling the quantity of dietary protein is prudent in the ageing pet, though increasing the quality of the protein that the food contains is equally important.

Protein **deficiency** can result from insufficient dietary protein or from a deficiency of a particular amino acid. Signs of protein deficiency include:

- Poor growth or weight loss, due to loss of lean muscle mass
- Dull hair coat
- Increased susceptibility to disease
- Oedema, due to low blood plasma albumin levels
- Death.

FAT

Dietary fat may be referred to as oils, lipids or fats and consists of mainly triglycerides, which are composed of one molecule of glycerol and three molecules of fatty acids.

The specific fatty acids present determine the physical and nutritional characteristics of the fat. Fats are required in the diet:

- To provide energy
- To aid absorption of the fat-soluble vitamins (A, D, E, K)
- To enhance palatability
- As a source of essential fatty acids.

Inadequate dietary fat may lead to fatty acid deficiency and/ or energy deficiency. Fats containing a high percentage of unsaturated fatty acids are liquid at room temperature and are called oils. Those with a low percentage of unsaturated fatty acids are solid at room temperature and are called fats.

Just as some amino acids cannot be synthesised by the body and must be provided in the diet, some fatty acids are also termed 'essential'. The three essential fatty acids are:

- Linoleic acid
- Linolenic acid
- Arachidonic acid.

Linoleic acid is an essential fatty acid required in the diet of all animals. It is common in vegetable oil and makes up 15–25% of poultry and pork fat but only 5% of beef tallow. Arachidonic acid is synthesised from linoleic acid in dogs, but not in cats, and so it must be present in the diet of the cat. Arachidonic acid is only found in fats of animal origin. Linolenic acid is synthesised from linoleic acid by both dogs and cats; therefore, neither species requires linolenic acid in dietary fat.

Fatty acids are needed as constituents of cell membranes, for the synthesis of prostaglandins and in controlling water loss through the skin. Essential fatty acid **deficiency** may result in impaired reproductive performance, impaired wound healing, a dry coat and scaly skin. This can predispose the skin to bacterial infection and eczema 'hot spots'. Essential fatty acid deficiency occurs most commonly in dogs receiving low-fat dry dog foods containing beef tallow or dry food that has been stored too long, especially under warm or humid conditions. Fatty acids become rancid due to the oxidation of their double bonds. Once rancid they lose their nutritional value. This oxidation is hastened by high temperatures and humidity. Oxidation of fats is prevented by the inclusion of substances called antioxidants such as vitamin E and ethoxyquin.

Certain fatty acids (such as docosahexaenoic acid [DHA]) have been shown to play an important role in neural development in puppies and kittens. DHA is one of the 'building blocks' of brain tissue during growth. Eggs, meat and fish, such as salmon, sardines and tuna, are rich in DHA. Bitch and queen milk is also rich in DHA, but once weaned puppies and kittens suffer a drop in DHA intake. Some premium pet puppy and kitten foods are now supplemented with higher levels of DHA and these foods have been shown to improve trainability and vision development of puppies and kittens.

Excess dietary fat, or a reduction in vitamin E intake, can lead to pansteatitis or 'yellow fat disease'. Signs include cutaneous pain, anorexia, pyrexia and nodular fat deposits within the skin, as the adipose body fat of the animal becomes inflamed. This can occur in cats eating a diet chiefly composed of red meat or tuna. Treatment involves correction of the diet and vitamin E therapy. Excess dietary fat may also lead to obesity, a serious condition that has many lifelong health consequences, including diabetes, heart disease, increased risk of joint disease and skin disorders. The majority of British pets are considered to be overweight and so educating clients as to the dangers of obesity and helping them choose the most appropriate diet for their pet are valuable skills for all veterinary nurses to learn.

CARBOHYDRATES

There are three main groups of carbohydrates:
- Monosaccharides – glucose, fructose (simple sugars)
- Disaccharides – maltose, sucrose, lactose
- Polysaccharides – starch, glycogen and fibre (complex carbohydrates).

Carbohydrates provide the body with energy and may be converted to body fat. All animals have a metabolic requirement for glucose, but, provided the diet contains sufficient glucose precursors (amino acids and glycerol), most animals can synthesise enough glucose to meet their metabolic needs without dietary carbohydrate. Sugars and cooked starches are an economical and easily digested energy source. Sugars increase palatability to dogs, but cats do not respond to the taste of sugar.

The value of certain carbohydrates is limited by the animal's ability to digest them. Digestion of disaccharides such as sucrose and lactose is controlled by the activity of the intestinal enzymes, i.e. disaccharidases sucrase and lactase. The activity of lactase decreases with age and so an excessive consumption of lactose-containing products in older animals can lead to diarrhoea.

DIETARY FIBRE

Dietary fibre, or roughage, consists of a group of indigestible polysaccharides such as cellulose, lignin and pectin. They are the main constituents of plant cell walls and are relatively indigestible within the gut of dogs and cats. In these species the role of fibre in the diet is to provide bulk to the faeces, regularising bowel movements and helping to prevent constipation and diarrhoea. Fibre also has therapeutic uses in the treatment of fibre-responsive diseases. Since fibre is largely indigestible, it decreases the energy content of the diet and so has a role in the correction and prevention of obesity. Fibres can be split into fermentable and non-fermentable and each has its own benefits in clinical nutrition; this is covered in Chapter 10.

MINERALS

The term 'mineral' is used to denote all inorganic elements in a food. Minerals are sometimes referred to on pet food labels as ash.

More than 18 minerals are believed to be essential for mammals. They are divided into macrominerals, which are needed in larger amounts, and microminerals, which are required in smaller amounts. Electrolytes are minerals in their salt form and are found in body tissues and fluids.

Minerals have many varied functions in the body. They are required for the maintenance of:
- Skeletal structure (especially calcium, phosphorus and magnesium)
- Acid–base and fluid balance (especially potassium, sodium and chloride)
- Cellular function
- Nerve conduction (especially potassium, sodium and magnesium)
- Muscle contraction (especially magnesium and calcium).

The absorption of different minerals is often linked, so that an excess intake of one mineral can lead to a deficiency of another. This is important since supplementation of one mineral can cause deficiency of another.

There are seven macrominerals. These are:
- Calcium
- Phosphorus
- Magnesium
- Sodium
- Potassium
- Chloride
- Sulphur.

1. **Calcium** and **phosphorus** are the major minerals involved in maintaining structural rigidity as components of the bones and teeth. The level of calcium and phosphorus in the blood is controlled by a complex series of reactions involving parathormone, calcitonin and vitamin D. It is the absolute concentrations of these minerals that are of most importance, but the ratio of calcium to phosphorus is also significant. The correct ratio for growth is 1:1. Imbalance in this ratio with either in excess leads to skeletal deformities. Calcium deficiency occurs most commonly in diets that are high in phosphorus (high meat and offal diets), and in lactating bitches it can cause eclampsia. Calcium excess occurs when high-calcium diets are fed, especially to large-breed puppies. It most

commonly occurs when calcium supplementation is given in addition to a growth type diet. Many skeletal abnormalities have been attributed in part to excess calcium, including osteochondritis dissecans (OCD), hip dysplasia and wobbler syndrome.

2. **Magnesium** is required for the normal function of heart and skeletal muscle. Foodstuffs containing bone, grains and fibre are rich in magnesium. Magnesium deficiency can cause muscular weakness but is very unlikely to be due to a lack of magnesium in the diet. Very high intakes of magnesium have been associated with feline lower urinary tract disease (FLUTD) and the formation of struvite crystalluria.

3. **Sodium** and **chloride** are the major electrolytes in the body water. They are needed for acid–base balance and for the regulation of the concentration of the body fluids. Chloride is a component of bile and hydrochloric acid. Fish, eggs, whey and poultry meal are rich in both sodium and chloride. A deficiency of these minerals can arise from excessive fluid loss, such as occurs in vomiting and diarrhoea. Signs include exhaustion, inability to control water balance, dry skin and hair loss. An excess will cause a greater than normal fluid intake and may predispose animals to hypertension, and therefore heart and kidney problems.

4. **Potassium** is plentiful within cells and has an important role in maintaining both acid–base and osmotic balance. Potassium is also needed to facilitate the transfer of nerve impulses and muscle contractility. Potassium is present in a wide variety of foods, including soya, rice bran, grains and wheat bran. A deficiency of potassium is termed 'hypokalaemia' and will cause anorexia, lethargy and muscle weakness. An excess of potassium is rare but may occur when potassium excretion is impaired, especially in cases of urethral obstruction, where it can prove to be fatal.

There are at least 11 microminerals, the most important of which are as follows:

* **Iron** is an essential component of haemoglobin, the oxygen-carrying pigment of the blood, and myoglobin, the oxygen-carrying pigment found within muscle. Most meat ingredients are high in iron and primary dietary deficiency is rare. It may arise as a consequence of chronic blood loss causing anaemia and fatigue, or occur in young puppies and kittens if milk is fed for too long a period, as milk has a low iron content.
* **Copper** is needed for the formation of red blood cells and in the normal pigmentation of the skin and hair. Most meat ingredients, especially ruminant livers, contain plentiful copper. Copper deficiency may occur when zinc and iron excess arise and causes poor reproductive performance, early foetal loss and hair depigmentation. Copper toxicity is very rare in dogs and cats with normal metabolisms, and it occurs mainly in Bedlington terriers, West Highland White terriers and Doberman Pinschers – these breeds are all prone to an inherited metabolic defect that causes liver cirrhosis.
* **Zinc** is required by all animals for maintaining a healthy skin and coat. Very high calcium diets can increase the animal's need for zinc. Zinc is relatively non-toxic and signs of dietary excess are rarely encountered in animals consuming normal commercial pet food. Signs of zinc deficiency have been reported in dogs fed cereal-based foods because of the presence of phytates that bind the zinc and prevent its absorption. The most common presentation of zinc deficiency is poor skin, hyperkeratosis and a sparse hair coat.
* **Manganese** is of little practical relevance in the dietary management of cats and dogs but is an essential component in the diet of all birds. Manganese is required for the activation of many enzymes and is thus involved in a wide variety of important metabolic processes. Fibre sources and fish meal are rich in manganese.
* **Iodine** is a major constituent of thyroid hormones, which are required for thermoregulation, reproduction, growth and metabolism. An animal's iodine requirement is influenced by its physiological state and diet. Lactating animals have a greater need for dietary iodine since about 10% of intake is excreted in the milk. Fish, eggs and poultry by-products are rich sources of iodine.
* **Selenium** is an important constituent of the body's antioxidant protective system, in which it functions in combination with vitamin E. Selenium deficiency will cause muscular dystrophy and reproductive failure in ruminants but has not been reported in dogs and cats.

VITAMINS

In order to be classified as a vitamin, a substance must have five basic characteristics:

* It must be an organic compound different from fat, protein and carbohydrate.
* It must be a component of the diet.
* It must be essential in minute amounts.
* Its absence must cause a deficiency syndrome.
* It must not be synthesised in sufficient quantities to support normal physiological function.

Not all vitamins are essential for all species: e.g. guinea pigs and primates must have a dietary source of vitamin C, whereas other species can synthesise it themselves.

Vitamins can be divided into two main groups, depending on whether they are soluble in fat or water:

* Water-soluble – B complex and C
* Fat-soluble – A, D, E, K.

Vitamins assist in regulating energy metabolism and are involved in many biochemical reactions. Most vitamins cannot be synthesised in the body and so must be present in the diet. Since the water-soluble vitamins are readily lost via the urine and are poorly stored in the body, a daily supply must be available. In animals suffering with polyuria, higher levels of the water-soluble vitamins are lost and therefore supplementation may be required. Fat-soluble vitamins are more readily stored and so a daily intake is not so important. Toxicity arising from excessive intake is much more common. There is no daily dietary requirement for vitamin C (ascorbic acid) in dogs and cats, since they can synthesise all they require from glucose.

Many factors influence an animal's individual requirement for vitamins. During growth and reproduction animals are making new tissues and so require higher levels of all nutrients, including vitamins. Various disease conditions also affect vitamin status through a reduced intake, e.g. following prolonged anorexia, or due to increased losses or decreased production, e.g. reduced synthesis of vitamin D during renal failure.

All commercial pet foods contain added vitamins both from synthetic and natural sources. It is therefore unnecessary and indeed contraindicated to supplement the diet of healthy dogs and cats with additional multipurpose vitamin formulations.

Water-soluble vitamins

Vitamin B complex – this includes thiamine, riboflavin, niacin, biotin, folic acid and cyanocobalamin. The water-soluble B vitamins are generally considered to be non-toxic. Since commercial pet foods contain plentiful supplies of B vitamins, deficiency states in pets fed such foods are very unlikely.

Deficiencies can occur as a result of overconsumption of certain foods that contain specific antivitamins: e.g. avidin in raw egg whites binds biotin; thiaminase in raw fish can lead to thiamine deficiency in cats. Water-soluble vitamin deficiencies can also be demonstrated in pets fed unusual home-prepared diets. Dogs fed exclusively on cereals such as porridge have been reported to develop niacin deficiency (termed 'pellagra'), which presents as dermatitis, diarrhoea, dementia and death.

Vitamin C – vitamin C mainly functions in the body as an antioxidant and free radical scavenger and is needed for the synthesis of collagen.

Fat-soluble vitamins

Vitamin A – also called retinol, is the most nutritionally important vitamin. It is required for normal vision and for healthy coat, skin, mucous membranes and teeth. Naturally rich sources of vitamin A include fish oil, liver, eggs and dairy products. Plants do not contain active vitamin A but instead are rich in provitamins called carotenoids.

Deficiencies are uncommon but cats require a source of preformed vitamin A, which is only found in animal tissue, and thus theoretically could become deficient if fed a vegetarian diet. Vitamin A toxicity is fairly common in cats receiving a diet high in liver or following oversupplementation with cod liver oil, since these foodstuffs contain abundant amounts of preformed vitamin A. Clinical signs of vitamin A toxicity include liver damage and painful bone disease, especially of the cervical vertebrae and long bones of the fore limb.

Vitamin D – this is required for the intestinal absorption of calcium and for the mobilisation and bone deposition of both calcium and phosphorus. It can be absorbed from the diet in the small intestine and also can be synthesised in the skin following exposure to ultraviolet B light. Marine fish and fish oils are the richest natural sources of vitamin D and can potentially be a source of toxicity. Vitamin D deficiency is very rare but can cause rickets in young animals and severe bone disorders in adults. Toxicity can occur due to oversupplementation and causes hypercalcaemia, soft-tissue calcification and ultimately death.

Vitamin E – this is an important antioxidant and the requirement for vitamin E increases with the dietary levels of polyunsaturated fatty acids (PUFA). Vitamin E is only synthesised by plants and the richest natural sources are vegetable oils, seeds and cereal grains. The clinical manifestations of vitamin E deficiency vary markedly between species. In dogs the main clinical signs are degenerative skeletal disease with muscular weakness and gestational failure. In cats deficiency can arise when diets that are high in PUFA, such as oily fish, are fed. The clinical signs associated with vitamin E toxicity in cats include the occurrence of painful subcutaneous nodules, termed steatitis, as well as myocarditis and myositis.

Vitamin K – this regulates the formation of several blood-clotting factors and can be found in green leafy vegetables. The

TABLE 9.7	The potential sources of free radicals	
Internal sources	**External sources**	
Mitochondria	Smoke	
Phagocytes	Pollution	
Reactions involving iron	Radiation	
Exercise	UV light	
Inflammation	Drugs	
Ischaemia	Ozone	
	Pesticides	

daily requirement for both dogs and cats is easily met in the healthy animal by synthesis from gastrointestinal bacteria and so a deficiency is unlikely.

ANTIOXIDANTS

The role of antioxidants in preserving fat in pet food is well known and understood; however, there is now a considerable body of evidence to suggest that dietary antioxidants can have a positive effect on health and disease prevention through preventing cellular damage by free radicals. Oxidation of dietary fat causes the food to go rancid, whereas oxidation of endogenous fat causes tissue damage termed 'lipid peroxidation' and the production of a continuous supply of free radicals.

Free radicals are reactive, unstable molecules that cause cellular damage to proteins, nucleic acids (DNA) and membrane lipids. Free radicals are unstable because they have a single unpaired electron in an outer orbit. Unpaired electrons attempt to regain stability by attacking and modifying other molecules. Free radicals can propagate damaging chain reactions within the body in an attempt to produce more stable atoms and molecules. This process of transferring electrons from one atom or molecule to another is called oxidation.

Free radicals are produced in the body by everyday metabolism and following exposure to adverse environmental conditions. Potential causes of increased free radical production are shown in Table 9.7.

An antioxidant is a substance that has the ability to scavenge free radicals (in reactive oxygen species) and reduce the overall number of oxidants in the system. The body has a complex antioxidant defence system that limits the effect of free radicals on tissues. This includes:

- Enzymes (catalase, superoxide dismutase)
- Free radical scavengers (vitamins A, C, E)
- Flavenoids.

Some antioxidants are made in the body and others are supplied by the diet. The main dietary antioxidants are:

- Vitamin E
- Vitamin C
- Carotenoids.

The role of vitamin E in preventing the oxidation of polyunsaturated fatty acids (PUFA) is well documented. Antioxidant defences are therefore highly dependent on adequate nutrition; indeed, inadequate ingestion of vitamins C and E mimics the effects of radiation exposure. Cells of the immune system are sensitive to changes in levels of antioxidants due to the very high percentage of PUFA in their cell membranes.

The best food sources of dietary antioxidants are fruit and vegetables. They are especially high in vitamin C and carotenoids but also contribute a significant amount of vitamin E and non-nutrient antioxidants to the diet. It is a well-held belief that people should try to consume at least five daily portions of fresh fruits and vegetables in an attempt to reduce their risk of degenerative diseases and cancer. Unfortunately, the typical diet for the majority of the population in the Western world falls far short of this goal.

Pet dogs and cats very rarely consume this type of diet. Many commercially available pet foods now contain added dietary antioxidants designed to protect dogs and cats against the risk of disease. These products have added levels of vitamin C, vitamin E and selenium to provide antioxidant protection.

Food and feeding

In order to recommend a diet or give general advice about diets it is important to be able to understand packaging/labels of diets, feeding techniques and how to calculate the energy requirements, and thus the feeding quantities of diets. Many owners will ask if a specific diet that they are currently feeding is good for their pet. In these cases it is not just the food that needs to be looked at but also the pet's overall body condition, energy levels and health status. One diet may suit one dog exceptionally well and another not so well. The best diet for the pet is the one that the pet does best on. Other factors such as availability of the diet, pack sizes that the diet is sold in, price and owner preferences also need to be taken into account. Owner preferences can include whether the food is 'ethically' manufactured, organic foods, wet foods rather than dry, and in some cases owners will specify that they want to avoid diets that contain artificial colourants and preservatives.

LABELLING OF DIETS

In order to correctly identify the diet of choice for an individual, evaluation of the diet needs to be made; this is achieved by analysis of the ingredients.

Diets which are fed for a clinical application are required to show further information relating to the particular purpose it is designed for and the species being fed. The type and levels of nutrients, additives and characteristics of the diet that have been modified to suit this purpose should be stated. Also stated is the length of time for which the animal should be fed the diet; this is normally 6 months. Many diets can be fed for longer than this period, but it is recommended that all patients on clinical diets on a long-term basis have a medical examination at least every 6 months.

FOOD COMPARISONS

The quality of the food cannot be assessed from the food label, especially the true digestibility of individual nutrients and the overall digestibility of the diet. The bioavailability of nutrients is not disclosed on the label, and this needs to be conveyed to owners when they compare foods. The typical analysis states the percentage of protein, oil (fat), fibre, ash and moisture (when over 14%). In the USA a guaranteed analysis is used, where percentages again are used, but minimum and maximum values of each nutrient are given.

The moisture content of the diet has a direct effect on the remaining ingredients, moist diets being more diluted than dry diets. Thus direct comparison of the typical analysis is

inaccurate when moisture contents differ (see Table 9.6). Comparisons should only be made when using dry matter basis (DMB) percentages or when based on energy content (e.g. per 100 kcal).

PROXIMAL ANALYSIS OF FOOD

The most common method of determining the nutrient content of the diet is through proximal analysis. This method calculates the percentage of water (moisture), protein, fat, ash and crude fibre in the diet. The percentage that is left (i.e., 100% − % moisture − % crude protein − % fat − % crude fibre − % ash) is carbohydrates or nitrogen-free extract (NFE). Crude protein levels are calculated on the basis that the protein contains 16 ± 2% nitrogen. The crude protein therefore equals nitrogen multiplied by 6.25, or nitrogen divided by 0.16. Errors can occur when non-protein nitrogen such as urea or ammonia is used with the product. Figure 9.2 demonstrates proximate analysis of foods.

TYPES OF PROPRIETARY DIETS

Proprietary diets are those which are commercial made, i.e. processed, and fall into two basic categories − complementary or complete.

Complete diets

Complete diets are those which provide a nutritionally balanced and adequate diet when fed as the sole source of food. All of the nutrient components are provided in the correct ratio, for the specific life stage, and do not require any additions from any another food source. In fact, adding other food sources to the diet in large quantities can make the overall daily intake of food nutritionally unbalanced.

Complementary diets

Complementary diets are those which do not provide a nutritionally balanced diet when fed alone. These diets are designed to be fed in combination with another diet, in order to form a balanced and adequate diet. All treats and snacks are labelled as complementary foods, and thus should only make up a small portion of the daily ration.

Home-made diets

It is still relatively common for cats and dogs to be fed home-made diets. If prepared well, and careful consideration has been made to ensure that they are balanced, home-made diets can serve some purpose in certain cases, e.g. in food trials. Many home-made diets contain excessive quantities of protein and carbohydrates and are limited in vitamins and minerals, especially calcium. If owners do wish to pursue the use of a home-made diet, examples of a diet should be obtained from the veterinary practice. It is also advisable that the animal has its BCS, weight and clinical health examined regularly, to ensure that the diet is balanced and no deficiencies are present. Aiding the owner in designing the diet is important, and there are six simple guidelines to follow when designing a diet. They are:

1. Do the five main food groups appear in the diet?
   - A multivitamin
   - A source of minerals including trace minerals − careful consideration should be given to calcium levels
   - A fat source

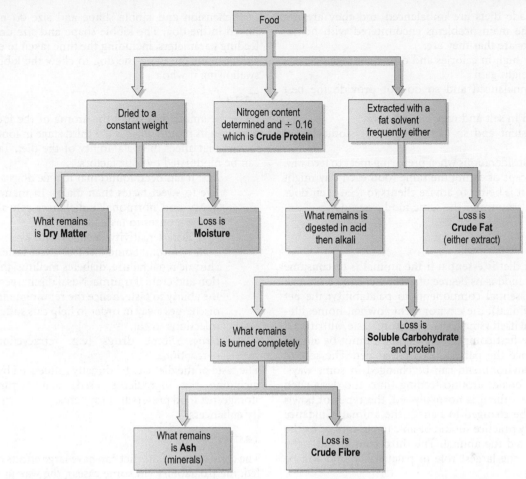

Fig. 9.2 Proximal analysis of foods

- A protein source – it is vital in feline diets that an animal source of protein is used
- A carbohydrate source – this includes fibre. Sources used should be from cooked cereals, grain or potato. (Potatoes and tapioca are an excellent carbohydrate source when performing food trials, as they are not commonly used in commercial diets.)

2. What is the quality and source of the protein?
   - The protein levels and the protein quality within the diet are two very different elements. A high protein level does not necessarily mean that the animal is receiving all of the necessary essential amino acids it requires. Skeletal muscle protein from different sources does contain similar amounts of amino acids, and there is therefore no great advantage of feeding one type of meat over another, unless it is for the purpose of food trials. Novel protein sources used include duck, venison, salmon and egg. Egg is an excellent protein source (BV 100%), and in cases where restricted protein levels are required, the inclusion of egg as a protein source in the diet is highly recommended, as you ensure a high protein quality.

3. What is the fat content of the protein source?
   - Cuts of meat vary greatly in their content of fat. Where the fat content is high, other fat levels should be reduced in order to compensate for this.

4. What is the carbohydrate-to-protein ratio within the diet?
   - The carbohydrate/protein ratio should be approximately 1:1 to 2:1 in cat diets and 2:1 to 3:1 in canine diets.

5. Is there a source of vitamin and minerals?
   - A home-made diet will be unbalanced in view of vitamins and minerals unless they are supplemented. When using home-made diets for food trial cases, the use of supplements is not recommended, as this will affect the trial. As the trial is not long term, short-term deficiencies can be tolerated in many cases.

6. Is there a source of other essential nutrients?
   - Other essential nutrients such as essential fatty acids (EFAs), taurine and other essential amino acids (EAAs) do need to be supplemented into the diet in order to ensure adequate levels. This can be achieved through the addition of oils and other supplements.

Home-made diets should be cooked, as this aids in increasing the overall digestibility of the diet and reduces the risk of food poisoning. Overcooking will result in a loss of nutrients from the diet, especially vitamins and the denaturing of proteins. A vast number of different home-made diets are available on the Internet, and can even be designed for a specific animal and/or clinical disease.

Most home-made diets are unbalanced and they are not recommended. The main problems encountered with home-made diets for pets are that they are:

- Often very high in calories and can encourage overeating and weight gain
- Usually unbalanced and so do not provide the best nutrition
- Often high in salt and may be addictive
- Not consistent and so can cause upset stomach and diarrhoea
- Hygiene considerations when preparing meat to feed raw.

Although the concept of eating the same food each day might appear dull to us, it is better to advise clients to feed their dogs and cats the same amount of the same food every day.

PALATABILITY

Palatability of any diet is essential if the animal is to consume it. Palatability of a food is its degree of acceptance to an animal. There are three essential components to palatability: the pet (species and individual), the environment (owner, home, lifestyle), and the food itself (smell, shape, texture, taste, nutritional composition). The first component, the pet, cannot be altered in order to enhance the palatability of the diet. The second component, the environment, can be changed in some ways. The habits of the owner around feeding time, the designated areas in which the animal is normally fed, the types of bowls used, etc. can all be changed to benefit the animal. Guidance from the veterinary practice should be able to be sourced by the client in order to aid the animal. The third component – the food itself – plays the largest role in palatability, and will be discussed further.

Food aroma and temperature

The temperature of the food plays a huge role in the acceptance of the diet. Cats prefer food that is near body temperature. This is a direct reflection of their natural diet in the wild. Food which is taken straight from the fridge can be less appealing, as can foods above 40°C (104°F). The aroma of the diet plays a significant role in the animal's acceptance to consume the food. Animals that have a reduced olfactory capacity, such as older animals, sick animals and those on medication that reduces olfactory senses, can have a marked decrease in the acceptation of the diet. Cleaning any mucus from the animal's nose will aid in this. The use of moist diets can be advantageous; this is due to these diets giving off stronger aromas.

Prehension

The way in which the animal picks up the food in its mouth and the way in which it eats it have a role in the palatability of the diet. Cats exhibit three different methods of dry food prehension. The most common method is labial prehension. In this method the cat grasps the kibble between the incisors, without the use of the tongue. The second method, supralingual prehension, involves the cat using the dorsal side of the tongue to lap up the kibbles. The third method, sublingual prehension, occurs when the cat applies the ventral side of the tongue to the kibble, turning the kibble backwards into the mouth. Sublingual prehension is commonly used in brachycephalic breeds, such as Persians. Different kibble shapes have been shown to suit certain types of prehension. For example, almond-shaped kibbles are best suited for cats that use sublingual prehension.

Prehension and kibble shape and size do not seem to be linked in the dog. The kibble shape and size does affect other feeding parameters, including the time taken to eat the diet and aiding in encouraging the dog to chew the kibble rather than swallowing it whole.

Taste

Once the animal has smelt the aroma of the food, and picked it up into its mouth, taste is the third stage in food selection and factors that affect the palatability of the diet. Taste perception can be modulated by four factors:

- *Sex:* It has been found that female dogs are more receptive to sweet tastes than males. In many species, pregnancy and hormonal imbalances can also affect taste and responses to taste and smells.
- *Age:* Taste sensitivity declines with age.
- *State of health:* Some diseases affect taste. These include chronic renal failure, diabetes mellitus, thyroid dysfunction and cranial trauma. Nasal discharges will also affect the ability to taste, hence the requirement to bathe nasal discharges away in order to help cats suffering from viral infections to eat.
- *Drugs:* Some drugs (e.g. tetracycline) alter taste perception.

The taste of the diet can be directly influenced by many factors, including the ingredients used, manufacturing practices, storage, pet food preservation systems, packaging and palatability enhancers.

Texture

The consistency of the diet can have large effects on the quantity fed, the palatability (in some cases), the way in which the diet is stored and packaged and the methods in which the animal is fed. Cats and dogs prefer meat-based canned products rather than dry expanded diets. This has been attributed to the higher moisture content, due to blood and fluids containing positive palatability factors.

MOIST DIETS

Moist diets contain 70–85% moisture and are extremely popular. Packaging for moist diets can range from cans to foil trays and pouches. These diets are very palatable and can lead to overeating and obesity. The moisture content of these diets can prove to be invaluable when trying to increase water content of the animal's diet, especially in cases of feline lower urinary tract disease (FLUTD). It is recommended that all cats have a portion of their diet made up of moist foods.

Semi-moist diets

Semi-moist diets contain around 30% moisture. The diet pieces are formed by the ingredients being cooked and formed into a paste. The paste is then passed through an extruder and shaped. Acid preservatives are then added in order to inhibit bacterial and fungal growth. Corn syrup can be used to coat the pieces to prevent drying out, and also removes the availability of the moisture for bacterial and fungal growth. The coating of the syrup makes the pieces very palatable, but totally unsuitable for diabetic patients. Semi-moist diets should not be fed to cats as they can contain propylene glycol. Propylene glycol is an approved food additive for dog food under the category of animal feed and is generally recognised as safe for dogs.

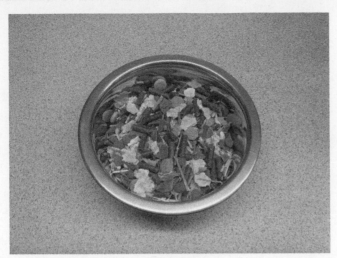

Fig. 9.3 Meal-type diets

Similarly, propylene glycol is an approved food additive for human food as well. The exception is that it is prohibited for use in food for cats.

Dry diets

Dry diets contain 10–14% moisture and can be made by a number of different methods. Using a mixture of dry flaked and crushed cereals and vegetables creates meal-type diets (Fig. 9.3). These diets can be beneficial when catering for large numbers of animals, as each individual animal's requirements can be met; this is a common method for feeding horses. Forming the ingredients into a paste and cooking creates extruded diets. This process involves steam and pressure-cooking. The cooking process can improve the digestibility of the diet, as some nutrients are broken down in the process. The extruded kibbles can then be coated in flavourings and packaged once dried.

Extruded diets tend to be complete and balanced for the life stage that they are designed for. In some species extruded and pelleted diets are preferred as they prevent selective feeding, a common problem in meal-type diets, especially in rabbits and small rodents. Extruded diets do increase chewing compared to pelleted diets, thus increasing palatability and increasing positive eating behaviour – no gulping etc. This eating behaviour also causes an increase in the production of saliva. Extruded diets are ideal for working/performance diets, for any species, as higher fat levels can be utilised.

Some food manufactures use a combination of extruded kibbles alongside semi-moist kibbles, as the semi-moist kibbles can aid in increasing the overall palatability of the diet.

Post-ingestion effects

Once food is consumed, the gastrointestinal tract provides many signals related to food ingestion. The distension of the stomach with food stimulates stretch receptors and chemoreceptors. These receptors send vagal signals to the satiety centre. Both positive and negative feedback mechanisms are responsible for regulating food intake. Negative feedback mechanisms such as insulin, serotonin, leptin, neurotensin and glucagons appear to attenuate food intake. Daily administrations of leptin have been shown to decrease food consumption and thus induce weight loss. Positive feedback includes the activation of the autonomic system during eating. Opioid and dopaminergic neurons are involved in the stimulation of food intake and aid in the positive reinforcement of food intake.

COMMERCIAL DIETS

Commercially available diets have undergone extensive research by vets and nutritionists at the pet food companies. The degree of scientific research that the diet is formulated on is dependent on the pet food company and its resources. They provide the best balance of nutrients combined with convenience and excellent value. Three main types of dog and cat foods are available: moist foods, dry foods and semi-moist foods.

PREMIUM FOODS

Premium pet foods are highly sophisticated foods that have been developed by specialist veterinary nutritionists. They are usually available in both moist and dry forms. Premium foods contain higher-quality ingredients than regular pet foods, and this makes them much more digestible. Premium foods may at first glance seem more expensive than economy brands, but they have several advantages:

- They are fed in smaller amounts so the cost per day compares favourably with other foods.
- The pet produces smaller firmer faeces, as the food is more digestible; this makes toilet training easier and less messy.
- The high-quality ingredients often lead to improved skin condition.
- They are complete and so no extra supplements are needed.
- They are always made to the same consistent recipe; this is called fixed formulation and reduces the likelihood of digestive upsets.
- They tend to be lower in potentially harmful nutrients such as salt.
- They are available in different life stages to suit the pet's age, body condition and lifestyle.

TREATS

Most pet owners like to buy treats for their pets, but if the pet is receiving a complete balanced diet then this is not necessary. Providing that the total number of calories eaten each day in treats is no more than 10% of the pet's daily intake, they can be safely fed. It is best to get owners to reduce the daily feeding amount by about 10% to compensate for the additional calories from the treats.

Most new puppy owners will use treats as a reward when they are training their puppies – the main meal should be reduced to compensate for this, or use a portion of the kibbles from the main diet.

Feeding puppies and kittens

PUPPIES

Puppies should start to be weaned at 4 weeks of age. Many puppies will start to eat solid food before this by exploring their surroundings and coming into contact with their mother's food. If the mother is fed a good-quality balanced puppy food during the latter stages of pregnancy and throughout lactation, then this is a suitable weaning ration for the puppies too. In the first few days the kibble can be soaked to allow smaller puppies to chew them more easily, but very soon puppies will learn to accept dry kibble. If a commercial balanced food is chosen, then no supplements should be needed and in fact adding other nutrients will only cause dietary imbalances.

The musculoskeletal system changes constantly throughout life but these changes are most rapid during the first few months of life. The exact point of maturity varies between breeds but is usually between 12 and 18 months of life. The skeletal system is most susceptible to physical and metabolic insult during the first 12 months because metabolic activity is heightened during this time. If damage occurs at this stage of development the structural soundness of the adult dog can be affected, leading to lameness or growth defects.

Optimum growth, including skeletal development, is dependent upon a combination of good genetics, the correct environment and balanced nutrition. The Kennel Club offers facilities on its website to ensure that breeders select the best breeding animals to maximise genetic potential, avoiding those with overt conformational defects. The environmental influences include litter size (and thus space available within the womb for development), activity level and housing conditions.

Nutrition is certainly one of the most important factors in optimal growth, and many scientific studies have shown that development can be adversely affected by both under- and over-nutrition. With the advent of modern commercial pet food, nutrient deficiency as a cause of developmental skeletal disease has been dramatically reduced. Today we see far more cases where the plane of nutrition has been too high because of over-feeding or oversupplementation. The main nutritional risk factors for puppies are:

- Obesity in smaller breeds, due to an excessive intake of energy
- Skeletal disease in larger breeds, due to a combination of excessive energy intake and/or high intake of specific nutrients.

Large-breed puppies are those that will weigh more than 25 kg when fully grown. Excessive nutrient intake has been shown to be a factor in the main developmental skeletal disorders of larger-breed puppies, including hip dysplasia, osteochondritis dissecans (OCD), wobbler syndrome, un-united anconeal process and panosteitis. The key nutritional influences on skeletal development are the:

- Energy content of the food
- Feeding method employed
- Specific nutrient content and ratios between nutrients, including calcium, phosphorus, protein, vitamin D and vitamin A.

Most dog owners are aware that puppies need relatively more energy, protein, calcium and phosphorus than adult dogs, i.e. in relation to their body weight, but many do not realise that too much of any one of these nutrients can be harmful.

The intake of too much calcium is more common than the intake of too little. This is because of the tendency of owners to overfeed and to supplement the diet with additional minerals and vitamins in the form of powders, tablets and capsules, as well as by adding high-calcium foods, e.g. milk, bone meal, treats and titbits, to the puppy food. This high intake of calcium has the effect of inhibiting the natural remodelling process of bone that has to occur during development in response to changing stresses on the skeleton. The consequences of this

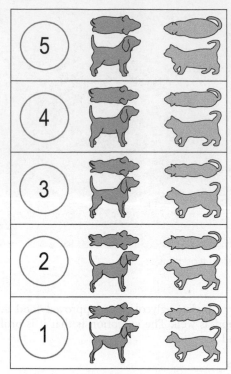

Fig. 9.4   Estimation of body condition score, 5-point scale

overnutrition are proportionately greater in puppies that grow more rapidly, i.e. the larger breeds, and this explains why the majority of the developmental skeletal conditions are diagnosed in breeds weighing 25 kg or more when adult.

New puppy owners have to digest a huge amount of information during their first few visits to the surgery. This information includes vaccination policies, worming regimens, flea treatments, neutering, insurance and training, as well as the correct way to feed their new family member. Completion of puppy growth charts can be invaluable for tracking growth rates and give appropriate guidance to owners (see Chapter 3).

To assess a puppy food for optimum development in growing puppies we must consider a number of factors.

Energy content

Growing puppies need twice as much dietary energy on a per-kilogram basis as adults. This need is greatest just after birth and then decreases as the dog grows and matures. Excessive dietary energy may support a growth rate that is too fast for proper skeletal development, which results in increased frequency of skeletal disorders in large and giant breeds. As fat has more than twice the calorific density of protein or carbohydrate it follows that dietary fat is the primary contributor to excess energy intake. Not only does excess energy result in rapid growth but also dietary energy in excess of the puppy's needs will be stored as fat and hence predispose to juvenile obesity. Puppies that are allowed to get fat will increase the number of fat cells they have (called fat cell hyperplasia) and are then predisposed to obesity for the rest of their lives.

Body condition scoring (BCS) evaluates body fat stores and therefore confirms if the energy intake is suitable (Fig. 9.4). Maintaining a proper BCS during growth not only avoids juvenile obesity but also helps control excessive growth rates and is a valuable practical step you can take to improve the long-term health of your clients' puppies. Limiting food intake (while avoiding deficiencies) to maintain lean body condition will not impede a dog's ultimate genetic potential; however, it will reduce food intake, faecal output and obesity and also lessen the risk of skeletal disease.

Protein content

Excess protein intake has not been shown to negatively affect the developing skeleton. Any protein in excess of what is needed for growth may be converted to energy and so may increase growth rate. Protein deficiency has been shown to be harmful. The minimum adequate level of dietary protein will depend upon the protein's:

- Digestibility
- Amino acid profile
- Ratio of essential amino acids
- Bioavailability – the amount actually utilisable by the body.

A puppy food should contain at least 22% protein on a dry matter basis (DMB) of high biological value. Once the puppy reaches maturity this level may be reduced.

Calcium content

It is the absolute level of calcium and the calcium-to-phosphorus (Ca:P) ratio that influences skeletal development. One study showed that young giant-breed puppies fed a food containing excess calcium (3.3% DMB) with a phosphorus level that was either normal (0.9% DMB) or high (3.3% DMB to maintain the correct Ca:P ratio) had a significantly increased incidence of developmental bone disease. Thus we cannot just increase the phosphorus to make up for the fact that the calcium is too high.

It was postulated that switching from a puppy to an adult food earlier than normally advised might help protect puppies from excess calcium intake, since the adult food would contain a lower level of calcium and should therefore lead to a reduced calcium intake. The puppy, however, must consume a greater volume of the lower-energy adult food in order to meet its higher calorie needs. This means that ultimately the puppy consumes a greater amount of calcium when eating the adult food. This reinforces the fact that puppies are not small versions of adult dogs but have unique nutritional needs that can only be satisfied by feeding a balanced growth food.

Feeding treats or giving supplements that contain calcium will further increase calcium intake. Two level teaspoons of a typical calcium supplement added to a growth food for a 15-week-old, 15 kg puppy would more than double the daily calcium intake. This would take the total calcium intake to a level much higher than has been shown to significantly increase the risk of developmental skeletal disease.

Studies demonstrate the safety and adequacy of 1.1% calcium (DMB) in the food. The Association of American Feed Control Officials (AAFCO) minimum recommended level of calcium is 1% DMB, and this should be with no supplementation, especially for at-risk puppies.

Other nutrients

- **Vitamin C** has been recommended in the prevention and treatment of several skeletal diseases; however, the relationship between vitamin C and disorders such as OCD and hip dysplasia has not been proved. Vitamin C (L-ascorbic acid) is required for the biosynthesis of collagen, a major component of ligaments and bones, but a study found that feeding puppies puppy diets totally devoid of vitamin C caused no skeletal problems and did not affect growth. There are no known requirements for dietary vitamin C in the dog.
- **Vitamin D** metabolites regulate calcium metabolism and therefore the skeletal development of growing animals. These metabolites aid in the absorption of calcium and phosphorus from the gut, increase bone cell activity, influence endochondral ossification and alter calcium excretion via the kidney. Unlike other omnivores, the dog seems to be dependent on a dietary source of vitamin D as well as that produced endogenously by the action of ultraviolet light on the skin. Commercial pet foods contain ample vitamin D, making vitamin D deficiency (rickets) very rare. Excess vitamin D can cause hypercalcaemia, hyperphosphataemia, anorexia, polydipsia, polyuria, vomiting, muscle weakness, soft tissue mineralisation and lameness. Vitamin D supplementation should be avoided in growing dogs since it may disturb normal skeletal development because of increased calcium and phosphorus absorption.
- The **trace minerals copper and zinc** are involved in normal skeletal development. In dogs, bone copper levels are not influenced by dietary supplementation. Long-term studies of the effects of dietary zinc on canine growth have shown no significant clinical influence on skeletal development. So, even though these minerals are required for normal skeletal development, their exact role in the dog has yet to be determined.

Feeding techniques for use in growing puppies

There are three basic methods:

- **Free-choice feeding** – this is when the daily allocation of diet is available throughout the day for the dog to choose when it wants to eat. Once the daily ration has been eaten, no further food is offered. This method is the most favourable for toy breeds that as puppies need to eat little and often, and for more timid or nervous dogs.
- **Time-limited feeding** – this can be used for most breeds. The food is only available for a set period two or three times daily, leading to a reduced intake in most breeds. This slightly reduced intake results in slower growth rates but does not diminish the adult size achieved. Close attention should still be paid to the total amount of food consumed, since certain individuals (very greedy feeders) are still able to consume large amounts of food during this limited time period. If this method is chosen, it is recommended to allow three 5–10-minute feeding periods for the first month after weaning, reducing to two per day after that.
- **Food-limited feeding** – this is the method of choice for feeding puppies to maintain optimum growth rate and body condition. Food-limited feeding involves giving a measured (weighed) amount of food based on calculated energy requirements. This will have been done by the manufacturer and is indicated by the feeding guide on the packaging. Clinical monitoring of growth and adjustment of the feeding amount are critical. Large- and giant-breed dogs grow rapidly and thus have steep growth curves. Their intake should be monitored closely and will have to be adjusted more frequently than for

dogs of smaller breeds. These 'at-risk' breeds should be weighed, evaluated and have their feeding amount adjusted every 2 weeks. Regardless of a food's nutrient profile and how it is fed, the ultimate measurement of appropriate intake is the physical condition of the puppy. The only way to reduce potentially harmful nutritional risk factors that can affect skeletal development is to assess body condition and adjust the amount fed to ensure lean, healthy growth. The ideal BCS of a growing puppy is represented by a score of 3 when using the 5-point scale (see Fig. 9.4). The ribs are palpable with a thin layer of fat between the skin and the bone. The bony prominences are easily felt, with a slight amount of overlying fat. Animals over 6 months of age should have a pronounced abdominal tuck when viewed from the side and a well-proportioned lumbar waist when viewed from above.

KITTENS

Growth problems in kittens resulting from unsuitable nutrition are very rare. Veterinary surgeons will sometimes see kittens with growth problems that have been fed on very unusual diets. These kittens have usually been fed home-made diets, especially 'all-meat' diets and diets high in liver.

All-meat diets are very high in phosphorus and very low in calcium. This mineral imbalance can upset the development of the skeleton and cause very thin, weak bones. The kittens may develop bone fractures after very minimal trauma, e.g. being dropped. Alteration of the diet to a more suitable balanced growth food can reverse the problem if caught early enough. Diets that are very high in liver are also very high in vitamin A. An excessive intake of vitamin A can cause abnormal bone development, leading to fusing of the bones in the neck, spine or joints. This condition is very painful and difficult to reverse even after the feeding is corrected.

Optimum growth in kittens is achieved by feeding a high-quality, complete, balanced kitten food. Supplementation with vitamin or mineral tablets and powders is unnecessary and could be harmful. Home-prepared diets for kittens are often unbalanced, containing very high levels of fat, protein and salt. They are best avoided.

The following points should be taken into consideration when recommending a kitten food:

- The product chosen should be complete and balanced for growth. All-purpose foods that claim to be suitable for pregnant and lactating queens, kittens, adult cats and senior cats should be avoided, since these different life stages have differing nutritional requirements.
- A fixed-formula product will reduce the incidence of gut upsets, including diarrhoea; this will make litter training the kitten much easier.
- A highly digestible product (made from high-quality ingredients) will result in smaller, firmer stools with less smell, again aiding litter training.
- The product should contain an increased level of protein, since more protein is needed during growth.
- The product should be high in energy (fat), since this means that the kitten can consume all the calories needed in a smaller amount of food – remember, a kitten's stomach is very small and so large-volume foods should be avoided.

- The product should produce naturally acidic urine; this has been shown to help reduce the incidence of bladder problems in cats. The natural urine pH for cats is 6.2–6.4.
- Milk should be avoided. Kittens do not need cow's milk and in fact lack the enzyme (lactase) needed to digest the milk sugar (lactose). Giving milk to a kitten can cause diarrhoea and will also upset the balance of the diet, since the milk also contains protein, fat and calcium. Kittens should be provided with an ample supply of fresh, clean drinking water.

Feeding during pregnancy and lactation

The aims of a good feeding programme during pregnancy and lactation are to reduce the number of matings needed to achieve pregnancy, i.e. to maximise conception rate and produce the very largest numbers of healthy puppies or kittens per litter. Good nutrition is also needed to maximise the growth rate of the newly born puppies and kittens and to ensure a healthy immune system in the early days of life.

Many of your clients seeking advice will be breeding from their pet dogs for the first time. These inexperienced hobby breeders will benefit from time spent giving sound nutritional advice and help with product selection.

As a general rule, only healthy adult dogs and cats in a good nutritional state, i.e. neither too fat nor too thin, should be considered for breeding. This is an important point, since often poor nutritional status prior to mating is only noticed once the puppies are born. Breeding from overweight bitches should be avoided since it has been shown that these dogs are at a greater risk of insufficient milk production as well as having an increased risk of difficulties giving birth. Breeding from thin animals should not be encouraged either as the strains of pregnancy and lactation can cause health problems for the already weak dog or cat.

THE PREGNANT AND LACTATING BITCH

Gestation in the bitch lasts on average for 63 days and is typically divided into three 21-day 'trimesters'. Adequately fed bitches will gain about 15–25% additional body weight between mating and whelping. After whelping the bitch should weigh no more than about 5–10% more than the pre-breeding weight. This weight gain can be explained mainly by the development of the mammary tissue. In the first 40 days of pregnancy the foetuses only gain about 5% of their final birth weight. This means that during the first two-thirds of pregnancy the energy requirements of the pregnant bitch are no different from those of the non-pregnant bitch. After day 40 the weight of the foetuses increases dramatically and energy intake should increase correspondingly during week 5 to reach a peak between weeks 6 and 8 (Fig. 9.5).

The following nutritional parameters are important during pregnancy.

Energy intake

This reaches about 30% above adult maintenance for bitches with small litters but may reach as high as 60% above maintenance if the litter size is large (Table 9.8). It may be

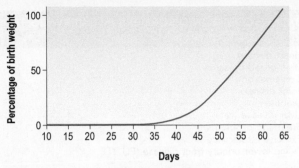

Fig. 9.5 Increase in weight of foetal puppies with time during gestation

TABLE 9.8	Target nutritional profile for pregnancy and lactation	
	Recommended level	
Nutrient	First 6 weeks of pregnancy	Last 3 weeks of pregnancy and during lactation*
Energy (kcal/g)	3.5–4.5	4–5
Protein (%)	22–32	25–35
Fat (%)	10–25	>18
Carbohydrate (%)	>23	>23
Phosphorus (%)	0.6–1.3	0.7–1.3
Calcium (%)	0.75–1.5	1.0–1.7

*Large-breed bitches may need this type of diet throughout pregnancy and lactation.

physically difficult for the bitch to eat sufficient calories in the final days since the abdomen will be filled with the large uterus containing the puppies. This means it is vital to slowly change the diet for a pregnant bitch so that by the last third of pregnancy, i.e. the last 3 weeks, she is eating a puppy diet. It is important to remember that large-breed puppy foods are not suitable for pregnant and lactating bitches since they have a lower energy level than that required for pregnancy and lactation. Giant breeds may sometimes need a higher-energy food throughout pregnancy and not just in the last 3 weeks. Food intake often decreases just prior to whelping and many bitches become totally anorexic. This may be a sign that whelping is imminent.

Protein intake

Just as the energy requirement of the pregnant bitch increases with the developing foetuses, so does the protein requirement (see Table 9.8). Foods for dogs in late gestation should contain increased levels of protein or the quality of the protein needs to increase. This can be achieved by switching to a ration formulated for small- or medium-breed puppies. A food containing 20–25% crude protein on a dry matter basis has been recommended. Protein deficiency during pregnancy may decrease the birth weight of the puppies and decrease their ability to survive.

Carbohydrate intake

Studies have shown that feeding a carbohydrate-free diet to pregnant bitches dramatically decreases the rate of survival of the puppies, as well as causing weight loss in the bitch. This is because the developing foetus obtains more than 50% of its energy from glucose. Bitches should have at least 20% of the energy provided by carbohydrate. This is important, since many raw meat diets will have very low carbohydrate levels. Inexperienced owners may choose to feed these foods, due to influences from friends and the Internet.

Calcium and phosphorus intake

In the last 35 days of pregnancy the requirement for calcium and phosphorus increases by 60%. This is because the skeletons of the puppies are developing and need calcium and phosphorus to form properly. Excessive intake of calcium at this time can, however, be detrimental since it may upset the delicate balance that controls calcium and phosphorus levels. It is recommended that the calcium intake during pregnancy is between 0.75% and 1.5% on a dry matter basis.

Lactation

Optimum milk production depends on several key factors, including:
- Breeding only from bitches in good physical condition
- Good nutrition during pregnancy
- Good nutrition during lactation.

During lactation the nutritional requirements are directly related to the amount of milk the bitch has to produce, which in turn depends on the number of puppies in the litter (see Table 9.8). Lactation puts the bitch under tremendous nutritional strain, more so than at any other stage of her life. The bitch must produce a huge amount of milk, since her puppies have to double their birth weight in the first 9 days of life. A German shepherd bitch with six puppies can produce up to 2 litres of milk per day. At peak lactation the bitch produces milk at a rate similar to that of a dairy cow. Bitch's milk is very rich, containing more than twice the fat and protein of cow's milk. This very nutrient-dense milk is needed to support such rapid growth rate in the puppies.

Water must be provided in large quantities. Always remind owners of lactating bitches to provide clean, fresh drinking water at all times – a 35 kg bitch at peak lactation may need up to 6 litres of water per day.

A summary of the dietary recommendation for pregnant and lactating bitches is:
- Complete adult food for the first 6 weeks of pregnancy
- Complete puppy food for the final 3 weeks of pregnancy and throughout lactation
- Complete puppy food may be required by giant-breed bitches, e.g. Great Danes, during the entire pregnancy and lactation
- Puppy large-breed foods should not be fed to pregnant or lactating bitches since they are too low in energy density.

Feeding adult dogs and cats

OBESITY-PRONE DOGS AND CATS

Obesity is the most common nutritional disease in the Western world in both pets and their owners. A staggering 50% of dogs and cats in the UK are considered to be above their ideal weight, with prevalence increasing. This means that every other dog and cat owner you speak to in your practice will have a pet that might benefit from a weight-management product. When

> ### BOX 9.1 DOG BREEDS THAT ARE COMMONLY PRONE TO OBESITY
>
> - Labrador retriever
> - Cairn terrier
> - Cocker spaniel
> - Shetland sheepdog
> - Beagle
> - King Charles spaniel
> - Basset hound
> - Dachshund

> ### BOX 9.2 COMMON DISORDERS IN OVERWEIGHT DOGS AND CATS
>
> - Heart disease
> - High blood pressure
> - Constipation
> - Joint disease
> - Diabetes
> - Liver disease (cats)
> - Breathing problems
> - Exercise intolerance
> - Feline lower urinary tract disease (FLUTD)

> ### BOX 9.3 COMMON DISORDERS IN OLDER DOGS AND CATS
>
> - Heart disease
> - Kidney disease
> - Liver disease
> - Constipation
> - Joint disease
> - Obesity
> - Impaired hearing
> - Impaired vision
> - Dental disease

discussing weight control it should be remembered that many owners might feel guilty that their pet has become overweight. You are as much counselling them as giving nutritional advice for their pet.

True obesity, where the pet is more than 15% over the ideal body weight, is considered to be a clinical condition and requires careful weight reduction under the guidance of a veterinary professional. This is important, since severe obesity can contribute to many other clinical conditions that would require veterinary attention.

THE CAUSES AND RISKS OF EXCESSIVE WEIGHT GAIN

The cause of weight gain is essentially very simple – a pet is given more calories to eat on a daily basis than it requires. Overeating results in the extra calories being converted to fat and then the fat is laid down in the body tissues. These extra calories can be from treats and titbits given by the owner or simply by giving too much of the pet's usual food.

The way in which the pet is fed also has an influence on whether or not it gains weight. Pets that are fed on an 'ad lib' basis are at a greater risk of weight gain.

Other factors that increase the risk of a pet becoming overweight include:

- **Breed** – certain pure-bred dogs seem to be more prone to becoming overweight than crossbreed dogs (Box 9.1); however, pedigree cats are less likely to develop obesity than crossbreed 'moggie' cats.
- **Age** – older dogs tend to be less active and if their feeding level is maintained, they will gain weight.
- **Sex** – neutered dogs and cats require fewer calories than entire animals. To prevent weight gain the energy intake for both dogs and cat should be reduced by about 15% after neutering; transition to adult light diets or diets designed for neutered pets needs to occur at the correct time-of-life stage.
- **Lifestyle** – pets with inactive owners often become overweight as a result of physical inactivity. Likewise indoor cats are more likely to gain weight than those that have access to the outdoors.
- **Body condition during growth** – it has been shown that puppies and kittens that are allowed to become overweight during growth are always more prone to becoming overweight adults. This is because, when an immature animal overeats, the additional calories not only cause an increase in the size of the fat cells but also an increase in their number – fat cell hyperplasia. This means that the pet now has more fat cells that when it was born, resulting in a greater risk of becoming overweight.

You may also find that clients seeking nutritional advice for overweight pets have a similar problem themselves. This requires tactful handling and careful choice of words. It is best to use technically correct clinical words such as 'obesity'; words like 'chubby' don't give owners the severity of the problem. Obesity is a chronic medical condition that needs to be managed for life.

Excessive deposition of body fat is damaging to both the quality and length of the pet's life. Overweight dogs and cats are at a greater risk of developing many conditions (Box 9.2) – see Chapter 3 for details on weight loss clinics and diets.

Feeding senior dogs and cats

You will often be asked for dietary advice regarding the optimum nutrition of the seemingly healthy older dog and cat. If at any stage you feel that the pet may have an illness, it is best to suggest that the client consult the veterinary surgeon, rather than attempting to make a feeding recommendation.

Senior individuals represent a significant, and increasing, proportion of both the canine and feline populations. Improvements in health care and nutrition have extended the average life span for pets as they have for humans. Approximately one-third of all dogs and cats owned by your clients will fall into the senior life stage, which is defined as being older than 8 years of age. These individuals are at a much greater risk of developing many disorders (Box 9.3) but, with appropriate dietary management and veterinary health care, the onset of such disorders can be delayed or even prevented. Most pet owners pay particular attention to quality as well as quantity of life for their pets and all you can do to help them in this will be much appreciated.

ADVISING ON SENIOR DIETS

The senior or geriatric phase of life starts at varying ages due to breed size and species. Toy and small-breed dogs enter the senior stage of life at approximately 8 years, medium breeds 7–8 years, with large and giant breeds entering a senior life stage at 5 years. Cats are deemed as senior from 8 years. Other factors such as nutritional status, environment, genetic makeup and clinical health will affect these ages and longevity of the dog and cat. Changes that occur with age include greying of the muzzle and slowing down in activity levels; less obvious changes include alteration in the physiology of the digestive tract, immune system, kidneys and other organs. Generally, the capacity to absorb and utilise nutrients is not decreased in older animals, but the body does become less able to tolerate excesses and borderline deficiencies, and the ability to respond to dietary changes may also be decreased. 'Geriatric' screening should be considered in all animals once reaching a senior age. A critical part of this screening should include evaluation of nutrition.

Nutritional changes in the diet of the cat and dog are aimed at supporting the physiological changes that occur within this life stage. Energy requirements for senior animals are reduced, due to a decrease in activity levels and expenditure. Some active senior animals may require an energy density higher than that provided by senior diets, and a compromise between senior and adult maintenance is required.

In cats, however, the maintenance energy requirements do not decrease as they get older. This could be due to cats remaining relatively inactive throughout their adult life. It is difficult to tell between an older and younger cat simply by looking at its activity levels, as cats spend a large portion of their day sleeping. The proportion of obese cats does tend to increase until the age of 7 years; after this it decreases, especially from the age of 10 years.

A reduction in renal function should be considered in all senior animals; a reduction in protein quantities within the diet could be beneficial if renal damage has occurred. The quality of the protein should be increased as skeletal muscle (lean muscle) mass reduces, which also reduces any protein or amino acid reserves if required. Some life-stage diets do not have a reduction in protein levels, as some views are that restricted protein levels are not required until there is direct evidence of renal impairment. In fact, protein requirements sufficient to support protein turnover actually increase in older dogs and cats. Protein

restriction in feline senior diets should be avoided. Cats are especially sensitive to reductions in protein levels within the diet. This is due to the inability to downgrade protein metabolism pathways. Reduced protein digestibility is also experienced in geriatric cats. In healthy adult cats, protein digestibility is typically 85–90%. In geriatric cats, this digestibility can be reduced to less than 77%. Diets which have a severely restricted protein level or proteins of a low quality/BV can predispose cats over 12 years to negative nitrogen balance and loss of lean body mass.

The restriction of phosphorus in the diet plays a significant role in the prevention of renal impairment. A reduction in kidney function can also lead to an increased loss of the water-soluble vitamins, due to the kidney's decreased ability to concentrate the urine. This can also lead to a reduction in hydration levels of the animal. Senior animals have a reduced sensitivity to thirst, and thus there is a greater risk of dehydration in these animals.

Most senior diets are formulated to have softer kibbles in order to accommodate any dental problems, possible reduction in number of teeth and a drop in musculature of the jaw. Moving to a moist diet can benefit the animal if it is having difficulties with mastication. A moist diet will also aid hydration levels.

The use of antioxidants for senior animals has been advocated, as free-radical production can increase with age; the diseases associated with ageing (cardiovascular, arthritis) will increase further production of free radicals. Older cats and dogs should be evaluated for vitamin and mineral deficiencies. Due to oxidative damage, demand is greater for the antioxidant vitamins. Geriatric animals, especially cats, have a reduced ability to digest fats. Due to the association with fat digestibility and the digestibility of other essential nutrients (fat-soluble vitamins), deficiencies can occur.

As the animal ages, smell is the first sense to decline. As the animal's sense of smell deteriorates, the animal may eat less. The aroma of the diet is particularly important in diets aimed at senior animals in order to encourage consumption.

BIBLIOGRAPHY

Hand, M.S., Thatcher, C.D., Remillard, R.L., et al., 2010. Small Animal Clinical Nutrition, fifth ed. Mark Morris Institute, Topeka, KA.

RECOMMENDED READING

Agar, S., 2001. Small Animal Nutrition. Butterworth-Heinemann, Oxford.
   Text written especially for veterinary nurses and covers all aspects of the syllabus as well as providing information for work in practice.

Cooper, B., Mullineaux, E., Turner, L. (Eds.), 2012. BSAVA Textbook of Veterinary Nursing, fifth ed. British Small Animal Veterinary Association, Gloucester.
   One chapter covers the normal nutritional requirements of a range of companion animals.

10

Clinical Nutrition

ALISON JONES | NICOLA ACKERMAN

KEY POINTS

- Nutrition assessment of all patients is required each time the animal is presented to the veterinary practice.

- Good nutritional assessment ensures the correct nutrition for the animal, in both quality and quantity of the diet.

- Certain disease conditions change the animal's nutrient requirement and are described as nutrient-sensitive diseases.

- Part of the treatment of these diseases involves dietary management or clinical nutrition.

- The diet for each of these disease conditions must still provide the correct balance of the essential nutrients.

Introduction

Many disease conditions may result in an alteration in the patient's nutrient requirement, and they are described as nutrient-sensitive diseases. Their treatment may be facilitated by dietary management and the use of these specialised diets is known as clinical nutrition, which has gained increasing importance in recent years. Clinical nutrition is an area in which veterinary nurses are heavily involved, and a thorough understanding of how diet can influence the patient's recovery is invaluable in modern veterinary practices.

Nutritional assessment

It is important that all animals undergo a nutritional assessment, in order to give good clinical advice regarding nutrition. Nutritional assessment can be based on visual observations, such as body condition score and muscle condition score, and specific measurements such as weight and plasma protein measurements.

Recording the animal's weight and body condition score (BCS) as a puppy or kitten and throughout the growth phase allows monitoring of the animal's body condition. Many practitioners take the animal's weight, which was recorded at the time of the first annual vaccination (around 1 year old), as the individual's ideal weight or lean body mass. This can be a true reflection, but if the animal was overfed during the growth phase this weight will be an overestimation. Conversely, in larger breeds maturity and full adult size would not have been reached, and the use of this weight will be an underestimation of ideal body weight. Use of breed guidance charts is not advised as there can be huge variations within breeds and this does not

take into consideration frame size. When calculating a lean body mass for an individual the animal must be visibly assessed and palpated. Advising an owner what his or her animal should weigh, if it has never been seen before, is not recommended. Use of the BCS index is the method of choice, but it cannot recommend an actual figure for the ideal body weight. The BCS can be based on a 5-, 7- or 9-point scale. Some breeds do not suit some aspects of the BCS index. For example, Whippets and Greyhounds in good condition have limited fat cover. A muscle condition score (MCS) should be utilised alongside the BCS. It is especially important to use the MCS when initiating a weight loss diet, as dramatic losses could be due to a drop in muscle mass and needs to be prevented. Owners should be taught how to BCS their own pets in order to assess adequate food intake.

All of these methods are subjective, but perform the job adequately. Other very sophisticated techniques are currently being used in human patients or in research work (e.g. multiple-frequency bioelectrical impedance, dual-energy radiographic absorptiometry [DEXA] and neutron activation).

'Overcoat syndrome' occurs when an MCS of 1 or 2 is present but the animal is carrying excessive amounts of weight. The large fat deposits mask the muscle wastage that is occurring. This can easily occur in animals that suffer from a dramatic decrease in food consumption, e.g. acute anorexia. Other aspects of physical examination of the patient should be taken into consideration. These aspects include hair coat quality and skin condition, evidence of peripheral oedema or ascites (which may indicate hypoproteinaemia) and clinical signs that indicate certain deficiencies in micronutrients (e.g. neck ventroflexion or tetany).

The use of BCSs can prove to be helpful with patients suffering from chronic conditions that can affect weight and body condition. Patients suffering from cardiac conditions can develop ascites, and this fluid collection can cause an overall gain in body weight. The patient's BCS can, however, actually be decreasing as lean body mass is lost. This highlights the importance of monitoring BCS alongside weight at each consultation.

MONITORING NUTRITIONAL INTERVENTIONS

Once an animal has been recommended a specific dietary regimen, the animal should be reassessed after an appropriate period of time. This depends on the animal, severity of disease (if any present), original nutritional status and the type of nutritional intervention received. Regular weighing of the animal, BCS, MCS and blood haematology and biochemistry parameters can all be utilised in these cases. Animals that are placed on diets that alter urinary parameters, for example pH, should have these parameters monitored regularly.

Animals that are hospitalised should be weighed at least twice daily, and depending on clinical health this may be required to be performed more often. All medications and fluid therapy flow rates are based on body weight, and if the animal is severely dehydrated dose rates will need to be adjusted accordingly as the animal is rehydrated.

Nutrigenomics

Nutrigenomics is a branch of nutritional genomics and is the study of the effects of foods and food constituents on gene expression. Extensive research has shown that specific nutrients can affect the gene expression of certain inflammatory pathways in dogs and cats, such as those involved in osteoarthritis. These nutrients have been refined and incorporated into diets and supplements. Other nutrigenomics work has shown that nutrients within tomato pomace, carrots, flaxseeds and coconut oil all help to maintain a higher metabolism in animals losing weight.

Nutraceuticals are products derived from food sources that are purported to provide extra health benefits, in addition to the basic nutritional value found in foods. There are varying amounts of clinical research in support of the vast amount of nutraceuticals that are available on the market.

Antioxidants are used to neutralise the ill effects of free radicals (reactive oxygen species [ROS]) within the body. Free radicals are produced as by-products of chemical reactions necessary to sustain life, e.g. cellular respiration. Damage caused is dependent on the balance between the antioxidants and free radicals within the body. Certain conditions are associated with an increase in oxidative stress. The influence of free radicals scavengers (vitamins E and C, caratenoids and selenium) is significant, and plays a role in the ageing process contributing to the development and/or exacerbation of a wide variety of degenerative disease. Many factors can contribute to excessive levels of free radicals being produced. These include exposure to ultraviolet light and radiation, air pollution (including cigarette smoke), residues from herbicides and pesticides, and illness and the medications used to treat it.

PREBIOTICS AND PROBIOTICS

Prebiotics are substances that are able to alter the gastrointestinal flora in a manner to benefit the microorganisms. Probiotics, however, are a live microbial feed supplement, which benefits the host animal by improving the gastrointestinal microbial population. Probiotics generally used are comprised of lactic acid bacteria such as *Lactobacilli*, *Streptococci* and *Bifidobacteria*. Probiotics have been shown to be beneficial following acute gastroenteritis or a course of antibiotics, especially in hindgut fermenters such as rabbits and horses. Live yoghurt has similar beneficial effects – the yoghurt reinforces the gastrointestinal mucosal barrier and helps stimulate gastrointestinal immunity. Questions have been raised about the ability of the bacteria to survive the acidic environment of the stomach. Hence the use of prebiotics has been stated to be more advantageous than probiotics. Probiotics need to be provided in large enough numbers and potentially on a daily basis. Yeasts have also been included in some probiotic preparations. Their role is to aid in improving the digestibility of fibre and other nutrients. Populations of yeasts do not seem to be maintained within the established gastrointestinal flora, and thus in order to maintain their effect administration on a daily basis is required.

The three main mechanisms of action for probiotics are:
- Competitive exclusion. Colonisation sites within the gastrointestinal tract and nutrients within the gut are utilised by the probiotics. This reduces the availability of resources to the potentially pathogenic bacteria. Chronic gut dysbiosis (when undesirable microorganisms take over in large numbers) can have detrimental effects on the immune system of the digestive system.
- Immunomodulation. A synergistic effect exists between probiotics and the stimulation and functioning of the immune system.
- Digestive efficiency. Probiotic microflora have an important role in aiding the breakdown of complex food nutrients.

Prebiotics are specific nutrients, which encourage the growth of beneficial bacterial populations (e.g. specific types of fibre). Benefits that the host will experience from this manipulation of the gastrointestinal bacteria include:
- Inhibition of potential pathogenic bacteria, which will cause a reduction in endotoxins, carcinogens and substances associated with putrefaction
- Stimulation of gastrointestinal immunity
- Increased synthesis of vitamins, especially B complex and K
- Increased absorption of nutrients
- Improved faecal consistency
- Increased production of volatile fatty acids (VFAs)/short-chain fatty acids (SCFAs).

VFAs benefit the animal by increasing available nutrients for gastrointestinal bacterial populations, which in turn aid in preventing nitrogenous waste materials from entering the bloodstream and causing azotaemia. This process is sometimes referred to as nitrogen traps in renal diets. Examples of prebiotics include manno-oligosaccharides, glutamine and fructo-oligosaccharides.

Manno-oligosaccharides (MOSs)

MOSs are prebiotics that also aid in increasing the populations of certain microflora that benefit the animal. Their unique structure also attracts pathogens and bonds them to the manno-sugars, rather than attaching to the surface of the gut villi.

Glutamine

Glutamine is an amino acid commonly included in critical care nutrition diets, due to its immune-enhancing properties and ability to enhance wound healing. Glutamine is utilised in rapidly dividing cells, such as epithelial enterocytes and mucosal immune cells. Glutamine acts as a prebiotic by maintaining the overall health of the gut lining, and therefore ensuring optimal nutrient absorption.

Fructo-oligosaccharides (FOSs)

FOSs act as a nutrient source for the beneficial bacteria of the gastrointestinal tract. FOSs also increase gut transit time and draw water into the faeces, increasing bulk and softness.

Gastrointestinal disease

There are many different types of gastrointestinal disease, and the clinical signs depend on which part of the gastrointestinal tract is primarily affected.

GASTRITIS

The term 'gastritis' refers to inflammation of the stomach. Dogs vomit readily as a protective mechanism due to their natural scavenging nature. If they eat spoiled or rancid food they are able to vomit and so prevent illness. Conversely, cats are naturally hunters and will kill and eat fresh food. They are therefore much less likely to eat spoiled food and so vomiting is a much more unusual occurrence in the cat.

Gastritis patients should be considered for parenteral fluids, depending on the frequency and severity of the vomiting and degree of dehydration. When enteral feeding commences the chosen diet should be low fat and highly digestible, i.e. low in fibre. Low-fat foods are recommended because high-fat diets delay gastric emptying and so remain for a longer period in the stomach, increasing the chances of the vomiting persisting.

GASTRIC DILATION (BLOAT)

Bloat is an acute-onset condition of the stomach and is often fatal if the dilation leads to volvulus (see Chapter 23). It commonly affects large, deep-chested breeds, especially Great Dane, Weimaraner, St. Bernard, Gordon setter, Irish setter and standard poodle.

The cause is unknown but risk factors include:

- Increasing age – dogs over 7 are twice as likely to succumb
- Obesity
- Body conformation, e.g. a narrow, deep chest
- Stress
- Aerophagia, i.e. swallowing air during eating
- Postprandial exercise, i.e. exercise just after eating.

It is controversial as to whether diet affects the incidence of recurrence. Avoidance of postprandial exercise and competitive feeding may also help reduce aerophagia. At-risk dogs should not be competitively fed, as this may increase the ingestion of air. Very greedy dogs should use feeding dishes that slow down the feeding rate. All food should be fed raised up in order to reduce aerophagia.

ENTERITIS

Enteritis means inflammation of the small intestine and the most common clinical sign is diarrhoea. Traditionally a period of starvation was initiated; we now know that this is detrimental to the patient. The gastrointestinal tract derives its nutrients from the lumen, from ingested food, and any period of starvation harms the recovery of the tract and in fact causes more deterioration and the possibility of bacterial translocation. Bacterial translocation occurs when the enterocytes deteriorate and the gastrointestinal tract can become 'leaky'; bacteria from the gut lumen translocate into the bloodstream and set up sepsis. Nutrition in these cases is small, frequent feedings of low-fat, highly digestible meals. As the diarrhoea improves, the animal can be slowly put back on to the normal diet (over a 5–7-day period).

COLITIS

Colitis means inflammation of the large intestine and the most common clinical sign is watery diarrhoea, often containing blood and mucus (jelly), with excessive straining and often a dramatic increase in the number of motions passed each day. The affected animal may be constantly trying to pass faeces, only achieving a small amount of blood-stained mucus. Animals with colitis often benefit from diets containing an increased amount of fibre. Some cases of colitis have been linked to food allergy so a strict elimination diet trial with a single novel protein source is recommended in cases that fail to respond to higher fibre levels alone.

CONSTIPATION

Animals are said to be constipated when too slow a passage of faeces through the large bowel causes difficulty in passing hard, dry stools. This may be more common in older dogs and cats partly due to decreased physical activity. Since fibre increases the rate of passage of stools through the large intestine, diets that contain higher levels of fibre have proven beneficial in constipation. Many senior pet foods contain a higher level of insoluble fibre in an attempt to help prevent constipation. In cases where megacolon has been diagnosed it is important that the animal is placed on a low-fibre, highly digestible diet that has a very low residue. Medications that help with gut motility are required.

Obesity

Obesity is the most common form of malnutrition in pet animals and occurs when there is an increase in body weight that is 15% over the optimum weight for the animal's breed, age and sex. Recent surveys suggest that as many as 40% of dogs and 15% of cats may be clinically obese and most owners are totally unaware of their pet's problem.

The diagnosis of obesity is simple, requiring no specialist equipment. To diagnose obesity a body condition score of the animal needs to be performed (see Chapter 3).

When embarking on a weight-reduction programme for a pet, it is important to remember that you are treating the owner as well as the pet. You should always consider a planned exercise programme as well, but any increase in exercise should be undertaken with caution, especially if the pet has an underlying condition such as joint or heart disease.

The aim of dietary management for obesity is to produce safe, effective weight loss, at the same time maintaining healthy levels of protein, vitamins and minerals. Many commercial low-calorie foods are available, but the best effects are achieved when used in conjunction with weight clinics to monitor weight loss. There are different diets available that can be fibre based, higher protein with lower carbohydrate levels, or those that aid in increasing the metabolism of the animal. Diets that are high in fibre provide bulk, which improves satiety while at the same time reducing the energy density of the food and in some way controlling the absorption of the other energy-containing nutrients. It is important that owners are made aware that a planned weight-loss programme is not a crash diet and that gradual weight loss is safer and more effective. A large dog should lose no more than 3% of its body weight per week and a cat no more than 2% each week. To achieve safe weight loss you should aim to provide 60% of the metabolisable energy requirement (MER) needed to maintain optimum body weight in dogs and 70% of MER in cats.

Osteoarthritis

Wear and tear on joints over the life of a pet can lead to osteoarthritis. Acute injuries such as a ruptured cruciate ligament or joint infection can also damage cartilage and cause arthritis in both dogs and cats. Osteoarthritis (OA) is a common condition that affects up to one in five dogs over 5 years old and as many as 70% of cats over 12 years old.

The clinical signs associated with OA are due to degeneration of articular cartilage, loss of proteoglycans and collagen, proliferation of new bone and inflammation. This leads to pain and disability; owners will recognise lameness, stiffness and reluctance to exercise as well as a reduced ability to jump, play and use the stairs. Many cats with OA go unnoticed, since owners believe the lack of mobility is just associated with 'old age'.

Recent nutrigenomic studies have shown that supplementing pet food with certain omega-3 fatty acids such as eicosapentaenoic acid (EPA) in dogs and docosahexaenoic acid (DHA) in cats can lead to a reduction in the clinical signs associated with OA by diminishing joint inflammation (and so controlling pain) and by a reduction in the activity of proteoglycan-degrading enzymes such as aggrecanase. The evidence supporting nutritional supplements (nutraceuticals) such as glucosamine and chondroitin is very mixed. Nutraceuticals and diets containing EPA for dogs and DHA for cats, however, have very supportive evidence for the positive effects of these nutrients and should be recommended in all patients with OA.

Skin disease

To achieve a healthy-looking coat requires good overall health and nutrition throughout the year. A period of poor skin and hair condition may take several weeks or months to completely recover. For hair to regrow after shaving may take 3 to 4 months in a short-haired dog and up to 18 months in a long-haired breed.

The skin and coat can influence nutrient requirements. Hair length, thickness and density affect temperature regulation in cold environments. The hair cycle is influenced by general health status, genetics, seasons, temperature, hormones and nutrition, as well as poorly understood intrinsic factors. Hair does not grow continuously, but in cycles. Each cycle consists of a growing period (anagen) during which the follicle is actively producing hair, and a resting period (telogen). During telogen, hair is retained in the follicle as dead hair, which is subsequently lost. Hair growth is maximal in summer and minimal in winter when up to 90% may be telogen. Illness, malnutrition and stress from reproduction may shorten anagen considerably and force many hair follicles to enter into telogen at the same time. Since telogen hair is shed easily, malnutrition can result in a visible thinning of the hair coat and cause a dull, lustreless hair coat through nutrient deficiency.

The skin and coat account for about 30–35% of the daily protein requirements of the healthy adult small-breed dog with a long coat. Nutrition is important in achieving and maintaining good skin and coat condition. Important nutrients include:
- Protein (especially sulphur-containing amino acids)
- Energy
- Fat
- Fatty acids
- Vitamin A
- Vitamin B
- Vitamin D
- Vitamin E
- Zinc
- Copper.

Irrespective of the nutritional cause of the disease, the skin usually only responds to nutritional imbalance in a limited number of ways. Skin changes that often indicate nutritional abnormality include:
- A sparse, dry, dull, brittle coat with hairs that epilate easily
- Slow hair growth or regrowth following clipping
- Abnormal scale (seborrhoea sicca)
- Loss of hair, crusting and erythema
- Decubitus ulcers
- Poor wound healing
- Loss of normal hair colour.

In healthy pets eating high-quality commercial pet foods, deficiencies of protein, fat, carbohydrate, vitamins and minerals causing skin disease are very rare. Nutritional deficiencies may be noted when animals have been anorexic for a period of time. Concurrent disease may reduce the ability of the animal to digest, absorb or metabolise nutrients. Animals fed home-made diets are more likely to develop nutrition-related skin and coat disease, since many of these diets are not balanced.

Nutritional imbalance may occur when owners overfeed a single food type. This is most commonly seen in cats fed on a liver-only diet which contains very high levels of vitamin A. Imbalances may also occur from the improper use of mineral supplementation. This can cause skin disease when the oversupplementation of one nutrient affects the levels of another nutrient that is important in maintaining skin and coat health. This is most commonly seen where oversupplementation of calcium gives rise to zinc deficiency.

Genetic factors may mean that the animal is unable to absorb or utilise a particular nutrient, causing skin or coat disease, e.g. zinc deficiency in Alaskan Malamutes.

The common clinical signs of skin and coat disease are:
- Pruritus
- Seborrhoea
- Alopecia
- Hyperkeratosis
- Pyoderma
- Otitis externa
- Slow hair regrowth after clipping.

Animals with non-specific skin disorders should be fed a high-quality, complete, balanced diet containing adequate levels of fat and essential fatty acids plus good-quality, highly digestible protein.

FOOD-ALLERGIC SKIN DISEASE

In rare cases the animal may actually be allergic to the protein within the diet. This is a true food allergy, but the term 'food allergy' is often misused. Many pet owners refer to the reaction their pet had to a particular food as an 'allergic' reaction when it may have just been food intolerance. A true food allergy must involve the pet's immune system and takes many months or even years to develop. A dog or cat that reacts to a new food the first time it is exposed to it probably has food intolerance.

Food allergy or hypersensitivity is an immunological response to one or more dietary proteins. It is considered the third most common skin hypersensitivity disease in dogs and the second most common in cats, accounting for up to 5% of all canine dermatoses and 6% of feline. The prevalence and severity of food hypersensitivity reactions are greatest in younger animals.

Clinical signs are predominantly associated with the skin and/or gastrointestinal tract. A high proportion of food allergies produce skin signs, primarily non-seasonal pruritus; the other skin signs mostly result from self-trauma. Cutaneous signs of food allergy include:

- Pruritus, generalised or localised – including pedal, perineal and facial areas
- Otitis externa
- Miliary dermatitis in cats
- Crusting/scaling
- Secondary pyoderma.

Studies have shown that in more than 65% of all the reported cases dogs were allergic to one of three main foods, i.e. beef, dairy products or wheat (or, more accurately, wheat gluten). Similar studies in cats have found that more than 80% of reported cases could be attributed to beef, dairy products or fish.

An elimination diet trial, for up to 10 weeks, is considered the only certain method of confirming food allergy and without it food allergy may remain undiagnosed. Diet trials can present difficulties and they have been eliminated by the use of protein hydrolysate technology. Major food allergens are proteins with molecular weights between 10 000 and 70 000 daltons. Hydrolysate technology uses digestive enzymes to break down these proteins to their components (peptides and amino acids), reducing their antigenicity up to 66 times. Hydrolysed protein components have an average molecular weight less than 6000 daltons, too small to trigger an immune reaction.

ESSENTIAL FATTY ACID DEFICIENCY

The epidermis depends on a supply of essential fatty acids (EFAs) derived either directly from the diet or via synthesis in the liver and transported to the skin in the blood. EFAs have a structural function in the lipoproteins of cell membranes. One of the most important functions of EFAs in the skin is to provide an essential barrier to prevent the loss of water and other nutrients through the epidermis. Linoleic acid must be provided in the diet of dogs and linoleic and arachidonic acids in the diet of cats.

Clinically, EFA deficiency can occur in animals fed low-fat dry or semi-moist commercial foods, or patients fed special low-fat therapeutic diets. Inexpensive or poorly stored foods and those with inadequate antioxidants are more likely to cause an EFA deficiency.

Skin changes have been described in dogs and cats with EFA deficiency. Skin abnormalities include:

- Scaliness (seborrhoea sicca)
- Matting of hair
- Loss of skin elasticity
- Alopecia
- Dry, dull coat
- Hyperkeratosis
- Interdigital exudation
- Otitis externa
- Lack of hair regrowth
- Extensive hair loss.

Fatty acid deficiency is rapidly reversible if the diet is supplemented with EFAs. Although the deficiency may take up to 6 months to develop, clinical signs often start to resolve within a few days of EFA supplementation and the skin is usually healthy within 6 to 8 weeks. Cats with EFA deficiency must be given pork or poultry fat as well as vegetable oils, since arachidonic acid is only found in fat of animal origin.

Diabetes mellitus

The diet chosen for the diabetic patient should:

- Be balanced to support long-term maintenance
- Help achieve and maintain normal serum glucose levels – this is important since it has been shown that good glycaemic control is important in preventing vascular and neurological complications that are often associated with uncontrolled diabetes
- Decrease postprandial glucose peaks
- Achieve as normal as possible metabolism of carbohydrates, fats and proteins
- Normalise body weight
- Be suitable for the senior life stage, since most cases of diabetes in dogs and cats are diagnosed in pets over the age of 7 years.

The key nutritional factors in diabetes are energy, protein, fat and carbohydrate, both soluble and insoluble.

PROTEIN

The chosen diet should contain sufficient protein to ensure normal development and maintenance of body functions. Diabetic dogs and cats have increased urinary losses of amino acids and this should be remembered when considering the optimum protein intake for the diabetic patient. A balance must be achieved between providing sufficient protein to meet daily needs and replace urinary losses while preventing an excess intake that may enhance renal damage or contribute to increased insulin secretion.

Protein levels for diabetic dogs should be approximately 15–25% on a dry matter basis (DMB) and more than 28% DMB for cats. The management of feline diabetes involves feeding high-protein (50% DMB), low-carbohydrate foods. These have been shown to increase tissue sensitivity to insulin and reduce cholesterol, leading to improved glycaemic control.

FAT

Dogs and cats with diabetes have abnormal fat metabolism. Many diabetic pets have increased serum levels of cholesterol and concurrent pancreatitis is a common finding. High-fat diets cause insulin resistance and decrease the number of insulin receptors; therefore high-fat diets should be avoided in dogs and cats with diabetes mellitus.

The supplementation of the diet with omega-3 fatty acids is controversial and in human diabetics there is conflicting evidence that these are beneficial. Omega-3 fatty acid supplementation has been shown to reduce the incidence of atherosclerosis, but not without other complications to glycaemic control. Since the risk of vascular damage is less in pets than in humans, the inclusion of omega-3 fatty acids does not seem to be desirable. The fat content of the diet should be restricted to less than 20% on a DMB.

SOLUBLE CARBOHYDRATE

Diabetic cats should not be fed diets containing fructose. Fructose is often found in commercial semi-moist foods as a humectant and as high-fructose corn syrup. Cats do not metabolise fructose, causing fructose intolerance, polyuria and potential renal damage. Some nutritionists believe that high-carbohydrate diets may be partly responsible for the onset of diabetes mellitus in cats. As a rule, soluble carbohydrates should make up no more than 30% of the total dietary carbohydrate level.

INSOLUBLE CARBOHYDRATE

Dietary fibre is one of the most important nutrients to consider in the management of diabetes mellitus in dogs.

FOOD TYPE

The physical presentation of the diet for dogs and cats with diabetes mellitus warrants some consideration. It has been shown that soft, moist foods (those marketed as individual meal-sized portions, usually in foil packets) have a hyperglycaemic effect compared to dry foods because they contain increased levels of simple carbohydrates (sugars) and the ingredients used as humectants (such as propylene glycol). These diets are unsuitable for diabetic pets and should be avoided. Providing the nutritional profile of the chosen food is within the desirable range, there is no advantage or disadvantage in using either canned or dry foods.

Dental disease

Dental disease is the most common disease affecting pet dogs and cats. It is so widespread that it could be thought of as an epidemic. Pet owners can easily identify the signs associated with dental disease, especially bad breath, but often do not link these signs with dental disease. Prevention is an important step in helping to keep pet dogs and cats healthy, since the presence of dental disease has been linked with an increased incidence of systemic diseases, including heart disease, kidney disease and respiratory disorders.

Dental disease begins with the accumulation of an invisible substance, called pellicle, on the surface of the tooth. Pellicle forms within a few minutes of tooth brushing and is formed from proteins found within saliva (Fig. 10.1). The natural development of pellicle encourages the deposition of plaque, which

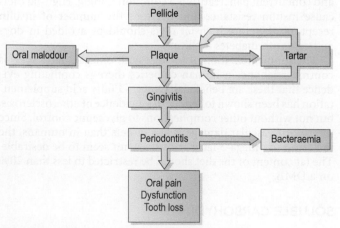

Fig. 10.1 Significance of the development of pellicle on the signs of periodontal disease (Adapted from Hill's Pet Nutrition.)

in turn becomes mineralised to form tartar (dental calculus) and also gives rise to halitosis (oral malodour). Tartar formation, by providing a rough surface, encourages further plaque deposition. The toxins from the bacteria in plaque, aided by the irritation caused by tartar, result in gingivitis (sore, red, inflamed gums that bleed). This is the beginning of periodontal disease and if this disease progresses, periodontitis results. Periodontitis causes the supporting structure of the tooth (the periodontal ligament) to become damaged and ultimately destroyed, leading to loosening, and finally loss, of the teeth.

The best way to keep teeth and gums healthy is to encourage your clients to brush their pets' teeth daily. Despite awareness that tooth brushing is how we keep our own teeth clean, most pets have never had their teeth brushed. This may be due to the temperament of the pet or simply due to lack of time or motivation on the part of the owner.

Life-stage diets are available that help to avoid the occurrence or recurrence of periodontal disease, by wiping away accumulated plaque and tartar when the pet animal chews. These foods are designed to allow a tooth to penetrate each piece of food (kibble) before the kibble splits. The fibres in the kibble are non-randomly aligned to clean the surface of the tooth as they come into contact with it and they wipe the accumulation of plaque, stain and tartar from the tooth's surface. By reducing plaque accumulation these dental foods may help to control bad breath.

Dogs and cats with severe periodontal disease require appropriate veterinary treatment to control bacterial spread and promote healing. The advanced nature of the condition, with severe inflammation and pain, means that they cannot chew effectively on affected teeth. Attempts at chewing might force food particles into exposed tooth sockets, causing bleeding and local irritation. If a pet has had extensive treatment for severe periodontal disease the veterinary surgeon and the client will need to monitor the healing and postoperative oral pain to determine when the feeding of an appropriate dental food can begin.

Cancer

Few diseases evoke as much emotion as cancer. A diagnosis of cancer is traumatic for both the owner and sometimes the veterinary practice team. Many owners already have some personal experience of cancer and they may approach cancer in their pets with some preconceived ideas, especially with regard to the use of chemotherapy. They may need considerable support and assistance during the initial weeks following the diagnosis.

Cancer cachexia may occur in dogs with seemingly good nutritional intake because the composition of the food is inappropriate for the canine cancer patient. The general metabolism of patients with cancer is forced to compete with the tumour for glucose and amino acids which are used for energy. The dog must therefore rely on fat as a source of calories since the tumour has a limited ability to use fat as an energy source. The following nutrients have been found to be vital in the management of cancer.

CARBOHYDRATE

Dogs do not have an essential requirement for carbohydrate in the diet. Most dogs have a remarkable ability to utilise carbohydrates for energy so they are often used by pet food manufacturers as a primary source of dietary energy. Dogs with cancer develop high levels of insulin and lactate, as the tumour uses glucose and produces lactate. High-carbohydrate foods should be avoided in dogs with cancer since they would add to this hyperinsulinaemia and hyperlactataemia. Carbohydrates should comprise less than 25% of the food's dry matter.

FAT

Dogs use fat as a source of energy and to aid in the absorption of the fat-soluble vitamins. Canine cancer patients must rely on fat as a source of calories, so to facilitate this and to reduce the loss of body fat stores, the ideal food should be high in fat. Dietary fat should make up 25–40% of the food's dry matter.

OMEGA-3 FATTY ACIDS

Dietary levels should be in excess of 5% of the food's dry matter, and research has shown that a food high in omega-3 fatty acids is beneficial to the cancer patient by:
- Inhibiting tumour growth and cancer spread
- Reducing cachexia by decreasing protein breakdown
- Enhancing immune function
- Reducing radiation damage to healthy cells.

PROTEIN

Normal healthy dogs use protein and amino acids to build muscles and organ tissue and to maintain immune status. In the dog with cancer the tumour is competing for these same amino acids. The ideal food for the canine cancer patient should therefore be higher in protein than a normal adult maintenance food. This is a very unusual profile for a canine senior food (many canine cancer patients will be in the senior stage of life), which would normally have controlled levels of protein. Dietary levels should be between 30% and 45% of the food's dry matter.

ARGININE

Arginine has been found to be essential in dogs with malignant tumours, and high levels improve both immune function and anabolism. Dietary levels should be in excess of 2% of the food's dry matter.

Chronic renal failure

Chronic renal failure (CRF) is a progressive deterioration of renal function that occurs throughout an animal's lifetime as part of the normal ageing process. In renal failure the kidney is unable to excrete metabolites at normal plasma levels under normal fluid loading or to retain electrolytes when the intake is normal. In the majority of adult dogs and cats, some degree of renal disease exists.

Clinical signs of renal failure include:
- Polyuria/polydipsia
- Weight loss
- Inappetance
- Uraemia/azotaemia
- Ulceration of oral/gastric mucosa
- Vomiting
- Dehydration
- Unkempt appearance.

The main problem facing the clinician is that changes do not occur in the blood of affected animals until 75% of nephrons have ceased functioning, i.e. the animal has lost the equivalent of one whole kidney and half of the other and these nephrons can never be repaired.

Early diagnosis of kidney disease can be made by considering urine specific gravity, daily water intake and urine chemistry. The animal with early renal problems will lose the ability to produce the most concentrated urine when about 66% of nephrons have ceased functioning. This stage is termed 'renal insufficiency' and it is now that dietary intervention should begin rather than waiting until the animal is uraemic and in renal failure.

The aim of dietary management in renal disease is to ameliorate clinical signs and slow down progression of the disease. Correct diet for an animal with renal compromise is critical. The animal still needs a nutritionally balanced diet that provides all the nutrients required for maintenance. By reducing the daily intake of phosphorus, renal deterioration can be slowed down, which is the most important element in the management of CRF. Moderate protein restriction can help to reduce the clinical signs caused by uraemia but adequate protein must be included in the diet to prevent the breakdown of lean body mass to provide essential amino acids. It is best if the protein source for animals with CRF is of very high biological value.

Dietary management is the cornerstone of the management of CRF in both the dog and the cat; however, other medical therapies can be beneficial to the overall well-being of the pet. Renal failure causes imbalances in minerals and electrolytes that can make the animal feel unwell:
- Hypokalaemia is common in cats with CRF. This causes muscle weakness, inappetance, anaemia and lethargy. Dietary supplementation is best but clinical cases can be treated with oral potassium gluconate and then maintained on a diet with adequate levels of potassium. Many renal diets have supplemented potassium levels in order to prevent this.
- Hyperphosphataemia can occur in CRF as a result of decreased ability of the damaged kidney to excrete phosphorus and reduced renal production of active vitamin D. This high circulating level of phosphorus stimulates the parathyroid glands to increase secretion of parathormone (PTH), leading to the development of renal secondary hyperparathyroidism. Excess levels of PTH have a deleterious effect on bone metabolism and result in pain and osteomalacia (termed 'rubber jaw', or renal rickets). Control of blood phosphorus levels is best attempted by dietary restriction of intake; however, some cases may benefit from oral phosphate binders if dietary restriction alone fails to correct hyperphosphataemia within 2–4 weeks. Intestinal phosphate binders can be administered with food at a dose rate of 60 mg/kg/day, increasing to 150 mg/kg/day if tolerated.
- As the animal is suffering from polyuria, there is an increased loss of water soluble vitamins. Renal diets are therefore supplemented in B vitamins.

The ideal nutrient profile for the management of renal failure is:
- Controlled protein, but of a high biological value
- Controlled sodium to help prevent hypertension
- Controlled phosphorus
- Buffered

- High fat
- Increased levels of B vitamins and potassium.

Liver disease

Liver disease is common in both dogs and cats. The liver has an enormous capacity to regenerate, so liver disease is not often diagnosed until the later stages of the disease process. In recent years significant new information has emerged concerning the metabolic changes that occur in patients with liver disease. These studies have also found that the correct nutrition is a vital step in helping to reverse these metabolic changes and facilitate recovery.

There is a vast array of supportive therapy for the liver patient in order to optimise regeneration; however, nutritional support is the cornerstone of therapy. A fine balance must be achieved between providing sufficient high-quality nutrients to allow regeneration, without overwhelming the metabolic capacity of the diseased liver, which may lead to the accumulation of toxic metabolites. The key objectives of dietary management are to:

- Maintain homeostasis
- Correct electrolyte disturbances
- Avoid accumulation of toxic by-products
- Support liver repair and regeneration
- Support storage and synthesis within the liver
- Prevent or reduce encephalopathy
- Improve the overall nutritional status of the animal.

The key nutrients of concern for the dog and cat with liver disease are as follows.

PROTEIN

Hyperammonaemia is a common finding in dogs and cats with liver disease because of the development of portosystemic shunts and the impaired activity of the urea cycle. This is the key metabolic abnormality that leads to hepatic encephalopathy. The clinical presentation of animals with hepatic encephalopathy can vary from mild lethargy to the severe classic central nervous system disturbances. Finding the correct level of protein in the diet for the liver patient presents a nutritional dilemma. A balance must be found between reducing the level of protein to control hepatic encephalopathy and at the same time providing sufficient protein to allow for adequate production of plasma proteins and for hepatic regeneration and repair.

The current recommendation is to provide a moderate level of high-quality protein containing a low level of aromatic amino acids. This will allow regeneration but limit the development of metabolic neurotoxins. Arginine is an essential amino acid for both dogs and cats. It is needed for the synthesis of protein and amino acids and is essential in the optimal function of the urea cycle. In patients with liver disease a high intake of arginine has been found to be beneficial by reducing blood ammonia levels and improving nitrogen balance.

ENERGY

Patients with liver disease have decreased glycogen stores and develop insulin resistance through increased glucagon levels. These metabolic abnormalities lead to the early onset of gluconeogenesis. This protein catabolism can be reduced by providing frequent small meals and by ensuring that sufficient calories are provided in the form of carbohydrate and fat.

CARBOHYDRATE

A very high carbohydrate intake must be avoided because insulin resistance commonly occurs in liver disease and can lead to glucose intolerance. This can be avoided by providing sufficient calories in the form of fat.

FAT

This is the most energy-dense nutrient, providing over twice as many calories per gram as either carbohydrate or protein. The provision of calories from fat supports protein synthesis and prevents gluconeogenesis. Fat also improves the palatability of the diet, an important fact in the liver patient where inappetance is very common. Fat also provides fatty acids, the major fuel for the liver, heart and skeletal muscles. The intestinal assimilation of fat is not compromised in dogs and cats with liver disease unless there is severe extrahepatic biliary obstruction, which is rare. This means there is no need to routinely restrict dietary fat in the liver patient; in fact, studies have shown a correlation between high-fat diets and increased survival in dogs with hepatic insufficiency.

L-CARNITINE

The final step in the synthesis of L-carnitine occurs in the liver and consequently it may be deficient in cases of liver disease. This deficiency may lead to the accumulation of free fatty acids in the cytoplasm and failure of the mitochondria, with impairment of the citric acid cycle, fatty acid oxidation and the urea cycle. This combines to cause an increase in blood ammonia levels. By supplementing the diet with additional L-carnitine this deficiency is avoided and thus the fatty acids provided from the dietary fat can be utilised as an energy source. Additional L-carnitine also decreases the risk of hepatic lipidosis, which is of particular concern in cats.

SOLUBLE FIBRE

Soluble (fermentable) fibre in the diet is fermented in the gastrointestinal tract to produce short-chain fatty acids, which provide an alternative energy source for enterocytes, stimulate intestinal motility and encourage bacterial proliferation and epithelial cell growth. These all combine to result in a significant reduction in the production and absorption of ammonia, which helps to reduce the degree of hepatic encephalopathy, as less is entering into the bloodstream. The use of fermentable fibres has been termed a 'nitrogen-fixing trap', and some renal supplements utilise them to add in the resulting reduction of uraemia.

COPPER AND ZINC

Copper toxicosis is a well-recognised syndrome in Bedlington terriers, West Highland White terriers, Doberman Pinschers and Skye terriers. Copper accumulates in the liver of all breeds in most forms of hepatobiliary disease, especially when a degree of cholestasis is present. The ideal diet for liver patients should be low in copper. Increased zinc intake decreases the intestinal uptake of copper and may also have a local protective effect against copper toxicity. Adequate zinc also helps to limit hepatic encephalopathy and may have an antifibrotic effect.

Critical care of the anorexic patient

Anorexia is defined as a loss of appetite. It is important to differentiate between an animal that is unable to prehend, masticate and swallow food (dysphagia) from an animal that is anorexic because of secondary systemic disease.

Many conditions cause a patient to become anorexic and these include:

- Alteration in taste or smell, due to profuse nasal discharge, old age, etc.
- Pain due to ulcers or foreign bodies, e.g. bones, needles
- Systemic disease, e.g. renal failure
- Trauma, e.g. head injury, jaw fracture
- Gastrointestinal tract dysfunction, e.g. intestinal obstruction, tumour
- Neoplasia.

When treating an anorexic patient consideration should be given to fluid and electrolyte balance as well as the calorie and protein content of the food. Water is the most important nutrient, since two-thirds of an animal's lean body mass consists of water and a 15% loss of body water would be fatal. An animal's water needs are met by drinking, by water in food and by water produced from energy metabolism in the body, but severe water loss may occur through vomiting, diarrhoea, salivation and burns. During periods of reduced water intake or increased water loss the kidneys attempt to conserve body water by producing more concentrated urine. If water loss exceeds water intake, dehydration occurs. All dehydrated critical care patients should have their fluid deficit measured and replaced as a matter of urgency via intravenous fluid therapy.

As well as fluid therapy, additional nutritional support is indicated if there has been recent weight loss of more than 10% or a history of anorexia for more than 2 days. The food chosen for the critical patient depends on the underlying issue, the clinical state of the patient and the life stage of the patient. As a general rule, if the gut works, then use it.

Protein makes up 15–20% of body weight. Initially an anorexic animal will use up all body glucose and then stored glycogen. After the first 4 days of food deprivation, muscle protein is catabolised. If this anorexic animal has malignant disease or burns, further protein losses will occur, leading to basal protein requirements increasing by up to 2–3 times depending upon the severity of the disease.

Animals will need extra protein as a source of calories and to support wound healing, maintain the immune system and reverse the hypermetabolic processes. When feeding a critically ill or anorexic patient you should aim to supply at least 4 g protein/100 kcal for the dog and at least 6 g protein/100 kcal for the cat. The total amount of both protein and calories needed will vary with the severity of the illness, e.g. a patient with a major burn will need twice the basal energy requirement (BER), whereas immediately after surgery the additional calorie needs will only be around 1.25 × BER (see Chapter 9). Animals with severe fluid loss may require supplemental water-soluble vitamins, especially B vitamins.

Some patients will refuse to eat voluntarily or may be too severely ill or injured to accept oral feeding. The enteral route is still preferred, since it is the most efficient and allows nutrition of the enterocytes. Failure to supply the enterocytes with their preferred fuel (glutamine) can result in defects in the intestinal mucosa and bacterial translocation from the gut into the bloodstream. If a patient refuses voluntary nutrition, tube feeding should be considered. Many different types of feeding tube are available, including:

- Naso-oesophageal tubes – simple to place and tolerated in most animals, although problems may arise if an animal sneezes or gags the tube out
- Oesophagostomy tube – may also be associated with gagging and local infection, but in most patients they are well tolerated
- Gastrostomy tubes – percutaneous endoscopic gastrostomy (PEG) tubes may be placed using an endoscope. There is also a piece of equipment called an ELD applicator that allows a gastrostomy tube to be placed without the need for an endoscope. The main advantage of a tube placed directly into the stomach is that it can be left in situ for considerably longer periods and it allows the use of larger quantities of food. When feeding through a tube, care should be taken not to exceed the maximum stomach capacity for the patient. This is 90 ml/kg/feed for an adult dog and 45 ml/kg/feed for a cat.

The diet used for tube feeding should be balanced, easily digested, easily assimilated and easily utilised. It should be in a form that does not block the tube.

Canine urolithiasis

Common forms of canine bladder stones and crystals include:

- Struvite – composed of magnesium ammonium phosphate (also known as triple phosphate). These crystals and stones are common in puppies, bitches and any dog with bacterial infection in the urine. Most cases of bladder stones and crystals in puppies are due to struvite formation. Bacterial infection is present in 95% of all cases and causes an increase in urinary pH, facilitating the formation of struvite, which forms in alkaline urine. One of the most important factors in preventing struvite crystals and stones is maintaining a normal, i.e. acidic, urine with a pH of 6.2–6.4. This can be achieved by dietary management.
- Calcium oxalate – tend to form in more acidic urine. They are more common in male dogs over the age of 8 years and in certain breeds, especially the Lhasa Apso, Shih Tzu and Yorkshire terrier. Calcium oxalate stones are more likely to also occur within the kidney. Dogs that consume high amounts of oxalate in their diets, e.g. vegetables, tea, nuts and chocolate, are at a greater risk of developing these stones. One of the most important factors in preventing their occurrence is reducing the calcium content of the urine and maintaining slightly alkaline urine. This means that the dog's urine should have a pH in the range 7.1–7.7, which can be achieved by dietary management.
- Ammonium urate – tend to form in more acidic urine. They are more common in certain breeds of dog, especially the Dalmatian and Yorkshire terrier. Dogs with liver disease are also more prone to the development of ammonium urate bladder crystals and stones.
- Cystine – tend to form in acidic urine. Most individuals affected with cystine urolithiasis are male bulldogs. It is assumed that they form as a consequence of a genetic defect in kidney function.

Dietary control is vitally important in the management of canine urolithiasis. Dietary management is useful both in the short-term treatment and in the long-term prevention of recurrence of the problem.

Struvite can be dissolved using a combination of drugs, including antibiotics if a bacterial infection is present, and diet. This is achieved by reducing the intake of the 'building blocks' of the stone. Struvite stones are composed of magnesium, ammonium and phosphate. Dissolution diets should therefore contain a controlled level of the minerals magnesium and phosphorus, plus an increased level of sodium. This increased sodium level encourages the dog to drink more water and produce a greater volume of urine, and so flushes the bladder out more frequently. The special dietary formulation also causes the formation of acidic urine, with a pH of about 6.0. At this level the formation of further struvite crystals is inhibited and those already present dissolve in the urine.

Disease caused by calcium oxalate uroliths can only be treated surgically, as these stones do not dissolve once formed. To prevent recurrence, provide a diet that contains a controlled level of the 'building blocks' of this stone type, plus one that produces more alkaline urine. The diet should contain controlled levels of both calcium and oxalate and produce a urinary pH of 7.1–7.7.

Feline lower urinary tract disease

Feline urinary tract issues may result from a number of different aetiologies, including infection, neoplasia, urolithiasis, neurological disorders, anatomical abnormalities and inflammatory conditions. The name 'feline lower urinary tract disease' may not be wholly representative of the condition; the role that stress has on the urinary system is starting to become more fully understood. Of the feline patients seen in first opinion practice approximately 7% present with urinary disorders. With increases of the prevalence of risk factors such as obesity there is the potential that more cases will be presented.

Feline lower urinary tract disease (FLUTD) is not a single disease but a group of conditions, many of which cause inflammation of the lower urinary tract. The most common presenting signs of FLUTD are:
- Difficulty passing urine – dysuria
- Altered frequency of urination
- Incontinence
- Haematuria.

Dietary control is vitally important in the management of FLUTD, especially in those cases caused by urolithiasis (most commonly struvite and calcium oxalate in the cat) and is useful both in the short-term treatment of FLUTD and in the long term to prevent recurrence of the problem.

Struvite can be dissolved using dietary management, environmental changes and increased water consumption (see Chapter 3). Dietary management is achieved by reducing the cat's intake of the 'building blocks' of the stone. Since struvite stones are composed of magnesium, ammonium and phosphate, the diet should contain a controlled level of the minerals magnesium and phosphorus. An increased level of sodium can be fed, as this increased sodium level encourages the cat to drink more water and produce a greater volume of urine and so flushes the bladder out more frequently. The special dietary formulation also causes the formation of acidic urine, with a pH of about 6.0. At this level the formation of further struvite crystals is inhibited and those present dissolve into the urine.

Dietary management is also important in the prevention of recurrence of FLUTD. In cases of struvite urolithiasis the diet should contain a controlled level of the 'building blocks' of the stone plus it should produce a naturally acidic urine (pH 6.2–6.4). Since obesity is a major predisposing factor in the development of FLUTD, calorie intake should be controlled in all overweight cats.

In cases of calcium oxalate urolithiasis, feed a diet containing controlled levels of both calcium and oxalate that produces a urinary pH of 6.6–6.9. This helps to inhibit the formation of calcium oxalate crystals. A dietary source of soluble fibre is also helpful, since the fibre will bind with calcium in the gut to further reduce the amount of renal excreted calcium. Every effort should be made to ensure that cats affected with FLUTD drink more water. Reducing the urine specific gravity will reduce the chance of recurrence.

Hyperthyroidism

Dietary management of feline hyperthyroidism relies on supplying a diet that has had all iodine removed. Without iodine the overactive thyroid cannot produce the thyroid hormones and the resulting clinical signs. Monitoring of the patient needs to follow the same protocol as all other hyperthyroid patients receiving other medical management. Dietary management only works when there is complete compliance from the owner in not allowing the cat to consume any other types of food or supplements.

BIBLIOGRAPHY

Hand, M.S., Thatcher, C.D., Remillard, R.L., et al., 2010. Small Animal Clinical Nutrition, fifth ed. Mark Morris Institute, Topeka, KA.

RECOMMENDED READING

Ackerman, N., 2012. The Consulting Veterinary Nurse. Wiley Blackwell, Oxford.
    Good reference book covering all aspects of clinical nutrition, and how to advise pet owners about dietary management.
Agar, S., 2001. Small Animal Nutrition. Butterworth-Heinemann, Oxford.
    Written especially for veterinary nurses and covers all aspects of the syllabus as well as providing information for work in practice.

Hand, M.S., Thatcher, C.D., Remillard, R.L., et al., 2010. Small Animal Clinical Nutrition, fifth ed. Mark Morris Institute, Topeka, KA.
    Very detailed coverage of the subject. Good reference text.
Kelly, N., Wills, J., 1996. Manual of Companion Animal Nutrition and Feeding. British Small Animal Veterinary Association, Cheltenham.

Good reference book that covers all aspects of nutrition in health and disease. Includes feeding of small pets and exotic species.

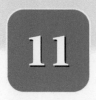

Equine Nutrition

CORINNA PIPPARD

KEY POINTS

- The anatomy and physiology of the equine digestive system is designed to deal with poor-quality food that is eaten throughout the day and digested slowly.

- A healthy horse must be provided with a similar range of essential nutrients to any other mammal, but the relative proportions of each depend on the type of horse and the 'work' it is undertaking.

- All food must be stored in such a way as to prevent deterioration and supplied to the horse using appropriate equipment.

Introduction

The genus *Equus* has evolved to roam large areas in search of its main food ingredient, grass. As a prey species, it has to be constantly aware of its surroundings and ready to flee instantaneously. As a result, the digestive system has evolved to deal with a poor-quality diet eaten over a long period of time and undergoing a slow but constant digestive process.

There are generally considered to be six species within the genus *Equus*, and a number of subspecies: *Equus przewalskii*, the wild horse; *Equus asinus*, the African ass; *Equus hermionus*, the Asian ass; and *Equus burchelli*, *Equus zebra* and *Equus grevyi*, the zebras. The origin of *Equus caballus*, the domestic horse, is something of a mystery, since it does not occur in the wild. The nearest relative of *E. caballus*, *E. przewalskii*, has one extra pair of chromosomes, 33 pairs compared with the 32 pairs of the domestic horse.

With domestication, many horses have to cope with being confined for large periods of time and fed two, three or four meals a day, a situation that is good for neither the mental nor physical health of the horse. The original purpose and design of the digestive system should always be considered when feeding horses, and care should be taken to ensure that a feeding system as close to nature as possible is chosen.

The digestive system

(See also Chapter 8.)

The digestive system of the horse can be divided into two parts:

- The foregut – comprises the mouth, oesophagus, stomach and small intestine; function is similar to these parts of the digestive system of other monogastric animals, e.g. dog and cat.
- The hindgut – comprises the caecum, colon and rectum; the caecum and colon fulfil a function analogous to the reticulo-rumen in ruminants, providing a region where extensive microbial fermentation of food can take place.

PRECAECAL DIGESTION

In this, the first part of the horse's digestive system, physical and chemical digestion take place as they would in humans, cats or dogs. Food is ingested and ground by the teeth before being swallowed and entering the stomach, where enzymatic digestion starts. Enzymatic digestion, followed by absorption, continues in the small intestine.

Mouth

Teeth. Adult dentition in the horse consists of a total of 40–44 teeth in the male (stallion or gelding) and 36–40 teeth in the mare. All horses have three upper and lower incisors on each side of the jaw, three upper and lower premolars, and three upper and lower molars. In the male, and occasionally the female, canine teeth known as tushes are found and many horses have extra premolar teeth, known as wolf teeth, which are frequently removed to aid placing of the bit. There is a large gap between incisor and premolar teeth, known as the diastema, which aids the separation of newly ingested and partly masticated food (Fig. 11.1A).

Foals are normally born without teeth, and the central incisors erupt during the first week of life, followed, at about 4–6 weeks and 6–9 months, by the lateral and corner incisors, respectively; premolar teeth also erupt at this time. Deciduous teeth are replaced by permanent teeth in the same order between the ages of about 2.5 and 4.5 years.

All the permanent teeth in the horse are constantly erupting and the grinding surface is made up of ridges of enamel and dentine (Fig. 11.1B). Since enamel wears more slowly than dentine and the horse subjects its food to a shearing and grinding movement, the surfaces of the teeth maintain a rough profile. They may develop sharp edges, which must be removed by a vet, or equine dentist, for efficient mastication of food. There is evidence that feeding from the ground leads to a more natural pattern of wear than feeding from a height (e.g. haynets).

The eruption of the deciduous and permanent teeth and the pattern of wear may be used as a means of determining the age of a horse; however, as the horse gets older this becomes less accurate.

Tongue. The tongue of the horse feels very soft because of the presence of shorter and softer filiform papillae than in other animals. Fungiform, foliate and circumvallate papillae are also present. Taste buds are present, and the horse can detect sweet, sour, bitter and salt flavours.

Lips. Lips are prehensile and very sensitive and are used by the horse to aid food selection and prevent the ingestion of potentially harmful material. A horse is capable of selecting individual ingredients out of a coarse mix or eating the last blades of grass from around a poisonous plant without touching it.

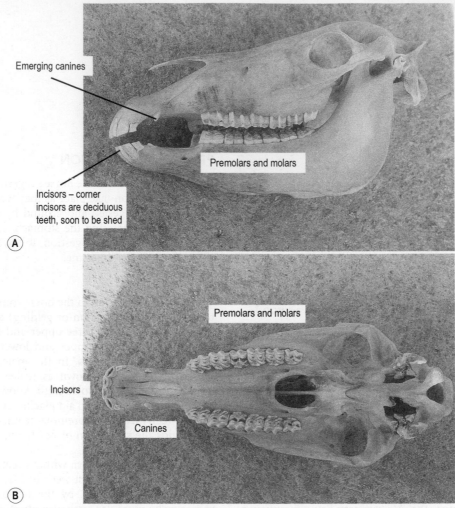

Fig. 11.1 (A) Dentition of a 4-year-old male horse. (B) The same horse, showing the ridges on the teeth that enable a rough surface to be applied to the food

Salivary glands. Horses secrete a large quantity of saliva (10–15 litres per day), the main purpose of which is to lubricate food. A small amount of salivary amylase is secreted but is probably of little importance. Bicarbonate is also secreted which has some buffering capacity.

Oesophagus

A muscular tube, similar to that found in other domestic animals, the oesophagus passes down the left side of the neck. The passage of food and water may easily be observed.

Stomach

The stomach of the horse is simple and digestion is monogastric as in the dog and cat. The stomach is small (7–14 litres) compared with the size of the animal and accounts for only about 7.5% of the total digestive tract. Living in natural circumstances the horse would normally graze for a large proportion of the day and food would continually enter and leave the stomach with little actual digestion occurring apart from the initial breakdown of protein. The horse is unable to regurgitate food. In the stabled horse the stomach fills rapidly when a concentrate meal is fed and then acts as a storage organ, enabling food to enter the small intestine in small quantities for maximum

digestion. The buffering capacity of the saliva may enable a limited amount of fermentation to take place in the first part of the stomach.

Small intestine

The small intestine is responsible, as in other animals, for the majority of enzymatic digestion of food and its subsequent absorption. In the horse the tract is long (about 16 m) and accounts for around 75% of the length of the gastrointestinal tract, but only 27% of its volume. As in other animals, it is divided into three parts, the duodenum, jejunum and ileum, and the ileum ends at the ileocaecal junction (Fig. 11.2). Digesta moves rapidly along the small intestine but, despite this, under normal circumstances digestion and absorption of soluble material are usually complete by the time it reaches the ileocaecal junction.

Large intestine

It is in the large intestine or hindgut that fibre digestion takes place, undergoing a microbial fermentation similar to that seen in ruminants and rabbits. The main areas involved in this process are the caecum and colon (see Fig. 11.2). The size and complexity of the hindgut in the horse are what makes its

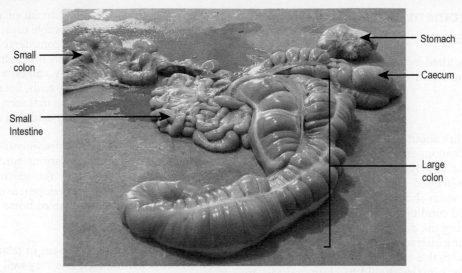

Fig. 11.2 Gastrointestinal tract of the horse

digestive system so different from that of other monogastric animals; the hindgut accounts for around 65% of the volume of the digestive tract.

Caecum. The caecum is a large (25–35 litres), blind-ending sac about 0.8 m long, running forwards along the base of the abdomen, and it is here that food entering from the ileum starts to undergo microbial fermentation. The digesta contains around 90% water but by the time defecation occurs the water content has fallen to about 60%, the largest proportion of water being reabsorbed in the caecum.

Colon. This can be divided into two parts: the large colon, mainly concerned with the digestion of fibre, and the small colon, where further water reabsorption takes place. Both are about 3–3.5 m long; however, parts of the large colon are up to 50 cm in diameter, while the small colon is only about 7.5 cm in diameter.

The large colon houses a considerable number of microorganisms, similar to the rumen in cattle and the caecum and colon of rabbits. It runs from the ileocaecal junction cranially towards the sternum – the right ventral colon, where it makes a turn – sternal flexure, back towards the pelvis – left ventral colon, then a sharp turn – the pelvic flexure, forwards again towards the diaphragm – left dorsal colon, and then backwards again – diaphragmatic flexure and right dorsal colon. Finally, the large colon makes another turn and crosses from one side to the other – transverse colon – before becoming the small colon. An important point to note, and a potential problem area, is the pelvic flexure, where the colon narrows from a diameter of about 25 cm to around 2 cm while undergoing a 180° turn. In the grass-fed horse this serves to slow down the passage of food, allowing ample time for microbial digestion; however, in the stabled horse fed a much drier diet and unable to move around freely, it can sometimes be the site of an impaction.

The small colon is approximately the same length as the large colon but of a smaller diameter (see Fig. 11.2). Microbial fermentation does not stop here; however, it is of less importance and the main function of the small colon is to slow the passage of digesta and reabsorb water to enable relatively dry faeces to be voided.

Rectum and anus

The rectum acts as a storage area for faeces, as in other mammals. Horses will defecate frequently throughout the day and night, maintaining a constant throughput of material through the gastrointestinal tract.

MICROBIAL ACTIVITY IN THE HINDGUT

Unlike many other monogastric species, the horse is capable of living on a diet solely composed of fibrous roughage and a large population of microorganisms is housed in the enlarged hindgut. These microorganisms consist of about $0.5–5 \times 10^9$ bacteria per gram of contents and $0.5–1.5 \times 10^5$ protozoa. Fungi are also present, but in much smaller numbers.

Microbial enzymes are capable of breaking the β-1,4 linkages found in cellulose, unlike mammalian enzymes, and produce end-products of volatile fatty acids (largely acetic, propionic and butyric acids) and lactic acid, which can be absorbed directly from the hindgut. Other products of microbial fermentation of potential use to the horse are amino acids and a number of vitamins.

The microorganisms in the hindgut are very specific to the type of food eaten by the horse and also to the pattern of meals eaten when the horse is fed concentrates. Changing the diet suddenly can result in the death of large numbers of microorganisms that were digesting the old foodstuff and an insufficient number capable of digesting the new foodstuff. Such changes in diet can result in impaction, colic, laminitis and swollen legs.

Unlike some other hindgut fermenters, such as the rabbit, the horse does not normally practice coprophagia, although foals may be observed eating the faeces of adult horses, usually their mother's. This may be done in an attempt to populate the hindgut with suitable microorganisms. As they do not generally eat their own faeces, horses probably make little use of the amino acids synthesised by their microorganisms, although some may be absorbed.

Dietary management

ESSENTIAL NUTRIENTS

The basic nutrients required by the horse are the same as for most other domestic animals. However, the form in which they are offered differs.

Water

An adult horse will drink about 25 litres of water a day, more in hot weather, after strenuous exercise or in the case of a lactating mare. For the horse at grass, much of or the entire water requirement may be obtained from its food. Although it is usually advocated that water should be available at all times, it is likely that, under wild conditions, horses only drink at dawn and dusk, thus increasing the distance that can be travelled in search of food during the intervening time. However, unless all food is fed damp it is advisable to make sure that water is regularly available. All water supplies should be clean and easy to reach. Dehydration in the horse will reduce performance, since the horse relies extensively on sweating as a cooling method and severe dehydration (loss of 10–12% bodyweight) can be fatal. Donkeys are much more resistant to water deprivation than horses.

Energy

This can be obtained from carbohydrate, fat or protein. In the horse, the largest proportion normally comes from carbohydrate. Energy deficiency in the diet will result in a thin and probably lethargic horse; too much energy will result in either an unmanageable horse or one that is overweight, which can lead to a variety of other problems.

Carbohydrate

The majority of the natural diet of the horse consists of carbohydrate and this can be divided into soluble and insoluble carbohydrate. Unlike many monogastric animals, the horse has evolved to make good use of insoluble carbohydrate by utilising microbial action in the hindgut. The gross energy (GE) content of carbohydrates is about 17.5 MJ/kg.

- **Soluble carbohydrate** – consists of sugars and starches. Grass, especially young grass, contains large amounts of sugars which are readily digested in the small intestine and will produce abundant energy quickly. Starch is found less in the natural diet but is a major component of commercial concentrate diets. It must always be remembered that the horse does not digest starch particularly effectively, although some starches are more easily digested than others with cooked starches being the most readily digested. Any soluble carbohydrates undigested in the small intestine will enter the large intestine where they may upset the balance of the microbial population and cause serious problems.
- **Insoluble carbohydrate** – like the ruminants, the horse is capable of digesting a large proportion of the fibre in its diet. The structural parts of plants are made up of a variety of celluloses, hemicelluloses, lignins and other materials. None of these are digestible by mammalian enzymes but, with the exception of lignin, can be digested by microorganisms. In the hindgut, these are broken down to volatile fatty acids and lactic acid, which are used by the horse for energy and produce a large amount of gas, which is either absorbed into the bloodstream or released via the anus. Unlike the digestion of soluble sugars, the process is a slow one and also produces a considerable amount of heat. Since the horse relies only partly on **glucose** absorbed from the gastrointestinal tract for energy, and obtains a large proportion of its energy from volatile fatty acids, the glucose concentration of a horse's blood is lower than that seen in other monogastric animals. The only volatile fatty acid that can be metabolised to glucose is propionic acid.

Lack of **fibre** in the diet is detrimental to the horse's health, both physical and mental. Various physical problems result from the lack of activity in the gastrointestinal tract, and boredom, with the possible development of stereotypical behaviour, may also occur in the stabled horse fed too little fibre.

Fat

Despite the fact that fat is present in relatively small quantities in the horse's natural diet, it is very well digested and utilised. Since fat contains about 2.3 times the GE (39 MJ/kg) of a similar weight of carbohydrate, it is an excellent energy source, especially where bulk intake or heat production must be restricted, e.g. in the endurance horse. The metabolism of fat also releases a considerable quantity of water, which the horse can utilise.

Protein

Like most animals, the horse has a requirement for amino acids, rather than protein, and 10 of these amino acids are believed to be essential (arginine, histidine, isoleucine, leucine, lysine, methionine, phenylalanine, threonine, tryptophan and valine). A high-quality protein will contain a good balance of these amino acids such that the horse can build its own proteins without a large wastage of unnecessary amino acids.

Protein cannot be stored in the body and any excess will be broken down in the liver. The carbon skeletons are then used for energy (protein contains about 24 MJ/kg GE), and the nitrogen is excreted as urea. Feeding excess protein is detrimental to horses since the deamination process requires energy and gives rise to considerable heat production. The urea produced requires water for its excretion, thus increasing water requirements, and in the case of the stabled horse, the urea breaks down to ammonia in the bedding and contaminates the stable air.

Protein deficiency gives rise to reduced protein and amino acids in the blood, resulting in reduced tissue synthesis. This is obviously of greatest importance in growing or reproducing animals but will also limit performance in the working animal.

Vitamins

Under normal conditions, the horse requires very few actual vitamins in its diet as it is capable of synthesising most of them itself. Vitamin A can be formed from β-carotene, which is abundant in grass. Vitamin A, along with vitamin D, is stored in the liver and a horse kept at grass during the summer can synthesise enough of both vitamins to avoid any deficiency during the winter. Vitamin D can be formed by the action of sunlight on the skin in a similar fashion to that seen in other animals. Vitamin E is found in many plants and, although not so readily stored, is rarely deficient in the horse's diet. Vitamin K is formed in the large intestine as in other mammals. Of the water-soluble vitamins, most of the B complex are formed by the microbes in the hindgut and a horse fed plenty of bulk is unlikely to suffer

TABLE 11.1	Approximate nutrient contents of some roughages			
Roughage	Dry matter (g/kg)	Crude protein (g/kgDM)	Fibre (g/kgDM)	Soluble carbohydrate (g/kgDM)
Grass	180–300	80–170	130–270	5–460
Hay	850–880	45–110	300–380	20–50
Haylage	500–650	80–100		50–90
Silage	200–350	100–190	230–340	10–100
Lucerne	230–240	170–220	240–300	60–80
Swedes	120	108	100	590
Carrots	115–130	100	95	
Sugar beet pulp (molassed)	876	90–120	130	300
Sugar beet pulp (unmolassed)	900	100	175–200	80
Oat straw	860	34	394	
Barley straw	860	30–40	390–410	

Roughages vary widely in their nutrient contents; these figures are a guide only.
g/kgDM, grams per kilogram of dry matter.

from any deficiencies of these. Vitamin C can be formed by the horse from glucose.

Minerals

The minerals required by the horse are similar to those required by other mammals, and are divided into macrominerals and microminerals, or trace elements. Since horses are often involved in heavy work that results in considerable sweating, electrolyte needs may be greatly increased at these times.

Common foodstuffs

ROUGHAGE

Grass

Grass is the most natural form of food for horses and the foodstuff around which the gastrointestinal tract has evolved.

Grass has a natural cycle of growth according to the seasons and as a result its feeding value varies. Growth starts in the spring when the ground warms up sufficiently and at this time the grass is low in dry matter but what dry matter there is, is high in sugars and proteins. As the season progresses growth rate increases, as does the dry matter and fibre content, and, as a result, protein and sugar levels fall.

During a very dry summer, and in the autumn as the soil cools, growth slows down and may cease altogether and what grass is available is very high in fibre and low in protein and sugar. Left to its own devices, a horse will put on weight over the spring and summer when grass growth and quality are at their maximum. Using the stored fat to carry it through the winter when there is little high-quality grass around. Foals are born in the late spring and early summer, allowing the mares to make best use of available foodstuffs at the end of pregnancy and during early lactation.

Domesticated horses, expected to perform throughout the year, will need their diets supplemented during the winter months to avoid the loss of too much weight. They are also generally confined to much smaller areas than their wild counterparts would have been and thus cannot rove in search of better pasture. Conversely, many animals, especially 'good doers' such as native ponies, need to have their intake restricted in the spring and summer to prevent them becoming overweight and possibly developing other problems such as laminitis.

All pastures for horses should be securely fenced, have a good water supply and be free of toxic weeds, especially ragwort. Many garden plants are toxic to horses and if a field borders a garden it is best double-fenced (this will also keep the owners of the garden happy).

Conserved grass

Since it is necessary to continue feeding throughout the winter despite the poor quality of grass, a number of methods of conserving excess spring and summer growth for feeding throughout the colder months have been developed.

Table 11.1 shows the nutrient contents of some forms of roughage that may be fed as replacements for grass.

Hay. Hay is the most common form of conserved grass fed to horses. Like the grass from which it is made, hay varies in quality according to the time of cutting and the care spent making it. It is always of lower quality than the grass from which it is made because of the inevitable losses which occur during the process of haymaking (see Table 11.1). The majority of hay used for horses is cured in the field and thus cannot be made until day length is sufficiently long and the weather sufficiently settled for the drying process to be carried out without fear of rain. As a result, much hay is made late in the season, when the grass is well past its best. The increased volume available is also a factor, and farmers may delay making hay in order to achieve more bales per hectare.

Hay can also be barn-dried in the UK, where the weather ceases to be a major factor, allowing hay to be cut much earlier. However, the cost of drying and the reduced quantity mean that the cost is prohibitive for most horse owners, although the resulting hay is generally of very high quality.

The dry matter content of hay is high (around 850 g/kg), but during the process of haymaking there is some loss of protein and sugar and a corresponding increase in the amount of fibre. Vitamin D increases, because of the action of sunlight on the cut grass, but carotene decreases dramatically. Contrary to popular opinion, the quality of hay cannot be assessed by its smell and appearance and analysis is needed. A good overall guess can be made if the source is known, together with the time of cutting, length of drying, weather conditions, etc., but these are no substitute for chemical analysis.

Two types of hay are generally available to the horse owner:
- Seeds hay – cut from specially sown grass leys. This tends to contain fewer species of grass, sometimes only one, and few other plants.
- Meadow hay – cut from permanent pasture. This will contain whatever was growing at the time, often a wide variety of grasses and broad-leaved plants, some of which may be toxic.

Opinion varies as to which is better for horses, but meadow hay has more variety and if hay forms the main bulk of an animal's diet throughout the winter it is more likely to fulfil nutritional requirements than hay made from a single grass species. Meadow hay is generally leafier and may have a higher nutritional value than late-cut seeds hay, which is sometimes little better than straw.

Hay is generally relatively cheap, although it will vary according to the harvest. Small bales are easy to handle (although still quite heavy, especially directly off the field) and easy to store in a watertight barn. Large bales, although otherwise satisfactory, require mechanical assistance to move them.

Hay can be fed off the floor, in a rack or in a net, and there are many new types of hayfeeders on the market. Many horses prefer to eat off the floor, as this is a natural position for them; however, this can lead to wastage, as some hay is trampled on. Nets and racks both raise the hay off the ground. Generally, nets are better, and can be filled in the barn and carried to the horse with little loss. A net with small holes will slow down the rate of consumption, which may be advantageous for the stabled horse.

One major disadvantage of hay is its potential dustiness and mould content. Hay that is obviously very dusty or mouldy should never be fed to horses, as the mould spores can be dangerous to both the horse and its owner. Low dust levels can be dealt with by damping the hay, either by steaming it in a bin or by immersing it briefly in water. Long soaking washes out nutrients and is not recommended. The quality of hay decreases during storage and hay should not be kept from year to year.

Haylage/silage. The popularity of haylage and silage for feeding to horses has greatly increased in the last few years. Neither is as dependent as hay on the weather for its satisfactory conservation, although better products will be made in good weather.

Silage is made by cutting a crop (generally grass, maize or cereals grown especially for cutting), packing it into a clamp or wrapping large bales in polythene and leaving it to ferment in an anaerobic environment. Once the fermentation process is complete, the silage will keep indefinitely provided no air is allowed in. The dry matter content of silage is relatively low, although it is very variable and generally a silage with a high dry matter content will be better than one with low dry matter. Silage for horses should always be made with great care, avoiding soil contamination, which can lead to detrimental fermentation and possible toxicity. The use of additives is generally not recommended. Little loss need take place during the process of silage making, so the conserved product will have the same feeding value as the grass from which it was made provided the process was carried out well.

Haylage combines the qualities of hay and silage and is made by allowing the cut grass to dry to a certain extent and then packing it into polythene, where a limited fermentation takes place. The resulting product combines the characteristics of hay and silage, having a dry matter content higher than silage but lower than hay. There will be small losses of protein and sugar, with an increase in fibre, but these are much less than in hay. Well-made haylage has a very sweet smell, and is extremely palatable to horses.

Both haylage and silage deteriorate on contact with air so, unless they can be obtained in small bales, are not really satisfactory for the one-horse owner. The bales, because of their water content, are much heavier than hay bales and will probably require mechanical handling. Recently there has been a large increase in feeding of haylage to horses, with the result that many contractors have started to produce it. Small bales are much more readily available and, as they are easy to handle, they suit the one-horse owner; however, they are relatively expensive.

Despite some problems, both silage and haylage are suitable feeds for horses and do not have the dust and mould problems associated with hay (although mould patches will sometimes be found in haylage if a bale has been damaged and these should be disposed of). Silage, because of its high water content, is probably best left to horses not expected to perform very strenuous work but haylage, with its higher energy content, is an ideal roughage food for the performance horse.

When fed by weight, more haylage or silage is needed than hay because a larger proportion of the weight is water, and it will usually be possible to cut down on concentrates because of the higher energy content. The horse owner should not be misled into feeding less because of the higher energy content – this may result in diarrhoea due to a reduced fibre intake.

Legumes

Legumes are plants that fix nitrogen by means of bacteria located in nodules in their roots. As a result they contain higher levels of crude protein than grasses. Several varieties of clover are frequently found in pasture and they have the capacity to increase the overall feeding value of that pasture, in terms both of its protein and mineral levels and the length of time the pasture is of high quality. This is because the nutrient content of legumes falls more slowly during the growing season than that of grasses.

Lucerne (also known as alfalfa) is a legume often used in horse feeds both as a source of roughage and to increase the protein content of the diet. In many countries lucerne is fed as hay; however, in the UK it is usually fed either as chaff or as pellets. Feeding lucerne will increase the protein content of the diet and also the calcium content, since it has a very high ratio of calcium to phosphorus. Lucerne also has a higher energy level than grass so, if fed dried by weight, it should be possible to decrease the concentrate intake.

Roots

Roots may also be fed to horses – mangolds, swedes, turnips, carrots and sugar beet, for example, are all suitable. Roots contain a high proportion of water and sugar as well as containing roughage. They are therefore succulent and a useful addition to the diet of the stabled horse. Sugar beet pulp is also available in dried form, both molassed and unmolassed, and after soaking makes a palatable addition to the diet as well as supplying a useful amount of energy and roughage. Since it absorbs three or four times its own weight in water, the amount to be fed should be weighed out before soaking.

Straw

Straw can be fed to horses. Wheat straw is best avoided, since it is very hard, although many horses bedded on wheat straw will happily eat it. Both barley and oat straw are suitable and may be particularly useful for adding bulk to the diet of animals that would otherwise get too fat. Some straw, fed at night to the stabled horse along with its hay and concentrate feeds, will keep it occupied once the higher-quality foods have been consumed.

CONCENTRATES

When a horse is expected to perform more than the lightest of work, a diet composed purely of roughage foodstuffs rarely provides sufficient energy, since the horse is restricted in the amount of food that can be consumed. To overcome this, concentrate foodstuffs in the form of a variety of grain-based diets are fed. Grains, although containing a higher energy level than grass and other roughage, contain poor-quality protein and thus if they are added to the diet it is usually necessary to add an extra protein source as well. Concentrate foodstuffs can be given either in the form of straights (single foodstuffs) or compounds (mixtures of two or more foodstuffs).

Straights

Any single foodstuff such as oats, lucerne or soya beans can be classed as a straight foodstuff. The addition of grain to the ration increases the starch content and care needs to be taken that the capacity of the horse's small intestine to digest and absorb starch is not exceeded. Excess starch reaching the large intestine is likely to give rise to rapid fermentation with a subsequent lowering of pH and possible serious results. Grains tend to be low in protein and have a poor balance of amino acids, being generally short of lysine and one or more other essential amino acids. They also tend to have a poor calcium : phosphorus ratio, which can lead to bone disorders.

These deficiencies in grain can be counteracted by adding other straight foodstuffs. For example, lucerne has an excellent calcium : phosphorus ratio, and contains a high level of good-quality protein. As it is a roughage, much of it is digested in the hindgut, which makes it an excellent foodstuff. Another good protein source is soya bean, which has the best level of lysine of any of the vegetable protein sources generally fed to horses. Table 11.2 shows the nutrient contents of some straight foodstuffs.

Oats. In the UK, oats have been the traditional foodstuff for horses and of all the cereal grains they are still probably the best for this purpose. Oats have a higher fibre content than other cereals, which, while lowering the energy content, also improves the texture of the grain in the stomach and aids digestion. Naked oats without the husk are also available. They have considerably higher energy levels than other oats and should be fed with great care. Oats are normally fed crushed, since, if a horse does not chew its food properly and the husk is not damaged, the oat grain can pass through the gastrointestinal tract undigested. However, whole oats can be fed to a horse that chews its food properly.

TABLE 11.2	Approximate nutrient contents of some straight foodstuffs			
Foodstuff	Energy (DE) (MJ/kgDM)	Crude protein (g/kgDM)	Fibre (g/kgDM)	Ca (g/kgDM)
Oats	10.9–13.4	100–140	100–125	0.5–1.1
Barley	12.8–15.4	100–130	50–65	0.5–0.6
Maize	14.2–16.1	90–105	24–25	0.2–0.5
Linseed	11.5–18.5	220–380	66–100	2.3–4.3
Soya bean meal	13.3–14.7	500–540	40–70	3.0–4.0
Sunflower meal	9.5–11.7	280–490	130–320	2.9–4.5
Field beans	13.1	275	75–80	1.0
Dried lucerne	9.2–10.0	156–220	240–290	11.3–15.1

DE, digestible energy; g/kgDM, grams per kilogram of dry matter; MJ/kgDM, megajoules per kilogram of dry matter.

Barley. Barley may be fed in the form of extruded rings. It can also be fed as a grain but it is best rolled, as it is very hard. Barley has a higher energy content than oats and is also denser, so care must be taken to feed by weight not by volume. Extruded barley is lighter and the cooking process makes the starch more digestible, so it is probably preferable to the uncooked grain.

Maize. Maize is fed extensively to horses in America and the UK. It is usually in a flaked form, although other forms are available, and the cooking process improves digestibility. Maize has the highest energy content of all the cereals and should be fed with caution to all but the hardest-working horses.

Compounds

Feeding a horse on straight foodstuffs is possible but these days the majority of horses are fed on compounds produced by animal feed companies. Although this is more expensive than feeding straights, compounds are usually more satisfactory because they are produced to suit all types of horse and pony and are nutritionally balanced, taking the onus off the owner to get the balance correct. They are available as cubes and mixes. Both consist of a range of grains with protein sources and usually some vitamin and mineral additives. Their palatability is usually high, not least because molasses is used in their manufacture. For horses doing less work, or those that put on weight easily, balancer cubes may be fed in small quantities, in order to overcome any deficiencies in their forage. Table 11.3 shows the nutrient contents of some typical types of compound foodstuff.

Cubes. The cubes fed to horses vary slightly in size but are usually fairly small with a diameter of about 5–6 mm. The ingredients used are generally the same as in coarse mixes but are ground up, mixed with molasses and forced through a die before being bagged up and sold. Although it is not possible to see the individual ingredients, if bought from a reputable firm there should be no reason to doubt them.

Coarse mixes. Many owners prefer coarse mixes largely because they look more appetising and it is also possible to see what has

TABLE 11.3	Approximate nutrient contents for different types of compound foodstuff		
Foodstuff	Energy (MJ/kgDM)	Crude protein (g/kgDM)	Fibre (g/kgDM)
Maintenance and light work	8.5–10.5	85–105	135–200
Hard work	11.5–13.0	120–140	60–140
Showing	10.0–12.5	100–150	95–190
Stud	11.5–12.0	140–160	65–100
Fibre replacer	8.0–8.5	100	200
Balancer	9.9–14.2	100–261	72–170

g/kgDM, grams per kilogram of dry matter; MJ/kgDM, megajoules per kilogram of dry matter.

gone into making them. One possible disadvantage lies in the ability of some horses to sort through foodstuff and they may become very adept at leaving certain ingredients, thus unbalancing the ration.

ADDITIVES

Where a reputable brand of compound is fed at the level recommended by the manufacturer, it is not generally necessary to give the horse any additives. Many horses, however, are given less than the stipulated amount or may have a particular problem such as poor hoof quality. These horses may benefit from certain additions to their diets. All additives should be fed with care: unnecessary additives are at best expensive and at worst toxic.

Molasses

Molasses is a by-product of the sugar industry used widely in the animal foodstuffs industry. For horses it can be obtained in liquid form and poured on to a feed to encourage a shy feeder. Most compound foodstuffs contain quite a high proportion of molasses, e.g. to bind cubes together and to reduce the dust in coarse mixes.

Herbs

Herbs are a popular addition to both human and equine diets. A large number of herbal supplements are produced to suit a variety of situations, e.g. oestrus problems, skin conditions and stiff joints. In its natural state the horse would have access to a wide variety of plants and would seek out for itself those required.

Vitamin and mineral supplements

A large number of vitamin and mineral supplements are produced for the equine industry. For many horses these are a waste of money, but some situations require them.

Prohibited substances

As with human athletes, equine athletes are subject to restrictions regarding diet and supplementation. Foodstuffs produced for the competition horse should be sold with a guarantee that they contain no prohibited substances. The owner must also make sure that the horse does not consume any of these substances in the form of titbits, topically applied substances or from the pasture.

Nutritional requirements

The nutritional requirements of the individual horse depend on a number of factors, e.g. age, workload, health. Although some horses are kept at maintenance levels, many are kept either for reproduction or to carry out some physical task. Requirements have generally been split into a requirement for maintenance and an additional amount that can be considered as production, in the form of either growth or work.

Whatever activity the horse is required for, it must be borne in mind that there is a physical restriction on intake, generally believed to be around 2–2.5% of bodyweight. In practical terms a horse of around 15.2 hands high (hh) (155 cm) weighing 500 kg can eat about 10–12.5 kg of dry matter a day, or the equivalent of approximately half a bale of hay. Hay alone may be sufficient for maintenance and, for a 'good doer' fed good hay, even this amount may be too much. For the horse in hard work there is a limit to the amount of concentrates that can be substituted for hay, since a certain amount of roughage must always be fed and this limits the potential energy intake.

MAINTENANCE

Maintenance requirements are considered to be the amount required by an animal to maintain its current weight and condition, with the addition of an allowance for essential movement such as foraging. Maintenance requirements allow the body to function, without any additional activity.

PRODUCTION

Working

Many horses are kept for work, which can vary from light hacking at weekends to the strenuous demands made by 3-day eventing or endurance riding. Depending on the level of work required, the energy requirements are considered to be maintenance plus an additional fraction of maintenance energy. The National Research Council (1989) considers that a horse in:

- Light work, e.g. gentle hacking, requires 1.25 × maintenance energy
- Medium work, e.g. show jumping, requires 1.50 × maintenance energy
- Hard work, e.g. eventing or endurance riding, requires 2 × maintenance energy.

However, opinions vary as to what can be termed light/medium/heavy work, and the condition of the horse in question must always be carefully monitored and feeding adjusted accordingly. Little extra protein is required for work and any extra is normally supplied by the increased rations fed without any further additions.

Horses in strenuous work (Fig. 11.3) sweat copiously and the fluid and electrolytes lost must be replaced if the horse is not to suffer from dehydration. There are a number of ways of doing this, but probably the most satisfactory is to administer an electrolyte paste via a syringe into the horse's mouth and then allow access to fresh water. Because the fluid lost in sweat is isotonic with blood, many horses will not feel significant thirst in spite of the water loss and will refuse to drink unless the electrolytes are first replaced.

Because the digestive system of a horse is designed for a poor-quality roughage ration, it does not take kindly to a high intake of concentrate foods with a consequent lowering of

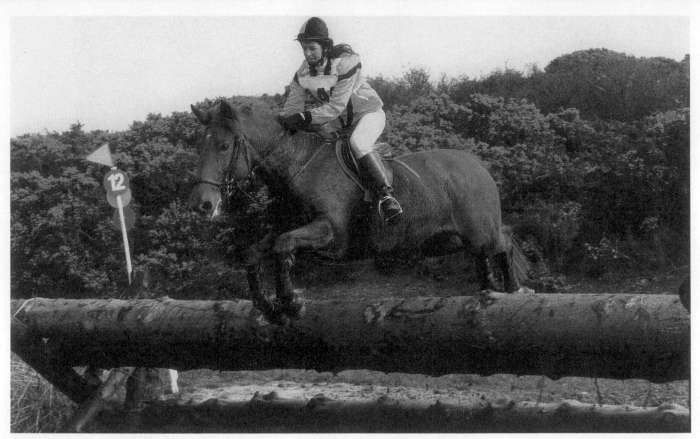

Fig. 11.3 Horse in work – eventing

roughage intake. Stabled horses may suffer from a number of physical and mental problems that are partly due to the nature of their feeding, and it should be possible to alleviate these with more turnout and adequate provision of roughage. The problem arises with the horse in hard work, which has a high energy requirement that cannot be met unless a large proportion of the roughage part of the diet is replaced by concentrates. This is further exacerbated by many horses in hard work being shy feeders, possibly because of the high-concentrate nature of the diet. Energy levels can be satisfactorily increased by the addition of oil to the diet, but care must be taken that sufficient protein is also fed since oil contains none.

REPRODUCTION

Reproduction or breeding is not an unnatural process for the horse and in fact the working situation is far more unnatural. Thus feeding the breeding horse should be easier than feeding the working horse. Problems arise when an exceptionally high growth rate is required of foals, to prepare them either for the show ring or for sale.

Stallions

Stallions during the covering season need a good all-round diet and their general condition and temperament should always be considered. Many stallions today are also used for work, especially for competition, where their natural presence gives them an edge over other horses, and these will normally be fed as any other working horse. For the stallion covering large numbers of mares, some increase in nutritional content of the diet is

required and the condition and mental attitude of the stallion should be a good indication of how much extra to give.

Pregnant mares

Pregnancy in the mare lasts for 11 months, and for the first 8 months the developing foetus is relatively small and makes few demands on the mare. A good all-round diet is recommended, and many mares continue to work during this period of their pregnancy.

During the last 3 months the foetus grows very fast and the mare needs some extra energy and quite a lot of extra protein. Feed manufacturers produce special diets for pregnant and lactating mares, usually with a protein level of about 16% (160 g/kg). These diets, combined with good hay, should be ideal, although if a mare is foaling late in the season a good grass paddock should supply all her needs. During the last month of pregnancy (Fig. 11.4), when the foetus is taking up a considerable amount of space in the abdomen, some mares will decrease their intake and may need a higher proportion of concentrates than would normally be the case.

Lactating mares

Like heavily pregnant mares, lactating mares have a high requirement for protein but energy needs are also greatly increased. A good stud diet should be fed unless ample high-quality pasture is available. Mares vary in their ability to produce milk. Some provide large quantities and sometimes lose their own condition in order to do so; others will produce less and use the extra food to build up their own fat stores. Figure 11.5 shows a 13-year-old mare with her first foal, both doing well on

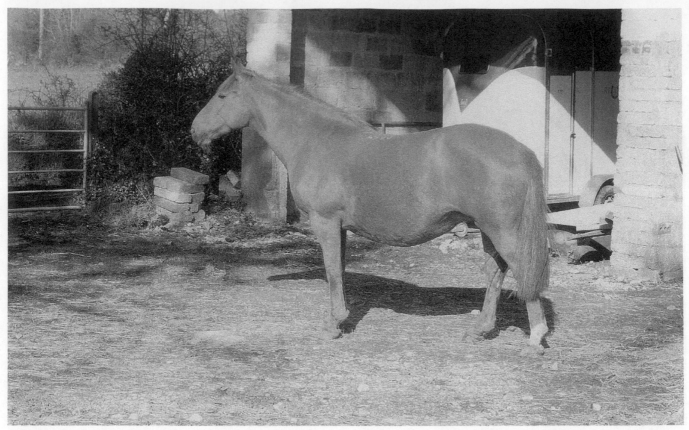

Fig. 11.4   Mare 1 week prior to foaling

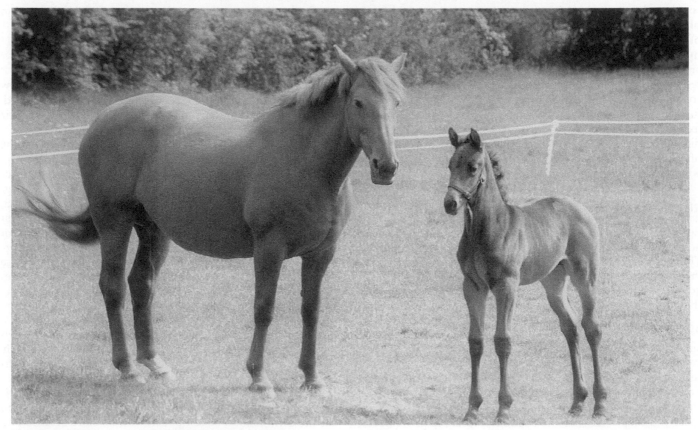

Fig. 11.5   Lactating mare with healthy foal at foot

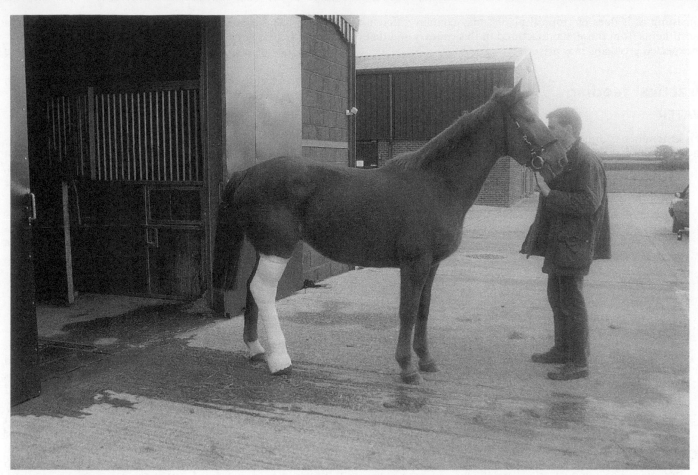

Fig. 11.6 A candidate for box rest

summer grass alone, an indicator of the feeding quality of grass at this time of year.

Youngstock

Most foals will start to investigate solid food within a week of birth. For a mare at grass, no extra feeding of the foal should be necessary at this stage. Where a mare is fed a compound food the foal will usually start to nibble it.

In the young foal, the hindgut is relatively small and undeveloped. As the foal starts to eat more solid food, especially roughage, the hindgut develops to cope with the new demands placed on it.

Many foals are weaned at 6 months old and it is important that by this time the foal has a good intake of solid food to compensate for the loss of its mother's milk. Creep feeding is often carried out, in which food is placed in such a way that the foal can reach it but the mare cannot. Generally, foals that have been creep-fed suffer less stress during weaning, since the gastrointestinal tract is accustomed to this type of food. Although foals have a higher need for concentrate foods than adult horses, good-quality roughage must always be fed to them alongside the concentrates. It is very important at this stage not to overfeed, since a variety of limb abnormalities can occur if this is the case. Foals do, however, have a considerably greater requirement than adults for both energy and protein in order to sustain growth, which can be at a rate in excess of 1 kg per day in the first months.

As the young horse grows, its requirement for high levels of protein falls, as does its need for higher levels of concentrate food. By the age of 3 years its diet will be the same as that of an adult horse. Most young horses are left to themselves during the spring and summer and fed extra food during the autumn and winter when grass growth is insufficient.

Sickness and convalescence

The horse on box rest does not have to move around in order to seek food and its energy requirements are therefore less than maintenance. Hay alone will generally suffice for these horses, but some supplementation may be necessary if the hay is not of good quality or the horse is under a particular stress, e.g. from surgery (Fig. 11.6).

Donkeys and exotic equids

Donkeys and zebras originated in the tropics. They are therefore not well suited to the British climate and may have nutritional requirements as yet unknown. It is often believed that donkeys digest fibre better than horses but this is not proven. Donkeys do conserve water better than horses and are able to withstand water deprivation for much longer, coming second only to camels in their ability to do this. Little is known about the requirements of zebras, and until further research has been carried out on these species it is probably best to treat them like horses at maintenance, remembering that a tropical diet, consisting as it does of tropical plants, may contain different constituents from those manufactured in this country and that unexpected problems may arise.

Practical feeding

WATER

It is generally recommended that water is available at all times, and there are a number of ways in which it may be provided:

- In the field, a self-filling trough is ideal. It should be situated away from trees and where it can be inspected regularly. It is worth bearing in mind that the ground around a trough usually gets very cut up, especially in wet weather, so having it too close to a gate is inadvisable.
- In the stable, water can be provided by self-filling drinkers. There is some evidence that horses drink less from self-filling drinkers and many people dislike them, since it is harder to tell how much a horse is consuming. The saving of labour is considerable, however, and the water is always fresh.
- Buckets allow the horse's consumption to be measured, but water in a bucket becomes stale and will absorb ammonia from the atmosphere. It is also liable to be kicked over or occasionally used as a foot bath. When a horse is stabled overnight and fed dry hay, it will usually drink the contents of two 15-litre buckets.

ROUGHAGE

The digestive system of the horse is designed to cope with a diet consisting of large quantities of low-quality roughage and all diets must be based on roughage. This can be difficult to achieve if the horse is performing hard work and has a greatly increased requirement for energy, since intake is limited and, as concentrate foods increase, so the roughage portion of the diet must necessarily decrease. This effect can be reduced by increasing the quality of the roughage fed, and generally at least one-third of the diet should be roughage.

Hay is the traditional conserved roughage feed for horses but recent years have seen a considerable increase in the use of other types of forage-based roughage, haylage being the most popular. Other roughage suitable for feeding to horses includes barley or oat straw for horses needing lower energy levels; silage or lucerne (alfalfa) for those needing higher energy levels; and roots, of which dried sugar beet pulp is the commonest and most convenient.

Roughage can be fed in a number of different physical forms:

- Long, e.g. hay, straw, and haylage; often given in a net which has the added advantage of keeping the horse occupied.
- Chaff, e.g. lucerne, hay and straw, chopped up into short lengths and mixed with the concentrate ration. Feeding chaff helps to slow down the rate at which concentrates are eaten and leads to better digestion, both through the slowing down the process and by making the food less dense in the stomach and so more readily available for enzyme activity.
- Pellets or shreds, e.g. sugar beet pulp. This must be soaked before use and it absorbs up to four times its own volume of water. It should never be fed before this

water has been absorbed, otherwise it will swell within the horse's stomach and, as the horse is unable to regurgitate its food, this could in extreme circumstances lead to rupture of the stomach. In hot weather, soaked sugar beet can start to ferment if left too long and it will then become unsuitable for feeding.

CONCENTRATES

Concentrates are fed as a concentrated source of energy and can either be in the form of straight, single foodstuffs, such as oats, or as a compound from a feed company made up of a number of different ingredients. Most horses today are fed manufactured compounds, either cubes or coarse mixes, which have the advantage of being nutritionally balanced for the different types of horse. For example, a low-energy cube can be obtained for a child's pony and a power mix for an event horse. Compounds are also produced for elderly horses, breeding animals, youngstock and invalid horses.

FREQUENCY AND TIMING OF FEEDING

When feeding a horse, remember that in nature it eats for about 16 hours a day and as far as possible this should be mimicked in the stable. It is rarely possible to give a horse constant access to food but a good supply of roughage should keep it occupied for some time. Concentrate feeds are usually given separately (although some feed companies are developing complete feeds) and, unfortunately, are rarely given more often than two or three times a day because of the owner's other commitments. An ideal feeding regimen would probably enable the horse to be fed a complete ration at hourly intervals throughout the day and night; however, without the development of sophisticated automatic feeding this is unlikely to be possible.

Stabled horses

The stabled horse is usually fed a concentrate food three times a day and hay two or three times daily depending on the working schedule, etc. It is possible with horses at maintenance or in low work to give large amounts of forage, possibly including oat or barley straw, thus occupying them for long periods of time. Horses in more strenuous work need more concentrate food, with a consequent reduction in roughage – this can lead to boredom and the development of stereotypical behaviour.

Horses at grass

Horses kept at grass are under the most natural conditions for the domesticated animal. The pasture should be well fenced and free from toxic plants, although a variety of plants other than grass are beneficial to the horse's health. Horses have a tendency to graze some areas of a paddock very closely and leave other areas rough and untouched. They will tend to defecate in the rough areas. Since horses are naturally herd animals it is best to keep them in consistent groups if at all possible – introduction of new animals to a group will cause some transitory disruption as the pecking order is re-established to accommodate the newcomer.

Combined system

This system allows for the animals to be at grass for part of the day or night and stabled for the rest of the time. During periods of stabling, horses are fed a roughage and concentrate ration suitable to their work and physiological condition but the quality and quantity of grass available to them should be taken into account and the ration varied accordingly.

FOOD STORAGE AND PREPARATION

Storage of foodstuffs should be considered as poor storage may have an effect on the efficacy of the contents and in particular the labile, readily oxidised pigments, unsaturated fats and fat-soluble substances are destroyed. Fat-soluble vitamins are all reduced during storage, as are unsaturated fatty acids, and rancidity of fats reduces acceptance. The synthetic forms of vitamins A and E are more stable than their natural forms but have little antioxidant capacity (see Chapter 9). B vitamins are relatively resistant to breakdown during storage, but riboflavin will be lost when exposed to light. Compound feeds may have permitted antioxidants added to them to guard against various forms of deterioration but these will not stop all forms of deterioration forever. Acceptability of all foods is reduced on deterioration.

Fungi may grow during storage and may produce toxins, as well as causing decay and lack of acceptability, and nutritional value will decline. Insects also cause deterioration and may carry fungal spores – some of these insects are visible to the naked eye but others are not. Rodent infestation leads to food loss and their droppings are dangerous to both man and animals.

Hay and straw are frequently bought off the field and stored throughout the winter to be used as required. This system is entirely satisfactory as long as the hay in particular has cooled down after making. Hay stored too early will heat in the stack, with a subsequent loss of nutrients. Both hay and straw can be obtained either in small or large bales. Large bales require mechanical handling, so unless they can be delivered direct to the barn small bales will be easier to deal with. Hay should not be fed before it has cooled down, since fermentation continues. Last year's hay should not be fed, as hay deteriorates gradually with time and by the following year will have little feeding value left. Hay must be stored in a dry place with plenty of air circulation, ideally in the dark to reduce the loss of carotene from the bales. Storing on pallets will prevent upwards seepage of damp, which can render the lowest layer of bales unusable.

Haylage, which is purchased in sealed bags, can either be bought in early in the season and used as required, or bought in as required. As long as the bags remain airtight there should be no loss of quality and the same is true of silage bought in big bales. Both silage and haylage can be stored outside, since the wrapping is also watertight, but bird damage can be a problem.

Concentrate foodstuffs and sugar beet pulp are usually purchased in sacks. They should be bought in as required, as the contents deteriorate with time. The purchase of a few weeks' supply at a time is generally satisfactory.

All foodstuffs should be stored at a low and uniform temperature, with low humidity, good ventilation and a dry environment. Metal bins are generally advised for concentrates as these prevent access by vermin, which not only eat the food but also contaminate it with their urine and faeces. The food should not be stored in direct sunlight as this can destroy some vitamins. If possible, rodents, birds and insects should be kept out. Opinion varies as to whether cats should be allowed in the food store – they will keep down vermin but may themselves cause some damage.

ALTERATION TO NORMAL FEEDING PATTERNS

Hospitalised or box rest

It is important to remember when feeding the horse on box rest that such circumstances are foreign to the horse's natural habitat. The inability to move around freely can in itself be detrimental to the digestive system, as movement aids the expulsion of the considerable quantities of gases produced in the hindgut (see Fig. 11.6). Provided that good-quality hay is available it may be best to cut out concentrate foods altogether. The requirement for energy is obviously diminished to below a normal maintenance level and some horses will actually refuse concentrates if they are offered. If the hay is not of sufficient quality to feed alone, a diet specially produced for the invalid horse should be used. This will have a low energy level but still contain adequate quantities of vitamins and minerals, etc. Succulent foodstuffs such as roots, apples or cut grass will be much appreciated by the horse on box rest.

In some cases it may be necessary to provide specific supplements such as B vitamins (B_{12} may be given by injection). If digestive function is impaired, partial or total parenteral nutrition may be necessary.

Overweight or obese

Many horses are overfed and this can put a strain on the limbs, especially in young animals. Food manufacturers' recommendations tend to err on the side of overfeeding and it should be remembered that feed companies, as well as providing foodstuffs, are in the business of making money! The showing world is notorious for its liking for overweight horses.

One common problem is an overestimation of the amount of work a horse is doing. The National Research Council (1989) considers that light work consists of Western and English pleasure riding, bridle-path hacking and equitation; medium work consists of ranch work, roping, cutting, barrel racing and jumping; and heavy work includes horses in race training. The recommendation is to increase the energy content of the daily ration by 1.25, 1.50 and 2.00 times the maintenance requirement, as appropriate. The horse doing a few hours of hacking a week can probably be considered to be at little more than maintenance, especially if stabled and not requiring any energy for foraging food in a field. Horses cannot be considered to be in medium or hard work until they are doing considerable amounts of fast work, such as regular hunting, endurance work or 3-day eventing. It is always better to err on the side of safety and keep the rations below what appears to be recommended. If the horse starts to lose weight, additional food can then be given.

The overweight horse should never be starved, as this will disrupt the digestive system and may cause problems such as hyperlipidaemia. Rather they should be fed a restricted diet in such a manner that it takes them as long as possible to eat it.

Underweight or too thin

Underfeeding is most likely to occur during the winter when animals live out, or in the case of older horses whose digestion is not as efficient as that of younger horses. The thick winter coat of horses overwintered outside can hide lack of condition very effectively. It must be remembered that, during the late autumn and winter, what grass there is will be very fibrous and contain little energy or protein. Horses and ponies neglected during these months with little or no supplementary feeding are likely to be underweight.

Older horses do not generally digest their food as efficiently as younger ones and as they get older may require extra food, especially protein. Horses, like people, vary widely in the age that they are considered old and some animals in their twenties may appear younger than those in their teens. Like dogs, larger animals tend to age faster and ponies living well into their thirties are common. Another problem encountered with the older horse can be loss of teeth, which will make the consumption of long roughages difficult. There are now many substitutes on the market and it should be possible to feed the rather toothless old horse without too much of a problem.

Should a horse be suffering from starvation, food should be introduced in small quantities at first, gradually building up the amounts given as the digestive system becomes more active.

BIBLIOGRAPHY

Bishop, R., 2003. The Horse Nutrition Bible. David & Charles, Newton Abbot.

Bone, J.F., 1988. Animal Anatomy and Physiology, third ed. Prentice Hall, Englewood Cliffs, NJ.

Frame, J., 2000. Improved Grassland Management. Farming Press, Tonbridge, Kent.

Frape, D., 2010. Equine Nutrition and Feeding, fourth ed. Wiley-Blackwell, Oxford.

Kerrigan, R.H., 1994. Practical Horse Nutrition, third ed. R H Kerrigan, Maitland, NSW.

McDonald, P., Edwards, R.A., Greenhalgh, J.F.D., et al., 2002. Animal Nutrition, sixth ed. Prentice Hall, Englewood Cliffs, NJ.

National Research Council, 1989. Nutrient Requirements of Horses, fifth ed. National Academy Press, Washington, DC.

Pagan, J.D. (Ed.), 1998. Advances in Equine Nutrition. Nottingham University Press, Nottingham.

Pagan, J.D., Geor, R.J., 2001. Advances in Equine Nutrition II. Nottingham University Press, Nottingham.

RECOMMENDED READING

Frape, D., 2010. Equine Nutrition and Feeding, fourth ed. Wiley-Blackwell, Oxford.

Geor, R., 2013. Equine Applied and Clinical Nutrition: Health, Welfare and Performance, first ed. Saunders, Oxford.

Behaviour and Handling of the Dog and Cat

JOCELYN LANDER | JANE WILLIAMS

KEY POINTS

- A thorough understanding of the behaviour of animals is essential for the safety of anyone working with them and to ensure that individual species are treated fairly and appropriately.

- Modern theories of the domestication of the dog are complex and still create much discussion among behaviourists. The most likely theory is that grey wolves were attracted to living near man because of the presence of food on waste dumps and that these individuals then became tame as a result of continuous proximity to man.

- Dispelling the myth of dominance hierarchy and alpha roles changes the way we think about our dogs and the methods of training them.

- The socialization period is critical in the behavioural development of both puppies and kittens, but the behaviour of any animal is subject to a multitude of factors and understanding these factors is vital in dealing with behavioural problems.

Introduction

Handling dogs and cats is an integral component of the veterinary nurse's role. To ensure safety in the working environment it is essential to have an understanding of the behaviour and body language of your patients. This chapter explores the history of domestication of the canine and feline species and how this relates to their behaviour. The concept of behavioural therapy is introduced and includes discussion of potential approaches to common problems encountered in these species in veterinary practice.

Handling dogs and cats

It is essential that the veterinary nurse knows how to assess and interpret the body language of dogs and cats to ensure a safe approach can be made. In turn your own body language, tone and pitch of your voice and self-assurance can influence how an animal reacts to you. Generally a reassuring voice with a low tone will put animals at ease. Never put yourself in a situation where you feel uncomfortable – it is always preferable to request assistance from a more experienced staff member than to injure yourself or your patient.

Animals require handling to allow:
- Grooming/bathing
- Clinical examination
- Administration of first aid
- Administration of drugs.

DOGS

All dogs are potentially aggressive so it is unwise to make assumptions about their nature, especially in a stressful situation of the veterinary practice.

Initial approach and restraint

It is advisable to talk to the owner prior to handling and to use the owner as much possible. Owners know their animal and their presence should reassure the dog. Owners can be particularly useful to fit muzzles without causing stress to their pets (Table 12.1). Aggressive behaviour can be the result of possessiveness over their owner or kennel, fear or pain, maternal behaviour, environmental factors (e.g. other barking dogs) or same-sex aggression.

Animals which are overtly protective of people or kennels should be examined in the absence of their owner and often the aggression will immediately be resolved. Kennel guarding can be reduced by leaving a form of restraint on the animal to allow ease of handling. Record cards should always be clearly marked with a warning for other staff members that animals may be aggressive.

- Approach the dog in a quiet but confident manner using the dog's name for reassurance.
- Lower yourself to the animal's level while maintaining your own safety.
- Offer your hand for the dog to smell using a sideways movement so as not to alarm the animal.
- Avoid handling animals in confined spaces as this can lead to anxiety and aggression if the dog perceives itself to be trapped.

In situations where the animal cannot be handled safely, the use of restraint equipment or drug therapy can be an invaluable tool.

All dogs should have a lead and collar fitted while handling occurs. Additional control can be obtained by using the following:
- Slip leads
- Haltis© or Gentle Leader©
- Muzzles
  - Wire or Baskerville© muzzles
  - Nylon or Mikki© muzzles
  - Tape muzzles
  - Box muzzles
- Dog catcher (not advised unless last resort)
- Chemical restraint
  - Pharmaceutical restraint includes medetomidine, butorphanol and diazepam and should only be administered under veterinary supervision.

TABLE 12.1	Restraint techniques in dogs
Method of restraint	**Procedure**
Muzzling	Ensure correct size muzzle is selected and straps are adjusted to fit the dog Approach from the side or behind the patient Prevent the head from moving from side to side by holding the scruff Pass the muzzle over the dog's nose and pass straps behind the head and fasten, then tighten to required length
Applying a tape muzzle	Select an appropriate length of non-conforming bandage to fit around muzzle, the head of dog and allow tying Form a loop with a square knot Use an assistant to restrain the dog Approach from the side and place the loop of the bandage over the dog's nose with the knot at the top Tighten and cross the free ends under the lower jaw of the dog, then pass back under the ears Tie the ends in a quick-release bow around the back of the head

All restraint equipment should be fitted correctly to avoid discomfort to the animal. Take care to avoid rubbing of the eyes or excessive tightening, and never leave a muzzled animal unattended. Never muzzle an animal which is dyspnoeic or suffering from emesis.

Lifting

- Perform a quick survey to ascertain if any injuries – if there are, avoid them.
- Grasp the animal around the front and hind legs, pressing it into your own body to prevent struggling.
- Lift with your knees bent and your back straight.
- For animals over 20 kg it is a Health and Safety requirement that another staff member assists.
- Smaller animals can be tucked under one arm to support the thorax with your body used to support the hind limbs.
- Larger dogs will require two people to lift – the first should support the front of the dog while restraining the head in an arm lock and the second supports the hind quarters and the abdomen (Fig. 12.1).
- Always ensure the head is safely positioned away from your face to prevent biting.

Restraint for examination – standing

Use a non-slip examination table in an area which is escape-proof. Ensure that all potentially necessary restraint equipment and examination equipment is close to hand.

- Lift the animal onto the examination table.
- Restrain by standing to one side of the animal, placing the near side hand around the animal's neck, and hold the head in a secure lock.
- The other arm is used to hold the animal's abdomen against the body or apply downward pressure on the dorsal neck region to prevent backwards movement.

This is a suitable position for administration of subcutaneous injections into the scruff or intramuscular injections.

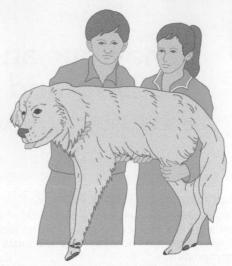

Fig. 12.1   Correct method of lifting a dog over 20 kg

Restraint for examination – lateral recumbency

Use a non-slip examination table in an area which is escape-proof. Putting a blanket on the table will sometimes make the animal feel more at ease. Ensure that all potentially necessary restraint equipment and examination equipment is close to hand.

- Stand beside the animal as it stands on the table.
- Place your arms across the back of the animal and grasp the off side front and rear legs at the level of the tibia and radius (Fig. 12.2).
- Gently pull the legs upwards and away from you using your chest to support the animal's body.
- The dog's body should gently roll down on to the table where it is restrained by applying downwards pressure to the limbs and using the elbows and forearms to hold down the head and body.

Lateral recumbency examinations may also be performed on the examination room floor, in which case you should lower yourself to the floor and support the body against your chest, restraining in a similar way.

Venepuncture

Cephalic vein. This is the most common site for both intravenous injections and placement of intravenous cannulas. The cephalic vein runs down the dorsal aspect of the lower forelimb.

- Restrain the dog in a sitting position. In active patients another assistant may be required to secure the rump, preventing backwards movement.
- Stand behind the animal and use the corresponding arm to the foreleg being sampled to raise and extend the leg.
- Cup the elbow in the palm of your hand, bringing the thumb across the crook of the elbow to apply gentle downwards pressure.
- Rotate the hand slightly outwards and maintain the pressure while the veterinary surgeon inserts the needle.
- If an intravenous injection is being given, the pressure can be released as the fluid is injected; if blood is being collected, maintain the pressure while the blood flows

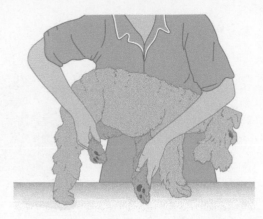
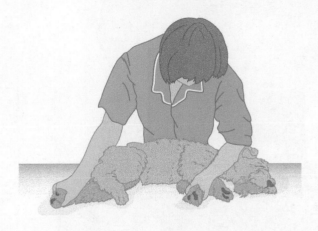

Fig. 12.2 Restraining a dog on its side

into the syringe. Blood should not be collected from the cephalic vein unless a very large dog, as the length of time to collect the sample causes clotting of the sample.
- As the needle is withdrawn, apply pressure to the injection site for approximately 30 seconds to prevent subcutaneous haemorrhage.

Jugular vein. This is the most common site for collection of blood samples. The jugular vein runs down either side of the neck in the jugular furrow.
- Restrain the patient in a sitting position or in sternal recumbency using an assistant to secure the rump, if required.
- Hold the head upright, extending the neck. The fore limbs can be preventing from being raised by placing your free hand across them.
- The person collecting the blood applies pressure to the base of the jugular furrow to raise the vein and collect a sample.

CATS

In general cats respond better to light handling and as little restraint as is practically possible.

One problem that can be encountered in cats within the veterinary practice is removing them from their kennels. Often cats are housed with or nearby other animals, especially dogs, which can cause stress or fear, resulting in aggression when the veterinary nurse attempts to remove the cat from its kennel. In this situation a towel can be used to cover the cat's head and body and then the cat can be scooped gently out. In extreme cases a cat grasper can be effective. Another method is to use a crush cage by placing it against the kennel entrance with the wire door removed effectively trapping the cat between the kennel and crush cage. A towel over the cage will make it more welcoming to the cat, and hopefully the cat will enter it; if not then gentle persuasion can be employed. Once the cat is in the cage quickly replace the wire door and secure the animal.

There is a variety of specialist restraint equipment available for cat restraint, including:
- Cat muzzles
- Cat bags
- Crush cages
- Chemical restraint
- Towels
- Cat graspers.

Restraint for examination

As cats are small animals, usually one person can safely restrain a cat for examination. Cats should never be scruffed for examination, because it causes more stress and aggression. Cats should be placed on the table, and the examiner should examine the cat with minimal handling, if any. If further restraint is required, this can be achieved by placing one hand over the animal's thorax while using the other arm to support the rear of the cat and hold the body into the handler's chest.

This position can be used for the administration of subcutaneous injections into the scruff or intramuscular injections into the quadriceps femoris muscle of the hind limb.

Lifting

Very few cats weigh over 20 kg, so one person can safely lift them. Place one hand over the animal's thorax to support the sternum and use the other arm to support the abdomen by placing it around the side of the cat and holding the animal into the handler's chest.

Venepuncture

Cephalic vein. A very similar method is used to that in the dog (Fig. 12.3).
- The cat is restrained in sternal recumbency or in a sitting position.
- Use the other arm to hold the body close to your side and using your hand extend the fore limb towards the veterinary surgeon.
- Support the fore limb in the palm of your hand, placing your thumb across the crook of the cat's elbow.
- Apply gentle pressure with your thumb to raise the vein and rotate your hand slightly outwards.
- Maintain the pressure while the other person inserts the needle into the vein.

Jugular vein. There are a number of methods used for jugular vein sampling in cats:
1. Hold the animal close to the handler's body using one arm to lightly restrain the thorax. This arm can also be

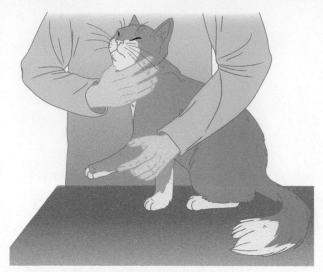

Fig. 12.3 Restraint for venepuncture using the cephalic vein in the cat

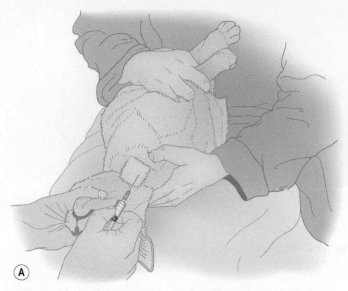

Ⓐ

Fig. 12.4A Dorsal restraint for venepuncture using the jugular vein in the cat

used to prevent the fore limbs from moving up. The other arm holds the head in extension with the hand softly grasping the mouth shut at the base of the jaws.

2. The handler seated holds the cat in dorsal or lateral recumbency often enclosed in a towel. The head is extended with one hand while the other keeps the body secure (Fig. 12.4).

3. While both methods can be successful it should be noted that often just raising the cat's head with minimal restraint applied is the most successful of all.

Evolution of the domestic dog (*Canis familiaris*)

It is thought that dogs and man first began to have a relationship in the Mesolithic period about 10 000 to 15 000 years ago. Until the start of the twentieth century the dog was largely unchanged, but in the last 100 years the need for dogs to have a specific function such as hunting, herding and guarding has declined and appearance has become more important (Fig. 12.5). It may be this shift in emphasis that lies at the root of physical and behavioural problems in our modern dog breeds.

FROM WOLF TO DOG

Our dogs are descended from the grey wolf (*Canis lupis*) and they share 96.6% of their genes, which supports this theory (Bradshaw 2011). However, the process of domestication must have been very subtle and not just a case of humans hand-rearing an orphaned wolf puppy and, from this, breeding generations of domesticated wolves. During the Mesolithic era, man adapted from a hunter-gatherer lifestyle to a more sedentary one. A result of this lifestyle was the formation of waste dumps outside the villages. This provided a rich source of food for wolves and other animals, especially when other food was scarce. Those wolves with less flight response to humans stayed around the dumps and bred successive generations of less fearful animals. In this way the animals with the least developed flight response to man naturally selected themselves and so the domestication process began. These dogs would have tolerated man and, over successive generations, they may have started

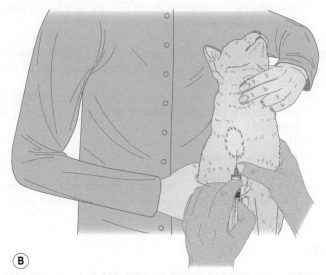

Ⓑ

Fig. 12.4B Restraint for venepuncture using the jugular vein in the cat

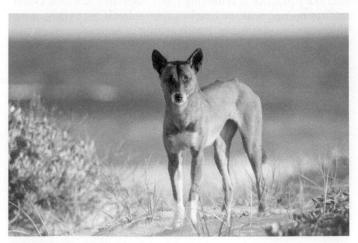

Fig. 12.5 A wild dingo

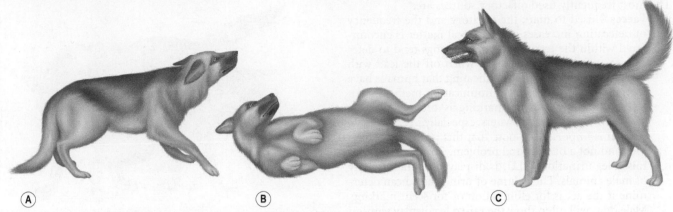

Fig. 12.6 Canine visual communication. (A) Fearful behaviour. (B) Appeasement. (C) Assertive posture

living within the villages. Man would have seen the benefit of having these animals around when they alerted him to danger and may even have used them as a protein source. The natural selection for tameness has been shown to change the species morphologically, as shown in the study done by Belyaev and his silver foxes (Serpell 1995). And so the wolf evolved into the 'village dog'. The dog has undergone huge physiological changes during its time with man and so to compare a dog's behaviour to a wolf's is unfair and dangerous. Ray Coppinger is an eminent scientist who writes: 'The popular dog press seems to feel that if dogs descended from wolves, they would have wolf qualities, but the natural selection model points out that the wolf qualities are severely modified. Dogs do not think like wolves, nor do they behave like them' (Coppinger and Coppinger 2001).

DISPELLING THE MYTH OF DOMINANCE

Most of us have grown up assuming that dogs are descended from wolves and therefore follow the same set of rules as a pack of wolves and adhere to a strict dominance hierarchy to keep the peace. For many years, behaviourists and scientists have questioned this unproven theory and even those scientists studying wolf behaviour cannot agree. Most of our knowledge of dog behaviour has been based on the study of captive wolves – a completely unnatural situation, much like a study on human behaviour being done in a prison.

Scientists have now realized that the way wolves live and organize their social structure is different to what was originally thought. David Mech is the leading authority on wolves and has been studying them for 50 years. He has found that a wolf pack consists of a male and female and their offspring – essentially a family group. Adolescents reaching 2–3 years of age leave the pack to form their own family packs and there is no fight for top dog, no linear hierarchy. Much like a father and mother are in charge of their children, the wolf parents are in charge of theirs. This does not constitute a dominance hierarchy.

After spending time with a wild wolf pack in the 1990s Mech felt compelled to dispel the myth of the alpha wolf, and this idea is very important in changing the way we view our dogs, how we train them and how we live with them. Education on the subject is vital, as most people who are using rank reduction techniques are merely following advice found in books and, unfortunately, on television. We are doing our dogs no favours by treating them like wolves and, in fact, we are creating more

problems. Dogs are a fantastic example of adaptability and opportunism and they deserve to be treated as individuals and as a species in their own right. The more people we can educate, the brighter the future for the domestic dog.

(Further information can be obtained from the Recommended reading at the end of this chapter.)

CANINE BEHAVIOUR PATTERNS

1. Communicative behaviour

Domestic dog populations show many of their wild relatives' social behaviour patterns although selective breeding by man has had an influence on modifying these patterns. Methods of communication tend to be via smell, facial expression and body posture, sound and physical contact.

Body posture. This is an important means of communication and it is vital that anyone dealing with a dog understands what the dog is 'saying':
- **Assertive postures** include standing tall with the tail held high, the ears erect and making direct eye contact (Fig. 12.6C). In extreme cases the dog may snarl and raise the fur along its back – the hackles. Beware of this!
- **Appeasement postures** include keeping the body low and, in extreme cases, lying on the back and presenting the inguinal region often in conjunction with urination, extreme tail wagging, nuzzling, licking, ears back and drooped and often showing an appeasement grin (Fig. 12.6B). Animals in pain or that are fearful often show extreme appeasement but care must be shown as they can still display aggression.
- **Fearful behaviour** is exhibited by the dog crouching low with its ears back, its tail held downwards and avoiding eye contact. The dog is uncertain whether to be friendly or to bite and is consequently unpredictable (Fig. 12.6A).

Olfaction. A solitary life within a household rather than in a pack may have resulted in domestic dogs relying more on olfaction than visual communication. Olfaction or the interpretation of scents is an important communication tool as scent remains in the environment, providing a long-lasting territorial marker and means of communication with other individuals of the same species.

The most frequently used olfactory sources are:

- **Faeces** – used to mark the territory and the frequency of defecation increases if alien faecal matter is encountered within the territory. Domestic dogs tend to defecate at an increased frequency when off the lead with no owner present, perhaps indicating that humans have interfered with inherent communication methods.
- **Urine** – excessive urine marking is often cited as a 'problem' behaviour by owners, especially in entire male dogs. It is important to note that this is normal behaviour and not a behavioural problem. Cocking the leg or raised leg urination (RLU) is displayed by the majority of male animals. The volume of urine passed can determine if the act is for elimination or for scent marking. Male dogs will often show the raised leg display without actually urinating, suggesting a communication role. Many males and some females will scratch and kick their back legs after urination or defecation, which is thought to spread scent. Another theory is that it is to leave scent from the sebaceous glands or interdigital glands in the feet, or it could also it be a visual means of communication.

In African Wild Dogs, double marking of male on female urine cements pair formation and improves courtship success and this is another behaviour that can be observed in their domestic cousins. Over-marking is common practice in packs but not in lone animals, suggesting territory marking.

Urine is also an important medium for communicating the readiness of a bitch to mate and the frequency of urination increases during the oestrus period.

- **Anal glands** – these are present in all species of *Canidae*. Analysis of the glandular secretions shows differences between groups and individuals. The glandular secretions are secreted on to the faeces as they pass through the anal sphincter.
- **Other glandular secretions** – these are used by all species of *Canidae*. Glands in the facial, tail, perineum and anal regions secrete social odours. There are two types of gland – the sebaceous glands, which produce oily secretions, and the suderiferous or sweat glands, which produce watery secretions and are used more commonly in social communication.

The anal region in dogs is used for postural communication – one dog will sniff the base of another's tail (Fig. 12.7). The most confident dog will present the anus to a subordinate individual and then it will check the other animal's anus. In very unconfident animals the anal region will be withdrawn, i.e. the tail clamped to prevent examination. This is more commonly seen in male animals but females do exhibit the behaviour during oestrus. Domestic dogs exhibit a similar behaviour between unfamiliar individuals and always follow the same sequence of behaviour or a 'fixed action' behaviour pattern – e.g. in the park dogs will:

- Inspect head and anal region
- Females tend to approach the head and males the anal region.
- Both try to reduce inspection by clamping.

Vocalization. This behaviour is more common in the domestic dog than its ancestors, and a broad repertoire of sounds have developed. Barking, grunting, growling and whining all have developed in dogs to assist with social communication and

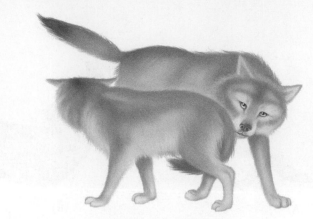

Fig. 12.7 Typical greeting behaviour of canids.

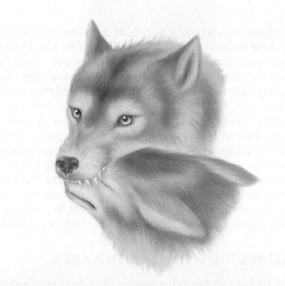

Fig. 12.8 Snout grabbing is part of precopulatory play

certain traits such as alarm barking have been selected for to meet our specific needs.

2. Reproductive behaviour

Domestic dogs are capable of mating at any time during the year while their wild relatives only produce sperm within a breeding season. The bitch (depending on her size and breed) will have a season every 6 months. The larger breeds tend to only have a season once a year. During the oestrus period the bitch displays visual signs of her season including a swollen vulva and gives off olfactory signals via vaginal discharges and an increased frequency of urination. Bitches may develop a preference for specific mating partners and appear to prefer animals with whom they are already familiar. Mating behaviour includes precopulatory play such as sniffing, snout grabbing (Fig. 12.8), nipping and chasing, all particularly seen in inexperienced pairings. This is followed by exploratory sniffing and licking by the male, mounting and the resultant tie, which is unique to the canine family (see Chapter 16).

3. Maternal behaviour

When near to term the bitch will be restless and may roam. She may tear up bedding to create a nest and some otherwise affec-

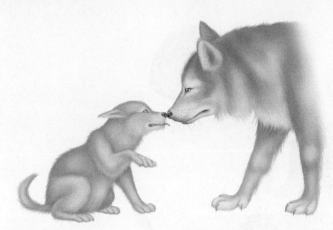

Fig. 12.9 A wolf cub using the paw raising and licking behaviours to solicit affection

tionate animals can become aloof. She will try and find a secluded area to nest, mirroring the wild situation in which the wild bitch will leave the pack and look for an abandoned hole to form her den. It is advisable to provide the bitch with a whelping box prior to her due date to allow her to acclimatize before the first stages of labour commence (see Chapter 16).

4.   Care-soliciting behaviour

In wild dogs care-soliciting behaviour is particularly seen when the pack return from the hunt to the pups within the den. The pups lick around the lips of their dam, trying to place their tongue in her mouth, which stimulates a reflex regurgitation of the food in her stomach that is then eaten by the pups. The domestic dog may also do this to its owner on his or her return to the house. Wild dogs will lift a paw when asking for affection or mutual grooming and this is often accompanied by a high-pitched whining noise (Fig. 12.9). The domestic dog will also lift a paw in a similar situation with the owner and this is often converted into an apparently learned 'trick' for the amusement of others.

The evolution of the domestic cat (*Felis catus*)

The domestic cat is most likely to have descended from the African Wild Cat (*F. libyca*) and not the European Wild Cat (*F. sylvestris*) as was originally thought. This is mainly due to the fact that the African cat is more easily tameable while his European cousin is not, and studies have also shown that the domestic cat is genetically almost identical to the African Wild Cat (Turner and Bateson 2000).

The earliest known records of the cat's relationship with man come from Egypt. Paintings on tombs dating back to 2300 BCE depict cats catching rats, indicating that they were living with humans around this time. It would seem likely that cats were initially encouraged into dwellings and villages to help control vermin, and those cats that were best at their jobs or more tameable were probably selected for breeding and so the process of domestication began. Cats soon began to exert their influence over the Egyptians and their position was raised from ratters to creatures with a god-like status who were revered as symbols of fertility and strength. The Egyptians were very protective of their cats and prevented the export of them outside Egypt.

Some did, however, slip through and cats made their way to Europe – Italy and Greece in particular – and they appear to have reached China around 200 BCE. With the beginnings of Christianity cats began to lose their exalted status and were seen as demons or agents of the devil and were horrifically persecuted. Modern attitudes are somewhat better, the cat having overtaken the dog as man's 'best friend', and it is now the most popular companion animal.

SOCIAL STRUCTURE

Cats are social creatures, not the solitary hunters we once thought they were. Most domestic cats seek out attention and enjoy interactions with humans and other species. In a feral colony, the females are the core of the colony and make up family groups with related females and their offspring. The size of the colony will depend on factors such as food sources and shelter (the resources) – the greater the food supply, the larger the colony; when food is more scarce the colony tends to become fragmented. Females also help to raise each other's young and siblings can form strong bonds which even persist to the juvenile stage. Young male cats tend to leave the colony and live on the periphery, waiting for the chance to reproduce. They often form their own social groups or coalitions of litter mates. Hunting is largely done alone and females will bring dead and live prey back to their kittens.

A cat's sociability is largely dependent on its individual temperament, genetics and its critical socialization during the sensitive period. Cats that like to live by themselves and hate all other cats are most likely to be the product of poor socialization, though lack of resources is the prime cause for conflict between cats. This is why it is so important that cat breeders are educated with regards to correct handling and socialization, ensuring that all our pet cats can enjoy a happy social life.

FELINE BEHAVIOUR PATTERNS

Generally, it has been observed that two broad types of social structure exist in feline populations and they are dependent upon food supplies:
1. **Solitary cats:**
   * Ranges overlap
   * Female ranges will be overlapped by larger male ranges
   * Thought to be food dependent
   * Male territories are bigger than females – need more food.
2. **Female social groups:**
   * Occur where there is sufficient food to sustain all
   * Males are usually loosely attached to group
   * Comprise adult females and their kittens
   * Cooperative kitten rearing/nursing
   * Structure is maintained by antagonism – strange females ousted and progeny recruited.

Pet cats are often forced to live in a group which can be well-tolerated but may also be a source of conflict and stress. They still have territories and ranges and those of the male cat are often 10 times larger than those of the female.

1.   Communicative behaviour

Cats use many methods of communication, several of which are able to transmit information over the long distances of the home range.

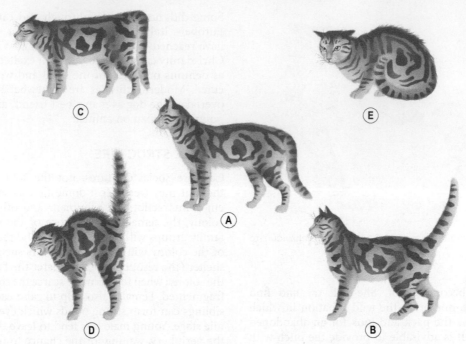

Fig. 12.10 Body postures used by the domestic cat. **(A)** Relaxed posture. **(B)** Greeting posture. **(C)** Aggression. **(D)** Fear. **(E)** Conflict

Visual. This relies mainly on body posture and facial expression:

- **Body posture** – a relaxed cat will walk around with its tail down but when greeting other cats or humans to whom it is friendly it will approach with its tail raised (Fig. 12.10). An aggressive cat will hold its tail close to its body while a frightened cat will arch its back and raise its tail. The hairs along the back and covering the tail will be erected to make the animal look larger and more formidable.

- **Facial expression** – the cat has a larger range of facial expressions than the dog (Fig. 12.11) and they rely on the position of the ears and whiskers and the pupil size. A relaxed cat carries its ears upright, whiskers on the side and the pupils of the eyes are moderately dilated. When alert the pupils dilate and the whiskers are tensed; an aggressive cat has erect ears turned back, and the pupils are constricted; if frightened the ears are held flat against the head, whiskers held stiffly out to the side and pupils are dilated while a cat in conflict will alternate the ear position between flattened and turned backwards.

- **Clawing and scratching** – cats will scratch trees, fence posts and furniture and this may have two functions. Firstly it is a visual sign of territorial boundaries and the scratches may be tainted with the odour of sweat glands present around the foot pads of the cat and it may also be used to maintain claw condition.

Vocalization. Sounds range from meows which change according to their demands – some owners will claim their cats talk to them – to loud, carrying yowls, particularly those associated with the queen in season. Purring, which is usually associated with contentment, may also be a sign of low-grade pain. Cats also use growling and snarling to accompany their threatening body posture and facial expression.

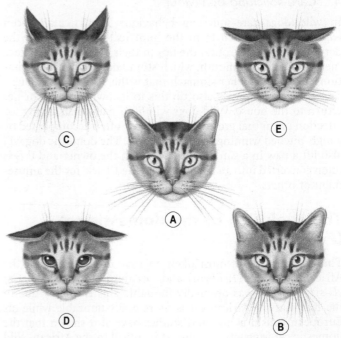

Fig. 12.11 Range of facial expression used by the domestic cat. **(A)** Friendly and relaxed. **(B)** Alert and inquisitive. **(C)** Threatening attack. **(D)** Frightened. **(E)** Conflict – cat may attack if cornered

Olfactory signs. The skin has many small glands, particularly on the cheeks, which deposit secretions when the cat rubs itself against objects in the environment, other cats or against its owner. The olfactory signals declare ownership of their territory. Cats also mark their territories using urine, which is sprayed backwards by the ventrally directed penis at the height of the next cat's nose. Urine also plays a role in reproduction, with males exhibiting the raised upper lip sniffing behaviour known as flehmen when they smell the urine of a queen in

TABLE 12.2	The characteristics seen in the different developmental phases of the dog and cat			
Neonatal	**Transitional**	**Socialization**	**Juvenile**	**Adult**
1–2 weeks	2–3 weeks	3–16 weeks	10 weeks to sexual maturity	Sexual maturity onwards
Born deaf and blind	Ears open and eyes respond to light	Critical learning period	Learning continues	Behaviours fully developed
Dependent	Can move around more easily	Teeth appear	Discovers sexual behaviour	
Reflex actions	More explorative	Exploring behaviour increases	Critical time to learn what is dangerous and what is not	
Can vocalize distress	Onset of weaning	Weaning occurs		
No hazard avoidance behaviour	No hazard avoidance behaviour	Hazard avoidance behaviour develops (respond to perceived danger)	Shows fear to unknown stimuli	

oestrus. Faeces is another significant territorial marker. Housed cats with an established territory will bury their faeces within the territory but may leave it on the surface at the boundaries – feral cats and wild cats, e.g. lions, do not bury their faeces.

2. Reproductive behaviour

Females or queens are seasonally polyoestrous and the beginning of the breeding season is determined by day length. Toms show increased activity during spring months, which then declines as the daylight hours decrease. A queen in oestrus will roll, rub herself over objects, yowl loudly (known as calling), and exhibit lordosis, i.e. crouching low with her backside raised and her tail to one side, all of which tell the male that she is sexually receptive.

3. Maternal behaviour

Queens make use of an improvised nest and many prefer solitude while others crave attention. Infanticide may be stimulated by disturbing the queen during kittening or during early neonatal life and may also be carried out by any male cat who is not the father of the litter (mirror of lion behaviour) and in feral colonies. Communal denning and nursing among related females has been observed.

4. Social interactions

Normal meeting behaviour begins with cats nose to nose with no touching. Then the head and neck are extended with the body slightly crouched to enable a quick retreat. The cat will attempt to sniff along the neck of the other to the flank and on to the anus while preventing the other cat from examining its own anal region. Cats also respond to 'model' cats in the same way and humans can trigger the greeting behaviour by using an outstretched finger to substitute for the nose. In social colonies individuals indulge in a great deal of social contact and aggression is rarely seen except between strange females and young males.

Behavioural development

DEVELOPMENTAL STAGES OF THE DOG AND CAT

It is widely recognized that there are five phases of development in puppies and kittens as shown in Table 12.2.

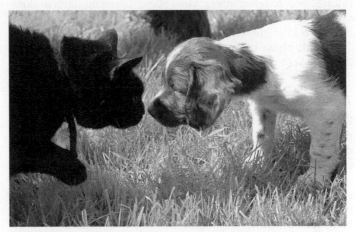

Fig. 12.12 During the socialization period puppies begin to explore new situations

The developing puppy

During the **neonatal** and **transitional** phases the puppy is completely dependent on its mother and at this time it is very important that puppies are handled, assuming that the mother is happy to allow this. Handled puppies have increased nervous system maturation, more rapid hair growth and weight gain, earlier opening of the eyes and enhanced motor development (Landsberg et al. 1999). Such puppies tend to grow up more confident, have improved learning ability and are emotionally more stable.

The **socialization** period is critical up to the age of 16 weeks. It is a period of rapid social behavioural development during which the puppies begin to explore more and respond to stimuli (Fig. 12.12). Most importantly, it is during this phase that puppies begin to show fearful behaviour to new objects and stimuli. They have to get used to these things and learn that they are not dangerous – a process called **habituation**. Whatever happens during this period will set the pattern for the puppy's behaviour in later life. Behaviours and responses learned now will be difficult to change. Positive social interactions with other animals and humans are paramount to ensure the puppy develops a balanced outlook on life. 'This appears to be period of extreme sensitivity to psychological stress. The sensitivity necessary to facilitate the formation of social relationships also seems to make the puppy vulnerable to psychological trauma' (Landsberg et al. 1999). It is around this time that an unsocialized puppy will become increasingly fearful of anything new and will overreact to sounds and stimuli. During socialization, puppies play with each other, learning important communication skills and what is appropriate behaviour and what is not. One of the most important things to learn during this time is bite inhibition.

Your role as an advisor to a new puppy owner is vital at this time. Stressing the importance of socialization and habituation within the correct time frame (up to 16 weeks) can mean the difference between a happy, confident puppy and a nervous, fearful puppy that could develop into an unhappy adult with a tendency towards aggression. The way in which this period is handled is very important (see later notes on puppy parties).

Basic behaviours and learning capabilities have fully developed by the **juvenile period**. Although exploration during this time increases, it is also a time of increasing avoidance of social interactions, so fewer interactions occur. Learning starts to slow down by 16 weeks: 'This is likely because previous learning begins to interfere with new learning' (Landsberg et al. 1999). The **adult phase** begins around 6–7 months of age and most dogs are seen to be fully mature by 18 months of age.

The developing kitten

Kittens follow the same developmental phases as puppies but the phases tend to be shorter in length. The critical period during **socialization** is from 2–7 weeks of age during which what they see, hear and experience will influence their behaviour in later life. Just as with dogs, sensitive handling will encourage more rapid development and reduce future fearfulness. Kittens removed from their mothers at 2 weeks of age or hand-raised kittens may show increased tendencies towards nervousness and aggression, although this also depends on inherited temperament and socialization by the foster mother. The most likely reason for this aggression is the inability of the human parent to teach the kitten how to cope with frustration – something the female cat does instinctively.

During the socialization period the mother will start to wean the kittens and bring live prey back to the nest. At this stage, their teeth are fully developed and kittens may even begin to hunt and kill their own prey by 5 weeks of age. They will also have full control over their elimination and will cover up urine and faeces. Most kittens will be fully weaned by 7 weeks of age. Social play also begins during this time and any interactions they have will influence their behaviour in the future. Kittens benefit from an environment that is full of different stimuli and objects to aid the habituation process. Too often we see cat breeders keeping kittens in an outdoor cattery until they are 9–10 weeks of age, resulting in a kitten that has not been socialized properly, only knows one environment and is often nervous and fearful in its new home.

By 6 months of age, most cats have reached sexual maturity and can begin to breed. They will now be self-sufficient hunters and able to care for themselves if need be.

Nature vs nurture

It is often debated whether behaviour in dogs and cats is the result of upbringing or is genetically based: i.e. 'nature or nurture.' Certain behavioural traits must be genetic or we would not have specialized groups such as pointers or collies; however, it is now apparent that behavioural development depends on two main factors:

- **Inherited or genetic factors** – these include temperament of the parents and certain innate behaviours specific to a breed of cat or dog.
- **Non-inherited factors or primary environmental influences** – these are very diverse and the list is long and includes the mother's health, nutrition, habitat and climate.

The significant thing to understand is that behavioural development is under the influence of a vast array of factors and they must all be taken into account when addressing any type of behavioural problem.

Behavioural therapy

INTRODUCTION

The science of animal behaviour is complicated with many differing opinions on the subject. We must try to understand how animals think and learn in order to interpret their behaviour as accurately as possible, and by doing this we can help resolve behavioural issues professionally and with the best interests of the animal at heart.

Behavioural problems are a very common occurrence in veterinary practice ranging from aggression and fear, to clients complaining of training issues or general unruliness. Many of these problems lead to pets being rehomed or even euthanized, and as veterinary professionals we are in a unique position to provide valuable assistance in resolving these issues. It is our job to identify these problems and try to help the client find a solution which will help maintain the pet/owner bond. Too often, behavioural problems can spiral into the client becoming resentful and frustrated, blaming the pet and not being able to rationalize the behaviour. Having the correct knowledge and skills can save this relationship and improve the lives of both the pet and the owner.

Veterinary surgeons are very busy people, and behavioural problems are often complex and can take a great deal of time to solve or manage. This provides an ideal opportunity for a veterinary nurse to develop new skills and to take over this role. An enthusiastic, motivated and knowledgeable nurse will be a huge asset to the practice, the animals and their owners.

LEARNING THEORY

The basic principles of learning

It is important to understand the basic concepts of how animals learn in order to give the best possible advice. Further details about learning theory are included in the Recommended reading list at the end of the chapter.

The basic principles behind animal learning can be divided into four different sections:

- **Reinforcement** – what animals are prepared to work for and what they want to avoid! Reinforcement occurs when a behaviour followed by a consequent stimulus is strengthened or becomes more likely to occur again. It can be divided into **positive** and **negative** reinforcement.
- **Extinction** (sometimes called **non-reward**) – ignore it and it will go away. Extinction occurs when a previously reinforced behaviour is no longer reinforced, resulting in the behaviour decreasing and eventually becoming extinct.

- **Punishment** – no! Punishment provides a consequence for a behaviour with the result that the behaviour is less likely to occur again.
- **Stimulus control** – this develops when a behaviour is only reinforced by the presence of a particular stimulus, e.g. a verbal cue.

NB. An animal will only repeat a behaviour if it finds it rewarding in some way – if it is not rewarding it is unlikely to want to repeat the behaviour.

Reinforcement

1. **Positive reinforcement (PR)** – most of us know that we should give treats to reward a behaviour that we want. It is important to find out what motivates the animal in order to be able to reward correctly: e.g. a Labrador will always find food rewarding but a ball-obsessed Collie may not try quite so hard for a piece of liver as he will for a tennis ball!
   - Timing is also crucial – for a reward to be effective, it must come within three seconds of the behaviour for the animal to make the association.
   - Using PR increases the likelihood of the behaviour occurring again: e.g. trainer holds treat in front of dog's nose → dog sits → dog is immediately rewarded with treat.
   - **Clicker training** is a very powerful PR training technique and one that has been around for a long time and has developed from the way in which marine trainers teach dolphins. Dolphins have to be trained from a distance so the trainers needed a way to let the dolphin know when they have correctly performed a behaviour. You cannot force a dolphin to do anything but, put simply, trainers use a whistle to which the dolphin has already been conditioned to understand that food is coming. When the dolphin performs a behaviour correctly, the trainer blows the whistle and the dolphin is rewarded with a fish. This technique ensures that the dolphin stays motivated and *wants* to perform. In dog training the whistle is replaced by the use of a clicker or other marker. More information on clicker training is included in the Recommended reading list.
2. **Negative reinforcement (NR)** – we use this more often than we care to admit! Most people equate NR with punishment, but these conditioning principles are very different. Put simply, NR is more frequently used to get the animal to do a behaviour by *removing* a negative stimulus, while punishment is to get the animal to stop doing something by applying a punisher – e.g. dog pulling on the lead → handler pulls back → handler releases tension on lead when dog stops pulling → dog is rewarded by the release. NR is a commonly used training technique, but is not advised as there are better ways to train.

Extinction or non-reward. The technique involves ignoring or not rewarding a previously reinforced behaviour until it becomes extinct. This is often used incorrectly as humans find it hard to stay disciplined. A classic example of extinction is shown by the dog that persistently sits begging at the dinner table. The behaviour has previously been reinforced by the children dropping food onto the floor for him. If he was then not given any more food ever again, he would eventually stop begging and the behaviour would become extinct. Something to note is that animals will show an **extinction burst** during which the behaviour will become worse or more extreme before it eventually expires. It is during this extinction burst that most humans feel the technique is not working and give up. This will only serve to reinforce the behaviour more and make it stronger! When using this technique, it is important to make sure that the animal is rewarded for showing an alternative behaviour: e.g. if the begging dog goes and lies down in his bed. This behaviour must be rewarded to help develop a new and more appropriate behaviour.

Punishment. 'Punishment involves the application of an aversive stimulus during or immediately following a behaviour to decrease the likelihood that the behaviour will be repeated' (Landsberg et al. 1999). Punishment is often associated with physical abuse or retribution, which gives it a negative connotation with respect to behavioural therapy and training. Its use is not recommended as the timing and the choice of the aversive stimulus must be precise and definite for it to be effective and for the punishment to be humane, it must be used correctly and only used once. This very rarely happens and can result in systematic abuse of the animal. Problems that may occur are that the pet does not associate the behaviour with the punishment and so learns nothing or that the pet learns to continue the behaviour in the owner's absence. It can also lead to an increase in the behaviour, or to an increase in fear or anxiety, compromising the bond with its owner. Punishment is not motivational and does not allow for new learning. It is the lazy trainer's technique in order to get a temporary quick fix. An example of punishment is dog chases deer → trainer uses electric shock collar → dog stops behaviour temporarily.

In the end, the only reinforcement in the learning of a particular behaviour is an emotional change. The rewards and punishments discussed are how those changes are induced. Techniques and stimuli have no learning value in themselves without a consideration of how each individual feels about them.

Stimulus control. A behaviour is said to be under stimulus control when there is an increased possibility that the behaviour will occur as a result of a specific stimulus: e.g. if we see a red light, we will automatically stop; if the light changes to green, we will automatically start to move off.

COUNTER CONDITIONING AND DESENSITIZATION

It is important to understand these concepts when dealing with and trying to solve specific anxiety- or fear-based behavioural problems.

Counter conditioning is used to counter or oppose an earlier negative experience: e.g. a young puppy becomes scared of a bicycle because his tail was once run over by one. He associates pain with the bicycle. Counter conditioning involves changing this association from bad to good for example, by feeding him his favourite treats every time he sees a bicycle and gradually getting him close enough to touch it. Eventually the puppy will see a bicycle and immediately think 'treat!'

Desensitization will occur when the dog eventually becomes non-reactive to the bicycle. Desensitization works best when done slowly and within the limits of the animal's capabilities: e.g. starting some distance away from the object that evokes fear, rewarding relaxed behaviour and then slowly working closer to the object over an extended period of time.

Flooding is the process in which the animal is exposed to the stimulus all at once and is the direct opposite of systematic desensitization. Flooding can result in overwhelming anxiety and fear and is not generally recommended to overcome fears. Animals can become aggressive and dangerous when put under such pressure – systematic desensitization is a far more humane method.

NEUROCHEMISTRY – IN A NUTSHELL

Animals, like humans, respond to stimuli in the environment. We have physiological systems in place to enable us to interact with and respond to all of these stimuli. The two most important systems are the **nervous system**, which affects the **endocrine system**, which coordinates all the chemical reactions in the body. These two systems are integrated and completely reliant on each other and in order to maintain homeostasis it is vital that these systems are functioning efficiently.

'Stress' is a word we use frequently in behavioural therapy but it is often misinterpreted. It is more than just a feeling of anxiety; 'stress is fundamental to almost all behaviours as it is about the demand for adaptation and the physiological response to that demand' (O'Heare 2003). What this means is that whatever stressor causes stress in the animal is causing it to make a change or adaptation to relieve the stress. Stress is at the core of most behavioural problems, e.g. aggression, fear, anxiety. Understanding the concept of stress and how it affects an animal is fundamental to recognizing the signs and dealing with it in a scientific way.

The mammalian brain is a complex organ (see Chapter 6) but for the purposes of this chapter it has been simplified. There are two major components involved in responding to our environment:

- The **amygdala** – this area deep within the cerebral hemispheres is responsible for the survival responses of fear, flight and fight. It helps the animal to 'act on instinct' to escape perceived danger. It is the most primitive part of the brain.
- The **cerebral cortex** – the more rational part of the brain responsible for cognitive function. 'Information is decoded and the brain analyzes the significance of the information based on previous learning and experience and then it goes to the frontal lobe where it is used to formulate a plan of action' (Strong 1999).

While the amygdala is active, the cerebral cortex cannot function properly. This is why most behavioural therapy is aimed at teaching animals or people to develop almost automatic coping strategies in anxious situations which enable them to gain control of their emotions and start rationalizing their fear using the cerebral cortex.

Information is conveyed from one part of the nervous system to another by **neurotransmitters**, which are chemical secretions produced at the synapses between nerve cells (see Chapter 6) and which ultimately affect the behaviour of the animal. It is important to have a basic understanding of how the brain works on a chemical level to understand why an animal behaves the way it does. Sometimes the behaviour is a result of a chemical imbalance and not the fault of the animal. This is where behavioural modification drugs can be useful, but they must always

be used with extreme care. Most behaviour modification therapy can help to correct any imbalances.

The main neurotransmitters are:

- **Dopamine** – this has an effect on the pleasure centre of the brain. Too much of it can promote agitation, impulsivity and over-reactivity; depleted levels can cause a lack of capacity to enjoy life. Dopamine is released after an 'adrenaline high' and is responsible for that sense of relief.
- **Adrenaline** – this is released as a result of a stressful event and prepares the body to respond to danger. Part of the 'fear, flight, fight' response.
- **Noradrenaline** – this is chemically related to adrenaline and is linked to an animal's energy levels. Trauma and chronic stress can deplete the levels of noradrenaline. High levels can result in aggression, over-arousal and impulsive behaviour, while decreased levels can cause lethargy and depression.

The effects of both dopamine and noradrenaline are regulated by an enzyme called monoamine oxidase, which deactivates them (O'Heare 2003).

- **Serotonin** – this regulates mood, controls sleep and arousal, regulates pain and controls eating. Decreased levels can lead to impulsive aggressive behaviour, impaired learning, anxiety and obsessive behaviour.
- **Gamma-aminobutyric acid (GABA)** – this is widely distributed throughout the brain and is the principal inhibitory transmitter. GABA is complex and has receptors that have three different binding sites – one for GABA, one for benzodiazepine drugs and the third for barbiturates and alcohol. When one of these binds to a GABA receptor it will amplify the effects of GABA and therefore increase neural inhibition.

Understanding emotions and their role in behaviour problems

(Centre of Applied Pet Ethology (COAPE) using the EMRA™ approach (emotional assessment; mood state assessment; reinforcement assessment)

Recent scientific studies have shown that animals do in fact have an emotional brain and are able to experience a wide range of emotions. This has transformed the way we look at animal behaviour and, more importantly, how we treat behavioural problems. Behavioural problems very rarely have an underlining clinical cause, and if they do, they usually present with other physical or neurological signs. It is the veterinarian's role to diagnose these conditions and present the correct treatment.

When investigating a behavioural problem, it is important to consider and try to understand the surge of feelings (*emotions*) the animal is feeling at that particular time, and also its baseline or average feelings (*mood state*) during the rest of the day, which might be contributing to the problem behaviour.

A human example might be as follows:

Imagine your 10-year-old son is playing football outside the kitchen window and you have already asked him, to no avail, to go and play in the garden so as not to kick the ball through the window. Sometime later, the ball smashes through the window. Your initial emotion might be one of anger at your son for not doing as he was asked. Now consider the same scenario, but this time you have flu, with a grumbling headache and feel irritable. The ball comes crashing through the window. 'What is your emotional reaction to this event this time? Explosive anger, probably, or resignation because you are too tired to bother' (Falconer-Taylor et al, 2014).

As individuals, we all have our own mood state that fluctuates during the day. This depends entirely on what sort of day we are having, what stresses we are under, whether we are suffering from an illness or depression. Someone who is carefree and positive will have a totally different emotional reaction to an event compared to someone with chronic depression or high stress levels. This same principle applies to our pets – a nervous cat that is stressed because there is a new baby in the house is likely to have a lower mood state than a confident cat that has 24-hour access to his own three-acre garden.

When assessing any behavioural problem it is important to assess the animal as an individual and take into consideration its personality, emotional state and circumstance.

First you should base an opinion on how the animal feels from two different perspectives:

a. **Emotional assessment** – this is a measure of the surge of feelings or emotions (good or bad) experienced before, during and after the problem behaviour.

b. **Mood state assessment** – this is the average, day-to-day feelings of well-being.

Then take into account:

a. **The hedonic budget** – this is an investigation into what the animal finds rewarding or pleasurable or what things are important to the animal. It also takes into consideration what things are missing from the animal's life that may be important to it. This is breed and species specific – e.g. a Greyhound and a Border Collie will have very different needs.

b. **Reinforcement assessment** – an investigation of exactly what factors, external or internal, are maintaining the problem behaviour.

EMOTIONAL ASSESSMENT

An animal can feel a range of emotions, from anger and frustration to fear and anxiety, from pleasure to extreme happiness and even depression. It is important to understand what range of emotions the animal is feeling at the time of the behaviour.

Case scenario: A young dog left alone at home, barks intermittently and chews up the sofa.

a. The dog could be **bored and frustrated** as it is left at home alone all day. Barking and chewing are innately rewarding behaviours that raise the dog's mood state. They help the dog to feel better and bring him relief from the boredom and frustration.

b. The dog could be **worried and upset** to be on his own as he has never been left before. He barks to try and make contact with his owners. The longer he is left, the higher his anxiety levels rise and he starts to panic. He turns to chewing as it brings him some relief from the stress of being home alone (raises his mood state while he is chewing) (Fig. 12.13).

In both cases, if the owner comes home while the dog is barking, the barking will be reinforced. In the dog's mind, the barking worked and brought the owner back. Punishment would not work as the joy/relief/excitement of having the owner home would far outweigh any punishment. The treatment of each of these cases would be different as the behaviours are driven by different emotional states.

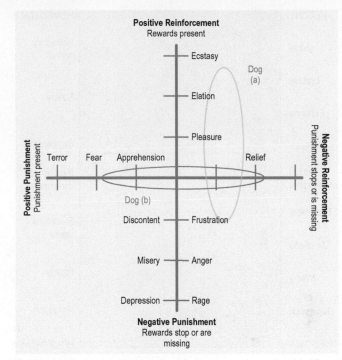

Fig. 12.13 Emotional Assessment Graph

MOOD STATE ASSESSMENT

This type of assessment measures the animal's mood state on a day-to-day basis. We know that our bodies and those of animals are regulated by complex homeostatic systems to maintain physiological equilibrium, e.g. pH and body temperature. In addition, both humans and animals experience a range of negative and positive emotions during the day and it is the feeling left after the ups and downs of the day have passed that we must assess. The emotional brain tries to maintain emotional homeostasis known as the hedonic set point (HSP), which aims to maintain the emotions at a 'normal' level.

Figure 12.14 demonstrates the relationship between mood state and HSP. Resting contentment (RC) is defined as having no particular emotion or feeling, such as just before you fall asleep. We would all love to be just above resting contentment every day (line A); however, to maintain this HSP we pursue normal everyday behaviours that are pleasurable and rewarding. If an animal is below the RC line (point B), it will partake in behaviours that help to raise its mood state, e.g. if a dog is tied up all day and very bored, he may bark a lot and run up and down on his chain. This behaviour is innately rewarding to him and will help to bring him some relief. If we can help animals to feel more contented (i.e. to raise their HSP towards RC) we can overcome a multitude of behavioural issues.

The hedonic budget

Animals have many different needs that must be met for them to feel contented. They need an outlet for instinctive and innately rewarding behaviours. Wild animals do not generally develop behavioural disorders as they are able to hunt, chase, mate and form social bonds in their natural environment. Our domesticated animals have been genetically manipulated and placed in unnatural environments and they often have no outlet for instinctive behaviour. Dogs, in particular, have been bred for

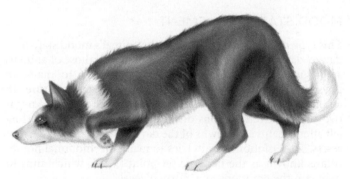

HEDONY — Mania — Ecstasy — Euphoria — Pleasure — Resting contentment — Discontent — Dysphoria — Misery — Depression — ANHEDONIA

HOMEOSTASIS — Refractory period — Satiety — Satisfaction — Resting contentment — Frustrative vigour — Energy — Motivation — HOMEOSTASIS

Ⓐ Ⓑ

Fig. 12.14 The relationship between mood state and Hedonic Set Point (HSP)

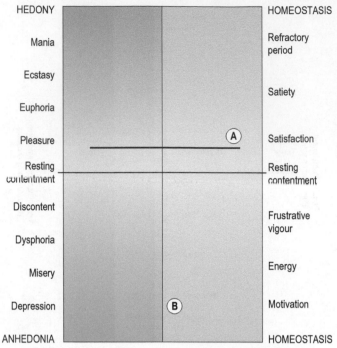

Fig. 12.15 Typical herding behaviour – a Border collie exhibiting eye stalking

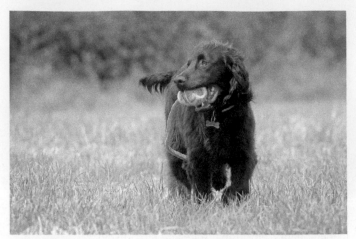

Fig. 12.16 A spaniel showing its innate retrieving instincts

many different disciplines and they all have different needs. They are descended from a predator but after much evolution and genetic manipulation, few breeds still have a full predatory motor pattern.

Example 1 – the hunting wild dog will **orientate → eye → stalk → chase → grab-bite → kill-bite**. During domestication we selected certain characteristics to suit our needs and culled any dogs that did not meet those criteria.

Example 2 – herding dogs would naturally **orientate → eye → stalk → chase**. We have removed the grab and kill part of the sequence by selective breeding as this is not a desirable trait. This is seen in breeds such as Border Collies or German Shepherds (Fig. 12.15).

Example 3 – dogs who guard livestock such as Anatolian shepherd dogs and Pyrenean mountain dogs would naturally **eye → bark**. These dogs have no tendency to chase or bite the animals they are guarding. All they are meant to do is bark when a potential predator is sighted.

Example 4 – dogs who hunt, such as spaniels, retrievers and pointers, will naturally **orientate → eye → stalk → chase →**

grab-bite. This sequence represents the ideal hunting/retrieving characteristic as the dog holds onto its prey but does not tear it up and eat it (Fig. 12.16).

It is important to understand the different breed characteristics in order to manage any behavioural problems. Certain breeds, like the gundogs, have a tendency to carry things around in their mouths and thus can also be more likely to guard things as they have an innate instinct to hang onto anything they grab. Herding dogs are likely to try and round things up, including children, and may be obsessive in their behaviour. They may be more orientated towards toys than food. Would it be that unusual if a herding breed nipped at a runner's heels in the park? You should always remain objective and try to see the situation from the dog's point of view. Such behaviour may be unacceptable to us, but it is completely normal for that breed of dog. We have to develop the skills to channel these behaviours into more rewarding, more appropriate behaviours. These behaviour sequences are 'hard-wired' in the dog's brain and performing them is innately rewarding and may be important in helping them to maintain their HSP.

When doing a hedonic budget assessment we need to first identify the behaviours that are typical or important for this breed or type of animal, then decide how well represented these behaviours are in the individual being assessed. After identifying which of the animal's behaviours are innately rewarding these can then be used in a behaviour modification programme. Using the behaviours that the animal is already programmed to do is a most effective method of dealing with the problem.

What dogs want! In any behaviour modification programme it is important that we not only stop the undesirable behaviour but also provide an alternative, more rewarding behaviour for the animal. There are many dog toys on the market that are designed to help to do this and they include:

- Interactive food toys – these include Kong®, Busy Buddies®, Buster Cubes® and other food-dispensing balls and food puzzle toys. These are important tools in helping dogs to feel contented and to ease frustration or boredom.
- Rawhide chews – these do need removing from the dog when they become soggy, as they present a choke hazard.
- Lots of exercise – this is by far the cheapest method and is both good for the dog and the owner.

- Training and stimulation – agility classes, clicker training, etc.

Reinforcement assessment

Reinforcement of behaviour can be both internal and external. Internal factors include problems with the animal's hedonic budget; external factors are less obvious but can be as simple as owners inadvertently reinforcing behaviours by paying attention to them: e.g. shouting at the Labrador that has chewed its owner's shoes. These reinforcers must be identified to help solve behavioural problems.

The EMRA™ approach is a concept used specifically by all COAPE behaviourists. For more information regarding this approach see the Recommended reading list.

Running successful puppy parties

A well-run puppy party can be very rewarding for both the individual puppy and for the practice. It bonds clients to the practice and is important in helping dogs to become less stressed when visiting the vet. It is also a huge responsibility because behaviours learnt at a puppy party can be carried through the rest of a dog's life. It is therefore vitally important that we take them seriously and ensure that we are equipped to give the best possible advice. A puppy party should be about educating the owner as to the importance of early socialization and training using sympathetic, positive reward-based methods.

Top tips
- Limit your class to a maximum of six puppies with two people per puppy.
- Puppies should be no older than 16 weeks. After this they start to lose their puppy teeth and social interactions are no longer on a par for the younger puppies.
- Match suitable breeds and sizes together if possible.
- Have plenty of interactive food toys and soft toys available to keep the puppies occupied while you talk to the owners.
- Keep your talk short and to the point. It is very difficult to keep the attention of an owner attached to a 9-week-old puppy that wants to do anything but sit still. As situations arise, this gives you the ideal opportunity to advise the owner on how to deal with the situation.
- Do not force puppies into interactions with other dogs. Allow them to sit somewhere safe to observe from a distance if that is what makes them feel comfortable. Make sure the owner does not overprotect them and reinforce fearful behaviour.
- Never let all six puppies off lead at the same time! This is a recipe for disaster, and many puppies have been scarred for life after a frightening interaction at a badly run puppy party.
- Mix and match two puppies at a time that you think may interact well, ensure that the off-lead time is closely supervised.
- Discuss the body language and behaviours you see with the client and help them to recognize signs of stress and anxiety and when to intervene. Be on the lookout for a puppy that is simply not coping. Remove it from the puppy party to a quieter area and see if you can get the owner to do some training/playing with it.
- Beware the overconfident puppy that tears around, trying to jump on and grab everything it sees! These puppies are best kept on a lead initially but allowed to interact with suitable puppies that can tolerate them. Letting this dog loose may cause him to learn how to be a bully and may frighten a less confident dog. This could result in a fear-based behaviour later on. Some people may not understand why they cannot all be off lead and it is important that the client understands that, just like children, puppies need to learn appropriate social skills.
- Start with a short training session to ascertain how well the owners are doing and what are their levels of skills. Demonstrate the basic principles of training. It can also be a good idea for owners to swop puppies at this point to see if they can get someone else's dog to sit!
- No puppy should be without a Kong® toy. These hollow rubber toys are ideal for teaching a puppy to be on his own, as playing with them is a rewarding experience. They are ideal for crate training and learning to be in the car. Stuff one with some tasty good-quality wet food and it will keep him occupied for a long time!
- Remember to have fun: e.g. teaching them to run through a children's play tunnel can be great fun for puppies and owners alike.

COMMON BEHAVIOURAL PROBLEMS IN YOUNG PUPPIES

The first few nights

We must remember this is a very traumatic experience for the puppy. The puppy suddenly finds that it has been taken from a secure environment with the comfort of its mother and siblings and put into an entirely new environment in which it is alone. Advise the owner to make sure they take time off work to devote to the first week of the puppy's new life.

- Plug in an Adaptil™ (dog-appeasing pheromone) diffuser or apply an Adaptil™ collar.
- Place the puppy in a bed or crate next to your bed so that if he cries in the night you can put your hand out to comfort him. Let him know you are there. This method is less traumatic than being left alone in the kitchen for example. Gradually you can move the bed/crate further away until it is outside the room.
- A hot water bottle can be comforting, but choose one that cannot be chewed and leak out.
- Have a play session before bed to tire puppy out.
- Put up baby gates so that puppy gets used to being on his own in a room without closing the door. Always give him something to do when you leave him – a Kong® stuffed with something tasty would be ideal or a new toy or chew.

Crate training

Teaching your puppy to feel safe and comfortable in a crate is very important. This can become his safe haven and will make leaving him alone much easier. It will also help with house training.

Do:
- Feed him in the crate
- Give him a tasty chew in the crate
- Keep the door open initially
- Make it comfortable with snuggly blankets
- Spray the blanket with Adaptil™.

Don't:
- Use the crate for punishment
- Close the door until the puppy accepts the crate
- Let the puppy become stressed and anxious in the crate.

Toilet training

Toilet training is entirely up to the dedication of the owner. Ideally, do not encourage owners to put paper or puppy training pads down, as this sets a precedent for urinating indoors.
- Take the puppy out after every meal and have a play session. Reward the behaviour with a treat. Start putting a command or key word to the behaviour such as 'Do your business' or 'Toilet'.
- Take the puppy out every hour if possible, thus reducing the chances of an accident happening indoors. By doing this you are setting the puppy up to succeed.
- Never punish toileting behaviour – the puppy will assume you are punishing him for toileting, not the toileting *indoors*. It will then start to toilet on the quiet to avoid the wrath of the unpredictable human. If an accident happens indoors the owner must be even more vigilant.

Mouthing

Dogs investigate with their mouths just as we do with our hands. By mouthing they learn how hard they can bite before there are negative consequences – this is very important for learning bite inhibition. If a puppy bites too hard, squeal in a high-pitched voice and end the game for a minute or two. Encourage the mouthing behaviour onto a toy instead of hands. Make sure that any child understands this rule too.

Food guarding

Certain breeds such as terriers and gundogs may guard their food. If a puppy starts to display this behaviour, advise the owner to feed small amounts by hand initially so the puppy sees the human as the giver not the taker. Do not under any circumstances take the food away and then give it back. By taking the food away, you are reinforcing exactly what the dog is afraid of and may make him even more wary (see Food or object guarding behaviour, later in this chapter).

Coprophagia

Coprophagia or eating faeces is a relatively normal behaviour in dogs, although obviously it is not recommended as it can lead to the puppy picking up worms or other pathogenic organisms. If the puppy is eating his own faeces recommend the following:
- Review the diet – the puppy may not be digesting his food correctly due to an underlying medical condition or to the type of diet. His own faeces will be palatable to him as they are relatively undigested.
- Always watch the puppy and clear the faeces up before he can get to it. Teach him a recall and reward him for coming away from it. If necessary have the puppy on a long line so that you have more control of the situation initially.
- Do not punish the behaviour – he won't understand and it may encourage him to eat it quicker!

Fearful or nervous behaviour in puppies

SOCIALISE, SOCIALISE, SOCIALISE using counter conditioning and desensitization techniques. Do not flood. Seek the advice of a good behaviour therapist. This will not go away as the puppy gets older and is likely to get worse if not dealt with correctly.

COMMON BEHAVIOURAL PROBLEMS IN ADULT DOGS

For the purposes of this chapter I have selected the most common complaints from owners that you may come across as a nurse in practice.

Jumping up

Jumping up to greet is a common problem and one which is not acceptable to humans.
Reasons:
- This is normal greeting behaviour for dogs and for this reason, it is advisable not to punish this behaviour as you may teach the dog that people will hurt it if it approaches them, changing a sociable dog to a fearful or anxious one.
- Reinforced with attention by owner, possibly encouraged.

Solution:
- Do not reinforce the jumping up with attention or touch.
- Reward all four feet on the ground.
- Make sure *everyone* the dog meets obeys these rules.
- Advise that the owner goes to a reputable trainer.

Pulling on the lead

Reasons:
- This is simply a training issue and has nothing to do with social hierarchy or dominance.
- The owner is probably reinforcing the behaviour or does not have the skills needed to retrain the dog.

Solution:
- Advise the owner to go to a reputable trainer.
- A Gentle Leader® or Halti® when fitted and used correctly will help with the training process. It is not advisable to use pain or force: e.g. choke chain or jerking on the lead to get a dog to walk next to you. You would rather have a dog that walks next to you because it is more rewarding than pulling.
- A training programme is required teach the dog to walk to heel; the head collars only allow the initial mechanism to direct the dog to stop or slow down, and reinforcement is then required. Once the dog has learnt to walk to heel, the head collar can be removed in stages, so that the dog walks nicely on a collar and lead.

Inappropriate elimination

1. **Indoors**
   Reasons:
   - Insufficient house training
   - Cognitive dysfunction – loss of previously learned behaviours in elderly dogs
   - The owner may be using harsh techniques causing the dog to try and eliminate out of sight of the owner – he equates owner + elimination with punishment.

Solution:
- Go back to basics with house training
- Ensure owners are using the correct techniques
- A full health check is recommended to ensure that there are no medical conditions that may be causing the problem.

2. **Excitement**

Reason:
- Young dogs often urinate when excited or anxious and it is normally related to fear or insecurity. It is thought that the smell of the urine may appease another dog by conveying certain messages regarding the dog's age, sex, etc.

Solution:
- Keep all greetings calm and try to distract the dog using training commands and treats to teach an alternative behaviour.
- Increase the dog's confidence.

3. **Marking**

Both male and female dogs exhibit this behaviour but it is more likely to be prominent in uncastrated males. The incidence will be reduced if castrated but it depends on the age of the dog and the learned component of the behaviour.

Separation-related problems

Reasons:
- Being left alone does not come naturally to our social dogs. It is important that puppies are taught from a young age that being left alone can be rewarding.
- Boredom/frustration.
- Fear/anxiety.
- Cognitive dysfunction.

Solution:
- Identify the underlying emotional behaviour using the EMRA™ approach as previously discussed.
- If the dog is genuinely anxious and shows severe signs of stress, such as panting, salivating, sweating from pads and destruction of doors, etc., refer to a behaviourist immediately. The longer the behaviour is unresolved the worse it will become.
- If the dog appears to be barking or chewing due to boredom or frustration, advise the owner to assess his hedonic budget discussed earlier.

Food or object guarding behaviour

This behaviour can be easily avoided if the right steps are taken as a puppy.

Reasons:
- Owner insists on 'being the boss' and takes the highly prized article off the dog. This is the very thing it was worried about. This behaviour has nothing to do with being dominant – it is natural for a dog to hold onto a prized possession. It is our job to make him understand that we are not a threat.
- Breed disposition to guarding resources – particularly in the gundogs.
- Being punished for guarding things.

Solution:
- If a dog is showing signs of food or object guarding behaviour, first identify its emotional state and review its hedonic budget.

- If the dog is very anxious or fearful because it has been punished for this behaviour before, refer immediately to a behaviourist.

Guarding behaviour may be seen:

1. When feeding:
- Do not feed from a bowl.
- Feed bit by bit – this way you are giving the food and the dog will eagerly anticipate you being near him during feeding time. Do this until the dog is more relaxed with you nearby and start to introduce a bowl.
- Always put small amounts of food out so that the dog does not have a lot to guard.
- Use this opportunity for training.
- Start teaching that a hand on the bowl means a treat.
- Never allow children near these dogs while feeding. No dog is ever 100% safe.

2. When playing with toys:
- While playing, always have another more desirable toy on hand that you can barter with. In this way you can teach the dog to relinquish the one toy and gain a better one. Teaching the dog to relinquish is the way to correct toy guarding behaviour. Don't leave desirable objects lying around.

3. Place guarding such as sofas or beds:
- These are highly desirable areas for some dogs. Make them less desirable by making the floor or other areas of the house more desirable. Use food or toys to lure them off and reward them when they come to you.
- Never physically try to remove them from the place they are guarding as you will force the dog to make an irrational decision.
- Be consistent with your training and make sure everyone in the house follows the same training principles to avoid confusion.

Aggression to people or other animals

This behaviour has serious ramifications for the dog and needs to be handled professionally and quickly. Refer to a reputable behaviourist immediately. The correct advice at this time may prevent a serious injury and a euthanized dog.

COMMON BEHAVIOURAL PROBLEMS IN CATS

Inappropriate elimination

Reasons:
- Unneutered male tom cats marking their territory
- Medical conditions such as cystitis, which may cause pain and negative association with the litter tray; cats may unable to access the outside as they are unable to get out of the cat flap due to arthritis or obesity
- Not enough litter trays per cat in the household (you should provide one tray per cat plus one extra)
- Fear, anxiety and insecurity, e.g. an aggressive cat outside, stressful multicat household; cats will urinate in the house to create a sense of security
- Poor litter training, the cat not liking the type of substrate being used, or the tray not be cleaned properly by the owner
- Cognitive dysfunction.

Solution:
- Rule out any medical conditions
- Identify the root cause of the problem using the EMRA™ philosophy
- Use pheromone diffusers (Feliway®) to create a less stressful environment
- Make sure there are an adequate number of litter trays in quiet areas
- Refer to a knowledgeable behaviourist
- Advise client not to use punishment as this will increase anxiety and possibly cause the urination/defecation to increase.

Scratching furniture

Reasons:
- Natural behaviour
- Absence of a scratching post
- Boredom
- Applying scent to objects to increase the feeling of security.

Solution:
- Provide cat gyms and a tall sisal scratching post; some cats do prefer horizontal scratching areas, especially if they are arthritic
- Ensure cat is stimulated and played with often
- Apply pheromone spray/diffuser to increase sense of security.

It is important that owners are aware that clipping a cat's claws has no impact on the amount of scratching that the cat exhibits.

Anxiety or fearful behaviour

Reasons:
- Poor socialization
- Inherited temperament
- Punishment applied for certain behaviours
- Inappropriate environment for the cat.

Solution:
- Seek advice of behaviourist
- Use EMRA™ approach to make the cat's environment better and more secure
- Avoid using punishment
- Use counter conditioning and reinforcement techniques.

Aggression

Reasons:
- Poor socialization
- Inherited temperament
- Hand-raised kitten
- Reinforcement from owner, e.g. playing roughly
- Fear and anxiety.

Solution:
- Seek advice of behaviourist.
- Determine the root of the problem using the EMRA™ approach.
- Advise owners not to reinforce aggressive play. Use toys and NOT hands to play with kittens.
- Use counter conditioning and desensitization techniques.

WHAT CATS WANT!

Cats are predators and there is no getting away from this. The first time our cute little ball of fluff brings in a half-mutilated bunny or bird, we are shocked and try and save the poor creature from further trauma. Some people punish their cats for this behaviour, but it is very important to educate owners that this is innate behaviour. It does not matter how much a cat is fed – he is not hunting because he is hungry, he is hunting because it provides him with an outlet for his instinctive, predatory behaviour. It is when cats are denied this opportunity to hunt that we start to see the emergence of behavioural problems. Cats find stalking, chasing, catching and plucking of feathers or fur very rewarding and will continue to do so if they can. Indoor cats are particularly susceptible to the build-up of frustration in the absence of a predatory behaviour outlet. These cats can become cantankerous, aggressive, reclusive, bored or depressed. Help your clients enrich the lives of their indoor cats by providing them with the following:
- Surfaces at various levels to sleep on (sisal cat gyms are ideal)
- Regular play sessions simulating hunting and stalking behaviour
- Large paper bags or cardboard boxes to hide in
- Catnip, which can encourage a feeling of well-being
- Possibly another feline friend to bond with and have a social interaction
- Make eating more challenging by introducing feeding toys that induce some frustration.

COGNITIVE DYSFUNCTION

In older dogs and cats, it is important to recognize behavioural changes that result from ageing of the brain. Clients should be educated to recognize these changes and seek advice and treatment.

Signs to look out for are:
- Confusion and decreased awareness
- Change in social relationships
- Change in activity levels – restlessness, repetitive behaviours, apathy, decreased responsiveness
- Anxiety
- Altered sleep cycles
- Loss of learned behaviours, e.g. house soiling, remembering commands
- Change in appetite
- Irritability.

EMPATHIZING WITH PATIENTS IN PRACTICE

It is vital that you as a vet or veterinary nurse are able to empathize with your patients and understand something of what they might be feeling. Put yourself into a dog's or cat's 'shoes' as they come through the door of the practice or the consulting room. Many animals are ill or in pain and as such are on the defensive. Treat them according to their temperament and individual needs. Learn to read their body language and adjust to each situation. This will make your job safer and the animal's stay with you less stressful. A bad experience in practice can make a normally amenable dog or cat difficult to handle, which can develop into a behavioural issue.

Look for the following signs of stress:

Dogs

- Yawning
- All-over body shake as if they have just come out of water
- Panting
- Sweating paws
- Dilated pupils
- Puppy-like, appeasing behaviour
- Barking.

Give fearful patients space and time to get used to their environments. Try not to approach them immediately and drop treats on the floor.

Cats

- Hiding in the back of the cage or carrier
- Dilated pupils
- Open-mouth breathing
- Sweaty paws.

Handle these cats gently and take time with them. Do not scruff as this will make a fearful cat very defensive. Use your thumb and forefinger together to create a greeting.

BIBLIOGRAPHY

Aspinall, V., 2008. Clinical Procedures in Veterinary Nursing, second ed. Butterworth-Heinemann, Oxford.

Bradshaw, J., 2011. In Defence of Dogs. Allen Lane, Penguin Publishing, London.

Burch, M.R., Bailey, J.S., 1999. How Dogs Learn. Howell Book House, Hoboken, New Jersey, USA.

Coppinger, R., Coppinger, L., 2001. Dogs – A Startling New Understanding. Scribner, New York.

Eaton, B., Falconer-Taylor, R.F., Neville, P.F., 2007. EMRA: dominance and the alpha dog: challenging traditional thinking. Veterinary Times 37 (5), 16–19.

Falconer-Taylor, R.F., Neville, P.F., 2004. EMRA: the brain reward system and therapy induced frustration. Veterinary Times 34 (38).

Falconer-Taylor, R., Strong, V., Neville, P., 2014. EMRA Intelligence. Cadmos Publishing Limited, Richmond, UK, pp. 13–15.

Landsberg, G., Hunthausen, W., Ackerman, L., 1999. Handbook of Behavioural Problems of the Dog and Cat. Butterworth-Heinemann, Oxford.

Lyon, H., Neville, P.F., Falconer-Taylor, R.F., 2006. Assessment and treatment of canine aggression problems using the EMRA approach. Veterinary Times 36 (3), 22–24.

Machell, B., Falconer-Taylor, R.F., Neville, P.F., 2006. Assessment and treatment of separation disorders in dogs using the EMRA approach. Veterinary Times 36 (16).

Mech, D., 2008. Whatever happened to the term alpha wolf? <http://www.wolf.org>.

Neville, P.F., Falconer-Taylor, R.F., 2004. EMRA: inappropriate elimination and impact of mood state assessment in a female long haired dachshund. Veterinary Times 34 (44).

O'Heare, J., 2003. Canine Neuropsychology, third ed. Behave Tech Publishing ebook.

Serpell, J., 1995. The Domestic Dog, Its Evolution, Behavior and Interactions with People. Cambridge University Press, Cambridge, UK.

Strong, V., Whitehead, S., 1999. The Dog's Brain – a Simple Guide. Alpha Books.

Turner, D.C., Bateson, P., 2000. The Domestic Cat: The Biology of Its Behaviour, second ed. Cambridge University Press, Cambridge.

RECOMMENDED READING

Aspinall, V., 2014. Clinical Procedures in Veterinary Nursing, third ed. Butterworth-Heinemann, Oxford.
Chapter One provides all details of cat and dog handling.

Bailey, G., 2002. The Perfect Puppy. Hamlyn, London.
Ideal for first-time puppy owners.

Beaver, B.V., 1980. Feline Behaviour: A Guide for Veterinarians. Saunders, Philadelphia.
Detailed description of cat behaviour.

Donaldson, J., 1996. The Culture Clash. James and Kenneth Publishers, USA.

Goleman, D., 2004. Emotional Intelligence. Bloomsbury, London.
This book will have a huge impact on how you view your own interactions and relationships in life.

Neville, P.F., Falconer-Taylor, R.F., 2004. EMRA: the new perspective in approaching companion animal behaviour problems (1). Veterinary Times 34 (29), 28–30.

Neville, P.F., Falconer-Taylor, R.F., 2004. EMRA: the new perspective in approaching companion animal behaviour problems (2). Veterinary Times 34 (31), 14–16.

Pryor, K., 1999. Don't Shoot the Dog. Bantam Books, London.
A detailed discussion on learning theory.

Semyonova, A., 2009. The 100 Silliest Things People Say About Dogs. Hastings Press, Hastings. <http://www.non-lineardogs.com>.
An enlightened new approach to understanding your dog.

Yin, S., 2009. Low Stress Handling, Restraint and Behaviour Modifications of Dogs and Cats. Cattledog Publishing, USA.
I would recommend every veterinary practice to have a copy of this book.

For more information regarding COAPE behaviourists and on behaviour education courses available:

<http://www.capbt.org> for details of local COAPE qualified, modern, fair and effective trainers and referral behaviourists.

<http://www.coape.org> for education courses in companion animal behaviour and training from basic to Diploma level.

The Indoor Cat Initiative at <www.indoorpet.osu.edu>.
An excellent resource for both pet owners and veterinary professionals for indoor cats.

Behaviour and Handling of the Horse

LISA ASHTON

KEY POINTS

- The wild horse is a sociable animal that lives in herds on open plains, and most of its behaviour patterns are based on the need to survive, eat, reproduce and socialise with others of its own species.

- It is important for your own safety when handling a horse in any situation that you understand the biology and the basic behaviour of the animal so that you can predict what it may do next.

- Transportation of horses may be unavoidable but can be distressing for the horse. Correct design of the vehicle, provision of correct travel clothing for the horse and adherence to the guidelines for welfare of the horse during the journey will all help to lower the stress levels.

- Effective training of horses, particularly foals and young stock, makes use of several different methods and is based on the horse's natural behaviour and the way in which it learns.

Introduction

Understanding horse behaviour is fundamental to being a safe, effective and ethical practitioner, the hallmarks of a twenty-first–century animal trainer. This chapter delves into behaviour and training through the lens of equitation science, the only evidence-based approach to horse training in the world. As a fast-emerging discipline, equitation science offers a 'road map' of horse behaviour, understanding what works, what does not, and why. In the past decade, evidence-based knowledge has shifted beliefs from traditionally 'naughty' horses to recognising confusion and re-training conflict behaviours. Veterinary professionals, owners, and riders have never felt more empowered, freely accessing 'training toolkits' brimming with safe, effective and ethical methods, always with the horse placed at the centre of every decision.

While every organism creates and reshapes its own world or *umwelt* (from the German word for environment), viewing today's world through the eyes of the horse highlights invasions, restrictions and inconsistencies in management and training. A horse experiencing inconsistent training, for example, may be more likely to be distressed by smaller frustrating aspects of his world such as limited friends and/or freedom. The UK Animal Welfare Act (2006) offers guidelines, a code of conduct for the responsible horse owner, known as the Five Freedoms (see Chapter 1). The code sets out essential requirements for a neutral welfare state for horses. Restricting and invading a horse's freedom, friends or forage is globally more recognised than a decade ago as having a negative impact on well-being, physically and mentally, of an individual horse. Cultural shifts towards welfare-driven animal husbandry (free-range chickens, pigs, etc.) during this same period may suggest a future spotlight on horse husbandry, training and performance. With animal scientists today identifying *positive* welfare states in animals, equitation science has commenced the journey towards positive welfare outcomes starting with environmental enrichment – flowers, olfactory triggers and music – measuring welfare parameters and cellular changes. Early findings demonstrate that environmental enrichment has a positive impact on both behavioural and cellular development in young horses.

Horse-human relationships

When did our two species become permanently and inextricably linked? Only 6000 years ago did we start to train horses to perform for transport, war, sport and more recently for our mental and physical well-being. Having to communicate non-verbally with a different species has demonstrated a positive impact on human health, emotionally and physically. Yet how have we humans affected horses?

Horse people mostly think about horses from a humanistic perspective. The use of 'nasty', 'stubborn' or 'lazy' and emphasis on a horse's 'attitude' can blur training so that when training does not work, the horse is blamed. These terms imply the horse is born that way and will never change. While horses vary in their genetic tendencies to behave in particular ways, these characteristics have significant *learned* components and can therefore be unlearned or suppressed, and better still avoided. Humanistic terms provide no useful answers for re-training the 'problem' or difficult horse. Worse, they lead to beliefs that place unfair expectations on the horse and often create further conflict through punishment and incorrect reinforcement strategies that are beyond the horse's mental abilities.

Applying evidence-based knowledge deepens understanding of innate behaviours, cognition and learning abilities, developing and improving optimal horse-human relationships.

Instinctive behaviour

Horses are all born with specific 'hard-wired' behaviours, in essence behaviours that are etched on the brain – feeding, flight response, play and reproduction. When two or more drives compete in the horses brain, the one with the greatest survival value will predominate. Extreme fear will prevail over mild hunger.

Equine survival relied on being cautious, fast and agile. The long nose ensured horses could graze while maintaining a lookout for predators. Grazing in pair bonds within family

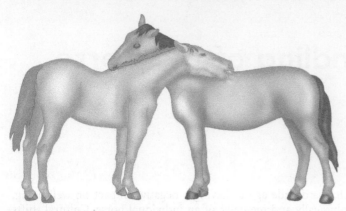

Fig. 13.1 Preferred grooming sites during mutual grooming

bands highlights the highly social nature of horses. A horse isolated is more likely to show separation anxiety and stereo-types (weaving, box-walking) than those kept in group housing conditions. So strong is the instinct for togetherness that grooming each other at the base of the neck is almost immediately relaxing. Research shows that grooming and scratching just in front of the withers causes a significant lowering of heart rate compared to any other region. By grooming there the heart rate lowers and it strengthens bonds; it is the optimal site to positively reinforce a horse with tactile rewards (Fig. 13.1).

While some training methods emphasise this predator-prey phenomenon, explaining that the horse needs to regard the human with respect and as a leader, with no tail, fixed ears, a short inflexible neck and only two legs, the concept that the horse must respect the leadership of the human is, at best, out-dated. More importantly, it is at odds with current knowledge and understanding of horse ethology. Dominance is not a personality trait; it focuses around drive or its reduction, and varies depending on the resource to defend. Research shows that even the most dominant horse is only dominant for 70% of the time. Equitation scientists know horses are only dominant for a specific resource or drive, such as food, water, sex and play, and that, as with dogs, social interactions are fluid. A 'bargy' horse is not dominant or trying to dominate a human relation-ship. It is easy to label a horse's behaviour as dominant and try to address it based on such. What is more helpful is describing the behaviour. A 'bargy' horse is simply a horse who has learnt a series of incorrect responses. If a horse 'walks all over' its handler, or 'does not respect your space', the problem is not one of attitude or lack of respect; it is simply because the horse does not lead straight. The crookedness could be further rewarded by the side-stepping behaviour of the handler. It is not cured by changing the horse's attitude, but by re-training the basic lead responses.

Equine intelligence and mental abilities

Understanding the horse's brain is important to handling and training as there are negative welfare implications in both over-estimating and underestimating the horse's mental abilities. In the past, underestimating has led to a lack of empathy with horses and unnecessary – and unhelpful – punishments. More common is the overestimating of higher mental abilities of horses. 'He knows what I am asking for, he's just being lazy', which also encourages delayed punishment – 'he knows what he did wrong'.

Horses do have outstanding mental abilities. Importantly, horses evolved the cognitive abilities needed to survive to be a horse. Think about it. With a constant supply of food and frequent watering, why would the horse have needed – and therefore evolved with – a more elaborate, complex pre-frontal cortex? Planning the next meal, reflecting on decisions, or thinking forwards about friends are redundant if you fail to be curious enough, fast enough or agile enough to survive to reproduce.

Living in the 'here and now' means the horse has an excellent memory of the physical world and associations. Remembering precise details of events is evolutionarily advantageous; it is the reason why a behaviour is context-specific. When training for routine preventative care – vaccinations, de-worming, teeth rasping or foot trimming – the association between the visual picture of the vet, farrier or dentist and the consequence (attrac-tive or aversive) results in a new memory. This new memory is triggered the next time the identical or similar visual surroundings appear. Associations between the environment (which includes the vet and other technicians) and the conse-quence rapidly establish new learnt behaviours. Before long the owner calls up the practice explaining that the horse 'does not do vets'.

With such precise memories, horses can remember these learned responses without practice for long periods of time. The powerful ability for horses to recall memories without distor-tion, altering or corrupting (humans constantly trawl through memories, reliving experiences personally and by storytelling) should steer our training practices to shape behaviours, which we can then 'proof' (test the horse's response to our signals anywhere and everywhere), generalising desirable behaviours for the horse.

Context-specific training is a hindrance to training if the horse learns to demonstrate flight-response behaviours in certain locations. Behaviours learnt with tense and fearful responses are learnt rapidly and become more permanent. These fear-memories can be suppressed and made less retriev-able with correct training, but in the right circumstances, the response can return with great speed and reaction (spontaneous recovery). An experienced rider – Ms Jayne Goodwin, 44 – sadly died after returning from an evening ride with friends on 9 January 2014. Her 6-year-old Friesian mare, Kali, bolted as she was trying to get back on after closing a gate. The coroner declared the mare had developed a habit of bolting while being mounted. With horses having the largest fear centre in the brain of all domestic animals, the amygdala (yet we don't ride dogs or cats), it is no surprise that equine vets have the highest injury risk of all civilian professions.

How horses learn

Horses are trained during every interaction we have, whether we are aware or not. This is significant because a person's action can have long-lasting consequences for the horse. If a vet/farrier handles a horse prompting fear and/or pain, the next time a vet/farrier attempts to handle the same horse, the horse may trial avoidance and/or escape behaviours (rearing, bucking, bolting, kicking, biting), both rewarding and reinforcing in removing the potential source of fear/pain.

IMPRINT TRAINING

- Learning to process stimuli rapidly, distinguishing similar stimuli from each other.
- Controversial non-associative training, prompting high levels of stress, yet unclear if this early stress can be justified in terms of later benefits found from early handling (birth, 12 hours, 24 hours and 48 hours after birth), as research has found no beneficial effect in behaviour at 1, 2, 3 or 6 months of age.
- Research demonstrates that aversives are just as traumatic for handled foals as for unhandled foals (fitting head collars and clipping).

HABITUATION

This is the mode of learning fundamental to handling and training and is interconnected at almost every stage of training. But why is learning to habituate important to the horse? It prevents horses from wasting energy in running away from or avoiding things in their environment that are harmless. Habituation is the result of frequent exposure to a stimulus whereby the horse learns not to react, e.g. girth, rugs, bit, clippers. With no consequence attached to a stimulus, it is the simplest form of learning. In the natural state, animals habituate to other harmless species, and to such things as wind blowing, trees and shadows. The *process* resulting in habituation is known as desensitisation. The aim of horse training and daily horse-human interactions is to habituate horses to some stimuli – humans, rugs, bits, girths, traffic, etc. – yet *sensitise* them to other stimuli, e.g. lead rope/rein pressure, lead ropes, leg aids, electric fences etc.

Sensitisation is the opposite of habituation. It occurs due to strong stimulation (habituation occurs due to weak stimulation) and can occur with a single stimulation (habituation requires repeated stimulation). Sensitisation increases behaviour (habituation decreases behaviour) due to exposure to a noxious stimulus.

Habituation methods

- Gradual habituation: occurs over time when the horse is free to escape. The horse practices his escape behaviour and gradually closes in on what he is afraid of until eventually he stops reacting to it. Trains running through fields horses graze upon and wind turbines are examples, and this habitualisation process takes time. The fear reaction expressed in the beginning can, however, return spontaneously (and unannounced) in the future, known as *spontaneous recovery*. Discovered in 1994 by neuroscientist Joseph LeDoux, fear responses are never forgotten; they are indelible (i.e. cannot be erased).
- Flooding: when you prevent the horse from escaping, presenting a fearful stimulus. Flooding the horse can be counter-productive and is thought to compromise welfare. Flooding can make the reaction to an aversive stimulus worse; any habituation method should only facilitate the lowest thresholds of fear.
- Response prevention: hold the horse still (restrain) while horse gets used to things. Restraint may be through stabling, stocks, tying up or restricting the horse's movements in-hand or under-saddle. It works because the horse is prevented from moving his legs and making distance, both of which reinforce fear.

The following are processes of operant conditioning to speed up habituation:

- Systematic desensitisation: using operant conditioning (positive and negative reinforcement) as a process to habituate to a stimulus.
- Overshadowing: when the horse is exposed to two strong stimuli at the same time (e.g. the clippers that make him want to run away, and the handler that makes him step forward and back), he can only listen to one of them. If the clippers are making him run away and you successfully make the horse step back, you tip the balance to a point where he is no longer showing a reaction to the clippers. That moment in time where the horse is responding to the handler is overshadowing. It's not about distracting the horse; it is a learning process of habituation where the horse diminishes his fear reactions very fast. It is also something that many horse trainers use, but they are not aware they are doing it. Another valuable aspect of overshadowing is that it accurately diagnoses the horse's level of fear. This is determined by noting how well the horse responds to the handler's signals in the presence of the fearful stimulus, i.e. how 'light' he is. The 'heavier' he is, the more driven he is by the clippers/needle/girth. As he becomes lighter, his fear is diminishing. Overshadowing *diagnoses* how a horse feels about a stimulus. Always keep the stimulus *below* his fear threshold, gradually increasing the proximity of the stimulus, only progressing to the next feature of the behaviour once the horse is 'light'. This can be used for injections, dental work and loading, and when introducing new stimuli.
- Counter-conditioning: desensitises the horse to things he was formerly afraid of. The process changes something fearful into something attractive, usually by becoming associated with the arrival of food or something else that the horse likes, e.g. placing feed inside a trailer or horsebox, or scratching the wither at the sound of clapping.
- Approach conditioning: the horse learns to make the fearful object retreat by chasing/accelerating towards the umbrella, quad bike, or ball. Shape the approach/retreat process of the stimulus by rewarding steps towards investigative behaviour (sniffing the ball) with a retreat of the stimulus. Within a few repetitions, the horse is now chasing the stimulus, getting close enough to touch it.
- Stimulus blending: blending a novel or fearful stimuli with another that the horse is already used to. Horses may be afraid of sprays or aerosols, and/or head shy. If you break down the features of an aerosol, for example, you will find there are three main characteristics:
  - The look of the bottle; this is probably the least important characteristic as most horses do not seem to mind the object much.
  - The sound of the aerosol – horses do mind that 'shh' sound. Hosing also has a sound, so by blending the two sounds together you get a much smaller reaction from the horse, and the habituation speeds up.
  - The feel of it – on dry hair the aerosol has a particular feel, but on damp hair it feels different; the horse has probably never felt that, which is why hosing is also useful.

CLASSICAL CONDITIONING

Occurs when a horse learns to associate an apparently unrelated event with another event because the first event actually predicts the second. The new, unrelated event or signal should come just before the known signal in order for the horse to learn the association. When a horse learns to associate an aversive environment or painful procedure – teeth rasped, routine vaccine, shoeing – the horse learns to associate the vet or farrier with the pain response, displaying arousal and possible anxiety.

OPERANT CONDITIONING

Operant conditioning is the most permanent form of learning and is how pressure-release works. It is also known as trial-and-error learning and explains much of these seemingly clever behaviours in horses. When a horse moves the stable door latch and the door opens, quickly the horse repeats the same behaviours to open the door, because of the consequence – freedom, food or friends. Horses are driven by their instincts to try various actions to resolve physical discomfort (rein or leg pressure). The action they give that immediately results in relief is the one they will remember and try next time. In training/handling horses, we hijack this learning mechanism, targeting the desirable behaviour, immediately followed by the release of pressure. Due to living in the 'here and now', whatever the horse did just before the release of pressure is the behaviour he remembers and associates as the solution to that pressure. Now the horse starts to increase that response whenever that pressure is presented in the future. So for some, the solution to being asked to step forwards into a confined space like a trailer or horsebox could initially be running backwards. Once the horse learns running backwards makes pressure cease (handler ends up releasing the rope), as horses have excellent associative abilities, coupled with operant conditioning, now the horse has solved the problem he faces. For some horses the solution to being squeezed in the ribs could be to buck the pressure off, just as he would a wild predator. Or perhaps the solution to constant metal and discomfort in the mouth would be to raise his head sufficiently high enough so the consequence is the removal of the bridle, disabling the fit of the bridle. This ability to solve problems should not be mistaken for reasoning. By trial and error, consequences from the behaviour make the behaviour more or less likely in the future. Through the lens of the horse, behaviour is not naughty or good, but more or less likely in the future depending on the consequence to the individual.

NEGATIVE REINFORCEMENT

Negative is not meant in the context of something bad. It is a mathematical definition, explaining the removal of something aversive to reinforce a behaviour. Negative reinforcement occurs when something the horse finds unpleasant, e.g. pressure, is applied to motivate a specific behaviour, followed by the immediate removal or release of the aversive stimulus. The removal of the aversive stimulus makes it more likely the horse will repeat the desirable behaviour in the future. Learning what to do, because of the removal of pressure, makes future behaviour more likely. Pressure on the lead rope towards the chin signals 'walk forward', and releasing pressure when the horse takes a step forwards trains the 'go' response from a lead signal.

Pressure and release is used to train acceleration, deceleration, line (straightness) and head and neck control (position).

Pressure and release from the rider's legs is used to train the horse to go forwards. When the horse lifts its head when you go to put the bridle/head collar on, or when you approach your horse to be caught, and he retreats, this increases the distance of your removal, thereby reinforcing his retreat. Very quickly retreating becomes a new habit. Pressure-release works because the pressure motivates the horse to give a response, and the release of pressure reinforces that the correct response was given. When this sequence of events is repeated, a habit forms and training has occurred.

There are three phases to pressure-release training:

1. Light aid – target the foreleg stepping back one step from your rein/rope. Using a light contact (100–200 g) place the rope/reins in the direction of the tail for 1 second. As soon as the horse steps back with one foreleg, release.

   If you release, but the leg has not stepped back, you will have trained immobility; or, worse, if the horse steps into the pressure, you have just trained an opposing response. Remember that whatever the horse does just before you release pressure trains this behaviour.

2. Stronger aid – increase the pressure if no response.

3. Release – remove pressure immediately when the horse starts the desired response.

Phase 1 – light aid

For welfare reasons, it makes sense to always signal a behaviour from a light aid through the learning process of classical conditioning; it also signals the immediate follow-up of greater pressure. With repetition the horse learns to avoid the stronger pressure by acting from the light aid. Remember that your pressures should be light enough not to cause conflict. Through repetition, the horse now starts to form habits from the light aids and – again through the process of classical conditioning (associative learning) – the horse begins to associate the light aids to more subtle influences such as arm position in-hand, seat position and/or weight under-saddle.

Phase 2 – stronger aid

This is the phase we eventually want to remove. It is the motivation for each response and applied if the horse does not immediately respond to the light aid (both qualities of obedience). Applying both the amount and speed of pressure directly correlates to the lack of response.

In foundation training, or for correcting only mild unwanted behaviours, only a slight increase motivates. For behaviours with a depth and duration of practice, pressures may need to be increased quickly. As soon as you identify the level of response, however, to motivate the behaviour, release. This is also the phase where if the horse is unmotivated in the next second for the response, we can use intermittent pressures such as rein vibrations or whip *taps*. (*CAUTION*: The whip is not used to create pain and fear. Use it as an extension of your arm. You never know – your horse might be surprised to find you can alleviate an itch.) There should be no gap greater than 1 second between pressures otherwise it serves to reward behaviours that might not warrant rewarding. The frequency to get a response should be approximately two taps per second and merely irritate the horse, not hurt or cause fear.

Phase 3 – release

An obvious release must happen at the first sign of every desired response. Why is it so important? Release rewards the response, telling the horse what *to* do, thereby training the response. Without the release, the best-case scenario for the horse is that habituation to pressures occurs, in-hand and under-saddle. The worst-case scenario is escalating conflict behaviour, as the horse has no controllability over the pressures, failing to remove them for any behaviours. Over longer periods horses can become ill through chronic stress; symptoms include ulceration, colic, supressed immune system and self-mutilation.

Do not wait for the horse to become light before you release – this is compromising the horse's welfare. Instead practice releasing the rein just as the horse is stopping or stepping back – then he will become light. It is easy to unintentionally reward heaviness in the mouth by maintaining pressure past the moment the horse stops, so that the response he learns is heaviness rather than stop. An opening mouth or a shortening neck during transitions usually means the rein release is not substantial or early enough.

POSITIVE REINFORCEMENT

Positive reinforcement occurs when a horse performs the desired behavioural response and as a consequence, a pleasant stimulus is added – e.g. scratching or receiving food. The addition of the pleasant stimulus makes it more likely the horse will repeat the desired response in the future. The reward is given when the horse performs the behaviour but there is no signal initially given. Rewarding a horse that approaches a handler with a scratch makes catching more likely in the future. Rewarding a horse as it stands relaxed makes relaxation more likely in the future.

SECONDARY POSITIVE REINFORCEMENT

Involves pairing a previously irrelevant stimulus such as a clicker or voice cue, e.g. 'good boy', with a primary reinforcer such as scratch or treat via classical conditioning. The secondary reinforcer marks the correct behaviour and is applied just before the primary reinforcer, rewarding the behaviour. When your horse lifts a leg to your signal or pressure cue, mark the leg lifting with a 'click' or 'good boy' and then treat. Very quickly your horse will associate the behaviour of lifting his leg to your marker (click), which is the signal food is about to arrive. Now you can gradually increase the holding of the leg before you click, training 'holding a leg' through secondary positive reinforcement. If you also train a horse to touch a target (the palm of your hand or an empty bottle on a stick) to receive a 'click and treat', before long the horse will associate the target to the marker (which always signals food is arriving) – now your horse will follow the target, even into stocks, stables or horse boxes.

POSITIVE PUNISHMENT

Positive punishment is the addition of an aversive consequence to *suppress* a behaviour. When a horse goes to bite the handler, pain from a whip may suppress biting. The addition of a punisher is to decrease a behaviour. In reality, pain triggers fear, associating the handler and all the components of the environment to the feelings of fear. The aim of punishment is to suppress or delete a behaviour; the punisher must be immediate, to avoid confusion and conflict (the result of delayed punishment).

NEGATIVE PUNISHMENT

Negative punishment is the removal of a reinforcing stimulus, withholding something attractive such as food, friends or freedom. As the horse lives in the 'here and now', this mode of learning is at best confusing for the horse, and at worst prompts conflict and, if endured, chronic stress.

SHAPING

Reinforcing the simplest behaviour of a more complex one is known as shaping. Effective trainers/handlers build behaviour piece by piece, then refine these into more complex behaviours. Training in small achievable steps/increments means the horse is more likely to offer the correct response. Training too fast and too far can result in the horse offering alternative behaviours, including conflict behaviours.

CONFLICT BEHAVIOURS

Consolidation describes the process of habit formation. The aim of training is to consolidate all of the horse's mobility in-hand and under-saddle into habits we desire. Optimal training is a result of training a specific signal to produce one specific response. A light pressure towards the horse's chin always means 'move forwards'. Bad habits arise when any random or undesirable behaviours from the horse are allowed/rewarded with the release of pressure; however, they also arise from unclear and inconsistent signals. The bad habits that arise from rewarding random behaviours and from confusion generally cause tension and conflict.

Expressions of the flight response

It is better for the welfare of horses if we can look through a lens of science, describing problem behaviours – bucking, rearing, spinning, shying, bolting, tense, cold-backed, etc. – as *expressions of the flight response*. From short, choppy steps, rigid body, tail swishing, teeth grinding, and head tossing, to the more dangerous behaviours often labelled as 'naughty', it is the flight response causing the release of specific hormones which override other perceptions in favour of flight. These behaviours are known as conflict behaviours and they arise because the horse is torn between at least two opposing responses. His instincts propel him to reduce the conflict and respond to only one stimulus. The flight response is usually the horse's instinctive choice, the evolved solution for a prey animal from the open plains.

Determining exactly what the horse is confused about is not difficult. It is usually about the horse not being able to solve his pressure problems. Consistency results in a predictable environment; remember, a relaxed horse finds his world predictable (light aid) and controllable (release of pressure). Not all horses, however, are able to resolve their problems; now it is inevitable that conflict escalates, until consistency of outcomes returns.

GETTING STARTED

Equipment and facilities

- Before you start, always use an approved safety riding helmet, boots, gloves and a long (dressage) whip – one that is stiff enough so it will clearly stop tapping when you do. Make sure you are in an enclosed area with safe footing. When you start a foal or young naïve horse's training use a normal webbed halter as they are learning everything from scratch, and they do not understand pressure and not to respond. Train using something stronger like a rope halter or a bit, if it is part of the equipment you will use eventually for medical interventions, or when re-training a horse. For the lead rope, use a nylon braided one that does not stretch (stretch makes the pressure/release less clear). Yachting-type rope is too heavy and makes it harder for the horse to feel a release clearly.
- At the most basic level, once your horse is habituated to human contact and to the equipment (the whip) teach him to 'go', 'stop', 'step-back' and 'park'. The one which is trained first depends on the horse. In the case of a foal, start from a standstill and target the 'go' response first as a single forward step from each front leg. Young horses tend to take one, maybe two steps and stop of their own accord, which is great as you can focus more on repetitions of 'go', keeping the lesson simple.
- In the case of re-training, you many not be able to train just 'go' or just 'stop' in isolation; you may need to work on both. If your horse is 'pushy', for example, start training the 'stop' first, or if he is what people call 'lazy' start with 'go'. *Training 'stop' is most important because the 'stop' deletes, and therefore allows you to correct any quickening and flight responses.*
- The muscles a horse uses to stop, slow down and reverse are all the same (retraction). The 'step-back' in fact is a deeper response to the stop, so training horses to step backwards to a light pressure from the halter or bit actually improves the stop. The step-back is itself very useful to correct any unwanted movements, and this also ties in with the 'park' response.
- 'Park' is essential for all medical interventions as well as loading, rugging and mounting.
- The 'park' teaches the horse to stand still until asked to move from the lead rope (not from your legs); he must not move even if you walk away. If the horse understands stop and step-back, park is easy to train.
- Keep training sessions short, especially with young horses. The most effective way to accelerate learning is by training in sets, with between three and five repetitions per set. Have a break between each set, aiming to finish each task (learnt response) with three consecutive, correct or improved responses. Young foals should be trained for very short periods.

Your position

- Stand facing the horse, level with his head (Fig. 13.2). In the early stages of training you want to face the horse so you can clearly see what he does with his feet. Hold the lead rope about 15 cm from the clip. Don't worry if your horse is looking around – don't try to control his head movements at this stage, concentrate only on what

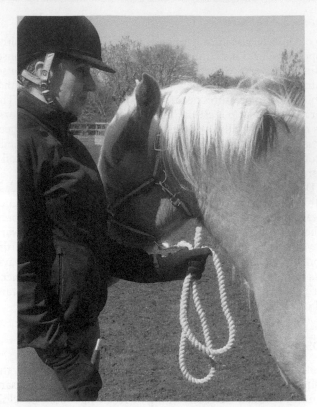

Fig. 13.2

his legs are doing. Looking around is just a sign that the horse is insecure (his world is unpredictable and uncontrollable); when he starts to understand his training, he will become more relaxed.

'Stop' response – basic attempt

- 'Stop' is first trained with a step-back as it is the same group of muscles used for stop and slow down, and stepping back actually deepens the response to stop (Fig. 13.3). You are aiming to get the horse to step back, even just one small step. This is known as a basic attempt (Australian Equine Behaviour Centre shaping scale), which must be rewarded with an immediate release of pressure. From here you can repeat the exercise until he takes a larger, clearer step, one step at a time.
- With all pressure signals, the basic rule is to apply a light pressure and if within 2 seconds you don't get a response, increase it with a vibration of the rein and release at the first sign of a basic attempt. Train one step at a time – make sure the horse has completed a single step-back before asking him to do another. Asking for multiple steps 'back-back-back' is likely to confuse him.
- As you work on each step from each front leg, you may notice that one leg takes a smaller step than the other one, or he is a bit heavier when responding with one leg (it takes more pressure to get him to step back with one leg than the other), so the next stage is to get him to take equal size steps with each leg, and to make him a little lighter. This is taking the response from a basic attempt to 'obedience' level but before you do that, work on 'go' at basic attempt level.

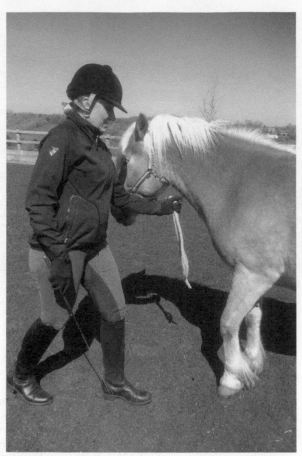

Fig. 13.3

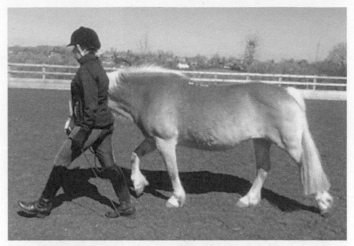

Fig. 13.4

'Go' response – basic attempt

- Once you have achieved a clear step-back from one leg then the other, start teaching 'go'. To train your horse to lead forward from pressure, you need to remain standing in the same position as before, facing the horse and with your shoulder level with his head, so you can watch what his legs are doing and so that you can clearly release the pressure at the exact right moment when your horse takes the step that you are asking for.
- Apply a light forward pressure on the lead rope; this will apply pressure to his poll and lower jaw. If he does not take a step forward straight away, you might need to pressure the lead rope to the side a bit or towards you (taking care to stay clear of his feet). Directing pressure sideways can make it easier to get that first attempt to step forward which you can reward by releasing the pressure.
- Repeat the exercise until your horse takes a single step forward from light lead pressure.
- Now take the 'step-back' and 'go' responses to obedience level.

Progress to obedience level

- At obedience level you are aiming for two clear steps (backwards or forwards) from light pressure. This is when the long dressage whip, used as an extension of your arm, is used. The whip is used to reinforce the lead rope signal. You only need to use it with light taps, but they need to be quite close together, using a 'tap-tap-tap' motion (this is so the horse does not interpret the interval between taps as a reward).

- Hold the whip as a signal – not how you ride with it but more how you would hold a tennis racket, with your index finger pointing down the shaft of the whip.
- Before introducing the whip as a signal, you must make sure you can rest the whip on your horse's body – that is, you need to habituate the horse to the contact of the whip on all parts of his body and legs.
- Start by gently resting the whip around his wither area and if he should move forwards you can use your stop aid while keeping the whip in contact with his body. It is important not to teach your horse that whip contact means 'move' – he should learn that the signal to move is a whip-*tap*.
- Make sure he accepts the whip on his shoulder area, on his rib cage, and even on his chest, correcting any steps forwards that he might take.
- If your horse is overly sensitive to the whip contact, make sure you spend enough time and be careful not to 'tickle' him or accidentally bump him with it; it is easiest to rest the whip quite firmly against his body. When you can repeatedly remove the whip and rest it on his body again, you know you can start to use the whip as an aid and train him to step back or step forward from the whip tap. With repetition you will soon be able to turn and face forwards (Fig. 13.4).

Step-back from the whip

- For the 'step-back' you will be tapping below the knee, on the front of the cannon bone area (Fig. 13.5). First, though, apply a backward and light lead pressure, and if the horse is delayed, or heavy, then start 'tap-tap-tapping' one leg until the leg steps back, and stop tapping the moment it does.
- Think about which leg he is likely to move first and target that one (normally the one which is slightly in front).
- If the horse tries to go forward you might have to correct him with the lead rein (you may need a small vibration) but keep tapping until he does take a step back, and stop tapping the moment he does.

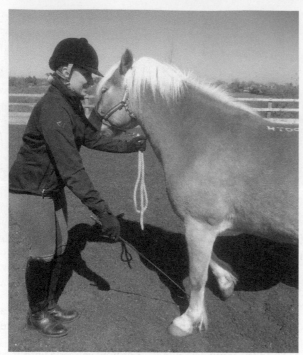

Fig. 13.5

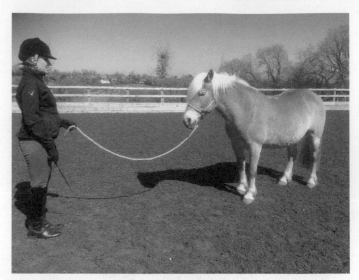

Fig. 13.6

- You are teaching your horse that when he feels light pressure on his nose, he should step back to avoid the 'tap-tap' on his legs, or the stronger vibration on his nose. If you are really consistent with timing the increase of pressure and the release of pressure, the horse will learn this very quickly.
- Remember to work just one step at a time with each leg – one foot, one complete step-back and release, and then the other foot.
- You can also operantly condition the whip taps without applying any initial lead pressure. This means you only tap without giving any other signal, until the horse attempts a step-back, and stop tapping when he does. This makes it very clear to the horse that the tap on the cannon bone means he should step back.
- Once your horse can do one step backwards from the whip with each front leg, you then aim to get two steps backwards from light pressure. When he takes a step back with one foot you tap the other so he takes that leg back and stop tapping to reward the complete two-step stride.
- When your horse responds to the light lead pressure with two clear even steps, you are at obedience level.

'Go' from the whip

- Start by resting the whip on the horse's rib cage, in the area where your legs will be when you ride him. Make sure you habituate him first by resting the whip on him while he stands, correcting any forward or backward steps he takes.
- Your dressage whip should be long enough (about 1–1.1 m) so you can rest it on his belly while you stand by your horse's head, holding the rein under his chin.
- Apply a light lead rein pressure on the rein forward, and if you feel there is no response, start tapping lightly until

the moment that he does take a step forward, when you immediately stop tapping and point the whip down to the ground. He may do more than one step forward – that's okay, you just ask him to stop.
- *It is important to train horses not to follow us,* but to only respond to the pressure, so we ask for the step forward *without walking* forward ourselves. As he learns that the whip taps mean go, he may not let you rest the whip on his body anymore, preferring to step forward, and here it is important that you go back to whip contact, asking him to stand still before you ask him to step forward again with a light tap. If you don't he will start moving as soon as he sees the whip coming, learning to be anticipatory of the tap.
- The acceptance of the contact of the whip is almost more important in the early stages than the response to the tapping. He must be completely relaxed about having the whip touch all over his body. Once he is relaxed he will find it much easier to discriminate between neutral contact and the aid/tap.
- With consistent timing, your horse will quickly learn to avoid the whip tap by responding to the light forward pressure of the halter, and this is when you have trained 'go' to obedience level. With repetition your horse will go forwards from a light hand signal (see Fig. 13.4).
- The time taken to train each response to obedience level depends on the horse and the situation. Often, horses are more controlled by the environment than their handler, and in that case it will take longer.
- Be aware that in the beginning, every time you change the surroundings, even if you turn him around and he sees a different view, he may again be more controlled by the environment and you may need to go back over what you thought he already had learned (shaping).
- If your timing is quite good this basic training in hand should not take too long.

Training 'park'

- Once you have reached obedience level in 'stop' and 'go' you are ready to train 'park' (Fig. 13.6).

- Park is a fantastic 'tool' in your training 'toolkit' to maintain and improve relaxation, and it also helps to consolidate the halt.
- You are aiming to teach your horse that once you have asked him to stop, he is not to move or follow you, even if you move away, unless you ask him to do so with your lead or reins. We only want the horse to follow us after we give him the aid to move.
- 'Park' is great for horses who tend to fidget, be anxious, push into you, or generally don't know how to stand still, but it is also important because standing still is a must for all sorts of routine and veterinary procedures, and these tasks are all a lot easier when the horse has been trained to 'park'.
- Many people wrongly expect the horse will know he is supposed to stand still in those situations, when in reality we should first train them thoroughly in easier settings and progress gradually.
- While some trainers specifically train their horses to follow them, there are many times when you need your horse to stand still while you move around, and it is too difficult for the horse to differentiate when he should follow and when not.
- Going around the off side to do up the girth, or perhaps closing a gate, you don't want your horse to follow you; for a start, he might be tied up. If you move towards his hindquarters, say to pick his feet, again you want him to stand still in one spot – you don't want him to be backing away from you or moving sideways around you. So train horses in your care to always stand still until you give them the lead signal to move.
- Start by facing your horse so you can see clearly what he does with his feet.
- Start your 'park' in an area where your horse feels reasonably comfortable. Lead him to the spot where you want him to park and give him the stop signal/aid (a light backwards pressure from the lead rein). He should stop in one-and-a-half steps (if he doesn't or he feels heavy, you may need to refresh the 'stop' lesson until you achieve obedience level again).
- Once he has stopped, move away from him, approximately 1 metre, still holding on to your rope but without applying any pressure, and have your dressage whip ready to correct any forward steps he may take.
- When you move away he will probably take a step towards you; the moment that he does, tap the cannon bone of the leg he has moved until he takes a step back and not just stop.
- He should step back to the position he was in. If he takes a step sideways with a front or hind leg, tap his cannon bone and ask him to take a step back.
- If he takes more than two steps, you may have to use your lead rein pressure to make him stop, and then use the whip again to make him step back to where he was. Teaching the horse to step back from the whip-tap allows you to correct any steps he may take during park training.
- We are asking the horse to step back using *only* the whip, and no rein pressure. This is because the whip allows us to reach the horse without having to move towards him.
- As the whip is an extension of our arm, from 1 metre away we can still use it effectively to achieve a step back.

If we were to use rein pressure, we would have to approach the horse first, and instead of learning to stand still, we may instead teach him to step back when we walk towards him.

- Once you have corrected him with a step back, move towards him again at least to where his head is, and then back away 1 metre again. He will probably take a step towards you again, so correct him again with a tap, making sure he does actually step back, and then move towards him again.
- Repeat this a few times. If you consistently achieve a step-back each time he moves a foot, he will soon learn to remove your tap by standing still and you will be able to progressively move away further and further each time, until you reach the end of the lead rein or the buckle of reins.
- You should be able to move anywhere the length of your rope allows, while your horse stands still, but be sure to never put any pressure at all on the reins and be ready to correct him if he moves (Fig. 13.7).

Making progress

- When your horse is parking well, turn around and face in the same direction as him and without putting any rein pressure, walk forward from his shoulder, being ready to correct any forward steps with the whip if he should follow you (Fig. 13.8).
- You should be able to walk past your horse without him moving and can even take it further by doing some small running steps, again making sure you don't accidentally put pressure on the reins. The reins must remain loopy at all stages (Fig. 13.9).

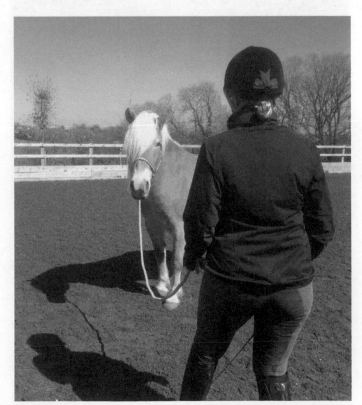

Fig. 13.7

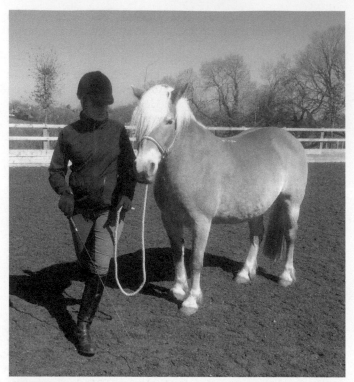

Fig. 13.8

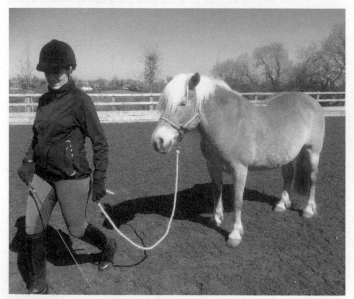

Fig. 13.9

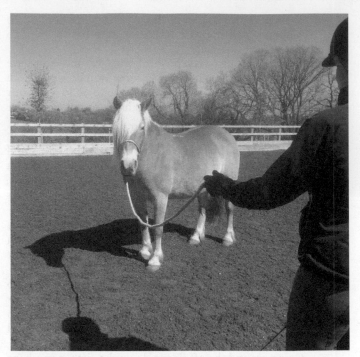

Fig. 13.10

without making him move his feet, which becomes very confusing to him. Be careful not to correct the horse's head from moving – once they understand the task, which is that their legs are staying still, they will relax and they will tend to look around less. Looking around is a sign of insecurity that will dissipate when he keeps his legs under your stimulus-control.

- Once you have your horse parking well in one area, you can progress by asking him to park in different places. You can start by turning him around so that he is facing in a different direction where he has a different view, then go and train him in other places and keep progressing until you can park anywhere and anytime (Fig. 13.10).

- Pawing while tied up is simply a symptom that your horse has never learned to 'park'. Horses that paw don't park, and are 'heavy in the mouth'. If you were to let go when he is pawing, he would walk or run away, which means that the training of his stop is poor enough that he can actually push through it to some extent, making the stop signal heavy by pushing forward into it.

- A thorough re-training in hand of 'stop', 'step-back' from a light aid, and of 'park' is required.

- Once you have a good stop and park in one situation practice in different places and teach him to stand still all over the place. With practice you will find that you'll not only be able to walk backwards away from him, but you will be able to move in all directions, even throw the reins over his neck and walk around him, and he'll stay parked in one spot.

- This training is essential for learning to stand while tied up. If tying up is a problem, go back and train/re-train the horse's 'park' response.

'Go', 'stop', 'step-back' and 'park' are the 'tools' to successfully train horses for routine and non-routine veterinary interventions.

- Another useful exercise is to ask the horse to park, and while he stands still, back away to the end of the reins, then ask him to move forward with light forward rein pressure until he comes up to you. When he does, ask him to stop and re-park, then back away again to the end of the reins.

- If your horse wants to look around, that's fine – he is allowed to look around as long as he doesn't move his feet. Many people have problems training their horses to stand still because they try to control the horse's head and they do so by putting pressure on the horse's mouth

Handling problems

- Failure to remove a reinforcer at the correct time can reward the incorrect response.
- Adding a reinforcer at the incorrect time rewards the incorrect response.
- Relentless pressure habituates the horse to pressure, failing to respond.
- Excessive pressures can result in a fear response, associating everything in the environment to fear, including the handler. Inescapable or conflicting pressures can cause confusion and result in the horse demonstrating conflict behaviours, e.g. tension, buck, bolt, spin, rear.
- Indiscriminate reinforcement, such as food, may result in an increase in anticipation of food, increasing the likelihood of a biting, 'mugging' horse.

AGGRESSION

- When fearful behaviour is experienced regularly, horses may develop long-term, chronic behaviour disorders. These may show up as aggressive or defensive behaviours or as insecurities. Biting, kicking, striking and threatening may become habitual, reinforced by the understandable retreat of people during these attacks. Horses with these behaviours should be treated with caution and only by experienced handlers.
- Interestingly, there is a correlation between aggression and having a poor *stop* response. Horses that bite rarely step-back from a light aid and are typically heavy in their leading response. After thoroughly re-training stop responses – stop, step-back, park, and downward transitions both in-hand and under-saddle – light responses will emerge, rapidly improving biting behaviour.

CATCHING

Horse owners are used to the concept of 'catching' a horse, yet dog owners universally train dogs to approach on command. Training horses to do this is no more difficult. Even in a large field the unhandled or nervous horse can be difficult to catch, but using learning theory, this can be changed. If a horse runs away whenever you approach him, his escape is rewarded by his running. After a few repetitions of this behaviour, you become the trigger for running. The horse has learnt to remove something (you), resulting in not being caught.

Approach and retreat

The most effective method of catching applies learning theory – negative reinforcement. Many practitioners know it as 'advance-retreat'. Start in a small field/area for quicker learning, if possible, but it is also a successful catching process in a large field. Because your approach causes the horse to retreat, you must retreat before the horse does.

1. As you approach the critical flight distance and you begin to notice the first sign that the horse might turn and escape, you take a backward step. Very quickly the horse abandons attempting to escape.
2. Now you can take two quiet steps towards him, noticing if you had taken a third step he would have turned and gone. If, as you take the second step, he is about to move, step back.
3. Stand a moment, then take another two steps, then step back before he moves. Remember, horses will look away, turn away, then run away, so retreat (step back) at the first sign – the look away. If you take time and remain quiet you will find that you will soon make contact with the horse.
4. The horse will sniff you and when he does, quietly withdraw your hand before he withdraws his nose.
5. Put your hand out again and repeat. Take a lot of time over this.
6. Leave a small pile of food and walk away.
7. Return and repeat the whole process.
8. When you have made contact again, touch his neck and area just in front of his wither (this is a known reward site of heart rate lowering and relaxation), working up towards his cheek.
9. If you sense your horse will withdraw, you must withdraw before he does. In learning theory terms you are negatively reinforcing the horse's lack of reaction and gradual habituation.
10. Alternate many of these sessions with you exiting and leaving food.
11. The more sessions you do, the more habituated the horse becomes to you.
12. When you can get to the point of touching his body all over, start the shaping process to place a head collar.
13. Open the nose-strap, and gradually working up from the neck, place the head collar around the highest part of the neck, possibly at the poll depending on your progress, and fasten the head strap.
14. Fasten the nose strap.
15. Quietly train leading basic-attempt 'go' and 'stop'.

If the horse is very afraid of the human approach and touch, he will be skilled at removing your hand, and that is counter-productive.

1. In a small enclosure it is useful to use a 'false arm' as your hand (stick with a glove filled with straw). Touch the horse on his neck; as soon as he is immobile, remove the false arm.
2. Gradually run the false arm over his body, removing the arm for longer and longer periods of immobility.
3. Replace the false arm with your arm and scratch his withers.
4. Use secondary positive reinforcement (marker before the scratch or treat) and reward him for allowing you to touch in more places.

Tying up

All horses should be trained at an early age to stand obediently or in effect 'park' until you signal otherwise. This will assist handlers for all routine procedures.

Select a suitable ring, post or rail – this should be firmly attached and should not be part of anything that will bang, rattle or fall over if the horse pulls away.

- Always use a quick-release knot (Fig. 13.11). A piece of string can also be incorporated into the lead rope to allow easy breaking or untying if the horse falls over or pulls backwards. This will prevent head injuries but may develop into persistent halter breaking and escape.
- Never leave the horse unattended.
- If the horse learns that pulling back makes the lead pressure stop and/or results in freedom, friends or

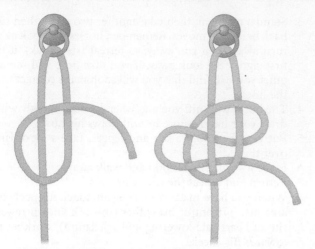

Fig. 13.11   A quick-release knot

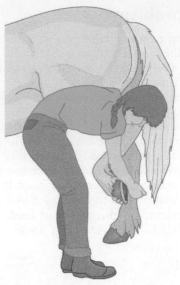

Fig. 13.12   Lifting a hind foot

forage, then pulling back from tying will be more likely in the future. You can re-train this unwanted behaviour by training to obedience-level stop, go and park responses.

Leading

- Horses are traditionally led from the left or near side but they should learn to respond to lead responses from both sides – it improves laterality and is useful when walking on the road towards oncoming traffic.
- If 'trotting up' to show a horse's paces or for the investigation of lameness, lead the horse away from the observer in a straight line for about 25 metres. Turn the horse around away from the handler, to reduce the risk of being trodden on, and walk past the observer. Repeat at a trot.
- For the purpose of diagnosing any gait abnormality the lead rope should be held in an open hand to allow free movement of the head, but you must be ready to apply pressure via the hand in a direction towards the tail to decelerate the horse's legs and do a downward transition; then repeat the exercise. Remember to use the go and stop signals to finish the trotting-up exercise.
- Young foals should be trained to lead correctly using negative reinforcement from a young age.

Picking up the feet

A horse should be trained to allow its feet to be picked up for daily cleaning, regular inspection and shoeing:
- Speak to the horse as you approach its shoulder.
- To lift a fore foot, stand facing the tail and run the hand closest to the body down over the elbow, back of knee and tendons until you reach the fetlock.
- Before squeezing with intermittent pressure at the fetlock use a verbal cue 'up'.
- As the horse lifts its foot up, catch the toe of the hoof and support it with your other hand. The horse should be encouraged to stand square, otherwise it may lean on you.
- Do not allow the horse to remove its foot away, as it will quickly learn how to train you to stop. You may also get injured if the limb comes down on your toe.

- To lift a hind foot (Fig. 13.12) run the same hand over the horse's back down the rump and back leg to the point of the hock.
- Move your hand over the anterior part of the cannon bone to the medial part of the fetlock.
- Before squeezing with intermittent pressure at the fetlock use the command 'up'. Do not release the pressure until the horse lifts its foot up.
- Foals should be trained early to get used to this procedure. Through repetition and correct use of negative reinforcement horses quickly associate the verbal cue with the pressure cue and soon lift their feet on your verbal cue.

Examination of the mouth

This may be necessary for examination of the teeth, for treatments such as tooth rasping and for determining a horse's age:
- Steady the nose with one hand and insert the other, palm downwards, into the diastema (space between the corner incisors and the first premolars).
- Grasp the tongue and gently pull it out sideways so that it is out of the way.
- In this position an oral medicine can be given; for tooth rasping it may be necessary to use a gag, which keeps the mouth open and leaves the hands free.

Use of the twitch

As the field of equitation science grows and the body of knowledge is continually expanding, embracing alternative practices to conventional methods of restraint, such as the use of the twitch, are now regularly and successfully employed by vets, nurses, owners and trainers. Instead of the twitch, which works by facilitating the release of natural endorphins by the brain, possibly causing an analgesic/anaesthetic effect, habituation techniques such as over-shadowing, counter-conditioning, approach conditioning and stimulus blending have proven as effective as, and more ethical than, the practice of twitching.

PERSONAL PROTECTIVE EQUIPMENT

It is important that personal protective equipment (PPE) is worn when handling horses. Those horses that are in discomfort or in unfamiliar surroundings can behave in an abnormal and unpredictable manner. Types of PPE include helmet (ASTM/SEI approved), correct safety shoes and body protection when riding. Gloves should be worn at all times when leading and handling horses. Difficult-to-handle horses can also be led out with a bridle rather than a head collar.

ASSESSING PAIN

Horses may not be able to say how much it hurts in words, but recent research is demonstrating that their face tells it all. Recognising pain and pain intensity in horses has been a challenge for veterinarians and anaesthetists, making it difficult to assess if horses are receiving appropriate pain relief. New research shows that, as with humans and other animals, certain facial expressions can indicate a horse is in pain, and that learning to recognise the signs is relatively easy and feasible for veterinary professionals and horse owners.

A team of researchers from Italy, Germany and the United Kingdom were first to publish a standardised pain scale based on facial expressions in horses, called the Horse Grimace Scale (HGS). Similar to the body condition scoring system, the HGS recommends scoring of different facial expressions to add up to a final pain intensity score. Researchers from Denmark and Sweden have followed up with a study suggesting that a pain face scale may not need to score all pain features separately. The study shows that it is possible to score a 'pain face' as a simple yes/no, and that the intensity of the expression may be sufficient and more applicable (Fig. 13.13). The researchers identified five key areas – ears, eyes, nostrils, muzzle and facial muscles – and showed that learning to recognise facial expressions of pain is feasible. After a 20-minute lesson, participants were able to successfully score a pain face (yes/no) and the pain intensity as 'low', 'medium' and 'high' with, on average, 82% accuracy.

It is vital that the veterinary nurse is able to recognise and assess the signs of pain in the horse. This is achieved by:

- **Observing body language** – a horse in pain, depending on severity of the pain, may be restless, be sweating, kick, stamp or bite at certain body areas, kick bedding around, grind their teeth and be vocal; horses can also become depressed, lose interest in their surroundings, hang their heads low and lose their appetite.
- **Measurement of clinical parameters** such as temperature, pulse and respiration.
- **Measurement of humoral factors** such as epinephrine (adrenaline), norepinephrine (noradrenaline), cortisol and endorphins in the blood can give an indication of the level of pain.

STEREOTYPICAL BEHAVIOUR

Is classed as a repetitive behaviour with no obvious goal or function and linked to suboptimal environments for animals:

- Inability to perform highly motivated behaviour patterns
- Inability to escape/avoid stressful situations
- Kept in confinement or social isolation
- Used as an indicator of poor welfare.

One study reported that 15% of all domesticated horses demonstrated stereotypical behaviour, with causes linked to boredom, stress, diet, housing, genetics, and a combination of genetics and management, strongly placing the spotlight on current housing practices and the uptake by individuals to recruit a coping strategy or sterotypy to manage an individual horse's environment. Comparing time budgets of feral and domesticated horses, findings demonstrate over a 10 km per day locomotion difference and increased forage intake while stabled horses exhibit long periods of standing. Undoubtedly this affects diet. Feral horses spend no more than 3–4 hours without feeding. This means the stomach almost always contains food and for that reason they constantly secrete gastric juice. When stabled, their natural feeding pattern is altered both in meal schedule and composition. Many times horses experience sustained fasting; when a 500-kg horse receives the last meal of 4 kg of hay at 6pm and is not fed until 8am the next day, with no other forage available, he will be fasting. When food is not available, the pH in the stomach becomes very low because the saliva's buffer is not present plus there is no food in the stomach. In particular, forage forms a virtual 'mat' between the mucosa and the acid and contributes to diluting the gastric juices. If your feeding schedule provides intermittent periods of food and quite long periods of fasting, the nonglandular mucosa is easily exposed to acid conditions. In comparison, in a horse with free choice of forage the stomach pH is higher, therefore lowering the amount of acid.

There are two types of stereotypical behaviour: oral and locomotive. Chewing, lip-licking, licking, wood chewing, cribbiting, wind-sucking, self-biting, head tossing/circling/shaking, and nodding are examples of oral stereotypies. Cribbing has been reported as early as 20 weeks with weaning typically between 16 and 24 weeks, suggesting possible links to a foal's motivation to suckle and/or dietary needs.

Risk factors of oral stereotypies

- Withdrawal of opportunities to suckle
- Breaking the mare-foal bond
- Altered feeding practices; feeding concentrate after weaning can induce a fourfold increase in rate of development of cribbing
- New social groupings
- Amount of human contact increased.

Interestingly, cribbing is not air being swallowed. The grunt stems from a rush of air into the cranial oesophagus (passage of turbulent air through the oesophageal sphincter, not the larynx). One theory is that the oesophageal distension is the source of gratification for the horse, or that cribbing stimulates the release of endorphins, therefore reinforcing the behaviour via reward mechanism. One certainty is that the behaviour of cribbing is a form of stress relief and is associated with a decrease in heart rate and changes in responsiveness to external stimuli, having a positive effect on affected horses. Cribbing, however, may cause colic, due to entrapment of the small intestines.

In a British study of cribbers, the stomachs of cribbing foals were significantly more ulcerated than non-cribbers, leading to the British hypothesising that cribbing is a consequence of stomach ulcers. Conversely, researchers in the USA hypothesise that horses crib, *causing* stomach ulcers. There is no evidence that horses can learn from observation, with lots of cribbers housed with non-cribbers, and that cribbers do not crib simultaneously.

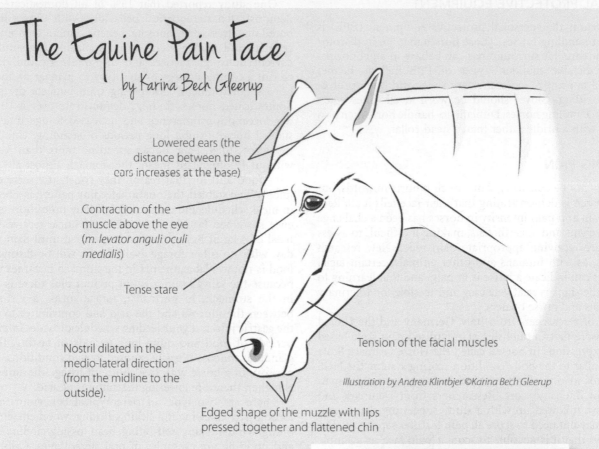

The Equine Pain Face
by Karina Bech Gleerup

Lowered ears (the distance between the ears increases at the base)

Contraction of the muscle above the eye (*m. levator anguli oculi medialis*)

Tense stare

Nostril dilated in the medio-lateral direction (from the midline to the outside).

Tension of the facial muscles

Illustration by Andrea Klintbjer ©Karina Bech Gleerup

Edged shape of the muzzle with lips pressed together and flattened chin

IMAGE ON RIGHT:

Can you spot the facial expressions of pain described in the illustration? This horse is in pain. (Photo courtesy Karina Bech Gleerup).

IMAGE BELOW LEFT:

The nostril dilated in the medio-lateral direction (from the midline to the outside) is one of the facial expressions of pain. (Photo courtesy Karina Bech Gleerup).

IMAGE BELOW RIGHT:

Can you spot the contraction of the muscle above the eye and the tense stare? This horse is in pain. Photo courtesy Karina Bech Gleerup).

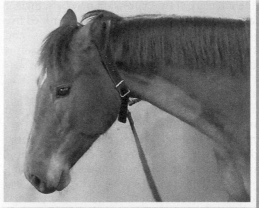

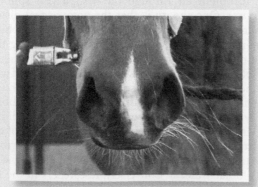

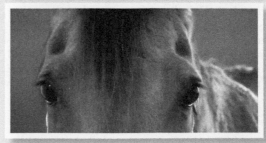

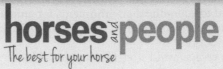

Fig. 13.13 Marketing poster demonstrating the 'Faces of Pain' (*Gleerup 2015.*)

Locomotor stereotypies include box-walking, weaving, pawing, tail-swishing, door/box kicking and rubbing self. The onset of weaving is 60 weeks of age and box-walking 64 weeks of age, placing the spotlight on both the motivation to move and social needs of the yearling. Risk factors of locomotor stereotypies include:

- Barrier frustration.
- Arousal.
  - Anticipatory behaviour
  - Feeding time
- Social interaction.
  - No visual and tactile contact
- Exercise routine.
- Stall walking with fast legs is a symptom of escape behaviour, or lack of it and separation anxiety, while slow-leg stall walking is a stereotypical behaviour. While weaving can be as a result of restricted social contact, both visually and tactile, stall kicking and pawing can have many causes: normal behaviour, learned, attention seeking, frustration, anticipation, impatience or aggression.

Research shows it is important when treating stereotypical behaviour to first make a diagnosis – do not just treat the symptom. Address the underlying causes, rule out medical causes and then find the motivation for the behaviour to consider any environmental and/or behaviour modification.

Identification and the use of horse passports

The Horse Passports (England) Regulations 2004 require all owners to obtain a passport for each horse they own. This includes ponies, donkeys, and other Equidae. Owners cannot sell, export, slaughter for human consumption, or use for the purposes of competition or breeding a horse which does not have a passport. Owners of foals must obtain a passport for each foal on or before 31 December of the year of its birth, or by 6 months after its birth, whichever is later. Passports can be issued from organisations authorised by DEFRA. Some organisations will issue passports for specific breeds of horses, while others will do it for any breed. Each horse is issued a Unique Equine Life Number (UELN) which will appear on the horse's passport and identifies it. The silhouette of the horse, used as a means of identification, must be completed by a veterinary surgeon or an approved representative of the Passport Issuing Organisation (PIO) approved by DEFRA. This is completed by the use of colour, breed and distinguishing features such as whorls, stars, leg markings, etc. Freeze marks can be noted on the silhouette.

Any medicines administered to the horse should be recorded in section IX of the passport for those animals intended for human consumption. Details of the medicines concerned are contained in the consolidated version of the Annexes I to IV of Council Regulation 2377/90. If the declaration that the horse is ultimately intended for human consumption is signed, the date when any medicines are administered that have substances not included in annexes I–IV of 2377/90 must be recorded on the section IX pages of the passport. This is to comply with the legislation relating to the withdrawal period of drugs within which a food-producing animal must not be slaughtered. Note: Annex IV drugs must never be administered to a food-producing animal.

Other forms of identification are possible and these include freeze marking, microchipping and tattooing. In all cases the owner's details are held on a database and it is important that these details are kept up to date. Freeze brands and tattoos can be easily altered and can fade over time, so microchipping is strongly recommended by veterinary surgeons. The microchip should adhere to the protocol set out by the International Organisation of Standards (ISO) so that the microchip can be read by all microchip readers.

Transportation of horses

Transportation can cause distress, leading to a loss of condition and even metabolic upset. Correct preparation of the animal prior to transportation is vital and can reduce stress levels. In the UK the Horserace Betting Levy Board issue guidelines on the transportation of horses. There are three legislative orders that govern the transportation:

- The Horse (Sea Transport) Order 1952 (amended in 1958)
- Transit of Animals (Road and Rail) Order 1975 (amended in 1979 and 1988)
- The Welfare of Animal Transit Order 1997; Transport of Horses came into force in July 1998.

Transportation out of the country is also included in the Horse Passports Regulations 2004.

These orders set out details of dimensions of transport vehicles, lengths of time in transport, rest periods and which animals can and cannot be transported, e.g. ill, unfit or pregnant mares may suffer unnecessary stress or harm. Transportation of pregnant mares should be avoided during the 20–45-day stage of gestation as during this stage there is a transfer from the yolk sac to chorioallantoic placentation and the risk of abortion increases.

When transporting horses over long distances it is important to seek veterinary advice and to have the horse's health checked prior to movement. Horses with respiratory disease should not be transported if possible. Clinical examination with the emphasis on subclinical respiratory problems should be done prior to lengthy trips. Horses transported in close proximity with little ventilation and dusty hay all predispose to respiratory problems such as 'shipping fever', the name given to respiratory disease linked to transportation. This manifests itself as depression and inappetence with the presence of a soft cough, shallow frequent respiration and a febrile response. Appropriate treatment can be effective but the condition may be life-threatening. The condition may be prevented by the use of dust- and mould-extracted hay and good ventilation. Horses should not to be tied up with their heads in an abnormally high position, as this can lead to commensal bacteria spreading to the lower respiratory tract.

Stress is an important factor in respiratory disease and in the welfare of the horse during transportation. Several factors should be taken into consideration to reduce stress while travelling:

- The number of animals being transported in one vehicle
- Provision of food and water
- Ambient temperature
- Ventilation
- Degree of movement, which is determined by the length of rope on the head collar; the horse must be able to

balance itself without undue effort and have enough room to urinate and defecate
- The presence of a stable mate or other companion
- Habituation to travelling.

Horses are sensitive to movement underfoot and are aware of the stability of the ground beneath them. This may help to explain why some horses are reluctant to cross bridges or traverse ramps and which may lead to an aversion to load for travelling. This may reflect increased arousal and/or anxiety levels or pain related to previous learning history during travelling, e.g. travelling too fast, poor balance or falling off the ramp during loading or unloading. A horse that does not load is simply a horse with poor lead responses. Go back to your in-hand training and deepen the go, stop and park responses. Take the time to train these responses anywhere and everywhere, including on and off ramps and into trailers and horseboxes.

TRAVEL BY ROAD

The method of transportation can have an effect on the horse:
- **Type of vehicle** – horseboxes, i.e. those with an integral cab, tend to be better ventilated and have more head and body room than trailers. They also provide a smoother journey than a trailer. Some horses prefer travelling facing backwards rather than forwards, or standing diagonally, as happens in a horsebox. Horses should not travel backwards in a trailer unless the correct modifications have taken place.
- **Ramps** – the incline of the ramp into the vehicle should be no greater than 25° and should provide secure footing.
- **Journey times** – may vary from an hour to a few days. The usual practice is for the horse to rest overnight in stables after every 24 hours of transportation. Long journeys create long periods when the horse is standing in one position. This can create muscle fatigue and associated myositis.
- **Ventilation** – poor ventilation can have a detrimental effect on the health of the horse. Exhaust fumes and fumes from excreta can affect the respiratory system, as can mouldy hay. It is advised that dust and mould particles be removed from hay prior to travelling. Exhaust fumes such as ammonia, carbon monoxide and nitrogen dioxide may disrupt the epithelial barrier between capillaries and alveoli in the lungs, which increases their permeability to bacteria. Also an altered rate of pulmonary aerosol clearance after travelling increases the bacterial numbers in the lower respiratory tract.

TRAVEL BY AIR

Transportation by air is becoming more common and utilises either an enclosed 'air stable' or an open-stall system. There are strict regulations concerning air travel. The ratio of personnel to horses should be one groom to every three horses, but this is not always possible because of the number of seats available on some aircraft. Most bloodstock shipping agencies arrange for an equine clinician to travel on long-haul flights. Air travel is expensive, so few horses are transported in this way. When travelling by air the horse should wear the same protective clothing as when travelling by road.

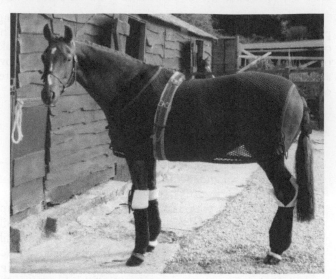

Fig. 13.14 Horse wearing protective leg wear, tail bandage, guard and sweat sheet ready for travelling. *(Image courtesy of Louise Moon.)*

CLOTHING FOR TRAVEL

The choice of travel clothing depends on the time of year and the weather on the day of travel, and no matter what the length of journey the protective clothing must always be of the same standard (Fig. 13.14). Protective leg bandages should always be worn. They may be either stable bandages with plenty of Gamgee padding or specially designed travelling boots, which must fit correctly and be non-slip. If the bandages do not cover or protect the knees and hocks, additional hock and knee boots must be worn. Over-reach boots can also add extra protection. A poll guard should also be worn to protect the head. The low headroom of the trailer or horsebox puts a head-shy or nervous horse at risk of injury. A tail bandage and tail guard will help protect the soft tissue in the tail and stops unsightly rubbing. It should be remembered that the horse will cool more quickly if it is moving and in a draughty environment and the horse that sweats while being transported may be anxious rather than hot. A combination of a sweat sheet and a warmer rug may be necessary.

TRANSPORTATION OF SICK OR INJURED HORSES

Sick and injured horses should not be transported unless authorised by a veterinary surgeon. If such a horse has to be transported it is still vital to provide protective clothing while it is travelling. Secondary injuries to any part of the body can be detrimental to the horse – if there is already an injury to one leg, a secondary injury to one of the supporting limbs may be disastrous. Additional stress to the animal should be prevented and care should be taken not to unbalance the horse.

In some cases transportation is unavoidable – e.g. disorders such as exertional rhabdomyolysis (tying up) require that the horse is not made to walk any distance at all as this exacerbates the condition, the degree of pain and muscle damage.

The transport should always be taken to the location of the horse; the horse should not be taken to the vehicle. If the ramp of the horsebox or trailer is steep, parking on a slope or in a loading bay can reduce the angle and benefit the horse. If support is required, straw bales can be used unless a modified ambulance is available.

All fractures should be immobilised and supported prior to transportation. If the horse has a fractured fore limb, travelling the horse backwards reduces the risk of it inadvertently putting weight on the fractured limb if the vehicle stops suddenly. If a hind limb is fractured, face the horse forwards. The head and neck should be left free to move and act as a counterbalance. There is great debate on the use of painkillers before moving and transporting horses that have fractures, and there is a belief that pain relief should not be given in order to discourage the horse from bearing weight on the fractured limb. A means of communication within the vehicle is important so that the handler can inform the driver of any problems. If an injured foal needs to be transported, two people can carry it or support it – one with hands around the neck and thorax and the other with hands around the abdomen and hindquarters. The mare should be allowed to remain close by.

Sedation for travelling should be avoided in all animals because the sedative creates problems with balance and thermoregulation, and when sedated the horse may overreact to certain stimuli, causing panic.

Use of equine ambulances

Equine ambulances attend most equine events and have been specially designed to cope with the types of emergencies that might happen there. The low ramp entrance is long to reduce the angle of incline into the ambulance. Internal partitions are easily positioned and moved around to allow access to different areas of the horse. Support can be provided from slings, and winches are available to drag unconscious patients into the ambulance.

TRAINING AIDS

There are many commonly used training aids – bits, reins, head collars, lunge reins, cavessons, etc. – yet with very little research in how the piece of equipment aids training a learnt behaviour as opposed to force. Any 'training aid' should provide a release of pressure if a horse is to learn the correct response. Constant or relentless pressure from training 'aids' or gadgets such as draw reins, side reins, etc. at best will deteriorate the horse's response to slow, stop and step back. At worst it will prompt active coping mechanisms such as rearing, bucking, bolting, spinning, or even spooking in an attempt to remove these pressures. If none of these behaviours actually remove the 'training aid' the horse is at risk from learning not to respond or switching off and dulling to all signals from the rider/handler. This behaviour is referred to as learned helplessness and results in symptoms of chronic stress – ulceration, suppressed immune system and self-mutilation. It is worth remembering an old adage: 'Only a good horseman should use a training aid. A good horseman never needs a training aid.'

Bits

There are several types of bit available and when choosing one it is important to remember that it must be:
- Of the correct length and thickness
- Properly fitted
- In good condition
- Mild in action to facilitate clarity of rider signals and rewards

- Permitted within the level or discipline at which you are competing.

Bits can be placed into 'families':
- **Snaffle** – considered to be one of the mildest bits but there are several different types and some can be very severe. A simple jointed snaffle has the action of flexing the poll and lower jaw and encourages the horse to raise its head. The bit acts on the tongue, on the outside of the bars of the mouth and on the lips or the corners of the mouth. Some snaffle mouthpieces have a nutcracker action on the tongue while other snaffles have double joints on the tongue – research has demonstrated that a double-jointed bit puts less pressure on the tongue, and therefore is milder than the nutcracker single-jointed snaffle. It is believed that the use of rings or keys can help stimulate saliva production, which may help to relax the jaw.
- **Double bridle** – combines a snaffle (Bradoon) with a curb bit (Weymouth) and chain (Fig. 13.15) and, in order to fit both bits into the mouth, both are finer and lighter than usual. The effect of the combination of bits is to add the action of the Weymouth, which has a lever action on the lower jaw. This leverage is dependent on the length of the cheeks of the bit and the curb chain. The curb bit should not be used without the Bradoon, with the same principles of negative reinforcement, releasing pressure for the correct learnt responses.
- **Pelham** – a single bit used with a curb chain (see Fig. 13.15). The bit is a combination of the curb and Bradoon in one mouthpiece. Two reins should be used so that the rider can facilitate the curb or snaffle action when required. Pelhams usually have an unjointed mouthpiece, which some horses prefer. It is commonplace to

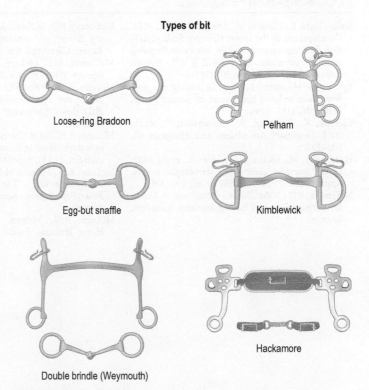

Types of bit

Loose-ring Bradoon

Pelham

Egg-but snaffle

Kimblewick

Double brindle (Weymouth)

Hackamore

Fig. 13.15 Types of bit

use leather rounders so that only one rein may be used. This can be an advantage for young riders but may act as a source of confusion to the horse.

- **Bitless bridle or Hackamore** – this bridle acts by exerting pressure on the nose and poll, which is achieved by the use of a single rein attached to long cheek pieces that create the required leverage. The Hackamore can be a useful means of regaining confidence in a horse that has suffered mouth injuries or biting problems in the past; however, it is severe and can cause a great deal of damage in the wrong hands.

Training aids, such as martingales, that have direct or indirect contact with the bit have recently been studied demonstrating the administration of small but constant pressures down the reins, at best habituating the horse to rein pressure and de-training the stop response.

Reins

The reins are the medium for a rider to apply pressure to the mouth and release it for the correct leg response. It is the rider who determines the intensity, duration and frequency of rein pressure and of course the speed of their reactions to release the pressure for the correct response to train desirable behaviours.

Head collars

The head collar is one of the most common ways of using pressure-release to train locomotion from a signal/aid by the horse. The head collar should fit well with different materials affecting how pressure is administered. Rope halters have a very thin surface area, applying pressure quickly over a smaller surface area than a webbed halter, dispersing pressure over a greater surface area and, it is believed, with less clarity for the horse when pressure is released.

Lunging and long-reining

Work from the ground includes lunging and long-reining and these training methods can be beneficial in the following situations:

- In the initial stages of training/breaking a young horse
- When the rider is injured and unable to ride
- When the horse cannot wear its normal tack, e.g. if it has a girth gall or a sore mouth
- In order to assess a problem that can be more easily seen from the ground, e.g. lameness.

When **lunging** the horse, the handler is positioned in the centre of the circle slightly behind the level of the horse's shoulder. The lunging cavesson should be worn with adequate padding to the noseband, providing protection to the delicate turbinate bones of the nose. Lunging is an opportunity to proof your in-hand training, testing your go and stop responses down the lunge line. Remember never to chase a horse – the act of chasing for most horses is arousing and could quickly place you at the centre of any arousal and/or fear. Remember that horses are associative learners, and if the practice of lunging becomes a fearful experience and you are associated to this practice (lunging), very quickly you will have trained your horse to express flight responses during the process of being lunged.

Long-reining provides an alternative to lunging and provides training for horses in the initial stages of breaking a horse to harness. Instead of a single rein, two reins are used and the handler is positioned behind the horse. The pressure of the reins against the side of the horse motivates the horse to accelerate.

RECOMMENDED READING

Dalla Costa, E., Minero, M., Lebelt, D., et al., 2014. Development of the Horse Grimace Scale (HGS) as a pain assessment tool in horses undergoing routine castration. PLoS ONE 9 (3), e92281. doi:10.1371/journal.pone.0092281.

Feh, C., de Mazieeres, J., 1993. Grooming at a preferred site reduces heart rates in horses. Anim. Behav. 46, 1191–1194.

Gleerup, K., Forkman, B., Lindegaard, C., et al., 2015. Veterinary Anaesthesia and Analgesia. 42, 103–114.

Hausberger, M., Muller, C., Gautier, E., et al., 2007. Lower learning abilities in stereotypic horses. Appl. Animal Behav. Sci. 107 (3–4), 299–306.

McGreevy, P.D., 2004. Equine Behaviour. A Guide for Veterinarians and Equine Students. Saunders, London.

McGreevy, P.D., McLean, A.N., 2007. Roles of learning theory and ethology in equitation. J. Vet. Behav.: Clin. Appl. Res. 2, 108–118.

McGreevy, P.D., McLean, A.N., 2010. Equitation Science. Wiley-Blackwell, Oxon, UK.

McLean, A.N., 2005. The mental processes of the horse and their consequences for training. PhD thesis. University of Melbourne, Victoria, Australia.

McLean, A.N., 2008. Overshadowing: a silver lining to a dark cloud in horse training. J. Appl. Anim Welf Sci. 11 (3), 236–248.

McLean, A.N., Mclean, M.M., 2002. Horse Training the McLean Way – The Science Behind the Art. Australian Equine Behaviour Centre, Victoria, Australia.

McLean, A.N., Mclean, M.M., 2008. Academic Horse Training. Equitation Science in Practice. Australian Equine Behaviour Centre, Victoria, Australia.

Mills, D., McDonell, S. (Eds.), 2005. The Domestic Horse. The Origin, Development and Management of Its Behaviour. Cambridge University Press, Cambridge, UK, pp. 23–32.

Mills, D.S., 1998. Applying learning theory to the management of the horse: the difference between getting it right and getting it wrong. Equine Vet. J. (Suppl. 27), 44–48.

Williams, J.L., Friend, T.H., Collins, M.N., et al., 2002. The effects of early training sessions on the reactions of foals at 1, 2 and 3 months of age. Appl. Animal Behav. Sci. 77, 105–114.

Williams, J.L., Friend, T.H., Collins, M.N., et al., 2003. Effects of imprint training procedure at birth on the reactions of foals at age six months. Equine Vet J. 35, 127–132.

Restraint, Handling and Administration of Medicines to Exotic Species

SHARON SMITH

KEY POINTS

- The exotic species commonly kept as companion animals do not appreciate excessive human contact or being handled and in many cases this may be a distressing experience that may affect their health. Handling should be avoided unless it is strictly necessary.

- For the welfare of the animal and the safety of the handler it is important that anyone dealing with these species is aware of the correct methods of handling and restraint.

- It is often important to determine the sex of an animal, e.g. to prevent or to encourage reproduction, prevent fighting, increase the value of the animal or simply to give the animal an appropriate name. There are different methods of sex determination that vary according to the species in question.

- An exotic animal under veterinary treatment is likely to need medicine. There are many routes of administration and the most appropriate methods depend on the species in care.

Introduction

In many practices it is no longer rare to be presented with an exotic animal requiring some form of veterinary care and nursing. The word 'exotic' may be taken to mean any animal that is 'out of the ordinary' and neither a cat nor a dog. The needs of these species vary widely and are certainly different from most of the patients in the kennels. It is therefore important for the welfare of the animal and your own safety that you understand a little about their biology (see Chapter 7), how they should be handled and how to give them the medicines prescribed by the veterinary surgeon.

Small mammals

Before handling any small mammal you must consider whether it is really necessary to handle the animal and, if you must do it, whether it is safe to do so. Ask yourself the following questions:

- Do you know how to handle this animal safely without doing harm to yourself or to the patient?
- Is the animal a well-handled, friendly pet or an aggressive one? Some ferrets can bite severely; chipmunks are fast and can harm themselves and you as they try to make a run for freedom.

- Is the animal debilitated in any way and is there any indication of respiratory distress? For example, in rats a nasal discharge may be shown by the presence of dried discharge on the forearms; rabbits with pneumonia may have a nasal discharge and dyspnoea. Always observe the patient quietly before handling and if you are in any doubt it is best not to handle it. Any excessive or rough handling could be fatal.
- Is there any reason to suspect metabolic bone disease? Has the animal got any fractures or a past history of having had one? Are their any signs of poor growth? What is the animal being fed? Is the diet lacking in calcium or vitamin D? This mainly occurs in young animals – often rabbits and sometimes guinea pigs.

Once you have decided that the animal must be handled you must consider the method of restraint – manual restraint is preferable but chemical restraint is occasionally necessary. Before removing any animal from its cage select a room that contains few objects behind which the animal can hide if it escapes and ensure that all doors and windows are closed.

RATS AND MICE

Rats and mice only have one means of defence and that is their teeth. Most of them are easily handled and not very aggressive but they can give nasty nips if handled roughly or incorrectly:

- Mice tend to bite if worried, stressed or handled by an unfamiliar person. The best way of handling a mouse is to grasp it firmly by the base of the tail, lift it up carefully and then place it on to a non-slip table (Fig. 14.1). Once it is on the table you should grasp the scruff at the back of the neck firmly between the thumb and forefinger. You now have the mouse securely restrained for examination or for administration of any medication.
- Rats tend not to bite unless roughly handled. The easiest way to pick up a tame rat is by picking it up around the middle with one hand just behind the front legs and putting the other hand underneath its bottom to support its weight (Fig. 14.2). If you have an unfriendly or aggressive rat then the safest way to handle it is in much the same way as the mouse. Grasp it by the base of the tail, lift it on to a non-slip table and then scruff it by the back of the neck with your thumb and forefinger.

A very important point to remember is that you should never grasp any mouse or rat by the end of the tail as the skin will slough off and cause severe damage, resulting in amputation of the tail.

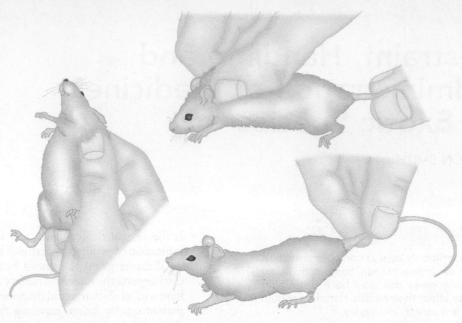

Fig. 14.1 Restraining a mouse

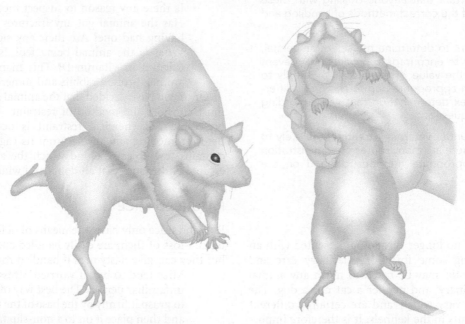

Fig. 14.2 Restraining a rat

Sex determination

The most common method of determining the sex of all small mammals is by measuring the anogenital distance, i.e. the distance between the anus and the tip of the penis in the male and between the anus and the vulva in the female (Fig. 14.3). There may also be other methods (Table 14.1).

HAMSTERS

Hamsters only have one means of defence and that is their teeth – they can give a very nasty nip.

The larger Syrian hamsters tend to be less aggressive than the smaller Russian and Chinese dwarf hamsters, who are known for having short tempers. These animals are nocturnal and do not take kindly to be woken up and handled during the day, especially by a stranger. For minor examinations or to move a friendly hamster, simply cup your hands around the animal and lift it up. For a more detailed examination or for an aggressive hamster firmly scruff it at the back of the neck, ensuring that you grasp a lot of scruff between your thumb and forefinger – if you do not take enough scruff the hamster will still be able to turn around and bite you. Make sure the scruff is pulled cranially to avoid pulling it too tight around the eyes as hamsters are prone to prolapse if roughly handled. If you have an extremely aggressive hamster that you just cannot get a hold of then scoop it up into a clear plastic box, which will enable you to see if there is anything obviously wrong. If a more detailed examination is required then a gaseous anaesthetic via an induction chamber may be necessary.

GERBILS

Gerbils are fairly docile animals, easy to handle if socialised well and will only bite if frightened or stressed by rough handling. They move fast and are very good jumpers – if they get worried they will escape by jumping away. To transport gerbils from one place to another, cup them in both hands underneath their bodies and gently lift them up. If a detailed examination is required or you have an aggressive animal then firmly but gently grasp the scruff between your thumb and forefinger, lift the animal up and support it underneath with your other hand and place it on a non-slip table for examination.

Never pick up a gerbil by the tail as it will slough the skin very easily, leaving only the vertebrae showing – known as a degloving injury. This will never regrow and would have to be amputated.

CHIPMUNKS

Chipmunks are very highly strung, fast-moving creatures that can leap extremely high to escape, so great care must be taken when handling them. Unless the chipmunk is correctly handled you are likely to be bitten. If you are lucky you may be able to grasp the scruff between the thumb and forefinger. If really well handled you may be able to cup a chipmunk in both hands and lift it out of the cage and then gently scruff it. If the chipmunk is in a large enclosure then the best way to catch it is by using a fine net. This is the safest way and will allow you to transfer it to a towel or restrain it on a non-slip table for examination. If manual restraint is not possible, gaseous anaesthesia via an induction chamber may be necessary. This is sometimes better for your safety and for that of your patient.

It is very important to remember that you should never approach a small mammal from above. To the animal your hands are like a bird of prey swooping down on them, which can make them very frightened, especially as they will already be worried by the strange environment. Always try to approach them from the side and at a low level.

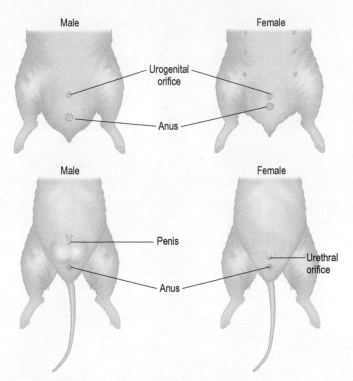

Fig. 14.3   General method of sexing small rodents

TABLE 14.1	Methods of sexing small mammals	

Species	Method of sexing
Rat	Examine the anogenital distance – it is longer in the male than in the female. Testes are large and obvious in adult males. Teats are present only in the female.
Mice	Examine the anogenital distance – it is longer in the male than in the female. Testes are large and obvious in adult males. Teats are present only in the female.
Hamster	Examine the anogenital distance – it is longer in the male than in the female. Large testes in the adult male make the hind end cone-shaped; in the female the hind end is rounded. Adult males have a pigmented scent gland on the point of each hip. Teats are present only in the female.
Gerbil	Examine the anogenital distance – it is longer in the male than in the female. Adult males have a scent gland on the ventral abdomen. Teats are present only in the female.
Chipmunk	Examine the anogenital distance – it is longer in the male than in the female. Testes are retracted during the non-breeding season and descend into the scrotum and enlarge at the start of the breeding season in February/March. Penis is visible and points caudally. Teats are present only in the female.
Guinea pig	Anogenital distance is less easy to measure. Gentle pressure placed on either side of the prepuce of the male will cause the penis to elongate. Testes are large. Female has a Y-shaped genital opening and a pale-coloured clitoris. Both sexes have a pair of elongated teats in the inguinal region.
Chinchilla	Female has a large urinary papilla, which you may mistake for the male's penis. She also has separate exits to the urinary and reproductive tracts, unlike most other small mammals. The male's penis resembles the female's urinary papilla, although it is larger and tends to point cranially. Pressure applied on either side of the prepuce may cause it to elongate. Both males and females have teats – one inguinal pair and two pairs of lateral thoracic teats.
Rabbit	Apply pressure on either side of the anal area to pop out the vulva or penis. The vulva is round, has a small slit in the middle and tends to point cranially. The penis is more cone-shaped and tends to point caudally. Adult males have large, obvious testes.
Ferret	The male has a very obvious prepuce on the ventral abdomen and large testes in the scrotum unless he has been castrated. The female has a vulval opening situated ventral to the anus.

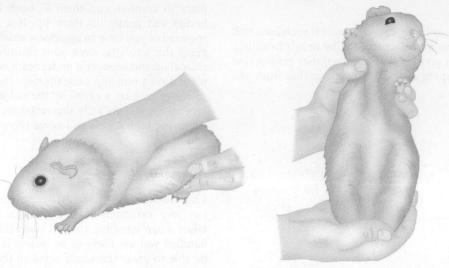

Fig. 14.4   Restraining a guinea pig

GUINEA PIGS

Guinea pigs are very sensitive creatures and do not like being away from their natural surroundings or from their companions. To reduce their stress it is helpful to dim the light and reduce the noise. To aid in their capture it is less stressful to catch them in a small box rather than chasing them around a large enclosure. The easiest method of restraint is to gently grasp them from behind under the front legs with one hand and with the other hand support the weight of the animal (Fig. 14.4). It is very important to support the guinea pig's weight as it has a rather large abdomen and a slender spine and surrounding bones and if there is not enough support spinal damage can occur.

CHINCHILLAS

Chinchillas are very timid and sensitive creatures that rarely bite. They are also easily stressed, so dimming the lights and reducing the noise is helpful when handling them. You must be very careful not to scruff or roughly handle them as a condition known as fur slip can occur in which clumps of fur fall out around the area being held, leaving a bald patch, which takes a few weeks to regrow. If a chinchilla is very stressed it will stand on its back legs and squirt urine at you – they have a very good aim. The best and safest way to handle a chinchilla is by quickly and gently picking it up, putting one hand around the body just under the front legs and the other hand to support the body weight. For young chinchillas, which are more wriggly than well-handled adults, it is sometimes easier to restrain them by using your fore and middle finger around either side of the head and your thumb and fourth finger under the front legs and then with your other hand support the body. You should also remember that they have powerful back legs, so you should always make sure you have a good grip of them.

RABBITS

Most domestic rabbits are very easy to handle and rarely cause injuries unless stressed or roughly handled. They are capable of using their teeth and claws, with which they can inflict deep

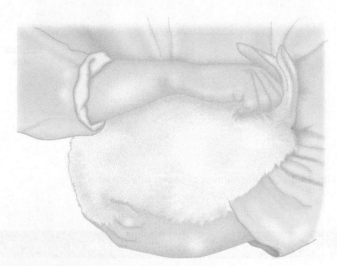

Fig. 14.5   Carrying a rabbit with the head tucked under your arm

scratches, and their back legs, which are very powerful. Some rabbits can be aggressive, especially males around the breeding season in the spring. Reducing the light and noise can help to reduce stress.

To handle a friendly rabbit it is best to pick the rabbit up by placing one hand under the thorax and using the first three fingers to gently grip the front legs by placing one finger either side and one in the middle. Using your other hand, you support the rabbit's weight. If you need to move the rabbit from one place to another, you can support the rabbit on one arm and place the rabbit's head under your arm (Fig. 14.5). Being in the dark under your arm or even covered in a towel or blanket will calm the animal. Ensure that you have a good grip, as a sudden noise can spook the rabbit and it may try and escape. You should quickly move it onto a non-slip table, as it may struggle. Never pick a rabbit up by the ears, or scruff a rabbit.

For examination it is sometimes useful to reduce the stress of examination by wrapping the animal up in a towel with the head sticking out (Fig. 14.6). It is important to remember that a struggling anxious rabbit may harm you and also harm itself.

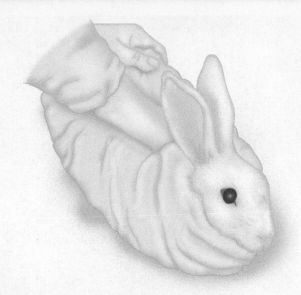

Fig. 14.6 Restraining a rabbit using a towel

Rabbits have very powerful back legs and if not properly restrained they can kick out and twist to get away, which can fracture or dislocate their spines. Another thing to remember is that severe stress can cause a cardiac arrest.

FERRETS

Some well-handled pet ferrets can be very friendly but others can be aggressive and fast, especially if not handled regularly. Working ferrets used for rabbit hunting and ratting are often not handled very much and can be aggressive. Ferrets have claws and teeth as sharp as those of a cat.

The easiest way to handle tame ferrets is to hold them from behind with one hand around the body under the front legs and support the body's weight with the other hand. The best way to restrain more aggressive ferrets is to firmly grasp the scruff behind the neck and pull them upwards. Then with the other hand, support the body by putting it around the pelvic area. It is sometimes useful to wear gauntlets for handling very aggressive ferrets.

Birds

Before handling any type of bird you must consider whether it is really necessary. Birds do not appreciate being handled in the way that dogs and cats do and some species may hurt you if handled incorrectly. Ask yourself the following:

- Is the bird a well-handled pet or is it a wild bird of prey or waterfowl?
- Do you know how to handle this bird safely without causing harm to you or the bird?
- Does the bird have any signs of respiratory distress that could be made much worse by restraint?
- Do you really need to handle the bird or can you just look at it through the cage to make decisions about its condition and its treatment?
- Does the bird require oral or injectable medication or could this be given in food or drinking water?

To perform a physical examination or to administer treatment, the bird will have to be restrained in some way. Before

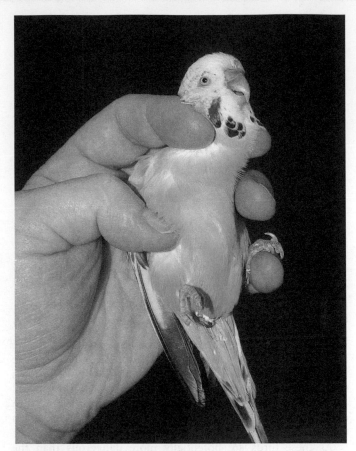

Fig. 14.7 Restraining a budgerigar

catching a bird always make sure all windows and doors are closed and that there is a warning sign on the door in case someone enters the room, allowing the bird to escape. There is nothing worse than having to tell an owner that you have lost their pet.

SMALL CAGED BIRDS, E.G. CANARIES, BUDGERIGARS AND FINCHES

These small birds cannot do much harm but they do have sharp little beaks and sharp claws, which you will need to avoid when examining them. Small birds may become stressed even if they are used to handling; to reduce this, dim the lights and reduce the noise. If the bird comes in its own cage with all its toys, remove them before trying to capture the bird – there is nothing worse than trying to avoid obstacles while chasing it around the cage.

To catch the bird, use a small facecloth or something similar to provide a greater surface area than your hand. It is also a protective layer between you and the bird to prevent you from being bitten. Once you have captured the bird, hold it very gently. Birds have no diaphragm and they rely on the outward movement of their ribcage for inspiration. If you grip too tight it can be fatal, especially if they are suffering from a respiratory disease. To examine the bird, hold it in the palm of your hand wrapped loosely in a cloth with its head out, placing your thumb under its beak to prevent it pecking you. It may help to allow the bird to grip your little finger, as these are perching birds and this may make them feel more secure. Unwrap small parts at a time for examination (Fig. 14.7).

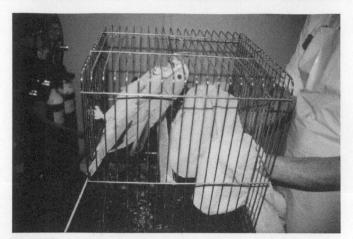

Fig. 14.8 Catching a small parrot with the aid of a towel

LARGE CAGED BIRDS, E.G. COCKATIELS, COCKATOOS AND PARROTS

The larger caged birds have powerful hooked beaks and can give a very nasty bite. They can become distressed, so dimming the light and reducing the noise will reduce this. Remove any toys or accessories from the cage to allow easier and less stressful capture. The use of a towel or small blanket will enable you to catch the larger birds, remembering not to hold them too tightly, as this can be fatal (Fig. 14.8).

As these birds are potentially more dangerous than the smaller birds, you must ensure that you grasp the bird carefully and quickly from the back. Once you have the bird out of the cage, restrain the head as this is the part that can cause you most damage. Wrap the bird gently in the towel with your thumb and forefinger positioned under the lower beak. This will enable you to push the beak upwards to prevent the bird from biting you. Once you have the bird in this position, ensure that the wings are securely restrained in the towel. If the bird is able to struggle and flap its wings there is a risk of it breaking its wings or damaging its plumage.

Once adequately restrained, unwrap parts of the body one at a time for examination. Handling aggressive parrots and cockatoos may require extra protection – leather gauntlets come in very handy. However, it is often difficult to feel much through them so you must be careful not to squeeze the bird too tightly. Once you have the bird restrained satisfactorily, remove the gloves to prevent any harm to the bird.

BIRDS OF PREY

Birds of prey can be broadly divided into the nocturnal species, i.e. owls, and the diurnal species, e.g. falcons, hawks and eagles. These birds have extremely sharp talons and powerful beaks, both of which can be very dangerous when handling them. The method of handling differs with each type.

Diurnal species, e.g. falcons

Most handled falcons will come in wearing a leather cap or hood, which fits over the bird's head (Fig. 14.9) covering the bird's eyes but leaving its beak exposed. This calms the bird and helps to reduce stress. These birds also have a very good sense of hearing, so reducing the noise in the room reduces the stress.

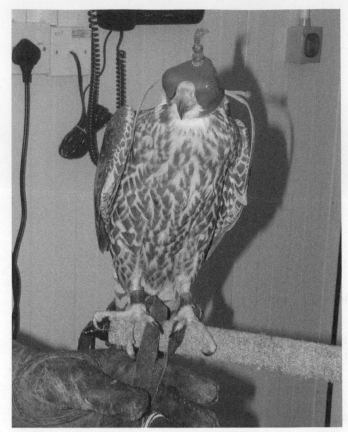

Fig. 14.9 A falcon wearing a hood and jesses – note the handler's leather gauntlets

Most falcons will also be presented wearing leather straps or jesses around their ankles, which enable them to be restrained while on their owner's arm (see Fig. 14.9). When restraining these birds, wear a leather gauntlet because it is extremely painful if they grip your arm without one.

If the bird has been transported in a box there are several ways to remove it:

- Ask the owner to remove the bird from the box, as it will respond to them better.
- If you are removing the bird yourself, place your gauntleted hand into the box beside the perch if it has one or beside the bird, grasp the leather straps with your thumb and forefinger and encourage the bird to step on to the glove. You must keep hold of the strap at all times. You can now remove the bird from the box and put the hood on if it is not already on. You should now be able to examine the bird safely. You must make sure that you always keep your arm up above the elbow, as otherwise the bird will attempt to climb up towards your shoulder, which can be painful.
- If the bird has no leg straps or hood and is not well-handled then you must take a different approach. Dim the lights and reduce the noise before you start. Some birds may be trained to perch on your hand and you may be able to encourage it to do this. If not you will have to grasp the bird from behind with a thick towel or blanket. Always make sure you know where the bird's head is. You must then grasp the bird over the shoulder

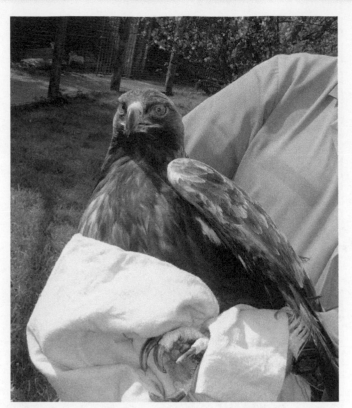

Fig. 14.10 A golden eagle with its talons wrapped in a towel to prevent damage to the handler

area facing towards you and place your thumbs under its beak to push it up out of the way. You can then place a hood on the bird's head if you have one. It is best to put the bird on your gauntleted arm, as gripping on to something makes it feel more secure.

When examining these birds it is sometimes necessary to hold their feet out of the way as they may try to grasp one foot, with the other causing puncture wounds and leading to serious infections (Fig. 14.10). This method really requires two people – one to hold the bird from behind, restraining the wings and body, and one to hold the legs from behind and away from the examiner.

Nocturnal species – owls

The overall technique is much the same but, as they are nocturnal, dimming the lights and wearing a hood has no real effect. Reducing noise will help reduce the stress. Owls have sharp talons but their beaks are not as large as those of falcons; however, they can still inflict a serious bite.

WATERFOWL

Most waterfowl are wild but you may encounter a few 'tame' ones that are kept on ponds in farms or parks. Most waterfowl are rarely handled.

Small waterfowl, e.g. various species of duck

Restraining these birds is fairly easy as they are moderately small and have blunt-ended beaks. Grasp the duck from behind by the neck, ensuring that your thumb is securing the back of the neck while your other fingers are gently curled around

the front of its neck. Make sure that you support the neck, as there is a weak area at the atlantooccipital joint. Control the wings as soon as you can by wrapping the bird in a towel and then tucking it under your arm, holding it close to your body. This position allows you to carry the bird safely. Examine one side at a time, keeping the other side restrained in the towel.

Large waterfowl, e.g. geese and swans

These species have large, powerful wings and can also be quite vicious with their beaks. The method of restraint is similar to that used for smaller birds. Restrain the head first, making sure that you support the neck, which may be difficult as they have long strong necks. The use of a swan hook or something similar may be useful. This is a pole with a smooth round hook that enables you to hook the neck of the swan or goose under the beak and gently pull it towards you to a point from which you can grasp its neck. Two people may be needed to restrain the bigger birds – one to control the head and one to control the large, powerful wings. Swan bags are available for restraining swans.

If any type of bird breaks free and tries to escape, dim the lights (unless it's an owl) and ensure that all exits are covered to prevent anyone from opening a door:

- Larger birds – throw a towel or blanket over it and wrap the bird up
- Very small birds – use a soft net, a small cloth or a light towel.

Always remember to be as gentle as possible and avoid restricting the bird's breathing whatever its size.

SEX DETERMINATION

Sexing birds can be difficult and there are several ways in which it can be done:

- **Sexual dimorphism** – the male's appearance is different from that of the female. Males tend to have much more colourful feathers; for example, in the mallard duck the male is a wonderful green colour and the female is a plain brown. In most budgerigars the adult male has a blue cere over the beak and the female has a brown one. Male cockatiels have bright orange cheek patches and have a solid colour underneath their tails. Females have paler orange cheek patches and horizontal dark stripes under their tails. Most female birds of prey are slightly larger than the males and are less coloured.
- **Examination of the pelvis** – requires experience. The pelvic bones of the female are wider than those of the male to allow eggs to pass through.
- **Endoscopic examination of the gonads** – the gonads, i.e. ovary and testis, of the bird are internal (see Chapter 7). Under a general anaesthetic a rigid endoscope is passed through a small incision into the body cavity to examine the gonads and thus identify the sex. This can be a dangerous and invasive procedure.
- **DNA sexing** – used for parrots and cockatoos, as, in many species it is impossible to determine the sex externally. A blood sample or pulp from a freshly plucked feather is collected and sent to a laboratory where the DNA from the tissue is used to examine the chromosomes of the bird.

Reptiles

Before handling any reptile you must ask yourself whether it is necessary to handle this reptile, whether it is safe to do so and whether you know what to do. Consider the following:

- Is the reptile a well-handled pet or is it aggressive, or even poisonous? For example, rock pythons, Tokay geckos and some green iguanas are aggressive; adders, cobras and Gila monsters are poisonous. If you are working with reptiles it is important to be able to recognise the poisonous species.
- Do you know how to handle this animal safely to prevent harm to you or your patient?
- Is the animal in any kind of respiratory distress? Is the animal mouth-breathing or is there mucus around the mouth, which may indicate that there is a problem?
- Is the reptile very delicate? Some of the members of the gecko family are very small and fragile and if stressed or handled roughly can shed their tails. Some of them are so small that handling is really not advised.
- Is the animal suffering from metabolic bone disease? Many lizards have this as a result of incorrect husbandry and if you are in any doubt, assume that they do have problems. Their bones can be very fragile and fracture easily, so care must be taken when handling them.

If the reptile must be examined or treated, then some form of restraint will be necessary.

Reptiles can be divided into:
- Lizards
- Snakes
- Tortoises and terrapins.

LIZARDS

The risk involved in handling lizards varies according to their species:

- Small lizards use their teeth for defence and can give a nasty nip if stressed or roughly handled.
- Larger lizards have teeth and claws and some of them have long powerful tails, which they use like a whip and which can be very painful. Some species, e.g. the green iguana, can be very aggressive: they have sharp claws, a long tail and sharp teeth, which can all cause damage. Male iguanas are more aggressive to women during certain phases of the menstrual cycle because they can detect human female pheromones, which are similar to the ones secreted by female iguanas during the breeding season.

Even if you are very experienced, handling any species of lizard can be difficult:

- **Tiny lizards**, e.g. anoles or some geckos, are not recommended for handling as they are very fast and very delicate; it is easier to place them in a clear plastic box and examine them by observation.
- **Small lizards**, e.g. leopard gecko. Grasp them from behind around the shoulder area with the thumb and forefinger and the other three fingers around the body. If the lizard is larger than your hand, gently support the back legs with your other hand to prevent them from wriggling.
- **Large lizards**, e.g. green iguana, water dragon. Restrain by grasping the lizard from behind the shoulders

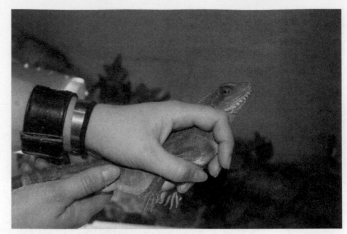

Fig. 14.11 Restraint of a water dragon

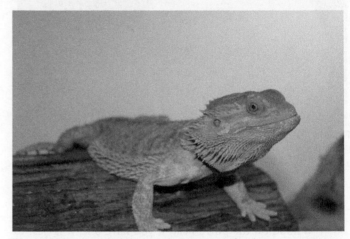

Fig. 14.12 A bearded dragon showing its spiky skin

(Fig. 14.11). With your thumb and forefinger, control one leg and use the middle and fourth finger to control the other leg. Using the other hand, grasp around the pelvic girdle from behind and use your thumb and forefinger to control one leg and your middle and fourth finger to control the other leg. Avoid holding the lizard too tight, as if it wriggles, this can cause spinal damage. If you have to move the animal, wrap it in a towel with its legs lying down by its sides. Then restrain the head and tuck the body and tail under your arm to prevent damage from the tail.

- **Spiky lizards**, e.g. bearded dragons (Fig. 14.12). If you restrain spiky lizards as described above, you will only injure yourself. Hold the lizard's back against your body with your hand held flat against the underside and under the front legs and gently restrain the head. The other hand restrains the tail and hind legs. Another method is to wrap the lizard in a towel, but this does not allow easy access for examination. It may be possible to get your fingers behind the spiky area on the head where there is a soft fleshy part and then restrain the lizard on its back – this may not be easy to do if the patient is wriggly or aggressive (Fig. 14.13).

The vasovagal reflex is useful for putting any lizard into a form of trance and may be used as a means of restraint for procedures such as radiography. This is done by putting firm but gentle digital pressure on both eyeballs, which stimulates the parasympathetic branch of the autonomic nervous system, resulting in a drop in heart rate, respiratory rate and blood pressure. This effect can last for 1–2 min if everything is quiet. The only problem is that any sudden noise will wake the lizard up and it will run off the table and escape. A useful tip is using two cotton wool balls and, placing them over the eyelids, bandage them firmly but gently in place. This is used instead of your fingers and keeps a constant pressure over the eyes for a prolonged effect. Sometimes putting lizards gently on to their backs will calm them and make restraint for examinations much easier (Fig. 14.14).

Another means of restraint for radiography is to bandage the front legs of the lizard gently along the body and the back legs along the tail. This enables you to get a clear image and keeps your patient still without you having to restrain it. This should not be done if you suspect any limb or rib fractures.

When restraining lizards it is very important not to grasp them by the tail as they can shed their tails – a process known as autotomy. Some species will also do this if they are really distressed or roughly handled. In most cases the tail will grow back but it will never look as good as the original and there are some species of lizard whose tail will not grow back, so you must be careful. Iguanas will not regrow their tails after the age of 3–4 years.

Sex determination

This is reasonably easy to do in a sexually mature adult but cannot easily be done in a younger reptile. Look for evidence of pores in the inguinal area of the lizard (Fig. 14.15):

- Male – obvious pores, i.e. anal, preanal and femoral pores that vary according to the species. In some species there may also be hemipenal bulges below the entrance to the cloaca. For example, the green iguana has femoral pores and hemipenal bulges; the leopard gecko has preanal pores and hemipenal bulges. Males are often slightly larger and have more body appendages, e.g. the male chameleon has horns.
- Female – very faint pores but no hemipenal bulges.

SNAKES

Most snakes are fairly docile if regularly handled but there are some species that are naturally aggressive, e.g. the rock python and the anaconda. Their main means of defence are their teeth

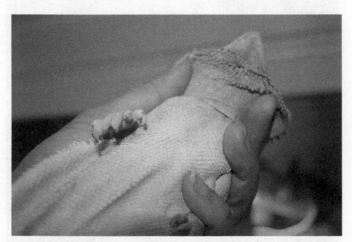

Fig. 14.13 Restraint of a bearded dragon

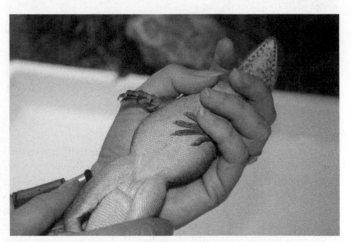

Fig. 14.14 Restraining a water dragon on its back

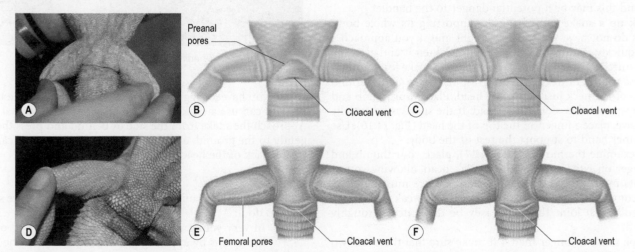

Fig. 14.15 Sexual differentiation in the lizard. (A, B, E) Male bearded dragon showing femoral pores. (D, C, F) Female bearded dragon showing lack of pores

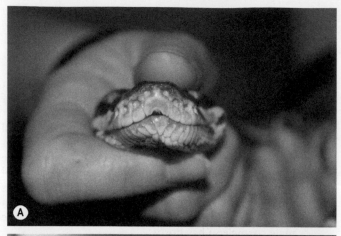

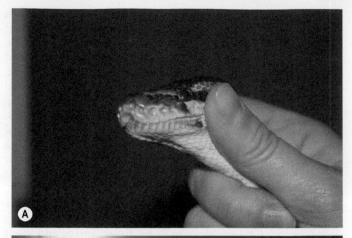

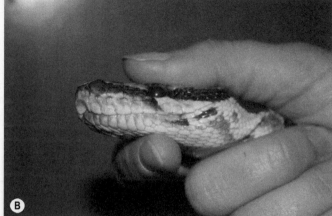

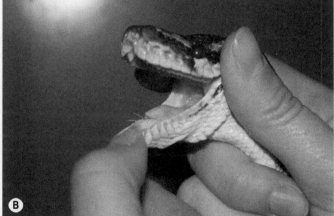

Fig. 14.16 (A, B) Restraining the head of the snake

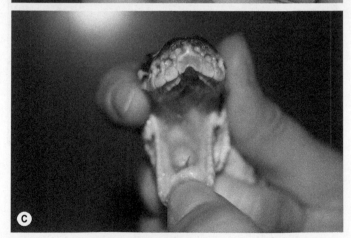

Fig. 14.17 (A–C) Opening the mouth of the snake

and the larger snakes can give a nasty bite. The teeth are curved and embed themselves in your skin – if you pull away you are likely to pull a large piece of skin off your finger or thumb. The best way to remove the teeth from your skin is by using a wooden spatula or credit card and pushing it between your skin and the teeth. Do not put the snake's head under water to make it let go – snakes can hold their breath for a very long time because they have air sacs at the end of their lungs that act as reservoirs. Some of the larger boas and pythons kill by constriction, and this may be a potential danger to the handler.

Pick up a snake from behind, supporting its whole body. Snakes do not have very good eyesight and if you approach a snake quickly from the front you will frighten it and even the best-natured snake may bite. To restrain the snake for examination, use your last three fingers to grasp the snake gently around the top of the neck just below the head. Place your thumb and forefinger on either side of the head. If the snake is potentially aggressive, place a finger on the top of the head (Fig. 14.16). Use your other hand to support the rest of the body.

To examine the mouth (Fig. 14.17), place your thumb and forefinger on either side of the snake's head, allowing you to open its mouth using a wooden spatula. Care must be taken when controlling snakes' heads, as they have a weak point at the atlantooccipital joint that can easily be dislocated if roughly handled.

If the snake is longer than 4 ft make sure that there are two people to handle it. Most snakes that are not poisonous are constrictors and they could squeeze a limb or even asphyxiate

you. If you have an aggressive snake that you are unable to pick up, you can use a snake hook, which is a smooth metal hook. Approach the snake from the side or behind and press the head gently to the ground, allowing you to grasp the snake carefully by the back of the head.

Sex determination

It is not easy to determine the sex of snake, but there are several ways to do it:

- In very young snakes you can sometimes pop out the hemipenis by applying gentle pressure from the tail to the cloaca. In a male the hemipenis should pop out but not in the female. This method requires experience.

- Measure the tail length by counting the scales between the cloaca and the end of the tail. In a male the distance from the cloaca to the tip of the tail is greater than in a female.
- Use of a snake-sexing probe – this is the most accurate method (Fig. 14.18). Lift the cloacal scale and insert the small, round-ended probe down inside the tail into the hemipenis of the male or the vaginal sac of the female. If you do not have a probe you can use a Jackson's urinary cat catheter (always remove the metal stylet). In the male the probe will go down a distance of about 8–16 subcaudal scales and in the female it will only go down about 2–5 subcaudal scales. Make sure that you lubricate the probe well before use and that you do not push the probe too hard, as you can perforate the vaginal sac.

TORTOISES AND TERRAPINS

Most tortoises are harmless but some of the terrapins and turtles can be aggressive and give a nasty nip with their sharp beak, e.g. snapping turtles, soft-shelled turtles and even red-eared terrapins. Terrapins also have sharp claws.

Restraint is usually fairly easy and is achieved by holding the shell on either side just behind the front legs (Fig. 14.19) which prevents the head and claws from causing damage. If a more detailed examination is required, the animal is likely to withdraw its head and legs into its shell. In some of the smaller species of mediterranean tortoise you may be able to pull the head and legs out gently. In larger species, especially the leopard tortoise, it is virtually impossible to get the head and legs to come out if the tortoise does not want to do it. Sedation may be necessary for a proper examination. If the animal is one of the more aggressive species, e.g. the snapping and soft-shelled turtles, holding any part of the shell is likely to result in you being bitten because these species have very long necks and they can reach right round to the back of their shell. You may be able to get them to snap at a piece of wood or cloth and then grasp the head, which is the dangerous part.

Note: You must wash your hands after handling reptiles, as they can carry zoonotic *Salmonella*, which occur naturally in their gut flora but are also found all over the reptile's body.

Sex determination

Sexing tortoises and terrapins is quite easy (Fig. 14.20):
- Males – have a longer tail, which is wider at the base, and the cloaca is further away from the plastron
- Females – have a short tail and the cloaca is closer to the plastron
- Some species of male terrapin, e.g. red-eared terrapin, have longer front claws than are seen in the female
- In some species of tortoise, e.g. leopard tortoise, the male has a concave plastron and the female has a flat plastron.

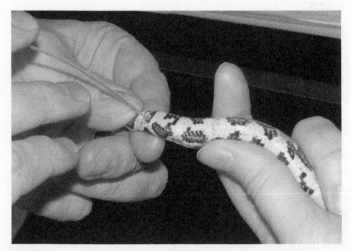

Fig. 14.18 Use of a probe to determine the sex of a snake

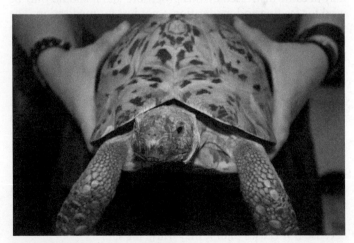

Fig. 14.19 Restraining a tortoise

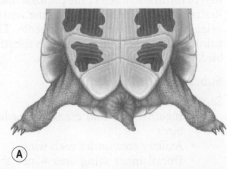
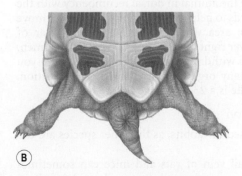

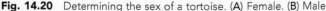

Fig. 14.20 Determining the sex of a tortoise. **(A)** Female. **(B)** Male

Administration of medication

The available routes and methods of administration of medication to most animals are as follows:

- Oral dosing
- Intramuscular injection
- Subcutaneous injection
- Intravenous injection
- Intraperitoneal injection
- Intraosseous injection – used for the introduction of fluids into the medullary cavity of the bone.

SMALL MAMMALS

Oral

This method is used most often in small animals as medication can be given by this route at home by the owners, reducing the stress to the animal. Medication for small animals mainly comes in a liquid form, which makes it easier to administer. Most small mammals will take the medication if you syringe it into the side of the mouth slowly. If the medication has a particularly nasty taste, mix it into some baby food and syringe it down. Rodents are able to close off the back of the mouth with the cheek folds, which may make oral administration difficult but is quite normal, as it allows them to gnaw at wood without ingesting it.

If oral administration is difficult, a feeding tube or straight crop tube can be used. Keep the patient firmly scruffed to prevent it from wriggling and keep the head and oesophagus in a straight line to allow the tube to pass down easily. The animal may become distressed by this procedure and it should only be used for feeding and medication – not just for medication. The use of naso-oesophageal or gastric tubes can be used in the larger animals like guinea pigs, chinchillas, rabbits and ferrets but rats and mice are too small.

Intramuscular injection

This route is not often used as the muscles of most small mammals are so small. Use the quadriceps femoris muscle in the hind leg or the muscle over the spine. Use 25-gauge needles or an even smaller gauge.

Subcutaneous injection

The scruff area is the most useful but the skin over the lateral thorax can be used in the larger animals. The use of a 25-gauge needle is recommended. Use this route with care in chinchillas because if it causes pain it may cause fur slip.

Intraperitoneal injection

Used for administering fluids, not medication, it is a relatively easy procedure. Place the animal in dorsal recumbency with the head tilting downwards to help the abdominal contents to move cranially, leaving the area where you are injecting clear of organs. Select the lower right quadrant of the ventral abdomen. Insert the needle and withdraw the plunger first to ensure you have not punctured any organs; then complete the injection. The best size of needle is a 23–25-gauge 5/8-inch needle.

Intravenous injection

Only satisfactorily used in rabbits, as the other species are too small.

- The lateral tail vein of rats and mice can sometimes be used, warming the tail first and applying local anaesthetic cream to help dilate the vein – use a 25–27-gauge 5/8-inch needle.
- The cephalic and saphenous veins may be used in guinea pigs, chinchillas and ferrets but they are quite difficult to locate and the procedure is not tolerated well, especially if a catheter is to be left in place.
- Cephalic and saphenous veins may be used in the rabbit and the lateral ear vein can also be used. The use of a 25–27-gauge needle or butterfly catheter is best for administration.

Intraosseous injection

This site is used for the administration of fluids rather than medication. It cannot be done in the small rodents as they have very fine bones with a small medullary cavity and there is no needle safe enough for the procedure.

In some larger rats, chinchillas, guinea pigs, rabbits, etc., the best site is the proximal femur in the fossa between the hip joint and the greater trochanter. The area must be surgically prepared as the needle would track bacteria straight into the medullary cavity, resulting in severe osteomyelitis. A 20–21-gauge needle or a spinal needle is screwed into the bone. Apply antibiotic cream around the needle to prevent infection. Cap the needle and bandage in place. This procedure is very painful and so requires heavy sedation or a general anaesthetic. The procedure should never be attempted if there is any sign of metabolic bone disease. A radiograph should be taken after the needle is placed to ensure that it is in the correct position.

BIRDS

Oral

This route is a useful method for administering medication, as many drugs can be added to food or drinking water for self-medication. It is an easy and less stressful method but you cannot be sure how much of the medication the bird has actually ingested.

A more accurate method is to use a crop tube (Fig. 14.21). Restrain the bird, maintaining its head tilted upwards to keep the head and oesophagus straight. Using a feeding tube or straight crop tube, carefully introduce it into the oesophagus until you reach the crop just below the base of the neck.

Medication may be given by simply syringing the medication straight into the mouth but the bird may choke. If the bird tolerates this method well you may demonstrate it to owners, who may not feel able to use the crop tubing method.

Intramuscular injection

This is probably the easiest and quickest method of administration of medication. Select the pectoral muscle in the breast area. Restrain the bird and inject into the ventral part of the muscle using a 23–25-gauge 5/8-inch needle. This route is relatively painless and as it is quick it reduces the stress of handling to the bird.

Subcutaneous injection

Several sites may be used:

- Inguinal skin fold cranial to each leg – useful in small birds
- Axillary area under each wing
- Dorsal inner wing area – not the best site to use. A 23–25-gauge 5/8-inch needle is best.

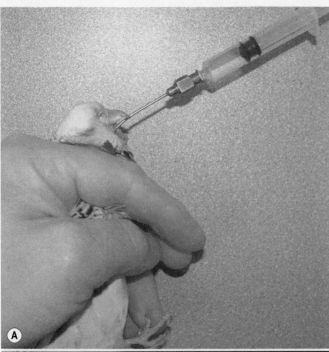

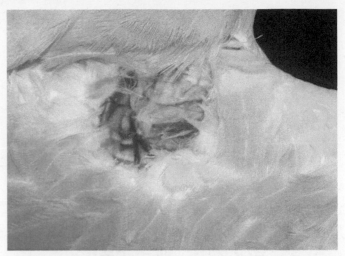

Fig. 14.22   Site for intravenous injection in larger birds: the basilic vein runs caudal to the humerus

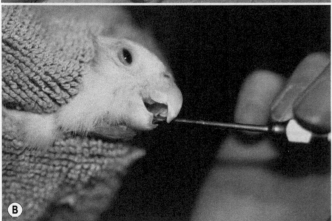

Fig. 14.21   Use of a crop tube. (A) In a budgerigar. (B) In a parrot

Intravenous injection

Mainly used for blood sampling and the administration of fluids:

- This is not easily done in smaller birds – use the right jugular vein and a 23–25-gauge 5/8-inch needle.
- In larger birds the basilic (or brachial) vein, which runs along the ventral part of the wing just caudal to the humerus, can be used, but it ruptures easily, causing large haematomata (Fig. 14.22).
- The ulnar vein, which runs along the ventral part of the wing just caudal to the ulnar bone, can sometimes be used but is very narrow and mobile. This vein can only be used in the larger raptors and waterfowl and it also ruptures easily.
- In larger geese and swans use the medial metatarsal vein on the leg.

Larger birds tend to tolerate repeated injections fairly well but many small birds will not and the use of a catheter is recommended. Sedation or a general anaesthetic may be required for this procedure: 23-, 25- or 27-gauge 5/8-inch needles or butterfly catheters are best for this procedure.

Intraperitoneal injection

This route should *never* be used in birds as their body cavity is full of air sacs, which are a vital part of the respiratory system. If a needle is introduced it may rupture the air sacs.

Intraosseous injection

Only used for the administration of fluids and can be performed in both small and larger birds. In small birds the best site is the proximal tibiotarsal bone below the stifle joint; in the larger birds the distal and proximal ulna can also be used (Fig. 14.23). The procedure is painful and the use of sedation or a general anaesthetic is advised.

The area must be surgically prepared before the needle is screwed in place to prevent osteomyelitis. After the needle is placed apply an antibiotic cream around the site before bandaging the needle in place. For the smaller birds use a 25–27-gauge needle or spinal needle and for larger birds a 20–23-gauge needle or spinal needle. It is useful to radiograph the site to ensure that the needle is in the correct position.

REPTILES

Oral

This is a good route to use as the glottis is clearly visible and can be avoided. It lies at the front of the oral cavity in snakes (Fig. 14.24) and at the base of the tongue in lizards, tortoises and terrapins. Some reptiles will tolerate medication by direct syringing into the mouth but there is a risk of inhalation and it is also inaccurate.

The most efficient method makes use of a feeding tube or a straight crop tube and with practice can be carried out by owners at home and is well tolerated by most reptiles. If prolonged medication and feeding is required, then the placement of a pharyngostomy tube is advised as this will reduce the stress of repeated tubing.

To locate the stomach you should always measure the tube against the outside of the body before placing it to ensure you really are in the stomach, preventing regurgitation. In snakes

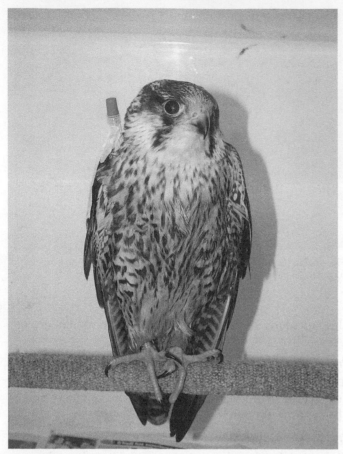

Fig. 14.23 Falcon with an intraosseous catheter placed in the ulna of the wing

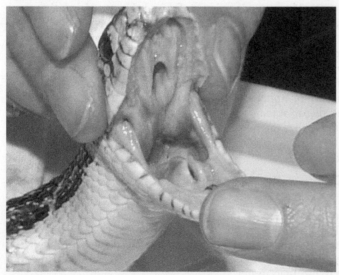

Fig. 14.24 Oral cavity of the snake showing the position of the glottis

the stomach is located about one-third of the way down the body; in lizards the stomach is located about halfway down the body; in tortoises and terrapins you measure from the nose to the line where the pectoral and abdominal scutes meet (see Chapter 7). Mark the position of the mouth on the tube using a biro – this is the point that the tube will reach when the end

is in the stomach. Open the mouth with a wooden spatula. Introduce a well-lubricated tube up towards the roof of the mouth and down the oesophagus, avoiding the glottis. Advance the tube until your marked point.

Intramuscular injection

Fairly well tolerated and easy to do:
- Snakes – inject into the caudal third of the snake, using the muscles that run parallel to the spine.
- Lizards, tortoises and terrapins – inject into the proximal part of the forearm. The hind limbs can also be used but be aware of the renal portal system. Tortoises and terrapins may withdraw their limbs into their shells, so you may have to use the pectoral muscles at the junction of the neck/forelimb with the body.

Use a 23–25-gauge 5/8-inch needle. Always clean the skin before injecting, as reptiles have very dirty skin. This is achieved by scrubbing the area with an iodine solution and a toothbrush. Always inject under the scales, never through them.

Subcutaneous injection

An easy route to use but may be less well tolerated with some drugs, as they can be painful:
- Snakes – use the first third of the body in the lateral dorsal area.
- Lizards – use the lateral thoracic area. There is a risk of the skin around the injection site becoming darkened – especially common in the chameleon family. The owner should be advised of this.
- Tortoises and terrapins – use the area cranial to the fore limbs and hind limbs. Strong tortoises tend to pull their legs in, making it very hard to inject. The use of a 23–25-gauge 5/8-inch needle is recommended. The area must be thoroughly scrubbed with an iodine solution, and you must inject under the scales, not through them.

Intracoelomic injection

Reptiles do not have a diaphragm and the entire body cavity is known as the coelom. The intracoelomic route is mainly used for fluid administration:
- Snakes – enter the body cavity within an area on the lateral part of the body just dorsal to the ventral scales, cranial to the cloaca in the caudal third of the body
- Lizards – place the lizard in dorsal recumbency with the head tilted downwards to encourage the organs to move cranially away from the injection site. Select a site in the lower right quadrant of the body cavity.
- Tortoises and terrapins – this is not the easiest route as it is difficult to reach an area cranial to the hind limbs. The bladder lies in this area and can be punctured very easily.

The injection site should be scrubbed with an iodine solution before injection is performed. Inject under the scales not through them. The plunger should always be drawn back before injection to ensure you have not punctured an organ. Use a 23–25-gauge needle.

Intravenous injection

This route is more difficult than the others as you cannot easily 'raise' the vein or see it through the thick skin:
- Snakes – use the ventral tail vein. Insert the needle in the midline about one-third of the tail length from the

cloaca at a 75° angle. Advance it slowly until you hit the vertebrae. Pull out slightly while drawing back on the plunger until you get blood back. Administer your medication. The palatine vein, which runs along the roof of the mouth, may be used in larger snakes when they are anaesthetised.

- Lizards – use the ventral tail vein. Insert the needle at a 75° angle about one-third of the way down the tail from the cloaca to ensure you avoid the male hemipenes in the caudal third of the body. Advance the needle until you hit the vertebrae. Pull out the needle while drawing on the plunger. When you get blood back, stop and inject the medication. You must be careful with some species of lizard as they are able to spontaneously shed their tails – this may occur if they are injected on a regular basis.
- Tortoises and terrapins – two routes are used:
  a. Jugular vein – this is the recommended route. Extend the head, tilt the body away and pull the neck towards you. Raise the vein on the right side by applying pressure at the base of the neck. The vein runs from the eardrum down the neck and can sometimes be seen when it is raised.
  b. Dorsal tail vein – more difficult. The vein lies midline on the dorsal aspect of the tail. Insert the needle at a 90° angle and advance it until you hit the vertebrae. Gently pull back while drawing back on the plunger. When blood comes back into the syringe, stop and administer the medication. Use a 23–25-gauge 1-inch needle.

Ensure that the area is scrubbed well with an iodine solution, and go under the scales not through them.

Intraosseous injection

This route is mainly used for fluid administration. This route is impossible in snakes as they do not have any legs:

- Lizards – use the proximal femur, distal femur and the proximal tibia. As this procedure is painful, the use of sedation or a general anaesthetic is required. The area must be scrubbed well with an iodine solution, as the needle could introduce an infection straight into the bone and cause osteomyelitis. Use a 23–25-gauge needle or spinal needle depending on the size of the lizard. The proximal femur is entered at the fossa between the hip joint and the greater trochanter. This is not an easy route to use as it is at a difficult angle. The distal femur is a bit easier to access as you enter at the stifle joint but it does restrict the movement of the leg. The proximal tibia is really only used in the larger lizards and is entered at the tibial crest.
- Tortoises and terrapins – there are two main sites:
  a. The area at which the plastron and carapace meet just cranial to the hind legs – this is easily accessed but can be very tough, especially in older tortoises. A 21–23-gauge spinal needle is screwed into the shell, ensuring that it is kept parallel to the side of the shell.
  b. The proximal tibia – this is accessed via the tibial crest.

After the needle has been capped, apply an antiseptic cream around the site to help prevent an infection. A radiograph should be taken of the area to ensure it is in the correct place. If you suspect that the reptile may be suffering from a metabolic bone disease you should never use this route, and to check this you should always radiograph the animal prior to this procedure.

BIBLIOGRAPHY

Anderson, R.S., Edney, A.T.D. (Eds.), 1991. Practical Animal Handling. Pergamon Press, Oxford.

Aspinall, V., 2008. Clinical Procedures in Veterinary Nursing, second ed. Butterworth-Heinemann, Oxford.

Cooper, B., Mullineaux, E., Turner, L. (Eds.), 2012. BSAVA Textbook of Veterinary Nursing, fifth ed. British Small Animal Veterinary Association, Gloucester.

Hotston Moore, A., Rudd, S. (Eds.), 2008. Manual of Canine and Feline Advanced Veterinary Nursing, second ed. British Small Animal Veterinary Association, Cheltenham.

RECOMMENDED READING

Aspinall, V., 2014. Clinical Procedures in Veterinary Nursing, third ed. Butterworth-Heinemann, Oxford.
  Step-by-step guide to handling the more common species of exotic pet.

Hotston Moore, A., Rudd, S. (Eds.), 2008. Manual of Canine and Feline Advanced Veterinary Nursing, second ed. British Small Animal Veterinary Association, Cheltenham.

  Detailed chapter describes all aspects of exotic animal care, including nutrition, anaesthesia and patient care.

15

Introduction to Genetics

DOROTHY STABLES

KEY POINTS

- Every living cell contains a set of chromosomes in the nucleus – a cell containing the normal two sets of chromosomes is called diploid. Gametes (ovum or sperm) have only one of each chromosome pair present and are haploid.

- Two mechanisms are necessary for cell division: mitosis, or the division of somatic cells; and meiosis, the production of gametes. During meiosis the chromosome complement is halved.

- Genes are arranged in a specific order, each in the same locus on the chromosomes in every member of a species. Alleles are alternative versions of genes at a locus. If an animal has two alleles alike at a locus, it is homozygous. If the alleles differ, the animal is heterozygous.

- DNA molecules consist of a double helix made up of two complementary chains of nucleotides composed of phosphoric acid, deoxyribose and four nitrogenous bases, two purines – adenine and guanine – and two pyrimidines – thymine and cytosine.

- The full complement of DNA is called the genome. The genetic makeup inherited by an individual animal is called the genotype. The outward appearance of an animal, or the phenotype, results from gene–environment interactions.

- A form of control of gene protein production to turn it on or off is by the attachment of chemical groups to specific sites on DNA without changing the underlying DNA molecule. Understanding these mechanisms is called the science of epigenetics.

- Congenital defects present at birth are not all inherited. They may occur because of genetic/chromosomal abnormalities, the action of environmental teratogens, multifactorial disorders caused by the interaction of environment and genes or idiopathic defects with no known cause.

Introduction

Genes are molecules within cell nuclei that control the development, structure, function and maintenance of living organisms. Like words in a book, genes can sometimes be 'spelled' wrongly, leading to abnormal development or to diseases. As genes are involved in cell division and in the manufacturing of antibodies, cancers and some immune disorders have a genetic basis. The actions of genes may also be influenced by environmental features, leading to disorders such as hip dysplasia in dogs. A knowledge of basic cell physiology helps us to understand both normal and abnormal gene function.

Characteristics of mammalian cells

Cells are the basic structural and functional units of living organisms (see Chapter 6) and are membrane-bound units filled with an aqueous solution of chemicals and organelles. Cells extract raw materials necessary for their function from their surroundings and expel waste products. Their structure and functions are governed by genetic information. Cells create copies of themselves.

CELLULAR ORGANISATION

A typical cell includes a single **nucleus, cytoplasm** and a cellular boundary known as the **cell membrane or plasma membrane**. The nucleus contains the genetic material and the cytoplasm is composed mainly of cytosol containing water, electrolytes, proteins, lipids and carbohydrates, and the organelles. The plasma membrane encloses the cellular contents and maintains the boundary between the cytoplasm and the extracellular environment. This chapter is concerned with the functions of the cell nucleus.

THE NUCLEUS

The nucleus is the largest structure of the cell and is its control centre. It is surrounded by a double nuclear membrane. The outer one is continuous with the endoplasmic reticulum of the cell cytoplasm. The nuclear membrane is penetrated by several thousand nuclear pores through which molecules pass. Most cells have only one nucleus, although skeletal muscle cells are multinucleated. Nuclei contain large quantities of **deoxyribonucleic acid (DNA)**, made up of **genes**. Several other structures are essential to the normal functioning of the nucleus, such as the **nucleoli** where ribosomal subunits are synthesised. DNA is found in a thread-like mass known as **chromatin**.

HISTONES

To fit it all into the cell, DNA needs compacting into a much shorter molecule and to accomplish this it is associated with proteins called **histones**. Each histone has a floppy tail called the histone tail. Histones are alkaline proteins found in the cell nuclei which package DNA into structural units called **nucleosomes**. Histones are globular shaped and there are four main ones – H2A, H2B, H3 and H4. Two copies of each of these four come together to form the histone octamer (composed of eight individual histones). These can be visualised as eight table-tennis balls stacked one on top of each other in two layers, around which the DNA coils to form nucleosomes. Each human cell has about 2 metres of DNA, but when it is wound onto the histones this is reduced to only 0.09 mm of chromatin. Prior to cellular reproduction, chromatin shortens and coils into rod-like bodies, forming **chromosomes**, the number of which varies between species.

CHROMOSOMES

When dividing cells are observed under a light microscope, the chromosomes are clearly visible. During cell division the chromosomes become condensed. At this time DNA replication results in an X-shaped structure consisting of two identical strands called **chromatids** joined by a constricted area called the **centromere.**

In **somatic** (body) cells, chromosomes are arranged in pairs. One of each pair originates within the maternal ovum and the other within the paternal sperm. A cell containing two sets of chromosomes is called **diploid. Gametes** (sex cells) are **haploid**, containing only one of each pair. In all but one of the pairs the chromosomes are identical and these pairs are called **autosomes.** The pairs that are alike are called **homologues.**

The other pair is the **sex chromosomes.** In mammals two X chromosomes are present in females and an X and a Y chromosome in males. In birds the sex chromosomes have different names – Z and W. Unlike the mammals, it is the female bird that has two different chromosomes, one Z and one W, while the male bird has two Z chromosomes. We will concentrate on mammalian inheritance.

Identifying chromosomes

Circulating lymphocytes are commonly used to study chromosomes. The cell samples are encouraged to divide. The process is stopped during mitosis (see the next section) by adding colchicine. The two chromatids have been formed from one chromosome and, if cell division had continued, the centromere would have split and each chromatid would have become a separate chromosome in a new cell.

A photograph is taken and the chromosomes are cut out and arranged in a standard fashion and then photographed again to produce a **karyotype** (Fig. 15.1). Chromosomes are usually referred to as pairs and the total number is called the $2n$ number, where n is the number of pairs. Chromosomes are identified by their size, light and dark banding patterns and position of the centromere. A chromosome is divided by its centromere into short and long arms. The short arm is referred to as 'p' and the long arm as 'q'. Chromosomes can be classified by the position of their centromeres. If located centrally the chromosome is **metacentric**, if intermediate it is **submetacentric** and if found at one end, **acrocentric**. It is common to use the term metacentric to cover metacentric and submetacentric (Nicholas 2009), as shown in Table 15.1.

CELL DIVISION – MITOSIS AND MEIOSIS

There are two mechanisms necessary for cell division. **Somatic cells** must replicate themselves with minimal mistakes. During **mitosis** each daughter cell receives a copy of all the chromosomes. Multicellular species replace cells damaged by wear and tear or lost during programmed cell death (apoptosis) by the cycle of somatic cell division. Where ill health, trauma or surgery occurs, loss and replacement of cells will increase. Where natural cell division is halted, for example, in exposure to a large dose of ionising radiation, the animal is likely to die within a few days because of rapid cell destruction. However,

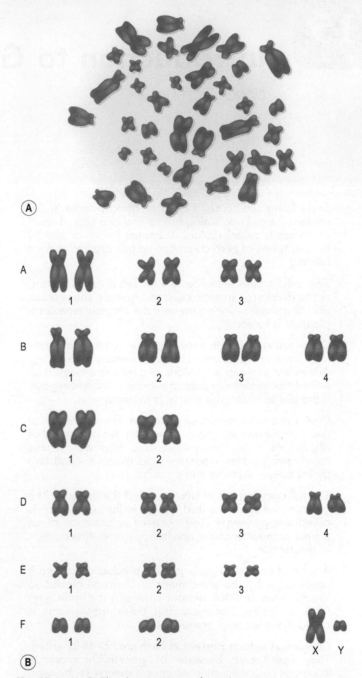

Fig. 15.1 (A, B) The chromosomes of a male cat

something special is required in sexual reproduction, where mother and father must contribute one of each pair of chromosomes to their offspring. During **meiosis** only one of each pair of chromosomes enters each **gamete** (sperm or ovum).

Replication of DNA

To produce a pair of genetically identical daughter cells, nuclear DNA in chromosomes must be precisely replicated and separated into two identical cells. At the same time most cells double their mass and duplicate all their cytoplasmic organelles. Cells must not enter mitosis or meiosis until the chromosomes have been replicated, otherwise they may lack a particular chromosome.

TABLE 15.1	Karyotypes of some domestic species		
Species	Total (diploid 2n)	Metacentric pairs	Acrocentric pairs
Cat, *Felis catus*	38	16	2
Dog, *Canis familiaris*	78	0	39
Goat, *Capra hircus*	60	0	29
Sheep, *Ovis aries*	54	3	23
Cattle, *Bos taurus*	60	0	29
Horse, *Equus caballus*	64	13	18
Rabbit, *Oryctolagus cuniculus*	44	19	2

Adapted from Nicholas 2009

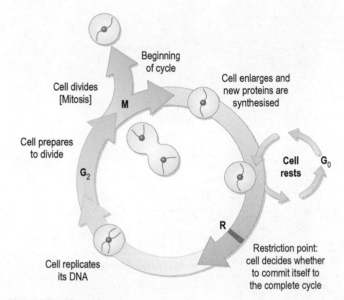

Fig. 15.2 The cell cycle

The duration of the **cell cycle** (Fig. 15.2) varies greatly from one cell type to another but always consists of three distinct phases, interphase, mitosis and cytokinesis. The standard cell cycle is fairly long, extending to 12 hours or more, the mitotic phase taking about one hour, a small fraction of the whole. The time between one mitotic phase and the next is taken up by interphase, which itself consists of three distinctive phases, G1 (gap1), S (synthesis) and G2 (gap2). During G1 phase the cell becomes committed to DNA replication, which occurs during S phase. The subsequent G2 phase appears to provide a safety gap, allowing DNA replication to be complete before mitosis.

Mitosis

During mitosis (Fig. 15.3) the nuclear membrane breaks down and the nuclear contents condense, forming visible chromosomes. The stages of mitosis are prophase, metaphase, anaphase and telophase:

- During **prophase**, the cell's microtubules establish the mitotic spindle, which will eventually separate the chromosomes.
- In **metaphase** the duplicated chromosomes align on the mitotic spindle, in preparation for segregation (see Fig. 15.3).

- During **anaphase** the chromosomes move to the pole of the spindle, where they decondense and establish new nuclei.
- During **telophase** the cell is pinched and gradually divided by a process known as **cytokinesis**, the critical point of mitosis that terminates the cell cycle. All phases of the cell cycle are variable in length but the greatest variation occurs in the G1 phase. If cells in G1 are not committed to DNA replication, they can enter a resting state known as the G0 phase for days, weeks or years before resuming proliferation.

Meiosis

During meiosis (diminution), the chromosome complement is halved. Meiosis involves two nuclear divisions rather than one. A mature haploid gamete produced by the divisions of a diploid cell during meiosis must contain half the original number of chromosomes. Only one chromosome from each homologous pair is present, ensuring that either the maternal or the paternal copy of each gene, but not both, is present. The homologues recognise each other and become physically paired prior to lining up on the mitotic spindle.

Meiosis consists of two stages (Fig. 15.4):

- **Meiosis 1** begins with each chromosome duplicating itself, giving rise to two identical chromatids joined at the centromere. The duplicated homologous pairs form a structure containing four chromatids. This close proximity allows recombination (crossing over of genetic material) to occur. Fragments of maternal chromatids are exchanged for corresponding fragments of homologous paternal chromatids. Next, the two centromeres are pulled to opposite sides of the cell, a process called **dysjunction**. The cell now divides into two new cells, one containing a recombined maternal chromosome and one containing a recombined paternal chromosome.
- In **meiosis 2** two chromatids in each new cell are formed and move apart and these cells divide into two, each containing one chromatid or new chromosome. The result is four haploid spermatozoa but only one functional ovum because of the loss of a set of chromosomes in meiosis 1 into a dark body called the first polar body and the loss again in meiosis 2 of one set of chromosomes into a second polar body. The union of a sperm and ovum at fertilisation results in a **zygote** with the normal diploid number of chromosomes.

FELINE AND CANINE CHROMOSOMES

Genes are arranged in a specific order, each in the same place or **locus** on the chromosomes, in every species such as the domestic cat (*Felis catus*), ensuring that any male cat can mate with any female cat. This is the defining feature of a species. Cats have 19 pairs of chromosomes. All domestic dogs (*Canis familiaris*) have 39 pairs of chromosomes (see Table 15.1).

Development of modern genetics

In 1865 a monk called Gregor Mendel presented a paper on his experiments on garden peas. He studied peas that differed in a single characteristic, such as tall and short plants or wrinkled and smooth seeds. He found that one of two characteristics, for

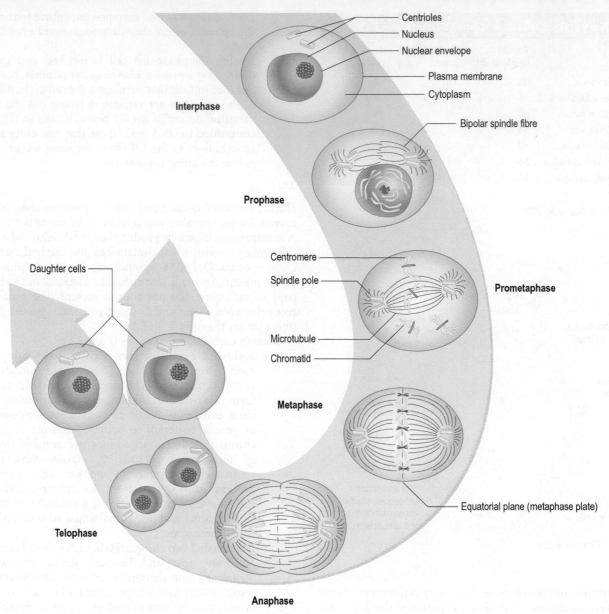

Fig. 15.3 Stages of mitosis

example, tall plants, seemed to dominate the next generation, the first filial (F1) generation, and these were called **dominant factors.** The opposite characteristic – short plants – disappeared, only to reappear in the second or F2 generation. These were called **recessive factors.**

Mendel proposed that each pair of characteristics was controlled by a pair of factors, one arising from each parent plant. Pure-bred pea plants were **homozygous,** inheriting two identical genes from their parents. The F1 generation that resulted from the breeding of a tall plant with a short plant were all tall plants. However, they inherited two different genes from their parents and were **heterozygous.** These factors were called genes by a Danish botanist, Johannsen, who shortened the term pangenia that Charles Darwin had coined for his unknown hereditary factors (Gould 2007). The alternative versions of genes at a locus are called **allelomorphs,** usually shortened to **alleles.**

For other useful definitions see Box 15.1.

> ### BOX 15.1 USEFUL DEFINITIONS
>
> - Chromosome – thread-like mass of DNA found within the nucleus of the cell
> - Gene – unit of inheritance; genes consist of short pieces of DNA which, when joined together in a sequence, make up specific chromosomes
> - Locus – the position of a gene on a chromosome
> - Allele – a gene on the same locus of a pair of homologous chromosomes
> - Homologous chromosomes – identical in size and shape
> - Homozygous genes – identical genes on the same locus of a pair of chromosomes
> - Heterozygous genes – non-identical genes on the same locus of a pair of chromosomes
> - Phenotype – outward or visible appearance of the animal; may be affected by the environment
> - Genotype – the genetic makeup of an animal

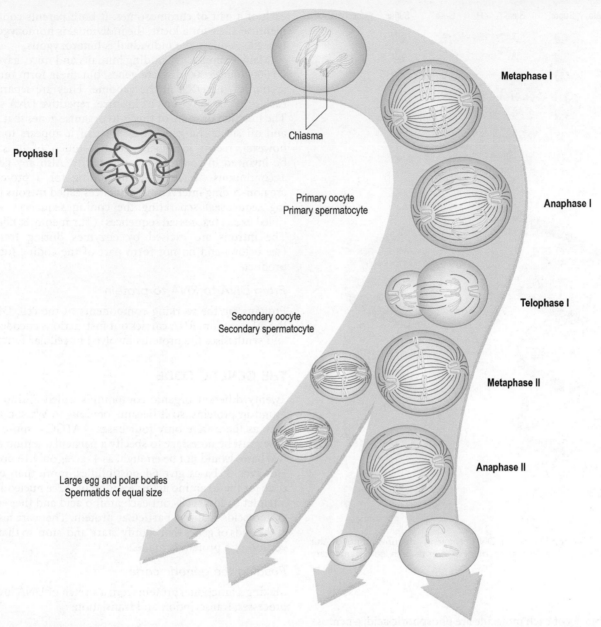

Fig. 15.4 Stages of meiosis

MENDEL'S LAWS

Three main principles developed from Mendel's work:

- **The law of uniformity** – when two homozygotes with different alleles are crossed, all the offspring of the F1 generation are identical and heterozygous. Characteristics do not blend and can reappear in subsequent generations.
- **The law of segregation** – each individual possesses two genes for a particular characteristic, only one of which can be passed on in the ovum or sperm to the next generation.
- **The law of independent assortment** – members of different gene pairs segregate to offspring independently of one another. This third law is not strictly true, because, if two genes are situated closely together on the same chromosome, they may be linked and inherited together during meiosis.

Mendel's findings were ignored until 1900, when thread-like structures were seen in cell nuclei. These were the chromosomes and in 1903 two people independently proposed that they carried the hereditary factors known as genes. It was only in 1952 that DNA was identified as the universal genetic material. In 1953 the structure of DNA was discovered by James D. Watson and Francis H. C. Crick. Without Rosalind Franklin, who developed the skills of X-ray crystallography, their discovery might not have occurred. The correct number of 46 human chromosomes was identified in 1956 (Jorde et al. 2006).

COMPOSITION OF DNA

The double helix

DNA molecules consist of a double helix made up of two complementary chains of nucleotides. These are composed of chemical compounds bound together in a regular pattern. The

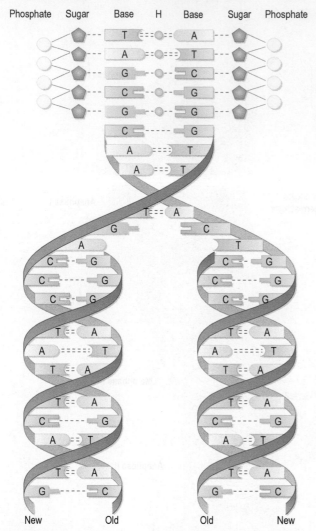

Phosphate Sugar Base H Base Sugar Phosphate

New Old Old New

Fig. 15.5 The replication of DNA, showing the unwinding of the double helix and the formation of new strands with complementary base pairs

building blocks of each molecule are phosphoric acid, a pentose sugar called deoxyribose, and four nitrogenous bases, two purines – **adenine** and **guanine**, and two pyrimidines – **thymine** and **cytosine**, identified by the single letters A, G, T and C. A second form of nucleic acid is ribonucleic acid (RNA). In RNA thymine is replaced by uracil (U). Two sugar-phosphate strands wind around each other and the base pairs are stacked between these strands, pointing inwards to the centre of the double helix. The two strands run in opposite directions and are complementary to each other. A purine always pairs with a pyrimidine and the pairs stack one above the other. The complementary chains are held together by hydrogen bonds, which are easily broken, a feature necessary for DNA replication (Fig. 15.5).

Genes

The full complement of DNA is called the **genome** and the study of it is called **genomics**. DNA is arranged in segments called **genes**. Genes code for proteins, which may act as hormones, receptors, structural tand regulatory proteins. Two alternative **alleles** of any gene are present at a specific **locus**, one on

each of a pair of chromosomes. If both parents contribute an identical allele for a locus, the individual is **homozygous**. If the two alleles differ, the individual is **heterozygous.**

Many mammals, including humans and mice, have between 20 000 and 25 000 discrete genes, but these form only a small section of the DNA in the genome. They are separated from each other by long runs of inactive, repetitive DNA sequences. The function of some of this is to organise genes that switch on and off structural genes, but most of it appears to be 'junk'; however, recent ideas suggest that much of it is likely to be involved in control of gene activity. Also any gene is not a continuous stretch of DNA coding for a protein. There are non-coding intervening sequences called **introns** (intervening sequences) separating the coding sequences which are called **exons** (expressed sequences) (Turnpenny & Ellard 2011). The introns are excised by enzymes during transcription (see below) and do not form part of the coding for the gene product.

From DNA to RNA to protein

Proteins are the working components of the cell. DNA stores the information. RNA carries out instructions encoded in DNA and synthesises the proteins involved in cellular function.

THE GENETIC CODE

Twenty different organic compounds called **amino acids** are found in proteins, so it became obvious to Watson and Crick that, as there were only four bases – ATGC – more than one base must be necessary to specify a particular amino acid. Even two bases would not be enough, as 4^2 gives only 16 possibilities. However, 3^2 bases give 64 possibilities, more than enough to code for the 20 amino acids. A group of three nucleotides called a **triplet codon** spells out each amino acid and the sequence of amino acids shapes a particular protein. There are also codons at the ends of genes that signify 'start' and 'stop' so that a correct version of a protein is made.

Reading the genetic code

Making a functional protein from a stretch of DNA involves two processes, transcription and translation.

Transcription. In a gene only one of the two DNA strands forming the helix acts as a template for a polypeptide. It must be copied by messenger RNA (mRNA) before it can be read. This is called transcription (Fig. 15.6). Every base in the single-stranded mRNA is complementary to the DNA but uracil replaces thymine.

Translation. Following transcription, mature mRNA is transported to the ribosomes for translation into a specific protein (see Fig. 15.6). In the cytoplasm a particular amino acid is bound to its transfer RNA (tRNA) for transporting to a ribosome where it is linked up with others to form a polypeptide chain to build the protein.

PATTERNS OF MENDELIAN INHERITANCE

There are four basic types of single-gene Mendelian inheritance – autosomal dominant, autosomal recessive, X-linked dominant and X-linked recessive. Recessive X-linked disorders are rare and will not be discussed.

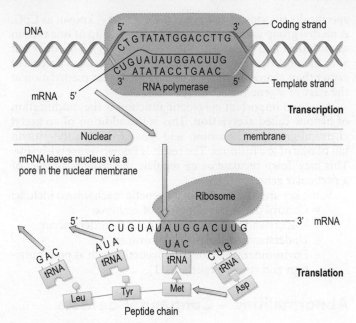

DNA

CTGTATATGGACCTTG — Coding strand
CUGUAUAUGGACUUG
ATATACCTGAAC — Template strand
RNA polymerase
mRNA 5'

Transcription

Nuclear — membrane

mRNA leaves nucleus via a
pore in the nuclear membrane

Ribosome

5' — 3' mRNA
CUGUAUAUGGACUUG
UAC

GAC AUA tRNA CUG
tRNA tRNA tRNA

Translation

Leu Tyr Met Asp

Peptide chain

Fig. 15.6 Synthesis of polypeptides in a eukaryote by means of transcription and translation

Dominant genes

- Only one copy is needed to affect the phenotype and manifests its effects in heterozygotes.
- The effect does not miss a generation.
- Every affected offspring with that particular phenotype has at least one affected parent.
- Where one parent is affected, offspring have a one in two chance of being affected.
- Normal offspring of an affected parent only produce normal offspring.

Recessive genes

- A recessive allele only affects the phenotype in homozygotes.
- Animals with one copy of the allele are carriers.
- The progeny of two carriers have a one in four chance of being affected or normal and a one in two chance of carrying the disorder.
- Matings between a homozygous affected animal and a normal homozygous animal produce normal offspring.
- The effect may be to skip generations until two carriers reproduce.
- An example of recessive inheritance is illustrated in Box 15.2.

Dominant X-linked genes

- The X chromosome carries a large number of genes involved in development and function.
- Males only have one X chromosome and are hemizygous for X chromosome genes.
- If there is an abnormal X chromosome gene, males will be affected by an X-linked disorder.
- Females are usually heterozygous for the X chromosome and will not be affected because of the opposing normal allele. They will be asymptomatic carriers.

BOX 15.2 INHERITANCE OF COAT COLOURS IN LABRADOR DOGS

The working of single genes can be illustrated by the inheritance of coat colour in Labrador dogs. Coat colour in mammals is brought about by the presence of pigment granules called melanins in a protein framework. Two varieties of melanin are converted from the amino acid tyrosine. One is called eumelanin and gives rise to dark coat colour and the other is phaeomelanin, which produces light colour – various shades of yellow from pale to red (Nicholas 2009).

PUNNETT SQUARE 1

Labradors come in three basic colours – black, chocolate and yellow. Chocolates can vary from light to dark in colour. Two alleles of the same gene are responsible for the black and chocolate colours. Black is dominant and is represented by the upper case letter B and chocolate is recessive to black and is represented by the lower case letter b. Therefore a dog with a black coat (phenotype) may be genetically either homozygous BB or heterozygous Bb. If a dog and bitch are both homozygous all their puppies will be black BB, as shown in Punnett square 1.

PUNNETT SQUARE 2

If a dog and bitch are both heterozygous Bb, three of their puppies will be black and only one chocolate, as shown in Punnett square 2. One of the black puppies will be homozygous BB, two will be heterozygous Bb. The chocolate puppy will be homozygous for the recessive gene bb.

PUNNETT SQUARE 3

The yellow colour is brought about by a second recessive gene, E, which functions to mask the dark colour by producing phaeomelanin instead of eumelanin. If the animal is homozygous for the dominant allele, i.e. EE or heterozygous Ee, there is no effect on the basic coat colour. Eumelanin will be produced and the coat colour will be black or brown. If the animal is homozygous for the recessive version ee, phaeomelanin will be produced and the coat colour will be yellow as shown in Punnett square 3. For simplicity of cell numbers in the Punnett square, both dog and bitch are shown as homozygous BB.

MITOCHONDRIAL DNA

- Each mitochondrion has its own circular double-stranded DNA called mitochondrial DNA (mDNA) inherited only from mothers because sperm mitochondria rarely enter the ovum and do not contribute to the embryo.
- mDNA codes for genes that are important in cellular respiration.
- mDNA disorders affect males and females but are transmitted only through their mothers. The disorders combine muscular and neurological features, affecting cells with high energy needs.

INACTIVATION OF THE X CHROMOSOME IN FEMALES

In females only one X chromosome is functional in each cell and the other is inactivated in the early embryo. This phenomenon is called lyonisation (Box 15.3). Laura Gould has written an interesting and informative book about her male calico (tortoiseshell and white) cat George, updated 2007. It is called 'Cats Are Not Peas' and she discusses how George came to be – he carried two X chromosomes (XXY) instead of one and therefore half his cells carried black and half red.

BOX 15.3   INACTIVATION OF THE X CHROMOSOME

In females one or other of the X chromosomes is randomly inactivated in cells early in embryonic life. Half the cells of a female will contain one activated X chromosome and half the other. All daughter cells of a particular cell line contain the same inactivated X chromosome. This effect is called lyonisation, after its discoverer, Dr Mary Lyon. Each female is a mosaic of half paternal and half maternal X chromosomes.

The tortoiseshell cat – in cats the orange gene (O) is responsible for the colour of the ginger cat. It is carried on the X chromosome. The O gene eliminates all black or brown pigment from the hairs. A tortoiseshell cat is a female heterozygote Oo. In any cell only one X chromosome functions. Two cell lines develop at random – one with O producing hair with orange pigment and the other with o, allowing normal pigment to colour the hair with whatever the animal has inherited (Fig. 15.7).

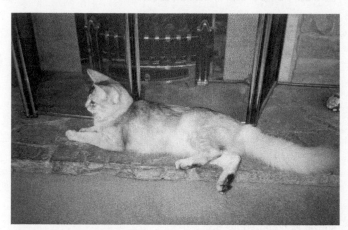

Fig. 15.7   A tortoiseshell silver Somali cat showing patches of red and black on a silver base

The role of the environment in gene regulation – Epigenetics

The full complement of genes inherited by an individual animal is called the **genotype**. The outward appearance of an animal, i.e. its physical, biochemical and physiological nature, is known as the **phenotype** and results from gene/environment interactions. Genes perform their functions in response to environmental changes. These may be internal, such as a response to fluctuations in hormone level, or external, such as the response to a meal.

Cells in the body contain all the genetic information but most of it is not needed in a particular cell. For instance brain cells do not need to make liver enzymes. The mechanism by which control of individual gene function without changing the underlying DNA is called **epigenetics** (around genes) and understanding of it began in the 1990s. Epigenetic modifications can dramatically change how well a gene is expressed or even if it is expressed at all. Any epigenetic modification must be able to be passed on so that control of gene expression is passed on from mother to daughter cell.

Many types of epigenetic modification have been discovered. One major is called **DNA methylation** which is the addition of a methyl group to the DNA base pair of cytosine-guanine, specifically to cytosine followed by a guanine – known as CpG. A methyl group is a very small molecule made up of one carbon atom linked to 3 hydrogen atoms (Carey 2011). This does not alter the underlying gene sequence as the C has been decorated rather than changed. Under most circumstances methylation at the start of a gene turns that gene off.

A second important epigenetic function is the modification of histone called **acetylation**. This is the addition of an acetyl chemical group to the amino acid lysine found in the protein tail of one of the histones. The result is known as **acetyl-lysine**. This may down regulate or up regulate the protein product of a particular gene.

Some key areas of interest in epigenetic mechanisms include:

- Control of the development of embryos
- Understanding how some genetic disorders occur
- Understanding the nature of cancer
- Environmental factors in epigenetics such as poor nutrition and stress (Francis 2011).

Abnormalities – Congenital defects

Congenital defects are present at birth. Some may be visible or they may be hidden, such as changes in protein molecules, e.g. haemoglobin. Not all congenital defects are inherited. Some result from environmental influences on the embryo. Congenital defects may occur because of the following factors:

- Genetic/chromosomal abnormalities may cause abnormality. Some genes (pleiotropic) support multiple functions and an abnormality may affect multiple systems. Some disorders may involve the interactions of many genes and are referred to as polygenic.
- Teratogens reach the foetus by crossing the placenta and cause DNA mutations. During organogenesis, the embryo is vulnerable to developmental disruption. Examples of teratogens are infectious agents such as feline panleukopenia virus, drugs such as griseofulvin and radiation.
- Multifactorial disorders are caused by the interaction of environment and genes, e.g. canine hip dysplasia.
- Idiopathic defects have no known cause; at present they are the largest group.

MUTATIONS

Genes usually produce their product faithfully but occasionally a mutation or alteration in the genetic material in a cell arises either naturally or because of the effects of environmental challenges called mutagens. These include radiation, chemical or physical stressors. Mutations can be minor changes in DNA or macromutations involving alterations of large amounts of a chromosome. Mutations often result in harmful or lethal defects. A few examples include:

- Point mutations of a single base cause amino acid substitutions resulting in faulty protein products, which may cause functional defects.
- Nonsense mutations involve the creation of a stop codon in the middle of a gene; the broken gene does not code for a protein product.
- In frameshift mutations additions or deletions of a nucleotide alter the reading frame of the DNA to the left or right so that triplet codons do not code for amino acids.

GENETIC DEFECTS

Slight differences in a protein brought about by a genetic mutation may cause devastating metabolic diseases such as **phosphofructokinase deficiency** in Cocker and Springer Spaniels. Not all diseases are due to alterations in metabolic pathways; some proteins have cellular structural roles while others control embryological development. Many feline and canine disorders have similarities to human diseases. Dogs share 85% of their genetic code with humans and over half of their genetic disorders mirror a human genetic disease (Guynup 2000), e.g. severe combined immunodeficiency disease (SCID) in Basset Hounds and Welsh Corgis.

Incidence

Research has identified many hundreds of inherited genetic defects in the cat. Many also afflict humans, including muscular dystrophy, polycystic kidney disease and retinal degeneration. Many genetic diseases have been identified in the dog and Donald Patterson, professor of medical genetics at Pennsylvania University, runs a 'canine genetic disease information system'. Over 500 genetic diseases had been recorded in dogs, with the poodle breed top of the list. Most inherited diseases are due to recessive genes (Ostrander & Ruvinsky 2012). The loss of genetic diversity in pure-bred animals means that most of these disorders have been found among specific breeds of animal rather than among the outbred mongrel or house cat. It is difficult to identify carriers of recessive disorders until affected offspring have been born from two apparently normal parents.

CHROMOSOMAL DEFECTS

Occasionally, whole chromosomes may be involved but such defects often result in stillbirth or spontaneous abortion. Numerical or structural changes may affect the autosomes or sex chromosomes.

Numerical chromosomal defects

Many of these numerical defects arise during failure of dysjunction, when sister chromatids fail to separate. This may result in too many or too few chromosomes:

- Polyploidy means the presence of multiples of the haploid number of chromosomes, i.e. three or more.
- Triploidy is the presence of three copies of each chromosome.
- Monosomy is when one of a chromosome pair is missing.
- Trisomy is the presence of an extra chromosome. Trisomy of the sex chromosomes is quite common and XXX females (triple X) or XXY males occur. This can lead to the unusual occurrence of a male tortoiseshell cat with the genotype 18XXY (18 pairs + X and Y and an extra X).
- Mosaicism results when the zygote develops into an individual with two genotypes or cell lines. The condition arises as a result of non-dysjunction during early mitosis.

Structural chromosomal defects

Pollution or radiation may induce breaks in chromosomes, resulting in macromutations. Two of these, inversion and translocation, may be transmitted from parent to offspring.

- Translocation is the transfer of a piece of one chromosome to another non-homologous chromosome. If the translocation is balanced, the normal complement of chromosomal material is received. There will be no abnormality. If the translocation results in extra chromosomal material, abnormality will occur.
- Deletion is the loss of part of a chromosome.
- Duplication is where a section of a chromosome is repeated; this is less harmful as there is no loss of chromosome material.
- Inversion occurs if a segment of a chromosome breaks free and becomes reattached in the reverse position.

Application to practice

THE GENOME PROJECTS

Over the last few decades identification of genes through the use of molecular genetics using DNA/RNA-based technologies has given rise to a new science of **genomics** or the study of the genome. Work has proceeded on various animal genomes, including feline and canine. Obtaining samples of DNA for study requires only a blood or saliva sample. Recent developments have greatly increased the speed at which DNA can be sequenced.

Researchers at Cornell University began sequencing the dog genome in 1990 and the genome of a female boxer dog called Tasha led the way. Similarly, Professor Stephen J. O'Brien began to study the genetics of the house cat in the 1970s. A low-resolution map of the feline genome was announced in 2005 when the DNA of an Abyssinian cat called Cinnamon was sequenced (Little 2008). As mentioned above, the domestic cat is known to have at least 250 genetic diseases, many of them having similarities to human diseases. Genome research is of importance not only to our cats and dogs but also to ourselves. Once an inherited trait has been identified to a specific location a DNA test can be created for it. The ethics of using the new technologies have to be considered and Meyers-Wallen (2003) discusses the problems clearly.

DIAGNOSIS OF DISORDERS

Although molecular genetics has provided sophisticated tests for identifying disorders there are other, more traditional ways of identifying risks for breeding animals and selecting against an inherited single gene problem. These are clinical screening, pedigree analysis and test matings. The technical methods include biochemical screening and DNA markers (Nicholas 2009).

Clinical screening

Although single-gene disorders give rise to serious problems such as inherited eye disorders in dogs and polycystic kidney disease in cats, they may not prevent animals from reproducing. Some disorders, especially dominant gene disorders such as feline polycystic kidney disease, can be identified by clinical examination and any affected animal prevented from breeding. The simplest way is to neuter them and sell them as pets.

Pedigree analysis

Breeders of pedigree animals are expected to keep meticulous pedigrees containing at least four generations. Studying the

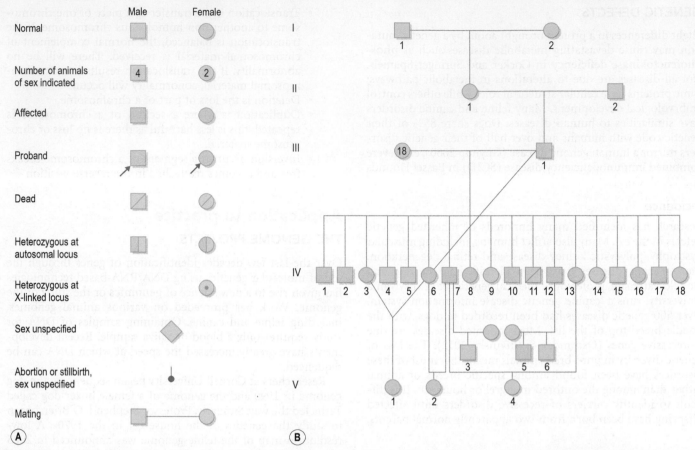

Fig. 15.8 (A) Symbols used in writing and interpreting pedigrees; a proband is an affected individual through whom the family came to the notice of an investigator. (B) BOA pedigree, showing the pattern of inheritance of multiple exostoses in horses. (*Reproduced with permission from Nicholas, F.W., 2009. Introduction to Veterinary Genetics, second ed. Blackwell, Oxford.*)

pedigree can help to estimate the probability that a prospective parent may be homozygous for a particular gene. There is also a retrospective use of pedigrees. When an animal has been born with a genetic disease, closely related parents who may be carriers can be identified and test matings may be carried out. Specific symbols are used to make interpretation of pedigrees universal (Fig. 15.8).

Test matings

These are time-consuming and may be expensive but allow the breeder to identify the source of an abnormal allele. The concept will be discussed more fully in Chapter 16.

Biochemical screening

Some diseases are caused by the lack of a specific protein that acts as a catalyst or an enzyme in a metabolic process. If the disease process leaves a biochemical marker in blood or other readily obtainable tissue, a biochemical screening test can be developed. Sometimes the heterozygote carrier of the gene has reduced manufacture of the particular protein and can be identified by the test.

DNA technologies

DNA technologies are being increasingly used to identify genes associated with defects. The techniques include the use of restriction enzymes, polymerase chain reaction (PCR) and

Southern blotting. Nicholas (2009) gives a good account of these techniques in Chapter 2 of his book.

Restriction enzymes. In 1970 scientists discovered that bacteria produce enzymes that can break down any foreign DNA that enters their cells. These enzymes restrict viruses from damaging the bacterium, hence the name restriction enzymes. They cut the foreign DNA at specific sites into pieces of varying lengths, and these fragments can be isolated and cloned (making multiple identical copies). If a fragment is inserted into a suitable vector, such as the small circular DNA found in some bacteria called plasmids, the resulting DNA is called recombinant DNA (rDNA).

Polymerase chain reaction (PCR). Cloning can produce many copies of a particular fragment to use in gene sequencing. Another use for cloning is the manufacture of a genomic library which could contain most of the DNA for that species. These libraries are then used to track down specific genes, including those causing inherited disease. PCR, developed in 1985, is widely used in the detection of particular genes. PCR rapidly produces more than a million copies of DNA. The original DNA can be from a cell or from any source: from a living cell, a museum specimen, a single sperm or a hair follicle.

Southern blotting. The technique is named after Ed Southern, who developed it in 1975. Depending on their length, fragments of DNA will travel different distances through a gel when an electric current is passed through it. This is called gel electrophoresis. The fragments are denatured into single strands, separated by size and blotted onto either a nitrocellulose or nylon membrane. The membrane is baked in an oven to fix the DNA and then bathed in a solution containing labelled (with a substance that fluoresces), denatured DNA probes. The strands will combine with any complementary strand in the solution. The unattached probes are washed off, leaving the matched DNA.

Examples of screening for specific canine and feline defects

KENNEL CLUB AND BRITISH VETERINARY ASSOCIATION

In the UK the Kennel Club (KC), together with the British Veterinary Association (BVA), currently have three screening schemes for inherited conditions. These are inherited eye conditions (including peripheral retinal atrophy), hip dysplasia and elbow dysplasia.

Generalised progressive retinal atrophy

Although there are different types of generalised progressive retinal atrophy (PRA) most forms are inherited as an autosomal recessive trait (Dekomien & Epplen 2003). The genetic cause varies between breeds, making a single diagnostic DNA test difficult. Homozygous animals develop degeneration of the peripheral retina, leading to night blindness and loss of visual fields. Typically the disease progresses to complete blindness. Genetic testing is available under the eye scheme for the Irish setter but the BVA maintain a list of other breeds indicating the approximate age at which the deterioration can be diagnosed by ophthalmoscope.

Canine hip dysplasia – a multifactorial problem

Unfortunately, some serious disorders are not caused by a single gene or even a combination of genetic effects (polygenic). There may also be an environmental factor predisposing animals to a disease, i.e. the disease is multifactorial. One of these diseases is canine hip dysplasia. Hip dysplasia is a major congenital canine health problem. Large pedigree dogs such as Labradors are more prone to it but smaller dogs and mongrels may also suffer. There is abnormal formation of the 'ball and socket' hip joint. Normally the head of the femur fits snugly into the socket. Dogs with a genetic disposition are born with normal hips but as they grow the structure of the joint becomes deformed so that the head does not fit into the socket and the joint does not rotate smoothly. The dog becomes lame and may have difficulty climbing stairs. It may walk with a waddle; the result is a painful, crippling arthritis.

Many factors work together to cause this disease. The dog must be genetically at risk, but environmental factors, especially nutrition and exercise, bring about the symptoms. There may be excess calcium in puppy food, obesity and high-protein and high-calorie diets. Incorrect levels of exercise (too much or too little) also produce symptoms, but the continued breeding of dogs with hip dysplasia is a major contributor.

Total elimination of the disease may be unrealistic but selective breeding of dogs with good hips can reduce the incidence. The BVA and the KC run a scheme to test for hip dysplasia, which helps the breeder to choose good breeding stock.

Radiographs from dogs more than 1 year old are submitted to ensure that skeletal maturity is sufficient. An overall hip score based on examination of specific sites for malformation in both joints is calculated. A list of breed mean scores (BMS) is published and breeders are recommended to ensure that their breeding stock has scores well below the BMS for their breed of dog.

Elbow dysplasia

Elbow dysplasia is a degenerative polygenic inherited disease of the elbow joint. The causes, diagnosis and management are similar to hip dysplasia. The Orthopaedic Foundation for Animals maintains an elbow registry and elbows can be graded from normal through grades 1, 2 and 3 as the severity of the radiographic appearance increases. Three main disorders may occur singly or in combination:

- Fragmented medial coronoid process
- Osteochondritis of the medial humeral condyle
- Ununited anconeal process.

Elbow dysplasia occurs mainly in larger dogs and is breed-related. The incidence ranges from 0% in Border collies to 47.8% in chow chows. Male dogs are more likely to be affected than females and in 20–35% of cases both elbows are affected. Affected dogs should probably be removed from the breeding programme, although the severity of symptoms is only loosely related to the radiographic signs.

International Cat Care (formerly the Feline Advisory Bureau)

International Cat Care organise a screening program for the autosomal dominant problem – **polycystic kidney disorder (PKD)**. In PKD a large number of fluid-filled cysts form within the kidneys. The cysts are present from birth but increase in size until they damage the surrounding kidney tissue and cause kidney failure (Fig. 15.9). The cat will eventually die, despite supportive treatment. The disease is peculiar to Persian cats and any breed of cat where they have been included, such as the Tiffany.

The problem has become widespread in these breeds because the disease is an unfortunate combination of an autosomal dominant gene, so that only one parent needs to be affected by

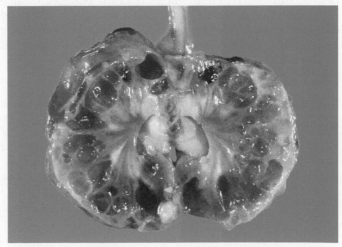

Fig. 15.9 Cross-section of a severely affected kidney showing cysts throughout. (Reproduced with permission of the Feline Advisory Bureau.)

PKD, and one in two of any offspring will be affected; also, it is a condition whose symptoms may not be obvious until the age of 7 or 8, by which time the cat may have produced several litters of kittens, 50% of whom would be affected.

International Cat Care provide a PKD screening scheme that relies on ultrasonography of the kidneys, looking for the presence of cysts. This is best done when the cat is more than 10 months old. This enables breeders to make informed decisions about which cats to use for breeding

Feline erythrocyte pyruvate kinase deficiency (PKDef)

Enzymes are proteins which speed up metabolic reactions. Genetic mutations may alter enzymes so that normal metabolism cannot occur. Pyruvate kinase (PK) is an enzyme involved in breaking down glucose to release energy inside intracellular mitochondria. During this glucose cycle, PK converts phosphoenol pyruvate (PEP) to pyruvic acid.

Mature erythrocytes (red blood cells) lose their mitochondria but can still produce enough adenosine triphosphate (ATP) to cope with wear and repair. PK deficiency, especially common in Somali and Abyssinian cats, prevents energy production, resulting in irreversible cell membrane injury and premature haemolysis that leads to anaemia. PKDef is recessively inherited and an affected cat inherits an abnormal gene from each parent. To summarise:

- Animals with one copy of the abnormal gene are carriers and show no signs of disease.
- The progeny of two carriers will have a 1 in 4 chance of being affected or normal, and a 1 in 2 chance of carrying the disorder.

There is now a diagnostic test available from Bristol University for detecting both carriers and sufferers. Obtaining samples of DNA for study requires only a blood or saliva sample.

PK deficiency can also affect various breeds of dog and is a very severe disease. Affected dogs die mainly before they are 4 years old. Cats do not generally develop severe problems and may have a normal life span; however, they may develop intermittent anaemia with variable symptoms. Some develop severe lethargy, weakness, anorexia and lose weight and they may have pale mucous membranes. Damaged red cells are removed from the blood by the spleen, resulting in an enlarged spleen, and the destruction of red cells results in the release of bilirubin, causing jaundice. However, the body is good at making new red blood cells so anaemia is often mild or occurs gradually. Occasionally a severe, life-threatening anaemia may develop. The problem has been eradicated in Somali cats.

Feline blood grouping

Incompatible blood groups between the stud tomcat and the queen can lead to the devastating loss of whole litters of kittens. This problem can be solved by screening the prospective parents' blood and avoiding the mating of incompatible animals. One scheme for the identification of feline blood groups by screening is offered at the University of Glasgow by Dr Diane Addie, who also maintains a register of blood-typed stud toms and queens (Addie 2004). This problem is discussed further in Chapter 16.

Future trends in biotechnology
CLONING OF ANIMALS

Genetically identical animals are produced naturally every time an early embryo splits into two or more to produce identical twins, triplets, etc. From the 1970s embryos have been split in the laboratory and each of the resulting embryos inserted into a different mother. This form of cloning has been widespread in livestock breeding (Nicholas 2009). Cloning by transferring the nucleus of a somatic cell into an unfertilised ovum was introduced in the 1980s, culminating in the birth of Dolly the sheep in February 1997. Since then many animals have been cloned in this way but the technology has major problems:

- The success rate is very low – only 1–2% of cloned embryos survive.
- Many die soon after birth.
- Survivors suffer from abnormalities, including abnormal enzyme expression and poor immunity.

If the technique can be perfected, gene replacement will be more effective, replacement organs and tissues could be grown and it could be used in the conservation of rare species.

TRANSGENESIS

Transgenesis involves the insertion of genes from one species to another, e.g. a human gene into a pig. As the genetic code is universal the transferred gene will work in its new environment. The new animal is described as transgenic. The first transgenic animals were mice produced in 1980. Pigs and sheep were produced to manufacture human growth hormone in 1985. The technique is mainly used in disease research. Another use is in the production of human polypeptides for use in pharmaceuticals. Financial and ethical considerations may limit the use of this technique.

GENE THERAPY

Therapeutic uses of recombinant DNA techniques include gene therapy, i.e. 'the deliberate introduction of genetic material into human somatic cells for therapeutic, prophylactic or diagnostic purposes' (UK Gene Therapy Advisory Committee definition quoted in Turnpenny & Ellard 2011). When the gene enters the new cell it may change the way the cell works or the chemicals that the cell secretes. The identification of many abnormal genes and their products has led to possibilities of treatments for some important diseases, both human and animal. It overcomes the major problem of transplantation, as genes work within the cell and are not affected by immune rejection. It is unlikely to be of use in animal therapy, where best practice would prevent breeding from any abnormal animals by carrier detection.

BIBLIOGRAPHY

Addie, D., 2004. What Are Feline Blood Groups? Available online at: <http://www.dr-addie.com/Blood%20groups.htm> (accessed 13.8.2015).

Carey, N., 2011. The Epigenetics Revolution. Icon Books Ltd, London.

Dekomien, G., Epplen, J.T., 2003. Evaluation of the canine RPE65 gene in affected dogs with generalized progressive retinal atrophy. Mol. Vis. 9, 601–605.

Dog Genetic Disease, 2009. RUF Dog Health Problems. <http://doghealthproblems. co.uk/dog-genetic-disease/weeeee>.

Francis, R.C., 2011. Epigenetics: How Environment Shapes Our Genes. W W Norton, London.

Gould, L.L., 2007. Cats Are Not Peas, second ed. A K Peters, Copernicus, New York.

Guynup, S., 2000. Genetic Testing for Dogs. Genome News Network, Rockville, MD. Available online at: <http://www.genomenewsnetwork.org/articles/07_00/genetic_testing_dogs.shtml>.

Jorde, L., Carey, J., Bamshad, M.J., et al., 2006. Medical Genetics, third ed. (updated) Mosby, St Louis, MO.

Little, S., 2008. Feline Genetics: What Technicians Need to Know (proceedings). <http://veterinarycalenfdar.dvm360.com/avhc/Veterinary+technicians/Feline-genetics>.

Meyers-Wallen, V.N., 2003. Ethics and genetic selection in purebred dogs. Reprod. Domest. Anim. 38 (1), 73–76.

Nicholas, F.W., 2009. Introduction to Veterinary Genetics, third ed. Blackwell, Oxford.

Ostrander, E.A., Ruvinsky, A., 2012. The Genetics of the Dog. CABI Publishing, Wallingford.

PetEducation.com. Hip Dysplasia in Dogs: Diagnosis, Treatment and Prevention. Available at: <http://www.peteducation.com/article.cfm?c=2+1569&aid=444> (accessed 11.5. 2009).

Turnpenny, P., Ellard, S., 2011. Emery's Elements of Medical Genetics, thirteenth ed. Churchill Livingstone, Elsevier.

RECOMMENDED READING

Jorde, L., Carey, J., Bamshad, M.J., 2010. Medical Genetics, fourth ed. Mosby, St Louis, MO.

This textbook on medical genetics presents its subject matter clearly and is illustrated by good diagrams. Although it is aimed at those interested in human genetics, the basic science is presented in a sensible progression to maximise understanding.

Nicholas, F.W., 2009. Introduction to Veterinary Genetics, third ed. Blackwell, Oxford.

This is an excellent textbook on veterinary genetics. The detailed contents pages make it easy to follow and it progresses information from the basic sciences to application to future developments.

Pet Education.com. Hip Dysplasia in Dogs: Diagnosis, Treatment and Prevention. Available at: <http://www.peteducation.com/article.cfm?c=2+1569&aid=444> (accessed 11.5.2009).

This paper is included because of its comprehensive and up-to-date data about hip dysplasia.

16

Practical Animal Breeding

DOROTHY STABLES | GARETH LAWLER

KEY POINTS

- Pedigree animals are the result of selective breeding. Inbreeding, line breeding and outbreeding are strategies used by breeders to select for traits such as hair colour, body type and behaviour.

- Breeding stock, i.e. the stud male and the breeding bitch or queen, must be selected with care using criteria based on health, temperament and adherence to the breed standard.

- The mating process usually takes place on the stud male's territory and must be carefully monitored to avoid injury to either individual.

- The dam must be cared for during pregnancy and consideration must be given to nutrition, exercise, vaccination and preventative worming treatment.

- Parturition takes place in three stages and knowledge of these will ensure the delivery of healthy offspring.

- In some cases the dam may need assistance or the neonate may need extra care in order to survive.

- Colostrum ingested within the first 24 hours of life provides protective antibodies for the neonate.

- All kittens and puppies should receive preventative health care (vaccination and parasite control) dependent on the offspring's age.

- All pedigree animals can be registered with the appropriate organisation.

Introduction

The aim of this chapter is to provide an insight into breeding pedigree animals from a breeder's point of view. The two authors, Dorothy Stables (cat breeder) and Gareth Lawler (dog breeder), are both experienced breeders and in the following two sections they explain how they produce healthy kittens and puppies.

Breeding pedigree cats

About 200 million years ago, mammals arose. They coexisted with the huge dinosaurs and were small, warm-blooded, covered in fur and fed their babies with milk but probably also laid eggs. By 65 million years ago there were many species but suddenly all the dinosaurs disappeared, as did the majority of birds and fishes. Something cataclysmic happened, possibly the arrival of an immense asteroid that landed in the Caribbean Sea. Clouds of dust cut out the light from the sun. The small, warm-blooded mammals could control their own body temperatures and were

at an advantage, so most survived. By 45 million years ago all the major groups of mammals alive today had evolved. True cats are found in the fossil records from about 25 million years ago.

Feline domestication may have begun in Egypt. The African wild cat (*Felis libyca*) began to live around the grain stores, catching small rodents. Gradually the more tame amongst them allowed humans to play with their kittens. Domestication led to selective breeding for favoured features such as hair colour and length.

SELECTIVE BREEDING

Pedigree animals are the result of selective breeding, where specific favourable traits are chosen to be perpetuated by the breeder. In the latter half of the 19th century people started to breed specific types of cat and over the last century about 30 recognised breeds have been developed (Fig. 16.1). Alterations in features occur because natural mutations are already present in wild cats. Generally, one of the two alleles for a characteristic such as coat colour mutates but is recessive. When two cats both carrying the mutated gene mate, a new characteristic appears (see Chapter 15).

BREEDING STRATEGIES

'The good and bad points of the individual cats (or dogs) should be assessed and weighed against each other before mating' (Vella et al 1999):

- **Inbreeding** is the mating of closely related individuals such as father and daughter or siblings. How closely these animals are related can be calculated using the mathematical concept of the inbreeding coefficient, which can be defined as 'the probability that the two genes present at a locus in an individual are identical by descent'.

- **Line breeding** is the mating of animals with shared ancestors but not as closely related as in inbreeding. The word 'line' is probably related to the term 'blood line'. Both strategies are used by breeders to select for desired traits, but there is a risk with mating related animals that they may both carry a harmful recessive gene and this would be expressed in the homozygous individual – a condition known as **inbreeding depression**. Advances in genetics should help breeders to identify and eliminate many harmful genes over the next few years.

- **Outbreeding** or the mating of two unrelated individuals is a method of reducing inbreeding depression. Cross-breeds, mongrels or simply 'domestic house cats' are the extreme form of outbreeding. However, Vella et al. (1999) quote Joan Miller, then vice president of the Winn Feline Foundation, as saying that 'In the majority

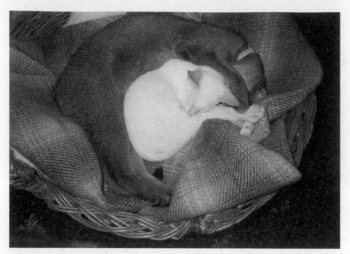

Fig. 16.1 Two short-haired breeds; a Usual Abyssinian neuter male cuddling a red point Siamese male kitten

of breeds it is now impossible to find two cats unrelated to each other because every pedigree is based on a few early founding cats'.

- **Gene linkage** is another problem associated with selecting closely related animals and is a situation where a desired trait may carry with it an abnormality – if the two genes lie close together on a chromosome they may be inherited together (see Chapter 15); for example, blue eyes are often associated with white coat colour and deafness.

Two inheritable feline characteristics, coat colour and behaviour, are briefly discussed to show why an understanding of genetics is important for cat breeders.

Coat colour

Pigment production – genes in the melanocytes at the base of the hair follicles influence the production of hair pigments. As discussed in Chapter 15 (Box 15.2), eumelanin is a black pigment and phaeomelanin produces a yellowish ground colour. The dominant gene that controls the colour deposition known as agouti (A) produces agouti protein 'A', which gives a hair that is black at the tip and yellow at the base. Its recessive partner, which codes for non-agouti, is designated 'a'. When the amount of agouti protein within the melanocytes reaches a certain level, production of eumelanin stops and that of phaeomelanin begins.

All cats have a second system of pigmentation superimposing a pattern of dark markings on the agouti coat. Some areas of skin have a poor response to agouti protein and then the hairs are coloured from base to tip by eumelanin and are black. Alternating bands of agouti and black produce the tabby pattern. In cats who are homozygous for the recessive mutation called non-agouti 'a/a', a defective agouti protein is produced that does not affect eumelanin production. The phenotype of these cats is the self (solid) black cat.

Coat colour genes – the three basic colours, black, chocolate and cinnamon, are coded for by the gene TYRP1 or tyrosine-related protein or mutants of that gene. This gene is called the B locus. The enzyme produced by TYRP1 is located in melanocytes, which produce the melanin that gives animal skin, hair and eyes their colour. TYRP1 may stabilise the enzyme tyranosinase, which is responsible for the first step in melanin production. Two different mutations of this gene give the two shades of brown known as chocolate (b-) and cinnamon (b^1/b^1 recessive) (Lyons et al 2005). Testing for these changes in the TYRP1 gene is now available at different laboratories and can determine which gene is present and therefore the colour of the cat if, as in the Somali cat, it may not be clear to the eye.

The three basic colours can be modified by the presence of other genes:

- The dominant inhibitor gene (I) suppresses the amount of pigment fed into the hair, resulting in the presence of white hairs with coloured tips.
- The recessive dilute gene (dd) causes pigment granules to be enlarged and deposited unevenly along the hair: the hair may be very lightly pigmented.
- The sex-linked orange (O) gene causes the production of phaeomelanin, resulting in a male ginger cat or female tortoiseshell.

Behaviour

Behaviour is partly instinctive (inherited) and partly learned. However, instinctive behaviour is fine-tuned by learning. Fogle (1991) believes that we can attribute human mental characteristics to cats because their brains are wired up like ours. Cats learn quickly and anticipate events such as feeding. My cat Filly remembers that she is fed separately from the other cats so she does not run into the kitchen with the rest of the cats, but goes to where her food is served.

Learning requires input from parents, littermates and humans (Turner & Bateson 2013). Socialisation is the breeder's responsibility (see Chapter 12). There is a sensitive period from 2 to 7 weeks when kittens need handling for at least 40 min a day if they are to interact with humans. Petting, playing with and talking to them (Fig. 16.2) is more important than feeding for their social development (Karsh 1983; Halls 2007). Behaviour must be considered when choosing a kitten for breeding or showing.

BREEDING PRACTICES

Rice (1997) suggests that professional cat breeders take cat breeding seriously, with 'carefully planned agendas and well-defined motives'. They may wish to develop a particular breed to enhance certain desirable features such as coat colour or head shape, or they may wish to breed for showing. Two examples of problems occurring in pedigree cats are outlined below.

Deafness in white cats

Congenital deafness is seen almost exclusively in white-coated cats. It is caused by degeneration of the auditory apparatus of the inner ear and may be unilateral or bilateral, linked to whether the cat has one or two blue eyes. Breeding studies have shown a relationship between deafness in white cats and blue eye colour. The responsible gene is dominant and pleiotropic (see Chapter 15). A number of breeds insist on white cats being checked for deafness (International Cat Care 2014).

Brachycephaly in Persian Cats

Brachycephaly refers to the abnormal short head shape with flattened face seen in Persian cats. It is associated with breathing difficulties, dental disease, difficulties in grooming and irritation and ulceration of the eyes and face, all long-lasting

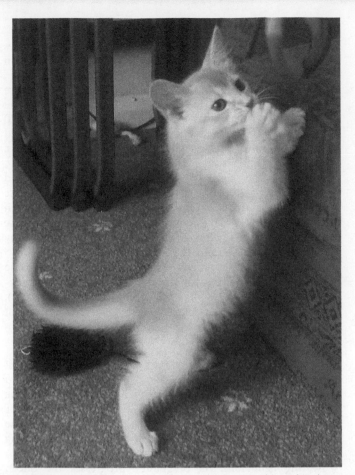

Fig. 16.2 Mistral, a red silver male Somali kitten aged 8 weeks, playing with an unseen human

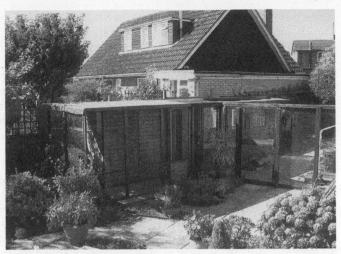

Fig. 16.3 Typical stud quarters

conditions that cause discomfort and pain. Schlueter et al. (2009) described four categories in head shape depending on the severity of the deformity. The condition has a genetic background but so far, no genes have been identified. In Germany there is already a ban on breeding from cats whose nose tip is higher than the level of the lower eyelid. It would be easy for the feline governing bodies to adopt a policy of banning registration, showing and breeding categories 3 and 4.

Buying a breeding queen

Before buying a breeding queen, consider the following:
- Is the home environment suitable for rearing kittens? Ornaments may not survive a healthy litter of kittens and trailing wires may be dangerous.
- Is the expense prohibitive?
- It is better to buy a kitten rather than an older queen so that there is time to develop a bond before the first litter of kittens comes along. The potential queen should be visited in her home and her siblings and mother should be observed for type and behaviour. If the stud is owned by the breeder he should also be looked at. The pedigrees of the animal should be checked to exclude potential problems:
  - Is there a suitable stud cat in the vicinity? Some of the rarer breeds of cat may be scattered around the country, requiring a lengthy journey with a howling queen!

- Although all kittens will have had a health check when they were vaccinated, new owners may wish their own vet to examine the kitten before purchasing it.
- The new owner should receive a receipt of purchase, a four-generation pedigree, a certificate of kitten registration and transfer of ownership with a suitable body such as the Governing Council of the Cat Fancy (GCCF), certificate of vaccination and advice on caring for the kitten.

The stud cat

Most breeders will not sell a stud tom to someone until they have been breeding for 4 or 5 years and own two or three queens. He will need his own quarters (Fig. 16.3) near to the house because of urine spraying. They will need to be airy in summer and heated in winter, with a run attached so that he can exercise. The owner should be able to sit in with the stud and play with him.

If he is to have visiting queens there should be suitable quarters where the queen can be kept near to him, but can be separated if the need arrives. He should be introduced to his stud quarters at about 16 weeks old so that by the time he matures he is happy and familiar with his own territory. A stud tom should be chosen with as much care as a breeding queen. His pedigree should be studied and discussed to avoid any relationships between the queens and the stud.

THE MATING PROCESS

The queen

Sexual maturity in a queen occurs between 5 and 12 months. However, she may not be physically or psychologically ready to have kittens and should be at least 1 year old before mating (Rice 1997). She could be allowed a breeding life of about 5 years during which she should have no more than two litters every 18 months.

Queens show few obvious physical signs of the oestrous cycle or being 'in heat' although some develop pinkness and a slight swelling of the tissue around their vaginal orifice. However, their behaviour can be quite dramatic, with vocalisation (calling) and posturing. Naïve owners have taken a queen to the vet because she was crying so loudly they thought she was in pain! Because a queen may be ready to mate without showing signs, no entire female should be allowed to go outside. The local tomcats from miles around will know she is ready!

Oestrus, which can last from 3–10 days, often begins with the queen rolling around on the floor and purring. She then shows lordosis, which involves lowering her chest, lifting up her bottom and placing her tail to one side while treading with her back legs. During this time the female will allow the male to mount and copulate. Oestrus is shortened if the queen is mated.

Cats are induced ovulators, which maximises the chance of fertilisation. Copulation releases luteinising hormone (LH), which stimulates ovulation (see Chapter 6). The level of LH increases with each copulation so that fertilisation and pregnancy are more likely to occur. As the penis is withdrawn from the queen's vagina the scratching of the papillae or spines covering the glans penis may stimulate a rise in LH levels.

The stud cat

A tom shows signs of sexual activity at about 7–8 months of age and may mate with a receptive queen. From about 10 months old he is capable of fathering kittens but this does not mean he is ready to work. The owner must allow time for him to mature.

Boy meets girl

The queen is usually taken to the stud for mating. Some males prefer their own territory, as it gives them confidence. A receptive queen should be introduced to him carefully. She may be left in her carrying basket to see how the two cats react. The journey may affect the queen and it may be 24 hours before she returns to being receptive. A maiden queen should be taken to an experienced tom and a young tom should be allowed a mature, experienced queen for his first mating. If all seems well they should be allowed to have physical contact with each other. She may show her willingness by calling, rolling and flirting. The tom will respond by making a low, throaty noise. He watches for signs of acceptance and, at an opportune moment, runs in and grabs the queen by the neck. He has to be quick as she may attack him. The queen responds to the neck grasp as a kitten does, by remaining still while he mounts her (Morris 1996). With a few thrusts, he deposits his semen before withdrawing his penis. At this point the queen often screams loudly and turns to attack him. Each act of copulation takes only about 10 seconds.

Experienced studs have their escape route planned and will only let go when they can safely run. Both cats now settle down apart and vigorously wash their genital regions. Cats will mate several times in a day. Matings rarely require human intervention but it is wise to be nearby. Occasionally a tom may be too rough or a queen attack too harshly and the cats may need to be separated for a while.

Aftercare of the queen

After mating the queen may continue to call for a few days, so other entire males should not have access to her. After this, her appetite, reduced during calling, and her behaviour will return to normal. Her neck should be examined for tooth marks and any damage should be treated. Puncture wounds extending through the skin should always be examined by a veterinarian.

Pregnancy

The average length of pregnancy in the domestic cat is 63 days or 9 weeks, but a range of 58–70 days is accepted. If parturition occurs earlier than this the kittens may not be viable and if later, size problems may occur, requiring urgent intervention. There is no accepted blood or urine test available for diagnosing feline pregnancy. A vet may be able to palpate the foetuses at 15–20 days of gestation, but this is dangerous if done by inexperienced people as too much pressure may cause the loss of the kittens. Ultrasound imaging can be used from 15 days.

At 21 days the queen's nipples become more vascular and turn a rosy pink. Later the nipples grow larger and a discrete area of hair loss occurs around them, often aided by the queen plucking hairs. By 35 days there should be a noticeable increase in abdominal girth and by 49 days the individual kittens may be observed and felt to move.

A queen who fails to conceive may call again any time between 28 days and towards the end of the anticipated pregnancy. Some develop a phantom pregnancy (pseudocyesis), during which their abdomens increase in girth and they do not return to oestrus.

Care of the pregnant queen

Nutrition. As pregnancy progresses beyond the second week the queen requires more calories. Her daily calorie intake should increase by 70% and her body weight will steadily increase due to the rapid growth of the foetuses and the storage of fat for lactation (Rice 1997). This can be achieved by increasing the number of times a day she is fed from two to four and by giving her free access to whatever dried food she enjoys.

Nesting behaviour. As pregnancy progresses the queen seeks out a secluded place in which to have her kittens. She can be provided with two or three alternative places, which she will inspect and rearrange. If this is not done she will choose her own place, which could well be the sofa. A cardboard box that can be disposed of after the event makes an excellent nest. Commercial boxes are available (Fig. 16.4), but a queen may not like them. Any box should be large enough to allow her to stretch out and accommodate mother and kittens for at least 5 weeks. It should be enclosed, with an opening big enough for the mother to go in and out but high enough to keep the kittens confined. Bedding should be smooth and flat at first so that the kittens cannot find their way beneath the layers. A piece of synthetic fleece (Vetbed) over which a piece of sheeting can be placed is ideal. Material such as towels and blankets with loops should be avoided, as they may trap the kittens' claws and damage their feet.

Parturition

Cats usually give birth without human interference and queens who have been given too much attention during delivery have been known to abandon their kittens (Rice 1997). However, breeding for different body shapes has increased birth problems in the modern Siamese cat and the Persian cat.

A breeder should be ready to give assistance if necessary. Equipment likely to be needed includes:

- Haemostat forceps, dental floss and blunt-ended scissors for dealing with the umbilical cords
- An antiseptic solution in a shallow dish for sterilising the instruments
- Warm, disposable cloths for receiving the kittens
- Cotton swabs

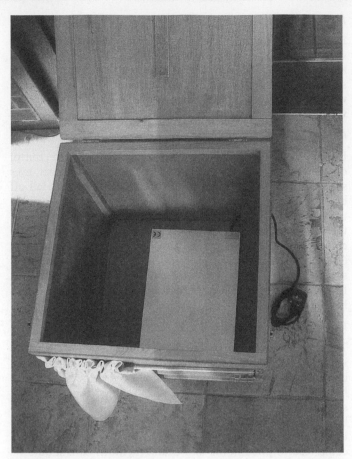

Fig. 16.4 A commercially made kittening box

- A 2 ml syringe without needle for neonatal resuscitation
- Bags for disposing of blood-stained articles.

Signs of parturition. The onset of parturition or labour can be predicted by taking the queen's rectal temperature every 8 hours for a day or two before the expected date of delivery (EDD). There will be a drop from the normal 38.5°C to 37°C about 12 hours before labour begins. Behavioural signs include reduced appetite, restlessness, pacing, making frequent visits to the nesting place, licking the genitalia and discomfort. My queens come for me when they are in early labour and insist on taking me to the delivery place! One young queen likes to get into a sleeping basket and cuddle up to her mother, an old neutered female.

During the first stage of labour, uterine contractions dilate the cervix and move the kittens towards the body of the uterus. There is usually a clear, odourless discharge of mucus, which may become tinged with blood just before delivery. Cats, though uncomfortable, rarely cry out but, in the presence of their owners, may purr loudly, which is thought to indicate low-grade pain. It is difficult to pinpoint the onset of the first stage but it probably is not necessary as long as the cat is not distressed. Normal progress is more important than length of time (Rice 1997).

The second stage is the delivery of the kittens, and the third stage, which usually follows immediately for each kitten, is the delivery of placenta and membranes. If the queen has been walking about she will now lie down in her kittening box. The uterine contractions become stronger and she will actively push. A bubble of amniotic fluid may appear at the vulva but this usually bursts and slightly blood-stained amniotic fluid escapes. It is not normal to see quantities of fresh blood.

Kittens may be born head first (anterior presentation) or tail and hind legs first (posterior presentation) but as long as progress is made it does not matter. This stage may take up to 1 hour for the first kitten and the length is best related to progress and frequency of contractions rather than time. It is shortened to about 5 minutes or less for subsequent kittens. Once the kitten is born the mother clears the membranes from its nose and mouth, chews and separates the umbilical cord and eats the placenta.

Following the birth of the first kitten there is usually a short delay of 10 minutes to 1 hour before the birth of the next kitten. This gives the mother time to clean the first kitten and for it to find a nipple and commence suckling. Occasionally labour is interrupted for a time and the mother rests happily with the kittens already born.

Assisted delivery. This is usually only necessary during the late second stage where a kitten has partially emerged but progress does not continue. Most queens will deliver themselves if time is allowed, as demonstrated by my own cat Scampy, who is small but progressed in labour very well until the time came to push. An hour went by and Scampy valiantly pushed with no obvious progress. I was about to call my vet when she suddenly leapt out of her box and wedged herself upright in the angle of a corner in a 'defecating position'. Two minutes later the first kitten popped out bottom first and the other three kittens followed quickly.

Normally, if the kitten is halfway out, gentle traction should be attempted. A dry cloth should be wrapped around the kitten and, taking care to avoid compressing internal organs, traction should be applied to complete the delivery. The direction of traction is important: it should follow the shape of the feline birth canal downwards towards the mother's feet and backwards away from her body.

Resuscitating a kitten. Newborn kittens soon establish regular respirations. If a kitten continues gasping or if bubbles of fluid are coming down its nose and out of its mouth, help is needed. The mouth and nostrils should be wiped and suction using a small syringe can be used to extract mucus. A vigorous drying with a warm towel may stimulate respiration.

If the kitten is still in difficulty, some suggest holding the kitten belly down wrapped in a cloth so it is not slippery. Vigorous rubbing of the kitten and removal of any fluids from the mouth by using cotton buds is required. Puppies and kittens should never be swung as this causes cerebral haemorrhage.

Completion of parturition. Ensure that all the placentas are delivered and that there is no heavy bleeding. The kittens should be warm, dry and vigorous and have found a nipple to suckle (Fig. 16.5). Following the birth the queen will clean herself and may even take a little food and water. She may not pass urine for 24 hours and will then pass a large quantity. She should resume normal defecation at the same time.

CARING FOR THE FAMILY

The kittens should only be checked to ensure that their condition is satisfactory. The family should be given a peaceful and

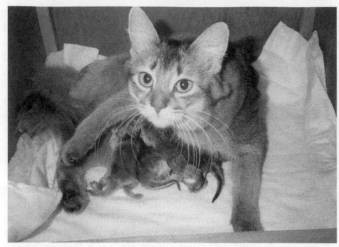

Fig. 16.5 Molly, a chocolate Somali, feeding her newborn kittens

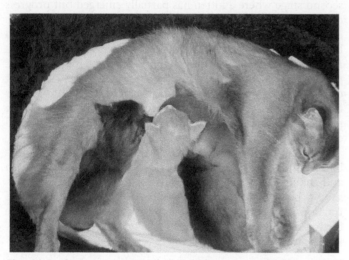

Fig. 16.6 Scampy, a tortoiseshell Somali queen, and her sex-linked kittens – a red male, a cream male and two tortie females

quiet environment to ensure that the queen accepts and cares for them (Fig. 16.6). After 3 days a confident queen will allow handling of her kittens.

The queen's milk provides all necessary nutrients. Colostrum provides all the antibodies the kittens need. The hair from around the nipples could be trimmed before birth if the queen has long hair. The first 6 weeks put a great strain on the queen's nutritional status: she may lose 25% of her body weight and will need extra food. Once the kittens begin to eat solid food the queen's food intake will decrease, although she will continue to suckle them until they go to their new homes. Her mammary glands should be inspected frequently for signs of sore nipples or mastitis and her milk will gradually reduce as the kittens eat more.

Most queens spend 90% of their time with their kittens during the first 2 weeks (Rice 1997). She will lick their urogenital area to stimulate them to pass urine and faeces and consume their excretions until they are weaned. If the queen is disturbed or if the bedding becomes soiled she may move her kittens.

Neonatal examination

Each kitten should be carefully examined for any abnormality such as extra digits or cleft palate. The sex and weight of each kitten are recorded. If the littermates are all the same colour some breeders identify them early by marking up a specific claw with nail polish. A spot of the same colour or notification of which toe is coloured is made in their records.

Ongoing development

Development proceeds in a craniocaudal manner, with control of the head, forelegs and hind legs developing in that order. Eyes should open between days 8 and 10 and cords usually fall off between the 3rd and 6th day. By 3 weeks the kittens wobble unsteadily around the inside of their box and a few days later they climb out and begin to explore. Specialised kitten food can now be fed to them. The aim is to wean them by about 6 weeks. As soon as the kittens begin to eat solid food they should be provided with a litter tray. They will play in this at first, digging holes. Shortly afterwards they will use it for its intended purpose.

Hand-rearing kittens

There are times when the mother is incapable of feeding her kittens or has so many she cannot cope. The young kittens must be kept warm, dry and clean and will need to be fed every 2 hours day and night for 3 weeks. It is important to obtain special kitten milk, as cow's milk is not suitable. It is possible to buy miniature bottles and teats but an eye dropper is equally useful. Care must be taken to avoid aspiration of milk, which could lead to pneumonia and death. As much care should be taken over sterilising the feeding equipment as would be used for a human baby, as infection is a great killer of young animals. If the queen is not caring for the kittens at all, their anal and vulval regions must be stimulated gently with damp, warm cotton wool to enable them to urinate and defecate.

Aftercare of the litter

Vaccination. Cats are subject to some dangerous pathogenic organisms and may become seriously ill or die, so all kittens should be vaccinated. In the UK the first vaccinations are given at nine weeks, followed by a repeated dose at 12 weeks. Typically a kitten is vaccinated against feline panleucopenia (feline infectious enteritis), feline respiratory viruses (cat flu) and leukaemia (International Cat Care 2008). Show cats may also be vaccinated against *Chlamydia*.

Worming. All kittens should be treated for the roundworm *Toxocara cati*. Although the lifecycle (see Chapter 29) of this worm means that the larvae do not cross the placenta into the foetal kittens, they do pass into the mammary glands so the kittens become infected when taking their first drink. Kittens should be routinely treated from 1 month old, repeated at monthly intervals until the kitten is 6 months of age and then every 3 months throughout life.

Registering and selling kittens

All pedigree kittens have to be registered with a formal organisation if they are to be sold as pedigree cats, used in a breeding programme or shown. In the UK the Governing Council of the Cat Fancy (GCCF) is the main organisation. Details of the kittens' parents and grandparents, their sex, colour and birth date are recorded.

It is essential to find a good home for the kittens and most breeders wish to meet the prospective purchasers before a sale is agreed. Some will deliver the kitten to its new home as a final check on suitability. The breeder must provide the purchaser with:

- A four-generation signed pedigree
- The vaccination certificate
- A certificate of transfer of ownership
- A receipt of payment.

Also recommended are:

- An advice sheet on caring for their kitten
- Insurance to cover the first 6 weeks following transfer
- Contact readily provided to discuss problems.

Showing cats

The first major cat show in the world was held at the Crystal Palace on 23 July 1871, organised by Harrison Weir. The shows are run by the official bodies such as the GCCF and certificates and titles are awarded. Kittens can be shown from 14 weeks and queens can be shown 12 weeks after they have given birth. Any cat that attends a show is 'vetted in' and may be excluded from the show if it appears ill, is pregnant, has dirty ears, fleas or other parasites or has a skin lesion of any kind. If a cat is taken ill during the show there is a duty vet to see to it and a room is set aside as a hospital. Cat breeding is challenging and rewarding as long as the breeder follows the rules.

Breeding pedigree dogs

SELECTIVE BREEDING

The artificial evolution of dogs into many different types with morphological diversity and variation in size, which is seen in few other species, is a direct consequence of years of selective breeding by man. This has resulted in the creation of a range of purebreds with individual traits and characteristics. Modern-day breeds are a standardisation of the desirable traits of some of the older breeds, especially those characteristics that have been useful over long periods of time. It is, or at least should be, the aim of dog breeders today to attempt to perpetuate those traits while simultaneously paying great heed to the maintenance of a friendly disposition, a characteristic so essential for a family pet, and a dog that will be healthy.

BREEDING STRATEGIES

For definitions of inbreeding and line breeding, return to the section on cat breeding.

The brood bitch

The most valuable asset for anyone striving to breed good stock is a good brood bitch. There is more to breeding dogs than just producing pretty-looking specimens and the aim is to produce puppies that are sound both mentally and physically. Consider the following factors:

- Health – avoid a bitch that has a history of ill health.
- Temperament and disposition – until the puppies go to their new homes, the pups continually learn from and even mimic the mother. Do not even consider a bitch as a breeding prospect if she shows any behavioural issues, including separation anxiety and noise phobias.
- Freedom from hereditary diseases – there is increasing awareness of breed-specific hereditary traits and many breeds now require certain health checks before breeding. By the time a breeder reaches this stage, they should be fully aware of the problems the respective breed may have and which tests are required prior to breeding. DNA testing and radiographs are both examples of some of the diagnostics that can be required.
- Breed standard – as well as exhibiting special traits of the lines concerned, she should descend from very good specimens of the breed and should not depart by any significant degree from the breed standard. Using the Mate Select tool on the Kennel Club website will enable breeders to establish whether their dog is suitable to breed from, and the likelihood of offspring suffering from any heredity disorders.
- Inheritability – the ability of the bitch to pass on desirable features to her offspring.

No expense should be spared in the acquisition of a suitable bitch for breeding, as she will prove her worth time and time again. The brood bitch is the key to the immediate future because she has much more influence on her puppies than just her contribution to their genetic make-up. You should never be tempted to breed from an immature bitch. Age of maturity differs between breeds and some breed clubs have introduced 'codes of ethics' pertaining to the minimum age for breeding from your bitch. It is essential that she is allowed to mature both physically and mentally so that she will have the confidence to cope with her own litter.

The bitch should be kept in the peak of condition, during her pregnancy and also prior to mating. She should be up-to-date with her vaccinations before mating, and she must also have been wormed regularly.

Some stud dog owners require all visiting bitches to have a vaginal swab tested as a precaution against any foreign bacteria or infections before they will use their dog. The veterinary surgeon will prescribe appropriate medication to clear any infection prior to mating, as long as the bitch is swabbed as early as possible during her season.

The stud dog

In a similar way to the brood bitch, whatever the breed, quality or even pedigree, the stud dog should satisfy some basic criteria before he is deemed suitable to pass his genes to the next generation. He must be sexually mature, entire and in good health, both physically and mentally, and, ideally, he should be mature in growth and development. It is unwise to use a young male before he has developed his adult characteristics, as he may depart from the breed standard as he matures. Some hereditary conditions, e.g. hip dysplasia and progressive retinal atrophy, are not always obvious until the dog is well into middle or old age. The older a dog is, and the more bitches he has covered, the smaller the chance of him producing an 'affected' puppy if he has not already done so.

The choice of stud dog should result from exhaustive research and breeders should be aware that no dog is suitable for every bitch.

THE MATING GAME

The bitch will normally come into season every 6 months, although some bitches, particularly in the larger breeds, cycle every 8–10 months. It is not uncommon for some bitches to go as long as 12 months between seasons. The period of oestrus or 'heat' usually lasts about 1 weeks, and the most notable sign is vaginal bleeding. Bitches vary as to the stage of the heat when they start to bleed, many starting almost at day 1 and others not until the end of the first week. Vaginal swelling is another sign of oestrus.

The optimum time to mate should be at the time the bitch ovulates. Bitches are spontaneous ovulators and textbooks indicate that the bitch ovulates on day 10 of the cycle; however, this can be variable and may be difficult to assess in some bitches. It is a fact that some bitches will ovulate as early as day 3 or as late as day 23. There are several tests available now to determine the exact time of ovulation and thus the optimum time for mating. These involve monitoring vaginal cytology and a hormonal assay. If the bitch has had a history of unsuccessful matings, it is advisable to seek veterinary advice and have, if necessary, daily or twice daily blood samples taken to determine an accurate ovulation time. It is as well to remember that, whatever the chosen method, conception and pregnancy, even when all eventualities have seemingly been covered, pregnancy can never be guaranteed.

The process of mating involves mounting by the dog and then the 'tie' during which the penis is locked into the bitch's vagina by the contraction of her vaginal muscles. The actual mechanics of mating are another potential pitfall. Some matings may take a matter of seconds before a 'tie' results, while others take rather longer. Some bitches will develop an exceptionally strong liking for a particular male, so strong that all other males may be rejected. Very often males will mount and dismount the bitch for a period of time before thrusting forward and penetrating the bitch. If the dog seems to be in position, and yet fails to get a mating, there is a possibility that the bitch has a stricture, something that will need veterinary intervention.

Once penetration occurs, there should follow a stage where the male lies on the female's back, and after a short time he will try and lift one leg over the bitch to stand rear to rear in a classic 'tie' position. It is thought by some that the purpose of the 'tie' is to prolong the mating time, as the ejaculate in a dog is dispensed in three fractions, but it would probably be rather more truthful to admit that nobody really knows why they do it – we just accept the fact that they do. The 'tie' position can last from just a few minutes to over 1 hour, and it is important to understand that it is a mutual action by the dog and the bitch, with the swelling of the bulb at the end of a dog's penis coinciding with constriction of the vaginal muscles of the bitch. It is still possible to get puppies produced in the absence of a 'tie' but most breeders feel more comfortable if a 'tie' has occurred. It is also worth noting that some dogs of certain breeds, e.g. West Highland white terriers, are well known for not 'tying' and yet are still able to produce normal litters.

Pregnancy

Pregnancy lasts for about 63 days on average but the length of gestation depends not only on the bitch and when she was mated in relationship to her cycle. The normal range is considered to be 57–68 days.

It is possible to determine pregnancy from as early as 28 days by careful palpation of the abdomen. At this stage, golf-ball-like structures can sometimes be felt. From 35 days, these structures will become less palpable as their weight pulls them down into the abdomen and after this time it may not be possible for another 2–3 weeks to determine whether the bitch is pregnant.

The growth rate of the embryo is very slow for the first 35 days and this is when organogenesis takes place, but after this stage the growth of the foetus should become increasingly rapid. This should enable the owner to tell if the bitch is pregnant, but again it has been known for bitches not to 'show' until a week before they are due, when they seem to 'blow up' overnight. Ultrasound is an accurate way to determine whether a bitch is pregnant but, although it is possible to see the puppies from about 3 weeks, partial reabsorption of the litter may occur and you may not get as many puppies as you thought you would.

Antenatal care

The bitch should be treated as normal for the first 6 weeks. After this time the amount of food should be gradually increased, so she is having about 1.5 times as much as normal by the time of whelping. It is also advisable to split the food into several smaller meals throughout the day, and a good-quality puppy food should be fed. Large-breed dogs should be fed a puppy diet for medium to small breeds. This is due to large-breed puppy diets having a lower amount of energy for growth, which is needed during pregnancy and lactation.

During pregnancy or prior to mating, the bitch should be given a booster vaccination. This will raise the levels of maternal antibodies that she will pass to her puppies in the colostrum or first milk. She should also be treated for roundworms (*Toxocara canis*) to prevent the transmission of roundworm larvae across the placenta into the developing foetuses.

It is essential that the bitch is given gentle exercise right up until the time of whelping so that she can retain the muscle tone necessary for a straightforward birth. Table 16.1 shows the developmental stages of the puppy during pregnancy (see also Chapter 6).

TABLE 16.1	**The development of the puppies during pregnancy**

WEEKS OF DEVELOPMENTAL STAGE GESTATION

1	Fertilisation occurs; two-cell embryos are in the oviduct; the embryo is fairly resistant to external interference in development
2	Embryo increases from 4 cells to 64 cells. Embryo enters the uterus
3	Embryo becomes implanted in the uterus on day 19
4	Development of eyes and spinal cord; faces take shape; foetuses grow from 5–10 mm to 14–15 mm. Organogenesis begins – foetuses are most susceptible to developing defects. Days 26–32 are the best to palpate for puppies
5	Development of toes, whisker buds and claws. Foetuses look like dogs and the sex can be determined. Eyes are closed. Foetuses grow from 18 mm to 30 mm. Organogenesis complete. Puppies are now resistant to external interference in development
6	Development of skin pigment. Foetal heartbeat can be heard with a stethoscope
7	Growth and development continues
8	Detection of foetal movement when bitch is at rest. Puppies may be safely born at 8 weeks
9	Growth continues until parturition at around 63 days

Parturition or whelping

Preparation. About 1 week before the whelping is expected, it is important that the bitch is moved to her whelping quarters. She should be allowed time to become used to her whelping box and surroundings, giving her time to adjust to the new routine and the new smells. Traditionally, the whelping box was wooden, with rails inside, about 10 cm above the base, so that the bitch was not able to 'crush' the puppies against the side. The more modern whelping boxes are made of uPVC, for hygiene purposes, or even disposable cardboard whelping boxes. Some breeders prefer a child's inflatable paddling pool – which obviates the necessity for rails and provides soft, cushioned sides.

Early signs. Many bitches will display nesting behaviour in the days leading up to the birth. Signs will include scratching up of the bedding and an attempt at burrowing. They may also become very restless and be rather 'clingy' to one or more people. A sudden drop in rectal temperature within 24 hours of birth may be a sign that the birth is imminent. Minor fluctuations in temperature are quite normal but when the temperature suddenly drops from about 39°C to around 37°C you may be sure that whelping is about to start. The majority of bitches may prefer to give birth at night.

Parturition in the bitch, as in other mammals, is split into three distinct stages of labour:

Stage 1. The cervix starts to dilate. During this time it is quite normal for the bitch to refuse food, become restless, start to pant and even vomit. You may also see external signs of very weak contractions. This stage can last from 1 hour to more than 1 day and it is often difficult to be certain when it started.

Stage 2. The cervix dilates fully, contractions become more obvious and the stage ends with the delivery of the puppy. As the urge to push becomes stronger the bitch's straining is very noticeable. It is quite normal for the bitch to shiver at this time. Before the first pup is born there is very often a greenish-black discharge or lochia, which results from the placenta separating from the uterus. It is important that the timing of this discharge is noted, as in an uncomplicated whelping the first pup should be born within the next 2 hours. Puppies may be born in anterior presentation, i.e. with the nose and front paws first, or in posterior presentation, i.e. with tail and hind feet first – either is quite normal. In the uterus each pup is surrounded by two sacs – the outer one, the allantochorion, tends to rupture as the pup enters the birth canal. The second sac, the amnion, may or may not rupture during birth. If it does not the bitch will break the sac to release the puppy, enabling it to begin breathing; if she does not, then the breeder will need to do this. She will also bite the umbilical cord and lick the puppy vigorously, stimulating it to breathe and to dry off.

The breeder may need to intervene at this stage to open the sac so the pup can start to breathe normally. If the breeder needs to break the umbilical cord it is essential that the cord is not cut too short and that it is torn rather than cut with a sharp blade, as this will cause haemorrhaging. The puppy must be rubbed quite vigorously with a towel, which will mimic the bitch's licking actions. Sometimes a maiden bitch is reluctant to start licking the pups. The bitch will normally suckle pups between births. This is something I always allow as the nursing will stimulate the release of oxytocin, increasing milk let-down and causing further contractions of the uterus.

Stage 3. The foetal membranes and placenta are passed. As the bitch is a litter-bearing (multiparous) animal, stages two and three very often alternate. The bitch may consume the placenta and this is quite normal.

Timing. There is no definite timescale between the second and third stages of parturition as some puppies are born within minutes of the previous one, and yet it is not unknown for a bitch to go several hours between puppies. The main criterion is whether or not the process is progressing and it is important to observe the bitch during this time. Although there is no need for alarm if there are extended periods between pups, it is very dangerous to allow the bitch to have continual contractions for a prolonged period without producing a pup. This is the time to request veterinary assistance. Sometimes a car journey to the vet will stimulate another birth and it is not unknown for people to arrive at the surgery with more pups than when they left home!

Dystocia. A difficult whelping, referred to as dystocia, is the main cause of puppies appearing rather weak at birth. An overlarge puppy, a puppy in the incorrect position or a small or abnormal birth canal through which the puppy must pass are the most common causes of dystocia. A bitch that is not in the best physical condition, through lack of exercise and corresponding poor muscle tone or through being overweight, may also result in prolonged labour due to inertia.

Inertia can be divided into:

- **Primary inertia** – a result of the uterus failing to contract effectively. This can occur when the uterus is so full of puppies and therefore so distended that there is little chance of strong contractions starting. Conversely, primary inertia may also be caused by the 'single puppy syndrome', when there is so little distension of the uterine muscle that there is no apparent stimulus to initiate contractions. It is imperative that bitches are kept fit and with good muscle tone and at an ideal body condition score, as an unfit bitch is more likely to develop primary inertia.
- **Secondary inertia** – a result of prolonged straining. There are many reasons why intervention is required, including exhaustion in the bitch, low calcium (hypocalcaemia) or low oxytocin levels.

Assisted delivery. Assisted delivery may be necessary when a puppy is lodged in the birth canal during delivery. The use of gloved fingers is the most reliable and safe way to pull a puppy through the birth canal. It should be noted, however, that in the smaller breeds this is very difficult and potentially dangerous. Under no circumstances should the breeder attempt to use any instruments to assist delivery as they can do great harm to the puppy and the bitch.

In larger breeds when assisted delivery is needed it is important to locate the puppy by firm but gentle palpation of the lower abdomen. Once the puppy has been located, apply gentle pressure to this area to prevent the puppy slipping back up the vagina (Fig. 16.7). Insertion of a clean lubricated finger into the vulva then allows the breeder to ascertain whether the puppy is presented head first or tail first.

When the presentation position of the puppy is known, it is possible, after the removal of any obstruction, to gently ease the puppy down the birth canal (Fig. 16.8). It is imperative that the

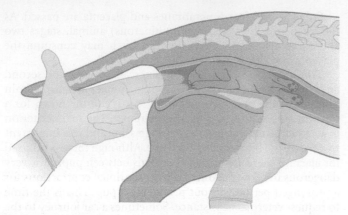

Fig. 16.7 Applying gentle pressure to the abdomen to prevent the puppy slipping back

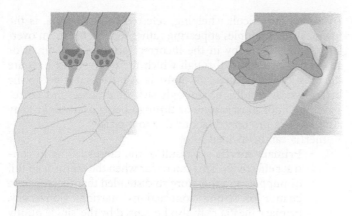

Fig. 16.8 Gentle pulling by the hind legs or head – only possible in a large breed

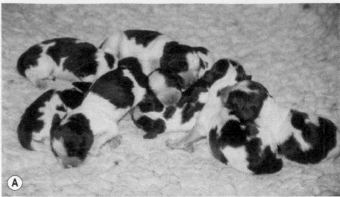

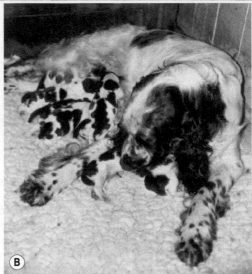

Fig. 16.9 (A) Newly whelped pups on a Vetbed. (B) Lying contentedly with mum

puppy is pulled gently in unison with the bitch's contractions. It should be noted that a breech birth is not when a puppy comes hind feet first – this is normal posterior presentation – but when the puppy is presented tail first with the hind legs curved underneath it.

Resuscitating a puppy. The most common cause of death in newly delivered puppies is hypoxia (low oxygen levels). It is essential when resuscitating a puppy that you complete the following steps:

- The puppy's airway should be cleared immediately and freed of any membranes, fluid and meconium (a puppy's first faeces).
- Excess fluid should be swabbed from the mouth and opening of the throat using a lint-free swab or the corner of a towel.
- Vigorous rubbing of the puppy can help stimulate breathing, alongside the use of Doxapram oral drops (Dopram-V).
- Warmth and oxygen are especially important in these cases.

'Never give up' is a phrase that has no greater relevance than when in this situation, and even after a couple of minutes when you may feel all is lost it is not unusual for a puppy to start breathing. For a while the puppy may appear to be gasping but usually this will cease after a short period.

Once the puppy is breathing satisfactorily it must be kept warm, either with the bitch or in a box warmed by dry towels placed over a lukewarm hot water bottle or heat pad.

Completion of parturition. The bitch will usually indicate when she has finished whelping and will appear to be more settled with her litter (Fig. 16.9). At this stage, I always give the bitch a thorough examination and palpate her abdomen to be sure there are no more pups inside. Do not be too alarmed if you can feel a hard lump inside, as very often this will be the uterus, which has yet to involute to its former state.

Once a puppy is born it will crawl around to find a teat and then begin to suckle. This may happen while others in the litter are still being born, or the breeder may remove the puppies to a warm box and return them to the bitch when parturition is over. It is vital that the puppies receive the first milk or colostrum within the first 24 hours of life. Colostrum is rich in maternal antibodies, which will provide protection against disease for about the first 12 weeks.

After whelping is complete the bitch will need to go out to go to the toilet, although you may find you have to put a lead on her to get her to leave the pups for the first few times. She will be tired and thirsty and probably hungry too. She should be allowed to rest at this point and apart from keeping an eye on the proceedings there should be as little interference as possible.

For a few days after whelping, there will be a vaginal discharge known as the lochia, which is greenish-black to start with, changing to a watery red/brown discharge as the days go by. It is important to check the bitch's teats for signs of inflammation or mastitis. If you are in any way concerned about this, veterinary advice should be sought immediately.

CARE OF THE NEWBORN

Examination of the puppies

As soon as the puppy is breathing normally and is clean it should be carefully examined and you should check for any obvious defects, e.g. cleft palate, umbilical hernia, absence of an anus. If an abnormality is found you should inform the veterinary surgeon and the puppy may be euthanised, depending upon the significance of the problem. In some congenital conditions there is virtually no hope of the puppy surviving, and it is irresponsible to prolong the inevitable.

It is very important that the temperature in the whelping quarters is kept constant at about 23.8°C for the first few days, as puppies cannot regulate their own body temperature. By the time they reach 10 days old their sensory systems are developing rapidly and they are able to withstand temperatures of as low as 15.5°C, although this is not recommended.

Unless there are obvious problems, keep interference with the bitch and her litter to a minimum but keep a close eye on the family at the same time. At this age, up until about 3 weeks, the bitch should be able to supply all the puppies' needs and as long as she is quite settled I tend to leave her to do the job that nature intended. The one time I do interfere is when the bitch returns to the puppies after going outside to relieve herself. I tend to lie the bitch on her side and place the puppies where they can get on to the teats. This is because sometimes, particularly with a younger or inexperienced bitch, an act of clumsiness at this stage can lead to the bitch unintentionally squashing a puppy.

Puppy development

The development of the puppies is very rapid and, compared to humans, the growth rate is exceptionally high. This gives us some indication of the nutritional demands of the puppies. In the early stages, the nutritional requirements of the bitch to be able to sustain the constant demand by the suckling litter are therefore also very high. It is quite usual for the puppies to be constantly 'twitching', especially when they are sleeping. This is known as 'activated sleep' and is thought to be the external symptoms of the full development of the nervous system. Puppies are born deaf and blind, and these senses, among others, are fully developed within the first 2 weeks of the puppy's life. Puppies are expected to open their eyes on the 10th day, though there can be differences of as early as 7 days to as late as day 20.

Hand-rearing puppies

If the bitch produces no milk and is unable to feed her own puppies, or if she rejects them, then it may be necessary to hand-rear them. There are special formulas available for feeding puppies, which have their own guides as to how much to feed. Various bottle and teat designs are available, depending on the size or age of the puppies, and these must be sterilised between uses.

The bitch will normally lick the area under the tail to stimulate the puppy to urinate and defecate. In her absence, you will need to clean this area with damp cotton wool or tissues after each feed to ensure regular toileting.

Diarrhoea is a common problem in hand-reared puppies and can lead to rapid dehydration and death. It is often caused by poor hygiene, so all equipment used when dealing with the puppies must be kept rigorously cleaned. Feed the affected puppies with milk diluted with cooled boiled water, but if the diarrhoea does not reduce within 24 hours or the puppy shows other signs of illness, consult your veterinary surgeon as soon as possible.

All puppies should be:
- Wormed against roundworms from 2 weeks of age at regular intervals depending on the dosing regimen clef the anthelmintic used. Puppies should then continue to be treated every month until they are 6 months old. The dosage depends on their weight, so regular weighing is required.
- Vaccinated at 8 weeks of age with a second vaccination given at around 12 weeks – timing varies according to which vaccine is used. There is a recommendation for a third parvovirus injection at 16 weeks of age. Some litters need earlier vaccinations if they have not received the important colostrum.

Registering and selling puppies

The breeder of a pedigree litter will undoubtedly want to register the puppies with the Kennel Club (KC). The KC does have a code of ethics and each person who registers puppies with them must undertake to abide by this general code. It covers the general daily care of dogs in registered ownership, the responsibilities of the owner of a bitch who is going to be bred from, and the responsibility that the breeder has to new puppy owners.

Showing dogs

The first recorded dog show was held in 1859 and, since that time, showing has become the most popular canine hobby in the country. Nowadays dog shows are held almost every weekend and have become large social as well as competitive events. All dog shows are licensed by the KC and held under their rules and regulations. At early dog shows all breeds of dog were judged together. At later dog shows the dogs were divided into sporting and non-sporting breeds.

Today's championship dog shows are organised into many more groups: i.e. hounds, terriers, gundogs, toy dogs, utility dogs, working and pastoral dogs. These distinct groups have developed throughout the history of the dog. In this way dogs are judged against dogs of similar characteristics before the best dogs of each group are judged. Finally, the best of each group compete against each other for the position of overall Best in Show.

If you want to compete:
- Your dog must be registered with the KC on the Breed Register.
- Your dog must be at least 6 months old.
- You will need to train your dog to stand still while a stranger (the judge) examines him. Then he must be able move at a steady trot so that his movement can be assessed.
- When your dog is ready you will need to find out when and where shows are taking place.
- You must have trimmed or tidied up your dog as appropriate for the breed.
- You must bathe your dog if appropriate for the breed.

BIBLIOGRAPHY

Abrantes, R., 1997. Dog Language. Wakan Tanka, Naperville, IL.

Caddy, J., 1995. Cocker Spaniels Today. Ringpress Books, Cheltenham.

Coppinger, R., Coppinger, L., 2001. Dogs – a New Understanding of Canine Origin, Behaviour and Evolution. University of Chicago Press, Chicago, IL.

Craige, P.V., 1997. Born to Win, Breed to Succeed. Doral Publishing, Sun City, AZ.

Evans, J.M., White, K., 2002. The Book of the Bitch. Ringpress Books, Cheltenham.

Fogle, B., 1990. The Dog's Mind. Macmillan, Basingstoke.

Fogle, B., 1991. The Cat's Mind. Pelham Books, London.

Gwynne-Jones, O., 1983. The Popular Guide to Puppy Rearing. Popular Dogs, London.

Halls, V., 2007. Cat Councellor; How Your Cat Really Relates to You. Bantam Books, London.

Harmar, H., 1974. Dogs and How to Breed Them. John Gifford, London.

Hollings, P., 1996. The Essential Weimaraner. Ringpress Books, Cheltenham.

International Cat Care, 2008. Vaccinating your cat. Available at: <http://icatcare.org/advice/vaccinating-your-cat>.

International Cat Care, 2014. Inherited deafness in white cats. Available at: <http://www.icatcare.org:8080>.

Karsh, E., 1983. The effects of early handling on the development of social bonds between cats and people. In: Katcher, A., Beck, A. (Eds.), 1983 New Perspectives on Our Lives with Companion Animals. University of Pennsylvania Press, Philadelphia, PA, pp. 22–28.

Lyons, L.A., Foe, I.T., Rah, H.C., et al., 2005. Chocolate coated cats: TYRP1 mutations for brown colour in domestic cats. Mamm. Genome 16 (5), 356–366.

Morris, D., 1996. Cat World, a Feline Encyclopedia. Ebury Press, London.

Muirhead, C., 1996. The Complete English Springer Spaniel. Ringpress Books, Cheltenham.

Rice, D., 1997. The Complete Book of Cat Breeding. Barron's Educational Series, New York.

Roberts, J., 1987. The Irish Setter. Popular Dogs, London.

Robinson, R., 1982. Genetics for Dog Breeders. Pergamon Press, Oxford.

Schlueter, C., Budras, K., Lugewid, E., et al., 2009. Brachycephalic feline noses. CT and anatomical study of the relationship between heads conformation and the nasolacrimal drainage system. J. Feline Med. Surg. 11, 891–900.

Serpell, J., 1995. The Domestic Dog – Its Evolution, Behaviour and Interactions with People. Cambridge University Press, Cambridge.

Turner, D.C., Bateson, P., 2013. The Domestic Cat – the Biology of Its Behaviour, third ed. Cambridge University Press, Cambridge.

Turner, T. (Ed.), 1990. Veterinary Notes for Dog Owners. Popular Dogs, London.

Vella, C.M., Shelton, L.M., McGonagle, J.J., et al., 1999. Robinson's Genetics for Cat Breeders and Veterinarians, fourth ed. Butterworth-Heinemann, Oxford.

RECOMMENDED READING

Allen, W.E., 1992. Fertility and Obstetrics in the Dog. Blackwell Scientific, Oxford.
  Covers all the scientific points associated with reproduction. Easy access bullet points throughout.

Cooper, B., Mullineaux, E., Turner, L. (Eds.), 2012. BSAVA Textbook of Veterinary Nursing, fifth ed. British Small Animal Veterinary Association, Gloucester.
  Long and detailed chapter covering reproduction in dogs and cats.

Evans, J.M., White, K., 2002. The Book of the Bitch. Ringpress Books, Cheltenham.
  Covers all aspects of dog breeding.

Harmar, H., 1974. Dogs and How to Breed Them. John Gifford, London.
  Useful guide to practical dog breeding.

Rice, D., 1997. The Complete Book of Cat Breeding. Barron's Educational Series, New York.
  This book on cat breeding is excellent. Although written for the lay person it is worthwhile reading so that the professional is aware of the knowledge base needed by the conscientious breeder to ensure the welfare of animals. It is very well illustrated.

Turner, D.C., Bateson, P., 2013. The Domestic Cat – the Biology of Its Behaviour, third ed. Cambridge University Press, Cambridge.
  This long-awaited update includes discoveries made over the last 10 years and is an excellent book about the biological nature of feline behaviour and how this impinges on their relationships with humans. It is well written and helps towards an understanding of the nature of pets and patients. It dispels some myths and may help us optimise the caring environment for our cats.

The Essentials of Patient Care

JESSICA MAUGHAN | CLAIRE CAVE | MICHELLE RICHMOND | NICOLA ACKERMAN

KEY POINTS

- While providing nursing care to an animal it is important to consider the whole patient rather than focusing on a particular disease or injury.

- On admission all hospitalised patients should be given a detailed clinical assessment in order to design an effective nursing strategy based on the individual needs of the patient.

- All animals perform certain daily activities that are essential to maintain a comfortable existence and, in some cases, to survive. These essential activities, e.g. feeding, drinking and elimination, must be provided for within a hospital environment if the patient is to recover.

- Certain types of hospitalised patient, such as recumbent or geriatric animals, require specific forms of nursing care.

Introduction

Every patient, procedure and disease process is unique. No two patients will respond to treatment, surgery or medical intervention in the same way, despite being the same species or even the same breed.

The foundations for providing exceptional patient care are built upon this understanding of patient individuality. The ability to appreciate patient uniqueness has a positive effect on every aspect of nursing care, ensuring that the care provided is tailor made to the patient's specific needs and not focused solely upon the reason the patient is admitted into the practice.

Admission

The veterinary nurse is involved with assessing patients' needs at the time of admission. Patients may be hospitalised for hours, day or even weeks and often the care that these patients require will change on a frequent basis. Initially, the veterinary nurse can gather information at the time of admission that provides an insight into the patient's general well-being. This information can be obtained from a variety of methods, such as simple observations in the waiting room, discussion with the patient's caregiver and the physical examination/assessment.

OBSERVATION

Simply watching the patient from afar can offer information about the patient's ability to adapt to being in the practice. Anxiety can manifest in a variety of forms, from excessive excitability in canine patients to open-mouth breathing in feline patients resulting from a stressful car journey (Fig. 17.1). Human interaction should also be assessed; for example, does the patient come into the practice willingly? Hides behind the owner? Resents being handled or not used to being handled (such as lagomorphs)? Does the patient have an enhanced bond to the owner? For example, guide dogs, medical alert dogs and pets used as therapy may experience considerable anxiety in the owner's absence.

Watching the canine patient enter the consulting room also provides information about the patient's ability to walk, signs of stiffness, ocular/auditory changes and demeanour/temperament. Feline patients often urinate/defecate in the cat baskets due to a stressful journey and smaller pets hide, with limited voluntary interaction. The initial observations can and often do change once the patient is admitted into the practice and the situation the patient is placed within alters.

A true insight into the routine and needs of the patient can be obtained during discussion with the owner.

CLIENT QUESTIONNAIRE

The aim of a client questionnaire is for the veterinary staff to gain as much information about the pet before being admitted into the hospital. The answers provide a vital link between what is 'normal' for the patient and what can be considered 'abnormal' behaviour by the owner. This information should be available for all the veterinary staff to access and attached to the patient's hospitalisation or consent forms for reference (Box 17.1).

ADMISSION INTO THE PRACTICE

Species-specific considerations – the environment

Every species have individual requirements during their period of hospitalisation and the degrees to which these requirements are met are dependent upon practice facilities. With careful planning and pre-emptive organisation, the environmental needs of many patients can be provided.

Separate canine and feline wards are now becoming standard in many veterinary practices. Having such facilities provides the gold standard in meeting the basic environmental needs of both species.

Cats are often solitary animals and their relationships with other species can be challenging; even the aroma of having dogs within close proximity causes additional stress which is compounded when cats can visualise and/or hear dogs in the same room. That said, having separate rooms next door to one another can still be stressful to the feline patient as the noise

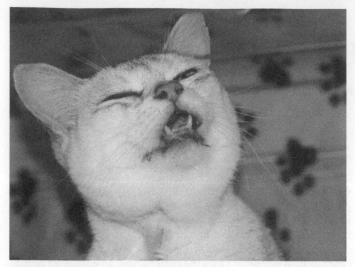

Fig. 17.1 Open-mouth breathing in a cat

level is still audible, but this solution is much better than both species being integrated into the same ward/kennel room.

Feline environmental considerations. The optimal cat cage is large enough to accommodate an appropriate hideaway (the client's carrier can be used as an ideal hideaway) and for the litter tray to be away from food, bedding and water. The cage should be at mid-level or higher. Side-by-side cages are preferable to cages facing each other so that the cats do not see each other and become visually aroused (Fig. 17.2).

Provide a safe haven with both hiding and perching places (e.g., sturdy cardboard box). If a cat shows less anxiety when in a darker area, cover the front of the cage with a towel or simply design a hideaway using a cardboard box.

Ideally the room should have controlled temperature and sound insulation. Fiberglass cages are warmer, less reflective and quieter than stainless steel.

Owners should be encouraged to bring in a towel and/or toys from home. Often providing the cat's preferred food and litter is helpful. (While this may not be possible with every patient, it may help those that are anxious or fearful.)

Manage odours by cleaning surfaces and washing hands between patients. Ventilate after all olfactory incidents (cleaning where another cat has walked or rubbed on furniture, emptying litter trays promptly).

Cats are macrosmatic – their sensitive sense of smell drives many of their behavioural responses. Some odours (such as air fresheners, disinfectants, rubbing alcohol, blood, deodorant, perfume) and unfamiliar clothing may cause anxiety or fear.

Consider using a synthetic feline facial pheromone (FFP) analogue. Studies show that a synthetic FFP may have calming effects in stressful environments, reducing anxiety, fear and aggression, and increasing normal grooming and food intake in caged cats.

Cats may benefit from diffusers placed throughout the hospital and a spray used about 30 minutes in advance on materials used for cats to lie on, in cages, as well as on towels used for handling. Use FFP only in addition to, and never as a substitute for, removing odours, washing, gentle handling and other provisions for creating a cat-friendly environment.

Manage visual and auditory input. Minimise visual cues that may lead to anxiety. Keep other patients away from the cat's line

of vision. When possible, provide a separate feline entrance and feline waiting room or area. Cover cat carriers with a blanket or towel.

Minimise harsh lighting and provide a quiet environment and speak softly. Minimise noise that might startle the cat, such as phones and fans. Consider using soothing background music and acoustic dampeners.

Canine environmental considerations. Dogs are social animals and often respond to human contact in a positive way, and this is reflected during their hospitalisation period. Some canine patients can show signs of anxiety and fear-related aggression related to being within the hospital environment,

---

BOX 17.1   EXAMPLE OF A CLIENT QUESTIONNAIRE

We would be grateful if you would take the time to fill in this questionnaire. Our aim is to gain as much information about your pet's daily routine to ensure that their stay with us is as comfortable as possible.

FEEDING

1. What is your pet's normal diet?
2. How often is he/she fed?
   Once, Twice, Thrice – other – Please provide further details if required.
3. Does your pet have any favourite food or treats?
   Yes/no If so please provide details.
4. Does your pet have any specific feeding needs?
   Type of bowl, hand feeding, shy eater.
5. Are there any types of food that your pet should not eat?
   Please provide details of any allergies/intolerances.

DRINKING

1. Does your pet drink from a bowl at home or prefers another source (such as water fountain)?

URINATION/DEFECATION

1. Does your pet suffer from urinary or faecal incontinence?
2. If your pet is a cat: Do they use a litter tray at home and if so do they have a preference for the litter used, such a wood/soil/clay types?
3. If your pet is a dog: Do they prefer to urinate/defecate on a particular surface? If so please provide details.
4. Will your dog willingly urinate while on a lead?
5. Do you use a specific command to encourage urination/defecation?

SLEEPING

1. Where does your pet usually sleep?
2. What type of bedding/surface does he/she use?
3. What are their normal sleep patterns?

GROOMING

1. Does your pet enjoy being groomed? Yes/no

GENERAL

1. How would you describe your pet's normal temperament at home?
   Placid/friendly/excitable/nervous
2. Does your pet have any mobility problems? Yes/No – please provide details
3. Does your pet like to interact with other people?
4. Does your pet have a favourite type of toy? Yes/No – please provide details
5. How do you normally give medication to your pet?
6. Is there anything else you would like us to know about your pet that might help the nursing staff during his/her stay with us?

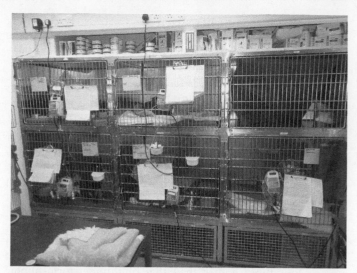

Fig. 17.2 Cages need to be assessable and at an appropriate height

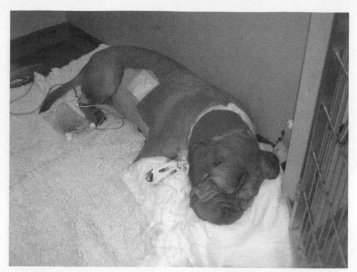

Fig. 17.3 Facilities for giant breeds can be difficult

but often this behaviour changes with compassionate handling and understanding the patient's individual needs.

Dogs can become overly stressed by the presence/odour of other dogs and relocating such patients away from vocal and excitable patients allows them the solitude to begin to settle. Dogs have an incredible bond to their owners and often separation anxiety can have a negative impact upon the patient's emotional well-being. Reducing this anxiety can require multiple alterations to the patient's environment.

Dogs have more than 220 million olfactory receptors in its nose, while humans have only 5 million. Dogs explore their environment via olfactory input and often become stimulated by new scents. This occurs on a daily basis when dogs are exercised by their owners. The need to explore and stimulate the olfactory receptors is just as important when the patient is hospitalised – fresh air and environmental smells can have a dramatic effect upon the patient's demeanour, and even recumbent/paralysed patients need to have exposure to the external environment. Being carried or stretchered outside has a positive effect on the patient's physiological well-being; if this is not possible then having the ability to open windows/doors into the ward/kennels allows the outside to come indoors.

Adaptil® is a synthetic copy of the natural canine-appeasing pheromone which has been scientifically proven to help support dogs in a range of stressful situations. The pheromone is available as a diffuser which can be plugged into an electrical socket on a permanent basis within the ward/kennel environment. This allows the pheromone to diffuse continuously in the room. Other forms of the pheromones are available and the spray form can be used in the kennel or on bedding prior to the admission of the patient into the hospital, and often patients benefit from having the pheromone sprayed onto a bandana which can then be placed around the patient's neck to provide additional support. If the patient is being hospitalised for a pre-planned procedure then consideration should be made of the use of the canine-appeasing pheromone within the home prior to admission.

Having a familiar item in the kennel from the home environment or item of clothing from the owner can aid in providing a form of reassurance in the owner's absence, but it is important that these items are not laundered during the animal's stay.

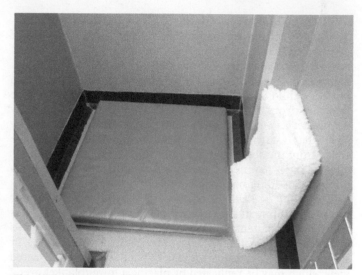

Fig. 17.4 Waterproof foam mattress

Dog cages should be large enough for the patient to adequately lay in a lateral recumbency with ease, to allow turning and to stand to full height. This can often be a challenge for the giant breeds as facilities may not be available to accommodate such patients (Fig. 17.3).

Careful selection should be made on the type of bedding material considering the patient's medical/surgical condition. Veterinary bedding provides the patient with an absorbent and comfortable contact layer. This comfort can be enhanced by the placement of a specific, waterproof mattress which conforms to the shape of the patient and can be vital for the nursing care of recumbent patients (Fig. 17.4). It must be remembered that veterinary mattresses are covered with a waterproof cover to protect the foam interior from soiling. This waterproof cover can also act as a form of insulation and some canine patients with thick fur can become hyperthermic due to the non-breathable material, lack of circulating air under the patient and a warm kennel environment. The ambient ward/kennel room temperature is 18–22°C, which requires daily monitoring to allow temperature adjustments to occur.

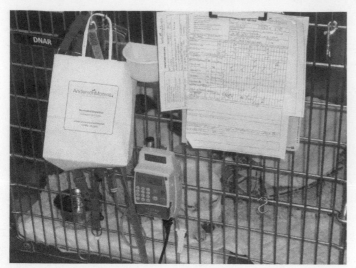

Fig. 17.5 Multiple items on the front of cages can obscure vital monitoring of the patient

The provision of incontinence pads should be carefully considered for recumbent patients or patients with any form of urinary/faecal incontinence. These absorbent pads are designed to trap liquid into the absorbent layer (similar in design to a baby's nappy), but it must be remembered that the sheets do not wick fluid away from the patient and do not prevent the moisture from coming into contact with the patient; they simply act as an absorbent layer. If they remain in situ when soiling has occurred then the patient can and often does become soiled from the absorbent sheets. Prompt removal of the sheets after soiling is required or their use is avoided and replaced with a suitable bedding material with wicking properties.

The front of kennels can become obscured with various pieces of equipment such as infusion pumps and patient folders which hinder patients' view of the environment and the nurse's ability to observe the patients (Fig. 17.5). Some anxious or scared patients feel more secure within a darkened or obscured view which may be replicated by placing a towel/blanket over a portion of the kennel front.

Smaller species. Lagomorphs and other small species are often more challenging patients to hospitalise. Both cats and dogs are prey animals and often they prey upon lagomorphs. Ferrets can also predate upon rabbits and both species should be housed as far away as possible. The odour of a ferret can be potent so pre-planning should be implemented to prevent having both species within the hospital environment on the same day.

Rabbits and other small species are often housed at home with companions. Stress can be reduced by allowing a companion to join the patient in the hospital environment for company.

Providing a suitable environment involves planning on a daily basis and can largely be influenced by the patients already hospitalised. Choosing a cage as far away from dogs and cats as possible is one of the important steps, and providing a dedicated staff member who is not in contact with dogs and cats to care for the patient helps to prevent stress from transferrable odours on clothing.

Smaller species benefit from having an enclosed area to hide within. Cardboard boxes are ideal with the addition of suitable bedding material – this prevents the stress of being out in the open. Clarification at the time of admission with the owner

should confirm the patient's preferences to bowls, e.g. providing a rabbit with a water bottle may not be suitable when at home the rabbit drinks from a bowl. Simple measures can dramatically alter the patient's ability to adapt to being hospitalised.

THE EFFECTS OF STRESS UPON HOSPITALISED PATIENTS

Traditionally patients' medical care has been prioritised over their stress levels within the hospital environment. This has now altered and stress has become recognised in its own right along with the effects on patients' health outcome. Reducing stress in patients is now becoming an important part of patient care.

The body's response to stress

- Cortisol levels in healthy dogs on their first night in a veterinary environment have been shown to be two to four times higher than that of thunderstorm-phobic dogs at home with their owners during a storm.
- Chronic stress can negatively affect the health outcomes in a multitude of systems.
- The immediate effect of stress can be seen on a complete blood count – 'stress leucogram' – which includes leucocytosis, neutrophilia, lymphopenia and related changes.
- As stress is prolonged and becomes chronic, leucocytosis may become leucopenia and with many other changes related to inflammatory cytokines results in immunosuppression. In humans this has been shown to result in an increased susceptibility to infection and neoplasia.
- Limited evidence is available for the effect of stress-induced immunosuppression on hospitalised veterinary patients, but they are not any less significant to any other species.

Studies in laboratory animals and humans also show that stress delays wound healing, an obvious concern for postoperative surgical or trauma patients. Chronic stress has been shown to negatively affect the gastrointestinal system, exacerbating large-bowel disease in humans and being associated with chronic idiopathic large-bowel disease in dogs. As for its effects on the cardiovascular system, chronic stress is prothrombotic, associated with hypertension, and has triggered atrial fibrillation in humans.

Stress in veterinary patients is very difficult to quantify. Unfortunately, there are no validated cage-side measurements for stress assessment by veterinary professionals, and behavioural measures are notoriously difficult to interpret. Recent work investigating stress behaviours in hospitalised dogs suggests that many behaviours frequently used by veterinary staff to identify stress, such as barking, do not correlate with elevated cortisol levels. While two behaviours did correlate with high cortisol levels (panting) or low cortisol levels (resting the head on the ground), 20 minutes of observation was necessary for these behaviours to be predictive; 2 minutes of observation was insufficient. These findings suggest that assessment of a patient's stress levels by veterinary personnel may be inaccurate simply because of inadequate time for thorough observation of the patient.

Patients' bodies are not our only nursing responsibly but also their minds, especially as the nursing care of both the body and mind are so inextricably entwined.

Noise

Noise is defined as any sound that is physiologically arousing, harmful, subjectively annoying or disruptive to performance and was described by Florence Nightingale in 1859: "Unnecessary noise or noises that create an expectation in the mind, is that which hurts a patient."

Studies have shown that the body has many harmful physiological responses to excessive noise levels.

Physiological responses
- Constriction of peripheral blood vessels
- Tachycardia
- Increased cerebral blood flow
- Skeletal muscle tension
- Increased cortisol and cholesterol levels

The noise level within a veterinary environment is an additional stress to patients. Veterinary nurses can become desensitised to the sound levels in the ward/kennel rooms due to being subjected to the various noise levels on a daily basis. The veterinary nursing staff have the ability to leave the room when noise levels become excessive and have a break from the ongoing noises at the completion of a shift. Many hospitalised patients are exposed to damaging sounds for a continual period of time – often hours through the day and night – with respite being provided only when patients are removed from their cage for exercise or examination.

Bothersome noises that are often considered 'normal' include staff conversation, radio noise, infusion pumps, equipment alarms, opening/closing doors and noise from other patients.

Exposure to noises with raised decibels over time will cause hearing loss. The volume (dBA) and the length of exposure to the sound will provide an indicator as to how harmful the noise is. In general the louder the noise, the less time required before hearing loss will occur. According to the National Institute for Occupational Safety and Health, the maximum exposure time at 85 dBA is 8 hours – 85 dBA is considered the same level as a toilet flush, lawn mower and heavy traffic/noisy restaurant.

At 110 dBA, the maximum exposure time is only 1 minute and 29 seconds. A large dog bark is 100 dBA, a single dog barking is 113 dBA and one of the loudest dog barks recorded was 124 dBA. This does not include the noise of multiple dogs and the additional environmental sounds occurring simultaneously. At this level the exposure time to the noise should be reduced and/or ear protection should be worn. Noise levels above 140 dBA can cause damage to hearing after one exposure. Not only does a good auditive environment facilitate patient recovery, it also leads to patients having a better sleep pattern and a higher level of patient and staff well-being.

Studies have shown that the bedside noise measured in human intensive care units (ICUs) is 70–76 decibels (light traffic is 50 decibels; light machinery is 90 decibels). ICUs within many veterinary universities can reach 120 decibels, which is the noise generated from rock music or heavy machinery. Sensorineural hearing loss can occur at 80–90 decibels.

So, what happens to hospitalised patients? Recumbent patients who are unable to be removed from the environment are often subjected to high levels of noise for prolonged periods. Often this can be in excess of 24 hours in larger veterinary hospitals where patient care is provided throughout the night. Auditory protection for recumbent/critically ill patients should be considered by the nursing staff.

This can be achieved by placing cotton wool into the ear canals to help muffle sounds. Ear defenders can be worn by the staff and can also be placed upon the ears of larger canine patients. Eliminating the controllable stressors may be possible, such as reducing staff 'traffic' within the wards, allowing only the ward staff to enter. Limiting conversation/patient discussion away from the patients can be achieved by simply leaving the room to discuss patient care. Metallic bins for clinical waste disposal are often used to hold clinical waste bags and are operated via a foot pedal to prevent hand contamination. The noise generated by repeatedly closing the lid can often be excessive due to frequent use and can be extremely stressful for feline patients. A simple measure of adding foam tape around the top of metallic bin lids or by using plastic swing lid bins can provide the patients with the sensory rest they need. The same result can be achieved on cupboard doors/room doors.

One of the most persistent sounds which affect the levels of stress in both staff and patients is barking dogs. Often these patients are considered healthy individuals, admitted or recovering from routine procedures and are day patients not requiring overnight care. Having the facilities to separate the day patients from the intensive care/critically ill patients would be considered the 'gold standard'. One recent study has shown that classical music has a positive influence upon cats, but had no effect on dogs, though previous research has showed positive effects for dogs. The music level still needs to be at an adequately low level.

The effects of listening to classical music have been widely studied in relation to humans. Playing classical music to children can help awaken parts of their brains; it can lower blood pressure, relieve pain after surgery and help combat insomnia.

Many other stressors can be reduced or eliminated by taking a step back from seeing the practice from a veterinary nurse's point of view, but rather the view of a patient. Training should be provided in low-stress handling techniques and support a go-slowly approach with some patients despite a loss of efficiency. Owners should be encouraged to visit their hospitalised pets.

Sleep

The importance of adequate sleep for hospitalised patients should not be underestimated by the veterinary nursing team. Sleep is an essential biological function; the body needs time to rest and heal and sleep provides the patients with the time to do so. Sleep deprivation has been shown to have considerable negative effects upon the body, all of which can delay patient recovery.

The effects of sleep deprivation on the body
- Immune function impairment – the patient develops an increased susceptibility to illness
- Reduces the tissue healing process – sleep provides a period of increased protein synthesis and tissue renewal
- Hormonal changes
- Changes to metabolism
- Pulmonary function and control of breathing.

Every patient requires hours of undisturbed sleep to allow the body to rest. For adequate sleep to occur the environmental decibels should not exceed 40 dBA, which is equal to the noise generated in a library. At night this noise level within a practice may drop to a level which permits the patient to sleep. During the day, patients' ability to sleep is suppressed. Patients need to feel secure and safe and once this security is achieved then active sleep occurs.

Veterinary nursing techniques to enhance patients' sleep patterns

- Reduce noise by adjusting environmental elements – e.g. staff traffic in wards, reducing conversation, barking dogs.
- 'Soundproof' the environment – place foam around the edges of bin lids, around doors, keep drip pumps charged to help reduce alarming.
- Group together nursing interventions, from walking patients, feeding and medicating.
- Between patient interventions, minimise patient contact.
- Create periods of artificial day and night – turn lights off at night – use a pen torch/torch during patient checks at night; this reduces the need to light the entire room.
- Consider other options for settling the patient – at night patients may settle better away from the kennel room. Consulting rooms provide a suitable alternative and can often be an area to have quiet time spent with nervous, timid, stressed or vocal patients.

Reducing sensory deprivation

Dogs and cats spend a considerable amount of time outside with stimulating odours, sound and interaction with other animals and people. Reducing patients' access to the outdoors has a negative impact upon their psychological/mental well-being.

Human hospital studies have shown that patients with a window by their beds and a view of trees had a much shorter hospital stay, took fewer moderate and strong analgesic doses and had lower scores for post-surgical complications. It has been suggested that the view of a natural scene and fresh air has therapeutic influences in humans.

With veterinary patients, access to the outdoors can often be a dramatic turning point in the recovery process. If the patient cannot go outside for safety reasons (e.g. feline patients), then options should be considered in bringing the outdoors inside (see later).

The length of time outside may, for some patients, be limited, but done frequently this allows the patient's senses to become stimulated. Recumbent patients (such as patients that have undergone spinal surgery) benefit from being stretchered outside and simply given time to 'watch the world go by.' Grooming, massage, physiotherapy and hand feeding can all be achieved in the open air and will allow the patient to have one-to-one relaxation time which is the foundation for the active sleep process.

Patients being hospitalised in the practice isolation facilities can be one of the most challenging environments for nurses to provide sensory stimulation. These patients are carrying potentially contagious/infectious disease. Contact with staff members is limited for these patients to reduce the risk of staff-to-patient transmission, and isolation kennels/wards can be located away from the main area of the practice.

Providing canine patients with a specific area outside to toilet and experience sensory stimulation should be considered as part of the care process for the patient's psychological needs in balance with the patient's medical/surgical requirements.

The considerations for this area should include the following:

- The surface the patient has access to should be easy to clean and disinfect. Avoid all grass areas where suitable disinfection is not possible.
- Cordon the area off – away from clients and other hospitalised patients.
- Clearly identify the area as an exercise area for isolation patients.
- Use biohazard cones and tape to enclose a suitable area.
- Ensure that the area is cleaned and disinfected promptly after urination/defecation.
- The area should be easily accessible without the patient coming into contact with other staff members or areas of the practice where patients have access/walked.
- The designated exercise area should be only used for one patient at a time and the entire area disinfected thoroughly once the patient has been discharged. A new area should be cordoned off for new patients admitted into isolation.

Bring the outside in

Taking a patient to the outside environment may not be a suitable option due to concerns over the patient's safety/health. Bringing the outside in has been shown to considerably improve the mental well-being of human patients; simple techniques such as opening windows, blinds and curtains allows for the patient to experience 'fresh air' and the warmth of the sun through the glass.

Veterinary patients that are unable to leave the confines of their cages can have the stimulation of the outside world brought into their cages. Feline patients that are used to toileting outside benefit from having soil/compost in their litter trays. Branches/twigs and leaves can provide stimulation for lagomorphs, and they would also benefit from litter trays with soil/sand or cat litter to encourage digging.

Opening windows and doors during quiet periods of the day/night when patients are secure provides continuous change of air flow and hence continuous olfactory stimulation.

TENDER LOVING CARE – THE POWER OF PETTING

Many research experiments have linked the positive medical effect of touching pets upon human health. Blood samples taken from humans before and while stroking a dog/cat measured positive changes in several neurochemicals found in the brain, including dopamine, oxytocin, prolactin and noradrenaline, which directly influence emotions of exhilaration, positive excitement, pleasurable experiences, social bonding, sense of well-being and contentment and feelings of comfort and security. Cortisol, which increases during periods of stress, is reduced.

Patients also exhibit similar neurochemical changes with the results reflecting those exhibited in humans. The power of touch can dramatically alter the patient's relationship with the caregiver (positively or negatively), and one essential aspect of patient care is implementing low-stress handling techniques.

Unfamiliar smells, sounds and sights and potentially threatening patients and people assault patients the moment that they enter into veterinary practices. Procedures are performed that are often unpleasant, painful and in some instances achieved by force. A single such experience can result in the patient experiencing a negative emotional response resulting in fear. This fear can result in fidgeting, fighting to leave the environment/person and/or aggression when subsequent handling/procedures are attempted.

The level of veterinary care provided to hospitalised patients can be heavily influenced by the patient's behaviour and response to medical/surgical intervention by the veterinary staff. Aggressive patients, for example, may be discharged from the veterinary practice before a complete return to full health has been achieved.

Patient treatment protocols are also designed to suit the individual and its ability to adjust to the environment. Some patients require sedation for procedures, which can be routine such as jugular blood sampling. Other patients will be comfortable to sit for more invasive procedures that can be intimidating such as ocular examinations. Many patients benefit from low-stress handling techniques, which work to condition a positive emotional response by pairing the experience with something that naturally elicits a positive emotional response from the patient.

One of the most powerful ways of providing this positive response is by using food. This can be useful for patients requiring repeated clinical examinations on a frequent basis where a particular food treat (this treat should only be fed during examinations) can help make the experience more relaxing for the patient.

UNDERSTANDING WHAT IS NORMAL AND WHAT IS ABNORMAL

Veterinary textbooks provide the veterinary nurse with the details of the physiological parameters for every species that enters into the veterinary environment. This information can be used as baseline for what is considered to be normal physiological values, such as heart rate and respiratory rate, but it should be remembered that every patient is different and may not conform to such values even when the patient is in good health. The respiratory rate and rhythm of a bulldog, for example, can appear abnormal, with increased respiratory effort and rate. This may be normal for that particular patient with brachycephalic anatomy. Understanding the concept and the importance of the use of baseline values of every patient as an individual (rather than a species) provides the nursing team with the indicator of the patient's health status and how the patient's status alters in accordance with the baseline values.

THE IMPORTANT PARAMETERS – THE PHYSICAL EXAMINATION (NURSING ASSESSMENT)

The physical assessment of the hospitalised patient should be part of the nurse's role as the caregiver and should not be considered to be exclusively the role of the veterinary surgeon. Frequent assessment can highlight subtle changes in the patient's parameters that can indicate a change in the patient's health status and in some situations can detect changes that, if left untreated, could become life threatening.

During a physical examination, the patient should be evaluated from the head to the tail, with a nurse's assessment of the body systems. Some systems can be palpated, such as lymph nodes and bladder diameter. Some systems require auscultating, so the correct technique of using a stethoscope for thoracic

and cardiac assessment should be mastered. Having a 'worth-it-meter' is helpful – i.e. is this procedure/part of the examination worth it? If the stress a procedure creates for the patient exceeds the benefit then it may not be a part of the routine examination but only on an as-needed basis. Some parts of the physical examination may fall into this category, such as rectal temperatures (changing this to aural readings can be a suitable alternative).

NURSING PHYSICAL ASSESSMENT OF THE HOSPITALISED PATIENT – EVALUATION PARAMETERS

Cardiovascular

- Heart rate – beats per minute
- Strong, regular pulse and palpable with normal rate and quality
- Absence of abnormal heart sounds and rhythm
- Heart rate within established parameters
- Mucous membranes pink, moist with suitable capillary refill time
- Absence of systemic oedema

Pulmonary

- Respiratory rate per minute
- Respiratory effort and rate within established parameters
- Observe chest expansion – should be visible, equal and bilateral
- Bilaterally clear lung sounds on auscultation
- Airway patent with absence of abnormal secretions

Gastrointestinal

- Absence of vomiting, diarrhoea, and constipation
- Normal abdominal palpation with absence of tenderness, pain and distension
- Normal faecal movement
- Oral cavity normal
- Eating and drinking

Renal/urinary

- Voiding clear, yellow urine with appropriate frequency and volume
- Passing with ease – no stranguria
- Non-distended, non-painful bladder
- Absence of discharge from penis or vulva

Musculoskeletal

- Equal strength and weight bearing bilaterally
- Absence of muscle weakness
- Normal gait
- Non-tender muscle and limb palpation with full functional range of motion
- Symmetrical muscle mass

Reproductive tract

- Absence of discharge from penis, vulva or teats
- Non-painful, normal mammary or testicular tissue upon palpation
- Mucous membranes pink and intact
- Able to contract penis into prepuce

Integumentary/lymphatic

- Skin warm, dry, clean and intact
- Normal skin turgor
- Hair coat symmetrical, clean and non-brittle
- Absence of external parasites
- Absence of lymph node enlargement upon palpation

Neurological/sensory

- Alert and aware of surroundings
- Exhibiting behaviours typical/appropriate for the species
- Eyes open spontaneously and respond to external stimuli (visual, tactile and auditory)
- Symmetrical movement with intact proprioception and appropriate gait
- Intact pain response

Incisions/wounds

- Intact suture lines
- Absence of erythema, swelling and discharge
- Absence of abnormal odours
- Bandages clean, dry, intact

Pain

- Patient has a low pain score on assessment
- Absence of clinical signs of pain

Self-care

- Ability to eat and drink, defecate, urinate and groom without assistance

Peripheral/invasive lines (catheters and drains)

- Absence of oedema, pain, heat and discharge at the site of entry
- Extremity distal to the IV catheter site is warm with no swelling
- Fluid line/urinary catheter drain patent, unobstructed
- Bandages/dressings clean, dry and intact

NEVER UNDERESTIMATE THE VALUE OF BASIC NURSING SKILLS

Advanced monitoring equipment has become widely available in veterinary practices. This technology provides the veterinary staff with the ability to monitor parameters that are unable to be assessed via a physical examination – e.g. pulse oximetry permits the measurement of the patient's oxygen saturation. (A crude assessment can be made by assessing the mucous membrane colour, but often by the time a colour change has been noted the patient's oxygen saturation is so low that it can be life threatening.)

Monitoring equipment can aid in providing optimal patient care; however, this technology should never replace the hands-on skills of observation, interpretation and monitoring of the veterinary nurse.

Monitoring machines provide numerical values, visual traces and a variety of data. How this information is interpreted is the responsibility of the veterinary nurse recording these values. Recording these values requires interpretation, e.g. could the tachycardia be related to inadequate analgesia and signal discomfort? Has the patient's posture changed? Does the patient need to urinate? Has the mentation of the patient changed?

Observation skills and the ability to interpret the observation and act upon it immediately are crucial for every patient. Sometimes a patient is admitted with what is considered to be a common condition and the significance of the clinical signs can be underestimated. Case one highlights a patient that was admitted into a hospital with subtle clinical signs awaiting diagnostic investigations.

Nursing the critical care patient requires a detailed understanding of the complex techniques that must be carried out if the patient is to survive. Many of these techniques are rarely seen within the day-to-day workings of a veterinary practice. It is important, however, to remember that, for all the highly skilled techniques we may employ and for all the equipment used, the veterinary nurse and his or her ability to observe and care for the animal is still the major contributing factor to a quick recovery and prolonged survival time. Never forget that the animal needs home comforts, comfortable bedding, a stimulating environment (unless contraindicated) and huge amounts of 'TLC'. Relationships that develop between the nurse, patient and owner can be rewarding and satisfying and the sense of achievement at seeing one of your patients recovered and going home can be immense.

RECORD-KEEPING

All observations must be recorded in a legible and accessible form. A daily summary sheet should be on each cage door recording patient and owner details, a problem list, a drug list and administration times, a monitoring list and times and resuscitation orders. Resuscitation orders should have been discussed with the owner and recorded, e.g. 'Do Not Resuscitate', or, if measures are to be carried out, to what level (closed or open chest). Critical care patients may also need records of other aspects of their care, including fluid therapy, nutrition and care of chest drains or tracheostomy tubes.

Patient monitoring and observation

Basic monitoring of temperature, pulse rate and respiratory rate is essential in the critical patient as it is for any other, although there are many types of extra monitoring equipment that can also be used.

TEMPERATURE

Metabolic rate is closely linked to temperature regulation and this is especially true in shocked patients or those that are anaesthetised or comatose. Hypothermia may affect the mechanics of respiration, cardiac function and the patient's coagulation state.

Body temperature is usually taken rectally using either a mercury or digital thermometer. In poorly perfused animals, the rectal temperature may not truly reflect the core temperature. Thermometers should be placed carefully against the mucosa to avoid measuring faecal temperature. Core temperature can also be taken aurally or via the oesophagus in unconscious patients.

In a critical care patient pyrexia or hyperthermia may indicate:

- Pain
- Infection
- Sepsis
- Convulsion activity.

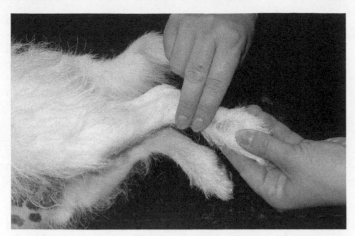

Fig. 17.6   Palpating the dorsal pedal pulse in a dog

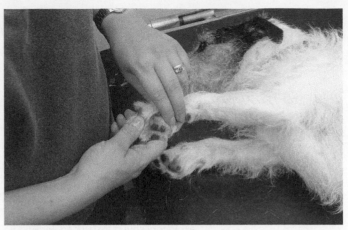

Fig. 17.7   Palpating the digital pulse in a dog

There are a variety of ways to cool an animal down but, in a critically ill animal, some methods may not be suitable, e.g. fluids can be administered at room temperature, but not chilled; a crushed ice enema may work in extreme situations where temperatures are approaching 41–42°C. Total body cooling is best accomplished by immersing the body in cool but not cold water; if the water is too cold, peripheral vasoconstriction may occur, which slows the heat loss process.

Hypothermia may indicate:
- Shock
- Hypovolaemia/circulatory collapse
- Moribund patient.

It is vitally important to try to warm these patients as quickly as possible. When the temperature starts to dip below 36°C, the patient must be actively warmed from the core. Administering fluids intravenously at a temperature of no more than 40°C may help.

The bladder may also be used to administer warming fluids – a urinary catheter is placed aseptically into the bladder and boluses of sterile saline no warmer than 38–40°C can then be administered. Optimal effect will be seen if the fluid is left in place for at least 30 minutes, removed and another bolus administered. You can see temperature increases of up to a degree at a time with this method.

In a patient that is in hypovolaemic shock, direct heat is contraindicated, because vasodilation will occur, encouraging blood flow to non-essential parts of the circulatory system such as cutaneous vessels. The body does not consider these to be important in times of circulatory crisis.

PULSE

The pulse rate can be felt at any place where an artery runs close to the surface of the body and is commonly felt at the femoral artery in the dog and cat. If a critically ill animal is in hypovolaemic shock, the peripheral pulses will be the first to be affected (Figs. 17.6 and 17.7). In these situations, palpating and reading the peripheral pulses can be a good indicator of circulatory state or response to any fluid therapy that may have been initiated.

A slow pulse rate may indicate:
- Hypothermia/low body temperature
- Circulatory failure
- Hyperkalaemia.

A rapid pulse rate may indicate:
- Pain
- Pyrexia
- Sepsis
- Disease process
- Shock
- Ventricular tachycardia.

Sinus arrhythmia

This occurs in relation to the respiratory pattern of the animal. During inspiration the pulse rate will increase, and during expiration it will decrease. This is a normal sequence of events.

Pulse deficit

This occurs when the pulse rate is slower or absent in relation to the corresponding heart sound. This indicates that, although the heart is pumping the blood through the chambers, it is not able to pump it around the rest of the circulatory system. It is a good idea to get into the habit of palpating a pulse at the same time as listening to the heart rate with a stethoscope.

Pulse volume

Pulse volume should be part of the assessment of the pulse and it is essential that you recognise what the normal volume of a pulse should feel like. The pulse wave should be felt over three fingers.

Pulse volume is also called pulse quality:
- An abnormally strong pulse can be described as **hyperkinetic**, **bounding** or a **water-hammer pulse** and can sometimes only be felt across one finger width.
- An abnormally weak pulse is called a **hypokinetic pulse** and almost flutters across your fingers.

Hyperkinetic pulse/bounding pulse is found in:
- Anaemia
- Fever
- Sepsis
- Cardiac disease
- Hyperthyroidism.

Hypokinetic pulse/weak pulse is found in:
- Hypovolaemic shock
- Dehydration
- Cardiac tamponade
- Left-sided heart failure.

TABLE 17.1	Classification of respiratory sounds
Respiratory sound	**Description**
Breath sounds	The normal airway and lung sounds that are audible during normal respiration
Stertor	Noise generated from the nasal passages
Stridor	High-pitched inspiratory sound generated from turbulent airflow in the extrathoracic airways
Rhonchus	Low-pitched, continuous inspiratory or expiratory sound associated with rapid airflow through the larger airways
Wheeze	High-pitched, continuous inspiratory or expiratory sound associated with narrowing of the airways
Crackle (coarse or fine)	High-pitched, discontinuous inspiratory sound associated with reopening of airways that closed during expiration

RESPIRATORY RATE

When assessing respiration it is important to count the rate, assess the pattern and depth and note any sounds associated with each breath:

- **Paradoxical respiration** – normally the chest wall expands during inspiration and returns to normal during expiration. Paradoxical respiration is usually seen when there is a flail chest present and happens because of a change in the intrapleural pressure, usually as a result of trauma. We see the fractured segment moving inwards during inspiration and outwards during expiration.
- **Abdominal respiration** – occurs when the animal uses its abdominal muscles to try and improve respiration and is a sign of respiratory distress. (Other signs of respiratory distress are listed later under Oxygen therapy.)
- **Respiratory sounds** – these are made during inspiration or expiration. A normal animal will breathe almost silently, so any sound may be abnormal and should be classified (Table 17.1) and reported to the veterinary surgeon.

MUCOUS MEMBRANES

Whenever basic monitoring is carried out, it is important to also check the mucous membranes. Check the colour, feel or texture of the membranes and the capillary refill time.

Colour

Cyanosis. This is generally recognised as a 'bluish' tone but the colour can range from a deep red-purple colour to a pale or dusky blue and is caused by excessive amounts of desaturated haemoglobin in the capillary blood. In cases where the mucous membranes are pigmented it will be necessary to look at other, non-pigmented, areas, e.g. vagina or prepuce. There may also be a difference in the appearance of the mucous membranes under natural or artificial light, especially under fluorescent lights. If the animal is found with cyanosed mucous membranes, supply with oxygen before calling the veterinary surgeon.

Hyperaemic (injected). Membranes are a deep brick red and look 'injected'. This change is most commonly seen in hyperthermia, sepsis and polycythemia. In hyperthermia, it occurs because of the massive vasodilation needed for heat loss so there is a huge amount of blood present at places such as the peripheral membranes. In a septic patient, there is pooling of blood due to the loss of vascular tone, giving a dark, brick-coloured appearance.

Icteric (jaundiced). This occurs when there is a build-up of bilirubin in the plasma and tissues (hyperbilirubinaemia) which causes a yellow discoloration of the skin, mucous membranes and also the sclera of the eye.

Pale. Varies from a pale pink to grey/white. It may indicate that the animal has a low packed cell volume (PCV) or that the animal has circulatory shutdown.

Texture. When the mucous membranes are touched, they should feel slightly moist. If they are dry or sticky to the touch, this could be an indicator of dehydration – described as 'tacky'.

CAPILLARY REFILL TIME

Using a finger, put a little pressure onto the mucous membranes of the gum. This reduces the capillary blood flow and causes blanching of the mucous membranes. Lift up your finger and the capillaries will refill. In a normal animal, capillary refill time (CRT) should be no more than 1–1.5 seconds. If it is slower than this it could be an indicator of heart failure, hypovolaemic shock or severe vasoconstriction. Sometimes, it may appear that no blanching occurs or that the CRT is extremely rapid. This may be due to severe vasoconstriction, e.g. in septic shock or pyrexia. When digital pressure is applied, there is nowhere for the blood to flow to, so no blanching occurs.

MONITORING EQUIPMENT

Equipment used in critical patients includes direct and indirect arterial blood pressure measurement, electrocardiograms, capnographs for the monitoring of carbon dioxide and oxygen-monitoring equipment such as pulse oximeters (see also Chapter 27). The measurement of central venous pressure can also be invaluable in the critical patient.

A multichannel monitor incorporates all the following pieces of equipment in one big bedside monitor, which makes life easier if space is limited (Fig. 17.8).

Central venous pressure

Central venous pressure (CVP) is an essential part of monitoring the effects of fluid therapy in critical patients. It is sometimes necessary to challenge animals with fluid boluses and, in patients that may have cardiac disease, it is important to know how the heart responds.

Method. A jugular catheter is placed into the jugular vein. The tip of the catheter should ideally reach the right atrium but often it is positioned at the junction of the right atrium and the cranial vena cava. The measurement that is obtained still reflects change within the right atrium and so it is a reliable estimate:

- The catheter is attached to a three-way tap via some extension tubing.

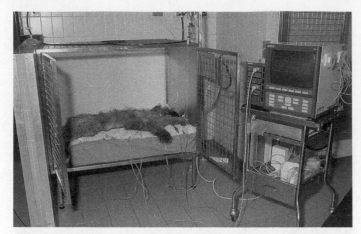

Fig. 17.8 A critically ill dog connected to a bedside monitor

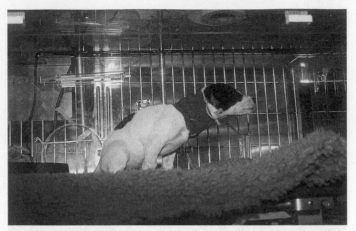

Fig. 17.9 A 4-month-old puppy showing classic signs of respiratory distress. Note the extended neck, abducted elbows and open-mouth breathing

- An intravenous giving set and a bag of fluids are attached to the opposite side of the three-way tap and a water manometer is attached to the upright opening of the tap. The zero of the manometer measure must be level with the sternum (approximate level of right atrium).
- The manometer must be filled with fluid from the bag (always make sure that the whole system is filled with fluids before the tap is turned on to the catheter) and will reach an equal pressure to the right atrium when the tap is turned on to the catheter. If correctly set up, the meniscus in the manometer will rise and fall with each breath that is taken.
- When not in use the tap can be turned off to the manometer and on to the fluids.
- When a measurement is required, the tap is turned off to the fluids and on between the catheter and the manometer. A measurement can then be read from the manometer measure.
- A series of three readings should be taken initially to ensure consistency and accuracy. A reading is taken in centimetres of water (cm H_2O).
- The normal range for CVP is 0–10 cm H_2O but the optimal range is 3–8 cm H_2O:
  - A low CVP is usually the result of hypovolaemia: a series of low readings would indicate that fluid rates could safely be increased.
  - A high CVP might indicate a volume overload or right-sided heart failure. If there is no other evidence to support this, the patency of the catheter should be checked. An occluded jugular catheter will give consistently high CVP readings and so regular flushing of the catheter will be necessary.

Blood pressure monitoring

Blood pressure can be measured directly and indirectly using invasive or non-invasive methods. Blood pressure monitoring is regularly used in critical patients, for animals that are in shock, have renal or cardiac failure, or may be suffering from diseases such as hyperthyroidism or hyperadrenocorticism, where blood pressure may deviate from normal levels. Direct measurement is the most accurate way of monitoring blood pressure but special equipment (a transducer and monitor) is required, together with the placement of an arterial catheter, making it costly.

Electrocardiography

The electrocardiograph (ECG) records the electrical potential of the heart muscle and is an invaluable piece of equipment. Its uses range from determining arrest rhythm during cardiopulmonary resuscitation (CPR) to monitoring cardiac arrhythmias caused by toxicity or poisoning, or to monitor the administration of medicines such as calcium in hypocalcaemic patients. There is usually an audible sound linked to each heartbeat, and this can be very useful if the nurse is looking after several animals at once. A change in tone or speed will automatically alert you to a change in the patient's condition.

Capnography

This is used to record end-tidal carbon dioxide concentration. It is commonly used in the anaesthetised patient but can be used for animals that are being mechanically ventilated. A detector is placed between the endotracheal tube and the anaesthetic machine and connected via tubing to the monitor.

Oxygen therapy

Oxygen therapy should be implemented at the very first signs of hypoxia. If an animal is showing signs of respiratory distress (Fig. 17.9), oxygen should be given and the veterinary surgeon should be called straight away. Oxygen delivery via a mask, an oxygen cage or 'flow-by', i.e. a gas tube that opens close to the patient's nose, would be the preferred methods of delivery in the first instance.

Signs of respiratory distress include:
- Abdominal effort
- Cyanosis
- Open-mouth breathing
- Flared nostrils
- Abducted elbows
- Extended neck
- Anxiety
- Tachypnoea
- Respiratory noise
- Irregular chest wall movement.

Supplementation of oxygen increases the oxygen content of the blood, increases the partial pressure of oxygen in the capillary system and improves tissue perfusion.

TABLE 17.2	Fraction of inspired oxygen (FiO₂) achieved by the different methods of delivering oxygen	
Delivery method	FiO$_2$	O$_2$ flow rate (l/min)
Flow-by	0.24–0.45	6–8
Face mask	0.35–0.55	6–10
Nasal catheter	0.30–0.50	1–6
Oxygen cage	0.40–0.50	Variable
Oxygen collar	0.30–0.40	0.2–0.5
Ventilation	0.21–1.00	10–15
Intratracheal catheter	0.40–0.60	50 ml/kg/min

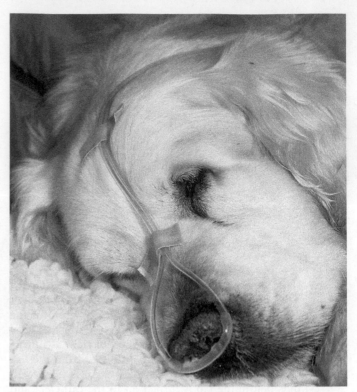

Fig. 17.11   A dog with nasal prongs placed for oxygen therapy

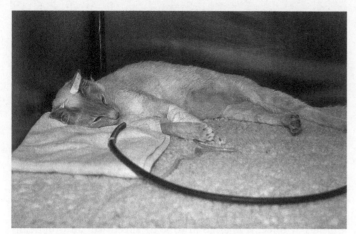

Fig. 17.10   A Siamese cat receiving oxygen therapy using the flow-by method. Note the lack of distress with this method

When oxygen therapy begins, ensure that as high a fraction of inspired oxygen (FiO$_2$) as possible is delivered:
- In room air FiO$_2$ is 21% or 0.21.
- In a patient intubated with a cuffed endotracheal tube on 100% oxygen, the FiO$_2$ would be 100% or 1.

In the methods of oxygen delivery listed in Table 17.2 it is only possible to reach an adequate FiO$_2$ by using appropriate levels of oxygen.

OXYGEN DELIVERY

There are various methods of delivering oxygen to the patient and they all have their advantages and disadvantages. When deciding which method to use the most important factor is patient tolerance, FiO$_2$ achievement and the equipment available.

1. Flow-by oxygen

This is mainly used in an emergency situation. It causes little interference and stress while enabling the clinician to stabilise the patient. The oxygen line is placed 1–3 cm away from the animal's nose and mouth and oxygen is administered at a rate of 5–8 l/min (Fig. 17.10).

The disadvantages of this method are that it requires an assistant to be present at all times. It also requires a high flow rate of oxygen, which is wasteful, and some patients can be distressed by the sound and the rapid airflow of the oxygen, which may cause them to avoid it.

2. Facemask

This is a quick method of delivering oxygen to a patient in an emergency situation. A mask is placed over the mouth and nose of the cat or dog and oxygen is administered at a rate of 3–10 l/min. A transparent mask seems to cause less distress to animals and makes it possible to observe the colour of the oral mucous membranes without removing the mask. Disadvantages include poor patient tolerance, leakage around the mask if it is poorly fitting and little or no removal of carbon dioxide.

3. Nasal catheter

For long-term use, this method produces good oxygenation with relatively low gas flow. The patient can also be examined without disturbance of the oxygen flow. Measure a 5–10-French gauge catheter (usually a nasal feeding tube) from the nostril to the medial canthus of the eye and mark accordingly. A small amount of local anaesthetic gel/cream can be applied to the end of the catheter and also to the external nares that is to be used. Carefully introduce the catheter in a ventromedial fashion up the nasal chamber until the mark is reached. Fix the catheter onto the skin at the nares using glue, suture or staple. A second attachment can be made on the top of the head. Connect the catheter to a source of humidified oxygen using an adaptor. It may be necessary to fit an Elizabethan collar to prevent patient interference.

As the oxygen is going directly into the nasal passages it must be used with a humidifier. Humidification should be carried out using sterile saline at room temperature, which should be changed daily if long-term use is expected.

If using a unilateral catheter the site should be changed every 48 hours to reduce the risk of damage to the mucosa. It is also possible to buy nasal prongs made of very soft silicone, which originate from human oxygen therapy (Fig. 17.11). The disadvantages of this method include poor patient tolerance, jet damage to the mucosa and increased expense.

4.   Oxygen cage

This is a non-invasive method providing a sealed and enclosed environment for emergency or prolonged use. It causes very little stress to the animal and is well tolerated. Some of the oxygen cages enable the control of humidity, temperature and FiO_2 and there is adequate removal of carbon dioxide. The patient can be observed at all times and there are ports for intravenous lines and monitoring leads.

Disadvantages include the fact that the patient is completely isolated from staff, it is expensive and a high flow rate is needed to enrich the cage adequately. There is also a danger of the patient decompensating whenever the cage door is opened and the oxygen-rich environment is lost. It takes a large amount of oxygen to resume adequate oxygen levels, which can be expensive and wasteful. The temperature within the cage must also be closely observed and adjusted accordingly.

5.   Oxygen collar

This is very effective way of delivering oxygen in an emergency situation or for temporary use. An Elizabethan collar is placed on the patient and clear cellophane is then used to cover two-thirds of the front and is taped to the sides. The opening acts as a vent for removal of carbon dioxide and any excess oxygen. The size of the opening will determine the oxygen percentage. The temperature of the patient and the temperature and humidity within the collar must be monitored. Oxygen can dry the mucous membranes and it is necessary to lubricate the eyes with an appropriate ointment such as Lacri-Lube (Allergan) or Viscotears (Novartis Ophthalmics). Disadvantages include poor patient tolerance in some instances, hyperthermia, oxygen leakage and high humidity.

6.   Intratracheal catheter

This method works by bypassing the anatomical dead space, i.e. the nasal chambers, pharynx, larynx and trachea, and allows continuous oxygen delivery at low flow rates. These catheters are placed between the fourth and fifth cartilaginous rings following full surgical preparation. A hole is made that is slightly larger than the catheter to be used. Select a large-bore, long, soft, preferably silicone catheter – it is preferable to fenestrate the end before application, which reduces the risk of jet damage. Place the needle of the catheter between the two cartilaginous rings in dogs and through the cricothyroid ligament in cats and small dogs. Feed the catheter through to the level of the fifth intercostal space. Withdraw the needle and, if appropriate, cover it with a needle guard and secure it to the animal's neck with a bandage. Connect the end of the catheter to a humidified oxygen source. This is a cheaper method of delivering oxygen as low flow rates are used. It is generally well tolerated by patients and allows easy access by the clinician or nurse.

The disadvantages include a risk of the catheter kinking at the site of insertion, subcutaneous emphysema, jet damage to the airways, tracheitis, bronchospasm, infection at the insertion site and possible airway obstruction.

Some animals may need sedating to carry out this procedure.

MONITORING OXYGEN THERAPY

Simple observation of patients may determine how well they are responding to oxygen therapy. Signs of improvement include decrease in respiratory effort and rate, an improved mucous membrane colour and reduced anxiety and stress. Cats will vocalise less. There are also pieces of equipment that indicate whether the oxygen therapy is sufficient.

Blood gas analysis

Blood gas analysis will measure the amount of oxygen (PaO_2) and carbon dioxide ($PaCO_2$) in the arterial blood.

Blood may be collected from the femoral artery or the dorsal metatarsal artery into a heparinised syringe, and it is then analysed by the appropriate machine. The results should be relayed to the veterinary surgeon, who will make an informed decision on the need for further oxygen therapy.

As a general rule:
- $PaO_2 < 70$ mm Hg and/or $PaCO_2 > 45$ mm Hg = need for supplemental oxygen
- $PaO_2 < 60$ mm Hg and/or $PaCO_2 > 50$ mm Hg = respiratory failure and need for ventilatory support.

During oxygen therapy the PaO_2 should be five times the FiO_2, e.g. FiO_2 of 40% = PaO_2 of 200 mm Hg. If it is less than this, there could be a problem with gas exchange and the veterinary surgeon should be informed at once.

A blood gas analyser is a vital piece of equipment, but they are expensive and not all critically ill animals will tolerate samples being taken frequently. For this reason it can be preferable to place an arterial catheter.

Pulse oximetry

This is a simple non-invasive method for monitoring oxygen saturation (SaO_2). It works by calculating the saturation of haemoglobin using the principle of spectrophotometry, i.e. an oxygenated haemoglobin molecule (oxyhaemoglobin) and a reduced or deoxygenated haemoglobin molecule (deoxyhaemoglobin) absorb different lights at different rates. The pulse oximeter shines red light and infrared light through an arterial bed and the microprocessor computes the difference (see also Chapter 27). If the SaO_2 falls to 93% or less, it signals the need for oxygen therapy. This is a less expensive piece of equipment than many others and the probes are well tolerated by the patient. However, the accuracy cannot always be relied upon and, as with blood gas analysis, should be noted in relation to the clinical observations.

HUMIDIFICATION

Where oxygen is supplied directly into the animal's airway, it must be humidified because the animal's own methods of warming and moistening the oxygen, i.e. within the nasal chambers, have been bypassed. Commercial bubble humidifiers (Fig. 17.12) are relatively cheap, but it is also possible to make one:
1. Take two lengths of piping.
2. Take a plastic bottle, sterilise it and half fill it with sterile saline.
3. Attach one length of tubing to the oxygen source. This should be long enough to go through the top of the bottle and into the saline.

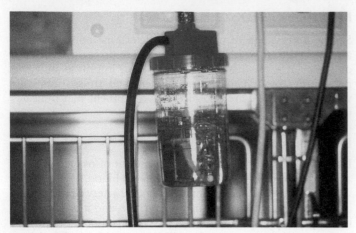

Fig. 17.12 A commercially available bubble humidifier

4. Attach the other tube to the animal – it should be out of the saline at all times.

Case one

A 6-year-old male neutered West Highland White Terrier was admitted into the ward environment with a cough. The patient was hospitalised pending thoracic radiographs. The ward environment was extremely busy, with an abundance of barking dogs.

The patient continued to cough while in the kennel and attempting to bark with the other dogs. A towel was placed over the kennel to help calm the patient and prevent barking. The coughing continued even with the kennel door covered.

The patient was monitored every 2 hours with the patient's vital signs being recorded. The patient could still be heard coughing. The last recorded nursing assessment was at 10.30am and the patient was found deceased at 1pm when no coughing had been heard for a prolonged period of time.

The cause of the death was cardiac arrest due to stimulation of the vagus nerves of the pharynx due to excessive coughing, gagging and retching; the coughing had become more persistent due to the additional stress of the ward environment.

This case also highlights the potential complications/dilemmas of obscuring the front of the kennel in attempting to alleviate stress and provide patient seclusion in a stressful ward environment. The question remains: If the patient had been visible, and coughing caused vagus nerve stimulation resulting in syncope, would the veterinary team have been able to prevent cardiac arrest?

THE POWER OF THE PEN – RECORDING INFORMATION

Excellent veterinary medical record-keeping protocols are the core to the ability to deliver quality care to patients. Computer systems provide a streamlined solution to handwritten clinical records but hospitalisation records for patients still remain as a paper format, requiring accurate, clear and complete details. Completing hospitalisation sheets/records can increase the workload for veterinary staff but the importance of record-keeping can never be overstated. Keeping poor records that are difficult to read, difficult to interpret and confusing can result in detrimental patient care.

It should be remembered that any form of documentation may be called upon if an owner considers taking legal action against a veterinary practice in regards to what the owner considers to be inappropriate patient care. The records should serve as non-verbal proof of quality of care – remember, 'if it isn't in the medial records then it didn't happen' (care not documented is care not given).

It should also be pointed out that no part of the records (such as hospitalisation/medication/treatment sheets) should be written over, erased with correction fluid or otherwise obliterated. A single line is drawn through the incorrect information and the word 'error' as well as the name of the person making the changes should be written next to the entry.

Medical records should be viewed as a ladder, with each rung of the ladder representing the patients' journey from admission to the top of the ladder being the point of discharge from the practice.

Every rung of this ladder needs to be documented and a plan in place for the next step. If at any point the plans become halted, unclear and without focus then the possibility of the patient reaching the top of the ladder becomes hindered and delayed.

A term often used by caregivers in human medicine is having the provision of an 'if I should die' file. This file provides all the information required to allow another professional, totally unfamiliar with the patient, to pick up medical records and immediately understand prior history, patient treatment, patient response and client consent or refusal for care (such as do not resuscitate orders).

Veterinary surgeons are often gathering patient information and devising patient care via the 'SOAP' style of equivalent detailed work-up.

- S = Subjective: Subjective information or data is observable but not exactly measurable, such as decreased appetite, pain level, colour of urine and degree of oedema.
- O = Objective: Objective information is data that can be measured or quantified, such as temperature, blood pressure, respiration and laboratory results.
- A = Assessment: Veterinary surgeon lists patient evaluations in order of priority.
- P = Planning: Plan of care for the patient. This plan usually reflects the medical model, with the patient being treated as a 'case' with the veterinary surgeon planning the diagnostic, medical, surgical and therapeutic details of the patient's veterinary needs.

Information that may be subjective may become objective under different circumstances, e.g. urine output is often subjective, based on observation such as urinary frequency and amount; however, when a urinary catheter is in place, the exact amount of urine can be measured and hence urine output becomes objective.

All the information/data collected should be recorded onto the patients' records and importantly even if the results are within normal limits as this indicates to subsequent caregivers that the examinations/test were carried out and provides the baseline for comparison.

NURSING CARE PLANS

Medical model or veterinary nursing model?

Veterinary surgeons follow a disease-orientated approach to the diagnosis and treatment of their patients which is derived from the human medical approach that focuses on the illness or malfunction of a particular part or system of the body and hence the use of a SOAP system.

Patients are often referred to by their diseases/conditions, such as 'could you take a blood pressure from the renal cat' or 'next in theatre is the bitch spay'. This terminology often experienced in veterinary practices highlights how patients simply become 'cases' referring to the condition/disease rather than the patient. Veterinary nurses play a vital role in providing a separate and distinct patient evaluation which leads to a patient-based approach to nursing care, assessing the individual needs of the patient rather than nursing the patient as a 'case'.

This approach has developed into veterinary nursing models adapted from knowledge and models from human nursing practice. Veterinary nursing care plans are designed to allow veterinary nurses to begin to adopt a more patient-focused, systemic approach to their patient care and allows for this model to be adapted into patient care plans. Adaptations and inclusions into nursing models should be strongly encouraged and should never be employed in an inflexible manner, and they should be regularly questioned for the suitability for each patient and assessed.

Nursing care plans may also be designed without the constraints of a nursing model, as the foundations can lead to a wide range of practice-led formats. There are three main recognised models of veterinary nursing practice:

- Orem Eight Self-care Requisites Model
- Orpet and Jeffery Ability Model – OJAM (Orpet and Jeffery 2007)
- 12 Activities of Living Model – Roper, Logan and Tierney (Roper et al. 2000).

There are a number of different nursing models present in human nursing, each having a range of philosophical assumptions and approaches. Of the range of human nursing models, the Roper, Tierney and Logan model (Table 17.3) appears to be the most compatible with veterinary nursing. This was devised by three British nurses in 1976 as part of a research study into human nursing education. It was developed initially as a conceptual framework for individualising patient care. In 1980 it was published as a theoretical model in a book called *Elements of Nursing* and 3 years later it was applied in clinical situations by human nurses. The authors were keen for it not to be a static model but for it to continue to evolve and develop as knowledge and technology advances.

THE CONCEPTUAL FRAMEWORK

There are five main concepts to the model:

- Activities of living (AOL)
- Life span
- Dependence/independence continuum
- Factors influencing AOL
- The nursing process – individualising care.

Activities of living (AOL)

These are a list of 12 activities that living animals have a need and a right to carry out on a daily basis. In context this may be used as a template for the nursing care plan discussed later in this section. The activities of living are all interrelated and influence one another, so it is important to look at all 12 as a whole. They are:

- Maintenance of a safe environment
- Communicating
- Breathing
- Eating and drinking
- Eliminating
- Personal cleansing
- Controlling body temperature
- Mobilising
- Working and playing
- Expressing sexuality
- Sleeping
- Dying.

These form the basis of the Roper, Tierney and Logan model. It can be argued that some of these activities hold little relevance to animal patients, e.g. expressing sexuality, while others only apply in a few specialist cases, e.g. most veterinary patients will not be working apart from police and guide dogs but they can actually become quite distressed when they are stopped from working.

Life span

This relates to the stages of a patient's time from birth to death – kittenhood/puppyhood, adolescence, adulthood and senior/geriatric stages. Knowledge, expectation and prediction are the key words in this concept and it is what we need to be good at as nurses. By knowing at which stage each patient is in its life span we can predict possible complications associated with each activity of living at that particular life stage and allow appropriate nursing care to be instigated, e.g. a newborn kitten and a geriatric dog will share many potential problems even though they are at two different life stages, such as maintaining personal cleanliness, controlling body temperature and maintaining a safe environment; however, there are big differences in how they are nursed and managed on a day-to-day basis and consequently their care plan should be designed individually.

Dependence/independence continuum

This part of the nursing model brings the previous two concepts together. In the case of a sick animal there will be times when it will not be able to fully perform all the activities of living. The dependence/independence continuum (Fig. 17.13) is used to assess the individual patient's level of competence in carrying out each activity of living. Effective nursing care may then be implemented to help achieve optimum competency for the

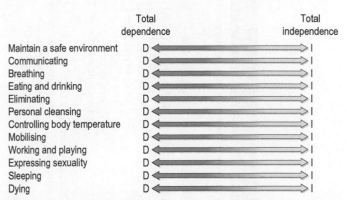

Fig. 17.13   Dependence/independence continuum

TABLE 17.3 The nursing process (adapted from Roper, Logan and Tierney model of nursing) – example of a nursing care plan

To be completed once daily or more often if dramatic changes in patient's status; evaluation to be completed prior to writing new NCP

Date: _____ Time: _____ Initials: _____ Case no: _____ Patient: _____ Client: _____

Ability	Actual problem	Potential problem	Short-term goal	Nursing intervention	Evaluation
Eat adequate amounts	Nothing by mouth (nil per os [NPO]) – due to dysphagia, unable to open mouth and oesophageal dysfunction Gastrostomy tube in place	Gastrostomy tube displacement: blockage; infection; regurgitation/vomiting Gastrointestinal hypo-/hypermotility, delayed gastric emptying Aspiration pneumonia	Check gastrostomy tube with clinician Follow nutritional plan – provide one-third total resting energy requirement (RER) today – day 1	Gastrostomy tube care twice daily (BID) and stoma care (follow designated protocol) Ensure correct feeding guidelines are followed – check with clinician	Clinician: change the non-adhesive dressings twice daily at stoma site as exudate present Patient tolerating enteral feeding very well
Drink adequate amounts	NPO Intravenous fluid therapy via peripheral vein	Dehydration, reduced urine output, risk of urinary tract infection (UTI), renal compromise Phlebitis, thrombophlebitis of cephalic vein due to intravenous catheter – localised/systemic infection	Maintain hydration via intravenous fluids Assess fluid balance for the initial 24 hr – measure urine output	Intravenous catheter care – redress BID Maintain intravenous fluid rate – 30 ml/kg/hr Measure urine output q2hr for 24 hours – calculate ml/kg/hr Use damp swabs to wipe around lips and mucous membranes	Phlebitis developed at 16.00 (clinician informed) Removed left cephalic catheter and replaced into right cephalic Cold compresses placed over cephalic for 10 min Urine output recorded (see below) initial 2 hr = see fluids in/out chart
Urinate normally	Able to urinate – urinary catheter placed to prevent urine scalding/measure urine output	Urinary catheter dislodgement, haematuria, UTI Urinary catheter occlusion, reduced urine outflow	Monitor urine outflow and measure	Follow urinary catheter care protocol Measure urine output q2hr –notify clinician if urine output drops below 2 ml/kg/hr Ensure urine collection bag is located below the patient	Catheter checked, cleaned and flushed 9am and 19.00 Urine output measured and recorded on chart Clinician notified at 19.00 – urine outflow 5 ml/kg for last 2 hr Flushed catheter – haematuria and urine outflow returned
Breathe normally	Intercostal muscle function reduced/fatigued due to tonic muscle spasms Aspiration pneumonia Tachypnoeic	Respiratory arrest Hypostatic pneumonia complicated by pre-existing pneumonia Dyspnoea, bradycardia, hypoxia, reduced oxygen saturation Cardiac arrest – death	Maintain patent airway and supplemental oxygen Maintain respiratory rate (RR) 38–45 Optimise patient ventilation by turning patient through lateral/sternal recumbency Reposition q4hr	Record RR q2hr Provide oxygen supplementation via nasal prong – 2 l/min Continuous SpO$_2$ monitoring, probe located on ear pinna – record values q2hr Suction oral cavity q4hr Thoracic auscultation q2hr Reposition patient q4hr from left, sternal and right recumbencies	Muscle spasms and head extension caused displacement of nasal prongs on two occasions – clinician notified Suctioning of oral cavity is tolerated very well by the patient Repositioning patient causes severe muscle spasms through tactical stimulation (21.30) Clinician informed and medication altered to provide muscle relaxation

Maintain body temperature	Muscular spasms result in intermittent hyperthermia (depending upon medical therapy used)	Persistent hyperthermia	Administer muscle relaxation therapy to elevate muscle contractor and hyperthermia Prevent visual, tactile, auditory stimulus which results in more spasms	Provide patient with verbal reassurance and limit tactile stimulation to patient rotation Monitor and record rectal or auditory temperature q4hr	Patient temperature fluctuates; hyperthermia occurs during muscle spasms – significant trend recorded on records Clinician notified at 23.10 that spasms are becoming more frequent (no further action required)
Pain free	Neurological/nerve/orthopaedic pain from hind limb amputation Intercostal muscle pain from tachypnoea and disease process Muscle pain due to muscular contractions and relaxation	Medical intervention not controlling pain from muscular spasms Inadequate pain control (patient discomfort, anxiety increases) Inability to accurately assess the patient's analgesic levels due to uncontrolled muscle spasms	Ensure opiate patch remains in situ Administer additional analgesics as ordered on medication chart Assess analgesia by using pain scoring system Notify clinician if patient's pain score rises	Pain score patient q2hr to coincide with other nursing procedures (measuring urine output) q2hr Ensure intravenous line remains patent to allow sedation and additional analgesia to be provided AVOID passive or active massage/physiotherapy of the patient as this stimulation results in muscle spasms Keep patient on the memory foam mattress to aid in preventing decubital ulcers and reduce tissue damage	Pain score value dropped considerably at 01.45am when ketamine CRI began (clinician DW) Additional intravenous catheter placed for continuous rate infusion (CRI) Discussed with DW if mattress could be insulating the patient and increasing patient's temperature (MR) No suitable alternatives available
Groom itself	Unable to groom	Faecal soiling Maceration of the skin Dermatitis Decubital ulcers Matted fur	To prevent faecal soiling due to recumbency Assess the patient's bony prominences for skin colour changes to prevent the development of ulcers	Clean perineal region with warm water, dry the skin and apply barrier spray and topical barrier cream BID or more frequently if faeces passed Assess skin integrity and colour by parting the fur and examining the skin; if in any doubt, clip the fur to provide clearer assessment Assess q4hr when patient repositioned Record skin examination on decubital ulcer prevention diagram	No faeces passed on this shift Perineal area cleaned at beginning of shift – to be done again at patient handover 7am Skin inflammation and erythema developing on medial aspect of the right elbow – notes made and photo taken for comparison for day staff 04.00am
Mobilise adequately	Non-ambulatory with muscular rigidity	Muscle atrophy Muscle fatigue due to muscle spasms Muscular pain Increase in calorie utilisation resulting in malnutrition/cachexia High risk for decubital ulcers	Provide passive physiotherapy and massage under the direction of the clinician to help provide analgesia Procedures not to be carried out if tactile stimulation results in spasms	Follow guidelines for preventing hypostatic pneumonia with patient rotation q4hr Passive physiotherapy and massage q6hr ONLY if no muscular spasms If patient requires removal from the kennel, lift with a stretcher Take patient outside when dark (preventing external stimulation) and allow time on the grass to provide some form of environmental stimulation/change	Passive muscular massage completed q6hr with no muscular spasms Patient taken outside on a stretcher at 1.00am to provide patient with an environmental change – patient response was promising, nasal flaring in the breeze and moving his eyes; no spasms occurred– remained outside for 30 min (MR)

Continues

TABLE 17.3   The nursing process (adapted from Roper, Logan and Tierney model of nursing) – example of a nursing care plan—cont'd

To be completed once daily or more often if dramatic changes in patient's status; evaluation to be completed prior to writing new NCP
Date: _____   Time: _____   Initials: _____   Case no: _____   Patient: _____   Client: _____

Ability	Actual problem	Potential problem	Short-term goal	Nursing intervention	Evaluation
Sleep/rest	Medications providing mild sedative effects Physically patient is exhausted due to muscle spasms which increase with stimulation Patient located into the isolation area to reduce visual, auditory and tactile stimulation and permitting environmental control – lights off, reduced sound – providing an environment which is optimal for relaxation	Complications of sleep deprivation include: • Immune system compromise – risk of the patient developing further diseases/conditions while hospitalised • Reduced tissue healing and risk of wound breakdown • Alterations in the patient's metabolism resulting in altered absorption of medical therapy • Patient fatigue	Environmental control to avoid excessive stimulation that could result in muscle spasms Adjust ALL potential stimuli in the ward environment – from noise, lighting, handling etc.	Lights out time from 10pm–6am with all patient interventions being completed using a spotlight if possible Avoid excessive noise and handling if possible If weather permitting, patient can sleep on the stretcher outside for a period of time (under the supervision of an animal nursing assistant)	Patient has not been outside all day due to the sunshine, noise levels and excessive number of people Patient taken outside as above for a period of time, then placed back into isolation (MR) Nursing interventions successfully completed with limited lighting and patient remained relaxed throughout (MR)
Express normal behaviour	Appears very anxious, with inability to express anxiety Normal behaviours associated with anxiety will not be seen due to muscle rigidity, discomfort	Patient will be misunderstood or his mental anxiety underestimated as he is unable to express any normal canine behaviour Pain scoring will be difficult to assess As a young puppy, this prolonged period of hospitalisation and social isolation could have a negative effect on the patient's social/behavioural development and his behaviour in the future	To provide the patient with the balanced care required to ensure that the medical status of the patient remains stable and the patient's mental well-being is continually assessed	Ensure that the pheromone bandana remains in place and refreshed throughout the day while the pheromone collar begins to take effect Pheromone diffuser is in place in isolation The patient is mentally aware so ensure that time is spent talking to him, touching and reassuring him; provide him with olfactory comforting smells (e.g. leave the owner's T-shirt by his head) Time spent with the patient should be assessed at end of shift highlighting patient's response to TLC	Patient appeared more 'relaxed' when placed outside for a period of time Frequent visits of a short duration for TLC are well tolerated (5 min) Muscle spasms increased when the duration of time spent with the patient increased (MR)

particular activity. The patient's level of competence should be plotted along the line of each activity to record the degree of dependence or independence for each activity of living. Once this is done, nursing goals can be set, alongside clinical intervention, in order to move the mark further towards independence.

It is important to note that most activities interact and influence one another and so all 12 must be looked at together as well as individually. It is also important to know the patient's normal status and routine at home, so as not to confuse it as an abnormality of the patient's current condition. To minimise disruption and delay in treatment, you must maintain effective communication with the owner to obtain relevant information about the patient's daily routine and any pre-existing conditions. At times this may be difficult to achieve, e.g. when dealing with a canine patient that will only eliminate on grass and the veterinary practice is surrounded by concrete and tarmac.

Factors influencing the activities of living

These factors may influence the nursing care given to the patient. They are:

- Biological
- Psychological
- Sociocultural
- Environmental
- Politico-economic.

Biological – veterinary patients are unique in that there are different breeds within the species which have physiological and anatomical differences and these must be taken into consideration: e.g. a Bulldog may not be able to breathe as well as a Labrador in its 'normal' state; a Siberian Husky may not be able to control its body temperature as effectively in the summer compared to a short-haired Terrier. This allows for the implementation of effective nursing care to maintain health and prevent further disease and deterioration of the patient.

Psychological – illness and injury are both stressful for the patient and owner and can sometimes lead to anxiety and unwelcome behaviour in the patient (and sometimes in the owner). As well as feeling unwell, the animal has been removed from its familiar environment and it may have also had a previous bad experience at the surgery. Some of the life stages, e.g. a geriatric animal that is blind and deaf, will also have increased anxiety over and above what might normally be expected.

Stress will affect the activities of living and this will present in a variety of manifestations. Cats may become withdrawn, inappetent, unable to relax or sleep or even eliminate. Dogs may become very aggressive and impossible to handle. This will undoubtedly affect the nursing care given and the chances of recovery, and some patients will be impossible to treat within the veterinary practice. A good nurse will anticipate a patient's state of mind, recognise the body language, and adapt the environment and care to suit the patient. A stressed cat will benefit from accommodation away from dogs, in a low-lit, quiet area with a familiar bed in the cage. Any visits from the owners will ultimately be dependent on the individual patient and the nurse is usually the best person to make the decision.

Sociocultural – different cultures have different attitudes to animals as pets and their pain thresholds. People have different ideas as to the perception of their animal in pain. You may recognise the owner who brings in their pet that has had an open wound for a week and it is only when it has stopped eating, because the wound is now infected, that they decide to get it treated. You may also recognise the Bichon Frise owner who instantly brings her dog in when it has cut its nail and is spotting blood. Our own perceptions as veterinary nurses influence our approach to the patient and its owner. Their opinions or ideas of their pet in pain may differ from what we recognise or have experienced as professionals in the field.

Our patients cannot tell us if they are in pain so we have to look for outward signs, which can be very subjective. As veterinary professionals we have all dealt with cases of the 'sensitive' owner, who may reflect their own feelings or even experiences onto their pet rather than the animal actually showing outward signs of pain. As veterinary professionals we also consciously or subconsciously relate different breeds to having different pain thresholds and this may also extend to the type of owner that may have these pets as well. This leads to an idea that sociologist Talcott Parsons put forward in 1966. He suggested that some human beings may adopt a 'sick role' and can 'act' or give the perception that they are in pain and discomfort in order to obtain a positive response. It may be that animals can adopt a similar role but as yet this has not been proven.

Different cultures and religions may hold ideas and values that extend to their pets: e.g. Jehovah's witnesses do not believe in blood transfusions and may prevent the use of a blood transfusion in their own animal. People also have different ideas about homeopathic medicine, spiritual healing and conventional medicine and may also have different perceptions of the doctors and veterinary surgeons themselves. Some may see them as God-like figures; others may not. All of these will ultimately affect the outcome for the patient.

Environmental – this is particularly significant as this tends to be under the complete control of the veterinary nurse. As nurses we need to be able to adapt the external environment to fit the patient's needs and allow all the activities of living to take place. Environmental factors pertain to light, noise, temperature, humidity and smell. It also includes cleanliness and the presence of any microorganisms in the environment, which is particularly significant in cases that require barrier nursing. The environment must be managed to make the patient as comfortable as possible, to increase the chances of it making a full recovery while also maintaining the health and safety of the other patients and staff.

Politico-economic – the veterinary industry is based almost entirely on private health care so the economic climate at the time has a direct influence on patient treatment and how much clients are able/willing to spend on their animal. In a recession a practice may see a reduction in spending by clients and an increase in debtors. Clients are less likely to invest in preventative health care, e.g. worming, flea treatment and vaccination. This in turn affects the level of investment a practice is able to put into staff and equipment. Animal charities will also suffer, with fewer donors and more people seeking financial help. Fewer animals are likely to be insured as monthly premium payments are usually the first thing people drop when tightening the purse strings. All these factors ultimately affect what treatment a patient receives and how effective or successful that treatment is going to be.

The care of the patient is also dependent upon cultural, financial and owner compliance considerations which are included in the Orpet and Jeffery Ability Model (Box 17.2). This model requires veterinary nurses to consider 10 patient 'abilities' on which to base patient assessment, planning, implementation and evaluation of their nursing care.

In conjunction with the OJAM the key stages of the nursing process should be incorporated and followed. The key stages are:

- Assessment
- Nursing diagnosis
- Planning
- Implementation
- Evaluation.

Clinical diagnosis is not in the legal or professional remit of anyone other than the veterinary surgeon. A veterinary nurse, however, needs to be able to make judgements about a patient's nursing needs based upon the information gathered during the assessment of the patient and to identify problems with any of the 10 abilities to help elevate them.

Example

A dog is brought in exhibiting laboured respiration, cyanotic mucous membranes and altered mentation. The veterinary surgeon is the only person that can diagnose the cause of the clinical signs, but the veterinary nurse can judge the animal's response to the physiological changes, such as decreased perfusion/oxygenation, cerebral and cardiopulmonary compromise, and immediately institute intervention – providing supplemental oxygen therapy and assessing the correct equipment for oxygen administration depending upon the patient.

In addition to making the nursing diagnosis about the actual or existing conditions, veterinary nurses also may make assessments about the future or possible conditions – e.g. a risk assessment for the above patient would include respiratory arrest and or cardiac arrest and plans can be in place if the patient's condition deteriorated (e.g. locating rapid response equipment by the patient's kennel which would allow intubation, tracheostomy tube placement and intervention to assist respiration and, importantly, knowing the resuscitation status of the patient – i.e. owner's consent).

Prioritisation

Human medicine patients often present with multiple conditions that may be interlinked to the initial disease process or that develop as a result of the underlying condition. Prioritisation is a methodical determination of the order in which each problem should be addressed. Using the OJAM, the abilities can be broken down into the needs of that particular patient from a veterinary nursing view.

It must also be remembered that the care of the patient is not just limited to one particular nursing model as other patients' needs must be met as well.

Chronic pain/acute pain (mild to moderate) – if the patient is in pain due to thoracic injury then the patient's ability to breathe will be impaired. Again this is not a diagnosis but an understanding of the complex jigsaw puzzle of nursing care. Address one nursing condition (pain score and administer pain medication under the direction of the veterinary surgeon), then the thoracic pain should reduce and allow the patient's respiratory rate and effort to improve. Prioritise the patient's need for analgesia over the need for grooming or feeding. The patient's needs are not placed in any particular order and prioritising one over the other does not make one less important, but simply indicates that that need will be addressed at a more suitable point in the patient's care.

Interestingly in human medicine other needs are placed into the model, such as oxygenation with the understanding that lack of oxygen will kill a patient more quickly than any other cause. Non-critical safety is added and includes factors and circumstances that affect the patient's well-being but are not immediately life threatening, such as minor wounds that can increase the risk of infection especially nosocomial multidrug-resistant infections.

Planning

The plan of care for an animal is about setting goals for the patient and working out how these goals will be met with nursing care and actions – nursing interventions. This then leads to the development of a care plan for the patient. In emergency situations, planning and implementing interventions may be almost simultaneous with very little written plan in place. Once the assessment has been made, then the number of actual and potential veterinary nursing concerns/problems would be identified.

The veterinary nursing assessment and evaluation then allow for discussions to be made regarding the goals for the patient and the nursing care and action required. The planning phase allows for the setting up and organisation of the equipment required for the nursing interventions. At this point the interventions can be prioritised.

This is the problem-solving stage and involves:

- Solving actual identified problems
- Preventing potential problems from becoming actual problems
- Alleviating problems that cannot be solved – effectively managing a patient and owner, allowing them to cope
- Preventing the recurrence of any problems
- Keeping the patient as comfortable as possible even if death is imminent.

Communication is important and should involve all members of staff. It is a good idea to record this as it may be constantly referred to especially in the evaluation stage.

Goal setting is also part of the planning stage and should involve:

- Long- and short-term goals
- Goals set to alleviate each actual and each potential problem
- Goals that may be measured, observed or tested in the evaluation stage.

All goals should be described in enough detail so that they may be used and understood by other nurses and members of clinical staff.

Implementation

Veterinary interventions should be communicated in a way that enables everyone involved in the care of the patient to fully understand and carry out what needs to be done. All interventions require specifying – the order of priority, how often it needs to be done and how much should be done.

Providing standard written protocols for practical procedures ensures that the correct techniques are followed by every care provider, and having written protocols allows for nurses to refer back to these for reference to ensure continuity of care.

A statement without explanation or vague details can lead to misinterpretation depending upon who is reading the information, e.g. 'Place nasal oxygen prongs and provide oxygen supplementation.' This intervention is vague. A more appropriate way would be to state, 'Place nasal oxygen prongs following the written protocol for correct placement. The patient will require 2 litres of humidified oxygen per minute and if the patient exhibits signs of distress/discomfort then the nasal prongs must be removed and flow-by oxygen provided at 4 litres a minute. Notify the veterinary surgeon for further instruction.'

It should not be assumed that all members of the nursing team will approach a particular patient with a particular condition in a similar way without written detailed planning. Providing a systematic approach to planning patient care does ensure that the patient experiences optimal nursing by the entire team.

Evaluation/reflection

Once a care plan has been developed and implemented, evaluation is an essential part of the process in ascertaining the extent to which the interventions and treatments are doing what they set out to achieve. For this evaluation to be made effectively, the veterinary nurse needs to assess the patient again.

Using a nursing care plan ensures that a systematic and holistic approach is used for continuous evaluation. The veterinary nurse will reassess each of the patient's abilities now, compared to what the patient could or could not do before, and in this way a judgement can be made as to whether the patient is responding to the nursing care better or worse than expected.

The evaluation or reflection can be an extremely difficult process. As a veterinary nurse the thought of not achieving the goals can be very demoralising and upsetting. Sometimes the goals are not achievable and the reflection is vital in understanding that different techniques/procedures are required.

This evaluation allows for the patient to be re-evaluated, which in turn may lead to the original care plan to be amended or a new care plan is completed.

'It is difficult to justify planning and implementation of nursing interventions if the outcomes cannot be shown to have benefited either the patient or the client in some way' (Jeffery 2006).

Evaluation is a crucial stage in the nursing process but not a critical one. It is a re-evaluation of how successful the whole process has been but should not involve criticising the nursing care given if the goal has not been achieved and the problem not resolved. The whole process is a learning one and can only help to improve nursing skills. This stage can be difficult to do and is dependent on a time frame – either hourly, daily or weekly. It is a comparative exercise and aims to look back at the goals set for each patient and the benefits that have been achieved. It needs to be done honestly by all members of the clinical team involved with the patient.

Some questions to consider at this stage are:
- Has the goal been fully achieved?
- Does it require input from another part of the team?
- Should the nursing intervention be changed or stopped?
- Is the problem unchanged or worsening?
- Is the goal to be achieved inappropriate or impossible? (In some cases the situation may have changed due to reduced funding or a change of diagnosis.)

Revision

The evaluation stage naturally leads us to revise our nursing plan, the goals we wish to achieve and the ways in which to achieve them. In other words the whole nursing process needs to start again beginning with reassessment of the patient.

Summary

Many nurses may see this approach to nursing as another time-consuming chore, to add to an already long list; however, some nurses may be doing all this in their heads on a daily basis. The aim of this process is to instil a mind-set rather than start a paper chase, although some stages do require staff to record information. Using this theoretical approach provides continuity of care as well as individual, finely tuned care and allows a gold standard to be set, to which all clinical staff may work.

The introduction of a theoretical approach to veterinary nursing only serves to compound the idea of veterinary nursing as a separate entity to veterinary medicine and surgery. While still working under and in conjunction with the veterinary surgeon, the two have completely different roles to play in achieving the continued welfare of individual patients.

PUTTING NURSING CARE PLANS INTO PRACTICE

Meet Tyke (Fig. 17.14)

Tyke, a 7-month-old Lurcher cross, initially presented with acute lameness of the left hind leg after slipping on laminate flooring.

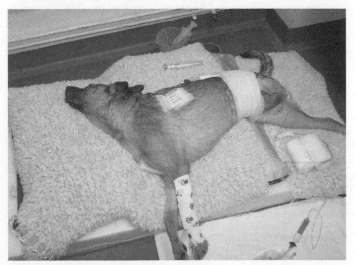

Fig. 17.14 Tyke

Radiographs revealed a transverse fracture of the tibia. Considering the patient's age, body size, athleticism, the affected limb and type of fracture, surgical intervention was considered unnecessary and financially not a viable option for the owner. A synthetic plaster cast was applied.

The patient was discharged and did not return to the hospital for a period of 10 days. On presentation the patient was anorexic, lethargic and vomiting. The patient had been chewing the distal end of the cast and the owner had noticed a pungent odour developing from his exposed digits. The fourth and fifth digits were swollen, erythema had developed and the patient was in obvious discomfort.

The patient was hospitalised and the cast was removed under general anaesthesia. A pressure sore had developed at the medial aspect of the hock. Circulatory compromise had caused oedema and necrosis on the fourth and fifth digits. The skin between the digits has become necrotic.

The wounds were lavaged and radiographs confirmed that a callus had formed at the site of the fracture, so a suitable daily wound management plan was devised and a Robert Jones dressing was applied.

On the third day of hospitalisation, Tyke had begun to salivate, he was reluctant to lie down and dysphagia was evident. His facial expression had altered with his facial muscles in spasm which had caused the retraction of his ears and lips resulting in a grinning appearance (*risus sardonicus*).

His condition deteriorated, with stiffness of his neck and back muscles. His mouth could not be opened manually and when he was placed into lateral recumbency all his limbs were in extensor rigidity. A diagnosis of tetanus (*Clostridium tetani*) was made.

Summary of his treatment/surgical and medical intervention

- General anaesthesia and hind limb amputation
- Percutaneous endoscopically placed gastrostomy (PEG) tube
- Intravenous antibiotics, supplemental oxygen therapy
- Placement of a fentanyl transdermal patch to provide analgesia
- Placement of an indwelling urinary catheter with a closed urine collection system
- Intravenous catheter placement and fluid therapy

The introduction and benefits of care plans into the veterinary nursing profession continue to be debated. The benefits of providing continuity of care and precise nursing care based solely upon the individual needs of each patient is without doubt a positive step in patient care and is considered the gold standard in nursing care. The one major disadvantage is the time required to complete a nursing care plan. The nursing care plan for Tyke highlights a patient requiring more intensive nursing care and hence the time to complete a concise care plan can result in time being spent completing the care plan and less time nursing the patient.

The details written on the care plan are also dependent upon the knowledge of the person completing the plan. Often care plans are written or overseen by qualified veterinary nurses to ensure that vital nursing interventions are not overlooked.

Patient care plans are an excellent learning tool for student veterinary nurses, with research often required to complete the plans and hence extending the knowledge/learning process of the student nurse.

ASSESSING THE PATIENT

The veterinary nurse is usually the person who spends the most time with each patient and so his or her observations are very important in assessing the condition of a patient and the progress of treatment.

When monitoring the condition the SOAP method may be used to ensure completeness. SOAP stands for subjective, objective, assessment and planning:

- **Subjective** – personal assessment of immeasurable observations, e.g. patient's behaviour, demeanour, posture
- **Objective** – factual assessment of measurable observations, e.g. temperature, pulse and respiration
- **Assessment** – a comparative exercise to assess the progress of the patient; may include both subjective and objective observations
- **Planning** – outlines the plan for each patient for that day, whether it is a specific treatment protocol or procedure to be carried out.

Subjective observation relies on the premise that one nurse will be assigned to a specific patient, as interpretation will differ from one person to the next. The assigned person will become familiar with the patient's behaviour and demeanour and any changes are easily identified. Objective assessment relies on the accurate use of equipment, e.g. ability to use a digital thermometer or to auscultate the patient's thorax using a stethoscope. In order to assess accurately and record the progress of a patient it is important to know the normal ranges of the various clinical parameters, e.g. pulse rate, respiratory rate, in healthy patients so that any abnormalities may be identified (Table 17.4). This is also true of behaviour, as in many cases this is the first observation made of a patient's condition or response to treatment.

Vital signs

The vital signs initially assessed in a hospitalised patient are temperature, pulse, capillary refill time and respiration. However, a general assessment should be made of the whole patient, to include eyes, nose, ears, anus, vulva or penis and coat condition. Lymph node enlargement and sensory status, e.g. presence of nystagmus, ataxia and anisocoria, should be assessed and findings should be recorded on a hospital sheet for each patient.

1. **Temperature.** Core body temperature is a useful guide to the health status of a patient. A patient may have a high temperature (pyrexia) if infection or sepsis is present or in cases

TABLE 17.4	Normal clinical parameters in the dog and cat	
Parameter	**Dog**	**Cat**
Temperature (°C)	38.3–38.7	38.0–38.5
Pulse (beats/min)	60–180	110–180
Respiration (breaths/min)	10–30	20–30
Mucous membrane colour	Salmon pink	Salmon pink
Capillary refill time (s)	<2.5	<2.5
Urine production (ml/kg/24 hr)	20	20
Fluid intake (ml/kg/24 hr)	50–60	50–60
Faeces production (ml/kg/24 hr)	10–20	10–20
Acid–base balance (pH)	7.27–7.43	7.25–7.33

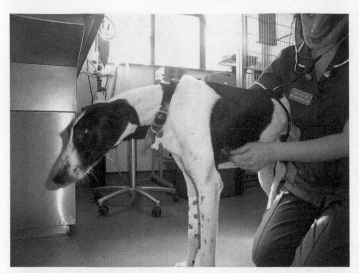

Fig. 17.15   Correct method of auscultation of a dog's heart

of heat stroke. A subnormal temperature may be recorded in patients who have undergone extensive surgery under general anaesthesia or in cases of hypothermia.

A digital or mercury-substitute style thermometer is used to take a patient's temperature. If using a mercury thermometer it is important to ensure that the mercury is shaken down to the base before use, though these thermometers are not commonly available. The thermometer is then inserted into the anus, using a lubricating gel such as KY jelly, and left in situ for 1 minute. The thermometer should be gently twisted as it is inserted and held at a slight angle so as not to record the temperature of any faeces within the rectum. Digital thermometers should be left in place until they beep. Different digital thermometers will state the ideal length of time between use, though most state 3 minutes before taking a temperature again.

2.   **Pulse.** This is a basic measurement of heart rate using a stethoscope to auscultate the thorax. This may be done by placing the stethoscope over the lateral aspect of the thorax, just behind and level with the bottom of the scapula (Fig. 17.15). Any irregularities in the heartbeat such as sinus arrhythmias or heart murmurs may also be picked up at this point. Palpation of peripheral pulses gives some indication as to the state of a patient's peripheral circulation.

The pulse may be palpated in several areas of an animal's body. In an anaesthetised animal the lingual pulse may be used. In conscious animals the most commonly used sites are the femoral pulse (medial femur; Fig. 17.16A), digital pulse (palmar aspect of carpus; Fig. 17.16B) and the tarsal pulse (medial aspect, mid tarsus; Fig. 17.16C).

A pulse oximeter may be used to assess pulse rate and the oxygen saturation of the blood. This small machine contains a pair of sensors that may be attached to a membrane or piece of skin such as the interdigital folds or the pinna of the ear. The tongue may be used in anaesthetised or comatose patients. The measurement relies on a degree of peripheral circulation in order for the sensors to obtain a reading and is of no use in patients with severe circulatory failure.

3.   **Capillary refill time and mucous membrane colour.** These may be used as a measurement of blood volume and circulatory status. Capillary refill time is taken by blanching the patient's gum with the tip of a finger and timing how long the gum takes to return to normal colour again. Mucous membrane colour is an observational measurement in which the gums or sclera may be used (Fig. 17.17). Pale mucous membranes may be observed in patients suffering from shock because of the redirection of blood to the body's vital organs. The capillary refill time would also be increased due to the reduction of blood volume in peripheral vessels.

4.   **Respiration.** Respiratory rate and pattern may be assessed by observation and auscultation of the thorax. Auscultation of the thorax is used to listen to a patient's lung to detect chest sounds: e.g. in the case of a chylothorax, the presence of fluid in the chest cavity may be heard. Respiratory rate is calculated by observing and timing the number of times a patient takes a breath over 1 minute.

It is important to note the pattern of respiration when observing patients. Dyspnoea is the term given to difficult and laboured breathing. Stridor is used to describe breathing associated with a shrill, harsh sound heard during inspiration. This is usually associated with upper airway complications such as laryngeal obstruction. Cheyne-Stokes or agonal respiration is a term given to a particular pattern of breathing that usually heralds the onset of death. There is usually a short period of very deep, convulsive breathing which suddenly changes to small shallow breaths or complete termination of breathing, the pattern of which occurs periodically.

KENNELLING HOSPITALISED PATIENTS

Depending on the layout and design of a kennel area cats and small patients such as rabbits, guinea pigs, rats and birds should be housed separately from dogs. Serious thought should be given to the patient's condition and the effect of the external environment around them: e.g. a dyspnoeic feline patient should not be placed in the kennel above a barking dog. A recumbent patient should not be hidden away in a kennel on its own but accommodated next to an area of activity so that it does not feel forgotten and can be closely monitored.

The size of the kennel should be relative to the size of the patient, and the patient should be able to fully stretch out. This is particularly relevant with recumbent and geriatric patients. Placement of equipment within the kennel is also important. A feline patient may be hesitant to eat if its food bowl is directly next to the litter tray. A geriatric patient with spondylosis or a patient with megaoesophagus may benefit from their food and water bowls being raised off the ground.

Essential activities

The needs of a patient encompass all the daily essential activities which a patient performs in order to maintain a comfortable existence and in many cases survive. These relate to the activities of living used in the nursing model discussed earlier and include:

- Elimination, i.e. urination, defecation, vomiting, coughing
- Food intake – maintaining nutritional status
- Fluid intake – maintaining hydration status
- Controlling body temperature
- Mobilisation or moving around

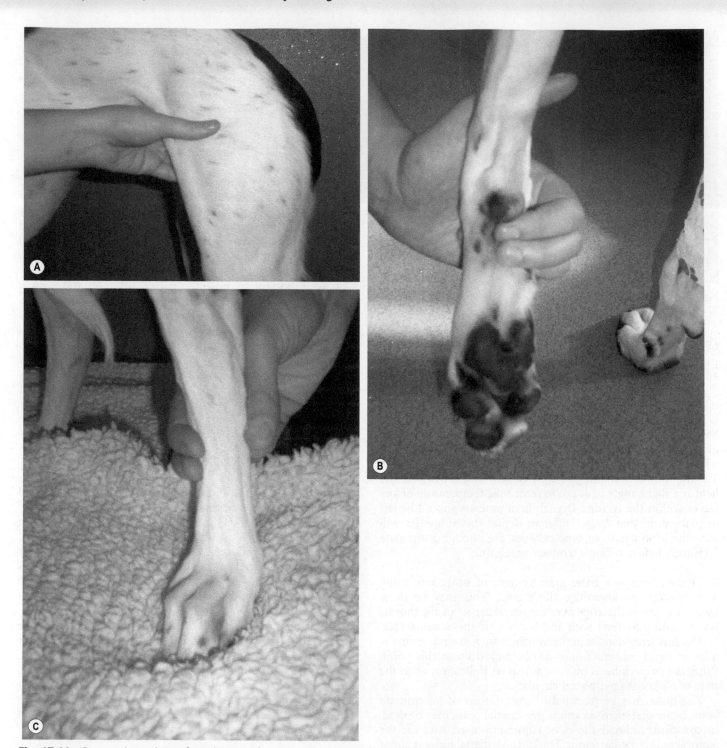

Fig. 17.16 Commonly used sites for palpation of peripheral pulses. (A) Femoral pulse. (B) Digital pulse. (C) Tarsal pulse

- Grooming
- Communication.

In providing nursing care it is important to consider the whole patient rather than focus primarily on a particular disease or injury. By recognising the ability each patient has to carry out these essential activities an effective nursing strategy may then be planned. Knowledge also plays an important role in the understanding of an injury or disease and the setting of realistic goals when reviewing patient recovery.

ELIMINATION

Urination

Conditions that may cause abnormal urine production include:
- Feline lower urinary tract disease (FLUTD)
- Diabetes mellitus
- Renal disease/failure
- Dehydration
- Bladder rupture.

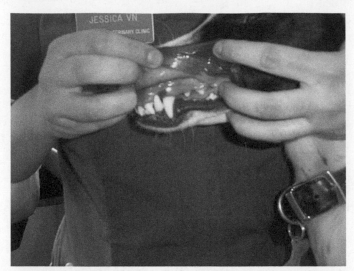

Fig. 17.17 Healthy pink mucous membranes in a canine patient

Useful terminology:

- **Oliguria** – reduction in daily production of urine
- **Anuria** – complete cessation of urine production
- **Stranguria** – passing of urine is painful and uncomfortable
- **Dysuria** – passing of urine is difficult and uncomfortable
- **Poikuria** – irregular passage of urine
- **Polyuria** – passing larger volumes of urine than normal.

Assessing urine production. This may be significant in conditions such as acute renal failure or a ruptured bladder. Note should be made on the hospitalisation sheet of when a patient has passed urine, together with volume and appearance of the urine and with a description of its passage, e.g. whether it was difficult or painful.

In cats, a litter tray may be placed in their cage, which also aids the collection of urine, particularly if it is empty of litter. Stressed cats, however, can deliberately not urinate and cease to pass urine for long periods of time, so manual palpation to check bladder size is sometimes necessary. Dogs should be taken outside to urinate regularly throughout the day as many will be reluctant to urinate in their kennel. Grass is an ideal substrate to encourage urination and a wall or fence is very helpful when encouraging male dogs.

Methods of urine collection

Cystocentesis (cysto- = bladder; -centesis = puncture and aspiration). Equipment required for this procedure includes:

- Sterile universal plain container (white lid) and/or a boric acid (red lid) container
- 23-G needle – use as small a gauge needle as possible and a 10-ml sterile syringe
- Sterile gloves
- Chlorhexidine scrub.

The procedure is carried out by a veterinary surgeon and is only usually carried out if the bladder is full, allowing the veterinary surgeon to identify its position. A sterile needle is inserted into the bladder via the patient's flank and correct restraint of the patient is required by one or more assistants. Sterility should be maintained throughout to avoid introducing bacteria into the bladder and to obtain as sterile a sample as possible.

The skin over the area of insertion should be aseptically prepared: the fur clipped and the skin scrubbed with chlorhexidine solution. Sterile gloves should be worn and all equipment used must be sterile. The needle is inserted at a 45° angle to the patient's flank. The urine is then aspirated via the syringe and placed straight into a sterile plain universal pot, identified with the patient's name. As the needle is withdrawn pressure is placed over the site for 10 seconds to seal the point of insertion.

The advantages of using this method are that the urine sample collected is relatively non-contaminated, useful for bacteriology and sensitivity studies, and can be used as a method of urine collection on patients that are unwilling or unable to pass urine normally, e.g. anaesthetised patient. The procedure is also relatively quick and simple and is usually well tolerated. Disadvantages include patient non-compliance, although sedation may be an option. There is also a risk of peritonitis, through poor technique, resulting in fluid leakage from the bladder into the abdomen.

Natural urination – litter tray/midstream sample. With regard to feline patients there are many commercial brands of litter substrate, e.g. Katkor, which may be placed in the tray to encourage urination but will not absorb the urine, allowing it to be collected from the tray via a syringe. The litter may then be disposed of or resterilised. Ideally the litter tray itself should be sterilised, using ethylene oxide sterilisation to minimise contamination of the sample.

The advantage of this method is that collection is quick, stress-free and non-intrusive. Disadvantages include poor patient compliance and an increased risk of contamination from passage through the prepuce/vulva and from the patient's coat, paws and collection tray affecting the accuracy of the results obtained. The litter substrate itself can be quite expensive and only a minimal amount of urine may be passed at any one time.

Collection of a canine urine sample requires a collection vessel such as a kidney dish or a sterile plain container. The sample should be collected midstream, which is easier with male dogs. The advantages and disadvantages are similar to those of feline patients. Patient cooperation is essential and gloves should be worn by the collector. Only a minimal amount of urine may be passed at any one time, which may be insufficient to carry out a full urinalysis.

Manual palpation. Gentle pressure is applied on either side of the abdomen in the region of the bladder. This method may be used on anaesthetised patients or those that are unwilling to urinate for no known medical reason. It must not be used if bladder/urethra patency is not known or a blockage is suspected, as excessive force may easily rupture the bladder. A full bladder is required to carry out the procedure and patient compliance is necessary, although it is generally well tolerated.

Urinary catheterisation. Not a commonly used method of urine collection as sedation or a full general anaesthetic is usually required for placement of the catheter to avoid damaging the urethra. It can be used in conjunction with contrast studies and indwelling catheterisation of hospitalised patients and its many uses include:

- Obtaining a non-contaminated urine sample for bacteriology culture and sensitivity
- Removing urethral blockages by hydropropulsion
- Allowing repeated bladder emptying via an indwelling catheter

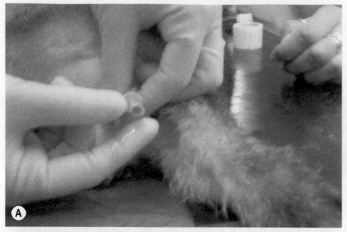

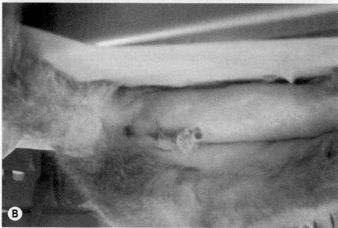

Fig. 17.18 Placement of a Jackson cat catheter into a male feline patient. (**A**) Inserting the catheter. (**B**) Catheter sutured in to be maintained as an indwelling catheter

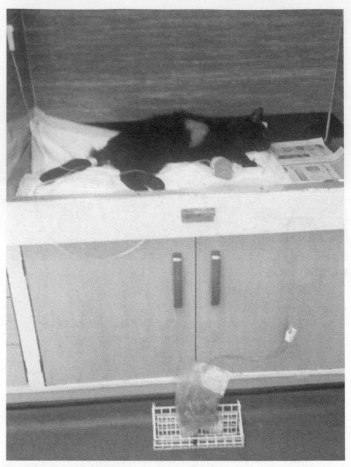

Fig. 17.19 A closed urine collection system

* Instilling contrast media and drugs into the urinary tract
* Preventing urine scalding in recumbent animals
* Emptying the bladder in anaesthetised animals prior to surgery.

Insertion of a urinary catheter should be as aseptic as possible to prevent introduction of contaminants into the bladder. A sterile catheter should be used and sterile gloves worn. This procedure may be carried out by a veterinary nurse.

The anaesthetised patient should be placed in an appropriate position. In male cats this is usually in dorsal or lateral recumbency, in female cats and bitches in sternal recumbency with legs hanging over the end of a table and in male dogs, lateral recumbency. A catheter may be placed in conscious dogs and bitches, in which case they may be standing.

In females a speculum may be used to expand the vaginal opening, giving a better view of the urethral orifice. Lubrication of the catheter tip aids easy passage into the urethra and reduces the risk of epithelial damage to the urethral tract during passage of the catheter. Depending on the type of catheter and its function, it may be sutured to the patient or the balloon inflated (Foley catheter) to keep it in place. A collection bag may be attached to an indwelling catheter to maintain kennel hygiene, measure the amount of urine production and reduce the risk of introducing infection via the catheter (Fig. 17.18).

Maintenance of indwelling catheters

* Keep the area around the catheter clean from faeces and urine unless a collection bag is used.
* For prolonged use it may be necessary to change the catheter. Commonly used materials are silicone or Teflon, which cause minimal mucosal irritation, making them useful for long-term use.
* In some cases prophylactic antibiotics may be administered to reduce the risk of ascending infection. This is especially important in post-surgical and hospitalised patients where indwelling catheterisation is expected. Frequent monitoring is required to check that the catheter is not blocked and in some cases daily flushing with sterile water may be necessary.

The use of a collection bag is advantageous as it creates a closed system, reducing the risk of ascending infection through an open catheter. The amount of urine produced must be monitored as part of good nursing care of the patient. The use of used intravenous fluid bags complete with giving set to make collection bags should not be advocated, as these are not sterile. Care must be taken that the bag is not increasing resistance to flow, especially in smaller patients, and that the urine is flowing freely. The urine may also be inspected to monitor for signs of trauma from placement of the catheter. Figure 17.19 shows a urine collection system.

Assessment of urine. Note the volume of urine voided and its appearance. Normal urine should be clear and have a slightly yellow colour. Cloudy or very turbid urine indicates presence of sediment such as white or red blood cells, calculi and casts. Dark red/brown colour urine indicates a large amount of haemoglobin or myoglobin present. A strong brown/yellow colour indicates the presence of bile pigments. See Chapter 31 for more details on urinalysis.

Defecation

Useful terminology
- **Diarrhoea** – the rapid expulsion of soft, non-formed material from the rectum
- **Constipation** – impaction of hard, dry faeces within the large intestine or rectum, which is difficult or may become impossible for the animal to pass
- **Tenesmus** – painful, ineffectual straining to pass faeces, seen in cases of constipation
- **Dyschezia** – difficult and painful passage of faeces
- **Melaena** – production of dark, tarry faeces with or without mucus: evidence of blood loss in the upper gastrointestinal tract
- **Haematochezia** – production of fresh, bright red blood in the faeces: evidence of blood loss in the lower gastrointestinal tract
- **Coprophagia** – when an animal eats its own faeces – usually a vice in a dog
- **Steatorrhoea** – passage of large volumes of pale, fatty faeces, usually associated with exocrine pancreatic insufficiency (EPI).

Diarrhoea. May occur in EPI, dietary intolerance/allergy, bacterial infection due to *Salmonella, Campylobacter,* etc., parasitic infection, viral disease due to parvovirus, etc., malabsorption, colitis.

Diarrhoea can be acute or chronic and can originate in either the small or large intestine. Some cases may be associated with vomiting, anorexia and water and electrolyte losses, particularly potassium, which, if not replaced rapidly, can be life threatening. Other associated signs can include depression and lethargy, abdominal pain, polyphagia (especially in EPI), anorexia and dyschezia. The presence of any of these clinical signs must be noted on the hospitalisation sheet when monitoring the patient, as well as colour, consistency, odour, amount and frequency of any diarrhoea passed. If you are unsure, a sample should be kept for the veterinary surgeon to examine. History and hospitalisation sheets are important in determining the origin and cause of the diarrhoea.

Nursing considerations. Plenty of opportunity should be given for canine patients to go outside to defecate as many will be unwilling to do so in their kennels. This is especially beneficial in paralysed recumbent patients, as appropriate support, movement and exercise will encourage normal bowel movement and faecal passage.

Maintenance of basic kennel hygiene is important when dealing with these patients. The bedding used should be washable, or disposable in cases of infectious disease, and incontinence sheets are very useful in these cases. Newspaper and towels are also useful bedding materials. Thick blankets and synthetic fleece (Vetbed) should be avoided as they increase the wash load and can harbour bacteria and viruses within the thick fibres. Long-haired patients benefit from having their perianal area clipped to prevent the accumulation of faeces in the surrounding hair, keeping the area clean and hygienic, and fluffy tails can be bandaged.

Barrier nursing may be indicated if an infectious disease such as parvovirus is present and all materials in contact with the animal's bodily fluids must be adequately sterilised or disposed of.

Intravenous fluid therapy is commonly administered in patients with diarrhoea because of associated losses of water and electrolytes, especially potassium and bicarbonate. Hartmann's solution (lactated Ringer's) is usually indicated to replace any losses, and further potassium supplementation may be required in severe cases.

The nurse will also play a role in the dietary requirements of these patients. The use of a short-term diet of easily digestible food, low in fat and high in good-quality proteins will be beneficial. For patients with a dietary intolerance or allergy, a low-sensitivity diet can be used.

Constipation. May occur in cases of dehydration, neurological disease/trauma, enlarged prostate, inactivity and obesity, and megacolon. Constipation can result in the patient becoming very restless and depressed. Opportunities should be given to canine patients to walk outside as movement and exercise aid the passage of faeces and the patient may be more willing to defecate away from the kennel.

Physical trauma, such as a fractured pelvis, will prevent defecation from occurring, resulting in the faeces within the rectum consolidating and becoming hard and impacted. Oral medication may be administered in the form of lactulose, a natural laxative, to help loosen the faeces, resulting in a relatively pain-free passage. It may also be given to some patients in cases where there is pain around the perianal region, such as after anal gland removal.

Enemas. In some cases where the impaction of faeces is particularly severe an enema may be given. This involves the introduction of a solution into the rectum to help break up the faeces and facilitate the passage of faeces from the rectum. Enemas may also be given preoperatively if surgery is concentrated around the perianal area or involves entering the lower gastrointestinal tract. Patients undergoing abdominal radiography may also be given an enema to allow clear visualisation of the caudal abdomen or to introduce contrast agents for lower gastrointestinal contrast studies.

Materials used for enemas include liquid paraffin or warm saline solution. Phosphate enemas or glycerine used in human enemas should not be used in cats as they are toxic; soapy enemas should also be avoided as they are an irritant (Fig. 17.20).

Administration of an enema – most patients will need to be sedated or under general anaesthesia in order to carry out the procedure as it is quite uncomfortable and a relaxed anal sphincter tone is preferable. The veterinary surgeon will usually ensure that there is no physical blockage, such as a foreign body or enlarged prostate, preventing the normal passage of faeces before carrying out an enema.

The warm solution is introduced into the rectum using a Higginson syringe, with one end placed in the solution and the other end inside the rectum (see Fig. 17.20). Water is then pumped by squeezing the bulb in the middle of the syringe, which allows the solution to travel one way only into the rectum. The impacted faeces is hydrated and broken down by the

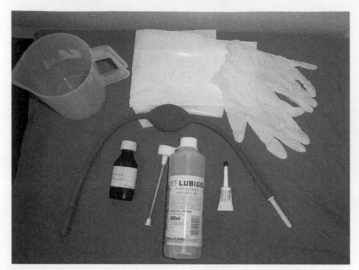

Fig. 17.20 Equipment required for administration of an enema

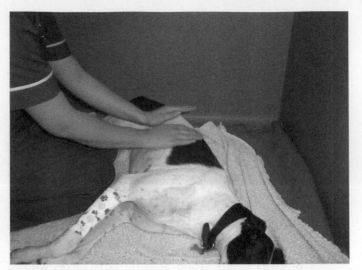

Fig. 17.21 Coupage being administered to a recumbent patient

pressure from the continual introduction of water into the rectum.

Vomiting

Conditions that can cause a patient to vomit include gastritis/gastroenteritis; viral infection, e.g. parvovirus or feline infectious enteritis; poisons/toxins; ketoacidosis as seen in diabetes mellitus; pyometra; bacterial infection, e.g. *Salmonella*; pancreatitis. Cases where regurgitation can occur include megaoesophagus and where there is delayed gastric emptying.

Useful terminology:

- **Vomiting** – an autonomic reflex in which the contents of the stomach are actively ejected via the mouth
- **Regurgitation** – passage of undigested food from the oesophagus out of the mouth
- **Haematemesis** – blood present in vomit; may be similar in appearance to coffee grounds or red and fresh
- **Emetic** – an agent that induces vomiting, e.g. apomorphine.

Nursing considerations. Intravenous fluid therapy is usually indicated because of the loss of water and electrolytes, e.g. hydrogen and potassium ions. Fluids containing sodium chloride (saline) or Ringer's solution are indicated as the replacement fluid of choice. Anti-emetics such as metoclopramide and maropitant, which inhibits the vomiting reflex and increases gastric motility, may be prescribed by the veterinary surgeon and administered to nauseous and vomiting patients, though it is contraindicated if there is a possibility of a foreign body. The anti-emetic Maropitant is a NK-1 (neurokinin) receptor antagonist for use in controlling vomiting in cats and dogs. As it only acts centrally, it can be used if a foreign body has not been ruled out.

Frequency, quantity and appearance of vomitus should be noted and recorded. Fresh or haemolysed blood with the appearance of dark coffee granules or bile, a yellow colour, may be present. Bedding should be easily washable or disposable, as with diarrhoeic patients. Barrier nursing should be applied in cases where an infectious disease has been identified or is suspected.

Nauseous patients are usually depressed and may intermittently lick their lips, and have increased hypersalivation (ptyalism). If indicated, they should be offered food but avoid leaving it in the kennel for a long period as this may make the patient more uncomfortable and increase food aversion. Many patients will be prescribed 'nil per os' (NPO; nothing by mouth) and all medication will be given parentally. Oral fluids (and micro-enteral nutrition) should be maintained unless directed by the veterinary surgeon.

Coughing

Coughing is an expulsive mechanism transmitted by the vagus nerve to the thoracic muscles to expel mucus or foreign bodies. Conditions that can induce a coughing reflex include bronchitis/tracheitis/laryngitis, kennel cough or infectious rhinotracheitis, left-sided congestive heart failure, pneumonia, foreign body, laryngeal spasm (in cats following endotracheal tube extubation), malformation, e.g. an overlong soft palate.

Nursing considerations. Initiate barrier nursing to isolate infectious patients such as those with kennel cough, though in most cases these are nursed at home. Offer warm, palatable food as in some cases the patient may be anorexic.

Ensure appropriate medication is administered. In most cases antitussives or cough suppressants (e.g. butorphanol), antimuscarinic or secretory inhibitors (e.g. atropine) and antibiotics or bronchodilator drugs (e.g. theophylline) may be prescribed. Coupage and nebulisation may be used to help loosen up secretions and encourage a more productive cough (Fig. 17.21). Cupped hands should be used to tap firmly on the chest wall, starting caudally and working forward.

MAINTAINING NUTRITIONAL STATUS

Conditions that may affect the nutritional status of the patient may be due to:

- Anorexia – e.g. cat flu due to calici/herpesvirus; patients with cervical spine damage or fractured jaw; hospitalised or postsurgical patients in pain; highly stressed patients, usually cats; geriatric patients often have impaired taste bud renewal; olfactory impairment; oncology patients following radiation treatment

- Gastrointestinal compromise – e.g. malabsorption/ maldigestion syndromes (e.g. EPI, following gastrointestinal surgery, megaoesophagus).

Useful terminology

- **Inappetence** – partial reduction in appetite
- **Anorexia** – loss of desire for food before calorific requirements have been met
- **Starvation** – long-term deprival of food, resulting in the appearance of associated physical effects such as reduction in fat/muscle mass, loss of skin turgor, lethargy and weakness and hypothermia
- **Pica** – cravings for unusual items of food, licking and eating at foreign objects; usually seen in animals with nutritional deficiencies
- **Coprophagia** – ingestion of an animal's own faeces; usually a vice in dogs or cats.

A compromised nutritional intake for whatever reason can seriously affect all body systems and is exacerbated in situations where the animal is also immunocompromised.

A reduction in all nutrients, particularly protein, can result in reduced heart muscle mass and function, compromised pulmonary and immune function and increased catabolism of the body's energy reserves. When applied to hospitalised patients this also results in reduced tissue repair and synthesis, reducing the chance of effective wound healing and recovery. There is also an increased risk of sepsis and altered drug metabolism, resulting in an increase in the risk of drug toxicity. The altered metabolism will also result in an increase in adipose tissue and muscle loss as increased demand for proteins and fat are not being met. Dogs are better at coping with starvation in comparison to cats, who may take up to 6 weeks to recover completely (Agar 2001).

It is vital to ensure that patients are provided with the key nutrients needed for tissue repair and to maintain adequate immune function. Depending on the needs of the individual patient, different forms of assisted feeding will be initiated by the veterinary surgeon to ensure that these nutrients are received. There are two main routes used for feeding:

- Enteral – administration of food or medicines using the gastrointestinal tract
- Parenteral – administration of food and medicines by a route other than that of the gastrointestinal tract, e.g. by intravenous injection (the term literally means the space between the outer surface or skin and the gastrointestinal tract)
- Enteral feeding.

Further information on nutritional support can be found in Chapter 25.

CONTROLLING BODY TEMPERATURE

Problems in controlling body temperature may be seen in the following conditions: hypothermia, hyperthermia, heat stroke, severe dehydration and/or starvation, systemic infection – pyrexia, underdeveloped thermoregulatory system in neonates, compromised thermoregulatory system in geriatrics, post anaesthesia – recovery phase, recumbent patients, laryngeal paralysis patients.

Nursing considerations

As part of the nursing care there may be cases, such as those outlined, in which the patient is unable to fully thermoregulate

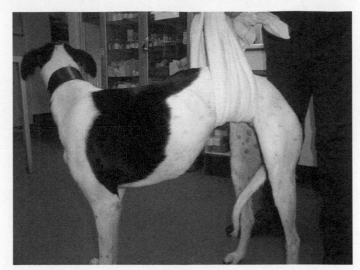

Fig. 17.22 Method of supporting a patient using a towel sling

its body temperature. It is therefore necessary to alter or adapt external temperature or conditions to maintain as normal a temperature as possible.

It is important to note, in patients with a subnormal body temperature, that conserving what heat they already have is insufficient and a direct source of heat is required:

- Heat lamps – care must be taken not to hang the lamp too near to the patient. This form of heating is best suited to small patients such as neonates, as the warmth from the lamp is focused in quite a small area. Larger lamps may be used for larger, walk-in kennels.
- Under-floor heating – some practice kennels have under-floor heating, which provides controlled, continuous warmth directly underneath the patient.
- Heat pads – various commercial heat pads may be warmed in the microwave for a specified length of time and placed under the patient's bedding. They lose their heat eventually and will need rewarming. Latex gloves may also be used by filling them with hot water, knotting them closed and placing them within the patient's bedding. Care must be taken not to place heat pads or gloves directly in contact with the patient.
- Space blankets may be used to conserve heat, and bubble wrap is often used, especially in neonates, to wrap up limbs and torso.

MOBILISATION

Conditions that can compromise mobility include neurological disease, spinal trauma, skeletal limb trauma, ligament and tendon trauma in limbs, e.g. cruciate ligament damage and vestibular disease.

Nursing considerations

Depending on the degree of immobility, various methods of support may be implemented to allow the patient to carry out normal activities as much as possible:

- In cases of hind limb paralysis or paresis, a long towel may be placed under the patient's caudal abdomen and held like a sling to give support to the hind limbs, enabling the patient to walk and toilet (Fig. 17.22). In male

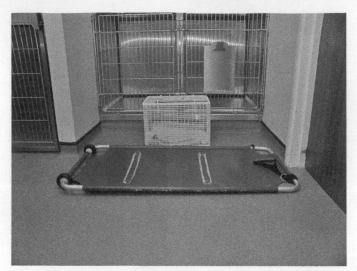

Fig. 17.23 Two methods of patient transport: a stretcher for larger canine patients and a basket for feline patients

dogs it is important not to occlude the penis with the towel. Specialist sling harnesses are available, which do the same job as the towel but are easier to handle.
- Crossed towels may be placed under the chest to support tetra/quadriplegics.
- Small patients such as cats and small dogs may be carried but it may be beneficial for them to use their limbs as much as possible to improve limb circulation and prevent muscle atrophy.
- Care must be taken when supporting large patients, and more than one member of the nursing staff may be required. It is important to use the correct physical posture when moving patients, keeping the back straight and taking the weight on bent knees. Do not be afraid to ask for help when lifting a patient, no matter how busy everyone else is.
- Cats may be transported in baskets. This is especially important when moving them within the practice, to prevent escape (Fig. 17.23).

GROOMING

Conditions that can compromise a patient's ability to groom include recumbency, cervical injury, cat flu (calici/herpes virus due to ulcerated tongue), feeding tube placement (usually due to the large bandaging around the neck), geriatrics with conditions such as spondylosis or arthritis, or orphaned neonates.

Principles of grooming hospitalised patients

Grooming is one of the basic activities of general nursing care that can be beneficial to the patient in many ways. Depending on the temperament and condition of patients, it allows the nurse to spend time with them, allowing a bond to be formed. It will also reassure the particularly stressed patient that the kennel door opening is not always associated with something unpleasant happening. It can help to relax patients, providing mental stimulation, and improve their general feeling of well-being, especially if they are unable to do it for themselves.

From a health point of view it allows the veterinary nurse to assess the patient's body and coat condition, allowing early recognition

of problems such as lump formation or reduction in body condition associated with weight loss. The presence of ectoparasitic infection may also be established. Removing dead hair and debris from the coat reduces mat formation and skin irritation while promoting new hair growth. Discharge should also be removed from the eyes and nose to prevent infection arising.

Grooming hospitalised patients also gives a good impression to the owner when a patient is discharged as its appearance portrays the care it has received.

COMMUNICATION

Effective communication with animal patients can be a rather difficult and misunderstood area and this may be a particular problem when the animal is in pain. Commonly recognised signs of pain in animals can be displayed in obvious behaviour patterns such as vocalisation and aggression and in some cases there are specific signs associated with certain diseases; for example, patients with anterior abdominal pain, as seen in cases of pancreatitis and portosystemic shunt, often adopt a noticeable 'prayer' position.

Behavioural signs of pain and discomfort include:
- Restlessness and pacing
- Frequent posture changes
- Paying attention to the site of pain
- Panting and tachypnoea
- Depression
- Appearing lethargic/comatose
- Inappetence
- Attempting to hide away/curl up tightly
- Hiding away the affected body part
- Attention-seeking.

There are also many clinical signs that will indicate a level of pain. These include:
- Tachycardia/bradycardia
- Abnormal body temperature
- Dehydration due to anorexia and lack of drinking
- Abnormal faeces – due to anorexia or gut stasis
- Loss of weight
- Twitching or convulsions
- Abnormal urine/faecal voiding and appearance.

In most cases it is necessary to assess both the behaviour patterns and the clinical signs a patient may be exhibiting, together with its clinical history, to obtain a full picture and a more accurate interpretation.

Nursing specific types of patient

RECUMBENT PATIENTS

Recumbent patients require a demanding amount of intensive care, often for a long period of time. Recumbency is associated with a number of complications, so an effective nursing strategy must be designed to deal with these problems before they arise, reducing the chances of secondary complications and improving the chances of a successful recovery.

Conditions that may cause a patient to become recumbent include neurological disease, spinal trauma, spinal disease (wobbler syndrome), fractures, spinal tumours and poisoning inducing a semi-conscious or comatose state.

Nursing considerations

In many cases the patient may be partly or fully dependent on the nurse to fulfil a number of essential activities, so you should consider the following:

- Mobility will be severely compromised. Depending on the condition and size of the animal it may be possible to aid mobility by using a towel or specialist support harness. Walking around will help improve circulation to the joints and prevent muscle atrophy, as well as improve the mental well-being of the patient.
- Feeding and fluid intake – intravenous fluid therapy will be initiated in all patients to provide maintenance fluid support. Water should be offered at least every 3 hours and may also be syringed into the mouth to moisten the lips and mucous membranes. Some cases will require assisted feeding through PEG, oesophagostomy or nasogastric tubes while others may be able to feed normally from a bowl. The type of food given should be a highly digestible diet. Energy expenditure can be reduced so nutritional assessment is required to determine calorific requirement for the individual.
- Constipation may be a complication and an enema or laxative may be beneficial if faeces have not been passed for more than 3 days. Enabling the patient to go outside will help to encourage natural defecation, as many patients will be unwilling to do so in recumbency.
- The patient's bladder function should be regularly monitored to assess whether voluntary control is present. Many patients will also be unwilling to urinate in recumbency, so supportive mobility to encourage natural urination should be carried out if possible. Gentle pressure on either side of the bladder may also be used to encourage urination but only if a blockage is not suspected.
- Cystitis is another common problem because of reduced water intake, reduced mobility and urine retention. An indwelling urinary catheter may be placed in patients that are difficult to mobilise or are incontinent. A closed urine collection system should be used to prevent urine scalding and reduce the risk of ascending infection. The amount of urine produced should also be measured on a daily basis.
- Self-grooming may be difficult in many of these patients. Grooming the patient will allow the nurse to spend some time with it as well as improve its physical and mental well-being. Some patients with longer coats may require clipping around the perineum or prepuce area to maintain cleanliness.

Potential complications

The successful recovery of these patients depends not only on specialised equipment and resources but also on being able to predict potential complications and implement the correct nursing care to reduce the risk of them occurring.

Skin problems. In recumbent patients common primary skin problems include decubital ulcers (pressure sores) and urine scalding.

Decubital ulcers are primarily caused by a combination of pressure from the weight of the animal, moisture from sweat, and friction caused by movement between the animal and the bedding. These can be difficult to treat once established and

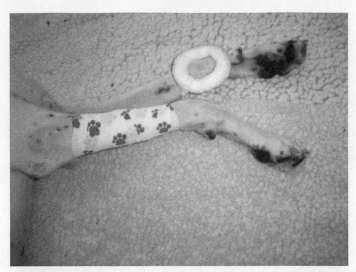

Fig. 17.24 Use of a doughnut bandage to pad bony prominences in a recumbent patient

common sites tend to be over bony prominences such as the elbows, tarsus/carpus, shoulders and hips. Thin-skinned animals such as greyhounds and lurchers are particularly susceptible.

The occurrence of decubital ulcers may be reduced by providing padded, clean, dry bedding and turning the patient regularly so the potential area is not always under pressure or in contact with the bedding. Waterproof mattresses are ideal as bedding and duvets may also be used. Towels and blankets are certainly not ideal. Synthetic fleece or Vetbed is useful for a contact layer, as it is soft and highly absorbent. Padded bandages may also be applied to risk areas but care should be taken that this does not put pressure on to other areas. Figure 17.24 shows how a doughnut bandage may be used to pad bony prominences in recumbent patients. The area is elevated without being directly in contact with anything, thus minimising further abrasion while allowing the air to circulate. This bandage must be secured to the area using adhesive tape.

Management of decubital ulcers includes clipping the area, bathing in dilute chlorhexidine solution and applying a soothing barrier cream.

Urine scalding is caused by repetitive soiling of the skin by urine. Fur or hair provides little protection and all areas should be protected. By initially applying and frequently reapplying a water-repellent barrier cream such as Vaseline, the urine is prevented from coming into contact with the hair and skin. Placing a well-fitting indwelling urinary catheter can also prevent urine scalding, as the urine is unable to come into contact with the skin.

Hypostatic pneumonia. This can be a complication in laterally recumbent patients, especially those that are geriatric or seriously ill. Pooling of blood and fluids can occur in the lower lung, i.e. the lung closest to the floor, and provides an ideal medium for the growth of bacterial microorganisms. This then reduces the viability of the lung, resulting in the development of pneumonia. Clinical signs include coughing, tachypnoea and a rapid shallow breathing pattern.

Preventative treatment includes turning the patient a minimum of every 4 hours (Fig. 17.25), if not contraindicated, preventing the lower lung from becoming non-viable.

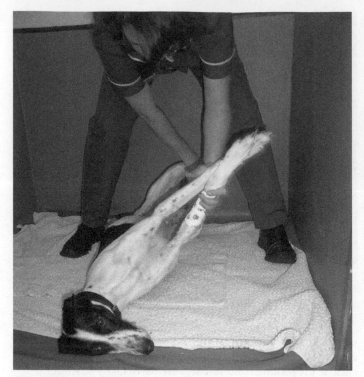

Fig. 17.25 Turning a recumbent patient

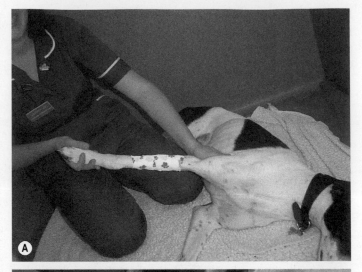

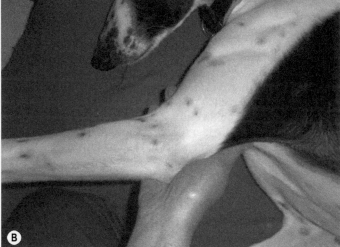

Fig. 17.26 A shoulder joint extended (**A**) and the shoulder joint flexed (**B**) in a recumbent patient as part of a passive physiotherapy routine

The patient can also be repositioned into sternal recumbency, allowing both lungs to inflate fully. Coupage may also be carried out to aid expulsion of secretions.

Muscle atrophy and joint adhesion formation. Muscle atrophy may be a potential complication through reduced limb use and can lead to joint adhesions and muscle spasms, which can be painful and cause permanent damage. Physical therapy under instruction from the veterinary surgeon, in the form of controlled passive limb movement and voluntary exercise, can help to reduce the risks of these complications occurring (see Chapter 18). Passive limb movement involves the nurse gently extending and flexing the joints in the limbs. Care should be taken not to overstretch the muscles and checks must be made to ensure that all limbs are fully functional and amenable to such activity (Fig. 17.26). Hydrotherapy may be of benefit, as the water provides much of the support for the patient.

Massage has also been shown to increase circulation in immobile limbs, as well as increasing fluid exchange, flushing toxins out of the tissues via the pulmonary and lymphatic drainage system and reducing the presence of oedematous fluid formation. Massage can prevent fibrous adhesions occurring between connective tissue in the limbs and provide mental relaxation for the patient. In spinal cases, massage has been beneficial in alleviating painful spasms associated with spinal disease and trauma (A. Sutton, unpublished work, 2002).

Psychological needs. In most cases the patient will be physically unwell, in pain or discomfort, and may become depressed. Bonding with the patient is important so that changes in behaviour or improvements or decline in its condition may be recognised quickly. Ideally, these patients should be kennelled in busy areas where they can observe people and other animals. Visits from owners can be beneficial and if a favourite toy or piece of

clothing can be left in the kennel with the patient it will provide additional reassurance.

NEONATAL AND JUVENILE PATIENTS

Neonates requiring hand-rearing by the veterinary nurse may have been abandoned or orphaned at birth. Their care can be very time-consuming but also extremely rewarding. The type and intensity of care varies greatly over a relatively small age range. A patient of 6 weeks and under will require a greater amount of care compared to that required by a 10- or 11-week-old patient, which will be more independent and able to carry out most essential activities by itself. Consider the following factors:

Feeding and fluid intake

From birth to 7 days healthy neonates will require feeding approximately every 2 hours. This will then increase to every 3–4 hours up to 5 weeks old. At this stage weaning should be actively encouraged by offering semi-solid, highly palatable, high-caloric-density food and allowing the patient to lap. Bottle-fed neonates can find this transition difficult and a syringe may be used initially.

Neonates born by Caesarean section should be reunited with their mother as soon as possible to enable them to suckle. This is important as they require the colostrum, rich in maternally derived antibodies, which may only be absorbed effectively by their gastrointestinal system within the first 24 hours of life.

Once fully weaned the young animal will benefit from frequent small meals especially prepared for their life stage. Close checks on weight gain should be made on a daily basis. If necessary, fluids may be administered subcutaneously in small quantities to very young patients. The intraosseous route may also be used for more rapid fluid administration. Intravenous access can be difficult in these patients as the veins are fragile and small.

Elimination

Up to about the age of 4 weeks stimulation is required to induce the neonate to defecate or urinate. A damp piece of cotton wool may be used to rub the prepuce or vulva and perianal area after each feeding. Juvenile patients may be partially, fully or not toilet-trained at all, so an initial assessment will need to be made as to what stage the patient is at so that it can be nursed accordingly.

Temperature regulation

A combination of an underdeveloped thermoregulatory system, minimal subcutaneous fat deposits and a high body surface area to volume ratio increases the potential risk of significant heat loss in the neonatal patient, so maintaining a warm environmental temperature is essential. The temperature for the first 7 days should be 29°C, decreasing to 26°C for the following 7 days and then 20°C until the animal is about 6 weeks of age. Hot water bottles and microwave heat pads can be used within the bedding to provide warmth. Heat lamps can be used carefully at the recommended distance.

Communication and behaviour

Neonatal and juvenile patients require a stimulating environment but they should also have a quiet area for sleep. They should be housed in an area of activity unless incubating a contagious disease, in which case they should be isolated. The kennel should be secure and free from draughts.

Toys and bedding from home should be provided to allow play and make them feel a little more secure and happy in a strange environment. An alarm clock placed under the bedding of orphaned neonates to simulate the heartbeat of the mother provides comfort and contentment.

Unfortunately, long periods of hospitalisation during the prime socialisation period between 8 and 14 weeks of age can have an effect on behavioural development, with resultant undesirable behaviour patterns emerging in these patients. This can be seen in puppies with canine parvovirus that have to be isolated for long periods of time, which restricts normal developmental interaction with other dogs and people (Hobbs, unpublished work, 2004). Hand-reared kittens can also become difficult to handle when they become adults because of their lack of discipline and teaching from the mother cat during kittenhood (Hewitt, unpublished work, 2004).

Nursing considerations

Neonatal and juvenile patients have an undeveloped immune system so, as with any other hospitalised patient, a high level of cleanliness and hygiene must be maintained. This is even more significant in sick neonates and juveniles, especially if the primary vaccination has not yet been given and levels of maternally derived antibody levels are waning, which usually occurs around 8–12 weeks of age. All feeding bowls and litter trays should be disinfected and sterilised. Barrier nursing should be implemented in the case of a contagious disease.

There are very few veterinary drugs licensed for use in neonates and juveniles because of their potential toxicity and low therapeutic index. It is therefore very important to obtain an accurate weight on which to base correct drug dosages.

Always check for potential congenital defects in neonates and juveniles, e.g. cleft palate, umbilical and inguinal hernias, heart problems such as patent ductus arteriosus, and overshot or undershot jaw. Most may be obvious and diagnosed in the early stages, but other complications, such as heart defects, may not become apparent until the patient is older.

GERIATRIC PATIENTS

Geriatric patients usually require intensive nursing because their ability to recover from disease or surgery will be significantly reduced compared to that of younger patients. There may also be some sensory deprivation in the form of blindness or deafness, which may make the elderly patient disorientated and anxious.

Common conditions in these patients include cancer, cardiac disease, cataracts, hepatic and renal disease, pulmonary disease, osteoarthritis, spondylosis, degenerative joint disease and dental disease. Consider the following factors:

Feeding and fluid intake

A significant proportion of hospitalised geriatric patients will be suffering with one or more conditions, so the history is a significant factor when formulating a nursing plan. Part of the treatment will be achieved through effective dietary management. Common examples include elderly dogs with heart disease or old cats with renal or hepatic disease (see Chapter 10).

Obesity may also be a problem, particularly in geriatric dogs, who usually take less exercise but their owners continue feeding the same amount and type of food the patient was fed when it was 2 years old. The energy requirements of a senior dog are approximately 20% less than its younger counterpart (McCune 2003). In some cases, owners in fact increase the food as a loving gesture. The resultant problems include the onset of joint disease such as arthritis, which, although a common condition in geriatrics, may be exacerbated by extra weight and strain on the joints. Palatability is an important factor in feeding geriatric patients because of the reduction in olfactory senses and impaired renewal of the taste buds.

Elimination

Reduced bladder or anal sphincter tone is a common condition associated with ageing and patients should be offered more frequent opportunities to defecate and urinate outside, as many will be reluctant to do so in their kennels. Defecating indoors in the kennel or on the bedding can be as a result of mental ageing and the onset of senility. These patients may benefit from disposable padded incontinence sheets over their bedding.

Nursing considerations

When preparing a kennel for a geriatric patient, well-padded bedding is essential, especially if the animal is suffering from joint disease. This will provide support and comfort and prevent further joint stiffness and the development of decubital ulcers.

Water should be available at all times, unless it is contraindicated and intravenous fluid therapy has been put in place. These patients are less able to deal with water deprivation, compared to adult patients, and it may result in severe renal compromise.

Drug toxicity can occur because a reduction in renal and hepatic function makes metabolism of the drugs less efficient and overdosing can become a significant risk. Accurate body weights should be taken to enable accurate dosage calculations to be made.

Sensory compromise may make these patients anxious and disorientated. They should be approached gently and attempts should be made to attract their attention before entering the kennel and touching them, as they may bite if startled. An item of the owner's clothing, a familiar toy from home or visits from the owner may make them feel happier; however, some patients may find the departure of the owner too upsetting and stressful and this should be taken into consideration when planning the individual nursing care of these patients.

Understanding compassion fatigue – a hidden consequence of patient care?

CARING THAT HURTS TOO MUCH TO CARE ANYMORE

In the human nursing field compassion fatigue has been recognised among nurses and doctors who struggle with the continued demands of caring for patient.

Compassion fatigue (CF) is a deep physical, emotional and spiritual exhaustion accompanied by acute emotional pain that overtakes a person and causes pervasive declines in their energy to feel and care for themselves and others. Nurses suffer from a myriad of stress-related illnesses, and eventually leave the profession from the deleterious effects of CF.

It is not pathological in the sense of mental illness, rather it is considered a natural behavioural and emotional response resulting from helping or desiring to help relieve another's

suffering or pain over a prolonged period, often not seeing patients get better. It is not simply from a busy workload and related issues.

Veterinary nurses by virtue of their caring natures and personalities are also at risk of developing compassion fatigue. Providing nursing care to cherished pets can become an emotional roller coaster, often with patients being hospitalised for days or weeks requiring immense care and considerable emotional input on a daily basis. Sadly, CF is confounded when patients lose their fight for life.

Individuals can begin to experience forgetfulness, shorter attention span, self-doubt and decreased self-esteem:

- Emotional: anger – rage out of proportion, less ability to feel joy, decreased sense of personal accomplishment
- Spiritual: pervasive hopelessness
- Interpersonal: projection of anger/blame
- Physical: headaches, fatigued, impaired immune system, stomach aches.

Often we 'forget' about the successful cases. These patients are the ones that against all the odds fight on and have a second chance in life. The patients that often remain in the forefront of our minds are the ones that sadly pass away and begin the cycle of CF. To help cope with the feelings of CF several tips are useful:

- Take time out for self
- Know when to take a break
- Develop a new talent – hobby
- Leave 'work' at work
- Learn to laugh, focus on positives
- Find 'joy in the journey'
- Rediscover your humanness
- Reflect on your practice regularly
- Nurture your hope!

My own personal philosophy is to learn something new from every patient that I nurse, analysing my role in the care of the patient – both positives and negatives. The patients that I have had an emotional connection with (often these are the patients that I have spent 12 hours a night nursing on a one-to-one basis) that sadly lose their life due to their illness/disease are the patients that continue to live on in a different way – as a veterinary nursing learning model, helping other nurses to enhance their skills in the essentials of patient care.

BIBLIOGRAPHY

Agar, S., 2001. Small Animal Nutrition. Butterworth-Heinemann, Oxford.

Blood, D.C., Studdert, V.P., 1999. Comprehensive Veterinary Dictionary. W B Saunders, London.

Cooper, B., Mullineaux, E., Turner, L., 2011. BSAVA Textbook of Veterinary Nursing, fifth ed. British Small Animal Veterinary Association, Cheltenham.

Jeffery, A., 2006. Moving away from the medical model. Veterinary Nurs. J. 21 (9), 13–16.

King, L.G., Boag, A., 2007. BSAVA Manual of Canine and Feline Emergency and Critical Care. British Small Animal Veterinary Association.

McCune, S., 2003. Nutrition. In: Lane, D., Cooper, B. (Eds.), Veterinary Nursing, third ed. Butterworth Heinemann, Oxford.

Mullineaux, E., Jones, M. (Eds.), 2007. BSAVA Manual of Practical Veterinary Nursing. British Small Animal Veterinary Association, Cheltenham.

Orpet H, J.A., 2007. Implementing the Ability Model, November 2010 ed. [Graduate Diploma in Professional and Clinical Veterinary Nursing course notes]. The Royal Veterinary College, London.

Roper, N., Logan, W.W., Tierney, A.J., 2000. The Roper-Logan-Tierney Model of Nursing: Based on Activities of Living. Churchill Livingstone, Ediburgh.

Williams, L., 1992. Care of the paraplegic patient. Veterinary Practice Nurse 4, 17–20.

RECOMMENDED READING

Agar, S., 2001. Small Animal Nutrition. Butterworth-Heinemann, Oxford.
  An easy-to-read and informative book covering all aspects of small animal nutrition. Good as a quick reference guide.

Aspinall, V., 2014. Clinical Procedures in Veterinary Nursing, third ed. Butterworth-Heinemann, Oxford.

Good step-by-step guide to all procedures involved in nursing patients.

Jeffery, A., 2006. Moving away from the medical model. Veterinary Nurs. J. 21 (9), 13–16.

Mullineaux, E., Jones, M. (Eds.), 2007. BSAVA Manual of Practical Veterinary Nursing. British Small Animal Veterinary Association, Cheltenham.

Orpet, H., Jeffery, A., 2006. Moving towards a more holistic approach. Veterinary Nurs. J. 26 (5), 19–22.

Orpet, H., Jeffery, A., 2010. Handbook of Veterinary Nursing, second ed. Wiley Blackwell, Oxford.

Physiotherapy Techniques

GILLIAN CALVO

KEY POINTS

- Rehabilitation is the process of restoring the maximum function, independence and quality of life following illness or injury.

- Physiotherapy may be indicated in a variety of clinical conditions associated with the musculoskeletal and nervous systems but by no means is restricted to this and may include some soft tissue conditions.

- Physiotherapy can be utilised in conjunction with a postoperative treatment plan but may also be implemented for patients undergoing conservative or palliative care of a disease process.

- The aim of physiotherapy is, by using a range of physiotherapeutic modalities predominantly in combination, to restore maximum functional mobility to allow the animal to perform all activities of daily living.

Introduction

Rehabilitation is the process of restoring the maximum function, independence and quality of life following illness or injury. The word comes from the Latin 'rehabilitare' meaning to make fit again. Physiotherapy uses physical approaches to promote, maintain and restore physical, psychological and social wellbeing. Physiotherapy is an integral part of the recovery of most spinal patients, especially following surgery.

The first step in the physiotherapy process is to identify if physiotherapy is indicated in the presented patient. Initial assessment includes a history and a thorough examination of the musculoskeletal system to identify any problems the patient may have. Based on these findings, treatment goals (short-term and long-term) are determined based on the abilities of the patient and the expectations of the owner and a treatment plan is established. Where possible, objective outcome measures are used to monitor progress. Depending on the practice, this discussion is done by a combination of veterinary physiotherapy, the veterinary surgeon, and the veterinary nurse.

Indications for physiotherapy

Physiotherapy may be indicated in a variety of clinical conditions associated with the musculoskeletal and nervous systems but by no means is restricted to this and may include some soft tissue conditions. Physiotherapy can be utilised in conjunction with a postoperative treatment plan for patients following surgery (e.g. cranial cruciate ligament injury or hemilaminectomy for intervertebral disc extrusion), but may also be implemented for patients undergoing conservative or palliative care of a disease process (e.g. osteoarthritis or degenerative myelopathy). To maximise the benefits, and the patient's response to physiotherapy, treatment should be started as soon as possible unless contraindicated.

Aim of physiotherapy

A range of physiotherapeutic modalities are used predominantly in combination to restore maximum functional mobility to allow the animal to perform all activities of daily living expected for that species. Some may also require the fitness level and function to be able to participate in activities such as agility or to fulfil their role as a working dog.

Ultimately physiotherapy will be utilised to:
- Reduce pain
- Reduce inflammation, oedema, swelling
- Promote the healing of musculoskeletal tissues
- Improve muscular strength
- Improve core strength and stability
- Improve joint flexibility
- Promote and restore functional movement ability
- Improve cardiovascular fitness and stamina
- Increase speed of recovery
- Positive psychological effect for the patient, owner and therapist.

Physiotherapy in small animal practice

The benefits of physiotherapy in small animal practice are becoming more widely accepted among the veterinary profession and human physiotherapy profession. It is now possible for chartered physiotherapists with a degree in the human profession to participate in a postgraduate diploma or master's degree in veterinary physiotherapy, allowing them to register with the Association of Chartered Physiotherapists in Animal Therapy (ACPAT) (Box 18.1). A qualified ACPAT physiotherapist is given the title of Category 'A' ACPAT Physiotherapist.

An ACPAT physiotherapist may work within a small animal practice on a full-time basis alongside the team of veterinary surgeons and veterinary nurses, providing a daily in-house service for patients (this is common in veterinary referral hospitals), or may be contracted to provide a clinic for outpatients on set days during the week/weekend.

The team approach

The team approach is a working relationship whereby all parties involved work collegially bringing their knowledge and

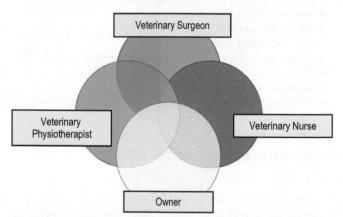

Fig. 18.1 Team approach to physiotherapy

experience together, providing a multidisciplinary team approach to patient management (Fig. 18.1).

ROLE OF THE VETERINARY SURGEON

Current veterinary surgeon degrees do not incorporate physiotherapy training; however, they will most likely become involved with patients throughout their career who could benefit from physiotherapy. As the primary responsible person for patients, they must gain a reasonable level of knowledge of the role of the veterinary physiotherapist and the physical therapeutic modalities available to allow them to seek intervention when required. In order to fulfil this, veterinary surgeons tend to participate in short CPD courses to improve their knowledge and understanding of the discipline, but more and more collaborate with local veterinary physiotherapists to provide a physiotherapy service in their practice.

ROLE OF THE VETERINARY PHYSIOTHERAPIST

Due to the unprotected title of 'veterinary physiotherapist', veterinary surgeons must be vigilant that they are collaborating with an appropriately trained, qualified, registered and regulated veterinary physiotherapist. Collaboration with a person acting as a veterinary physiotherapist without the above status could have a wide range of implications for the veterinary surgeon responsible for patient care. When entrusting the care of a patient to a veterinary physiotherapist, it is the veterinary surgeon's responsibility to ensure that the veterinary physiotherapist is suitably qualified and registered to perform veterinary physiotherapy.

ROLE OF THE VETERINARY NURSE

Veterinary nurses have a very important role in physiotherapy, especially when managing patients postoperatively. Postoperative nursing care plans should incorporate basic physiotherapy techniques, e.g. cold or heat therapy, massage, passive range of joint motion, and simple therapeutic exercises (all of which will be outlined later in the chapter). All of these physiotherapeutic techniques can be performed by registered veterinary nurses and trainee veterinary nurses as long as they have been trained to do so, are confident to do so, and it is within their capabilities. All undergraduate veterinary nurse training programmes now incorporate learning outcomes for basic physiotherapy techniques, and there are many CPD courses or postgraduate courses that nurses can participate in to improve their knowledge and skill sets of physiotherapy. It is important to understand that any patient you have been providing physiotherapy for still remains the responsibility of the veterinary surgeon and both you and the veterinary surgeon should remain vigilant as to when referral to a veterinary physiotherapist is appropriate.

ROLE OF THE OWNER

Owners usually respond very positively to their pets receiving physiotherapy, but they have the right to know that the physiotherapy is being performed by a suitably trained and qualified person so may request referral to a veterinary physiotherapist if it is a service outside the remits of your practice or if the treatment required is complex. Most owners are happy for basic postoperative physiotherapy to be carried out by veterinary nurses within the practice for the duration of their pet's hospitalisation period, and then continue ongoing physiotherapy guidance in simple-to-manage patients on an outpatient basis.

Many owners are required to perform physiotherapy techniques at home following discharge of their pet. It is normally the veterinary nurse's responsibility to demonstrate and ensure competency of the owner in the absence of a veterinary physiotherapist. It is important that owners are not only able to physically perform the physiotherapy required but must also have the time and dedication to provide their patient with the exercises they require on a regular basis. This leads to the benefits of a nurse-led mobility clinic within veterinary clinics. Some referral veterinary hospitals may have such clinics running on an outpatient basis through a contracted veterinary physiotherapist on specific days of the week or full time through an in-house physiotherapy and rehabilitation clinic or centre.

The practicalities and logistics of running a mobility clinic or physiotherapy/rehabilitation clinic are similar to a greater or lesser extent depending on who is responsible for the clinic – i.e. a veterinary physiotherapist will be able to provide a more comprehensive service than a veterinary nurse with basic skills, and a veterinary physiotherapist will have more dedicated time without interruption from other duties than a veterinary nurse will have.

As long as you know your limits as a veterinary nurse and recognise when the patients' best interests outweigh the treatment you can provide and require a veterinary physiotherapist's intervention, it is possible to provide a basic physiotherapy service to your patients and clients. There are, however, a number of things you must be aware of before venturing to setting up a mobility clinic.

The remainder of this chapter introduces various physiotherapy techniques and exercises that can be incorporated by you, a veterinary nurse, but also introduces some more specialised physiotherapy equipment that may be used by a veterinary physiotherapist. But first things first – you must understand the effects of immobilisation and disuse on musculoskeletal tissues.

The effects of immobilisation and disuse on musculoskeletal tissues

The tissues most affected by immobilisation are:
- Cartilage
- Muscle
- Ligaments and tendons
- Nerves
- Bone.

Tissues must be challenged to enhance and influence recovery and healing, but if tissues are over challenged it may result in damage and delayed recovery.

CARTILAGE

Articular cartilage problems lead to debilitating conditions that are commonly seen in veterinary practice by veterinary surgeons, e.g. osteoarthritis. Problems within articular cartilage arise when there is a combined decrease in range of motion within a joint and reduced loading.

Articular cartilage has a matrix formation and is supported by the flow of synovial fluid through the complex matrix giving it a viscoelastic property to withstand loading and dynamic forces. In the incidence of abnormal loading on the articular surface, abnormalities begin to form in the cartilage matrix leading to degeneration caused by the breakdown of normal cartilage constituents, especially collagen.

Factors affecting collagen breakdown include:
- Direct trauma
- Obesity
- Immobilisation
- Excessive repetitive loading.

Cartilage thickness may be reduced significantly if immobilisation techniques are implemented in the management of disease processes. The effect of the position of the limb during immobilisation on blood flow to the joint must be considered in every patient. Remember that loading and unloading of articular cartilage permits the transport of nutrients and water into the articular cartilage.

Cartilage response to disuse and immobilisation:
- Atrophic or degenerative changes
- Reduction in matrix and cellular components
- Disorganisation of cartilage
- Potential irreversible damage if prolonged immobilisation
- Reduction in synovial fluid
- Reduction in cartilaginous nutrition.

Immobilisation of a joint in extension:
- Decreased muscle interaction with the joint leading to increased muscle contraction against the immobilisation device, e.g. a splint, cast or external skeletal fixation device
- Changes in articular cartilage similar to osteoarthritis.

Immobilisation of a joint in flexion:
- Cartilage atrophy.

The effects of a 6-week immobilisation period are generally reversible with several weeks of gentle remobilisation; however, if immobilisation extends beyond 11 weeks more rigorous and prolonged rehabilitation is required and it is unlikely that full remobilisation will be achieved without having residual deleterious effects.

If high levels of repeated loading are exerted on articular cartilage immediately following a period of immobilisation then it is possible to cause more damage to the areas of cartilage that have become softened as a result of the immobilisation process. Following a period of immobilisation the introduction of gentle and prolonged load-bearing exercises is far more beneficial to, and protective of, the cartilage than aggressive load-bearing exercises – e.g. 10 minutes of gentle underwater treadmill therapy will be far more beneficial than 10 minutes of off-lead, high-impact exercise in the park since the underwater treadmill therapy provides buoyancy and therefore gentle reintroduction of loading during exercise.

Massage is a useful method of rehabilitation for dissolving adhesions that may have formed in muscles that span the associated joint during the period of immobilisation. Massage followed by joint range of motion is also beneficial to increase nutrition of the cartilage since the 'pumping' action encourages replenishment of synovial fluid in the joint.

MUSCLE

Immobilisation results in a decrease in the cross-sectional diameter of a muscle and a rapid decrease in its strength, especially in the first week, and becomes atrophic. If muscles are immobilised in a lengthened position then atrophy is less pronounced.

When a patient is undergoing a healing process involving immobilisation then the connective tissue in the belly of the associated muscles develop degenerative changes because contraction and extension within the muscles are no longer present. This results in collagen fibres moving closer together forming crosslinks, or 'knots', and an overall reduced muscle mobility occurs resulting in muscle shortening and fibrosis. In the hind limb especially, immobilisation of the stifle or reduced range of motion in the stifle, for example, has deleterious effects on the quadriceps femoris muscle group that spans the stifle joint resulting in shortening of the quadriceps and overall shortening of the limb. This is commonly a result of an excessive immobilisation period and is referred to as contracture of the quadriceps. If such changes occur for a prolonged time, they can be irreversible and have significant consequences on the patient's hind-limb mobility. Fortunately, most of the changes that occur during an immobilisation period are reversible and it is generally expected that a remobilisation period of twice the immobilisation period is required to return the limb circumference to normal values and reverse the effects of immobilisation.

Massage increases local blood flow and mobilises adhesions. It is important to eliminate any crosslink formation, encourage muscle lengthening and restore normal muscle contraction by promoting gentle weight-bearing exercises and use of the limb.

In patients who are unable to bear their weight – e.g. pelvic trauma or spinal injury – the best treatment to hinder muscle contracture is electrical stimulation because muscle cells are depolarised by electrical stimulation resulting in muscle contraction, allowing reproduction of physiological muscle activity without placing load onto the limb(s). Induced muscle contraction mobilises adhesions and increases local blood flow resulting in improved tissue structure and reducing the risk of atrophy and contracture.

LIGAMENTS AND TENDONS

Repair of ligament or tendon injuries, e.g. Achilles tendon avulsion, requires a period of immobilisation to aid the healing process in the bone–tendon/bone–ligament interface. Unfortunately, the period of immobilisation has a negative effect on the structural and material components that make up each of the aforementioned tissues. Thankfully the remobilisation period restores the mechanical properties (tensile strength and mobility) of the ligaments and tendons to nearly normal with time; however, recovery of the bony insertion site can take far longer. Unlike in repair of muscles, a remobilisation period of three times that of the immobilisation period is necessary to restore many structural properties but as long as 12 months may be necessary to achieve complete recovery.

Massage mobilises adhesions and increases blood flow within the ligament and tendon and especially encourages blood flow to the bony insertion site, thus encouraging healing. Gentle passive range-of-motion exercises and active extension of the affected tendon triggers the reorganisation of the healing tissue. Transcutaneous electrical nerve stimulation (TENS) and underwater treadmill therapy with partial weight-bearing are also beneficial in the recovery period. Tendons absorb tensile stresses during stretching and muscle contraction and each tendon must be used regularly to maintain load capacity. The information and stimuli each tendon receives aids in tendon regeneration.

NERVES

Remember that a nerve can move freely in its surrounding tissues and this is important for nerve mobility. The nerves are normally surrounded by fatty tissue, which acts as a lubricant. Nerve degeneration is caused by structural changes in the connective tissue. Increased pressure on a nerve or nerve root can cause circulatory impairment and demyelination, reducing its function. Massage and passive exercise help to improve nerve mobility and circulation through mobilisation of the surrounding connective tissue.

Electrotherapy is often used to treat muscle and damaged nerves and this helps the damaged nerve to return to its normal function since muscle plays a large part in nerve healing by activating feedback mechanisms. The targeted tissue is stimulated and conduction along the nerve course stimulates the nerve cell to become activated.

BONE

Recovery of bone following a period of immobilisation, both in its mechanical properties and its morphological properties, is very much reliant on the type, intensity and duration of immobilisation and the age of the animal.

As we know, recovery from injury is far quicker in younger animals than older animals. A short period of recovery with minimal exercise and cage rest, e.g. 6 weeks, is usually sufficient in animals of an adult age to allow bone healing. This is evident on a daily basis if you work in a veterinary referral hospital when patients who have had a dynamic procedure – e.g. tibial levelling osteotomy (TPLO) or tibial tuberosity advancement (TTA) to repair a cranial cruciate ligament rupture – are usually rested for 6 weeks postoperatively and then undergo re-examination radiographs at this time to ascertain the progression of bone healing. A 6-week period of immobilisation can usually be remobilised within 2–3 months.

Physiotherapy treatments

THERMOTHERAPY

Cold

Cold therapy, also known as cryotherapy, is predominantly used in patients with acute inflammation.

Indications
- Postoperative pain and associated inflammation
- Trauma
- Acute osteoarthritis (may be an acute flare-up of chronic osteoarthritis)
- Tendonitis
- Prevention of exercise-associated inflammation.

Effects
- Cryotherapy leads to vasoconstriction of superficial blood vessels leading to a reduced blood flow to the area
- Reduces swelling associated with inflammation or trauma
- Reduced pain
- Reduced muscle spasm.

Cautions and contraindications
- Circulatory compromise
- Impaired sensations
- Open wounds
- Patient sensitivity to the cold.

Therapy options
- The **Game Ready System** combines intermittent compression with circumferential cold therapy in one fully adjustable, easy-to-use application. RICE (Rest, Ice, Compression, and Elevation) has long been used to treat acute and chronic injury and to assist in the recovery and rehabilitation after orthopaedic surgery. The Game Ready System continuously circulates cold water from the control unit's ice reservoir, via a connector hose, through an inner chamber of the anatomical wrap (this chamber is located

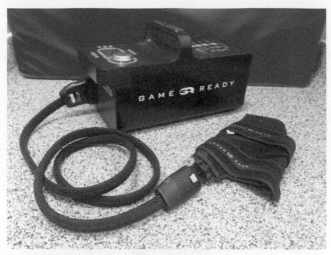

Fig. 18.2 Game Ready

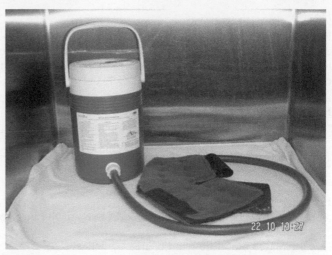

Fig. 18.4 Alternative ice compression system

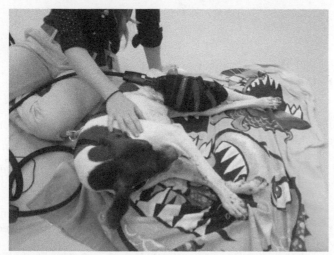

Fig. 18.3 Anatomical wrap for Game Ready

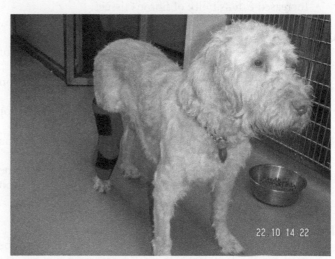

Fig. 18.5 Anatomical wrap for the stifle

closest to the body) before returning to the ice reservoir (Fig. 18.2). As a complete loop, the cold water is refreshed through the ice before returning through the anatomical wrap, thus delivering continuous cold therapy to the body part, allowing heat to be removed from the treatment site. Simultaneously, the control unit pumps air into the separate, outer chamber of the anatomical wrap (Fig. 18.3), intermittently inflating and deflating according to the pressure setting that is selected. The compression not only assists in preventing or limiting swelling, but also conforms the anatomical wrap to the contours of the body. This increases the surface contact and aids the delivery of the circumferential cold therapy.

- **Ice therapy and compression devices** are readily available and are far less expensive than the Game Ready System. Such devices have similar properties to the Game Ready by combining the ice chamber with a hose system connected to an anatomical wrap (Figs. 18.4 and 18.5). The system is not mechanical and needs manual input to replenish the iced water from the chamber to the patient, and the temperature within the ice chamber cannot be regulated.

- **Commercial ice packs or crushed ice** in a waterproof sealable bag. It is important that the ice pack can be conformed to the body to ensure optimum efficiency and is wrapped in a light cloth material to prevent ice burns.

Treatment duration and frequency

- Cold therapy should be applied for 15–25 minutes. If your patient shows any signs of distress or discomfort at any point during the treatment it should be ceased immediately.
- Frequency of treatment depends on the purpose of application and the desired therapeutic effect.
- Examples:
  - **Postoperative:** 3–6 times daily in the immediate postop period once the patient is normothermic until 48 hour postop (can be extended to 72 hours if required); do not apply over any incision initially as this may impede healing
  - **Arthritis flare-up:** 2–3 times daily
  - **After exercise:** apply to affected joint/joints after exercises such as passive range of joint motion or any active exercises.

Heat

Heat therapy is most commonly used in patients with chronic degenerative disease processes and should be performed prior to massage, passive joint range-of-motion and stretching exercises.

Indications

- Osteoarthritis (unless acute flare-up incident)
- Chronic lumbosacral disease
- Muscular tension/spasm
- Prior to exercise.

Effects

- Heat triggers the superficial blood vessels of the targeted tissues to vasodilate
- Increased blood flow to the area
- Muscle relaxation
- Reduction of pain
- Reduction in muscle spasm/muscle tension
- Increased extensibility of fibrous tissues.

Cautions and contraindications

- Must not be used in the acute inflammatory phase of injury or healing (0–48 hours)
- In any areas with an open wound, skin irritation/infection or chronic skin disease
- Areas of bruising or in patients with active bleeding or with known blood clots or coagulopathies
- Patients with circulatory compromise (e.g. trauma patients)
- Abnormal/reduced sensation in the treatment area (the patient is unable to respond if application device is too warm).

Therapy options

- Commercial 'hot packs' or wheat bags (Fig. 18.6) can be used for the treatment of small body areas but are not usually available in a large enough size to treat a large area.
- Infrared heat lamps are most appropriate for heating large areas of the body and are usually placed above a confined space to which you can direct the lamp to the treatment area of choice. It is immensely important that patients are supervised during treatment sessions to ensure they do not alter position resulting in direction of treatment to an inappropriate area.
- Aquatic therapy such a warm water spa tubs can be utilised to provide an all-over heat treatment similar to us taking a hot bath. Spa tubs allow you to submerge your patient in warm water (usually greater than the 32°C [89.6°F] that is standard for hydrotherapy pools) and some tubs may have the additional facility to apply a bubble or whirlpool effect enhancing the treatment with a 'therapeutic massage' type feeling.

Treatment duration and frequency. Heat therapy should be administered for 15–20 minutes within the patient's tolerance level. It is important to test the temperature of your warming device on your own bare skin for a minute or two to check that it is not too hot prior to applying upon the patient. If your patient shows any signs of distress or discomfort at any point during the treatment it should be ceased immediately.

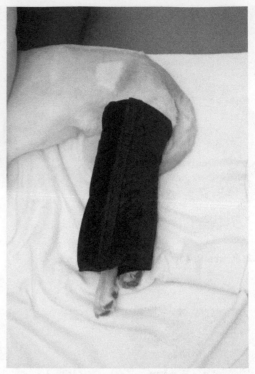

Fig. 18.6 Wheat bag used for heat therapy of the hind limb

Frequency of treatments depends on the purpose of application and the desired therapeutic effect.

Examples:

- **Arthritis:** 2–3 treatments per day before walks. Long-term treatment may be necessary in patients with a more progressive stage of disease.
- **Lumbosacral disease:** 1–2 treatments per day. Treatment may be best prior to exercise or following a prolonged period of rest (e.g. first thing in the morning).
- **Before exercises** as outlined above for 15–20 minutes.

MASSAGE THERAPY

There are arrays of massage techniques that can be learned by you and can also be taught to your clients when they are providing physiotherapy to their dog or cat at home. Principally massage techniques should only be performed on your patient when you are in the correct frame of mind to do so, and the patient is in the correct frame of mind to receive. This involves access to a designated room or area in your practice or hospital free from excessive noise, traffic and disturbances. Your patient should be given the opportunity to use massage sessions as a time to recuperate and relax. It will also do wonders for you, the therapist.

Indications

- Muscle tension
- Reduced blood flow to tissues
- Reduced elasticity of ligaments and tendons and therefore joint and muscle flexibility
- Tissue congestion
- Adhesions within musculoskeletal tissues
- Abnormal muscle tone
- Abnormal sensory awareness.

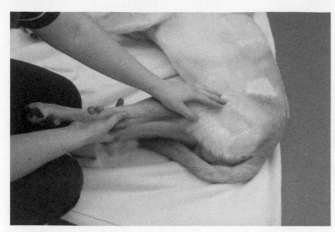

Fig. 18.7 Stroking (effleurage)

Effects

- Alleviate muscular tension and associated pain
- Prolonged muscle contraction in states of tension reduces blood flow to the associated tissues
- Tension and reduced blood flow reduces oxygen and nutrient availability to the tissues resulting in a build-up of metabolic waste and toxins
- Increased blood flow to tissues
- Improved oxygenation and nutrients to tissues
- Excretion of metabolites and toxins from tissues
- Stimulation of tissues resulting in endorphin release
- Increased musculoskeletal tissue temperature and elasticity
- Mobilisation of adhesions
- Increase/decrease muscle tone depending on the technique used
- Builds trust and bond between patient and therapist or owner.

Cautions and contraindications

- Skin infection
- Skin irritation
- Chronic skin disease
- Open wounds
- Tumours
- Cardiovascular or circulatory compromise
- Pyrexia
- Bleeding disorders.

Techniques

Stroking (effleurage). Should always be performed at the beginning of the massage process to make your patient relaxed and then at the end of the session to finish (Fig. 18.7).

- Superficial massage technique motion to increase blood flow and promote lymphatic drainage
- Long sweeping motion
- Stroking in a distal to proximal direction of the limb or caudal to cranial if treating muscles of the spine using slow and gentle pressure to promote lymphatic drainage in the first stroke and then from proximal to distal and cranial to caudal for the second stroke; alternate for the duration of massage
- Pressure can be slowly increased as the massage progresses

- Maintain physical contact for the duration of the technique when moving from one part of the body to another
- Can be performed with the patient standing or while in lateral recumbency
- Continue until your patient becomes relaxed.

Kneading (petrissage). Begin once your patient is suitably relaxed following stroking. Kneading pressure can be applied superficially or deeply for deep tissue treatment, e.g. large muscle groups along the back or in the hind limbs.

- Similar to how you would knead bread, gently grasp the roll of superficial skin and lift from underlying tissues.
- Once grasped, roll between fingers and release. Move forward to the next segment of skin and repeat. This technique stretches and mobilises the superficial tissue.
- Kneed distal to proximal when treating the limbs and caudal to cranial when treating along the back.

Rubbing (friction). Friction is alternated between kneading and stroking for treating both generalised and/or focal areas with particular tension or swelling and can be performed superficially or deeply by altering pressure. Stroking should always be performed after a friction treatment.

- Friction increases blood flow to the affected area and therefore promotes tissue oxygenation and nutrition by eliminating metabolites and toxins from the tissues.
- Rubbing (friction) breaks down adhesions.
- Treatment of a small focal area involves using slightly curved but extended fingers to slide over the small area in circular motions beginning with gentle pressure and increasing to more firm pressure to treat deeper muscles. Pressure can be further increased by placing one set of fingers over the other.
- Treatment of a large area involves positioning your hands as outlined previously. Position one or both hands on the muscle group of choice with your fingers slightly bent and use a sliding motion back and forward in the direction of the muscle fibres to diminish adhesions. Using both hands will exert more pressure. Care must be taken not to cause the patient discomfort but must be firm enough to achieve the desired effect.

Circular pressure. This technique is used to complement friction as outlined previously and is very effective at treating adhesions or relieving tension in very tight tissues. It is a similar technique used by a masseuse to rid your shoulders of knots. Using small circular motions with the tips of your fingers manipulates deeper tissues over a small area and rids the tissues of difficult adhesions. Your fingers or thumbs can be used (Fig. 18.8).

Shaking. Shaking is exactly what it sounds and involves shaking an entire limb or particular large muscle group to encourage relaxation of that specific region.

- To perform shaking of a particular muscle you must grasp the muscle group, e.g. quadriceps femoris, in one or both hands depending on the size of your patient and gently move it back and forth, almost like picking the muscle from the bone surface and rocking it back and forth over the surface of the bone.
- To perform shaking of an entire limb the limb must be gently lifted distally and supported in one hand

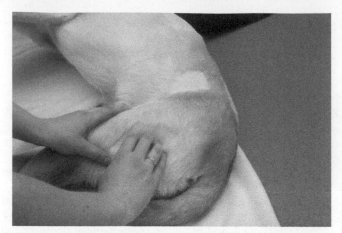

Fig. 18.8 Circular pressure

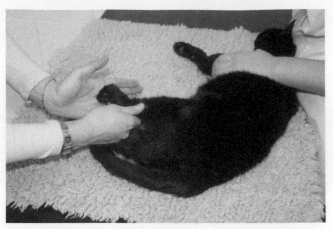

Fig. 18.9 Flexion of digits

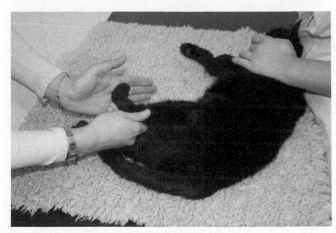

Fig. 18.10 Extension of digits

perpendicular to the body. The limb is then gently shaken to promote relaxation.

Percussion (clapping/hacking). Percussion is most frequently used in tense muscles to encourage relaxation. It is also a very important massage technique for breaking up secretions in the lungs in patients with pneumonia. Clapping, also known as 'coupage', indirectly treats the lungs by applying the technique over the thorax creating a vibrating type of effect on the thoracic wall which reverberates to the lungs.

- Performing clapping involves positioning your hands in a slightly 'cupped' position and the technique must be performed with loose wrists and in a rhythmical manner creating a hollow sound as the hands strikes the skin surface.
- Hacking involves positioning your hands in extension with the edge of the hand contacting the patient. The technique should be performed with loose wrists and in a rhythmical manner.
- Increasing the stiffness of your wrists will create a more forceful massage technique.
- Care must be taken that you do not use so much force that you cause discomfort to the patient but enough that the outcome is achieved.

Therapeutic exercises

Therapeutic exercises are an important aspect of any patient rehabilitation plan to improve not only the rate of recovery but also the quality of movement that can be achieved by the patient as well as improving stamina and cardiovascular fitness.

Therapeutic exercises can be implemented for any patient at any stage of the patient's rehabilitation journey, be it a patient day 1 postop or an agility dog getting back into competing. What differentiates these dogs is the type of exercise you use, the intensity, and the frequency at which it is implemented. Each patient's rehabilitation plan should not be stagnant but should be adjusted depending on the individual's response. It is important to remember that if patients are not fulfilling the goals or achieving the best performance from the exercise prescribed then maybe it is not the most appropriate for them, or maybe you are challenging them sooner than they are capable of. Evaluate your patient's performance on a daily basis and amend the rehabilitation plan accordingly.

GOALS OF THERAPEUTIC EXERCISES

- Improve muscle mass and strength
- Improve core stability and balance
- Improve active pain-free range of motion in the joints and limbs overall
- Improve flexibility
- Reduce lameness
- Improve limb use
- Improve ability to perform activities of daily living
- Prevent further injury though owner education.

PASSIVE EXERCISE

Passive range of motion (PROM)

PROM exercises are performed to improve joint range of motion and flexibility of the associated musculoskeletal tissues.

- PROM exercises must be performed with your patient comfortably in lateral recumbency.
- PROM exercises are most often performed following heat therapy and massage and essentially involve moving each joint associated with the limb or limbs through full flexion and full extension.
- The limb must be supported in a comfortable position perpendicular to the body; then, beginning at the joint most distal in the limb, gently flex, hold for a few seconds to allow tissues to respond, and then extend and hold for a few seconds (Figs. 18.9–18.16).

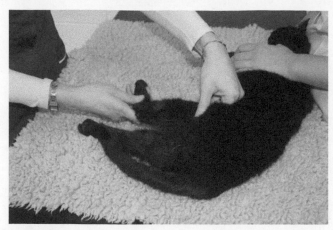

Fig. 18.11   Flexion of hock

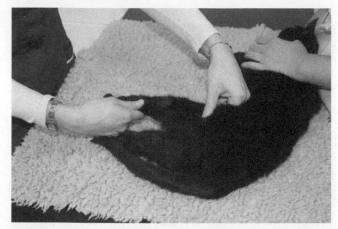

Fig. 18.12   Extension of hock

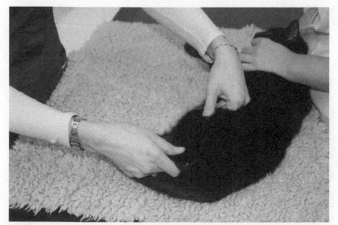

Fig. 18.13   Flexion of stifle

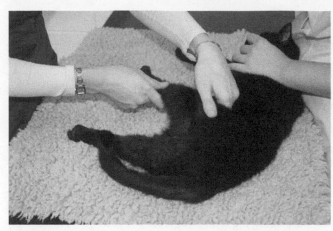

Fig. 18.14   Extension of stifle

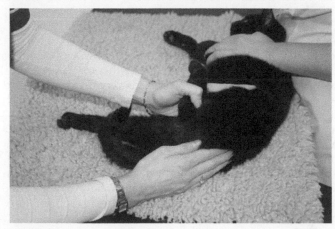

Fig. 18.15   Flexion of hip

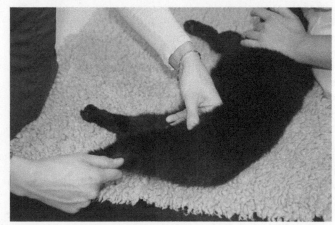

Fig. 18.16   Extension of hip

- Repeat PROM 10–30 times 3–6 times daily, depending on your patient's reaction.
- The point at which you stop flexing or extending is when you feel natural resistance. The 'pause', or 'hold', allows time for the tissues to respond, hopefully allowing them to be more extensible and therefore improve the range of motion in the joint.
- Perform the same technique in each joint moving distal to proximal if a complete limb is to be treated.

- Your patient should never show any signs of pain during PROM exercises. If the patient does show signs of pain, *STOP* and seek advice from a veterinary physiotherapist or veterinary surgeon.

Stretching

Stretching is usually combined with PROM exercises to improve musculoskeletal tissue extensibility associated with joints that have reduced range of motion or stiffness. The physical motion of joint flexion and extension remains the same. What changes is the length of time the joint is maintained in a flexed or extended position with an active gentle increase in the pressure at the end point. The 'hold' should increase to 30–90 seconds and the number of flexion and extension repetitions can be reduced to between two and five. Repeat stretching exercises 1–3 times daily.

Flexor reflex exercise

The flexor reflex exercise is extremely useful in neurological patients with reduced voluntary motion and reflexes. By achieving active muscle contraction this exercise is beneficial for maintaining muscle mass or preventing disuse atrophy. The flexor reflex involves pinching the toes to initiate a withdrawal reflex, i.e. pulling the limb away from the pressure. This actively encourages muscle contraction, and therefore the pressure should be maintained for a few seconds during the withdrawal to challenge the muscles more.

Bicycle motion

Bicycle motion is exactly how it sounds, and involves manipulating the limb through a bicycle motion either in lateral recumbency or while standing. This exercise is very useful when gait training and improving joint range of motion in neurological patients since you are stimulating or reminding all the musculoskeletal tissues how they work together as one unit, or network. The exercise is performed by grasping the patient's paw and gently moving the limb in a bicycle motion in an exaggerated fashion to encourage flexion and extension of all the joints in the limb. Be careful not to teach your patient how to walk backwards. The exercise can be repeated 5–10 times in each limb 3–6 times daily.

ASSISTED THERAPEUTIC EXERCISES

Assisted therapeutic exercises comprise a group of exercises that revolve around standing and can be utilised to help patients that have some ability to bear weight but are too weak and do not have the strength to bear 100% of their weight. It is important at this point to become familiar with various support devices that can be used to facilitate standing exercises and mobility in these patients as required. Some devices provide more or less support depending on the strength and weight-bearing ability of the patient. Examples are shown in Figures 18.17–18.19.

Assisted standing exercises

Assisted standing exercises are beneficial in all patients, orthopaedic or neurological, who need to improve their overall strength and endurance, and prepare them for some of the more challenging exercises outlined below. Standing exercises are exceptionally beneficial in neurological patients requiring proprioceptive training (awareness of paw position in relation to space and the rest of the body) and neuromuscular awareness enhancing.

- Position your patient on all four feet with or without a support device as outlined previously. Have the limbs positioned squarely beneath the body creating a normal standing position.
- Allow your patient to independently bear as much weight as the patient can manage.
- As the patient weakens and begins to crouch, gently correct the patient back into the standing position as before.

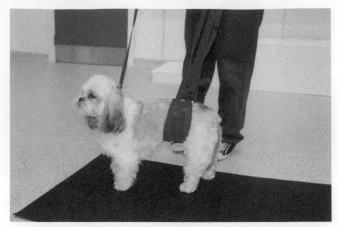
Fig. 18.17 Minimum support – abdominal support sling

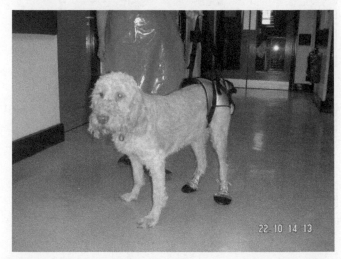
Fig. 18.18 Moderate support – pelvic support sling with additional foot-protecting boots

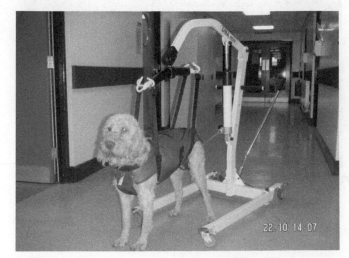
Fig. 18.19 Maximum support – mechanical hoist

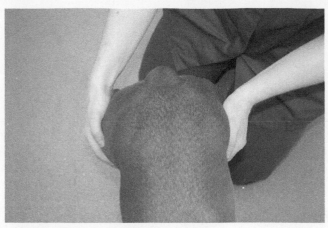

Fig. 18.20 Hip swaying in a dog

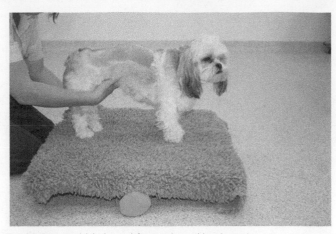

Fig. 18.22 Wobble board forwards and backwards

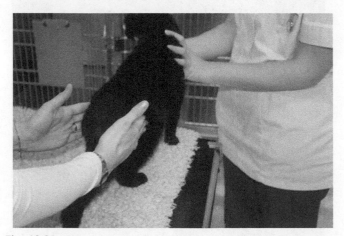

Fig. 18.21 Hip swaying in a cat

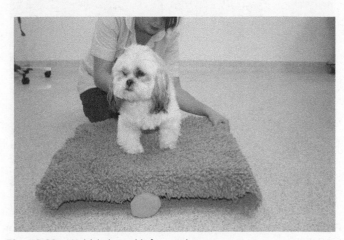

Fig. 18.23 Wobble board left to right

- Begin with short repetitions, from 5–15, depending on your patient's ability. Repeat 2–3 times daily.
- In more competent patients, standing sessions can be increased to 5 minutes per session.

Weight-shifting. Positioning your patient as outlined previously (using a support device if required), place your hands on either side of the patient's hips and gently apply pressure from left to right and vice versa to encourage a subtle 'hip sway' effect (Figs. 18.20 and 18.21). The same manoeuvre can also be performed on the shoulders. The force you use should not be so strong that it causes patients to fall over, but it should be forceful enough that it causes them to lose balance and they have to respond by correcting their position. As your patient becomes stronger and the patient's proprioception (paw-placing ability) improves, it is possible to increase the pressure you use causing the patient to lift and reposition limb placement to regain balance.

Downward pelvic/shoulder pressure. Have your patient stand squarely as outlined previously and gently apply 'bouncing' pressure over the patient's pelvis or shoulders, encouraging the patient to resist the pressure. The aim is to have your patient push against the pressure and not collapse beneath it. The bouncing and resistance should be in short sharp bursts.

Side bending. Again, having your patient standing squarely as described previously, challenge the patient's core stability and balance by encouraging the patient to bend from left to right and vice versa using treats. You are aiming for the patient to maintain balance during each movement.

Cervical flexion and extension. This manoeuvre is similar to side bending but uses treats to encourage patients to lift their head to the ceiling and down between their elbows without losing balance.

Balancing/wobble boards. Having patients standing squarely you can have them standing on the balancing board with all four limbs, the fore limbs only, the hind limbs only, the right fore limb and right hind limb only, or left fore limb and lift hind limb only. Once balanced appropriately, gently rock the board from side to side or back and forth to initiate a loss of balance (Figs. 18.22 and 18.23). The aim is for your patient to maintain balance during the rocking motions.

Physioball/'peanut'. Peanuts are very useful devices for encouraging neurological patients to support a proportion of their body weight by placing the peanut across the width of the patient between the fore limbs and hind limbs (Fig. 18.24). The

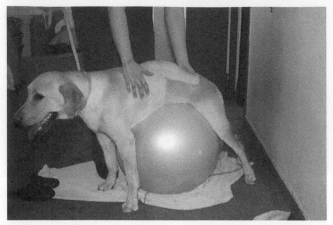

Fig. 18.24 Aided standing using a physioball in a neurological patient

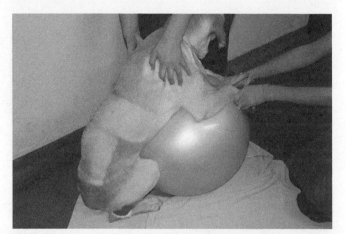

Fig. 18.25 Assisted sitting position using a physioball in a neurological patient

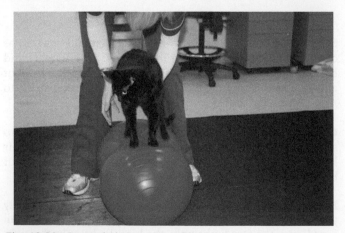

Fig. 18.26 Peanut balancing in a cat

peanut can also be used for transition training in dogs by placing the patient's fore limbs over the peanut while supported in a sitting position (Fig. 18.25). Then, by rolling the peanut forward, the patient can be transitioned from a sitting to standing position. Balancing on the peanut is also another very useful exercise for core stability training in neurological patients as this challenges not only core stability overall but also the fine-tuning of muscular strength in the limbs (Figs. 18.26 and 18.27).

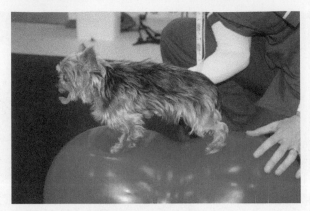

Fig. 18.27 Peanut balancing in a small dog

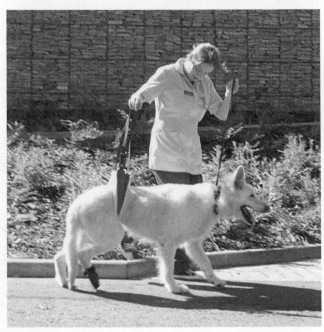

Fig. 18.28 Supported walking using an abdominal support sling in a large dog recovering from spinal injury

ACTIVE THERAPEUTIC EXERCISES

As suggested, active therapeutic exercises are beneficial for patients who are able to exercise with very little or no support. The exercises are directed to improve your patient's strength, cardiovascular fitness and overall functional ability.

Supported walking

Supported walking involves walking your patient on a short lead, in a controlled manner, to encourage functional use of the limbs. An abdominal or pelvic support sling may be required (Fig. 18.28). Deciding which support sling to use depends on the weight-bearing ability and proprioception ability of your patient (see the guidelines outlined previously). The pace of the walk should be slow or quick enough to obtain the best possible functional movement and placement of the limbs from the patient.

Sit-to-stand

Sit-to-stand exercises are exactly as they suggest. It involves using a treat to encourage your patient to transition from a

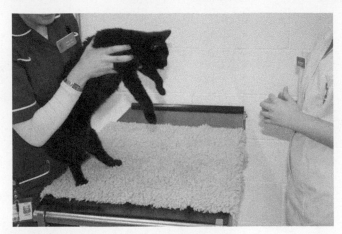

Fig. 18.29 Dancing exercise in a cat

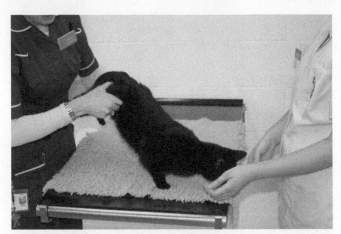

Fig. 18.30 Wheel-barrowing exercises in a cat

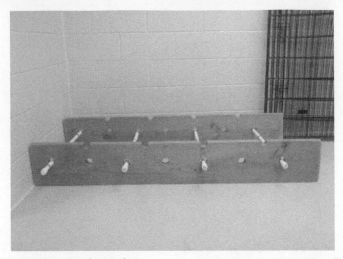

Fig. 18.31 Cavaletti poles

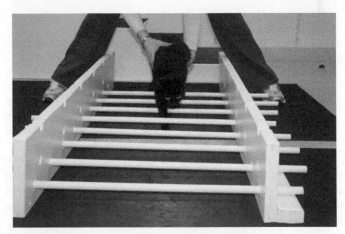

Fig. 18.32 Encouraging joint flexion and extension in a cat

sitting to standing position and vice versa with the optimum functional movement of the pelvic limbs, i.e. the limbs tuck normally beneath the pelvis at the end of the sit movement. If your patient has a tendency to 'kick' one of the limbs out to the side in the sitting position, try performing the exercise with the patient positioned against a wall which inhibits the ability of the limb to 'kick out'. Begin with 5 transitions and increase to 10–15 as your patient becomes stronger. Sit-to-stand exercises can be repeated 2–3 times daily.

Dancing exercises

Dancing exercises are very beneficial in patients with reduced hip extension and are a standard exercise used postoperatively for patients who have undergone femoral head and neck excision. The exercise involves having your patient standing squarely on all four limbs and gently lifting your patient's fore limbs from the ground. Encourage the patient to stretch in an upright position bearing all body weight through the hind limbs with the hips fully extended (Fig. 18.29). Then gently encourage your patient to take a few steps forward and then backward. This can be repeated 5–10 times 2–3 times daily.

Wheel-barrowing

Wheel-barrowing exercises are exactly the same as dancing exercises except you lift the patient's hind limbs from the ground and encourage the patient to walk forward and back on the fore limbs (Fig. 18.30). It is important that you do not lift the patient's pelvis too far from the ground, which can make the patient feel unsafe.

Cavaletti poles

Cavaletti pole exercises involve placing poles at set distances directly on the ground or raised depending on your patient's ability and the desired outcome (Fig. 18.31). If you are aiming to increase hip flexion, for example, you would position the poles a few inches from the ground, encouraging your patient to step up and over the pole (Fig. 18.32). To begin with, your patient should be slowly walked over the poles, but as the patient improves the pace can be increased to trotting.

Weaving poles

Navigating your patient around weaving poles placed vertically into the ground encourages spinal flexion and extension, challenges proprioception and if combined with cavaletti poles also challenges gait and joint range of motion.

ELECTRICAL STIMULATION

Electrical stimulation is the generalised term used to explain electrotherapeutic methods used for the treatment of acute and

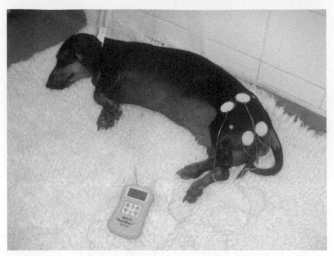

Fig. 18.33 Electrical stimulation in a Dachshund recovering from spinal surgery

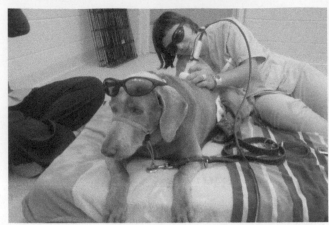

Fig. 18.34 Class IV laser therapy on the lumbar muscles of a Weimaraner

chronic pain and muscle atrophy associated with orthopaedic and neurological conditions. Electrical stimulation includes:

- Electrical nerve stimulation – direct stimulation of a denervated muscle via its muscle fibres
- Neuromuscular electrical stimulation (NMES) – electrical stimulation of a target muscle or tissue via an intact nerve
- Transcutaneous electrical nerve stimulation (TENS) – a form of NMES especially used for pain management.

Electrical stimulation involves the application of adhesive pads (electrodes) to the skin of the desired area from a handheld unit which features programmes that stimulate or send impulses to the desired areas via the electrodes (Fig. 18.33). The process is painless and well tolerated by patients.

LASER THERAPY

Non-invasive use of a class IV laser (light) energy generates a healing response in damaged or dysfunctional tissues. Laser therapy is used to alleviate pain, reduce inflammation, accelerate recovery and facilitate improved function and mobility.

Conditions that benefit from laser therapy are wounds, poor bone healing, soft tissue strains and painful swollen joints. Treatment sessions are relatively short and are well tolerated in the conscious patient (Figs. 18.34 and 18.35). Most often patients require one to two sessions of laser per week for up to 4 weeks, but this can vary between patients.

THERAPEUTIC ULTRASOUND

There are a broad range of indications for therapeutic ultrasound such as treating structures within the joint and aspects of joint disease. Some muscular diseases may also benefit from therapeutic ultrasound. The benefits of treatment include a reduction in pain, improved elasticity of fibrous structures, increased circulation to the treated area and therefore increased nutrition to the region. Therapeutic ultrasound should not be performed near tumours, infected/inflamed/irritated skin, or directly over the heart, eye or over epiphyseal plates that have still to close in young patients. Treatment frequency can be similar to laser therapy until desired effects are achieved.

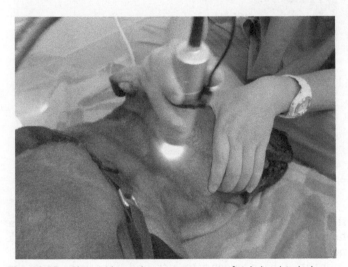

Fig. 18.35 Class IV laser therapy on a superficial decubital ulcer on the side of the face of a recumbent dog

Treatment is comfortable and can be performed while your patient is conscious.

EXTRACORPOREAL SHOCKWAVE THERAPY

Extracorporeal shockwave therapy (ESWT) provides accelerated healing similar to laser therapy but by means of high-energy pulses (shockwaves) penetrated into the tissues (Fig. 18.36). The ultimate effect is similar to the laser in that the body's normal cellular response to healing has increased efficiency.

Extracorporeal shockwave therapy can be uncomfortable; therefore most patient require heavy sedation or general anaesthesia for treatments to be performed. Most patients only require 2–3 sessions to achieve the desired effect but may require 'top-up' treatments at set intervals.

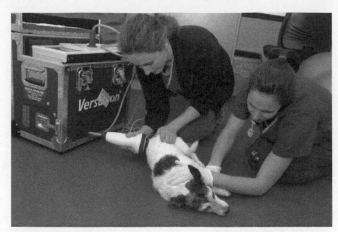

Fig. 18.36 ESWT in the lumbar region of a Jack Russell Terrier

BIBLIOGRAPHY

Bockstahler, B., Levine, D., Millis, D. (Eds.), 2004. Essential Facts of Physiotherapy in Dogs and Cats. Babenhausen, BE Verlag.

Goff, L., McGowan, C., Stubbs, N. (Eds.), 2007. Animal Physiotherapy. Assessment, Treatment and Rehabilitation of Animals. Wiley Blackwell Ltd, oxford.

Lindley, S., Watson, P. (Eds.), 2010. BSAVA Manual of Canine and Feline Rehabilitation, Supportive and Palliative Care: Case Studies in Patient Management. BSAVA, Gloucester, UK.

Millis, D., Levine, D. (Eds.), 2013. Canine Rehabilitation and Physical Therapy, second ed. Saunders, Oxford.

19

Fundamental Pharmacology

SALLY BOWDEN

KEY POINTS

- When a drug is administered to the body it moves through the tissues to its designated site of action – this is the study of pharmacokinetics.

- The speed at which a drug reaches its site of action is determined by the route of administration.

- The body metabolises drugs, mainly in the liver, during which process the drug is converted into a form that can be excreted.

- Different types of drugs have varying effects, depending on their formulation, and this determines their therapeutic use.

- Drugs and other chemicals in the body may interact with each other, resulting in unpredictable and sometimes adverse reactions.

- The production of drugs by pharmaceutical companies, the dispensing of drugs by veterinary surgeons to their clients and the subsequent disposal of surplus drug are subject to much legislation. This is all designed to protect the patient, the owner giving the drug, the general public and the environment.

Introduction

This chapter aims to provide veterinary nurses with a broad, basic understanding of various aspects of pharmacology. It encompasses a range of subjects, from general pharmacokinetics and pharmacodynamics, through the classification of commonly used drugs, to practical aspects of handling and dispensing medication.

WHAT IS PHARMACOLOGY?

Pharmacology is the study of the properties of drugs and their effects on living organisms. It is derived from the Greek word *pharmakon,* meaning 'drug', and the suffix *-logy*, meaning 'study of'. Clinical pharmacology, or pharmacotherapeutics, is concerned with the effects of drugs in treating disease. The term 'drug' may be defined in various ways but, put simply, describes any substance that, when administered, has a specific effect on the body.

THE ORIGINS OF DRUGS

Drugs have been used for religious, recreational and medicinal purposes throughout the course of history. Alcohol and opium are among the earliest examples of drugs. Other plant-derived drugs such as tobacco, strychnine, digitalis and atropine, to name but a few, have also been used for several hundred years.

More recently, around the beginning of the 19th century, scientists discovered methods of modifying natural substances, or synthesising drugs, to provide safer, more predictable and more effective treatment. Drugs from animal and mineral sources began to be used. In the modern age, genetically engineered drugs are the latest pharmacological development in a burgeoning pharmaceutical industry.

Pharmacokinetics

The word *pharmacokinetics* literally means 'drug movement'. It pertains to what happens to a drug when it enters the body, i.e. what the body does to the drug. This section traces drug movement through the body and examines how it gets in, where it goes, what happens to it along the way and how it leaves. Pharmacokinetic processes are often categorised into four main areas: absorption, distribution, metabolism and elimination.

DRUG ABSORPTION

The route of administration, the disease status of the patient and the formulation of the drug affect drug absorption into the body.

Route of administration and its effect on absorption

There are many routes of drug administration, but the most commonly used ones in veterinary medicine are the oral, topical, subcutaneous, intramuscular and intravenous routes. Generally, in order for a drug to reach its site of action and have an effect, it must enter the systemic blood circulation. The exceptions to this are drugs that act locally, i.e. in the area they are applied. An example of a locally acting drug that does not need to enter the circulation in order to reach its site of action is lidocaine hydrochloride.

The amount of drug that reaches the circulation intact (i.e. unaltered) determines the drug's **bioavailability.** For example, if the entire administered dose reaches the circulation intact, that drug has 100% bioavailability. This is also known as a bioavailability of 1. Consider the intravenous route of drug administration – drugs given by this route have a bioavailability of 1 as the drug enters the bloodstream directly and there is no absorption phase. Drugs given by all other routes of administration are said to have a bioavailability of less than 1, as less than 100% of the dose will reach the circulation intact.

Bioavailability is affected by the rate at which the drug is absorbed and also the ease of absorption. Generally, the better the blood supply to an area, the quicker the rate of absorption (Fig. 19.1). Drugs administered intramuscularly are usually absorbed quickly. Of the commonly used parenteral routes of administration, subcutaneously administered drugs have the lowest bioavailability because the skin is a less vascular part of

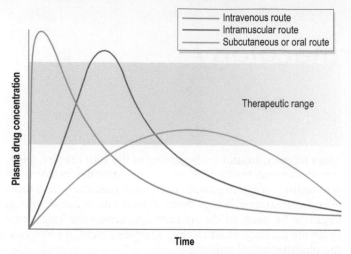

Fig. 19.1 Plasma concentrations following intravenous, intramuscular and subcutaneous injections *(Redrawn from Bill 1997)*

the body, and some drugs are absorbed/bound into the subcutaneous fat.

Orally administered drugs travel through the gastrointestinal tract and most are absorbed in the small intestine. Solid oral preparations, including tablets, capsules and granules, undergo a process of dissolving known as dissolution prior to being absorbed. Liquid preparations do not need to undergo dissolution and so are usually absorbed more quickly than the solid oral preparations. Some drugs are formulated as a 'sustained release' preparation, where dissolution and subsequent absorption is slowed down. Note that this is not the same as an 'enteric-coated' tablet, which has a protective coating to prevent the destruction of the drug in the highly acidic environment of the stomach.

Once absorbed across the intestinal wall, orally administered drugs enter the hepatic portal circulation and are routed directly to the liver. One of the roles of the liver is to remove potentially toxic substances before they reach the systemic blood circulation, and drugs may be partially or completely broken down because of this mechanism; this is known as the first-pass effect. The first-pass effect is one reason that some drugs cannot be administered orally, or that the dose rate of an oral preparation when compared with a parenteral preparation of the same drug is much higher. Due to the need for dissolution, time taken to reach the site of absorption and the first-pass effect, orally administered drugs tend to have a comparatively low bioavailability.

Other factors also affect the rate of absorption:

Tissue perfusion. Tissue perfusion directly affects the rate of absorption; for example, a drug injected into an active, well-perfused muscle will be absorbed more quickly than one injected into an inactive muscle, which will have a poorer blood supply. Vasoconstriction or vasodilation will cause reduced or enhanced blood flow to an area so, when injecting subcutaneously, exposing the patient to cold or hot environmental temperatures will affect the absorption rate. Disease conditions affecting perfusion or those animals in shock and having peripheral vasoconstriction have the same effect.

Drug formulation. The drug formulation can also have an effect on absorption. Drugs that dissolve more easily in water are termed hydrophilic, which literally means 'water-loving'. Drugs that dissolve more easily in fat are termed lipophilic or 'fat-loving'. Drugs administered intravenously or intramuscularly enter the extracellular fluid and, in the case of the intramuscular route, must diffuse through it to reach the circulation; therefore hydrophilic drugs are more readily absorbed via these routes. Drugs administered via other routes, e.g. orally or subcutaneously, must diffuse through cell membranes in order to reach the circulation. As cell membranes are mostly made up of phospholipids, lipophilic drugs are able to diffuse through them more readily.

While most drugs are formulated to facilitate absorption, there are some drugs deliberately designed to provide a 'slow-release' or 'depot' formulation. An example of this is nandrolone laurate, which is lipophilic and so not easily diffused into the interstitial fluid surrounding muscle fibres. Some drugs are formulated for slow absorption because they exert their effect where the drug is introduced. A prime example of this is piperazine, which is hydrophilic and therefore is not easily absorbed from the gut, as it must cross the cell membranes of the intestinal wall. This means that sufficient concentration remains in the gastrointestinal tract for the drug to be effective at this site. The pH of the drug and of the environment can affect absorption because it can affect the drug's hydrophilic or lipophilic tendency. Manufacturers sometimes advise that orally administered drugs should be given with food to improve absorption – an example of this is trilostane.

DRUG DISTRIBUTION

The movement of drug from the systemic circulation into the body tissues is known as **distribution.** Most drugs must reach a specific area or target tissue in order to have their desired effect, known as the **therapeutic effect**.

When a drug enters the systemic circulation, drug molecules attach themselves to a certain site on plasma proteins (notably to albumin); this is called **protein binding**. Once attached, the drug molecule is inactive, i.e. unable to move into the body tissues. In order for a drug to be active, it must become unbound or 'free' – in other words, detach itself from the plasma protein. The amount of bound drug in the circulation is always the same as the amount of unbound drug in the circulation, so, as free drug molecules move into the body tissues, more bound drug molecules are released to maintain this balance. Likewise, the amount of unbound drug in the circulation and the amount of drug in the tissues will always equalise along a concentration gradient.

Factors affecting drug distribution

Some drugs bind more strongly to plasma proteins than others – these are termed highly protein-bound. The more highly protein-bound a drug is, the less free drug is available to distribute into the body tissues. This means that it is often necessary to give high doses of drugs that are highly protein-bound in order for them to have a therapeutic effect. Disease conditions that cause a decrease in blood plasma protein levels, e.g. hypoalbuminaemia due to liver failure, can mean that a higher than normal amount of free drug is available for distribution and this can result in toxicity. Some drugs bind to the same site on plasma proteins. If administered together, this can result in the less highly bound drug lacking binding sites and, again, a higher than normal amount being available as free drug for distribution, so toxicity can occur. For this reason, some drugs, e.g. methotrexate and phenylbutazone, must not be administered together.

Natural barriers to the circulation exist in the body. These are the blood–brain, placental and testicular barriers. They are present to protect these areas of the body from dangerous toxins in the blood circulation. The capillary walls in the brain have a different structure from others, which means that only highly lipophilic drugs are able to cross into the brain tissue. Drugs that must reach the brain to have an effect, e.g. general anaesthetics, must be sufficiently lipophilic to be able to cross the blood–brain barrier. The placental barrier is not as efficient at preventing drugs passing into the foetal circulation and so caution must be exercised when treating pregnant animals.

Tissue perfusion in the target organ or organs will also affect distribution. Well-perfused organs will receive the drug quickly. After a time, the drug will also distribute into the poorly perfused areas and drug concentration levels will drop in the blood plasma. As distribution of drug occurs along a concentration gradient, this can cause the drug to leave the well-perfused organs and re-enter the circulation, then move into a less-well-perfused area until equilibrium is reached. This is called **redistribution**. An example of this is the anaesthetic thiopental, which is lipophilic and redistributes to the adipose tissues, causing the animal to regain consciousness (Fig. 19.2). Reduced blood flow to an organ or ischaemia caused by disease must be taken into consideration when monitoring the effects of drug therapy.

DRUG METABOLISM

The body will metabolise or biotransform drugs as it would attempt to do with any foreign substance in the circulation. The resultant product of metabolism is known as a metabolite. Biotransformation mainly occurs in the liver, although sometimes other organs, including the lung and the kidney, can be involved.

Biotransformation does not simply mean that the body turns potentially harmful substances into less harmful ones – it is the process by which drugs are changed into a form that is more readily excreted by the body. In some cases, the metabolite can be more active in the body than the original drug molecule. This can be an advantage if it is not possible to give the active form of the drug in the first place, and is known as giving a prodrug; for example, the corticosteroid prednisone is metabolised into prednisolone. Alternatively, the metabolite can be as active as the original drug, or even more toxic than the original drug.

The metabolic process

As elimination of drugs from the body occurs via body fluids, this means that drug metabolites must be hydrophilic to be excreted. There are two phases of drug metabolism:

- **Phase I metabolism** – enzymes act on the drug to transform it; the processes that occur are hydrolysis, reduction and/or oxidation.
- **Phase II metabolism** – the metabolite is joined with another molecule to make it more hydrophilic. This is known as conjugation.

Most drugs undergo both metabolic phases but some only undergo phase II.

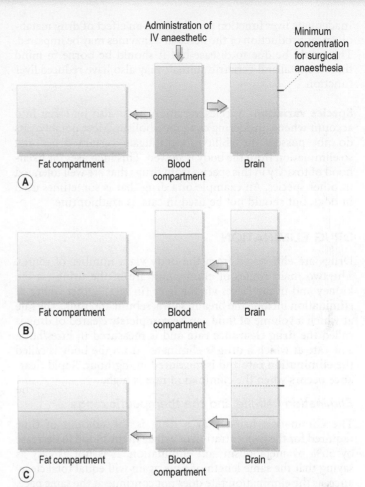

Fig. 19.2   Redistribution of an anaesthetic drug from the brain to other tissues. (**A**) The drug moves quickly from the blood to the brain, causing anaesthesia. (**B**) The brain concentration of anaesthetic then drops until it is too low to maintain anaesthesia. (**C**) When the animal begins to awaken (*Redrawn from Bill 1997*)

Factors affecting drug metabolism

Metabolic systems.   A key metabolic system found in the liver is known as the mixed function oxidase system. The enzyme involved, cytochrome P450, is induced by the presence of one or more of the drugs it metabolises. This means that persistent exposure to drugs metabolised by P450 will increase the rate of metabolism and result in ever-increasing doses being required to have a therapeutic effect. An example of this is the drug phenobarbital, used for controlling epileptic seizures. Other drugs affected by P450 would also be metabolised more quickly, so the dose rate of these would also have to be increased. Conversely, some drugs may suppress the release of P450, which can lead to toxicity of others administered concurrently if they are metabolised by the same system.

Drug interaction.   There are other enzyme systems that are not induced by the presence of the drugs they metabolise, resulting in a fixed amount of enzyme available at any one time. If two or more drugs are administered that use the same enzyme system, this can cause a delay in drug metabolism, resulting in drug toxicity if the doses are not altered.

Some drugs cause the inhibition of certain enzymes, which could result in the metabolism of that drug, or another drug, being slowed (see cytochrome P450 in the previous section).

Inadequate liver function can also have an effect of drug metabolism, as production of the necessary enzymes may be impaired. This could be due to disease but it should be borne in mind that neonatal and geriatric animals may also have reduced liver function.

Species variation. Species variation must also be taken into account when considering drug metabolism. Most notably, cats do not possess the ability to conjugate certain drugs and so elimination from the body is slowed. This increases the likelihood of toxicity in this species from drugs that are well tolerated in other species. An example of a drug that is sometimes used in dogs, but should not be used in cats, is azathioprine.

DRUG ELIMINATION

Drugs are eliminated from the body via a number of routes. The two main routes of elimination are in the urine via the kidney and in the faeces via the liver (in bile). Other routes of elimination include the breath, saliva, sebum and milk. The rate at which a volume of fluid can be completely cleared of drug is called the **drug clearance rate** and is measured in litres/hour. The rate at which a drug is eliminated from the body is called the **elimination rate** and is measured in mg/hour. Rapid clearance occurs when the elimination rate is high.

Elimination half-life and the therapeutic range

The elimination half-life of a drug is the amount of time required for the concentration of a drug in the blood to decrease by 50% by metabolism and elimination. It is not as easy as saying that the same length of time again will equal total clearance, as the elimination rate does not continue at the same pace, although it is usually constant. For example, if a drug had a blood concentration of 40 µg/l and after 2 hours blood concentration was 20 µg/l, that drug's half-life is 2 hours. In a further 2 hours, the blood concentration would be 10 µg/l; in another 2 hours it would be 5 µg/l and so on. The symbol for elimination half-life is $T_{1/2} \beta$ (Fig. 19.3).

Elimination half-life is important because it can be used to determine when repeat doses of a drug are required in order to maintain the drug concentration in the blood at a sufficiently high level to ensure that enough is available for distribution to the tissues for there to be a therapeutic effect. Giving repeat doses too frequently will result in drug levels climbing too high, causing toxicity. Leaving too long a time interval between repeat doses means that the blood concentration levels will drop too low to have a therapeutic effect in the tissues. Maintaining optimal amounts of drug concentration in the blood so that neither toxicity nor ineffectiveness is created is known as keeping the levels within the therapeutic range or margin. Some drugs have a wide therapeutic range – this means that a large overdose would have to be administered before toxicity occurred. An example of a drug with a wide therapeutic range is amoxicillin. Drugs with a narrow therapeutic range are those that cause toxicity with even the smallest overdose, such as digoxin. Therapeutic range can be measured by using the following calculation and this is termed the **therapeutic index**. The greater this figure, the safer the drug:

$$\text{Therapeutic index} = \text{Toxic dose/Effective dose}$$

When drug therapy is initially instigated, peak and trough blood concentrations are relatively low. After approximately 5

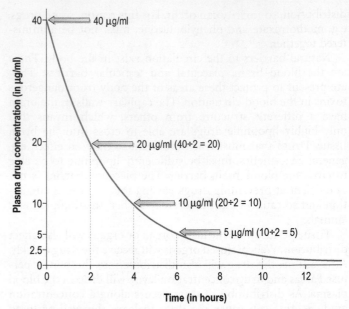

Fig. 19.3 Decrease in plasma concentrations of a drug with a half-life of 2 h (*Redrawn from Bill 1997*)

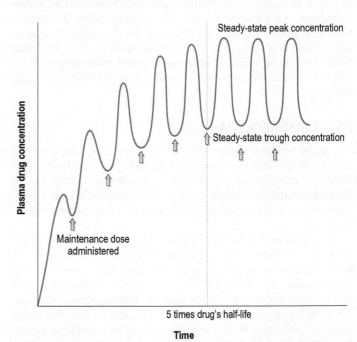

Fig. 19.4 Steady-state concentration (*Redrawn from Bill 1997*)

half-lives the rate of administration is equal to the rate of elimination and so the peak and trough levels increase and remain more constant. This is known as the steady state (Fig. 19.4). When monitoring drug concentrations in the blood, it is important that the steady state has been reached to ensure that peak and trough blood plasma concentrations are within the therapeutic range. Thus, knowing the elimination half-life of a drug is important. A common example is monitoring blood concentrations of phenobarbital. As this drug has an elimination half-life of 2 days, the steady state is not reached until day 10. Measuring blood plasma concentration prior to day 10 of treatment would give an inaccurately low measurement.

Some drugs with very long half-lives will not reach the steady state, and therefore are not fully effective, for many days. To combat this problem a higher than normal amount of drug is given initially, which is known as a **loading dose**. An example of a drug initially given at a loading dose is potassium bromide, which has a 24-day half-life.

Drugs licensed for use in food animals have a **withdrawal period**, which is the clearance time calculated using the elimination half-life of the drug. Withdrawal periods are present on all drug labels of products licensed for use in food-producing animals and state the period of time after the last dose of each drug that the animal or its produce, e.g. milk, cannot be used for human consumption. Withdrawal periods prevent drug residues entering the human food chain.

Factors affecting drug elimination

Renal elimination. Renal elimination, in which a drug is carried to the kidney by the blood and excreted via the urine, is dictated by the glomerular filtration rate (GFR), among other factors. Conditions causing reduced blood flow to the kidney, e.g. hypotension and hypovolaemia, will decrease elimination rate, which could result in toxicity. Geriatric animals often have a degree of renal compromise and the dose rates of renal excreted drugs may need to be reduced to allow for this.

Hepatic elimination. In hepatic elimination a drug is secreted into the bile by the liver. It is then emptied into the gastrointestinal tract and excreted in the faecal matter. Disease conditions affecting liver function can decrease the elimination rate via this route in addition to affecting metabolism. Some drugs are lipophilic after emptying into the gastrointestinal tract – this means that they may be reabsorbed through the gut wall and into the hepatic circulation, then return to the systemic circulation, where they can exert an additional therapeutic effect. This is known as enterohepatic circulation.

Pharmacodynamics

The word pharmacodynamic literally means 'drug action'. It pertains to what effect a drug has on the body systems, i.e. what the drug 'does' to the body. This section traces drug movement through the body and examines how drugs exert their effects.

The basic principle of drug therapy is to maintain concentrations within the therapeutic range. The higher the dose, the greater the pharmacological effect – too small a dose and the concentrations will be subtherapeutic; too great a dose and the concentrations may cause toxicity. The lowest level at which concentrations are therapeutic is termed the minimum effective concentration (MEC). The highest therapeutic level is usually the same concentration at which toxicity could occur. This is sometimes termed the maximum safe concentration (MSC) or minimum toxic concentration (MTC) (Fig. 19.5).

RECEPTOR-MEDIATED PHARMACODYNAMICS

The main mechanism of drug action is via receptor sites, which are specific protein molecules on a cell membrane. There are several different receptors, differentiated by their molecular structure or shape. Cells do not have all receptor types – different cells have a different range and number.

Agonist and antagonist effects

Receptors normally interact with natural substances called endogenous ligands, e.g. neurotransmitters and hormones that

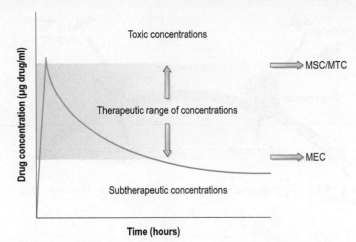

Fig. 19.5 Therapeutic range of plasma drug concentrations (*Redrawn from Bill 1997*)

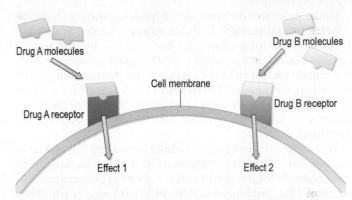

Fig. 19.6 Drug molecules have specific shapes that allow them to combine with specific receptors on the cell membrane surface (*Redrawn from Bill 1997*)

have an effect on the cell. When a drug is present in the body tissue it combines with the receptors into which it 'fits'; in other words, the molecular shape of the drug is similar to certain endogenous ligands and therefore compatible with its receptors (Fig. 19.6). Combining with the receptor causes a change in the activity of the cell – this is how the drug actually exerts an effect. The effect it has may be to stimulate the cell in a similar way to the endogenous ligand – this is known as an **agonist effect**. Conversely, it may combine with the receptor site and 'block' the endogenous ligand but produce no effect itself – this is known as an **antagonist effect**.

Some drugs 'fit' poorly but still partly combine with a receptor site. The effect of this is to block the endogenous ligand but not necessarily produce a particularly strong effect itself. This is known as **partial agonism**. There are drugs that have an agonist effect at some receptor sites and an antagonist effect at others – these are known as agonist/antagonist drugs.

Affinity and competitiveness

The majority of drugs combine only temporarily with receptor sites and when present in sufficient quantity they 'win' the competition with the endogenous ligand for the receptor site. As soon as the concentration diminishes, the endogenous ligand 'wins' the competition and the drug comes off the receptor site. In other words, competitive drugs have **reversible** effects. There are some drugs that do not come off the receptor site once they

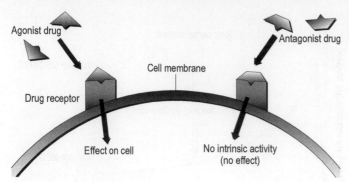

Fig. 19.7 Agonist and antagonist drug reactions *(Redrawn from Bill 1997)*

have combined with it – these are termed **non-competitive or irreversible.** Their effects do not diminish until the drug actually breaks down.

For a drug to combine with a receptor site, it must be attracted to that receptor. This attraction is known as **affinity.** Drugs with a strong affinity for the receptor site are usually highly effective and produce a good therapeutic response. They may remain on that site for a long time and therefore the potential for toxicity is higher. Drugs with a weak affinity for a receptor site tend to have a weaker therapeutic response as they leave the receptor site more quickly. These drugs, however are less likely to cause toxicity.

When more than one drug is administered that 'fits' the same receptor site, they may compete (Fig. 19.7). The drug with greater affinity for the site, or that is present in greater amounts, will 'win'. This could mean that the drug with weaker affinity or that is present in smaller amounts does not exert a therapeutic effect and is one reason why some combinations of drugs, e.g. morphine and buprenorphine, cannot be administered together. This mechanism is sometimes used to control the effects of drugs; for example, atipamezole is used to antagonise the effects of medetomidine.

Down-regulation and up-regulation

Continual and prolonged exposure to agonist drugs can cause the number of receptor sites to decrease – this is known as down-regulation. The result of this is that there is a decrease in therapeutic response. This is one reason why drug therapy should not be continued unnecessarily. Continual and prolonged exposure to antagonist drugs can cause the number of receptor sites to increase – this is known as up-regulation. The result is that, if the drug is suddenly withdrawn, the endogenous ligand that was being blocked by the antagonist suddenly has an excessive number of binding sites and its effect is enhanced. This is the reason why some drugs, e.g. beta-blockers, must be withdrawn slowly after a course of treatment.

Specificity, potency and efficacy

Drug specificity or selectivity relates to the ability of a drug to act on a small number of receptors. Generally, it is desirable to have a highly selective drug as it is possible to target and treat the affected tissue or organ without affecting receptor sites in other parts of the body, which could cause side effects.

Potency refers to the amount of drug that has to be present to produce a therapeutic effect. Efficacy refers to the ability of the drug to produce the therapeutic effect. It is easy to confuse

these two terms, but they do have different applications. Potency would be used to compare two drugs of the same type: for example, the one required in a smaller amount is more potent. Efficacy is used to compare two drugs of different types that produce a similar response: i.e. the drug that produces the more satisfactory response is more efficacious.

NON-RECEPTOR-MEDIATED PHARMACODYNAMICS

Not all drugs exert their effects via receptors. There are several other pharmacodynamic mechanisms. Antimicrobial drugs exert their action on the pathogenic microorganisms in the body and, unfortunately, sometimes on the commensal microorganisms too. Chelating agents act by combining with metals to create less-harmful substances. An example is EDTA, given for lead poisoning. Some drugs work by chemical action, e.g. antacids. Some drugs work by physical action, e.g. charcoal, used in poisoning cases to adsorb toxins, or mannitol, used as a potent osmotic diuretic for brain oedema.

Drug interactions and adverse reactions

Drugs or other chemicals can combine so that one has an effect on the other or so that they each affect one another; these occurrences are known as **interactions**. Drug interactions can occur outside the body, after administration or at any stage in the pharmacokinetic process.

Most drugs, if administered correctly, will have a predictable effect on most patients; on occasion, however, drugs will not have the usual effect. This may be because of the drug, because of its administration or because of the patient. When a drug has a harmful effect on the body it is known as an **adverse reaction**. This is not the same as a side effect, which is a predictable but unwanted effect of normal drug administration, usually related to its actions in parts of the body other than the area being treated.

DRUG INTERACTIONS

Using a combination of many drugs to treat a patient is known as **polypharmacy**. As the possibility that a drug interaction will occur increases with the number of drugs administered to a patient at any one time, polypharmacy should be undertaken with extreme care.

The use of interactions to treat patients

Sometimes, a known drug interaction is deliberately employed as it has therapeutic value. Two drugs with a different action can be given together to increase the therapeutic response – this is known as **synergism** (Table 19.1). If the response is the same as the sum of the two individual drugs, the effect is known as **summation**. In some cases however, the response is greater than the sum of the two individual drugs. This effect is known as **potentiation** – an example is acepromazine, which when administered with an opioid agonist (e.g. pethidine), potentiates the analgesic effect of the opioid. Another therapeutic interaction is when the rate of metabolism or excretion from the body is altered to prolong the therapeutic effect, or conversely to increase clearance rate.

TABLE 19.1 Definitions of drug interaction terminology

Definition	Numerical explanation
Summation – response is equal to the combined responses of the individual drugs	1 + 1 = 2
Synergism – response is greater than the combined responses of the individual drugs	1 + 1 = 3
Potentiation – one ineffective drug enhances the effect of another drug	0 + 1 = 2
Antagonism – one drug inhibits the effects of another drug	1 + 1 = 0

TABLE 19.2 Classification of adverse reactions

Reaction type	Description	Details
A	Augmented – enhanced drug effect	Predictable, dose-dependent, common, low mortality
B	Bizarre – allergic reactions	Unpredictable, not dose-related, high mortality
C	Chronic – due to continuous therapy	e.g. iatrogenic Cushing's disease from long-term prednisolone therapy
D	Delayed – occurring a long time after treatment	e.g. teratogenicity of griseofulvin, carcinomas
E	End of treatment – occurring on withdrawal of therapy	e.g. seizure after phenytoin withdrawal; adrenocortical insufficiency after prednisolone therapy

Unwanted drug interactions

Drug interactions often have an unwanted effect. This may be to inhibit the effect of the drug (antagonism) or to cause toxicity due to potentiation or alteration in the rate of metabolism or excretion. For example, meloxicam administration in an animal already receiving methotrexate will slow the elimination rate of the methotrexate, therefore increasing the plasma levels of methotrexate and the risk of toxicity.

Interactions can occur before the drug has entered the body. Sometimes, a drug can react with the carrier substance it is combined with in order to create the formulation, known as the excipient, or even the packaging. Drug manufacturers must be very careful to ensure that any changes to the excipient or packaging do not cause an interaction. On the pharmacy shelf, drugs exposed to inappropriate light levels, moisture levels or temperature extremes can alter in their effect.

Some drugs interact with certain foods to cause an unwanted effect. For example, oxytetracycline should never be given with milk or cheese as it binds to calcium and will not be absorbed from the gastrointestinal tract. Drugs can also interact with other drugs even if they are of different types and have been administered via different routes.

ADVERSE REACTIONS

Adverse reactions may be the result of a number of factors. The dose given to the patient may be inappropriate, either because it has been miscalculated or because the patient's MTC level is reduced because of concurrent drug treatment or disease. Other drug reactions are not dose-dependent – these are known as idiosyncratic reactions. Idiosyncratic reactions are far less common but are more dangerous as they are unpredictable and do not tend to be proportional to the dose. Adverse reactions are often classified according to their suspected cause (Table 19.2).

Patients prone to adverse reactions

In common with drug interactions, the possibility that an adverse drug reaction will occur increases with the number of drugs administered to a patient at any one time, so polypharmacy should be undertaken with extreme care (Box 19.1). Patients who are underweight, and therefore have less adipose tissue for drug distribution, are more prone to type A reactions, as are hypoproteinaemic animals, which have less plasma protein for the drug to bind to in the circulation. Dose rates for such patients should be reduced accordingly.

BOX 19.1 REDUCING DRUG INTERACTIONS AND REACTIONS – THE IMPLICATIONS FOR NURSING PRACTICE

NURSES SHOULD ...

- Be familiar with common interactions and reactions to the drugs frequently used in the practice
- Instigate appropriate patient observation and monitoring systems to ensure early detection of a reaction
- Report suspected drug reactions or ineffective treatment to the veterinary surgeon immediately and ensure that these are reported to the Veterinary Medicines Directorate
- Store drugs according to the manufacturer's instructions
- Ensure that stock is rotated correctly
- Monitor the environmental temperature in the pharmacy
- Vary parenteral administration sites for different drugs
- Consider staggering oral dosing intervals for different drugs
- Prepare drugs for administration immediately prior to use and not in advance, e.g. the night before
- Use separate equipment for each drug – do not mix drugs in the same syringe
- Ensure the case notes clearly indicate any history of a drug reaction
- Advise owners to keep a note of any prior drug reaction or have a collar disc engraved with the necessary information in case of straying or illness on holiday

Toxicology

Toxicology is the study of the harmful effects of chemicals. Any substance that has a harmful effect on the body is known as a poison or toxin. We often think of poisons as substances that have been accidentally ingested or absorbed by an animal, e.g. metaldehyde or slug bait. However, toxicity can also be caused by therapeutic substances, i.e. a drug used to treat one or more conditions in animals, if the dose rate is too high, the animal's response to the drug is not usual or a drug interaction has occurred.

Toxicity can be acute, i.e. when symptoms develop quickly after exposure and are severe. Chronic toxicity can result from repeated exposure of small amounts of a toxin over a long period of time. An example of chronic toxicity is prolonged, uninterrupted use of mavacoxib.

THE EFFECT OF TOXINS ON THE BODY

Most chemicals introduced to the body have some sort of physiological effect – this is the basis on which therapeutic drugs work. Toxins tend to have an extreme effect on the body, resulting in an unwanted alteration in function that can be life-threatening.

All organs in the body are susceptible to toxins, because of their role in drug metabolism and excretion, the liver and kidney are most at risk from damage. The mechanisms of action vary but include interfering with cellular function, alteration or destruction of vital enzymes, or competing for receptor sites, preventing the endogenous ligand from binding. Drug interactions can cause toxicity in this way, increasing the plasma concentration levels of the drug with less affinity for the binding site.

As there are many factors to take into consideration, the effect of an individual toxin on the body is only predictable to a certain extent. These factors are outlined in Table 19.3.

TREATMENT PROTOCOLS

(For further details see Chapter 20.)

Similar methods of treatment can be grouped together to give an overview of the management of poisoning cases:

- Prevention of absorption – washing, clipping, emesis, adsorbents
- Prevent action by using chelator/antidotes
- Increase clearance by inducing diuresis, dialysis
- Palliative and symptomatic treatment, ABC – life support.

Drug formulations, names and commonly used drugs for specific conditions

Once a condition has been diagnosed, the veterinary surgeon must decide the type of treatment necessary. This involves three stages:

1. The type of drug must be prescribed.
2. The formulation to be administered must be selected.
3. The dose rate must be decided.

It is essential for veterinary nurses to have a sound understanding of the various categories of drugs available, their mode of action and common side effects, in order to manage patients and support owners effectively. It is also vitally important that nurses can calculate drug dosages accurately in order to safely interpret the veterinary surgeon's instructions (see Appendix 1).

TABLE 19.3	Factors affecting the toxicity of a substance	
Substance-related factors	**Animal-related factors**
Time between exposure to toxin and treatment of toxicity	Species
	Age
Formulation of drug or substance	Genetic individuality
Action of drug or substance	Disease status
Dose or amount animal has been exposed to	Fitness/activity levels
Route of administration, metabolism and excretion	
Quality and age of drug (if applicable)	
Concurrent treatment	

There are so many drugs on the market that a comprehensive knowledge of all of them is not realistic. With experience, nurses tend to develop a good understanding of the commonly used medications, but must always refer to the veterinary surgeon, senior nursing staff or the drug's Summary of Product Characteristics (SPC) if they are unsure of anything relating to a patient's medication. Failure to do so may jeopardise patient safety and could constitute a breach of the RCVS Code of Professional Conduct.

DRUG FORMULATIONS

There are several factors to take into account when considering in which formulation a drug is to be used. Drug manufacturers must calculate what a drug can actually achieve – for example, some drugs would be ineffective if given orally because of the first-pass effect; others may be inactivated by the additives needed for certain forms of medication. The target species must also be considered, as it may be easier to administer certain formulations to some species than others, e.g. oral tablets for hamsters. In recent years drug manufacturers have become more aware of the need to increase the ease of administration, especially for owners, in order to improve compliance. Many medicines indicated for long-term use are now offered in palatable or easy-to-give formulations (Table 19.4).

What else is in a medicine apart from the drug?

All formulations are made up using the correct amount of drug, plus certain additives used for various reasons. As most drugs are divided into very small quantities, another substance is added to render the drug visible and easier to handle; this is called the **excipient**. Tablets also contain a **binder**, which is a substance that holds them together until they are administered. Once ingested, they must be able to dissolve in the gastrointestinal tract, so tablets often contain a substance such as starch, which aids disintegration. Consider the colourful array of drugs on the pharmacy shelf – most drugs also contain colouring and some sort of **preservative**. Drug manufacturers must be very careful to ensure that all of these substances are inert, i.e. have no pharmacological action. Sometimes a substance is combined with a drug to enhance its effect – this is known as an **adjuvant**. Pharmaceutical adjuvants are those used in drugs that treat disease; immunological adjuvants are those used in vaccines.

Oral tablets may have an outer coating, which is often added to protect the tablet prior to use, or disguise a bitter taste to ease administration. Coatings are also used on some tablets to delay disintegration until they have passed through the stomach. This may be because the contents will irritate the gastric mucosa, or because gastric acid would destroy the drug. These medicines are called enteric-coated. Drugs are sometimes given in capsule form; the capsule is usually made of gelatin.

DRUG NAMES

Most drugs have several names. On discovery, a drug is given a **chemical name**, which describes its atomic or molecular structure. The chemical name is usually too long and complicated for general use, so an abbreviated code name or number is often used by researchers. When a drug is issued with a Marketing Authorisation (MA), it is given a **generic** (official) name and a **trade** (proprietary or brand) name. The trade name is chosen

TABLE 19.4	Drug formulations and nursing considerations		
Formulation	Variations and routes of administration	Description	Nursing considerations
Tablets	Non-palatable oral tablets	Powdered, compressed discs. May be coated. Many different shape, size and colour combinations	Never crush or split an enteric-coated tablet, as this will expose the drug prematurely. If tablets are split, round off any sharp edges prior to administration to prevent scratching the patient's mouth or throat and wear protective equipment to prevent absorption, inhalation or ingestion of the drug when handling
	Palatable oral tablets	Flavoured, shaped tablets often made to look like treats	Ensure these are stored carefully to prevent patients helping themselves.
Capsules	Hard capsules for oral administration	Made up of two halves containing the drug in a powder or granule form. Many different colours and sizes	In some cases, it is possible to open or puncture the capsule and give the contents on food, or mixed with water as a paste. Check the drug SPC to ensure that this is not contraindicated and wear protective equipment to prevent absorption, inhalation or ingestion of the drug when opening the capsule
	Soft capsules for oral administration	Sealed pouches containing liquid	Handle the pot carefully as torn or punctured capsules can leak and cause the remainder of the capsules to stick together
	Sustained-release capsules for oral administration (see section on Pharmacokinetics for further detail)	Hard gelatin capsules containing individual granules of drug	Never open or puncture a sustained-release capsule as this will affect the absorption of the drug. Sustained-release preparations licensed for humans only do not always have the same effect because of differences in transit time. There is more likelihood of the drug not reaching therapeutic levels in the bloodstream and in some cases more likelihood of toxicity
Solutions	For parenteral injection	Available in single- or multiple-dose vials	Many drugs are unstable in solution so they need to be reconstituted from a powder immediately prior to use. Care must be taken when undertaking this task to use the correct volume of liquid and to adopt an aseptic technique. Never keep reconstituted solutions longer than the recommended time
	Linctus (syrup) for oral administration	Drug dissolved in a sugar solution	There are few veterinary-licensed products of this nature in the UK
	Elixir for oral administration	Drug dissolved in an alcohol solution	Never dilute elixirs with water as the alcohol and water will not mix together
Suspensions	For parenteral injection	Available in single- or multiple-dose vials or bottles	Must be shaken thoroughly before use to ensure that the particles are fully and evenly distributed throughout the liquid
	For oral administration		Suspensions must never be given intravenously as they contain solid particles
Long-acting solutions or suspensions (see Pharmacokinetics for further detail)	For parenteral injection	Either the drug or the carrier contents are not readily absorbed from the injection site	Sometimes referred to as LA, depot or repository injections. Suspensions must never be given intravenously as they contain solid particles
Creams	For topical administration	Water and oil emulsion base	Designed to liquefy at body temperature
Ointments	For topical administration	Oil base	Ensure gloves are worn when handling as absorption through the skin is possible with many drugs
Gels	For topical administration	Alcohol base	Some patients may need Elizabethan collar or similar to prevent them licking the medication
Pastes	For oral administration	Usually available in a pre-filled dosing syringe	If dosing several animals with the same syringe, disinfect the outside of the syringe to avoid cross-infection. Clients may need careful instruction on how to set the dial to the correct dose
Powders and granules	For topical administration	Often available in single-dose sachets	Now infrequently seen – many lost their product licences because of operator health and safety concerns, as inhalation and absorption of the products during administration is difficult to avoid
	For oral administration		Ensure that the correct dose is administered and ingested within a short time period or therapeutic levels may not be reached

Continued on following page

TABLE 19.4	Drug formulations and nursing considerations—cont'd		
Formulation	**Variations and routes of administration**	**Description**	**Nursing considerations**
Aerosol sprays	For topical administration	Pressurised or non-pressurised multi-dose bottles	Ensure that correct protective equipment is used to prevent inhalation or absorption of airborne drug particles. Use in a well-ventilated area
	For administration via inhalation	Liquids administered via a nebuliser, or using an inhaler and specially designed inhalation chamber (like a 'spacer' for asthmatic people)	Ensure a quiet and calm environment to reduce stress levels when administering medication via nebulisation or inhalation chamber
Shampoos	For topical administration	Usually presented in plastic bottles	Clients may need careful instruction on the safe use of these products and must also be made aware of the difference between medicated shampoos and cleansing or cosmetic shampoos
Drops	For oral administration	Usually solutions or suspensions presented with a precalibrated dosing syringe or dropper bottle	Some oral drops need to be reconstituted prior to use (see notes under solutions). Some drops require refrigeration once opened and/or reconstituted
	For administration to the mucous membranes	Unusual method of administration with limited applications	May be used to administer desmopressin, ketamine or buprenorphine (see section below). The most common sites are the conjunctival sac or oral mucosa.
	For topical administration	Usually single-dose vials contained in a multipack for sale to clients	An increasingly common method of administering antiparasitic agents. Most commonly used to treat ectoparasites, but some products also treat endoparasites
	For administration to the eyes or ears	Dropper bottles containing aqueous solution	Often have a short use-by date once opened – some need refrigeration. Bottles should not be shared between patients because of the risk of cross-contamination
Patches and Transdermal Gels	For transdermal administration	Unusual method of administration with limited applications. Gel impregnated with the drug is placed on skin. Protective cover may be placed on top	May be used to administer fentanyl or glyceryl trinitrate. Methimazole gel is available for application to the inner aspect of the pinna
Rectal bolus or suppository	For rectal administration	Unusual method of administration with limited applications	May be used to administer diazepam to control seizures

TABLE 19.5	Example of the names given to a drug during its development			
Chemical name		**Generic name**	**Trade names**	**MA holder**
RS)-5-amino-1-[2,6-dichloro-4-(trifluoromethyl)phenyl]-4-(trifluoromethylsulfinyl)-1H-pyrazole-3-carbonitrile		Fipronil	Dicrolin™ Effipro™ Frontline™	Alfamed Virbac SA Merial Animal Health

by the company holding the MA for the drug and identifies it as the exclusive property of that company. Protection from competition is afforded to the company for a time, providing the opportunity for scientific innovation to be rewarded by a financial return on their investment. Once this period has expired, legislation permits competition from other manufacturers – providing they can demonstrate their product is equivalent to the pioneer product. Other companies filing for approval to market the drug must use the same generic name but can create their own trade name. As a result, the same generic drug may be sold under either the generic name or one of many trade names (Table 19.5). It is standard practice to use the generic name when referring to drugs in text.

DRUG TYPES

There are hundreds of drugs available to treat animals in the UK, most under EU licence. The following list is not exhaustive but describes drug groups that are commonly used in modern veterinary practice. The drugs have been categorised into groups depending on their action.

Anaesthetics

Anaesthetics are drugs that induce loss of sensation in all or part of the body.

- **General anaesthetics** involve the central nervous system (CNS) and cause unconsciousness. Injectable barbiturates, such as thiopental, have largely been superseded in small animal practice by non-barbiturate drugs, such as propofol and alfaxalone, although thiopental is still commonly used in equine practice. Inhalational general anaesthetics include halothane, which has been largely superseded by isoflurane, although sevoflurane and methoxyflurane are increasing in popularity (see Chapter 27).

- **Dissociative anaesthetics** derive their name from human patients describing a feeling of being separated from their body. These also affect the CNS but do not cause muscle relaxation and loss of reflexes to the same extent as general anaesthetics. Ketamine is a dissociative anaesthetic.
- **Local anaesthetics** cause loss of sensation around the site of administration. The most commonly used local anaesthetic is lidocaine.

Analgesics

Analgesics are drugs that prevent or relieve pain without loss of sensation. There are two main types of analgesic:

- **Narcotic analgesics** are so-called because they tend to cause narcosis (sleepiness). They are opium-related agents and are sometimes called opioid analgesics. Narcotic analgesics, e.g. morphine and pethidine, exert their analgesic effect primarily by occupying the endogenous opioid receptor sites in the brain. They also occupy receptor sites elsewhere in the body, which can cause side effects. Buprenorphine is also a narcotic analgesic, although it is a partial agonist rather than a pure agonist like most others. Narcotic analgesics can be combined with a sedative to produce a state of semi-consciousness and drowsiness known as neuroleptanalgesia. Buprenorphine combined with acepromazine is a commonly given neuroleptanalgesic combination.
- **Non-steroidal anti-inflammatory drugs (NSAIDs)** work in a different way from narcotic analgesics. Instead of affecting the central nervous system (CNS), they have a pharmacological action at the site of the pain. Most work by inhibiting the production of cyclooxygenase (COX). Two types of COX have been discovered to date, known as COX1 and COX2. COX1 mainly plays a role in the normal functioning of a wide variety of body tissues, including the kidneys, stomach and intestine; COX2 mainly plays a role in the inflammatory process. NSAIDs that are not selective for COX2 (e.g. aspirin, phenylbutazone) can induce certain side effects, including gastric ulceration and diarrhoea. COX2-selective NSAIDs (e.g. firocoxib, and robenacoxib) are thought to be safer and have less effect on other body tissues.

Antacids

These are agents used to reduce acidity in the stomach, in order to prevent, manage or reverse damage to the intestinal tract. There are two types of antacids:

- **Non-systemic antacids** – work locally in the stomach to raise the pH of gastric juices. Examples are calcium carbonate and magnesium carbonate, although there are limited veterinary licensed products available. Some human formulations also contain alginic acid which, when exposed to stomach acid, forms a gel-like barrier on the surface of the stomach contents, preventing oesophageal reflux; these are called 'raft' antacids. Due to the alteration of pH in the stomach, all of these products can affect the dissolution and absorption of other drugs such as corticosteroids, tetracyclines, acepromazine and digoxin. Allow a 2–3-hour interval between doses.
- **Systemic antacids** – there are several types, and they act in a number of different ways; all aim to reduce gastric acid secretion. The most common example is cimetidine, which is an H2-receptor antagonist. These drugs block the effect of histamine in the stomach, which is to increase gastric acid production. (Do not confuse with antihistamines, H1-receptor antagonists, which are used to treat allergies.) Proton pump inhibitors, such as omeprazole, reduce gastric acid production. Other systemic antacids affect more than gastric acid production – the prostaglandin misoprostol also increases mucus production and increases blood flow to the gastric area, thus promoting healing.

Antiarrhythmics

These are agents used to treat arrhythmia, an abnormality in the rhythm of the heart. There are many types and causes of arrhythmia and the choice of drug depends on the diagnosis:

- **Beta-blockers** – work by blocking stimulation of the $\beta1$ receptors in the heart, which decreases the heart rate and strength of contraction (drugs that cause the latter are also known as negative inotropes). A commonly used example is propranolol. Due to up-regulation, animals treated with beta-blockers may need increasing doses to maintain the therapeutic effect. For the same reason, treatment should not suddenly cease: the sudden availability of $\beta1$ receptors to endogenous $\beta1$ stimulators such as epinephrine (adrenaline) could have a serious effect on the patient.
- **Calcium channel blockers** – reduce the rate of impulse generation and conduction across the heart; examples are amlodipine, verapamil and diltiazem. The latter is also used to treat hypertrophic cardiomyopathy in cats.
- **Sodium channel blockers** – these are drugs with local anaesthetic action, which act to reduce contractions from occurring outside of the normal heartbeat (ectopic beats or extrasystoles); an example is lidocaine, which must be administered by slow intravenous injection. The presentation containing epinephrine (adrenaline) that is available for use as a local anaesthetic is not suitable to treat arrhythmias, and using it for this purpose could be life-threatening for the patient.

Anticonvulsants

These are drugs used to prevent or control convulsions. The most commonly used drug for this purpose is the barbiturate phenobarbital, which stabilises the brain cells, making them less likely to begin abnormal activity, and also tends to lessen the severity of convulsions if they do occur. It is sometimes used in conjunction with potassium bromide to reduce the dosage of phenobarbital required.

Phenobarbital is metabolised by the mixed function oxidase system, so animals on long-term treatment develop tolerance and may need increasing doses in order to achieve the same therapeutic effect. Periodic testing of blood plasma levels will provide the necessary information to increase the dose safely.

Phenobarbital acts too slowly to be used in emergency situations, when diazepam may be used intravenously. Diazepam can also be administered rectally, which is a useful route for owners to use if the animal convulses at home. Imepitoin has been recently licensed to control primary seizures in dogs.

Antidepressants

Relatively new to veterinary pharmacology, three main types of antidepressant are used – tricyclic antidepressants, selective serotonin reuptake inhibitors (SSRIs) and monoamine oxidase inhibitors (MAOIs). All work by increasing the amount of neurotransmitter chemicals, e.g. serotonin, at the synapses. Clomipramine, nicergoline and l-deprenyl are examples of each type, respectively.

Separation-related problems, anxiety, feline idiopathic cystitis, stereotypies and geriatric cognitive dysfunction are sometimes treated with antidepressants. With these problems and other behaviour-related conditions, accurate diagnosis and a holistic approach, e.g. educating clients, altering routines and modifying animal and human behaviour, are usually needed for satisfactory results.

Antidiarrhoeals

These are drugs that combat diarrhoea. Diarrhoea is a symptom caused by an underlying condition or toxic substance and the drug of choice will depend on the cause of the diarrhoea. There are four main types of antidiarrhoeal drug:

- **Adsorbent/protectants** – these adsorb bacterial enterotoxins that cause hypersecretion of intestinal fluid and prevent them from contacting the intestinal lining; examples include charcoal, bismuth and montmorillonite. Some formulations, e.g. kaolin and pectin, also coat the gut wall, although this formulation has questionable efficacy. It should be borne in mind that adsorbent drugs may also adsorb or bind other drugs given concurrently, and therefore reduce their bioavailablity.
- **Intestinal motility modifiers** – opioid drugs increase segmentation (mixing) movements and decrease peristaltic movements of the gut. Low doses of oral codeine, morphine combined with kaolin and diphenoxylate are all used to slow the passage of intestinal contents. Loperamide, a commonly used human medicine, falls into this category.
- **Anti-inflammatory drugs** – these are most commonly used for treating the chronic diarrhoea caused by inflammatory bowel disease. The antimicrobial drug sulfasalazine is used as it is not well absorbed through the gut wall and has an anti-inflammatory effect on the colon. Sometimes, corticosteroid therapy is instigated. It should be remembered that a diarrhoeic patient may not absorb any orally administered drugs to the same extent as a healthy patient, so parenteral routes of administering drugs may be preferential. Some antidiarrhoeal agents, particularly the adsorbents and protectants, may also affect the constitution and absorption rate of other drugs, so should be given at 2–3-hour intervals.

Antiemetics

These are agents used to prevent or decrease vomiting. Vomiting is a symptom caused by an underlying condition or toxic substance. Examples of antiemetic drugs are metoclopramide, maropitant and mirtazepine. Metoclopramide works by affecting the vomiting centre in the brain – it causes an increase in oesophageal and gastric muscle tone, relaxes the pyloric sphincter and increases intestinal motility.

Antihistamines

Histamine is a substance present in large quantities in the gastrointestinal, lung and skin tissue and plays a role in the immune response. In humans, this response is triggered by certain antigens, e.g. pollen, to cause allergic symptoms and in extreme cases, anaphylaxis. In contrast, histamine does not appear to play a major role in many of the allergies seen in animals, with the exception of certain feline and equine respiratory conditions. In these cases antihistamine drugs may be used to combat the bronchoconstriction caused by histamine in the lungs. These drugs work by antagonising the H1 receptors in the smooth muscle of the bronchioles. So-called 'first-generation' antihistamines such as chlorpheniramine and cyproheptadine are sometimes used effectively, although they may cause sedation as a side effect. 'Second-generation' antihistamines, such as astemizole and terfenadine, are more expensive and some have been linked to heart problems, but they do not have a sedative side effect.

Antimicrobials

These are drugs that destroy, or facilitate the destruction of, microorganisms. The term antibiotic is sometimes used instead, although this is not strictly correct terminology as an antibiotic refers to a substance produced by one microorganism that affects another and most modern antimicrobials are synthetically produced.

Antimicrobials are broadly divided into two categories – those that destroy the target pathogen, defined by the suffix -*cidal*, and those that inhibit the growth of the target pathogen, defined by the suffix -*static*. They are further defined by the type of microorganism they affect – this may be bacteria, viruses, fungi or protozoa. For example, a substance that inhibits the growth of bacteria is called bacteriostatic, a substance that destroys fungi is called fungicidal, etc. Some drugs have a -static effect at a certain dosage, which becomes -cidal at a higher dosage. Table 19.6 describes the way in which antimicrobial drugs work.

Acquired resistance to antimicrobial drugs is an increasing problem, brought about by changes or mutations to the DNA of the microorganism in question. This allows the microorganism to survive in the presence of a drug designed to destroy it. Inappropriate use of antimicrobial agents may exacerbate this problem and much attention has been focussed on this issue recently in both human and veterinary medicine. The Veterinary Medicines Directorate (VMD) monitors antimicrobial sales and resistance trends throughout the UK and publishes its findings. Responsible use of antimicrobial drugs is vital to safeguard availability of a wide range of these drugs in the future. Table 19.7 identifies key points to consider when using such products to reduce the problem of acquired resistance to a minimum.

Antineoplastics

These are drugs used to treat neoplastic or cancerous tissue; most of them are cytotoxic, meaning that they kill cells. The term 'chemotherapy' is often reserved for this type of treatment, although this term literally means 'drug therapy' so it could be

TABLE 19.6	Mode of action of antimicrobials	
Mode of action	Description	Example
Inhibition of cell-wall synthesis	Prevent bacterial cell wall forming correctly	Penicillins, e.g. ampicillin, amoxicillin Cephalosporins, e.g. cefalexin Terbinafine
Disruption of microbial cell membrane	Change membrane permeability and so affect transport in and out of microorganism	Polymyxin-B
Inhibition of protein synthesis	Affect either protein synthesis in the ribosomes or in the nucleus, preventing effective replication of the microorganism	Tetracyclines, e.g. oxytetracycline, doxycycline Aminoglycosides, e.g. gentamicin, neomycin, streptomycin Metronidazole Erythromycin Quinolones, e.g. enrofloxacin
Interference with metabolic processes	Many microorganisms must manufacture folic acid in order to replicate – they cannot obtain it from food sources as animals can. These agents either interfere with or inhibit folic acid production	Trimethoprim, sulphonamides, e.g. sulfadiazine

TABLE 19.7	Actions to be taken to reduce the risk of antimicrobial resistance
Key area	Nursing implications
Implement and partake in effective infection prevention and control measures	Ensure practice protocol within and without the practice limit the opportunity for animals to be exposed to pathogenic bacteria. Measures include: • Operating stringent surgical theatre and sterilisation procedures • Reviewing and updating infection control measures on hospital wards • Educating clients so they understand how to reduce the chances of infection in their pets or livestock
Identify the pathogen in order to select the most appropriate drug to treat	Nurses may be involved in undertaking sample cultures and/or sensitivity testing. Ensure this is accurately carried out and interpreted
Veterinary surgeons should select the drug carefully	Where there is a choice, they should select narrow-spectrum drugs of least importance to human medicine Monitor the volume of broad-spectrum antimicrobial drug used – report excessive use to relevant person or authority
Start treatment early	Where treatment is necessary, it should be instigated without delay
Select the lowest optimal dose	Ensure adequate availability of suitable literature to access recommended doses – keep drug SPCs and data sheets within easy reach. Calculate drug dosages carefully
Select route carefully, ensuring that an adequate dose can reach the affected site	Ensure adequate availability of suitable literature to access recommended routes
Always complete the prescribed course of treatment	Ensure clients are fully aware that they should always treat the patient at the prescribed dose, route and time and should always complete a course of treatment even if the symptoms have gone
Religiously observe drug withdrawal times in food-producing animals	Ensure adequate literature is available in order to advise clients accurately
Do not use antimicrobial drugs unnecessarily	Discourage clients from retaining unused medication to use on another occasion or for another animal – consider an 'easy disposal' system in the practice to encourage them to return unused medicine
Limit the use of new products	Consider the stock of drugs in the pharmacy carefully and select new products on the basis of need
Report treatment failure	Monitor the use of antimicrobials in the practice as part of clinical governance and audit The VMD monitors antimicrobial resistance, so it is important to report any cases as a Pharmacovigilance event under lack of efficacy
Maintain currency and keep knowledge up to date	Disseminate any new information amongst staff Ensure all veterinary staff have access to current guidelines and that recommendations are incorporated into practice policies and standard operating procedures

used to describe any type of drug therapy. The aim of an antineoplastic agent is for it to be selectively toxic towards the neoplastic cells while sparing the normal healthy cells. It is the property of accelerated reproduction of neoplastic cells that allows this to happen. Unfortunately, other healthy cells in the body that tend to divide fairly rapidly, e.g. hair and bone marrow, can also be affected by the agent, which is why these types of drugs have so many side effects (e.g. suppression of bone marrow cells).

Veterinary nurses must be aware that accidental ingestion, absorption or inhalation of cytotoxic drugs can seriously affect their health. Local health and safety rules for dispensing and administering this type of medication must be observed at all times and clients must be made fully aware of the dangers of

TABLE 19.8	Methods of reducing the risk of contamination when using cytotoxic drugs
Action	**Method of reducing the risk**
Preparing, dispensing and administering	Prepare and administer these medicines in a quiet, calm environment away from areas of high human traffic. Ideally, use a safety cabinet if it is available and/or closed system drug transfer and administration devices
	Always wear gloves, apron, mask and eye shields. Keep a separate 'cytotoxic kit', so all personal protective equipment is readily available – replenish after each use, as gloves, masks and apron should be single-use only. Clear away spillages carefully
	Never cut or break tablets, unless the dose rate makes it necessary. Do not expect the client to do this at home
	Provide clients with a verbal and written explanation of the dangers of their pet's medication and how to reduce the risks to them
Nursing a patient	Hospital accommodation should be clearly marked with a sign if the animal is receiving cytotoxic treatment
	Remember that body fluids, vomit and faeces will sometimes be contaminated with the cytotoxic drug. The patient should ideally urinate and defecate in an area that is easily cleanable, although urine splashes are more likely on hard surfaces so a segregated grass or earth-covered area, or use of a disposable absorbent substrate could be considered preferable
	Ensure that the client understands the dangers of this route of contamination if they are nursing their pet at home.
Disposal	Clear away all empty packaging and excess drug carefully and dispose of it according to health and safety guidelines and legislation. Encourage clients to return any empty packaging or unused drug to the surgery for correct disposal

these drugs (Table 19.8). Vincristine, cyclophosphamide, doxorubicin and mastinib are all examples of antineoplastic agents.

Antiparasitics

These are drugs used to treat infection by parasites. There are several categories, which are divided according to their action:

- **Endoparasiticides** – agents that treat internal parasites, and are divided into anthelmintics – agents that treat helminths (roundworms, tapeworms and flukes) and antiprotozoals – agents that act against protozoa. Anthelmintics can be further divided into antinematocides (act against roundworms), anticestocides (act against tapeworms) and antitrematocides (act against flukes). Not all drugs will kill every parasite in a group but, conversely, some drugs have action against more than one group of helminths and are termed broadspectrum anthelmintics. Anthelmintics may act as either a vermicide, which kills the parasites, or a vermifuge, which paralyses the parasite, which may then be passed out of the host's body alive; some drugs are both vermicidal and vermifugal. Piperazine, fenbendazole, febantel, praziquantel, oxantel, moxidectin, milbemycin and levamisole are all commonly used anthelmintics.

  It is important to understand the life cycle of the parasites (see Chapter 29) being treated, as most anthelmintics act mainly in the gut lumen and may not treat migrating larvae or eggs elsewhere in the body.

  Antiprotozoals are often antimicrobials, e.g. sulfadimidine, although fenbendazole, an anthelmintic, has also been proved to be effective against the protozoan *Giardia* spp.

- **Ectoparasiticides** – agents that treat external parasites. May be acaricidal, i.e. act against acarids such as mites and ticks, or insecticidal, i.e. act against insects such as fleas, or have both properties. In the past, organophosphorus products such as dichlorvos and pyrethroid products such as permethrin were commonly used as insecticides but, more recently, products such as fipronil and imidacloprid have become the treatments of choice because of their relative safety compared with the former and efficacy compared with the latter. Products that interfere with insect functioning, growth and development have become popular as a useful adjunct to insecticides to treat fleas in dogs and cats. Examples include S-methoprene, spinosad and lufenuron.

Antitussives, mucolytics, expectorants, decongestants

Antitussives are used to suppress coughing. In veterinary medicine, these are centrally acting, i.e. act on the 'cough centre' in the brain; examples include butorphanol and codeine. Locally acting antitussives work by soothing the mucous membrane in the respiratory tract – they are not appropriate for use in veterinary medicine, as animals will not suck lozenges or gargle liquids as human patients will. Mucolytics and expectorants, e.g. bromhexine and eucalyptus oil, break down and thin out respiratory mucus. Decongestants, such as phenylephrine, act by causing vasoconstriction and a subsequent reduction in oedema and mucus production of the nasal mucous membranes. Care should be taken as this drug can have cardiovascular effects, which may prove deleterious to animals with pre-existing cardiovascular or respiratory disease.

Astringents and keratolytics

These agents are usually available as medicated shampoos, lotions or drops. Astringent products, such as zinc oxide, harden and protect the skin by causing proteins to precipitate on its surface. Keratolytics such as benzoyl peroxide enhance desquamation, and are therefore used to reduce scaling on the skin surface.

Bronchodilators

These are agents that cause the smooth muscle of the terminal bronchioles to relax, thus counteracting broncho-constriction and narrowing of the airway diameter. Two main types of bronchodilator are used in veterinary medicine:

- **Beta-agonists** – stimulate β receptors. There are two types of β receptor – $\beta1$ and $\beta2$. The former are found elsewhere in the body, including in the heart, so non-selective beta-agonists may have unwanted side effects, such as arrhythmias and tachycardia. $\beta2$ receptors are found in the smooth muscle of the bronchioles. Their stimulation causes bronchodilation. The more

TABLE 19.9	Side effects of glucocorticoids
Side effect	**Nursing considerations**
Inhibition of fibroblasts can cause delayed healing	Ensure that records of animals on corticosteroid therapy are clearly marked to prevent this fact being missed. Clients may need advice on temporary cessation of corticosteroid therapy prior to surgery
Immunosuppression due to inhibition of T cells and immune responses	Advise clients of patient's increased risk of infection. Take extra care not to expose hospitalised patients to infection
Increase of gastric acid and decrease of gastric mucus production	Advise clients never to give concurrent NSAID therapy. Do not give premedication on admission to hospital if it contains an NSAID
Catabolic effects – protein breakdown	Ensure adequate bedding for patients with thin skin and haircoat. Those with muscle atrophy may need physical support if standing for long periods. Do not use corticosteroid preparations on ulcerated tissue, e.g. corneal ulcers
Prolonged continuous use may cause hyperadrenocorticism – iatrogenic Cushing's syndrome or diabetes mellitus	Observe patients closely for symptoms of these iatrogenic diseases. Ensure that clients understand that a higher dose of corticosteroid every other day is safer than a lower dose of daily therapy, so they do not revert to the latter without consultation with the veterinary surgeon
Exogenous sources of corticosteroid suppress the endogenous release from the adrenal cortex	Ensure that clients taper doses at the end of treatment to prevent hypoadrenocorticism
Polyphagia, polydipsia and polyuria	Advise clients of these potential side effects and how to manage them to prevent obesity and inappropriate elimination

β2-selective agonists such as terbutaline minimise cardiac side effects and are usually preferred over the non-selective drugs such as epinephrine (adrenaline)

- **Methylxanthines** – work on the smooth muscle cells by interfering with their chemical composition, discouraging bronchoconstriction. They are not selective, so can cause a range of stimulatory side effects as they affect many other cells in the body; an example is theophylline. As methylxanthines are metabolised by the mixed function oxidase system, the dose may need to be increased in patients concurrently being treated with other drugs metabolised by the same system.

Central nervous system stimulants

These agents are commonly used to reverse the action of a sedative or anaesthetic, or to stimulate respiration in a patient. Two of the most commonly used CNS stimulants are atipamezole, an α2-agonist, and doxapram, a drug that works primarily in the medulla oblongata to stimulate respiration (e.g. resuscitation of puppies and kittens following Caesarean delivery). The methylxanthine drugs are also CNS stimulants.

Corticosteroids

Corticosteroids are hormones that are naturally produced by the adrenal cortex. They are divided into two main groups depending on the main action they exert: **mineralocorticoids** mainly affect the mineral balance of the body and **glucocorticoids** mainly exert an anti-inflammatory effect on the body, as well as affecting glucose metabolism. The mineralocorticoid fludrocortisone is used in animals to treat Addison's disease, which is atrophy of the adrenal cortex, resulting in hypoadrenocorticism.

Glucocorticoids are far more widely used, and they can be divided into three groups depending on their duration of action:

- Short-acting, e.g. hydrocortisone – commonly found in topical formulations; these have a 12-hour duration of action
- Intermediate-acting, e.g. prednisolone – commonly given as an oral medication; these have a 12–36-hour duration of action

- Long-acting, e.g. dexamethasone – duration of action is more than 48 hours.

Glucocorticoids are mainly used for their anti-inflammatory actions. They affect many of the body's cells and so, although they are useful for a variety of inflammatory diseases, they also produce a wide variety of side effects. Table 19.9 describes some of these side effects and the nursing considerations that arise from them.

Diuretics

These are agents that promote water loss by increasing urine production. They are usually used to reduce fluid retention caused by congestive heart failure, but are also indicated for certain respiratory diseases and acute renal failure. There are several types of diuretic, which are classified according to their action:

- **Loop diuretics**, e.g. furosemide, act on the loop of Henle to prevent the reabsorption of sodium, so that water remains in the urine by osmosis. Sodium is later exchanged for potassium; thus long-term use of loop diuretics can result in hypokalaemia.
- **Potassium-sparing diuretics,** e.g. spironolactone, work by antagonising the action of aldosterone. As the name suggests, they do not cause potassium loss.
- **Osmotic diuretics**, e.g. mannitol, are sugar-based substances that work by increasing the osmotic pressure within the renal tubule, thus drawing water into the urine from the plasma and increasing its volume. They are used to reduce cerebral pressure after head trauma and to increase elimination of a toxin from the body.
- **Carbonic anhydrase inhibitors**, e.g. acetazolamide, are used to treat glaucoma.
- **Thiazide diuretics**, e.g. chlorothiazide, are infrequently used as they are less potent than the loop diuretics yet can still cause hypokalaemia.

Hormones

Endogenous hormones are substances produced by endocrine glands that reach their site of action via the bloodstream. Exogenous hormones (natural or synthetic in origin) are sometimes used to test for or treat disease of the endocrine gland that has caused an imbalance of one or more of the endogenous hormones. In addition to the use of corticosteroids, several other hormones are used for therapeutic reasons:

- **Adrenocorticotrophic hormone (ACTH) and thyroid-stimulating hormone (TSH)** – are both anterior pituitary hormones. They are used diagnostically to measure the response of the adrenal cortex and thyroid gland, respectively.
- **Desmopressin** – this is a synthetic version of the posterior pituitary hormone antidiuretic hormone (ADH) and is used to treat central diabetes insipidus.
- **Insulin** – there are various types of insulin derived from various sources and available to treat diabetes mellitus. Each type has a different duration of action, allowing regimens to be tailored to individual patients depending on their blood glucose responses.
- **Oestrogens** – used in some species to induce oestrus, this group of hormones also includes diethylstilboestrol, which is sometimes used to treat misalliance and urinary incontinence.
- **Progestagens** – this group of drugs are progesterone-like in their activity. They can be used to suppress oestrus but should be used with caution as they predispose entire females to uterine disease.
- **Levothyroxine (thyroxine)** – also known as T4, this synthetic product replaces the naturally occurring thyroxine normally produced by the thyroid gland but lacking in cases of hypothyroidism. The drug methimazole, used to treat hyperthyroidism, works by blocking the ability of the thyroid gland to produce natural thyroxine.
- **Anabolic steroids** – this term relates to a group of drugs that promote increased mass of body tissues. They are most frequently used in convalescing, geriatric or chronically ill patients. In food-producing animals they have been used to increase the animal's weight and muscle condition. A commonly used example is the testosterone derivative nandrolone, but some progestagens and oestrogens also fall into this category.

Laxatives

These are agents used to facilitate defecation. There are four main types of laxative:

- **Bulk-forming laxatives** – these increase the bulk of faeces, which stimulates the musculature of the gut wall. Indigestible fibre such as bran or isphagula (psyllium) husk are examples
- **Osmotic laxatives** – these draw water into the faecal mass by osmosis; examples include lactulose and phosphate salts
- **Lubricant laxatives** – these products, e.g. liquid paraffin and glycerine, may be useful to soften faeces or facilitate their passage following pelvic trauma
- **Stimulant laxatives** – these products tend to have a stronger effect than other laxatives and can be irritating, so should be used with care. They work by increasing local gut motility, e.g. dantron.

'Natural' supplements

Increasingly, clients are showing a preference for products that they perceive to be 'natural', such as fish oils, garlic and chondroitin. Some of these products are proving extremely useful as a treatment or adjunct to certain conditions. However, clients should be advised to exercise caution as the fact that they do not fall within the definition of veterinary medicines and may be freely available does not necessarily mean that they cannot cause harm if incorrectly administered. It is not unusual for a client to use the same product (and dose) that they take themselves – remember that not all products safe for use in humans are equally safe for animals. In addition, instruct the client of the correct methods of handling these products as they may be easily absorbed, ingested or inhaled. This is particularly true of essential oils, which can have serious effects if incorrectly handled and administered.

Recently, there has been a lot of interest in the use of nutrients with therapeutic properties, which may be given as powder, tablets, capsules, etc., and may be included in a commercial diet or presented as a food product. These products are known as nutraceuticals. Examples of nutraceuticals include glucosamine, essential fatty acids and probiotics.

Herbal and homeopathic remedies are generally considered to be entirely discrete treatment systems. Many herbal and homeopathic remedies are defined as veterinary medicines and as such are subject to regulation and licensing legislation. Homeopathic remedies are listed in the *British Homeopathic Pharmacopeia*.

Parasympathomimetics and parasympatholytics

These are agents that mimic the effects and inhibit the effects of the parasympathetic nervous system, respectively. An example of a parasympathomimetic is the miotic (pupil constricting) drug, pilocarpine; an example of a parasympatholytic drug is atropine.

Sympathomimetics and sympatholytics

These are agents that mimic the effects and block the effects of the sympathetic nervous system, respectively. They are also known as adrenergic agonists and antagonists. They are used for conditions where sympathetic stimulation is excessive or inadequate and causes problems. Examples of sympathomimetic drugs are those used to stimulate the $\beta 1$ receptors in the heart, to increase its rate and contraction (known as positive inotropes). This group includes isoprenaline and pimobendan. An example of sympatholytic drugs is the β-blocker.

Tranquillisers and sedatives

This encompasses a range of drugs that have some effect on the animal's awareness or perception of its surroundings. There are several terms used in relation to this group of drugs that may appear confusing as some are interchangeable. Many drugs of this type can produce a variety of effects depending on the dose given.

Tranquillisers or ataractics tend to reduce anxiety (have an anxiolytic effect) and produce a mentally relaxed state.

Drugs that produce a more profound drowsiness are termed sedatives. Potent sedatives that induce sleep or reduced consciousness are termed hypnotics or narcotics.

Neuroleptic drugs produce a state of mental detachment. Commonly used tranquillisers and sedatives are the phenothiazine, acepromazine, benzodiazepines such as diazepam and midazolam and $\alpha 2$-agonists such as medetomidine and xylazine.

Urinary pH modifiers and antiseptics

The pH of urine can cause or precipitate certain conditions, most notably urolithiasis. The use of agents that modify urinary pH is often indicated in the treatment of such conditions and to prevent recurrence. Modern veterinary practice makes full use of diets that have been formulated to maintain a certain pH but it is also possible to achieve this using drugs. Urine acidification can be achieved using ascorbic acid (vitamin C) and alkalinisation can be achieved using sodium bicarbonate. Excessive use of these products can cause metabolic disturbances.

Vaccines, toxoids, antitoxins and antisera

A vaccine is a substance given to stimulate active immunity against a known disease or diseases (see also Chapter 21). Vaccines may be live, containing microorganisms that are similar to the pathogen, or the pathogen may have been manipulated to render it safe for use (attenuated) so that it stimulates a suitable immune response but does not cause the disease.

Killed or dead vaccines contain inactivated pathogen – these tend to be less effective than live vaccines and may contain an adjuvant to enhance their effect. Some inactivated vaccines contain purified versions of toxins produced by the pathogen in question, in order to stimulate immunity to that toxin. These products are called toxoids.

In certain circumstances, it may be necessary to give immediate protection against a disease rather than waiting for the animal's own immune system to respond to a vaccine. This type of passive immunity is achieved by administering antibodies to an animal that have been produced by another animal (usually of the same species). These antibodies are known as antitoxins, and they are administered in fluid known as antiserum. Although passive immunity is immediate, it does not last long.

Vasodilators

Certain conditions, e.g. congestive heart failure, cause vasoconstriction or a decrease in the diameter of blood vessels. This increases the resistance of blood flowing through the vessels and increases strain on the heart. Vasodilators increase the diameter of blood vessels, thus decreasing resistance and making it easier for the heart to pump blood around. These drugs exert their action by relaxing vascular smooth muscle – some on arterial vessels, e.g. hydralazine; some on venous vessels, e.g. glyceryl trinitrate; and some on both, e.g. the angiotensin-converting enzyme (ACE) inhibitor enalapril. This group of drugs is commonly used in animals with cardiac disease as it blocks the formation of the hormone angiotensin II, a potent vasoconstrictor. Other commonly used ACE inhibitors include benazepril and ramipril. Vasodilators can cause hypotension or low blood pressure, so ataxia and syncope may be seen, especially when initiating treatment.

Vitamins and minerals

Nutritional science is so well advanced today that dietary supplementation is rarely necessary for healthy animals. Careless addition of vitamin and/or mineral supplements to the diet could cause dangerous imbalances or excesses. However, there remains a role for certain vitamins and minerals in the veterinary pharmacy:

- Exotic animals, e.g. reptiles in particular, may require certain supplements (e.g. calcium dusting powder) in order to maintain their health. It is possible to buy proprietary powders and liquids in suitable combinations.
- Calcium gluconate should always be available as it is necessary to administer this mineral immediately in cases of hypocalcaemia, e.g. in eclampsia or damaged parathyroid glands.
- Potassium chloride supplementation may be necessary for patients receiving treatment for dehydration and anorexia and those on loop diuretics.
- Many phosphate binders used in the management of chronic renal failure are mineral salts.
- Vitamin B_{12} is used in the management of inflammatory bowel disease in cats.
- Vitamin K (phytomenadione) is used as an antidote for warfarin poisoning.

DOSAGE CALCULATIONS

Veterinary professionals must be able to calculate drug dosages correctly. Inaccurate calculations could lead to under- or overdosage of medication, with disastrous consequences. Most drug calculations are based on one or more commonly used formulae. Once the concept of these formulae has been mastered, drug calculations are relatively straightforward. It is, however, important to recognise your own limitations, and if in doubt, calculations should be checked by an experienced person (see Appendix 1).

Licensing, prescribing and dispensing medication

INTRODUCTION TO VETERINARY PHARMACEUTICAL LEGISLATION

There are two main pieces of legislation governing the use of drugs in veterinary practice. These are The Veterinary Medicines Regulations (VMR) 2013 and The Misuse of Drugs Act 1971 (with associated Regulations). The Supply of Relevant Medicinal Products Order 2005 also specifies some legal aspects of prescribing and supplying veterinary medicines. Table 19.10 describes these pieces of legislation and which area is covered by veterinary pharmaceutical practice. Other significant legislation includes:

- The Health and Safety at Work Act 1974, The Management of Health and Safety at Work Regulations (amended 1999) and The Control of Substances Hazardous to Health Regulations 2002 (COSHH), which relate to safe storage, transporting and handling of medicines
- The Control of Pollution Act (1974), The Controlled Waste (England and Wales) Regulations 2012/The Waste (Scotland) Regulations 2012 and The Environmental Protection Act (1990), which relate to safe disposal of medicines.

The Royal College of Veterinary Surgeons (RCVS) Codes of Professional Conduct also specify some requirements with which registered veterinary nurses and veterinary surgeons must comply. Failure to do so could result in disciplinary action being taken.

Changes in veterinary pharmaceutical legislation

For some years, there has been a drive towards producing a uniform approach to drug legislation for all European Union

TABLE 19.10	Legislation covering the use of veterinary medicines		
Legislation	**Function**		**Areas covered**
The Veterinary Medicines Regulations 2013 (VMR 2013)	• Sets out the legal controls in the United Kingdom required by EU Directive 2001/82/EC (as amended), to which all European Union Member States must adhere • Governs the manufacture, licensing, prescribing, supply and labelling of veterinary medicinal products in the UK		Issue and review of marketing authorisations (MAs) to manufacturers Exemptions for the requirement for medicines used to hold an MA (e.g. small animal exemption scheme) Use of unauthorised ('unlicensed') products (the prescribing cascade) Provisions for wholesale supply of veterinary medicinal products Provisions for retail supply of veterinary medicinal products, including prescribing classes and issue of prescriptions Restricts the advertising of POM-V, POM-VPS and NFA-VPS products
The Misuse of Drugs Act 1971 (Including The Misuse of Drugs Regulations 2001 and The Misuse of Drugs (Safe Custody) Regulations 1973)	• Controls the production, supply, possession and storage of dangerous drugs • Deals with controlled drugs (CDs), a special category of POM-V medicines • Refers to 'classes' of drug, i.e. Class A, Class B, Class C. These classes are not referred to in veterinary medicine • Also promotes education and research into drug dependency and addiction		Place CDs into one of five schedules (which are different from the drug prescribing classes) Relate to the storage of CDs. States that a locked car is not considered an acceptable place to store CDs
The Supply of Relevant Medicinal Products Order 2005	• Implements the recommendations of the Competition Commission in their 2003 'Report on the supply of prescription-only medicines for veterinary use (POMs)'		Prohibits discrimination of charges between clients who request prescriptions and those who do not for other veterinary services (see section on 'writing prescriptions')
The RCVS Codes of Professional Conduct	• Outlines the agreement between the RCVS and the Office of Fair Trading (OFT) relating to the supply of veterinary medicines		Ensures adequate information on the prices of medicines are accessible to clients

(EU) member states. In addition to this, there have been changes to the rules governing the supply of medicines against a prescription issued by another veterinary surgeon and also the supply and costs of prescriptions themselves.

These changes were first incorporated into the VMR in 2005 and this legislation has been regularly updated ever since; the current legislation is the VMR 2013.

Licensing of veterinary drugs in the UK

Veterinary medicines must only be administered to an animal if they have a product 'licence', called a Marketing Authorisation or MA, for the treatment of that particular species and condition. These regulations apply to both food-producing and non-food-producing animals. There are exceptions which are discussed in the next section.

Obtaining an MA requires the undertaking of a series of pharmacological and toxicological tests and clinical trials. This process is known as registration. The drug manufacturer must be able to prove by scientific means the product's safety, quality and efficacy. MAs are issued for a period of 5 years, after which time the granting of the MA is reviewed. In certain situations provisional, or 'exceptional', MAs are issued. This would be in circumstances where a new disease was discovered or the existing treatment was no longer effective or available. These are issued annually.

Manufacturers wishing to obtain an MA can apply through one of three routes, though the majority of MAs are centralised:

• Centralised – via the European Medicines Agency. MA would be valid in all EU member states.

• National – via the Veterinary Medicines Directorate. MA would be valid in the UK only.

• Mutually Recognised/Decentralised – the holder of an MA in another EU member state can apply for identical MAs in one or more other member states.

There are stringent packaging requirements for authorised veterinary medicines; sufficient information about safe and effective use must be printed on the packaging and where there is insufficient space a product leaflet must be included. All authorised veterinary medicines are also legally required to have an accessible Summary of Product Characteristics (SPC), which provides evidence-based information about the medicine, such as the dose rate, indications, special precautions, side effects and adverse reactions. Note that an SPC is different from a data sheet, although they often contain similar information.

PRESCRIBING VETERINARY DRUGS

When an MA is obtained the drug will be placed into one of four main categories, which have varying restrictions placed on the product with regard to who may supply it. The category they fall into will be determined by the potential of the drug to cause harm, the type of animal (food-producing vs non-food-producing) and the importance of receiving regular veterinary attention to prevent harm and/or suffering to the animal concerned. The prescribing categories are detailed in Table 19.11.

Veterinarians and suitably qualified persons (SQPs) supplying veterinary medicines may only do so from registered premises. The Register of Veterinary Practice Premises is held by the RCVS on behalf of the Veterinary Medicines Directorate

TABLE 19.11	Drug categories under the Veterinary Medicines Regulations 2013			
Abbreviation	Category name	Prescribing and supply restrictions	Notes	
POM-V	Prescription-only medicine – veterinarian	To be prescribed only by a veterinary surgeon following diagnosis for an animal under his/her care*	Another veterinary surgeon or pharmacist may dispense the medicine against a prescription but only from registered premises.* Advertising is restricted to veterinary surgeons, veterinary nurses, pharmacists and professional keepers of animals (e.g. farmers)	
POM-VPS	Prescription-only medicine – veterinarian, pharmacist, suitably qualified person** (SQP)	To be prescribed only by a veterinary surgeon, pharmacist or SQP. The animal need not be under his/her care*	Relates to livestock. Mainly antiparasiticides. Advertising is restricted to veterinary surgeons, pharmacists, professional keepers of animals and other veterinary professionals, including RVNs.*** Another veterinary surgeon, pharmacist or SQP may dispense the product against a prescription* but only from registered premises	
NFA-VPS	Non-food animal – veterinarian, pharmacist, SQP	To be supplied only by a veterinary surgeon, pharmacist or SQP*	Relates to companion animals, including horses, who are registered in their passport as not intended for human consumption. Mainly antiparasitic products. Can only be supplied from registered premises	
AVM-GSL	Authorised veterinary medicine – general sales list	May be supplied by any retailer	Veterinary medicines deemed to be extremely safe. Includes some shampoos and other products with very small amounts of active ingredient	

*Those prescribing or supplying veterinary medicines must provide advice on safe administration and warnings or contraindications. They must also be satisfied that the person supplied is competent to use the product safely and intends to use it for its authorised purpose.
**A suitably qualified person (SQP) is one deemed to have successfully undergone a course of training approved by the Animal Medicines Training Regulatory Authority (AMTRA). Currently, this does not include the RCVS veterinary nursing syllabus, although qualified veterinary nurses (VNs) are eligible for a partial cross-credit.
***RVN, Registered Veterinary Nurse.

(VMD). Registered premises are subject to inspection to monitor compliance (these inspections are incorporated into RCVS Practice Standards Scheme inspections where applicable).

Controlled drugs

Drugs that have the potential for abuse are placed in a sub-category of POM-Vs, known as Controlled Drugs (CDs). There are five schedules of CDs, which have controls that decrease in stringency. Table 19.12 shows the five schedules, their requirements and provides some examples of CDs that may be used in veterinary practice. A veterinary surgeon has the authority to supply Schedule 2, 3, 4 and 5 CDs, under the Misuse of Drugs Regulations 2001. Schedule 1 drugs require a prescription from persons with a Home Office license so these are not applicable to general veterinary practice and would only be used in research facilities. Examples include hallucinogenic drugs such as Ecstasy and LSD, raw opium and cannabis resin. Note that the *Classes* are not the same as the *Schedules*. Drug Classes (A, B and C) relate to the punishment for inappropriate use of these drugs, with those in Class C thought to have the least capacity for harm, so the Act demands more lenient punishment. This increases for Class B, and Class A carries the highest penalties for illegal possession or use. Examples of drugs falling into these categories are:

- Class A – morphine, fentanyl, pethidine
- Class B – codeine, ketamine
- Class C – buprenorphine, midazolam, tramadol.

In 2006, ketamine became a Schedule 4 CD, and in 2014 was upgraded to a class B drug. There are special storage requirements set out in the legislation; the RCVS and VMD both recommend that ketamine should be stored in a secure receptacle and have its usage recorded in a formal register. Consultation currently in progress, as of 2015, may result in ketamine being

rescheduled into Schedule 2, which will change these recommendations to legal requirements.

The prescribing 'cascade'

There are occasions when the veterinary surgeon is faced with a diseased patient for whom no product exists that is authorised in the United Kingdom (UK) to treat that species and condition; this probably happens most frequently in the treatment of exotic animals. The VMR 2013 allow for such circumstances by setting out the rules of the prescribing 'cascade' (Fig. 19.8). Use of unauthorised medicines for food-producing animals have additional restrictions; only substances approved for use in food animals can be used and minimum withdrawal periods apply.

It is a criminal offence for a veterinary surgeon to prescribe an unauthorised product where one that is authorised in the UK for that species and condition exists without valid clinical reason (subject to exemptions, e.g. Small Animal Exemption Scheme). The legislation does not allow the cost of the medicine to be taken into account, so it is not permissible to use an unlicensed medicine (e.g. a 'human' licensed medicine) purely because it is cheaper. VMD inspectors have the power to seize unlicensed products without compensation.

A veterinary surgeon can only prescribe unauthorised products to animals that are his or her direct, personal responsibility and to avoid causing unacceptable suffering to that animal. If such products are to be used, it is a professional requirement of the RCVS that the veterinary surgeon should inform the owner and obtain informed consent in writing.

Records must be kept for a minimum of 5 years and must include:

- Date of examination of the animal
- Name and address of the owner
- Identification and number of animals treated

TABLE 19.12	Classification, restrictions and examples of controlled drugs				
Schedule	Requisition restrictions	Storage restrictions	Dispensing restrictions	Nature of drugs included	Examples
S1	Veterinary surgeons are not generally authorised to possess S1 drugs – the only exception is for research purposes, when a special licence must be obtained	–	–	Highly addictive substances with no therapeutic indication in veterinary practice	Cannabis LSD Raw opium
S2	Can only be obtained with a written requisition signed by the veterinary surgeon. All requisitions must be entered into a bound register (commercially available). Entries must be written in indelible ink and made in chronological order, with a separate section for each drug. Mistakes should not be written over – a marginal note should be made, dated and signed	Most must be stored in a locked receptacle secured to the fabric of the building and can only be opened by a veterinary surgeon or person authorised by them to do so (Secobarbital is exempt from this requirement)	Each time a drug is administered and dispensed, a record must be made in a bound drug register S2 recording requirements are as stated in 'supply restrictions'. The register must be kept for a minimum of 2 years S2 drugs used in the practice cannot be destroyed, except in the presence of a person authorised by the Secretary of State	Substances with significant potential for abuse, but have a therapeutic indication in veterinary practice, e.g. some opiate analgesics	Morphine Methadone Fentanyl Secobarbital
S3	Can only be obtained with a written requisition signed by the veterinary surgeon. All requisitions must be entered into a bound register (commercially available). Entries must be written in indelible ink and made in chronological order. Mistakes should not be written over – a marginal note should be made, dated and signed	Most S3 drugs commonly used in veterinary practice are not subject to special storage requirements, although buprenorphine, temazepam, flunitrazepam and diethylpropion must be kept in a locked receptacle. The BSAVA recommends all S3 drugs are securely stored	Administration and dispensing does not have to be recorded in a drug register	Barbiturates and opioid analgesics with less potential for abuse	Buprenorphine Phenobarbital Pentobarbital Tramadol
S4	No special requisition requirements	No special storage requirements (except ketamine, which should be stored in a locked receptacle in accordance with the Codes of Professional Conduct)	No dispensing restrictions, although to comply with RCVS Codes of Professional Conduct, ketamine use should be recorded n an informal register	Anabolic substances and benzodiazepines	Diazepam Nandrolone Ketamine
S5	No special requisition requirements, although invoices of purchase should be kept for 5 years	No special storage requirements	No dispensing restrictions	Preparations containing less than a stated volume of substance, e.g. less than 0.2% morphine	Kaolin and morphine Codeine Cough linctus

- Diagnosis
- Trade name of the product if there is one
- Batch number if there is one
- Name and quantity of active substance
- Dose administered or supplied
- Duration of treatment
- Withdrawal period if applicable.

There are also specific labelling requirements if the medicine is to be dispensed for a client to administer at home.

Writing prescriptions

A prescription may be needed to obtain a supply of drugs, or may be made out in order that owners can obtain medication elsewhere. This commonly happens when owners use online pharmacies, which can offer competitive pricing on some products.

A prescription may be oral or written, but it must be written if the medication is to be obtained elsewhere. In many cases, recognised abbreviations are used which are often based on Latin (see Table 19.13). The VMR 2013 allow another veterinary surgeon, pharmacist or SQP to dispense against a veterinary prescription, but only from registered premises. According to The Supply of Relevant Medicinal Products Order 2005, it is permitted to levy a reasonable charge to supply a prescription, but there should be no discrepancy between those issued with a prescription and those not issued with a prescription with

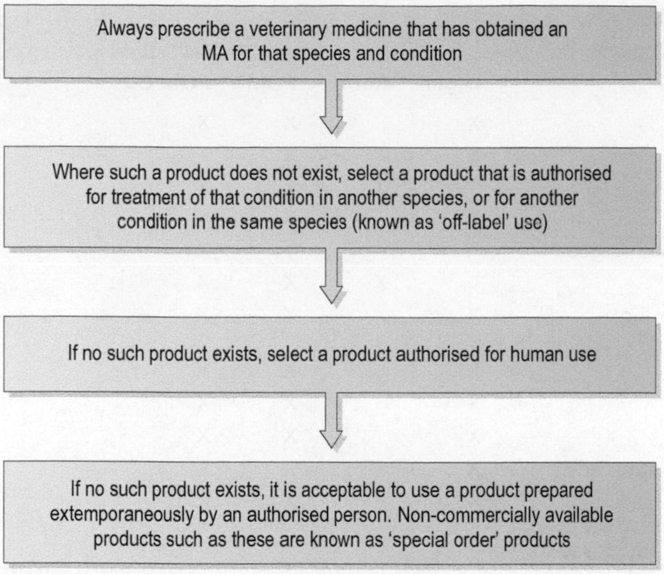
Always prescribe a veterinary medicine that has obtained an MA for that species and condition
Where such a product does not exist, select a product that is authorised for treatment of that condition in another species, or for another condition in the same species (known as 'off-label' use)
If no such product exists, select a product authorised for human use
If no such product exists, it is acceptable to use a product prepared extemporaneously by an authorised person. Non-commercially available products such as these are known as 'special order' products

Fig. 19.8 The prescribing cascade (MA – Marketing Authorisation)

TABLE 19.13 Abbreviations commonly used in dispensing and prescription writing

Abbreviation	Meaning
ad lib.	Take freely
b.i.d.	Bis in diem – take twice a day
o.m.	Omni mane – every morning
o.n.	Omne nocte – every night
p.c.	Post cibum – after food
p.o.	Per os – by mouth
p.r.n.	As required
q.i.d.	Quattuor in diem – take 4 times a day
q.4h	Every 4 hours
t.i.d.	Tres in diem – take 3 times a day
cc	Cubic centimetre
mg	Milligram
ml	Millilitre
a.c.	Ante cibum – before food
t.d.s.	Ter die sumendum – 3 times a day
q.d.s.	Quater die sumendum – 4 times a day
o.d.	Omni die – once daily
u.d.	Ut dictum – as directed
s.i.d.	Semel in die – once daily
q.q.h	Quater quaque hora – every 4 hours
s.o.s	Si opus sit – if necessary

regard to costs of other services (in other words, one cannot simply increase the consultation fee for one or both groups of people to recover the cost of prescription writing).

Table 19.13 demonstrates some commonly used prescription abbreviations. Prescriptions for POM-V and POM-VPS products have specific legal requirements and those for CDs have additional requirements over and above those for other POMs. In addition, there are some recommendations regarding prescription writing, which it would be good practice to take into account. Table 19.14 demonstrates legal and recommended guidelines for prescription writing. Prescriptions for POM products should not be dispensed any more than 6 months from the date of issue. Prescriptions for CD products should not be dispensed any more than 28 days from the date of issue, are non-repeatable and can only be dispensed against the original document (i.e. not a facsimile or email copy). Under the VMR 2013, it is a criminal offence to alter a written prescription unless authorised to do so by the person who signed it.

DISPENSING VETERINARY DRUGS

Dispensing procedure

In many veterinary practices, the veterinary nurse plays a key role in dispensing medicines to clients. It is important that this procedure is carried out accurately and carefully, in order to avoid mistakes by both the nurse and the client. According to The VMR and COSHH regulations, the prescribing veterinary surgeon, pharmacist or SQP must be satisfied that the owner is competent to administer the medicine and has a duty of care to ensure that the owner using the product knows how to do so safely, informing them of any contraindications and dosaging requirements. The prescriber must also check that the prescription is intended for use in the UK, and that the recipient of the medicine will use it for the purpose for which it is intended. If they are not personally dispensing the medication, they must also be satisfied that the person handing over the medication is competent to do so.

Each practice should have a standard operating procedure, designed to minimise the number of errors, maximise client and animal safety, and comply with legislative requirements. This should incorporate a mechanism whereby dispensed medication can be double-checked, either by a second person or by a computer. Clients not only need to fully understand how to dose the patient but they also need to be given sufficient information regarding contraindications, adverse reactions, storage, handling and safe disposal of medicines. The original product packaging and/or product leaflet insert will contain information, but it may be necessary to provide it by alternative written means where the product is not dispensed in the original packaging, or for other reasons, such as to facilitate client understanding of complex technical language or to highlight species-specific information. Table 19.15 identifies the routes by which those dispensing and administering medication may become contaminated (see also sections on handling and use of cytotoxic drugs and on pharmacy management).

When dispensing, ensure that the client is confident to administer the medication and has fully understood the instructions given by the person prescribing the medication. In some cases, a practical demonstration may be advisable, asking them to repeat the procedure after the demonstration. Clients must be made fully aware of any restrictions regarding the medication, e.g. only give with food, do not crush, give at a separate time to other medications, etc.

Occasionally, it may be necessary to send medication by post. This is permitted by Royal Mail, provided that the medication has been sent by or at the request of a veterinary surgeon, is not hazardous to the public, e.g. corrosive to the touch, has been packaged using a strong inner container and wrapped in sufficient outer layers to absorb any leakage. The total volume of any aerosol must not exceed 500 ml. The sender's name and address should be on the outside of the packaging. It is not

TABLE 19.14 Legal and recommended guidelines for prescription writing	Legal	Rec'd	POM	POM CD
In indelible format	X		X	X
Name and address of prescriber (may be headed paper)	X		X	X
Registration number of the prescriber		X	X	X
Prescriber's signature and professional qualifications	X		X	X
Declaration that the animal is being treated under the care of that veterinary surgeon	X			X
The wording, 'For animal treatment only'		X	X	X
For unlicensed medicines, the wording, 'The medicine is to be used under the prescribing cascade'	X		X	X
Date	X		X	X
Name and address of client or keeper	X		X	X
Premises where animal(s) is/are kept if different from owner's address	X		X	X
Species, name/identification and number of animal or group of animals (if applicable)	X		X	X
Name(s) and amount(s) of drug (Note: It is a legal requirement to normally prescribe only the minimum quantity required for treatment, unless the actual supplier of the medication is not legally authorised to break the packaging.)	X		X	X
Amount to be prescribed written in words and figures	X			X
Strength of drug where more than one is available	X			X
Form of drug to be dispensed	X			X
Dosage and administration instructions	X		X	X
Specific dosing instructions (i.e. 'give as required' is inadequate)	X			X
Any necessary warnings	X		X	X
Withdrawal period if relevant	X		X	X
Use leading zeros, e.g. 0.5 instead of .5, but avoid trailing zeros such as 5.0 as this can be mistaken for 50		X	X	X
Names of drugs should be written in English without abbreviation		X	X	X
Directions should be written in English without abbreviation (except the standard Latin abbreviations – but use these with caution and write clearly if handwritten)		X	X	X
Quantities of less than 1 g to be written in milligrams		X	X	X
Millilitres to be used instead of cubic centimetres		X	X	X
Number of times the prescription is to be repeated if more than once	X		X	X (repeats are illegal for S2 and 3 CDs)
Original prescription must be available at the time of supply (i.e. not a facsimile or email)	X			X (for S2 and 3 CDs)

permitted to send CDs, narcotics or psychotropic substance by post.

Packaging and posting a drug should not contravene any storage requirements as stipulated on the SPC, e.g. it would not be acceptable to post a drug that requires refrigeration unless you could guarantee that the product would kept at the required temperature during transportation.

Dispensing containers

According to The VMR 2013, any specific packaging instructions supplied by the MA holder on the SPC must be adhered to by the dispensing premises. If there are no specific instructions, the RCVS Codes of Professional Conduct dictate that the containers must be 'appropriate'. The British Small Animal Veterinary Association (BSAVA) issues guidelines for suitable containers. Box 19.2 outlines their recommendations.

Labelling medication

According to The VMR 2013, there must be sufficient information on the label to enable the product to be used safely, and any additional labels applied to packaging must not obscure the manufacturer's product information, e.g. a dispensing label must not be stuck on packaging over the top of storage instructions. There is currently no other legal restriction regarding labelling a product in a veterinary practice, i.e. when it is dispensed to a client, with the exception of medicines prescribed under the 'cascade' (see relevant section discussed previously). However, the RCVS Codes of Professional Conduct dictate that labelling must be 'appropriate' and it may be wise to include the same details regardless of whether a product is prescribed under the cascade, or as an authorised medicine. BSAVA guidance regarding this subject is a good source of information. Table 19.16 incorporates this guidance.

SAFE DISPOSAL OF MEDICINES

Clients should be discouraged from keeping medication indefinitely and made aware that any surplus or unused medication should be disposed of carefully to avoid risk to themselves, other people, animals or the environment. The ideal system is

TABLE 19.15	Health and Safety recommendations for safe handling of medication		
Route of contamination	**Method of prevention**	**Note**
Via skin	Always wear gloves when handling drugs	Some people have idiosyncratic hypersensitivity or allergy to a specific drug, e.g. penicillin allergy. However, even if this is not the case, it should be remembered that some drugs are very effective at entering the body via the transdermal route. Some may have an accumulative effect, so constant contact with the drug over a long period of time may cause problems
Via mucous membrane or by inhalation	Wear goggles and a mask. Dispense in a draft-free room, but ventilate the area thoroughly after use. Damp dust surfaces. Wear gloves and wash hands thoroughly after use. Do not rub face or eyes	This particularly applies to powders, but could also occur with very dry tablets that tend to accumulate loose powder in the bottom of the container
Open wounds	Cover open wounds with an appropriate waterproof dressing	More likely to occur when dispensing liquids or semi-solid medication such as cream
Ingestion	Do not eat or drink in the dispensary. Do not wipe face with hands. Keep work surfaces tidy and do not dispense medication on top of books, records or other equipment	Drug residue could be left on another object, then transferred to another part of the building, e.g. the restroom, where it could come into contact with food
Accidental injection	Observe strict rules relating to use of needle guards and swift disposal of sharps	It is unlikely that large quantities of drug could be accidentally injected, but residues in the needle, or trauma from the sharp point, could cause a nasty reaction or injury

BOX 19.2 BSAVA GUIDELINES FOR SUITABLE MEDICINE CONTAINERS

- Medicines should be stored in their original packaging with the lid tightly closed.
- Where possible, medicines should be dispensed in their original container.
- If a medicine is repacked or prepared extemporaneously, it should be placed in a container suitable for the medicine and the user.
- All containers should be stored in such a way that they remain free from contaminants.
- Child-resistant containers must be used unless otherwise requested.
- Tablets and capsules must be dispensed in crush-proof and moisture-proof containers.
- Sachets and manufacturers' strip or blister pack medicines should be dispensed in paperboard cartons, wallets or paper envelopes.
- Liquid preparations should be dispensed in amber bottles.
- Bottles containing topical preparations should be fluted to allow recognition by touch. This requirement does not apply to containers over 1.14 litres or to pre-packaged eye/ear drops.
- Some tablets or capsules are adversely affected by moisture and are supplied with a desiccant. This desiccant should not be dispensed; the quantities and packaging of such medicines should be such that deterioration after supply is prevented.
- Medicines sensitive to light should be supplied in suitably opaque or coloured containers.
- Creams, ointments, powders, granules, dusting powders, etc. should be dispensed in glass or plastic wide-mouthed jars.

to request that they return unused medication to the veterinary practice and some SPC sheets and packaging will stipulate this. Returned medication should not be redispensed as appropriate storage conditions in the client's home cannot be guaranteed. Clients who will generate sharps and other hazardous waste, e.g. owners of diabetic animals, should be supplied with an appropriate bin or clinical waste bag which can be returned at suitable intervals.

In a situation where Schedule 2 CDs that have never been dispensed to a client (i.e. have remained 'in stock') require disposal, e.g. they have passed their expiry date or have been spoiled, very specific requirements apply. Firstly, they must be destroyed in the presence of an authorised witness – these include inspectors approved by the VMD, a witnessing veterinary surgeon who is independent of the practice concerned (this excludes family members or any other relationship that may pose a risk of collusion), or another person authorised to witness the destruction of controlled drugs under the Misuse of Drugs Regulations 2001 or the Misuse of Drugs Regulations (Northern Ireland) 2002 such as a Police CD Liaison Officer. Destruction of these drugs can be achieved by using a commercially available denaturing kit. VMD guidance notes state that alternatively, solutions may be placed into sawdust or cat litter and tablets may be crushed and mixed with soapy water. A record must be made of the date of destruction and the quantity destroyed, which the witness must sign. It is good practice to also record the name of the controlled drug, form, strength and quantity and the name of the person destroying it. Returned Schedule 2 CDs (i.e. those that have been dispensed for treatment and returned unused or partly used) are not subject to the same legislation, although the VMD recommends that the same procedure be followed.

Once destroyed, Schedule 2 CDs may be disposed of following normal clinical waste regulations.

Pharmacy management

As in many areas of a veterinary practice there are a multitude of health and safety risks inherent in the veterinary pharmacy. Thorough assessment, evaluation and reduction of these risks is important. Apart from the health and safety considerations, there are other aspects of pharmacy management to consider: minimising drug error, wastage of stock (and therefore money) and providing an efficient service to the client. With the introduction of tighter regulation on the storage and supply of

TABLE 19.16	Recommendations for labelling medication (incorporating BSAVA guidelines)	
Item	**Recommended method/information**
Type of printing or writing to use	Must be indelibly and legibly printed or written. Mechanically printed lettering is ideal. Pencil and non-water-resistant ink are not acceptable
Expiry date	The label should not obscure the expiry date
Instructions on the product packaging	Product information printed on the packaging by the manufacturer must not be obscured. There must be sufficient information visible so that the product can be used safely
Manufacturer supplied product information sheets, inserts and leaflets	These should be passed on to the client. The VMR 2013 state that the user must be informed of administration method/s, risks, warnings and contraindications so omitting the leaflet could be illegal if no other information is given. Alterations to any instructions may only be made by the veterinary surgeon, or pharmacist acting on their instruction
Recommended information (legally required if the medicine is used under the 'cascade')	Name and address of veterinary surgeon Date of dispensing Initials of person dispensing Name and address of owner/keeper Animal/group name and species Drug name Drug strength and quantity Dose and administration instructions Special precautions and warnings related to administration Instructions for storage and disposal The wording 'For animal treatment only' and 'Keep out of the reach of children' or similar The wording 'For external use only' where relevant Expiry date of the medicine if this is not already clearly marked on the packaging The withdrawal period, where relevant (even if it is nil) for food-producing animals if this is not clear on the manufacturers label

medicines, including the registration and inspection of veterinary practice premises, those involved with pharmacy management must ensure they are up to date with the latest requirements in order to keep within the boundaries of the law.

KEY CONSIDERATIONS FOR EFFECTIVE PHARMACY MANAGEMENT

It is unlikely that veterinary nurses will be able to design a pharmacy from scratch and, quite frequently, they must 'make do' with the basic environment and position of the pharmacy. It is, however, still possible to undertake a full review of the pharmacy and make changes in order to improve this area of the practice. Table 19.17 illustrates some of the key considerations when reviewing pharmacy facilities and practice.

Client compliance

WHAT IS CLIENT COMPLIANCE?

Client compliance is the extent to which the actions of the owner coincide with the instructions of the veterinary team with regard to the care of an animal. It can be used to describe any aspect of treatment but is most commonly referred to when discussing drug therapy, and the likelihood that the owner will give prescribed medication correctly. More recently, the use of the word 'compliance' has been replaced by 'adherence' and 'concordance', as the former implies that people are being ordered to do as they are told, rather than following a course of treatment that has been negotiated and mutually agreed upon.

THE IMPORTANCE OF CLIENT COMPLIANCE

Studies in human medicine (Russell et al. 2003; Vermeire et al. 2001) show that patient non-compliance is a major cause of

ineffective treatment. The limited studies undertaken in the veterinary field (AAHA 2008; Adams et al. 2005; Barter et al. 1996; Boda et al. 2011; Grave and Tamen 1999) appear to demonstrate that the situation here may be similar. Ensuring client compliance will improve the health and welfare of the patient and the veterinary professional should facilitate this. Table 19.18 provides the details of factors that affect compliance.

THE NURSE'S ROLE IN IMPROVING COMPLIANCE

The veterinary nurse is ideally placed within the team to play a major role in increasing compliance and, in doing so, improving the well-being of patients (also see Chapter 3). The following lists some suggestions as to how this can be achieved:

- Ensure that clients clearly understand the recommendations that have been made for their pet by using effective communication skills
- Nurse consultations for patients diagnosed with long-term conditions
- Demonstrate how to give medication and encourage the owner to repeat the dosing technique while on the premises
- Offer medication aids such as reminders and pill givers
- Use written instructions and take advantage of commercially produced literature and videos
- Assure clients that they can return to check progress or discuss treatment at any time
- Consider a system of allocating a named nurse to each chronically ill patient to encourage confidence
- Check that repeat prescriptions are being ordered at the correct time intervals
- Ask clients if they are able to manage the treatment programme easily when they call for a repeat prescription.

TABLE 19.17	Considerations in designing and running a pharmacy
Area/issue	**Suggested action**
Environmental conditions	Purchase a maximum-minimum thermometer and hygrometer to monitor the environmental temperature and humidity. Additional heating or a dehumidifier may be necessary. Check the refrigerator temperature daily. Keep records of all temperature and humidity readings and review them regularly. Review the ventilation system to ensure that minimal dust and particles enter. Windows present a security risk and not desirable in a pharmacy, but if present they should be shuttered if possible. Heavy blinds could be used as an alternative, to reduce excessive heat, draughts and light entering the pharmacy. Ensure that light-sensitive drugs are kept in dark containers and stored in a light-proof receptacle.
Shelving	Check that there is adequate shelving to hold all stock. Cluttered shelves are difficult to keep clean and may interfere with stock rotation, as well as making it hard to locate drugs and increasing the risk of a dispensing error. Install additional shelving if needed or reduce the volume of stock kept.
Position of stock	Drugs should be kept in alphabetical order on the pharmacy shelf. Ensure that all personnel involved with the pharmacy are familiar with the system so they can locate drugs easily. Heavy items should not be stored on very high or low shelves. Controlled Drugs (CDs) must be stored according to legislative requirements. No foodstuffs can be stored next to pharmaceuticals.
Stock rotation	Ensure that stock is appropriately rotated. Only have one bottle or packet open at a time and mark each product 'OPEN', with the date of broachment when in use (as stipulated in the RCVS Codes of Professional Practice). Ensure that there is an effective system for recording batch numbers of stock once opened. Despite effective rotation, packaging often gets dusty and it is important to vacuum, damp dust or clean regularly to avoid spoilage of stock. Monitor stock usage – drugs tend to fall in and out of 'favour', so the types and amounts of each type will change as time goes by. Avoid stocking duplicate products, i.e. the same drug made by two different manufacturers. Unused drugs from an open pack or bottle should be discarded within 28 days of opening, unless the product information stipulates a shorter time frame.
Dispensing	Ensure that an adequate supply of Personal Protective Equipment (PPE) is within easy reach of those dispensing drugs. It is advisable to assemble a 'cytotoxic kit' especially for dispensing these drugs. Ensure that suitable waste bins are within easy reach. Ensure that clients are supplied with PPE as practice policy or medicine administration instructions dictate. It may be necessary to supply written instructions to accompany these.
Prevention of contamination	Never allow food or drink into the pharmacy. Remove unnecessary equipment and literature. Ensure that hand-washing facilities, first aid kit and eye-washing facilities are easily accessible. Ensure that staff clean the outside of drug containers (including swabbing the tops of multi-dose vials) as necessary. The premises must be vermin free.
Prevention of theft	Stock should not be kept where the general public can gain access to it. Ensure that pharmacy desks or serving hatches are staffed at all times when the surgery is open. CD receptacles should be out of sight of the public and kept locked at all times. Ensure that clients pay for their treatment prior to collecting it from the pharmacy.
Record keeping	Annual audit is a legal requirement. This must include a reconciliation of all incoming and outgoing stock, including disposal of out-of-date and damaged items. An efficient system of recording batch numbers is also required to conform with legislation. The exact requirement varies, depending on the type of animals being treated, i.e. food-producing or non-food-producing. Keep documentation relating to the RCVS registration of the practice premises updated and ensure fees are paid on time. Ensure all records of stock, material safety data sheets, SPCs, risk assessments and suspected adverse reaction report forms are kept up to date and in an orderly fashion. Store Controlled Drug (CD) registers securely as they contain confidential information, but ensure they are accessible when required.
Minimising dispensing errors	Ensure that adequate literature is available to enable staff to check dosages, etc., e.g. VMD Specific Product Characteristics, Veterinary Data Sheet Compendium from the National Office of Animal Health, and Small Animal Formulary from the British Small Animal Veterinary Association. Clearly differentiate between drugs of similar names and strengths, e.g. by placing them in different-coloured outer receptacles, especially if the manufacturer's packaging is similar. Ensure that staff dispensing medication are adequately trained and, if necessary, supervised. Introduce a system of 'double-checking' dispensed medication. Request that staff initial the labels of dispensed drugs, so that errors may be traced. This is not to apportion blame but to enable any problems to be identified and rectified. Encourage staff to be open and honest about mistakes – remember that this may prevent the death of a patient and that 'honesty and integrity' is also a requirement of the RCVS Code of Professional Conduct. Drug dispensing errors should be investigated as part of the clinical governance protocol of the practice.
Minimising administration errors	Produce client handouts about drug administration – these may be generic or specific to certain drugs, e.g. cytotoxic drugs or those with complex administration regimes. Produce these in other languages if the client base includes significant numbers of people who do not use English as a first language. Ensure an adequate supply of effective administration aids, e.g. pill crushers. Schedule patient discharge procedures when a nurse is available to demonstrate medication administration.
Adverse events and reactions	Ensure all veterinary surgeons, SQPs and other relevant staff are fully aware of the action to take in the event of a suspected adverse event or reaction to a veterinary medicine, i.e. report to the VMD. Note that this includes suspected lack of efficacy of a veterinary medicine, particularly applicable to antimicrobials.
Prescription tampering	Report all suspected cases of prescription tampering to the VMD.

TABLE 19.18	Factors affecting client compliance
Factors	**Description**
Relationship with the veterinary team	A clear recommendation for the client about the patient's treatment from the veterinary team is crucial. A good relationship with the veterinary team will enhance the possibility that clients will return for assistance if they encounter difficulty in adhering to a treatment regimen.
Patient characteristics	The patient's temperament and lifestyle – animals who are aggressive or spend time away from the house may be less likely to receive regular treatment.
Treatment regime	The complexity of the treatment regimen – frequent dosing intervals and polypharmacy may reduce compliance.
Disease nature	There is evidence from human studies that prophylactic treatment regimens and treatment regimens for chronic or terminal patients may be less likely to be administered as instructed (Russell et al 2003; Vermeire et al 2001)
Client characteristics	Aged clients or those who have disabilities or illnesses may be less likely to comply with treatment regimens.

REFERENCES

AAHA, 2008. Compliance: Taking quality care to the next level. Available from: <http://www.aahanet.org/protected/ComplianceExecutiveSummary0309.pdf> and discussion at: <http://veterinarynews.dvm360.com/aaha-unveils-details-client-compliance-study?rel=canonical>.

Adams, V.J., Campbell, J.R., Waldner, C.L., et al., 2005. Evaluation of client compliance with short-term administration of antimicrobials to dogs. J. Am. Vet. Med. Assoc. 226 (4), 567–574.

Barter, L., Watson, A.D.J., Maddison, J.E., 1996. Owner compliance with short term antimicrobial medication in dogs. Austral. Vet. J. 74 (4), 277–280.

Boda, C., Liege, P., Reme, C., 2011. Evaluation of owner compliance with topical treatment of acute otitis externa in dogs: A comparative study of two auricular formulations. Int. J. Appl. Res. Vet. Med. 19 (2), 157–165.

Grave, K., Tanem, H., 1999. Compliance with short-term oral antibacterial drug treatment in dogs. J. Small Animal Pract. 40 (4), 158–162.

Russell, S., Daly, J., Hughes, E., et al., 2003. Nurses and 'difficult' patients: Negotiating non-compliance. J. Adv. Nurs. 43 (3), 281–287.

Vermeire, E., Hearnshaw, H., Van Royen, P., et al., 2001. Patient adherence to treatment: Three decades of research. A comprehensive review. J. Clin. Pharm. Ther. 26 (5), 331–342.

BIBLIOGRAPHY

Antimicrobial resistance and sales surveillance information, 2013. Available at: <https://www.gov.uk/government/publications/veterinary-antimicrobial-resistance-and-sales-surveillance-2013>.

Bill, R., 1997. Pharmacology for Veterinary Technicians, second ed. C V Mosby, St. Louis, MO.

British Homeopathic Society, 1876, 2010. British Homeopathic Pharmacopeia. Kessinger Publishing, Montana, USA.

BSAVA Guide to the Use of Veterinary Medicines. Available at: <http://www.bsava.com/Resources/BSAVAMedicinesGuide.aspx>.

European Medicines Agency website. Available at: <http://www.ema.europa.eu/ema/index.jsp?curl=pages/regulation/landing/veterinary_medicines_regulatory.jsp&mid=>.

Galbraith, A., Bullock, S., Manias, E., et al., 2007. Fundamentals of Pharmacology, second ed. Routledge, Oxon.

Guide to Marketing Authorisation Process for Veterinary Medicinal Products in Europe. Available at: <http://www.noah.co.uk/issues/ma_dossier.pdf>.

RCVS advice on fair trading requirements. Available at: <https://www.rcvs.org.uk/advice-and-guidance/code-of-professional-conduct-for-veterinary-surgeons/supporting-guidance/fair-trading-requirements/>.

RCVS Code of Professional Conduct for Veterinary Nurses. Available at: <https://www.rcvs.org.uk/advice-and-guidance/code-of-professional-conduct-for-veterinary-nurses>.

Silverman, J., Kurtz, S., Draper, J., 2004. Skills for Communicating with Patients, second, rev. ed. Radcliffe, London.

Veterinary Medicines: A report on the supply within the United Kingdom of prescription-only veterinary medicines. Volumes 1 and 2. Archived at: <http://webarchive.nationalarchives.gov.uk/+/http:/www.competition-commission.org.uk/rep_pub/reports/2003/478vetmeds.htm>.

Veterinary Medicines Directorate Guidance Notes. Available at: <https://www.gov.uk/government/collections/veterinary-medicines-guidance-notes-vmgns>.

VMD Product Information Database. Available at: <http://www.vmd.defra.gov.uk/ProductInformationDatabase/Default.aspx>.

RECOMMENDED READING

AAHA, 2008. Compliance: Taking quality care to the next level. Available from: <http://www.aahanet.org/protected/ComplianceExecutiveSummary0309.pdf> and discussion at: <http://veterinarynews.dvm360.com/aaha-unveils-details-client-compliance-study?rel=canonical>.

Bill, R., 2006. Clinical Pharmacology and Therapeutics for the Veterinary Technician, third ed. C V Mosby, St Louis, MO.

BSAVA Guide to the Use of Veterinary Medicines. Available at: <http://www.bsava.com/Resources/BSAVAMedicinesGuide.aspx>.

Carpenter, J., 2012. Exotic Animal Formulary, fourth ed. Elsevier Saunders, St. Louis, MO.

Galbraith, A., Bullock, S., Manias, E., et al., 2007. Fundamentals of Pharmacology, second ed. Routledge, Oxon.

Jevring, C., 2005. Compliance in veterinary practice. EJCAP 15 (2), 205–209. Available at: <http://www.fecava.org/sites/default/files/fecava_15.2.pdf>.

Pawar, M., 2005. Five tips for generating patient satisfaction and compliance. Am. Fam. Physician 12 (6), 44–46.

Ramsay, I., 2014. BSAVA Small Animal Formulary, eighth ed. British Small Animal Veterinary Association, Gloucester.

Rock, A., 2007. Veterinary Pharmacology: A Practical Guide for the Veterinary Nurse. Butterworth-Heinemann, Oxford.

Silverman, J., Kurtz, S., Draper, J., 2004. Skills for Communicating with Patients, second rev. ed. Radcliffe, London.

Wanamaker, B., Massey, K., 2014. Applied Pharmacology for the Veterinary Technician, fifth ed. Elsevier Saunders, St. Louis, MO.

USEFUL RESOURCES

Animal Medicines Training Regulatory Authority (AMTRA) website. Available at: <http://www.amtra.org.uk>.

Antimicrobial resistance and responsible use of anti-microbials leaflet. Available at: <https://www.vmd.defra.gov.uk/pdf/leaflet_antimicrobials.pdf>.

Antimicrobial resistance and sales surveillance information. Available at: <https://www.gov.uk/government/publications/veterinary-antimicrobial-resistance-and-sales-surveillance-2013>.

BSAVA Guide to the Use of Veterinary Medicines. Available at: <http://www.bsava.com/Resources/BSAVAMedicinesGuide.aspx>.

Compendium of Data Sheets for Veterinary Products, 2014. National Office of Animal Health, Enfield. Available at: <http://www.noahcompendium.co.uk/Compendium/Overview/-21789.html>.

European Medicines Agency website. Available at: <http://www.ema.europa.eu/ema/index.jsp?curl=pages/regulation/landing/veterinary_medicines_regulatory.jsp&mid=>.

Guide to Marketing Authorisation Process for Veterinary Medicinal Products in Europe. Available at: <http://www.noah.co.uk/issues/ma_dossier.pdf>.

PROTECT antibacterial use poster. Available at: <http://www.bsava.com/Portals/4/kvsecure_publications/PROTECT%20poster_Nov_2014_2916.pdf>.

RCVS advice on fair trading requirements. Available at: <https://www.rcvs.org.uk/advice-and-guidance/code-of-professional-conduct-for-veterinary-surgeons/supporting-guidance/fair-trading-requirements/>.

RCVS Code of Professional Conduct for Veterinary Nurses. Available at: <https://www.rcvs.org.uk/advice-and-guidance/code-of-professional-conduct-for-veterinary-nurses>.

SPVS veterinary medicines information: What's available? Available at: <http://www.spvs.org.uk/sites/default/files/Vet%20medicines%20-%20Andrea%20Tarr.pdf?dm_i=OES>.

Veterinary Medicines Directorate Guidance Notes. Available at: <https://www.gov.uk/government/collections/veterinary-medicines-guidance-notes-vmgns>.

VMD Product Information Database. Available at: <http://www.vmd.defra.gov.uk/ProductInformationDatabase/>.

VMD Small Animal Exemption Scheme. Available at: <https://www.gov.uk/government/uploads/system/uploads/attachment_data/file/364479/PCDOCS-_406746-v3-VMD_VMGN_012_A_-_Exemption_Scheme_for_Small_Pet_Animals.PDF>.

20

Emergency and Intensive Critical Care

LOUISE O'DWYER

KEY POINTS

- Understand how to perform an effective triage.

- Improve understanding and knowledge in the assessment and monitoring of emergency and critical patients using a variety of techniques and equipment.

- Enhance understanding of metabolic derangements.

- Improve understanding of common poisons and toxicities and their effects.

- Identification and treatment of urinary tract and reproductive emergencies and disorders.

- Improve knowledge when dealing with paediatric emergencies.

- Up-to-date information and knowledge of how to perform effective cardiopulmonary resuscitation (CPR).

Introduction

Emergency patients can present with a wide variety of life-threatening problems, and there may only be a short time window in which intervention will be successful. Effective stabilisation and management of the emergency patient requires a coordinated team of well-trained caregivers who all understand the major priorities of emergency patient care.

Telephone triage

In theory, telephone triage requires clinic staff to determine the urgency of a pet's problem and to provide advice based on that determination. As the client may not possess the training to give an accurate account of the pet's problem(s), it is generally safest to recommend the client take the pet to a veterinary surgeon. Particularly, any patient experiencing breathing difficulty, inability or unwillingness to rise, inability to urinate or traumatic injury should be seen immediately without the need to ask further questions.

At the beginning of the telephone conversation staff should establish the animal's signalment (breed, sex, age and weight) if possible. The types of questions asked of the owner should be basic and simple, remembering the majority of pet owners are not medically trained. They should address the level of consciousness of the patient, whether or not the patient is breathing, and whether the patient is experiencing seizures or has broken and exposed bones. Based on the information, advice can be given on first aid, assuming that the problem can be clearly defined and is simple (Box 20.1). See Box 20.2 for a list of problems requiring veterinary attention without delay.

Information gathered during the phone conversation can aid veterinary staff in the preparation for the arrival of the patient at the hospital. Knowing information such as the animal's breed or weight can enable staff to select the appropriate intravenous (IV) catheter size, volume of fluids, endotracheal tube size etc.

Owners should be provided with information about safe transportation of their pet to the clinic.

Prep/treatment area

Initial management of the emergency patient begins with preparation to treat the emergency patient. The treatment area should ideally have enough room for the emergency team and be stocked with appropriate equipment. An oxygen source should be readily available and good lighting is essential, as it will aid endotracheal intubation, visualisation of veins and observation of the patient. The emergency cart/kit is essential as it make the management of trauma patients more efficient by having all the supplies (catheters, drugs, fluids, airway management supplies, tape and bandages, surgical kit, sterile gloves and skin prep supplies) readily available. An emergency kit may be as simple as a Tupperware tub or as elaborate as a mobile tool chest. If a cart is used additional equipment may be mounted on the cart such as suction machine, electrocardiograph (ECG) and capnograph. The emergency cart or kit should be checked at the beginning of each shift and restocked immediately after each use.

Patient assessment and management

For a busy emergency service to operate effectively all team members should be skilled at patient assessment. In order to make patient assessment as simple and reliable as possible a standardised approach should be used. Ideally all members of the team should use the same approach on all patients. There are numerous triage protocols available; the one most commonly referred to is the airway, breathing and circulation (ABC) approach. This approach is effective and most easily recalled in an emergency situation.

INITIAL OBSERVATION

An initial observation of the patient provides important information, and a brief 'look' at the patient before any hands-on contact is made should be performed. In this time two major issues are addressed. First, how serious does the situation look? Obviously the animal that can maintain sternal recumbency and is aware of its surroundings is far less concerning than the animal in lateral recumbency with no apparent response to external stimuli. Second, are there any obvious life-threatening problems that will require attention at or before the time you can evaluate the ABCs? Problems such as arterial haemorrhage or an open chest wound are likely to require immediate intervention.

The ABC patient assessment is performed within 1–2 minutes, and if there are multiple staff members dealing with an individual patient, then numerous parameters can be evaluated simultaneously. Ideally flow-by oxygen should be provided until the assessment is complete and the requirement for ongoing oxygen therapy has been adequately evaluated.

A – Airway

Assessment. All emergent and critically ill animals should have the patency of their airway evaluated. This involves assessment of the gag reflex and ensuring no airway obstruction is evident. For many patients this is a cursory examination as they show obvious swallowing and resistance to opening of their mouth and there is an absence of signs of obstruction (Box 20.3). Recumbent animals that have reduced jaw tone should be closely evaluated for the presence of a gag reflex.

Therapy. Any patient without a gag reflex should be intubated immediately. If there is a foreign body airway obstruction evident, it should be removed immediately. If an airway obstruction cannot be readily removed and it is preventing intubation, an emergency tracheostomy is likely to be required.

B – Breathing

Assessment. Following evaluation of the airway, it is necessary to confirm that the animal is making breathing efforts. Is the effort normal, decreased or increased? Are breath sounds normal, diminished or increased? Can the breath sounds be characterized (crackles, wheezes)? By observing the patient breathing and listening to breath sounds, you may be able to localise the breathing difficulty to the pulmonary parenchyma (Box 20.4), pleural space (Box 20.5) or thoracic wall (Box 20.6).

Therapy. If there are no respiratory efforts evident the animal should be intubated (if not already performed), and manual ventilation commenced. Severe respiratory abnormalities such as gasping, excessive respiratory effort and cyanosis despite oxygen therapy may also warrant immediate intubation and ventilation. If pleural space disease is suspected then thoracocentesis should be performed; this will often be diagnostic as well as therapeutic. If multiple thoracocentesis are performed over a short period of time or negative pressure cannot be achieved then a chest tube is warranted. Thoracocentesis should always be the first line of action ahead of thoracic radiographs in the dyspnoeic patient where pleural space disease is suspected following clinical examination.

C – Circulation

Assessment. There are six physical examination parameters that allow a rapid evaluation of the circulatory status or perfusion:

a. Mentation
b. Mucous membrane colour

c. Capillary refill time (CRT)
d. Heart rate
e. Pulse quality
f. Extremity temperature.

These clinical findings should be evaluated in combination; an abnormality in a single parameter does not have the clinical significance of multiple abnormalities.

Common clinical findings of circulatory shock are:

• Reduced mentation
• Pale or white mucous membranes
• Slow CRT
• Tachycardia
• Reduced pulse quality
• Cool extremities in comparison with core body temperature.

(Patients with vasodilatory shock can have red mucous membranes, rapid CRT, bounding pulses and warm extremities. As these animals are likely to present with concurrent hypovolaemia these signs of vasodilation may not be evident until after adequate fluid resuscitation.)

1. Mentation. Decreased mentation is indicated by a lack of interest in the surrounding environment, and diminished or absent responses to stimuli such as noise and touch. This can be described as obtundation or depression. As depression implies an assessment of the animal's emotional state, obtundation may be a more appropriate term. If there is a loss of consciousness it is considered to be either stupor or coma. Stupor refers to a patient that is unconscious and only responsive to noxious stimuli. Coma refers to a completely unconscious, non-responsive state. Most unconscious animals will require intubation to protect their airway.

An altered level of mentation can be the result of primary intracranial disease or significant systemic abnormalities such as hypoperfusion or hypoglycaemia. Any abnormality in mentation should be considered serious and a complete triage examination is warranted immediately.

2. Mucous membrane colour. Pale or white mucous membranes are a consequence of a reduced quantity of red blood cells perfusing the capillary beds of the mucosal tissue. This can be due to vasoconstriction in compensation to circulatory shock or severe anaemia. This abnormality in combination with other evidence of poor perfusion or inadequate tissue oxygenation warrants emergency intervention (Fig. 20.1).

Vasodilation will increase the flow of blood through the mucous membranes making them a deep pink to red colour. Vasodilation may be an appropriate response as seen in a hyperthermic animal after exercise or it can be pathological as seen in vasodilatory shock. Patients with vasodilatory shock commonly present with concurrent hypovolaemia and on presentation will have pale mucous membranes, and it is only after adequate fluid resuscitation that red mucous membranes are noted. Septic patients will also present with bright red mucous membranes due to a loss of vasomotor tone, but despite this these patients are still often hypovolaemic.

3. Capillary refill time. Capillary refill time (CRT), the time it takes for mucous membranes to regain their colour following blanching by digital pressure, is a reflection of local blood flow. When perfusion is normal CRT is 1–2 seconds. Vasoconstriction will reduce the flow of blood through the mucous membranes via arteriolar and precapillary sphincter contraction and it will take longer for the colour to return to the tissue after blanching. In severe vasoconstriction when the

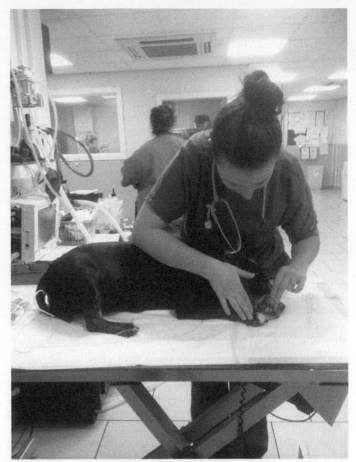

Fig. 20.1 Assessment of mucous membrane colour and capillary refill time in an emergency patient

mucous membranes appear white it is often impossible to appreciate any CRT. In patients with vasodilation the CRT can be more rapid than normal as there is less resistance to blood flow and the capillary beds rapidly refill with blood after the digital pressure is removed. A slow CRT is always a concern and suggestive of poor perfusion. A rapid CRT in conjunction with other perfusion abnormalities can suggest vasodilatory shock.

4. Heart rate. The normal heart rate of an animal varies with body size to a certain extent. In general, large-breed adult dogs have resting heart rates of 60–140 beats per minute (bpm), medium adult dogs 70–160 bpm and small dogs, puppies and cats are in the range of 100–220 bpm. There will be some variation depending on the fitness and activity level of the individual animal. When arterial blood pressure is threatened either by a drop in stroke volume, or as a result of vasodilation, there will be a baroreceptor-mediated increase in sympathetic tone resulting in a reflex tachycardia. As tachycardia is a normal response to anxiety, excitement and exercise, it is a common physical examination finding. The presence of a tachycardia in conjunction with other signs of abnormal perfusion (vasoconstriction or vasodilation) is suggestive of hemodynamic compromise.

Tachycardia is the appropriate and expected response to circulatory shock. The presence of normocardia or bradycardia in canine shock patients (i.e., patients with abnormalities of the other five parameters) is of concern as it suggests decompensated shock and is associated with greater severity of illness and a poorer prognosis.

Auscultable arrhythmias may or may not require immediate medical therapy. Femoral pulse evaluation should be performed simultaneously with auscultation for both time efficiency and recognition of pulse deficits. Arrhythmias without any other signs of poor perfusion are far less concerning but these patients should always be prioritised for a secondary evaluation including an ECG, as the clinical evaluation of these abnormalities is considerably limited.

5. Pulse quality. Pulse quality is subjectively determined by the digital palpation of the femoral pulse. Obvious abnormalities in pulse quality are concerning and if present in conjunction with other signs of poor perfusion the patient should receive immediate medical attention. Unfortunately patients can have considerable hemodynamic compromise without palpable changes in pulse quality. As a result the palpation of an adequate femoral pulse cannot be used to indicate a stable patient.

The pulse quality is determined by the difference between diastolic and systolic arterial blood pressure as well as the duration of the pulse and the size of the vessel. The greater the diastolic-systolic difference the 'stronger' the pulse will feel. A normal arterial blood pressure, for example, would be a systolic blood pressure of 120, a mean of 85 and a diastolic of 70 mm Hg. The systolic-diastolic pressure difference (pulse pressure) is 50. If there is a fall in blood pressure such that the patient is hypotensive with a systolic pressure of 90, mean of 55 and diastolic of 40 mm Hg the pulse pressure would still reflect a systolic-diastolic difference of 50 mm Hg. The examiner may be challenged to detect the change in pulse quality.

Vasoconstriction will tend to diminish palpable pulse quality, the 'thready pulse'. In contrast vasodilation will increase vessel size and compliance. In addition vasodilated patients usually have an elevated stroke volume such that the pulse quality is often appreciated to be normal or exaggerated (bounding) in these patients.

6. Extremity temperature. The sympathetic-mediated vasoconstriction that occurs in response to a fall in cardiac output will tend to shunt blood from venous capacitance vessels to the central circulation, preserving blood flow to vital organs at the expense of less vital tissue. This reduction in peripheral circulation will cause a fall in extremity temperature in comparison with core body temperature. If the patient is generally hypothermic, cool extremities that are essentially the same temperature as the rest of the animal do not indicate an abnormality in perfusion. For this reason the temperature of the extremities (evaluated by digital palpation of the paws and distal limbs) should always be interpreted with reference to the measured core body temperature.

Vasodilation will be associated with warm extremities if the patient is fluid resuscitated.

Therapy. All cardiovascular emergencies will require venous access for the administration of medications and fluids. A peripheral venous over-the-needle catheter is usually the easiest and quickest to insert in the first instance. Peripheral insertion sites include the cephalic, lateral and medial saphenous, and the auricular vein. Primarily the radius but also the length of the lumen determines the maximum fluid flow rate of a catheter. A large-gauge catheter is required if fluids are to be administered rapidly, e.g. severely hypovolemic patient. If a slow

TABLE 20.1	Guidelines for shock doses of intravenous fluids in dogs and cats	
	Total shock dose*	
Fluid type	**Dogs (ml/kg)**	**Cats (ml/kg)**
Isotonic crystalloids	80–90	50–55
7.5% hypertonic saline	4–6	3–4
Synthetic colloids	10–20	5–10

*Fluids should be given in increments and the total dose determined by the individual response.

infusion is acceptable then a small-gauge catheter might be appropriate. In the event an IV catheter cannot be obtained the establishment of an intraosseous line is a reasonable alternative. Fluid or drugs administered by this route are rapidly taken up into the circulatory system. The most common sites for access include the trochanteric fossa of the femur, the greater tubercle of the humerus, the wing of the ilium and the crest of the tibia.

If the patient is assessed as having poor perfusion the rapid initiation of fluid resuscitation to improve perfusion is important. The goal is to fully resuscitate the patient in 10–20 minutes.

There are three main types of fluids that may be used for fluid resuscitation (Table 20.1); they include isotonic and hypertonic crystalloids and synthetic colloids (also see Chapter 25).

Isotonic crystalloid fluids are mixtures of sodium chloride and other physiologically active solutes (K^+, Ca^{2+} or Mg^{2+}, glucose and buffer). They are generally isotonic to plasma and have sodium as the primary osmotically active solute. Balanced (compensation resembles ECF) crystalloids are generally given when the nature of fluid losses are not known, are due to trauma, and/or electrolyte measurements are not available; an excellent replacement solution is lactated Ringer's (Hartmann's) or its equivalent.

Hypertonic crystalloids such as 7.5% saline have been recommended for use in shock therapy; much smaller volumes are given when compared to balanced crystalloids. Hypertonic saline causes fluid shifts from the intracellular space to the extracellular (including intravascular) space resulting in improved venous return and cardiac output. Because of the fluid 'steal' that occurs with the administration of hypertonic saline, it will be necessary to replenish the interstitial space with a balanced crystalloid. It is indicated in cases where it is difficult to administer large volumes of fluids rapidly enough to resuscitate the patient, e.g. giant-breed gastric dilatation and volvulus patients. It is also thought that hypertonic saline may be beneficial in the treatment of traumatic brain injury by reducing brain oedema.

Colloids are large-molecular-weight solutions that do not cross capillary membranes readily and increase the serum colloid osmotic pressure. Intravascular colloid oncotic pressure (COP) is important in maintaining intravascular volume. Colloids are better blood-volume expanders than are isotonic crystalloids; 50–80% of the infused volume remains in the intravascular space when the capillary membrane wall is uncompromised. Colloids should be administered when crystalloids are not effectively improving or maintaining blood volume restoration or if oedema develops prior to adequate blood volume restoration.

D – Dysfunction (neurological). Any obvious neurological abnormalities usually require urgent attention even if the patient is otherwise stable. Animals with evidence of spinal trauma, for example, such as Schiff Sherrington posture, should receive immediate spinal stabilisation by taping the animal to a backboard. Seizures and other significant central abnormalities should also be prioritised as the neurological status can deteriorate if left untreated. Some ocular abnormalities may also require urgent attention such as prolapse of the globe.

Body temperature. Body temperature is not addressed in the standard ABCs and may not be required for the assessment of every patient. Extremes of body temperature are an indication for urgent medical attention, and as a result the temperature of at-risk patients should be measured during assessment. Any recumbent, poorly responsive patient should have its temperature measured, especially in small patients who are extremely prone to hypothermia. Animals that are rapidly panting or have obvious signs of exertion such as tremors or seizures should also have their temperature evaluated.

Severe hypothermia less than 34°C (93°F) requires immediate active warming. Temperatures less than 28°C (82.4°F) can cause arrhythmias and coagulopathies. Rewarming of the severely hypothermic patient should be gradual (1–2°C per hour), as rewarming will cause vasodilation and subsequent hypotension can develop. For this reason these patients require constant monitoring and appropriate cardiovascular support.

Temperatures greater than 42°C (107°F) can cause direct thermal damage to proteins, lipids and DNA. Cell damage, coagulopathies and neurological abnormalities can result. If severe, multiple organ dysfunction can occur. Immediate active cooling of these patients is essential in combination with appropriate cardiovascular support.

Monitoring of the emergency patient

RESPIRATORY SYSTEM

Much as monitoring the respiratory system of any patient is vitally important, when dealing with the dyspnoeic patient, this can be a life or death situation, and one should remain acutely aware of the fragility of such patients, as even the stress of a clinical examination can prove fatal, particularly in cats. With this in mind, the risks of any diagnostic tests must be carefully weighed against the potential benefits and treatment may have to be instituted prior to a definitive diagnosis. Most dyspnoeic cats will benefit from a period of 100% oxygen in an oxygen cage prior to a complete major body system evaluation and repeated assessment.

Initial evaluation of the respiratory system comprises respiratory rate, effort and respiratory auscultation, and this should be continued when monitoring the patient. A normal animal should have a respiratory rate of 15–30 breaths per minute and (because the majority of a resting inspiration is due to diaphragmatic contraction) there should be very little apparent chest movement. During normal inspiration, diaphragmatic contraction pushes abdominal viscera caudally and as a result, the abdominal wall moves out passively; therefore contraction of the abdominal muscles can only assist with expiration. With worsening dyspnoea, increased intercostal contraction pulls the diaphragm cranially on inspiration and the abdominal wall moves inwards. Additional postural adaptions may also be seen.

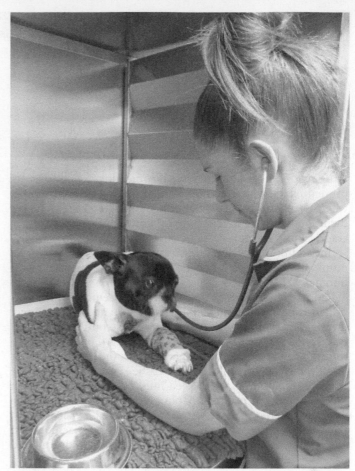

Fig. 20.2 Thoracic auscultation on a patient with aspiration pneumonia

Such changes in posture include straightening of the neck, and open-mouth breathing can be seen in both dogs and cats, but dogs prefer to stand with abducted elbows (orthopnoeic breathing) while cats tend to sit in sternal recumbency. Patients should be observed for changes in their body position, as a constantly changing body position in cats suggests a worsening of dyspnoea. Lateral recumbency in a dyspnoeic dog should be viewed seriously and can often indicate impending death in a cat.

The patient's respiratory pattern should also be observed, and this can yield valuable information alongside the clinical examination, as it can help to localise the level of the respiratory tract affected in two common situations. Upper airway obstruction is normally associated with prolonged inspiration with inspiratory stridor or stertor (noise), followed by a short expiration. In patients with small airway disease, such as feline asthma, a longer expiratory phase with increased abdominal effort on auscultation is often noted.

Pulmonary auscultation is also vitally important in the monitoring of respiratory patients. In order to ensure complete auscultation of all lung fields, it is useful to divide the chest into a noughts and crosses board, then auscult each square. It is normal to hear slightly louder and 'coarser' lung sounds in the cranioventral lung fields when compared to the dorsocaudal fields, due to increased turbulence in these smaller airways. The areas should sound symmetrical when comparing both sides of the chest, with the exception of the area of cardiac dullness in the left cranial fields (Fig. 20.2). Pleural space disease causes

TABLE 20.2	Hypovolaemia table		
Clinical parameter	Mild hypovolaemia	Moderate hypovolaemia	Severe hypovolaemia
Heart rate	120–140	140–170	170–220
Mucous membrane	Normal, or pinker	Pale pink	Pale/white/grey
Capillary refill	Brisk (less than 1 second)	Normal (1–2 seconds)	Slow or not detectable
Pulse amplitude	Increased	Decreased	Very decreased
Pulse duration	Mildly reduced	Reduced	Very reduced

muffling of lung sounds, as there is something, e.g. fluid or air, preventing the lung sounds reaching the bell of the stethoscope, whereas small airway or parenchymal disease usually makes them louder; these louder lung sounds are often described as crackles or wheezes.

In addition to physical examination, the use of other monitoring equipment can be used to supplement physical findings.

Pulse oximeters can be used to estimate haemoglobin saturation in critically ill animals; however, they do not give any direct information about tissue perfusion, cardiac output or oxygen delivery. Pulse oximeters use light-emitting diodes (LEDs) to transmit two wavelengths of light – one in the red and another in the infrared band – through tissue. When using a pulse oximeter a pulsating arterial bed must be positioned between the LED and the detector. A photodetector is placed on the opposite side of the tissue bed to measure the intensity of light that makes it through the tissue. Oxygenated haemoglobin absorbs less red light and more infrared light than desaturated haemoglobin, and this principle forms the basis of calculation of percent saturation. As arterial blood pulses through the tissue bed separating the LED from the photodetector, the path length increases slightly and the tissue absorbs more light. By analysing the ratio of absorption of red to infrared light and detecting the cyclic variations associated with pulsatile blood flow, pulse oximeters can accurately calculate the percent saturated haemoglobin. There are a variety of pulse oximeter models marketed for use on the fingers or earlobes of humans and so some imagination is sometimes required in order to use these devises in dogs and cats. The ear, tail or foot (in small dogs and cats) may be suitable locations for probe placement. Newer commercially available veterinary technology utilises digital sensors that greatly reduce signal loss and interference.

Arterial blood gas determination is used to evaluate pH of the blood, the respiratory contribution to acid-base balance and the oxygenating function of the lung. Blood gas evaluation is rapidly becoming more commonplace in veterinary practice as 'bedside monitoring' technology has decreased in price and automated most of the calibration and maintenance chores associated with these tests. Small, portable, automated units are now available for veterinary use (e.g. I-STAT, EPoc) that perform not only blood gas analysis but also other tests including electrolyte, lactate and glucose concentration measurement. Arterial blood is typically collected from the dorsal metatarsal or femoral artery using a heparinised syringe and a 25- or 27-gauge needle. The devices directly measure pH, pCO_2 and pO_2, and calculate H_2CO_3, TCO_2 and haemoglobin saturation. A venous blood sample may be satisfactory substitute for arterial when evaluating only the pH and pCO_2. The arterial pO_2 measured directly may be used to confirm the accuracy of pulse oximetry on any given patient.

CARDIOVASCULAR SYSTEM

Cardiovascular assessment and monitoring is aimed at identification of hypoperfusion as a result of hypovolaemia. Significant blood loss can occur into body cavities and fracture sites following trauma, without any visible haemorrhage, and this is particularly relevant in cats. The response to hypovolaemia is initially tachycardia, vasoconstriction and increased myocardial contractility as a result of adrenergic stimulation. With continued blood loss these compensatory measures fail to maintain tissue perfusion and signs of decompensated hypovolaemic shock ensue.

Dogs have a fairly predictable response to blood loss, and the degree of hypoperfusion can be estimated from the severity of their clinical signs (see Table 20.2). Cats, however, are less predictable and can be more difficult to assess. Their higher resting heart rate also means there is less room for an increase in heart rate. As a result we need to be more reliant on palpation of pulse quality for assessment in these patients. It is this assessment of the severity of hypovolaemia that should be used to guide fluid therapy.

Other common conditions that change the clinical haemodynamic parameters are anaemia, sepsis/inflammatory response syndrome and abnormal cardiac function. Most animals with abnormal perfusion have some component of hypovolaemia so recognising uncomplicated hypovolaemia is the rational starting point. In uncomplicated hypovolaemia, mucous membrane colour, CRT and vigour, pulse profile (height and width), heart rate and cardiac auscultation provide the means of intravascular volume assessment. A normal animal should have pink mucous membranes with a vigorous capillary refill that takes 1–1¾ seconds. Pulses (femoral and metatarsal) should be carefully palpated to allow assessment of their height (to estimate pulse pressure) and their width, i.e. the length of time the pulse lasts. Assessing the height and width of the pulse together allows an estimation of pulse volume and can generate a mental image of the pulse profile. There will be some normal variation in pulse profile from patient to patient. A normovolaemic animal that is stressed or painful will have slightly higher and narrower pulse profile than a resting animal.

In the compensatory stages of hypovolaemia dogs will develop a moderate tachycardia of 140–160 beats per minute. The increased heart rate, reduced blood volume and increase in cardiac contractility produces a pulse, which is narrower and higher than normal. This pulse profile is often referred to as being 'snappy' or 'bounding', but such terminology can be confusing.

With compensatory hypovolaemia the metatarsal pulses should still be palpable. Mucous membranes should be pink to pinker than normal with a rapid CRT of less than 1 second duration.

The increases in heart rate seen in dogs with hypovolaemia are surprisingly independent of body weight; this means that severe hypovolaemia results in a heart rate of 180–220 bpm in most dogs. Heart rates in excess of this should raise suspicions of a primary arrhythmia rather than just a sinus tachycardia in response to hypovolaemia and an ECG should be performed. Heart sounds are often very quiet due to the severe hypovolaemia (as are heart murmurs which will become apparent during volume loading). Mucous membranes have little or no red coloration (white, muddy or grey), and CRT is prolonged or absent. Femoral pulses are extremely weak (referred to as thready) and metatarsal pulses should not be palpable.

The ability to estimate intravascular volume status using clinical signs is an invaluable skill and particularly useful when then assessing the patient's response to acute volume replacement. In general, during successful volume replacement perfusion parameters will gradually and predictably return to normal through the same stages in reverse. This allows rapidly detection of an inadequate response to volume resuscitation and this should prompt detection of the underlying cause.

As with respiratory monitoring, in addition to physical examination, the use of other monitoring equipment can be used to supplement physical findings.

An **electrocardiograph** (ECG) records the electrical activity of the heart and is the method by which cardiac arrhythmias are defined. Continuous ECG monitoring is commonly used in patients with known arrhythmias and in animals at known risk for development of arrhythmias, e.g. post gastric dilatation and volvulus (GDV). It should be remembered that the ECG does not measure myocardial function or cardiac output and in fact may appear perfectly normal in the face of potentially fatal reductions of heart function.

Prolonged ECG monitoring is commonly required for critically ill patients, and as such requires atraumatic electrodes; therefore, alligator clips should not be used. Instead, disposable adhesive ECG patches are applied to clipped skin. Precise placement of electrodes and standard body positioning are not essential.

ECG characteristics relevant to critically ill patients include rate, rhythm, segment intervals, T wave size, and S-T segment positioning:

a. *Rate*: Abnormally fast or slow heart rates may indicate significant problems that require intervention. The heart rate in quietly resting dogs should not exceed 120–140 bpm. The most common abnormality seen in critical patients is sinus tachycardia caused by hypovolaemia, hypoxemia, depressed myocardial function, anaemia, hypotension, hypercapnia, pain, drugs and hyperthyroidism.

b. *Rhythm*: Is the rhythm regular or irregular? Do the PQRST waves appear normal? Irregularity of widths or intervals often signifies conduction abnormalities or arrhythmias, respectively. Remember sinus arrhythmia is a normal 'abnormal' finding in dogs – this is the regular increase in heart rate seen in inspiration, and decrease on expiration. This is not a normal finding in cats.

c. *T waves*: T waves may be large relative to the R waves during hypoxemia or hyperkalaemia. Hyperkalaemia may cause tall, symmetrical T waves with a narrowed base (Fig. 20.3).

d. *S-T segment*: The S-T segment may be depressed or elevated. The most common change seen in critical

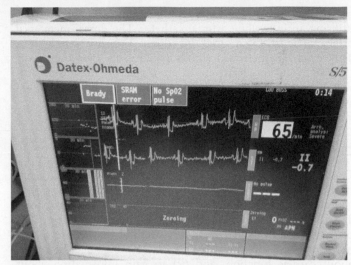

Fig. 20.3 Elevated T waves in a patient with urinary obstruction, resulting in hyperkalaemia

patients is ST segment depression due to ischaemia of the subendocardial muscle of the left ventricular free wall during hypovolaemia or hypotension.

Arterial blood pressure monitoring is critical to successful management of many patients. Maintenance of a mean blood pressure high enough to support tissue perfusion is essential for survival. An animal, however, can have lethal reductions in cardiac output while maintaining relatively normal pressures. Animals in hypovolaemic shock may not become hypotensive until all compensatory mechanisms are exhausted and they are near death. In contrast, septic shock may cause marked reductions in total peripheral vascular resistance and severe hypotension in the face of relatively well-preserved heart function.

Normal blood pressure in dogs has been reported as:
- Systolic: 148 ± 16 mm Hg
- Diastolic: 87 ± 8 mm Hg
- Mean: 102 ± 9 mm Hg.

Arterial pressure may be conveniently measured by indirect (external) techniques including ultrasonic Doppler instrumentation, e.g. Ultrasonic Flow Detector (Parks Medical Electronics) and by oscillometric devices, e.g. Dinamap®, Critikon. Both techniques rely on the use of cuff occlusion of arterial blood flow in a limb or tail. The Doppler method requires use of an ultrasonic probe to detect blood flow distal to the cuff as pressure is gradually released from the cuff. The blood pressure is read off a manometer attached to the cuff, and systolic pressure is read when the flow returns as the pressure is released. Oscillometric devices use a cuff in the same locations, but blood pressure is measured by machine detection of minute oscillations in cuff pressure as cuff pressure is released. One advantage of the oscillometric monitors is that they will obtain readings without constant operator involvement and may be programmed to repeat measurements at frequent intervals. The Doppler technique requires active operator participation in each reading, and reliably measures only systolic blood pressure. Both of these external techniques are technically difficult in animals with small limbs (cats and small dogs), hypovolaemia, or hypotension. The Doppler technique is generally more reliable in small animals, patients with arrhythmias and at low blood pressures. The oscillometric method is often inaccurate under those circumstances. Consequently, many critically ill patients must be monitored by direct (invasive) techniques, utilising an indwelling arterial catheter. The dorsal metatarsal artery is most often used for direct pressure monitoring. The vessel is catheterised with a 20–22-gauge over-the-needle type of catheter. Electronic arterial pressure monitors provide direct measurement of diastolic, systolic and mean blood pressure.

CENTRAL VENOUS PRESSURE MEASUREMENT

Central venous pressure (CVP) measurement is a useful diagnostic procedure for the management of fluid therapy in general, and is essential to the management of refractory shock. The CVP is the blood pressure within the intrathoracic portions of the cranial or caudal vena cava. Central venous pressure is measured clinically for two reasons: (1) to gain information about cardiac function, and (2) to gain information about intravascular blood volume.

Materials necessary for CVP measurement using a water manometer include:

- Central venous catheter in place
- Water manometer
- 1–30-inch IV extension tubing set if needed
- Three-way stopcock if needed
- 20 ml syringe filled with saline solution or fluid bag
- 20-gauge needle.

Once the patient has been placed into the desired position (sternal or lateral recumbency, with lateral recumbency preferred), the water manometer is connected to the central venous catheter and the syringe/fluid bag. With the stopcock turned 'off' to the manometer, the fluid line should be primed along with the extension set, ensuring no bubbles are present. In order to be able to repeat the measurement, the stopcock should rest on the kennel floor. The patency of the central catheter should be assessed by allowing fluid from the syringe/bag to flow freely into the catheter. If a multilumen central line is used, infusions of fluids through other lumens should be discontinued before obtaining the CVP reading, as they may artificially increase the measurement.

Before the CVP can be measured, the zero point on the manometer needs to be identified; the zero point needs to correspond to the patient's right atrium. This measurement will need to be subtracted from the reading in order to obtain the correct CVP. When the animal is in lateral recumbency, the cranial vena cava lies near the midline, and the manubrium is a good reference point. In sternal recumbency, the cranial vena cava is approximately level with the point of the shoulder (scapulohumeral joint). To find the zero point on the manometer, draw a perpendicular line from the reference point on the patient to the manometer, using string or a tape measure (Fig. 20.4).

To obtain a measurement, fill the manometer with saline significantly above the expected patient CVP. Turn the three-way stopcock so that the column of saline in the manometer is continuous with the central catheter and the stopcock is 'off' to the saline bag or syringe. The saline in the manometer will decrease until the hydrostatic pressure in the column equilibrates with the hydrostatic pressure of the blood at the tip of the central catheter. Once the saline in the manometer stops falling, it has reached the equilibrium point, which reflects the blood pressure inside the vessel at the point of

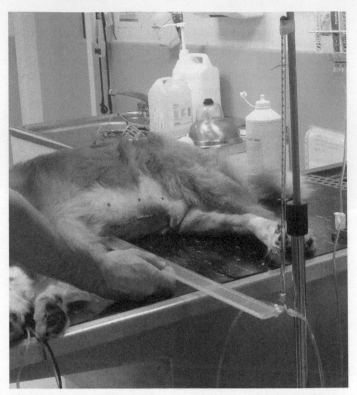

Fig. 20.4 Measurement of zero point for CVP monitoring

the catheter tip. The measurement is expressed in cm H_2O. Normal reference ranges are reported to be 0–10 cm H_2O in cats and dogs.

Electronic measurement of CVP is a more convenient (and potentially more accurate) method of measurement made feasible by the widespread availability of ECG monitors with dual electronic pressure ports. Materials needed in addition to the monitor itself include a pressure transducer (disposable or multiple-use), a sterile fluid path connected to the transducer ('pressure dome') and a sterile tubing set to connect the pressure dome to the catheter. This may be an IV tubing extension set or an arterial pressure tube.

Measurement of CVP in animals during fluid challenge yields important information about cardiovascular status. As intravenous fluids are administered and the intravascular blood volume expands, venous return and CVP will begin to rise. A rapid (less than 5 minutes) infusion of 10–20 ml/kg of crystalloid into a euvolaemic animal with normal cardiac function will result in a modest increase in CVP (2–5 cm H_2O or 2–4 mm Hg) that returns to baseline within 15 minutes. A minimal increase or no increase in a patient's CVP implies that the vascular volume is markedly reduced. If the CVP rises and returns to baseline rapidly (less than 5 minutes), this implies that there is reduced vascular volume and that the initial volume load has been accommodated by rapid changes in vasomotor tone. A large increase in CVP (greater than 4 cm H_2O or greater than 3 mm Hg) implies reduced cardiac compliance or increased venous blood volume or both. A slow (15 minutes) return towards baseline indicates that blood volume is close to normal. A very prolonged return to baseline (longer than 30 minutes) suggests that the intravascular blood volume is elevated relative to cardiac performance.

URINE OUTPUT MEASUREMENT

Urine output is technically easy to measure and provides useful information about renal perfusion. An indwelling urinary catheter should be placed and maintained with a closed collection system. This procedure is not without risk. Any catheter left in place will cause mechanical urethritis and allows the potential for bacterial colonisation of the urinary tract. The catheter should therefore be inserted using sterile technique, and removed as soon as possible.

The catheter is aseptically connected to a sterile closed collection system and is never elevated above the level of the patient, as this would allow retrograde flow of urine and bacteria into the patient. The catheter is anchored to the vulva or sheath with a single suture. The collection tubing is anchored to the tail (in bitches and cats) or a rear limb or belly wrap (in male dogs) to prevent traction on the catheter suture.

Urine production should be measured hourly in unstable patients. Urine production should be at least 0.5–1 ml/kg/hr, and is frequently much higher than this following adequate resuscitation of an animal with circulatory shock. The catheter should be removed as soon as possible to minimise the risk of bacterial infection.

TEMPERATURE

Skin temperature is generally not considered a diagnostic indication but its measurement allows estimation of the adequacy of circulation. Dogs in cardiogenic or hypovolaemic shock divert blood flow away from their skin and skin temperature falls. This is particularly evident in skin at the ears and extremities, where there is little underlying tissue mass to keep the skin warm. The temperature of the skin at the interdigital webbing of the feet is particularly labile and changes rapidly with changes in cardiac output. This can be determined by measuring the temperature of the skin at the interdigital webbing between digits 3 and 4 of a pelvic limb, and comparing this to rectal temperature. Normal dogs should have a rectal–toe web gradient of less than 4°C, and values above this signify reduced skin perfusion.

In pyrexic patients we should not attempt to reduce fevers unless the rectal temperature becomes worryingly high (above 41°C), at which point the veterinary surgeon should be alerted. Forced cooling is avoided at all costs, as this simply forces the animal to divert more energy towards restoring the fever.

METABOLIC MONITORING

Routine laboratory evaluations that should be performed at least daily in critically ill animals include packed cell volume (PCV), plasma total protein (TP), serum glucose and blood urea nitrogen (BUN). Changes in PCV and TP may indicate changes in hydration status, blood loss, or protein loss. The colour of the serum in the haematocrit tube should be observed for signs of icterus or haemolysis. The buffy coat may be examined for crude appraisal of the white blood cell (WBC) count. Other important tests include measurement of serum electrolytes and urinalysis.

Coagulopathies are common in critically ill animals and warrant aggressive monitoring. By the time an animal develops clinically obvious evidence of coagulopathy secondary to disseminated intravascular coagulation (DIC), it is usually too late to prevent death. Tests that are helpful to diagnose DIC and other causes of coagulopathy include activated clotting time (ACT), partial thromboplastin time (PTT), prothrombin time (PT), platelet count, fibrin degradation product (FDP) assay and complete blood count (CBC). The PT, aPTT, and ACT may be evaluated with a hand held device (SCA2000™, Synbiotics). Evaluation of red cell morphology as of a CBC may reveal the presence of red cell fragments and schistocytes that suggest microangiopathic red cell injury as a consequence of DIC.

SUMMARY

Critical care monitoring is tailored to identify relevant areas of concern and observe for changes in the patient's condition over time. To be useful, identification of significant trends in monitored variables must prompt appropriate therapeutic responses, and it can be useful to identify 'trigger points' or values on the patient's hospitalisation chart.

Oxygen therapy

There are some conditions that can be addressed immediately with emergency oxygen therapy, and oxygen therapy is warranted as soon as respiratory distress is suspected or observed. Common conditions include upper airway foreign body obstructions, pleural space disease due to air or fluid, abdominal distension due to ascites or GDV, asthma and cardiogenic pulmonary oedema. A chest tap may be considered not only as treatment but also a diagnostic procedure in the emergent setting that can preclude radiographs.

Oxygen therapy may be administered via 'flow-by', hood/Elizabethan collar, intranasal, intratracheal, facemask or oxygen cage systems. These systems start with a source of either portable tanks connected to a regulator or a central liquid, compressed or generated source piped to connections throughout the hospital. They should ideally be run through a humidifier before being delivered to a patient.

EVALUATION OF OXYGENATION

- **Respiratory rate and effort:** Even though all patients breathing hard and fast are not hypoxemic, all patients presenting tachypnoeic or dyspnoeic should be considered hypoxaemic until proven otherwise. Positive response to oxygen and return of distress when oxygen therapy is removed supports hypoxaemia.
- **Cyanosis** is a blue tinge to the capillary beds caused by deoxyhaemoglobin. Perception of this blue tinge is dependent on ambient light, observer, and patient pigmentation, and circulation in that capillary bed besides the absolute deoxyhaemoglobin concentration. Nevertheless, cyanosis indicates hypoxaemia. The converse is not necessarily true as cyanosis is generally seen at an arterial partial pressure of oxygen (P_aO_2) of 40 mm Hg while severe hypoxemia is considered anything below 60 mm Hg and below normal at 80 mm Hg.
- **Pulse oximetry (SpO₂):** Pulse oximetry measures light absorbance through a pulsating capillary bed to determine the degree of oxygen-haemoglobin saturation (SaO_2 but abbreviated SpO_2 when measured by pulse oximetry). It is non-invasive and provides real-time and continuous measurements. However, obtaining reliable

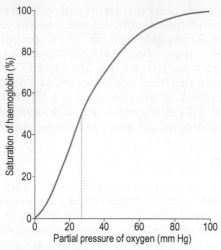

Fig. 20.5 Oxygen-haemoglobin saturation curve

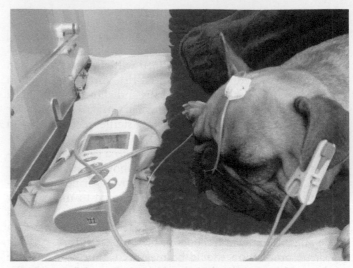

Fig. 20.6 Nasal catheter placed in a French bulldog

measurements especially in awake, poorly perfused or hypoxemic patients with pulse oximetry can be challenging. The microprocessor requires light transmittance through a pulsating capillary bed, and this may be difficult to obtain in those patients. Additionally, referring to the oxygen-haemoglobin saturation curve, a pulse oximeter does not possess the ability to accurately differentiate a patient on oxygen supplementation with a PaO_2 of 120 mm Hg versus 400 mm Hg as both would be expected to have a SpO_2 greater than 98. While this supports that adequate oxygen saturation is present at that time, one cannot accurately assess pulmonary function or its progression. Despite these limitations, pulse oximetry does provide valuable information as it can alert if the patient is hypoxemic despite oxygen therapy. A SpO_2 of 90% corresponds to a PaO_2 of 60 mm Hg, and a PaO_2 of 80 mm Hg corresponds to a SpO_2 of 95% (Fig. 20.5).

TECHNIQUES FOR OXYGEN ADMINISTRATION

- **Flow-by** oxygen is administered by placing the end of a tube directing oxygen flow to the mouth and nose of the patient. It yields a fraction of inspired oxygen (FiO_2), with room air being 0.21, a FiO_2 of 0.25–0.45 on 6–8 L/min of oxygen flow can be achieved. This method should be used with caution as it may upset an already stressed patient but is simple and less annoying to many patients than other methods.
- **An Elizabethan collar with plastic wrap** covering the opening except for a small dorsal vent space will provide a FiO_2 of 0.30–0.40 at 0.2–0.5 L/min of oxygen flow. A zip-lock kitchen storage bag can provide a good temporary means of administering oxygen in cats and small dogs ensuring the nose and mouth are kept away from the walls of the bag. Overheating may become a concern and an assistant must be in attendance at all times.
- **Intranasal** administration of oxygen is achieved through the placement of a catheter approximately one-half the diameter of the nostril placed in the ventral meatus and advanced to the level of the lateral canthus (Fig. 20.6).

FiO_2s of 0.30–0.55 can be accomplished with unilateral flows of 50 ml/kg/min increasing to bilateral catheters at 100 ml/kg/min. Some patients will not tolerate the catheters or jetting of oxygen; the use of topical anaesthetics and advancing the catheter into the pharyngeal area may address these concerns.

- **Intratracheal** administration of oxygen can be accomplished by advancing the nasal cannula (nasotracheal) into the trachea on inspiration with the neck dorsally extended. Radiographs are warranted to confirm appropriate placement, and this limits its use in the emergent setting. Alternatively, placing a catheter as one would for a transtracheal wash can also be used for delivery of oxygen directly into the trachea. As oxygen is delivered further downstream, a FiO_2 of 0.40–0.60 is accomplished with 50 ml/kg/min of oxygen flow. Airway irritation leading to clinically significant inflammation, kinking of the tube, insertion site complications plus the potential need for sedation for placement are considerations for its use.
- **Facemask** FiO_2 values range from 0.35–0.95 depending how tightly fitting the mask and the delivery system are, i.e. tube vs. anaesthetic circuit. Patient tolerance is variable and requires assistant attendance.
- **Oxygen cages** ranging from plastic-wrapped caged doors of stainless cages to ones costing in excess of £10K that scrub carbon dioxide and maintain temperature and humidity. They will provide a FiO_2 of 0.40–0.90. Oxygen cages are usually least stressful to patients but require interruption in oxygen supplementation for any hands-on dealings.
- **Patients that are unresponsive to or worsening under oxygen therapy** (as assessed by pulse oximetry, blood gases, or observation of a respiratory effort that will likely result in exhaustion) are often simply denied positive pressure ventilation (PPV). Other than a closed pneumothorax, all of the problems discussed will benefit from PPV. Sedating a patient with an exaggerated increased respiratory effort in the hopes of decreasing this effort is contraindicated outside of a dynamic upper airway obstruction as discussed earlier.

Electrolyte imbalances

Electrolyte imbalances have an impact on both mortality and morbidity of critically ill patients and can present a range of issues that often requires the efforts of a multidisciplinary team approach. Just as fluid imbalances can affect the patient's electrolyte balance, electrolytes themselves can result in fluid imbalances. Electrolyte imbalances may present as simple routine therapy and intervention addressed every day (e.g. intravenous fluids and potassium supplementation). Electrolyte imbalances may present as a minor problem or represent a life-threatening emergency (e.g. severe hyperkalaemia), requiring immediate intervention.

Electrolyte laboratory testing in the emergency and critical care setting should include sodium, potassium, chloride, ionised calcium, ionised magnesium and phosphorus.

SODIUM

Sodium is the primary cation of the extracellular fluid (ECF) and it aids in maintaining the osmolality of the ECF. Osmolality (mOsm/kg) is the concentrations of osmoles in a mass of solvent. Osmoreceptors in the hypothalamus detect changes in the osmolality of the plasma and induce mechanisms to keep plasma osmolality in check (with a variance of only 2–3 mOsm/kg). Thirst and the antidiuretic hormone (ADH) system are the primary two systems that aid in controlling this. Sodium is also essential in the development of membrane potential, which is fundamental in specialised cell functions such as muscle contraction and nerve impulse transmission. Sodium level in the body is controlled by intake and output of aldosterone.

HYPERNATRAEMIA

Increased levels can be due to high salt intake, protracted vomiting or diarrhoea, severe hyperthermia, adipsia or hypodipsia, rapid ventilation or urinary obstruction. Acute elevation in extracellular sodium leads to intracellular dehydration. A patient is considered to have hypernatraemia when sodium levels are less than 160 mEq/L. Clinical signs of hypernatraemia occur with sodium levels in excess of 170 mEq/L and become severe over 180 mEq/L, causing profound neurological signs. Clinical signs include anorexia, polydipsia, weakness, myoclonus, depression, dementia, confusion, seizures, coma and death. Historical or clinical findings of high salt intake, protracted vomiting or diarrhoea, severe hyperthermia, adipsia or hypodipsia, rapid ventilation, chronic nasal discharge or urinary obstruction should direct evaluation of sodium levels.

Acute elevations of extracellular sodium concentration lead to intracellular dehydration. High sodium concentration occurs in the cerebrospinal fluid (CSF) and interferes with the Na^+/K^+-ATPase pump. Sodium is trapped within the CSF and profound neurological signs (depression, weakness, confusion, seizures, coma and finally death) can occur due to dehydration of neurons. When sodium elevation is chronic, the nervous system is initially protected by production of intracellular idiogenic osmoles that counterbalance the hyperosmolarity of the serum. This protective mechanism can be overwhelmed and, in time, neurological abnormalities become apparent.

Rapid volume replacement with a low sodium-containing fluid causes water to move from the vasculature into the CSF. In the acute patient, this causes extracellular volume overload, and in the chronic patient it causes intracellular hypervolemia. Either mechanism can elevate intracranial pressure and lead to neurological compromise. Volume deficits should be replaced slowly over 12–24 hours using normal saline, a balanced isotonic crystalloid, or half-strength saline once adequate perfusion has been restored.

Hypernatraemia commonly involves the loss of water greater than the loss of sodium from the ECF. Routes of substantial water loss include gastrointestinal (vomiting and diarrhoea), renal (diuretic therapy), glycosuria, post renal obstruction, and acute or chronic renal failure; respiratory (hyperventilation); and loss of fluids into a third body fluid space (uterus, peritoneal cavity, pleural cavity or muscle tissues). Patients losing water greater than sodium are hypovolemic when unable to maintain oral water intake.

Hyponatraemia should always be treated, regardless of severity of clinical signs. Treatment of hypernatraemic patients is often misunderstood and is always difficult, and importantly must be done slowly, requiring close monitoring in the changes in plasma osmolality throughout the duration of treatment in order to prevent negative effects in the central nervous system (CNS). The goals in treating hypernatraemia are to replace the water deficit and restore electrolyte balance.

HYPONATRAEMIA

Hyponatraemia is a sodium level less than 130 mEq/L. Decreased levels can be due to excessive water intake, inappropriate reabsorption of water in proportion to sodium or failure to reabsorb sodium by the kidneys. Clinical signs occur when sodium concentrations fall below 120 mEq/L and are severe below 110 mEq/L. Severe signs include depression, weakness, dementia, myoclonus, seizures, stupor, coma, adipsia, ileus, anorexia, vomiting, hypotension and shock. In a normal patient, the body will decrease the amount of ADH released when there is excessive sodium loss, which will aid in the dilution of urine and return of normal plasma osmolality. If there is volume loss significant enough to result in water depletion, then the above mechanisms will be overridden and ADH will be secreted. The body will reabsorb water and sodium levels will decrease further.

TREATMENT

Diagnosing the underlying disease or process, as well as increasing the serum sodium content and plasma osmolality, and normalising the fluid volume, are all goals of treating hyponatraemia. If the hyponatraemia is chronic, the treatment can be more dangerous than the imbalance. Severe, acute-onset hyponatraemia (less than 24–48 hours) requires prompt treatment due to the life-threatening conditions that can result from it, but these cases are rare. Sodium levels can be corrected at a rate of less than 10–12 mEq/L/day (0.5 mEq/L/hr). Brain dehydration that may result in osmotic demyelination may result from too rapid a correction, especially in chronic cases. Use of isotonic replacement fluids, such as 0.9% NaCl, is recommended. Serial sodium serum measurements should be performed. If the patient is hypovolaemic, restoring fluid volume often will stop the ADH response and the sodium levels will normalise so sodium levels should be closely monitored. Free water should be restricted in normovolaemic patients, and drugs causing a diuretic effect should be stopped if possible.

Chloride

Chloride is a major extracellular anion, accounting for approximately two thirds of all anions in the ECF. Normal plasma concentrations of chloride are 110–120 mEq/L in dogs and cats respectively. The intracellular content of chloride is quite variable and dependent on the resting membrane potential of that particular cell. Initial chloride production and absorption initially occurs in the gastrointestinal (GI) tract with the production of gastric juice containing large amounts of chloride. The jejunum and colon play a particularly important role in the absorption of the chloride from this gastric juice, the latter reabsorbing 90% of the chloride that enters the colon. Chloride is the primary anion concentrated and filtered in the glomerulus and is linked to sodium reabsorption by both passive and active means, with 80% of sodium being coupled with chloride during reabsorption. Once chloride is reabsorbed by the kidney, it is returned to the systemic circulation. Chloride is often an overlooked electrolyte in the critical care setting, but it is significant in different ways. Particular changes in chloride levels are consistent with particular disease processes and may help aid diagnosis, and chloride also has a major influence in acid-base status. Close attention should be given to fluids and medications administered as they, along with other factors, can affect chloride levels, and therefore acid/base status.

Potassium

Potassium is the primary intracellular cation with levels of around 140 mEq/L. Potassium concentration in ECF is only around 4 mEq/L (range 3.5–5.5 mEq/L). Therefore 98% of potassium is intracellular with only 2% existing extracellularly, so plasma levels of potassium do not reflect intracellular. Normal potassium concentrations in both the ECF and ICF are vital to maintain proper resting potential of muscle cells. The gradient between the ECF and ICF of potassium is maintained by the sodium-potassium ATP-ase pump. Potassium levels are balanced by dietary intake, distribution throughout the body, and excretion. The kidneys are ultimately responsible for maintaining this balance by excreting amounts equal to those absorbed through ingestion, but there is some regulation in the GI tract as well. From 90–95% of potassium will be excreted through the kidneys and the remaining 5–10% will be excreted through the colon. The majority of potassium is reabsorbed in the proximal tubule and loop of Henle of the kidney. Approximately 10–15% of potassium will reach the distal convoluting tubule (DCT), which will further regulate excretion of potassium. Potassium concentrations in the ICF of the cells within the DCT are similar to the levels in the rest of the body cells. Therefore when there is a total body deficit of potassium and ICF levels are low, potassium will be reabsorbed in the DCT. Alternately, when potassium levels are high in the ICF, the DCT will excrete potassium. Dietary potassium after being absorbed through the GI tract is initially translocated from the ECF to the ICF. This movement is facilitated by insulin and catecholamines. Renal excretion will then normalise these levels over the following 2 days. The flow rate in the distal tubules affects the excretion and uptake of potassium as well. When flow in the DCT decreases, the uptake from the DCT increases, leading towards hyperkalaemia. Increased flow rate in the DCT leads towards hypokalaemia. If hyperkalaemia is present aldosterone will stimulate the colon to excrete potassium. In cases of hypokalaemia, aldosterone will not be stimulated and excretion

of potassium in the DCT will be decreased, allowing more potassium to be reabsorbed. Cellular concentrations will be decreased in the skeletal muscle first, protecting the brain and cardiac muscle concentrations so that they will be minimally affected by hypokalaemia. The colon can also adapt by decreasing the secretion of potassium in the faeces.

Hyperkalaemia

Hyperkalaemia results when potassium levels become higher than normal. It is considered uncommon if the patient has a normal renal function. Cases of haemolysis, thrombocytosis or leucocytosis may result in a pseudohyperkalaemia, where serum sodium levels are elevated due to restriction of these potassium-containing cells. Hyperkalaemia due to excessive intake is unlikely since potassium is quickly redistributed by insulin into cells until the kidneys can excrete the excess. It is possible to have an iatrogenic cause of hyperkalaemia in cases where potassium supplementation is given in excessive amounts, or too rapidly. Metabolic acidosis can cause serum potassium levels to elevate due to potassium shifting out of cells in exchange for H^+ ions entering the cells for buffering. Hyperkalaemia is most commonly seen in patients with acute, anuric, or oliguric renal failure, urinary obstruction, urinary bladder rupture, hypoadrenocorticism and some GI diseases. Certain drug therapies can also cause hyperkalaemia, e.g. angiotensin-converting enzyme (ACE) inhibitors, angiotensin receptor blockers, cyclosporine, potassium-sparing diuretics (spironolactone) and non-steroidal anti-inflammatory drugs (NSAIDs). These drugs cause decreased potassium excretion.

Clinical signs. Clinical signs of hyperkalaemia are generally seen when serum potassium levels exceed 8 mEq/L. At this level muscle weakness and ECG signs can be noted. The signs seen are due to the changes in the resting membrane potential of muscle cells. The higher the potassium concentration the less negative the resting potential, becoming closer to the threshold potential. This makes the cellular membrane more excitable with a weaker action potential when the threshold is reached. If the hyperkalaemia is severe enough then the resting potential can actually drop below the threshold, leaving the cell unable to depolarise, or contract. This is clearly very dangerous considering that the cardiac muscle is especially sensitive to these effects. These are classic ECG changes noted due to hyperkalaemia, the first being peaked, narrow, high T waves. Prolongation of the PR interval can also be seen, as well as shortening of the QT interval. Changes with the T waves and QT interval are due to the abnormally rapid repolarisation in these excitable cells at mildly increased potassium levels. With increasing hyperkalaemia, the prolongation of the PR interval and widening of the QRS complex can be seen due to the conduction through the atrioventricular system being slowed. As hyperkalaemia continues to progress, flattening and widening of the P wave occurs, until potassium levels are high enough that they disappear altogether due to the cessation of atrial conduction. This leads to bradycardia with a sinoventricular rhythm. Eventually ventricular fibrillation or asystole may occur. Other effects of hyperkalaemia on muscle cells can result in diarrhoea, abdominal pain or even flaccid paralysis.

Treatment. It is always necessary to treat the underlying cause of the hyperkalaemia as of the treatment (i.e. relieving urinary obstruction). Any drugs that may be contributing to hyperkalaemia must be discontinued. If hyperkalaemia is at a non-life-threatening level (6.0–8.0 mEq/L) treatment with intravenous (IV) fluids, as well as treatment of the underlying cause, is often enough to correct the imbalance. When levels are greater than 8.0 mEq/L, or any time cardiac effects are noted (even if levels are less than 8.0 mEq/L), then further treatment should be initiated immediately. Treatments other than treating the underlying cause include IV fluid therapy, calcium gluconate 10%, dextrose/insulin administration and sodium bicarbonate (HCO_3^-). IV fluid therapy is necessary for all patients with hyperkalaemia. Use of potassium-free fluid may be indicated although the levels in most replacement fluids are still lower than serum levels, and will still help dilute potassium levels. Calcium gluconate 10% can be administered (50–100 mg/kg over 10–20 minutes) while continually monitoring the ECG of the patient. If bradycardia occurs during administration of calcium, then it should be discontinued. Calcium works quickly by antagonising the toxic effects of the hyperkalaemia on the cardiac muscle by normalising the distance between the resting and threshold potentials, allowing the cells to have normal excitability. Calcium has no direct effect on the potassium level and the beneficial effects of calcium only last for approximately 1 hour or less, so additional actions to lower potassium levels must be taken. The administration of glucose, with or without insulin, is an effective means of lowering serum potassium levels. Giving glucose stimulates insulin secretion which will move glucose, and along with it, potassium, into the cells. Glucose can be given at levels of 0.5–1 g/kg. If the patient is already hyperglycaemic, then the patient's current available endogenous insulin may be exhausted and administration of insulin should be considered. Insulin can be given at doses of 0.5–1.1 IU/kg of regular insulin as an IV bolus, directly following glucose administration, or in the patient's IV fluids. It is necessary to closely monitor the patient for hypoglycaemia following insulin administration. Administration of glucose alone will aid in lowering potassium levels within an hour. Adding insulin to this therapy will result in more of an immediate effect. Sodium bicarbonate helps potassium to shift into body cells as they replace H^+ ions moving out of cells to be buffered by the HCO_3^-. Bicarbonate therapy works within 1 hour, with effects continuing for several hours. The dosage may be 0.5–2 mEq/L IV, or in the presence of concurrent metabolic acidosis, may be calculated using the following formula:

$$\text{Measured base deficit} \times \text{Body weight (kg)} \times 0.3$$

Starting with low-dose boluses (over 10–15 minutes) that may be repeated, if necessary, is recommended in order to reassess the patient's potassium level, ECG and acid/base status. Care must be taken with HCO_3^- administration in patients with renal compromise or dysfunction. Additionally a loop diuretic may be administered (non-potassium sparing).

Hypokalaemia

Hypokalaemia results when potassium levels fall below normal levels. There are many potential causes of hypokalaemia. Increased dietary intake, increased losses through GI or renal routes and intracellular translocation can all result in hypokalaemia. Hypokalaemia can have an iatrogenic cause due to lack of administration in supplemental potassium during IV therapy. Metabolic acidosis can result in potassium translocating into cells, causing low serum values. Administration of insulin/glucose can result in potassium shifting into cells. Hypothermia

or overdosage of albuterol may also result in shifting of potassium as well. Losses from vomiting, diarrhoea, chronic renal failure losses, post-obstructive diuresis, hyperadrenocorticism or certain drug therapies (loop diuretics, penicillins) are all potential causes of hypokalaemia. The majority of critical patients will develop some degree of hypokalaemia.

Clinical signs. Clinical signs seen with hypokalaemia are mostly related to the effects on the cardiac and skeletal muscle and kidney. Muscle weakness is a common sign that develops with potassium levels that decrease to less than 3.0 mEq/L. Ventroflexion of the neck is one of the most commonly observed sign of this weakness. These patients may also have weakness in the hind end or a stiff gait. Creatinine kinase levels will elevate if potassium levels fall below 2.5 mEq/L. Rhabdomyolysis can occur when potassium levels are less than 2.0 mEq/L. Low potassium levels result in the resting membrane potential of cells becoming more negative, increasing the distance between the resting and threshold potentials. Cells have decreased excitability and repolarisation becomes prolonged. ECG changes can occur including depression of the ST segment and low amplitude of T waves. QT intervals can become prolonged and both ventricular and supraventricular arrhythmias develop. Cardiac muscle may not be responsive to Class 1 antiarrhythmic drugs such as lidocaine and procainamide. Potassium levels should be checked in patients that are unresponsive to antiarrhythmic drugs.

Treatment. Treatment for hypokalaemia involves supplementing either orally (mild hypokalaemia) or intravenously. Oral dosing of potassium gluconate (2–4 mEq/day canines; 2.5–5 mEq/L felines) divided into 2–3 doses may be effective in mild cases. It may take 7–14 days to see resolution of clinical signs. Once the imbalance is corrected it may be necessary to continue maintenance doses of potassium at 1–2 mEq/day. Some felines with chronic renal failure may require maintenance doses of 2–4 mEq/day. Serial serum potassium levels should be checked regularly. IV supplementation in fluids is necessary for patients that are anorexic or vomiting, as well as patients receiving fluid therapy for correction of dehydration or treatment of disease. Potassium chloride (KCl) is generally given diluted in IV fluids. KCl rates should not exceed 0.5 mEq/kg/hr and must be diluted prior to administration or it will result in fatal cardiac bradyarrhythmias.

Calcium

Calcium is a vital ion for many functions within the body. Processes such as muscle contraction, blood coagulation, activity of various enzymes, the excitation of neurons and secretion of various body hormones require calcium. The majority of the calcium contained in the body is in the bone (99%). The remaining 1% is in both ECF and ICF spaces. Ionised calcium (iCa^+) comprises 50% of the calcium in the ECF spaces. The remaining 40% is bound to protein and 10% chelated to lactate, citrate and bicarbonate. Intracellular calcium exists in ionised form. Body pH, levels of protein, and amounts of available chelators all affect the distribution of calcium. Acidosis will move calcium bound to proteins to an ionised form and in alkalosis this process reverses. Parathyroid hormone (PTH) influences these processes as well as vitamin D_3. PTH will increase plasma calcium levels by mobilising calcium from bone. The kidney will normally reabsorb 98% of the calcium filtered within the proximal convoluted tubule and ascending loop of Henle with the remainder being absorbed by the distal convoluted tubule as regulated by PTH. PTH can also stimulate the bone to mobilise calcium as well as inducing synthesis of calcitrol. Calcitrol primarily acts on the GI tract, stimulating it to absorb calcium. Calcitrol also provides feedback in order to limit production of itself as well as PTH. In normal patients the amount of calcium excreted each day equals the amount of calcium ingested. Calcitonin will inhibit bone reabsorption and increase the amount of calcium excreted in urine.

Hypercalcaemia

Patients with hypercalcaemia require further diagnostic testing. The majority of patients with hypercalcaemia have an underlying chronic disease. Hypercalcaemia may occur spuriously in young growing animals, in laboratory samples with haemolysis, lipaemia, due to laboratory error, or contamination of the sample. Hypercalcaemia may be found transiently in some cases of hypoadrenocorticism, with hyperproteinaemia, or haemoconcentration. Disease processes such as acute or chronic renal failure, osteomyelitis, or other skeletal disorders, toxicities of oversupplementation or rodenticide, hypoadrenocorticism, or primary hyperparathyroidism can all be causes of hypercalcaemia. Neoplasia or malignant processes of various types can also cause hypercalcaemia; the most common of note is lymphosarcoma. Multiple myeloma, anal gland adenocarcinoma, prostatic adenocarcinoma, squamous cell carcinoma, and bone neoplasia may also cause hypercalcaemia.

Clinical signs. Clinical signs of hypercalcaemia include polyuria, polydipsia (early signs), anorexia, dehydration, lethargy, weakness, vomiting, pancreatitis, chronic renal failure, constipation, cardiac arrhythmias, hypertension, twitching, seizures, acute renal failure, calcium urolithiasis and death. Symptoms vary dependent upon the duration and severity of the hypercalcaemia.

Treatment. Treatment of hypercalcaemia is based on the underlying cause of the disease; supportive care is administered for organ malfunction, as well as normalising calcium levels. The patient's condition should guide how aggressively treatment is. IV fluids are essential in aiding dilution of calcium levels, but calcium-containing fluids should be avoided. The use of loop diuretics can be helpful in promoting diuresis and promoting the excretion of calcium by interfering with its reabsorption in the loop of Henle.

Hypocalcaemia

Hypocalcaemia is more commonly seen than hypercalcaemia. Serum total calcium concentration of less than 8.0 mg/dl in dogs and less than 7.0 mg/dl in cats and ionised calcium levels of less than 1.25 mg/dl in dogs and less than 1.1 mg/dl in cats are considered to be hypocalcaemia. Low serum albumin levels can cause artificially low total calcium levels since total calcium measures both ionised (free) and protein-bound calcium. If the ionised calcium is found to be normal in a patient with a low total calcium level, there should not be any clinical signs of hypocalcaemia present. Hypocalcaemia can be seen in a number of conditions: chronic renal failure, puerperal tetany (eclampsia), acute renal failure, acute pancreatitis, hypomagnesaemia, repeated blood transfusions (citrated anticoagulant), sepsis and furosemide diuresis.

Clinical signs. Clinical signs of hypocalcaemia vary dependent on the duration and severity of the deficiency. Hypocalcaemia leads to increased cell membrane excitability. In patients with concurrent disease, the other electrolyte abnormalities present may mask the signs of hypocalcaemia. Muscle tremors, hyperexcitability, restlessness, tetany, seizures, hyperthermia, panting, anorexia, vomiting and diarrhoea can all occur. These symptoms may be episodic.

Treatment. Treatment of hypocalcaemia involves the administration of parenteral calcium in addition to any supportive care the patient may require, dependent on underlying disease and condition. Calcium gluconate or calcium chloride should be given initially IV, slowly over 10–30 minutes (0.5–1.5 ml calcium gluconate 10% slow IV). Dosing should be stopped if bradyarrhythmias occur. Initial IV doses will abate symptoms of tetany for about 1–12 hours, dependent on the underlying cause. Additional doses may be required and some patients require a Continuous rate infusion (CRI). Calcium gluconate can be given subcutaneously for repeat doses. Serial ionised calcium levels should be checked at regular intervals and supplementation stopped once the iCa^+ level is just below normal, in order not to overcompensate. Dependent on the underlying disease, the patient may require continuous vitamin D supplementation along with oral calcium supplementation.

Phosphorus

In the intracellular space, phosphate is the major anion present. Phosphorus also plays multiple vital roles in the function and structure of the cells. It is a component of ATP so it is vital for energy production, as well as other metabolic processes within the cell. Cell membranes are composed of phospholipids, so clearly phosphorus is integral to maintain cell membranes as well as being involved in oxygen delivery to the cells. Phosphate also works as a urinary buffer, regulates various enzyme activities, and more. The majority (80–90%) of total body phosphorus is present in the bone as of the bone matrix. The remaining 10–15% is in the soft tissues. Less than 1% of total body phosphorus exists in the serum. In the serum phosphorus exists in protein-bound forms (10–20%), free anionic forms, and complexed forms with sodium, magnesium or calcium. Gradual changes in phosphorus can go unnoticed as the body will compensate. Normal serum levels of phosphorus range from 2.5–6.0 mg/dl. A wide number of factors can affect the phosphorus concentration in a patient including age, diet, timing of sampling, acid/base status, presence of haemolysis, thrombocytosis, hyperproteinaemia and hyperlipidaemia.

Hyperphosphataemia

Although it is not possible to calculate total phosphorus levels in the body, serum phosphorus appears to correlate well. In some cases, serum levels may appear normal or even elevated when there is a total body phosphorus deficit. Serial levels should always be monitored. Increased phosphorus intake due to vitamin D overdose, phosphate enemas, or excess IV administration may also result in hyperphosphataemia. Most commonly it is seen in cases of renal failure, either acute or chronic, although it is more commonly seen in acute cases, due to lack of time for compensatory mechanisms to develop. Hyperphosphataemia will also develop with chronic renal failure when the glomerular filtration rate is below 20% of normal. Reduced excretion of phosphorus is also seen with uroabdomen, urethral obstruction, hypoparathyroidism and hyperthyroidism. It should also be remembered that the influences of growth hormone in young animals and laboratory error may also be the cause of hyperphosphataemia.

Clinical signs. Signs seen are dependent on the underlying cause of the hyperphosphataemia, as well as how quickly it developed. Hyperphosphataemia can result in a compensatory hypocalcaemia and clinical signs may be related to the low calcium (tetany). Hyperphosphataemia can stimulate a secondary hyperparathyroidism, which will speed the progression of renal disease. Soft tissue mineralisation can also occur.

Treatment. Identification and treatment of the underlying cause is required. Sources of phosphorus intake should be limited, e.g. low-protein diet. IV fluid therapy with 0.9% NaCl will aid in diluting the phosphorus in the ECF and will enhance renal excretion. Administration of glucose, with or without insulin, can be given in order to temporarily reduce serum phosphate concentrations via the same mechanisms as potassium. Administration of phosphate binders with meals should be utilised, as this will reduce phosphate absorption from food.

Hypophosphataemia

Serum phosphorus levels less than 2.5 mg/dl are considered hypophosphataemic. When levels drop below 1.5–1.8 mg/dl clinical signs can appear. Hypophosphataemia can occur due to a variety of mechanisms. Translocation of phosphorus can occur during treatment of diabetic ketoacidosis, increased carbohydrate loads, insulin administration, respiratory acidosis or hyperventilation, refeeding syndrome or hypothermia.

Clinical signs. Clinical signs of hypophosphataemia depend on the underlying disease process. The rate and severity of development of the hypophosphataemia will also affect the clinical signs that are seen. Signs include muscle weakness, seizures, collapse and coma.

Treatment. Ideally hypophosphataemia should be anticipated in at-risk patients. Patients being treated for diabetic ketoacidosis (DKA) and refeeding syndrome should be closely monitored. If serum phosphate levels drop to 1.5–1.8 mg/dl or less, and/or if the patient demonstrates signs consistent with hypophosphataemia, then IV phosphorus supplementation should be initiated. Malnourished patients should have food gradually reintroduced over several days. DKA patients and those receiving phosphate binders should be monitored closely. IV phosphorus supplementation is given in the form of potassium phosphate, but care should be taken not to cause iatrogenic hyperphosphataemia or hypocalcaemia. Oral administration can be considered for at-risk patients with borderline low levels using oral phosphorus supplements.

Magnesium

Magnesium is often overlooked as an ion, but in more recent years its clinical significance has been recognised. Imbalance of magnesium is now thought to be one of the most common electrolyte abnormalities encountered in small animals, if its values are measured. Magnesium is the second most abundant intracellular cation, playing an important role in multiple cellular functions. Magnesium (Mg) is an essential co-factor in a host of important biochemical processes such as enzymatic

reactions, cellular permeability and the maintenance of neuromuscular excitability. Mg and potassium homeostasis are closely related, and intracellular and extracellular concentrations of these two ions tend to change in the same direction. In the critical care setting, hypokalaemia is frequently found in association with Mg deficiency. Magnesium is important for maintenance of intracellular potassium and is second only to potassium in intracellular cation concentration. Serum and tissue magnesium levels do not correlate well but serum measurement is the most clinically useful method of magnesium evaluation. Approximately two thirds of the serum magnesium is ionised while the remainder is bound to albumin. Magnesium functions as a co-factor in many enzymatic reactions involved in the hydrolysis or transfer of phosphate groups. It participates in activating amino acids and synthesising protein, in stabilising nucleic acid, in muscle contractility and in neuronal transmission.

Hypermagnesaemia

Hypermagnesaemia is not as common as hypomagnesaemia, and generally does not have the same clinical significance. Increased levels of serum Mg can arise due to excessive intake of magnesium products (antacids and laxatives), renal failure and severe dehydration in the presence of oliguria.

Clinical signs. Clinical signs observed include CNS depression, lethargy, coma and bradycardia. Clinical signs include peripheral vasodilation, hypotension, nausea, vomiting, drowsiness, depressed deep tendon reflexes, respiratory depression, skeletal muscle paralysis, cardiac arrhythmias, coma and death. It is primarily associated with renal failure or with excessive magnesium intake.

Treatment. Therapy involves discontinuing magnesium administration and/or treating the underlying renal insufficiency. When renal function is normal, isotonic saline volume replacement and diuresis with furosemide is of benefit. Intravenous infusion of calcium will temporarily neutralise the neuromuscular effect of hypermagnesaemia.

Hypomagnesaemia

Hypomagnesaemia can result from a wide variety of factors, e.g. reduced intake due to starvation or extended IV fluid therapy and reduced absorption due to small bowel disease, chronic diarrhoea, post-intestinal resection, pancreatic insufficiency or cholestatic liver disease. Renal factors that result in increased losses of magnesium may also play a role in the development of hypomagnesaemia. Renal losses can be induced by renal disease, post-obstructive diuresis, the administration of loop diuretics or drugs with renal toxicity. Hyperthyroidism or hypoparathyroidism, osmotic diuresis, hypercalcaemia or hypophosphataemia may also increase tubular losses. Insulin administration can result in shifts of magnesium from the ECF to the ICF spaces in a manner similar to potassium and phosphorus. Shock, sepsis, trauma or hypothermia can also cause shifts and chelation of magnesium, resulting in hypomagnesaemia.

Clinical signs. Patients may not demonstrate clinical signs of hypomagnesaemia, or they may demonstrate multiple signs. Deficiency of magnesium may alter function of the Na^+/K^+-ATPase pump. This results from intracellular potassium levels decreasing, which decreases the resting membrane potential and predisposes the cardiac muscles to arrhythmias. Atrial and ventricular arrhythmias may be seen. Hypokalaemia or hypocalcaemia may remain refractory to replacement therapy in the presence of hypomagnesaemia. Hyponatraemia may also occur. Signs include muscle weakness, twitching, hyperreflexia, ataxia, mental depression, seizures, coma, anaemia, anorexia, nausea and ileus.

Treatment. Supplementation of magnesium is recommended when levels are less than 1.2–1.5 mg/dl. It may also be considered if there are clinical signs supportive of hypomagnesaemia, or other electrolyte abnormalities that suggest it. Milder cases may resolve on their own with treatment of the underlying disease process. Magnesium should be administered IV in a CRI. Lower doses should be administered for several days after the initial dose, as it is impossible to replenish the total body quickly. Patients with life-threatening arrhythmias should have a slow IV bolus of magnesium in order to raise the threshold for ventricular fibrillation.

Trauma

URINARY TRACT TRAUMA

Urinary tract trauma is a relatively uncommon occurrence; however, missing it may be life threatening, and it pays to remain aware of the possibility of this as signs of urine leakage are easily missed. These patients often appear very well initially but then show deterioration due to acute renal failure 2–3 days after the initial episode.

Urinary tract trauma should be suspected if there is:

- Pelvic injury, particularly if there is involvement of the pelvic canal
- Blunt abdominal trauma
- Bite wounds involving the caudal abdomen
- Progressive abdominal distension
- Skin necrosis or abdominal distension and swelling in the perineal area.

Most commonly urinary tract trauma involves the lower urinary tract, particularly the bladder and urethra. Fortunately injuries to the kidney and ureters are rare.

If urinary tract trauma is suspected the following protocol can be followed:

- Blood sample for electrolytes, urea and creatinine. Urinary tract trauma is usually associated with azotaemia (which can be severe; creatinine greater than 1000 mmol/L) and hyperkalaemia. In the early stages, however, these changes may not be present.
- Abdominocentesis for cytology and creatinine. Diagnosis of uroabdomen can be made by evaluating abdominal fluid for creatinine levels, as abdominal fluid (creatinine) gradient is diagnostic for uroabdomen. If the abdominal fluid has an increased creatinine level compared to blood creatinine concentrations, it is suggestive of uroabdomen (creatinine is a relatively large molecule, and as such does not equilibrate across the peritoneal membrane, whereas urea – being smaller – rapidly crosses) (also see Chapter 31).
- Cytology is usually inflammatory, and the fluid appears blood tinged but can on some occasions look like blood.

- Survey abdominal radiographs – look for retroperitoneal fluid that may suggest ureteral injury, presence of a bladder, pelvic injuries. General anaesthesia and sedation must not be undertaken until the patient is stable. A diagnosis of urinary tract trauma should be made before any further diagnostics or invasive procedures are performed.
- Stabilise the patient – see later.
- General anaesthesia may be necessary for contrast studies to identify area of leak.
- Surgical intervention may be necessary depending on cause.

Stabilisation of patients with urinary tract trauma

All patients should have an IV catheter placed and be started on isotonic crystalloid fluid therapy. Fluid should be given in boluses depending on the severity of hypoperfusion (see earlier). Not all patients will be hypovolaemic, but most of them will have some degree of dehydration and electrolyte derangements.

Patients that are hyperkalaemic will require stabilisation prior to anaesthesia. Patients with urinary tract trauma have no capacity to increase urinary tract potassium excretion (an intervention used in most cases of hypokalaemia) and so other methods of decreasing serum potassium concentration are needed.

Clinical signs associated with hyperkalaemia include bradycardia, hypoperfusion and ECG abnormalities. If the patient is showing severe compromise relating to hyperkalaemia, calcium gluconate 10% 0.5–1.5 ml/kg IV is given first. This does not lower potassium concentrations but it stabilises the threshold potential of the myocardial cells; the effect lasts for 20–30 minutes.

Neutral insulin and glucose can also be used for hyperkalaemia. Administration of 0.2–0.5 IU/kg neutral (soluble) insulin IV will lower potassium levels by 2–3 mmol/L in 20–30 minutes but will also increase the uptake of potassium and glucose into cells. There is a high risk of hypoglycaemia with this protocol; therefore all patients should be maintained on a 2.5–5% glucose infusion (made up in 0.9% saline or Hartmann's) and have their glucose concentrations monitored for at least 8 hours after administration of insulin.

Radiography

The radiographic technique will depend upon the suspected site of injury. The most useful technique is a retrograde urethrogram, as this will evaluate the whole of the urinary tract. If ureteral injury is suspected, an intravenous urogram (IVU) will be required to identify the site of leakage.

Surgery

In cases of urinary tract trauma, a useful technique is the placement of a cystostomy tube. These can be placed if there is urethral injury and can be useful in severe bladder injury. A routine caudal midline laparotomy is performed. The bladder is exteriorised and manipulated using a stay suture in the bladder apex. A mushroom-tipped catheter may be used instead of the cystostomy tube. A stab incision is made into the abdominal wall and the tube passed through it into the abdominal cavity. A purse-string suture is pre-placed in the bladder, avoiding the ureters and blood vessels. The tube is placed into the

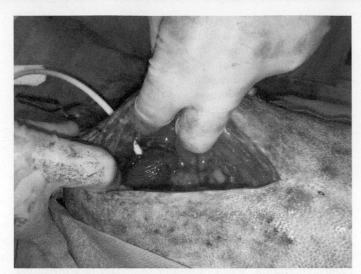

Fig. 20.7 Tube cystostomy placement

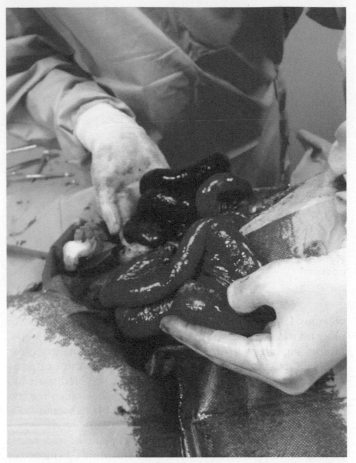

Fig. 20.8 Mesenteric torsion in a Labrador. Note the severely ischaemic large intestine

bladder via a stab incision and the purse string gently tightened to keep it in place (Fig. 20.7). A cystopexy is performed between the bladder and lateral abdominal wall; four mattress sutures usually achieves this. Finally, a Chinese finger trap suture is placed to hold the tube securely between the skin and the tube.

Cystostomy tubes should be maintained cleanly to prevent ascending infection. During the healing phase it is preferable to have them attached to a closed collection system to prevent bladder distension. Once the bladder or urethra has healed (around 14 days postoperatively), the tube can be removed by traction.

Ureteral injuries are difficult to repair and unilateral ureteronephrectomy is indicated in traumatic ureteral injury. Stenting techniques are becoming available in referral practices and may play a role in the management of these injuries in the future.

Urethral injuries may heal without surgical intervention if a urinary catheter can be placed into bladder. A cystostomy tube is necessary here as repair may take time. There is a high risk or urethral stricture formation.

Acute abdomen

Acute abdomen is the sudden onset of abdominal pain and may be caused by a wide variety of abdominal pathologies. A rapid, accurate assessment of the patient is vital in order to provide prompt treatment and prevent complications and deterioration of the patient.

Abdominal pain may arise due to displacement, inflammation, obstruction, distension, perforation, rupture or ischaemia of an intra-abdominal component. Abdominal pain can be mechanical or chemical. Mechanical causes of abdominal pain include rapid distension of hollow viscous (GDV, intestinal obstruction), rapid stretch of solid organ serosa or capsule (neoplasia, hepatic congestion, renal outflow obstruction), and mesenteric tension or traction (intestinal volvulus, gastric dilatation/volvulus, intussusception, bowel incarceration). Chemical pain usually stems from inflammatory or infectious causes such as haemorrhagic gastroenteritis, feline panleukopaenia, parvovirus, pancreatitis, haemoperitoneum, pyelonephritis, uroperitoneum or rupture of an organ within the abdominal cavity.

Differential diagnoses for acute abdominal pain include gastrointestinal pathology (ulcers, gastric dilatation/volvulus, gastritis/gastroenteritis, perforation, obstruction, intussusception, mesenteric volvulus [Fig. 20.8], acute pancreatitis or pancreatic abscess, or toxin ingestion), urinary system pathology (pyelonephritis, urethral or ureteral obstruction, urolithiasis, neoplasia, rupture), reproductive system pathology (labour/dystocia, pyometra, uterine torsion, testicular torsion), haemolymphatic or hepatic pathology (splenic torsion or rupture, biliary obstruction, acute hepatic congestion) or peritoneal cavity pathology (haemoabdomen, peritonitis, uroabdomen or blunt or penetrating abdominal wounds).

DIAGNOSTIC PLAN

Many aetiologies of acute abdomen are in danger of causing tissue necrosis and loss of function, so it is vital that the underlying cause be identified quickly in order to institute treatment and minimise more serious complications and relieve pain.

The diagnostic plan begins with a good history. The patient's signalment may be helpful in narrowing the list of rule-outs. Young animals may be more prone to foreign body ingestions or infectious diseases. GDV or splenic torsion is more likely to be seen in older, deep-chested, large-breed dogs. Pancreatitis might be suspected if the patient is an obese, middle-aged female dog or a schnauzer. German Shepherd dogs and other large or giant breeds are more likely to present with a mesenteric

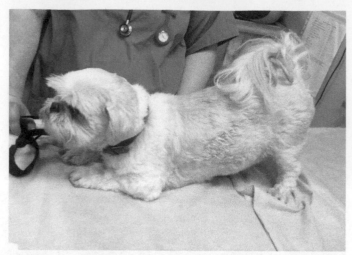

Fig. 20.9 A Lhasa Apso with pancreatitis demonstrating 'pray' position

volvulus. Linear foreign bodies are common findings in cats. An older intact female will be more likely to present with pyometra, uterine rupture, uterine torsion or dystocia, whereas older intact males should be suspected of having prostatitis or prostatic abscessation. Male cats and Dalmatians are predisposed to urolithiasis. Finally, older German Shepherds, Golden retrievers, and Labradors are more prone to present with haemoabdomen secondary to haemangiosarcoma.

Patient history should include the timescale of abdominal pain: time of onset and progression of symptoms. Evidence of GI signs should be ascertained. Distinguish regurgitation from vomiting and learn the frequency, character, duration and association with eating. Characterise diarrhoea as small or large bowel. Other symptoms should be inquired about including polyuria or polydipsia, anorexia, restlessness, panting, coughing or sneezing. The clinician should ask about the animal's dietary history, including changes in quantity or type of diet and most recent meal. Exposure to toxins, foreign objects or garbage, history of trauma, vaccination status, reproductive status, past pertinent medical history, and type, dose and duration of any medications, including owner-prescribed medications, should all be ascertained.

A thorough physical examination should be performed. The general examination should include temperature, pulse and respiration, peripheral perfusion parameters (pulse quality, mucous membrane colour, capillary refill time), respiratory effort, demeanour and posture of animal (kneeling, praying, splinting or abdominal guarding, tucked-up/arched back), hydration status, examination of oral cavity (ulcers, petechiae, string foreign bodies), musculoskeletal examination (evidence of trauma, penetrating wounds, bruising, herniation), urogenital examination (vaginal discharge, undescended testicle) and a rectal examination (prostate gland, pelvic urethra, sublumbar lymph nodes, presence of diarrhoea/melena/haematochezia) (Fig. 20.9).

The abdominal examination should include inspection, auscultation and palpation. The inspection is performed to evaluate for distension, deformity, displacement, and bruising. Clip the hair coat if needed to visualise wounds. Examine the umbilicus for red discoloration, and inspect the inguinal rings, body wall and scrotum for hernias.

Auscultation may reveal increased borborygmus (acute enteritis, acute intestinal obstruction, toxicities), decreased borborygmus (ileus, chronic obstruction, peritonitis, peritoneal fluid), or ectopic gut sounds outside the abdominal cavity (diaphragmatic hernia, body wall or inguinal ring hernias).

Palpation of the abdomen is used to detect pain, distension, organomegaly, fluid, foreign bodies, or masses. A superficial palpation should be performed first to localise pain to a region of the abdomen. This is followed by a deep palpation for detection of foreign bodies, abdominal masses, distended bowel, organomegaly or a fluid wave. Percussion and ballottement may be done for detection of abdominal fluid, fluid lines or gas-filled distended organs.

Diagnostic tests may include laboratory evaluation, radiographs, abdominocentesis or Diagnostic Peritoneal Lavage (DPL), ultrasonography, and computed tomography. The unstable patient should have a blood pressure checked to evaluate perfusion. Shock can occur secondary to acute blood loss, sepsis, endotoxaemia, fluid loss to a third body space, hypovolaemia from vomiting or diarrhoea, or GDV. In these cases, it may be pertinent to run an ECG or a pulse oximeter to evaluate for life-threatening abnormalities that often accompany acute abdominal pathology. Any life-threatening complications should be addressed aggressively and early.

Laboratory evaluation includes an immediate determination of the patient's PCV, total solids, BUN, blood glucose, serum electrolytes and blood lactate. Hypoglycaemia may be an indicator of sepsis, whereas hyperglycaemia may be seen with pancreatitis, some toxicities or patient stress. An elevated PCV may be seen with dehydration or Haemorrhagic Gastro Enteritis (HGE), and a low PCV may indicate haemorrhage (splenic rupture, severe GI haemorrhage or ulceration, hepatic neoplasia). Low protein concentration can be due to lack of production or loss due to haemorrhage or to GI, renal or peritoneal disease.

A complete blood cell count may help determine the presence of infectious or inflammatory diseases. Leucocytosis may be seen in these cases, and bands indicate a more severe process. Leucopaenia can follow decreased production, sequestration, or a viral infection. Platelet count should be evaluated, as a low platelet count can be an indication of DIC or other primary haemostatic abnormalities.

Electrolyte abnormalities are common secondary to vomiting, third spacing, anorexia and diarrhoea. Hyperkalaemia may be associated with urinary tract obstruction or rupture, or acute nephritis.

Serum biochemical analysis can help diagnose specific organ involvement. Hepatic enzyme concentration may be increased because of hepatic injury, hypoxia, pancreatitis, GI disease or sepsis. Increased amylase and lipase may raise suspicion of pancreatic disease or renal disease. Azotaemia may be pre-renal, renal, or post-renal (pyelonephritis, ureteral or urethral obstruction, ruptured urinary tract, GI bleed).

A venous blood gas may reveal a hypochloraemic metabolic alkalosis associated with stomach or upper GI obstruction. Often a metabolic acidosis is present due to lactic acidosis from hypoperfusion or diarrhoea. A urinalysis should be performed to look for casts, renal tubular cells, infection, crystalluria, and concentration ability. Other tests to consider could include arterial blood gas analysis, coagulation studies, and blood or urine cultures.

Radiographs should be obtained in any animal with acute abdominal pain. Examine all the intra-abdominal organs for density, shape, size and location. Examine the abdominal walls for integrity to rule out herniation or rupture. Also evaluate for retroperitoneal pathology, including streaking ventral to the lumbar vertebra. Free gas in the peritoneal cavity suggests intestinal rupture or the presence of gas-forming organisms. Intestinal obstruction should be suspected if there is segmental gaseous or fluid distension of the small bowel. Generalised small bowel distension suggests ileus or a very low GI obstruction. Other radiographic abnormalities may include generalised loss of abdominal detail that may indicate lack of fat, free abdominal fluid, pancreatitis, or large masses. Pancreatitis might be suspected if there is loss of detail in the right cranial quadrant with lateral displacement of descending duodenum.

Contrast radiography can also be performed. Tests may include double contrast gastography, positive contrast studies of the GI tract, barium enema, excretory urography or cystourethrograph. Water-soluble contrast agents should be used if bowel perforation is suspected. Upper GI contrast studies should be avoided if vomiting or aspiration is likely. Thoracic radiographs should be performed, especially if there is any suspicion of neoplasia.

Abdominocentesis or diagnostic peritoneal lavage may be indicated if there is loss of serosal detail on abdominal radiographs, penetrating abdominal injury without obvious peritoneal entry wounds, signs of abdominal injury after blunt trauma, persistent abdominal pain of unknown cause or postoperative complications.

Reproductive emergencies

Many of the reproductive abnormalities that present as emergencies are relatively straightforward and fairly easy to resolve. Effective treatment of these diseases, however, does require knowledge of the underlying pathophysiology as well as the options available for dealing with such emergencies.

DYSTOCIA

Appropriate management of dystocia requires that the client be well educated and able to recognise signs of impending problems. Once dystocia does occur, there is typically a small window of opportunity in order to save the unborn puppies and kittens.

Signs of foetal distress

- **Vaginal discharge:** Off-coloured discharge (green, red or brown) from the vagina prior to whelping is a sign of foetal distress. If discharge is seen an emergency Caesarean section should be performed if the goal is to have as many live puppies as possible.
- **More than 2 hours between stage 1 and 2 labour:** If a bitch takes longer than 2 hours between the initiation of labour and the birth of the first puppy. Veterinary attention sought and then cesarean.
- **A puppy becomes lodged in the birth canal:** A small birth canal can result from healed pelvic fractures, vaginal strictures, vaginal prolapse, etc. The puppies may be too big to pass through a normal-sized canal. In some breeds, such as the bulldog, the conformation of the breed is such that the wide-bodied, wide-headed pups frequently cannot pass through the pelvis. Bulldogs also have poor uterine contractility. Caesarean

section is routinely done in these breeds. When litters are very small (one or two pups) the pups may become too large to pass easily through the canal. Foetal monsters and anasarcous foetuses may also cause problems.
- **More than 1 hour passes between puppies:** If a bitch is in active labour and more than 1 hour passes between puppies, the bitch should be examined to determine if a puppy is malpositioned or any other problems exist.

A physical examination of the bitch should be performed in order to identify any systemic illness that might contribute to a difficult birthing such as anaemia from torn uterine vessels or sepsis from a uterine rupture. A digital vaginal examination should then be performed in order to detect obstructions or the presence of a wedged foetus. Radiographs may be helpful to evaluate foetal size and number, and any possible abnormalities of the pelvic canal. Although an uncommon cause of dystocia, serum calcium and glucose should be measured to detect low concentrations, which may prevent adequate contractions.

Dystocia due to failure of the uterus to push the foetus into the birth canal can be divided into primary uterine inertia and secondary uterine inertia. Primary uterine inertia is recognised by lack of abdominal straining. In some instances when the litter is small, parturition does not occur normally. It is thought that this may arise because there is not enough hormonal stimulation from the small number of foetuses to induce the normal process of parturition. Diagnosis of primary uterine inertia is based on the failure of parturition to occur within the expected period. Secondary uterine inertia follows a period of apparently normal labour, which then ceases. Diagnosis is based on the lack of labour, without problems involving the birth canal (no impingements, no stuck puppies).

Treatment

If there is absolute foetal oversize or inadequate pelvic diameter, a Caesarean section should be performed. If there is only one large pup wedged in the canal, manipulation can be attempted. In some cases gentle traction and the addition of lubrication will allow the foetus to pass. In many cases, however, this approach is unsuccessful.

In cases of secondary uterine inertia plasma glucose and calcium should be measured, if possible, to find whether there is a deficiency. Supplementation should only be given in cases with a documented deficiency. Treatment is administration of oxytocin. If no active contraction is seen within 20 minutes the dose can be repeated. If no puppy is born after two doses of oxytocin then a Caesarean section is indicated. Oxytocin should not be used in cases of narrowed birth canal, foetal malpositioning and foetal oversize.

PYOMETRA

Pyometra is an endocrine-related disease in the bitch. Although a bacterial infection is involved, it is the presence of progesterone (during dioestrus) that has allowed the disease to occur. Pyometra occurs almost exclusively in bitches in the 2 months following oestrus (during the luteal phase). The cause is related to progesterone-induced excess glandular activity, low myometrial activity and cervical closure, causing accumulation of secretions that allow bacterial overgrowth. The most common bacteria involved is *E. coli*. The source of infection is probably the vagina, as this is a common inhabitant. Oestrogen enhances the effects of progesterone and in this way may increase the chances of pyometra.

History and clinical signs

Pyometra is most commonly seen in older bitches, but may occur in young bitches. The pertinent history is that the bitch was in heat within the last 2–3 months. Signs can occur as early as the end of oestrus. Bloody or purulent discharge is usually noted by the owner. In some cases there is no discharge (closed-cervix pyometra). In these cases the bitch presents not as a reproductive problem (vulvar discharge) but as a systemic medical problem. The most common clinical sign is polyuria/polydipsia. Pyometra should always be ruled out in any intact female that is ill. Systemic signs of disease may not be demonstrated, but commonly depression, anorexia, polyuria, polydipsia or vomiting is observed. Clinical signs of illness are more common in a closed-cervix pyometra. Untreated, pyometra leads to worsening dehydration, endotoxaemia, shock, coma and ultimately death.

Diagnosis

Ultrasonography is diagnostic; a fluid-filled uterus is seen dorsal to the bladder and extending into the abdomen. Radiology is less sensitive, but may document the shadow of a large uterus. WBC count is usually elevated; however, in some cases of open cervix pyometra, the WBC count can be normal.

Treatment

Fluid therapy should be instituted in order to correct dehydration or shock, if present. Ovariohysterectomy is the treatment of choice. In the severely ill animal, the uterus is the source of the endotoxaemia, and it must be removed as soon as possible. Surgery should be performed as soon as the animal is rehydrated and is cardiovascularly stable.

If the bitch's reproductive potential is of great importance to the owner, medical management may be attempted. Medical management should not be attempted in the severely ill bitch. Additionally, medical management is not as successful and has a higher complication rate in bitches with closed-cervix pyometra. It is generally recommended to limit medical management to those bitches with open cervix pyometra that are not systemically ill.

MASTITIS

Mastitis occasionally occurs in lactating bitches and rarely in queens. The condition may range from hard, painful, enlarged mammary glands due to galactostasis to abscessed or gangrenous mammary glands with accompanying septic shock. In general, pups should be allowed to nurse unless the infected glands are necrotic or the bitch is systemically ill. Continued nursing will avoid galactostasis and will aid drainage. Hot packing the affected glands will also promote drainage. In severe cases, the pups should be removed and necrotic glands should be surgically lanced, drained, flushed and debrided.

UTERINE PROLAPSE

Uterine prolapse occurs during parturition when the cervix is open. It is more common in cats than dogs. External reduction should be attempted as soon as possible, because the longer the tissue is exposed, the more likely that severe oedema and

tissue necrosis will occur. The patient should be anaesthetised and sterile lubricant applied liberally to the exposed tissue. The uterine horn is flushed with sterile saline under pressure. Mannitol or hypertonic saline can be used to reduce oedema if necessary before attempting reduction. Once the uterus is replaced, the animal should be given 5–10 units of oxytocin intramuscularly to cause uterine involution. If the uterus stays in for 24 hours, further risk of prolapse is unlikely because the cervix should be closed. If the tissue is damaged or necrotic, ovariohysterectomy is recommended. Internal reduction of the prolapse can usually be achieved through a ventral abdominal incision. In some cases, reduction is impossible due to extreme engorgement of the prolapsed tissue. In these cases, the external segment can be amputated followed by ovariohysterectomy.

Paediatric patients

Paediatric patients (puppies and kittens) are often presented as emergencies and it is our task to recognise rapidly the underlying problems so that stabilisation can be promptly initiated. It is often easy to forget that crucial differences exist between a neonatal/paediatric patient and an adult patient in regards to the evaluation and interpretation of the cardiovascular, respiratory and neurological parameters, in the haematology and biochemistry parameters and in the drug therapy metabolism. It is therefore vitally important for veterinary staff to have the ability to recognise and be aware of these differences when dealing with neonatal or paediatric patients.

In veterinary medicine the term 'neonate' usually encompasses birth to 2 weeks of age and the term 'paediatric' refers to animals less than 6 months of age.

In the foetal circulatory system the blood is shunted past lungs that are non-functioning via the ductus arteriosus, located between the left pulmonary artery and the ascending aorta. During intrauterine life foetal respiration occurs via a blood-gas exchange process across the placenta. Only in the last days before birth is the production of surfactant in the lungs stimulated. When the umbilical cord is separated at birth, great changes occur in the respiratory and cardiovascular system; the navel circulation stops and this event creates a state of severe hypoxia. At the same time there is an increase in peripheral resistance in the peripheral vessels of the neonates. The sense of dyspnoea will allow the first chest contraction and the creation of a negative pressure within the lungs that will allow air to enter the lungs. The increase in oxygen tension will allow the ductus arteriosus to narrow and the pulmonary vessels to dilate. The closure of the ductus usually occurs 2–5 days after birth.

Normal puppies and kittens spend the majority of the day sleeping. When awake they should be able to respond to odour, touch and pain. They should demonstrate a strong suckle reflex, as well as rooting and righting reflexes. Withdrawal reflex should be present, although it may be slightly delayed. Pupillary light reaction should be present around 10–20 days of age and vision is normal by 30 days. Paediatric puppies and kittens have a more developed neurological system and neurological examination can be performed around 6–8 weeks of age, when the postural reaction should be present.

Normal heart rate for a neonate is usually around 200–220 bpm in the first week of life. In comparison to an adult, a new born has a decreased stroke volume and peripheral vascular resistance and a lower blood pressure (around 49 mm Hg at 1 month of age; it normalises around 9 months of age). It maintains its perfusion by having a much higher heart rate, cardiac output, plasma volume and central venous pressure.

The baroreflex control of the circulation is not fully developed because of incomplete autonomous innervations of heart and vessels; myocardial contractility is also limited. The neonate's heart rhythm is usually a normal sinus as the vagal reflex develops only around 8 weeks of age. It is important to remember that in the first 4–5 days of age neonates respond to hypoxemia with bradycardia (up to 45 bpm) and hypotension: for this reason a heart rate around 150 in a neonate should be suggestive of a serious underlying disease.

Paediatric patients have an increased heart rate compared to adult cats and dogs and a much lower blood pressure. The heart rate decreases around 4 weeks of age as soon as the parasympathetic system fully develops. Normal respiratory rate in a neonate is around 15–35 bpm. The respiratory rate is similar to that of an adult's at 4 weeks of age. The neonate is susceptible to relative hypoxemia because of a large metabolic oxygen requirement and immaturity of carotid body chemoreceptors. Furthermore the neonate requires a much higher work of breathing in order to maintain a normal tidal volume when compared to an adult, because of a higher compliance of his thoracic wall. This factor is important to remember as any respiratory disorder that shortens inspiratory duration has a potential to negatively affect gas exchange.

At birth, the GI tract is sterile and characterised by a neutral gastric pH and a time-dependent increased permeability of the intestinal mucosa, which decreases dramatically after 10 hours. The motility of the GI tract is affected by the presence of food and especially by body temperature; temperature less than 34.4°C is associated with GI stasis and paralytic ileus.

The kidney function and development is not complete in neonates, and nephrogenesis continues for at least 2 weeks after birth. Glomerular filtration rate (GFR) is decreased, as is rate of tubular secretion, reaching adult level at 8 weeks of age. Autoregulation of renal blood flow (RBF) and GFR in neonatal puppies appears to be relatively inefficient in response to rapid changes in systemic arterial blood pressure. In the adult dog, the renin-angiotensin system is an important regulatory mechanism; however, in the neonate RBF is directly correlated with arterial pressure and does not seem to be altered by inhibition of the angiotensin until approximately 6 weeks of age. Caution must be exercised when administering renally excreted or metabolised antimicrobials (penicillin, ampicillin, cephalosporins, fluoroquinolones and aminoglycosides) to neonates and paediatric patients.

Neonate puppies and kittens have an immature liver function; they have limited glycogen stores and their gluconeogenesis is impaired. Hepatic stores will be depleted after 24 hours and hypoglycaemia will ensue. Furthermore neonates have poorly developed microsomal and P450 enzyme activity until 4–5 months of age; caution must be exercised when using medications that require hepatic metabolism or excretion.

Normal body temperatures in the neonates are 35–37.2°C (week 1) and 36–37.8°C (weeks 2 and 3). At weaning, rectal temperature approaches that of the adult.

Thermoregulation in neonates is also difficult as they are unable to shiver and they show poor peripheral vasoconstriction in response to hypothermia. Neonates are also unable to pant; they have a poor blood flow to the periphery and little body fat, therefore they are unable to respond properly to hyperthermia.

When approaching a sick neonate or paediatric patient, a good physical examination is paramount, as in an adult dog, following the ABCD approach, but bearing in mind the important differences in heart rate, blood pressure and respiratory rate.

Sick neonates and paediatric patients should also be checked for body temperature, congenital defects, presence of open fontanels, and presence and patency of the anus and urinary tract.

A minimum database should include evaluation of the haematocrit, total protein, blood glucose, urine specific gravity and electrolytes. When interpreting haematological and biochemistry parameters, care should be given not to use the same reference range as in adult dogs and cats.

HAEMATOLOGY

Packed cell volume (PCV) tends to be high at birth, decreases over the first weeks of life, and then increases again to reach the adult values. Due to changes from foetal to adult haemoglobin and from a transplacental to a pulmonary respiration, in puppies PCV drops from 47.5% to 29.9% over the first 4 weeks of life, then increases to reach adult values at 12 weeks of age. In kittens, PCV drops from 35% at birth to 27% at 4 weeks and has reached the normal 35% by 16 weeks of age. In both puppies and kittens, haemoglobin concentration is roughly one third of the PCV value in adults. Because of the small blood volume (due to the patient's small size) and the fact that anaemia is often present, it might be advisable to administer a blood transfusion before the haematocrit reaches critical levels (at or below 15%), particularly if frequent sampling is anticipated. Given the small size of these patients, the volumes needed are usually small, and one should avoid raising the PCV well over the expected normal value. Platelets are fully functional from birth, and their numbers are similar to those seen in adults. In puppies, leucocyte count stays stable at around $12\,000 \times 10^9$ cells/l for the first 8 weeks, with lymphocytes peaking on day 21, believed to be related to increased antibody formation. In kittens, leucocyte count increases from 9600×10^9 cells/l at birth to $23\,000 \times 10^9$ cells/l at 8–9 weeks of age and then decreases to $19\,700 \times 10^9$ cells/l at 16 weeks of age.

SERUM BIOCHEMISTRY

There are several differences in biochemistry values between paediatric and adult patients. Albumin concentration is low at birth and gradually increases to reach normal levels by 8 weeks of age. During this gradual increase in concentration, its effects in colloid oncotic pressure and drug binding will also change. Globulins are low at birth, and during the neonatal period are mostly maternal in origin (ingested as colostrum). By the end of the infant period (8 weeks) they have reached adult levels. Alanine aminotransferase, γ-glutamyl transferase and bilirubin are elevated during the neonate and infant period and should be within adult reference levels by the end of the juvenile period. Cholesterol, on the other hand, will be low and gradually increase to reach adult levels before 12 weeks of age. While liver function and therefore bile acids are expected to be normal at 8 weeks of age, the presence of increased bilirubin may preclude their use as a diagnostic tool. Blood urea nitrogen and creatinine are low at birth and gradually increase as the kidneys mature, reaching adult levels at the time of full development by 8–12 weeks of age. Hypokalaemia is a common finding due to increased potassium losses by the immature kidneys. During skeletal development, puppies and kittens have increased calcium and an increased calcium/potassium ratio. The increases will be more significant in ionised calcium than in total calcium. Alkaline phosphatase also tends to be elevated during skeletal growth, increases that can last until full body growth has been achieved (over 1 year in large-breed dogs). In dogs, lactate is higher in neonates and infants, and concentration falls to reach the adult levels at approximately 2 months of age. There are no published data for kittens, although it is thought that the same phenomenon may occur. Nevertheless, the magnitude of the increases is small, so, from the clinical perspective, adult reference values can be used in most instances.

Differences in acid-base balance exist between puppies/kittens and adults. Neonatal puppies, but not kittens, have an impaired ability to increase renal ammoniagenesis in response to an acid environment when compared with adults. By 3 weeks of age, most amino acids are reabsorbed in puppies, and by 7 weeks of age adult patterns of amino acid reabsorption are evident.

Coagulation assessments are limited in neonates, but seem to fall within the normal adult reference ranges for prothrombin time (PT), activated partial thromboplastin time (aPTT) and fibrinogen in animals as young as 8 weeks of age.

URINALYSIS

Urine is isosthenuric until approximately 9–10 weeks of age (1.006–1.0017), and the detection of protein, glucose and various amino acids because of the immaturity of the proximal tubule is normal. By 3 weeks of age, urine protein and glucose concentrations approach those of the adult dog, and urine concentration is expected to compare with that of the adult dog by 6–8 weeks of age.

Toxicities

Accidental toxic exposures are common presentations in small animal practice, and it is important that veterinary staff are familiar with the effects of common toxicities.

When an owner calls with a patient that has a suspected toxin ingestion, it is vitally important to obtain as much information as possible. This should include the estimated weight of the patient, and have the owner bring the packaging (or ideally inform you of the toxin details over the phone ahead of arrival), so a drug and estimated dosage can be calculated. Many common medications and chemicals have a telephone number you or the owners can call for toxicological information.

The general approach to any toxin ingestion should include the following:
  a. Treat the life-threatening problem.
  b. Obtain your samples/database.
  c. Eliminate further exposure (varies depending on route of exposure).
  d. Promote excretion, or metabolism to a non-toxic compound.
  e. Administer antidote if available.
  f. Provide supportive care.
As with any emergency presentation, it is critical that you perform a primary assessment when the patient arrives. The primary assessment includes airway, breathing, circulation, level of consciousness and level of pain. Any abnormalities in

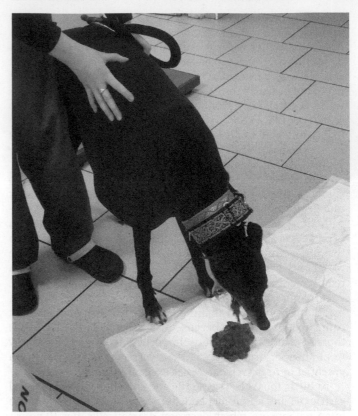

Fig. 20.10 Emesis in a Greyhound following chocolate ingestion

these should be treated first, regardless of the toxin ingested. Life-threatening problems may include respiratory difficulty, shock, seizures, arrhythmias and many other signs, all of which should be treated immediately.

Ideally, it is important to obtain your emergency database and laboratory samples prior to any treatment that is performed – although this is not always possible. This is important as some treatments interfere with testing (as an example, diazepam is suspended with propylene glycol which will cause a false-positive ethylene glycol test).

Eliminating further exposure should include bathing the pet if it is a topical medication (e.g. permethrins in cats). For ingested toxins, induction of emesis may be performed (Fig. 20.10).

Emesis can be a dangerous procedure, and it should be induced under the direction of the veterinary surgeon. Contraindications to emesis are noted later. Emesis itself may result in a vasovagal response that may require intubation, ventilation, IV fluids and parasympatholytic agents. Emesis may also result in aspiration pneumonia. Apomorphine is an effective agent to induce vomiting in the dog, but emesis is much more difficult to induce in cats. In cats xylazine can be administered IV, but can cause profound sedation, potentially increasing the risk for aspiration pneumonia. Yohimbine should be available as a reversal agent. Hydrogen peroxide and salt solutions are sometimes recommended but have toxic principles themselves, including mucosal injury and salt toxicity, respectively, so are not recommended.

Contraindications to inducing emesis include:
  • **Patient-related factors,** e.g. respiratory distress, seizures, neurological impairment, bradycardia, weakness,

rabbits/rodents, inability to protect airway, oesophageal and/or GI disease (including recent surgery or foreign body ingestion)
- **Toxin-related factors,** e.g. caustic substances, acids and alkali agents.

Gastric lavage can be performed but requires general anaesthesia and intubation to protect the airway. Gastric lavage also carries the risks of damage to the GI tract and aspiration pneumonia. Finally, charcoal and cathartics may be used to eliminate further absorption of the compound. For some toxins, charcoal should be repeated several times due to entero-hepatic recirculation; for other toxins, charcoal may not be effective.

Enhancing elimination should be performed as well through a forced diuresis (if the compound is excreted through the kidneys). If a specific antidote is available, then this should also be administered.

Finally, supportive care for the patient should be instituted; this can vary substantially based on the toxic agent involved and the clinical signs demonstrated by the patient. Examples may include IV fluids, anti-emetics, oxygen, gastro-protectants, etc.

COMMON TOXICITIES

Chocolate/methylxanthines/theobromines

Theobromine is the toxin found in chocolate; it is a xanthine derivative. The higher the cocoa solids content of the chocolate, the higher the levels of theobromine. A fatal dose is 100–250 mg/kg; this represents 6 g/kg of plain chocolate. Common systems affected include GI (vomiting/diarrhoea), cardiovascular (tachycardia/ventricular premature contractions [VPCs]/tachypnoea/hypertension) and CNS (hyperactivity/restless/tremors/seizures). Clinical signs include hyperactivity, tachycardia, convulsions and arrhythmias. Absorption is slow, so emesis is useful even a few hours after ingestion.

Treatment involves emesis, charcoal, IV diuresis (with or without urinary catheter to decrease resorption) and specific treatment for muscle tremors and arrhythmias. Seizures may be controlled with diazepam or for refractory cases, phenobarbital, pentobarbital or propofol.

Non-steroidal anti-inflammatory drugs (NSAIDs)

NSAIDs are a commonly seen toxicity within veterinary practice, either via ingested human medication, e.g. ibuprofen, or from accidental overdose or ingestion of veterinary preparations. NSAIDs inhibit the cyclooxygenase (I and II) of the arachidonic acid pathway, resulting in a decreased blood flow to, and mucous production in, the GI tract and kidneys, and can result in GI ulceration, perforation and renal failure. Aspirin additionally inhibits the formation of thromboxane, which results in decreased platelet function. Acetaminophen in cats results in methemoglobinaemia and liver failure from toxic compounds binding to cellular macromolecules.

The most common signs are related to the GI tract (vomiting, gastritis, gastric and duodenal ulceration) and nephrotoxicity (interstitial nephritis, papillary necrosis, acute and chronic renal failure).

Treatment typically involves gastric decontamination (induction of emesis), the limiting the absorption (administration of activated charcoal), and a 48-hour forced diuresis. Gastroprotectants (proton pump inhibitors, H2-receptor antagonists) should be administered as indicated. For acetaminophen intoxication, N-acetylcysteine and cimetidine are indicated to decrease formation of toxic metabolites. Aggressive supportive care is often indicated in acetaminophen toxicity in cats, such as oxygen, and administration of transfusions and/or haemoglobin-based oxygen carriers (HBOCs).

Rodenticides

Ingestion of anticoagulants is commonly seen within veterinary practice. The owner may observe the animal eating the bait, or may notice the bait is missing, or some cases will be presented due to clinical signs of coagulopathy 1–3 days after ingestion.

Rodenticides inhibit the coagulation factors II, VII, IX and X as well as the anti-coagulation factors protein C and protein S. This inhibition results in coagulopathies. Clinical signs vary based on the location of haemorrhage, and usually take more than 2 days after the ingestion to develop. Coagulation profiles should be run if possible (it is preferable to use peripheral veins, and caution should be used when drawing blood from jugular veins as haematomas and haemorrhage may result). Emergency management varies depending on the location of haemorrhage (pharyngeal, intrathoracic, abdominal, etc.). To control haemorrhage, frozen or fresh frozen plasma (or whole blood if necessary) should be administered. A specific antidote, vitamin K_1, should be administered as well, and its administration may need to be continued for weeks. With presentation of patients with recent ingestion (less than 6 hours), emesis, charcoal and monitoring of coagulation profiles (in 48–72 hours) is an acceptable alternative to treating with vitamin K_1.

Many rodenticides are commercially available, so it is important to determine whether the toxin is a first-generation drug (e.g. warfarin) or a more modern (and more effective) second-generation drug (e.g. brodifacoum).

Ethylene glycol

Ethylene glycol is a major constituent of antifreeze; toxic doses in the cat are as little as 1.5 ml/kg, and 4–6 ml/kg in the dog. It is relatively rapidly absorbed, metabolised and excreted. Classically, there are three stages of clinical signs. In the first stage (30 min–4 hours), signs include ataxia, incoordination and Polyuria/Polydipsia (PU/PD); usually the patient recovers from these. The second stage (12–24 hours) involves anorexia, depression, GI signs, hypothermia and coma from metabolic acidosis (in humans, cardiovascular signs predominate). In the final stage (greater than 24–72 hours), oliguric or anuric renal failure ensues. Diagnosis can be difficult as it can mimic other multi-system illnesses such as acute renal failure, acute gastroenteritis, pancreatitis and DKA. The animal will often be azotaemic with a low calcium level (oxalate is a metabolite of ethylene glycol and will combine with available calcium to form calcium oxalate). Ethylene glycol can be detected using specialised assays, but many other compounds can cause false positives (ethanol, propylene glycol, sorbitol [in many charcoal products]). Treatment includes induction of emesis for recent ingestions, supportive care (IV diuresis), dialysis and drugs that decrease toxic metabolism of ethylene glycol which include ethanol in the UK (dogs and cats) or 4 methylpyrazole, available in the USA (dogs only). Ethanol is an antidote if given within 24 hours of ingestion – as ethanol has a much higher affinity for alcohol dehydrogenase, it blocks the metabolism of ethylene glycol into its harmful metabolites. If continued for 2 days, this allows the body to excrete the ethylene glycol unchanged. Antiemetics and other supportive care are also indicated.

Grapes/raisins

An emerging toxic agent in dogs that has resulted in renal failure with as little as 3–57 g/kg is grapes or raisins. The toxic principle is not known at this time but possible causes include tannins, mycotoxins or excess vitamin D intake.

Early signs are diarrhoea, anorexia and lethargy followed by acute renal failure up to 24–72 hours after ingestion. Treatment includes GI decontamination (digestion of raisins is slow), followed by activated charcoal. A 48-hour forced diuresis is recommended. Supportive care for renal failure is indicated if it develops.

Xylitol

Xylitol is a common sweetener used in sugar-free chewing gum, cakes, sweets, medications and other products, which can result in an insulin release in dogs and subsequent hypoglycaemia (and hypokalaemia). Treatment involves decontamination (emesis, with or without activated charcoal, more for its cathartic ingredients rather than the charcoal itself) with a recent ingestion, and support for hypoglycaemia (which clinically rarely lasts longer than 12–24 hours) should include glucose (infusions) and frequent feedings. Hepatic necrosis has been seen in dogs with several proposed mechanisms so liver function should be monitored (often with a recheck of liver enzymes or chemistry panel) and treated as necessary. The patient may also develop a coagulopathy that will require infusion of fresh frozen plasma.

Wounds

Definitive wound management may need to be delayed as the treatment of life-threatening injuries takes priority. Emergency management should prevent any additional injury and minimise contamination. Open wounds may be covered with a sterile dressing until the patient is stabilised. Many patients may be in pain from their injuries, so appropriate analgesia is important. Fractious patients may require sedation or general anaesthesia for wound evaluation to be performed.

WOUND CLASSIFICATION

The following parameters can be used to classify wounds:
- Aetiology
- Nature and extent of the skin deficit
- Degree of bacterial contamination
- Extent of the trauma to the surrounding tissues.

TYPES OF WOUNDS

Abrasions

Abrasion wounds are the result of friction applied approximately parallel to the external surface of the skin. This friction usually results in the removal of variable amounts of the epidermis, dermis and hypodermis. In small animal practice these wounds are commonly seen as a result of road traffic accidents, e.g. where the animal has become trapped between the road surface and the moving vehicle. Such wounds are consequently frequently heavily contaminated with bacteria, and the frictional nature of the injury means that the bacteria and debris from the road surface are deeply embedded within the upper layers of the wound. Abrasion wounds may also be seen as a result of poorly fitting casts and bandages, or from the abnormal wear of the patient's pads following prolonged contact with rough surfaces or due to a patient weight bearing on areas other than the pads.

The effective debridement of these wounds is of paramount importance. As previously mentioned the debris from the debriding road surface is often deeply embedded within the wound combined with the fact that abrasion wounds frequently result in an extensive tissue deficit. These wounds are often located on the distal limbs resulting in reconstruction being challenging with skin grafting or open wound management being the only options for closure.

Degloving wounds

Degloving injuries are caused when the skin is torn from the underlying tissues, usually from a limb.

Mechanical degloving occurs where the overlying tissue is torn from the subdermal plexus, e.g. following road traffic accidents. Physiological degloving occurs when the skin is sheared from the subcutaneous tissues therefore resulting in damage to the local blood supply and ischaemia of the area; this results in necrosis and sloughing of the skin over the following days. Secondary bacterial contamination frequently occurs with this physiological sloughing.

Avulsion injuries

Avulsion injuries refer to the forcible separation of tissues from their underlying attachments. Avulsion injuries frequently occur following dog bite wounds or road traffic accidents where the skin and subcutaneous tissue is avulsed from the mandible, resulting in the exposure of the underlying bone.

Shearing

Shearing injuries have a similar aetiology to degloving wounds. They represent a combination of degloving and abrasion injuries and are frequently seen following road traffic accidents, with the wounds usually located on the patient's distal limb, particularly on the medial aspect of the carpus, phalanges and tarsometatarsal joint.

Shearing injuries tend to be deeper than abrasion injuries and may involve the underlying joints. Like abrasion injuries, large areas of tissue may be involved and will be heavily contaminated with foreign material, e.g. gravel and bacteria.

Shearing wounds tend to be extensive, deep and as a result a prolonged period of open wound management is often necessary. There may also be concurrent damage to the underlying joints and supporting soft tissue structures (tendons and ligaments) which may require external support of the joint during this period and ultimately prosthetic and replacement of ligaments.

In severe cases, salvage of the joint is not possible and therefore arthrodesis (surgical fusion of a joint) must be performed. In more severe cases, salvage of the limb is impossible and amputation will be necessary.

Incisional

These wounds are most commonly seen in practice as intentional surgical wounds but they can also be caused by trauma. These wounds may be caused by a sharp object, e.g. piece of glass or a metal shard moving in a plane parallel to the skin surface. These wounds typically have clean, regular edges, which will gape open because of the inherent elasticity of the adjacent skin.

There is often relatively little involvement of the skin, either side of the wound, but the incision itself may be long and there may be extensive damage to the deeper tissues, e.g. muscle and tendons, nerves and blood vessels, which may not be detected on first inspection. This highlights how important it is to surgically explore these wounds for signs of further damage.

Contamination of such wounds is likely to be less than for abrasions. In addition sharp trauma results in more bleeding, which will have an irrigating effect, thereby reducing contamination.

These wounds may be suitable for debridement and primary closure. However, delayed primary closure may be preferable if the wound is more than a few hours old or contamination is a concern.

Puncture wounds

Puncture wounds are caused by a sharp object, e.g. stick or metal railing, moving in a plane perpendicular to the skin surface. Penetrating wounds refer to those which have an entrance wound only, whereas perforating injuries refer to those with both an entrance and an exit wound.

The typical bite injury comprises the obvious, small puncture wound, which is usually of little significance, and the trauma to the deeper tissues, which is unseen and of much greater significance.

Animal bite wounds, in which the skin is punctured primarily by the canine teeth of the aggressor, are the most common puncture wound. The puncture wound, which is often the most obvious manifestation of the trauma, is not the only consideration. The mobile superficial layers of the skin may be subjected to a laceration injury, as well as the puncture wound, and the deeper more fixed tissues may be subject to crushing from the teeth. If the bite wound has been inflicted by another dog, the powerful masticatory muscles have the potential to crush tissues with a force of 150–450 psi, with the tips of the canine teeth puncture and lacerate the skin. Movement and shaking actions will result in additional tears and avulsion of the tissues from their attachment to deeper structures, possibly resulting in devitalisation of tissues and the contamination of the wound with bacteria, deep into the subcutaneous and muscle tissues predisposing bite wounds to infection.

All bite wounds therefore should be considered as contaminated wounds. If these wounds are left untreated, or are not treated using appropriate antibiotics, the wound may become colonised by pathogens which may ultimately lead to an infected wound. A wound is classified as infected when the bacterial load of the wound is greater than 105 bacteria per gram of tissue.

Firearm wounds and snakebites are also technically puncture wounds, but have additional complications over and above the initial puncture wound.

Puncture wounds are generally treated by lavage using copious volumes of saline or lactated Ringer's solution, debridement and drainage. Puncture wounds which arise as a result of animal bites generally have pockets of dead space which should be flushed and a dependent drain placed or the wound closed using walking sutures to eliminate this dead space if the wound is then considered sufficiently clean. It may also be worth obtaining a bacterial swab which may be sent to a laboratory for culture and sensitivity should wound healing not progress in a satisfactory manner. Dog bite wounds are generally allowed to heal by secondary intention using appropriate wound management dressings, but occasionally *en bloc* debridement may be performed to allow partial primary closure where there is sufficient tissue and skin available to perform this technique successfully.

Occasionally dog bite wounds may not heal successfully and studies have indicated that this may be due to inadequate lavage, debridement and drainage, which highlights their importance in wound management.

Penetrating wounds to the thorax may result in pneumothorax and those to the abdomen may damage viscera. Penetrating bite wounds to the thorax which go unnoticed may eventually result in the formation of a pyothorax.

Burns

Burns may be classified according to the depth and the surface area of the skin affected. The classification according to the depth of the burns is:

- First degree: epidermis only
- Second degree: epidermis and variable portion of the dermis
- Third degree: epidermis, dermis and variable proportion of the hypodermis.

Both local (wound associated) and systemic complications include the loss of a large area of skin and wound infection.

Systemic complications include hyper-/hyponatraemia, hyper-/hypokalaemia, metabolic acidosis, pre-renal azotaemia, anaemia and septicaemia.

Burns are often extensive and reconstruction of the large skin deficits often presents a challenge. Eschar formation invariably results in large tissue deficits, and it is important to remove this eschar in order to get back to a healthy granulation bed. Secondary bacterial contamination is common in burn wounds but septicaemia is uncommon.

First degree burns will often heal by secondary intention, but second degree burns may result in significant scarring with possible compromise of function if the burn is situated close to a joint or natural body orifice (e.g. mouth or anus). Third degree burns will require surgical reconstruction, i.e. flaps or grafts.

Burns may be thermal (hot or cold), chemical (acid or alkali), electrical or radiant in origin.

Thermal burns are caused by extremes of heat, generally heat rather than cold. Hyperthermic burns may be caused by exposure to hot water (scald), contact with hot surfaces (e.g. car exhaust during road traffic accidents) or exposure to burning materials.

Unfortunately, a common cause of thermal burns is the use of electrical heating pads placed under an animal, particularly during or after anaesthesia or in reptiles lying on a heat mat or beneath a heat lamp, which is not connected to a thermostat to regulate heat output. Burns from external heat sources are more likely if the heat mat is used for prolonged periods or at too high a temperature in recumbent patients who cannot change position. Animals with poor cutaneous blood flow arising from hypothermia may be at particular risk.

First aid treatment for thermal burns is aimed at stopping the burning process. Because the skin is slow to cool, the burning process may continue for some time after the patient is removed from the heat source. For this reason burned areas should be cooled with running water for up to 30 minutes (ideally by the client prior to transportation to the surgery). Current recommended first aid treatment includes cooling the wounds with cold tap water (15°C [59°F]) for 20–30 minutes. Cold water or ice should also not be used as this can rapidly decrease the patient's body temperature and may contribute to increased wound depth by inducing vasoconstriction. The temperature of the patient should be monitored closely while cooling burn wounds to avoid hypothermia. To avoid hypothermia during transport, the patient should be wrapped in several clean, dry sheets or blankets.

Hypothermic burns may result from exposure to a cold environmental temperature, i.e. frostbite. Environmental hypothermic injury usually affects the extremities, such as the toes, tail and ear tips, but damage as a result of contact with cold objects may affect any of the body. Hypothermic injuries are not commonly seen in the UK.

Chemical burns are caused by exposure to acid or alkali. These wounds often involve the pads, although oropharyngeal burns may occur in cases of ingestion. Depending on the chemicals involved, the treatment of chemical burns can vary greatly, and so veterinary advice should always be sought.

Electrical burns may be direct (contact) burns, where the animal touches a low-tension electrical source such as domestic electrical cables, or indirect (flash or arc burns), where the animal comes too close to a high-tension electrical source, e.g. railway lines.

Contact burns result from the current passing through the body and are often caused by the animal chewing through an electrical cable. Flash burns are more superficial injuries.

Snakebites

Snakebites are a particular subset of puncture wounds, complicated by the injection of the snake's venom. The adder is the only venomous snake found naturally in the UK, and snakebites are occasionally seen in dogs exercised outdoors on areas of heath or moor land. In other countries there are a large variety of poisonous snakes found in both urban and rural areas. The snake's venom results in local and systemic effects. Local effects cause tissue necrosis and damage to blood vessel walls leading to ischaemia and tissue sloughing.

These wounds usually involve an extremity or the ventrum. The wound is usually grossly swollen and initially oedematous. Later there is progression to ischaemia and necrosis of large areas of tissue around the site of the puncture.

Firearm injuries

The response of tissues to ballistic injuries is complex. The basic wound is a perforating or penetrating injury, but with extensive damage to the underlying tissue as the projectile moves on its trajectory.

The bullet will cause stretching, compression and laceration of tissue. Entry wounds are typically small, but the exit wounds may be large. Damage to tissue along the path of the projectile is likely to be more severe than the cutaneous wound. The pattern of trauma is determined by the velocity of the missile. As velocity increases then the kinetic energy imparted to the tissues increases exponentially. Shotguns, airguns and handguns are classed as slow velocity (where the bullet travels at less than 300 metres/second). Deeper tissues are damaged by a compression wave which moves ahead of the bullet and it is this compression wave that damages the tissues.

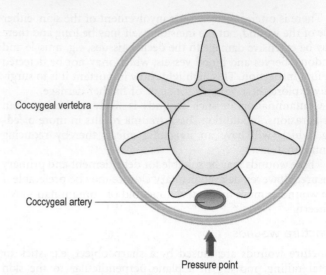

Fig. 20.11 Cross-section through a tail – site of the pressure point on the ventral aspect

Treatment of wounds

Bleeding should be controlled. Direct pressure is applied using sterile swabs or by bandaging. Addition of diluted adrenaline to swabs may help by causing vasoconstriction, but should not be used on extremities or in the presence of cardiac arrhythmias. Pressure can be applied to brachial or femoral arteries if arterial haemorrhage is present (Fig. 20.11).

A tourniquet can be applied above the wound if it is on a limb. Narrow elastic tourniquets put significant pressure on neurovascular structures and should only be used for up to 5 minutes. Bands 5–10 cm wide can be used for up to 30 minutes. Blood pressure cuffs can be placed proximal to the wound and inflated to 20–30 cm H_2O higher than arterial pressure and can be left in place for up to 6 hours. Ligation may be needed for larger vessels.

After achieving haemostasis, the wound should be covered with a sterile dressing. Using aseptic techniques, the wound is packed with sterile gel or soaked swabs and hair clipped from the wound outwards. The wound can then be lavaged with copious saline or lactated Ringer's solution (Hartmann's) and a protective bandage applied.

In traumatic and infected wounds, antibiotics should be administered as soon as possible. A first-generation cephalosporin or clavulanic acid potentiated amoxicillin are good first-line choices.

Once the patient is stable a more thorough evaluation may be carried out. Appropriate chemical restraint may be required for examination. Prior to their administration, it is important to evaluate distal neuromuscular and motor function. Diagnostic imaging may be used to check for foreign material, penetrating injuries, associated fractures, dislocations and tendon or ligament damage. A management plan should take into account the wound's location, size, damage to local structures and the amount of tissue loss.

Lavage reduces the number of bacteria present and helps to loosen necrotic tissue and debris. Lavage solutions containing antibacterials or detergents should be avoided; they can cause cell damage, slow wound healing and may result in bacterial resistance. Lactated Ringer's solution (LRS) is the best choice, it is the least cytotoxic and has a near-neutral pH. In heavily contaminated wounds tap water is adequate. The initial tap water lavage should be followed by sterile LRS.

The pressure for lavage solution needs to exceed the adhesive and cohesive forces of the contaminant, yet avoid pushing debris into the tissues and causing damage to vital tissues. The suggested force is 5–10 psi. In practice this can be achieved by using a bag of fluid with an 18–20-gauge needle fitted to the end of an attached giving set. The volume of lavage solution is equally important. For small, superficial wounds, 0.5–1 l is generally used; for larger wounds several litres of sterile lavage solution may be needed.

Any traumatic wound will require the debridement of devitalised tissues and foreign material in order to prevent infection and necrosis and to promote optimal wound healing. Debridement may be performed using a number of different methods.

Sharp debridement involves the use of a scalpel blade or scissors and may be carried out carefully in stages in order to preserve as much healthy tissue as possible. Subcutaneous tissue, fat, skin, fascia and muscle can generally be freely debrided. Tendons, vessels, nerves and bone should be debrided much more conservatively. In some situations necrotic tissue close to vital structures may be left in place until there is a line of demarcation.

Mechanical debridement involves the use of dressings (e.g. wet to dry), irrigation or hydrosurgery. Wet to dry dressings are commonly used in veterinary practice but their use requires sedation or anaesthesia as removal is painful. Autolytic debridement involves the use of wound dressings and solutions, e.g. hydrogels, and is not recommended in infected wounds.

Following debridement, a decision needs to be made about wound closure. In clean and clean-contaminated wounds, surgical closure to allow first intention healing may be the best option. If there is any doubt about the tissue viability or the risk of infection, the wound should be allowed to heal using open wound management. Damage to underlying structures such as tendon and bone may delay the healing of the overlying tissue and require specialist treatment. If there has been significant skin loss then skin flaps or grafts may be needed.

WOUND DRESSINGS

Wound dressings play a vital role in creating the optimum environment for wound healing to occur. Wound dressings have advanced greatly since moist wound healing was first pioneered in the 1960s by George Winter. A wide, and often confusing, variety of wound dressings are currently available on the veterinary market. These wound dressings have all been specifically created according to the wound type and its stage of healing. Advanced wound dressings have been designed to actively rehydrate wounds or to remove and retain excess fluid from wounds and also to protect the wound from further trauma.

Dressings are selected according to the patient's needs, wound classification, stage of healing, underlying conditions and anatomical site. Some wounds will require just a protective layer whereas deeper wounds may require a primary dressing with a secondary dressing to cover and protect the wound. Combining two or more dressings in the treatment of a wound provides greater flexibility in treating the symptoms of the wound.

Dressings should be specifically selected in order to manage the local wound environment and to achieve optimum wound healing – this is achieved by:
- Creating a moist, not dry or overly wet wound environment
- Eliminating debris, slough and necrotic tissue
- Reducing bacterial contamination
- Keeping the wound warm
- Protecting the wound from abrasion or contamination
- Preventing adherence to newly formed tissue
- Reducing disturbance of the granulating wound to a minimum.

Further considerations include:
- Minimising pain
- Achieving a good cosmetic outcome.

It is important to be able to recognise the stage in the healing process which the wound is at in order to know whether a wound is not following the normal progression in healing.

As mentioned there are currently a very wide, and sometimes confusing, array of dressings available on the veterinary market and the appropriate selection of dressing for a specific type of wound can be impossible without knowledge of the methods of action of these dressings.

Even those dressings which we consider to be 'advanced' are based on Winter's research that a moist environment will maximise the rate of healing. Many of these new dressings have been designed to either absorb excess fluid or exudate or to donate moisture in a wound that is producing insufficient fluid. There are also a range of products available designed to manage wound infection or contamination by being antimicrobial as well as creating the optimal environment for wound healing.

Perforated polyurethane membranes

These dressings consist of a thin perforated polyurethane membrane, which is coated with an absorbent backing layer, e.g. Melolin (Smith & Nephew). These dressings should be described as low adherence when compared to wet or dry-to-dry dressings, but strictly speaking are not non-adherent. As these dressings are permeable they will allow wounds to dry out and therefore their use should be restricted to the protection of an elective surgical wound from contamination and trauma, and some of these products (e.g. Primapore and Meopore) have adhesive edges making them ideal for this purpose. These dressings, if applied to open wounds, have the disadvantage of adhering to the wound if the exudate is allowed to dry out. Another disadvantage is that capillary loops and exudate can get into the pores or holes of these dressings and increase the adherency of the dressing; this will result in damage to the tissues upon removal of the dressing.

One of the mistakes frequently made in practice is the use of such perforated polyurethane membrane dressings in combination with hydrogels, e.g. Intrasite (Smith & Nephew). These dressings are often used together to treat granulating wounds as the operator does not fully understand the way in which the various dressings work and how they should be applied. Once such a dressing is applied to a wound, over a period of a few hours the hydrogel begins to dry out and forms a 'crust', which is often partly adhered to both the dressing and the surface of the wound. In combination with capillary loops adhering to the dressing, this results in a well-adhered dressing which will be particularly painful to remove and will do very little to improve the rate of wound healing.

Hydrogels

These are used in wounds that are thought to be at risk of drying out. These gels are composed of 70–95% water in combination with variable quantities of hydrophilic polymer base such as carboxymethylcellulose or alginate. The main role of hydrogels is a fluid donator as they are ideal for use in dry wounds but they can be used as an aid to debridement in fragile wounds. Hydrogels have the ability to both donate and trap water; this means they have the ability to absorb wound exudate as well as hydrating and debriding necrotic material within the wound.

A secondary dressing is required in order for these hydrogels to work efficiently, and this should ideally be a foam or dressing with a semi-permeable film backing in order to maintain humidity and a moist wound environment.

Hydrocolloids

These dressings are usually used in wounds that require additional moisture and natural debridement. These dressings actively stimulate wound healing and encourage debridement as they degrade on interaction with wound exudate. These dressings can be difficult to apply in animals. They are best used in dry to semi-dry wounds requiring maintenance of an optimal moist environment. The dressings consist of polymers suspended in an adhesive matrix; the dressings adhere to the normal skin around the wound edges and are left in place for several days where they provide a nearly ideal wound environment. Users should be warned that on initial removal the wound can look much worse; this is because they dressings swell and liquefy as the exudate is absorbed, as well as giving the wound a yellowish appearance. This, however, is normal and once the wound has been lavaged it should look much improved.

Polyurethane foam dressings

Foams have a highly absorbent capacity and act by drawing excess exudate away from the wound, maintaining some moisture conservation through humidity to keep the wound moist. These dressings are commonly applied on top of other products, e.g. hydrogels, honey. The ability of the dressing to absorb exudate is dependent upon the viscosity of the exudate and also the dressing's moisture vapour transfer rate. This semi-permeable membrane backing allows oxygen exchange and controlled evaporation, resulting in a moist wound environment. Foam dressings are now available with antimicrobial properties. Kendall's AMD Antimicrobial foam dressing is a new polyhexamethylene biguanide (PHMB) impregnated hydrophilic polyurethane foam dressing; PHMB works as an antimicrobial agent exhibiting broad-spectrum activity against bacteria and fungi. The PHMB within the dressing attacks bacteria in wound exudate as it is absorbed. The AMD foam dressing is effective against staph infections including methicillin-resistant *Staphylococcus aureus* (MRSA), *Pseudomonas*, *Proteus* etc. The dressing itself creates a moist wound environment as well as inhibiting pathogenic organisms from growing in or penetrating the dressing.

Alginates

Alginate dressings are fine fibrous dressings used to absorb moisture. They are presented as either a rope or flat form. These dressings are derived from kelp and consist of varying proportions of guluronic and mannuronuic acids. The wound exudate interacts with the alginate to release cations that actively stimulate wound healing via the inflammatory cascade, allowing the release of endogenous growth factors into the wound. These dressings can be useful in the treatment of wounds that have become stationary – in this case they should be moistened before use.

Super-absorbent dressings

Wounds which produce vast quantities of exudate can be very difficult to manage. Historically nappies have been used to manage such wounds; however, recent dressings have been designed to cope with very high volumes of exudate by incorporating polyacrylate crystals into the dressings in combination with silicone adhesives to make them very 'wearable'. These dressings are very useful when used on patients with Penrose drains in place.

ANTIMICROBIAL DRESSINGS

Honey

Manuka honey is currently the first choice in wound management due to its excellent antimicrobial effects. Manuka honey is derived from Manuka plants and requires a Unique Manuka Factor (UMF®) of 10 or more in order to be used in wound management to ensure its potency and antimicrobial effects are adequate, and also to ensure it is effective against common wound pathogens including *Pseudomonas* spp., MRSA and *E. coli*. Honey manufactured for medical use is prepared specifically involving high-level filtering to remove debris and beeswax as well as gamma sterilisation.

Silver dressings

Silver and its salts have antiseptic and antibacterial properties. Historically, silver has been used as a paste for the treatment of burns; however, the introduction of silver dressings has made a huge impact on wound management in recent years.

The silver in the dressings ionises to release active silver ions into the wound. Nanocrystalline silver has been developed as a product that rapidly releases high concentrations of silver into an infected wound. Dressings are available that can be left in place for up to 7 days. The dressings require activation prior to use by moistening with water for 10 seconds. Silver has a similar antimicrobial effect to Manuka honey and is effective against *Pseudomonas* spp., MRSA, *E. coli* and common yeasts and fungi, including *Candida*.

It should be remembered that holistic assessment and treatment of the patient is essential in order to ensure that the healing potential is optimised.

BANDAGES AND DRESSINGS

The ongoing management of the wound to allow secondary closure, delayed primary closure or second intention healing involves protection of the wound surface by bandaging.

Bandaging aims to achieve the following:
- Immobilisation of the wound surfaces, ensuring that the capillary buds and migrating epithelial cells are not disrupted and therefore maximising the rate of wound healing.
- Protection of the wound from trauma and contamination (including self-trauma and bacteria migrating through the dressing onto the wound).
- Pain relief for the patient.

- First aid – bandaging of a wound may be a temporary first aid measure to protect the wound from further contamination and aid haemostasis while a trauma patient is stabilised. The wound should be covered with a non-adherent dressing and an absorbent secondary layer. At this stage, ointments, antiseptics or wound powders may only serve to cause chemical damage and complicate debridement later on.

The most important layer of the dressing in terms of wound healing is the primary contact layer which should be chosen according to the condition of the wound. In the early stages, if the wound is still producing exudate and necrotic debris, debriding dressings are indicated. As the wound improves and granulation tissue is evident, a semi-occlusive non-adherent dressing may be used which will allow exudate to be drawn away from the wound into the secondary layer of the bandage, while keeping the wound surface moist and protected. New tissue is not damaged on removal. Petroleum gauze products allow excess fluid through, but may allow slow epithelialisation. Smooth non-adherent dressings, such as Melolin (Smith & Nephew), may be used as the exudate reduces.

Occlusive dressings are indicated once there is no infection and the wound is healing well. They keep the wound bed moist and warm and protect the new epithelium from abrasion. The hydrocolloids are a suspension of starch polymers in an adhesive matrix. They absorb fluid from the wound and form a moist gel. The edges of the dressing overlap with normal skin and form a seal, so that secondary dressing layers are not needed. This stimulates granulation tissue, allows rapid epithelialisation and also has some analgesic effect. Hydrocolloid dressings may prove expensive if dressing changes are frequent, but can be left in place for up to 5 days. These dressings will cause maceration of the tissue if the wound is exudative and they do not allow debridement. Furthermore, the adherence of the dressing at the wound edges may 'splint' the wound and prevent contraction. Intrasite gel (Smith & Nephew) is a hydrocolloid gel that may be used in a concave wound to allow the advantages of the moist environment but without being completely occlusive. The gel should be covered with a non-adherent dressing and a secondary absorbent layer.

Alginate dressings (e.g. Kaltostat; BritCair) also form a gel after absorbing wound exudate, and encourage epithelialisation in the same way. As they are not occlusive, they may be used as an alternative to the hydrocolloids if there is any doubt as to the state of the wound. Kaltostat may be useful for the transition from debriding dressings to hydrocolloids in the management of open wounds. The wound should be irrigated with sterile saline to remove the dressing.

All of these primary layer dressings are only as good as the bandage holding them in place. They must be changed regularly. It is important that the owner appreciates that if the bandage becomes wet it should be changed immediately.

Generally bandages are composed of three basic component layers:

- Primary (contact) layer
- Secondary (intermediate) layer
- Tertiary (outer) layer.

Primary layer

This involves the various dressings available for use as the contact later.

Secondary layer

It is essential that all layers of a bandage are correctly and meticulously applied in order to avoid the common complications that can arise from inadequate, unskilled or incorrect application. The role of the secondary layer in wound management, in addition to providing support and comfort, is absorption. It acts as a 'trap' for exudative fluids from the wound; evaporation from this layer helps to prevent bacterial strikethrough. To aid its absorptive role this layer needs to have good capillarity and should be thick enough (single or preferably multiple layered) to collect the fluid and pad the wound. The intermediate layer must be in close contact with the primary dressing but it should not be applied so tightly as to limit exudate absorption. Suitable materials are hospital-quality absorbent cotton wool or synthetic materials.

Tertiary outer layer

The outer layer serves to hold all the other layers of the bandage in place. In a multi-layered bandage (e.g. modified Robert Jones), an intermediate layer of conforming gauze and absorbent material may be used prior to applying an outer covering such as an adhesive wrap or preferably a self-adhering dressing. It is important that the outer layer allows evaporation of fluid but minimises external fluid absorption. Plastic bags which may be placed over the distal dressing should only be left in situ for a minimal period to prevent excessive fluid retention, with the increased risk of bacterial strikethrough and tissue maceration.

TIE-OVER (BOLUS) DRESSING

Tie-over (bolus) dressings are a useful method of securing contact layers to all parts of the body, where conventional bandaging techniques are of limited value, e.g. the greater trochanter. The most common method of securing such a dressing is to use several loops of 3 metric (2/0) monofilament nylon sutures placed approximately 2 cm from the wound edge. Umbilical (nylon) tape is passed through these loops to secure the dressing; the tape is laced across the dressing through the skin sutures. Alternatively, long strands of suture material may be stapled 2–3 cm from the wound edges all around the wound; these sutures may then be tied over the dressing to hold it in place. The entire area should then be covered with an outer bandage.

Non-adherent dressing is applied to the wound and cotton wool is then placed in the centre of the dressing. The edges of the dressing are then folded over and secured with either sutures or umbilical tape.

PRESSURE RELIEF BANDAGES

Pressure relief dressings are indicated for the prevention of decubital ulcer type lesions or treatment of superficial ulceration secondary to bandages or casts. Generally, doughnut-shaped and pipe insulation are employed to protect the area concerned by avoiding pressure over bony prominences. Care should be taken when using doughnut-shaped bandages as they can in some instances be counterproductive as they produce a 'halo' compression of the skin around a bony prominence. This compression can occasionally be severe enough to compromise the circulation and therefore delay wound healing.

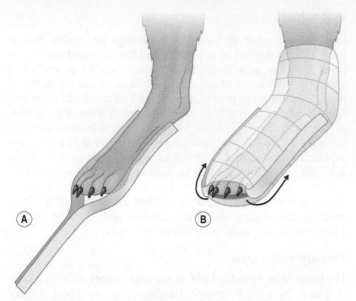

Fig. 20.12 The Robert Jones bandage *(Aspinall 2003.)*

Soft foam pad (pipe insulation) can be used parallel to the lesion so as to not encircle the wound so that the circulation is not compromised.

ROBERT JONES BANDAGE

This bandage was named after a famous orthopaedic surgeon, Sir Robert Jones (1858–1933); this type of bandage is used to support fractures of the limbs distal to the elbow or stifle. It is frequently used as a first aid measure or in combination with other methods of fixation. It is also highly useful in the prevention of or reduction of oedema, and in restricting the movement of a limb.

Placement

Any wounds which are present on the limb should be suitably dressed. Two 2.5-cm adhesive, non-elastic strips, e.g. zinc oxide, are attached to the limb (Fig. 20.12). These tape strips should be long enough to continue for 10–15 cm distal to the limb; these extended strips are later used to create the 'stirrups' which are used in order to prevent the bandage from slipping down the limb. The padding material is then applied evenly over the entire surface of the limb until the limb is approximately three times its original width. This padding layer should extend from the level of the toes and should extend proximally to include the joint proximal to the fracture. The most widely used and readily available material is cotton wool; this is cheap, easy to compress and will tear into suitable widths to allow for the natural angles and contours on the limb.

When placing such dressings on the hind limbs, the leg should be slightly flexed before the padding layer is applied, so that the limb will not be dragged when the bandage is finished, as it is effectively longer than the opposite limb.

At least two layers of conforming or white open weave bandage should then be firmly applied over the cotton wool layer, working from the toes proximally. Conforming bandage is bandage which takes the shape of, or conforms well to the shape of, the area in which it is being applied. The bandage should be unrolled in short sections, always keeping the flat surface towards the limb; with each turn the bandage should overlap the previous turn by one-half to two-thirds. The aim of this is to achieve an even, firm compression over the entire surface of the bandage. Any irregularities in the first layer of the bandage may be flattened by the second layer of the bandage. The tape stirrups are then folded back and stuck down on the bandage – these tape stirrups will assist in preventing the dressing from slipping down. If there is any excess cotton wool around the toes then this should be carefully removed and finally a protective layer of either adhesive elastic or cohesive bandage should then be applied. Ideally it is said that the finished dressing should be resonant when flicked and sound like a ripe watermelon. The central two toes should just protrude so they can be easily checked for their colour and temperature. Leaving two toes exposed also helps to encourage the patient to use the limb and allows for some weight bearing on the limb.

An alternative method of applying a Robert Jones bandage is to alternate several layers of cotton wool and bandage. Such dressings are frequently applied in various thicknesses; thicker if external support is required for a fracture or lighter if light support, to control swelling or to hold in place a primary dressing which may be placed higher up the limb. Such modified support dressings may also include splints which may be incorporated in between layers of padding material in order to prevent areas of pressure or rubbing, which may occur if the splint was placed beneath the padding layers. Sufficient padding should be placed at the proximal and distal ends of the splint to prevent trauma to the patient's skin.

Such dressings should be checked approximately 2 hours after application to ensure that the toes are not swollen. The temperature and sensation of the digits can also be assessed. If the toes do begin to swell, then the distal end of the bandage should be loosened slightly or a pressure bandage applied to the foot for 12–24 hours. The bandage must be kept clean and dry. The dressing should be checked regularly and may be left in place for 7–14 days.

Care should be taken that such dressings are kept dry as the cotton wool will act as a 'wick' on contact with moisture. The owner should be made aware of this and the bottom of the dressing should be covered with a plastic bag, old drip bag or specifically made bootee whenever the animal goes outside. It should be ensured that this covering of the bandage is removed once the animal returns to a dry environment, as long-term covering of the bandage with plastic would result in major skin complications.

HEAD AND EAR DRESSINGS

The majority of head and ear dressings are placed to protect an ear that may be haemorrhaging due to trauma or post-surgery (Fig. 20.13). Similar bandages may be modified to cover the patient's eye following surgery or trauma.

Placement

The ear which is to be dressed should be reflected upwards over the patient's head. Any wounds which are present on the ear/head should be covered with a suitable sterile dressing. A pad of cotton wool should be placed on top of the patient's head, with the ear then being reflected back onto the cotton wool pad; a further cotton wool pad should then be placed on top of the ear. It may also be useful to place a further cotton wool pad beneath the patient's throat, to prevent pressure from

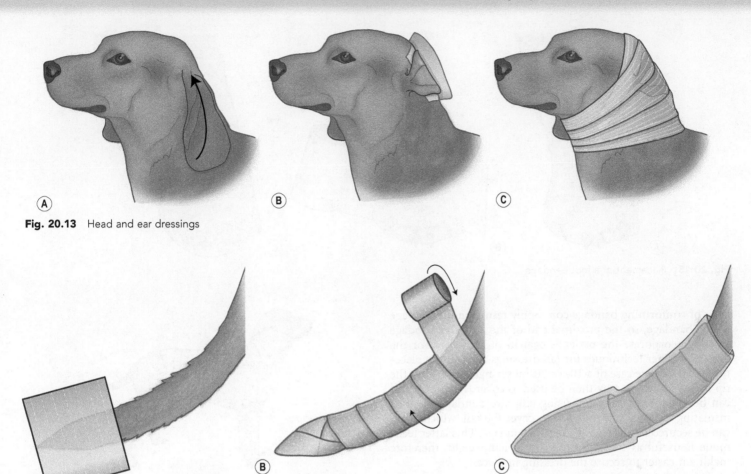

Fig. 20.13 Head and ear dressings

Fig. 20.14 Placement of a tail bandage

the conforming bandage and tertiary layer. A conforming bandage should then be used to secure the bandage in place. The bandage layer should start on top of the head, passing under the chin, in a figure-of-eight pattern. The patient's free ear should be used as an anchor, with the bandage passing around the free ear and over the head. It may require several layers of conforming bandage in order to secure the padding. A final tertiary layer of adhesive or conforming bandage should be placed in order to secure the dressing. If adhesive bandage is used then it may be useful to stick some of this bandage to the patient's hair in order to prevent the entire bandage from slipping forwards or backwards. A note should always be made on the bandage to show the position of the ear inside the bandage, to prevent laceration or even amputation of the pinna upon removal.

Whenever applying a head/ear bandage it is vitally important to ensure that the patient can still open its mouth and that respiration has not been impaired by the bandage being applied too tightly. It is particularly important that the adhesive layer is unwound prior to application; this is even more important if cohesive bandage is used, because if this bandage is applied under any tension, it can quickly become very tight, especially if more than a couple of layers are applied. If there is any cause for concern then the dressing should be removed and reapplied. Special care must be taken if the bandage is applied while the patient is anaesthetised, with an endotracheal tube in place, as

problems may only be detected once the endotracheal tube has been removed. A correctly applied head bandage should allow for the insertion of two fingers between the bandage and the chin to allow room for neck flexion without obstructing the airway. If the bandage is too tight then an incision can be made way across the bandage, under the chin.

If the patient is very persistent in its attempts to remove the dressing, it may be useful to extend the tertiary layer to include the cranial aspect of the chest, to prevent the removal of the dressing by anchoring it more securely around the shoulders, in a figure-of-eight pattern, like a chest bandage.

TAIL BANDAGE

This type of bandage is commonly applied following trauma to the tail tip, or postoperatively following amputation of the tail tip (Fig. 20.14).

These bandages are commonly difficult to keep in position and can be very frustrating to place, especially if the patient wags its tail immediately following placement and removes the dressing.

Placement

A suitable sterile dressing should be applied to any wounds. Many nursing texts advise the application of a layer of conforming bandage, covered with a layer of adhesive bandage, but the

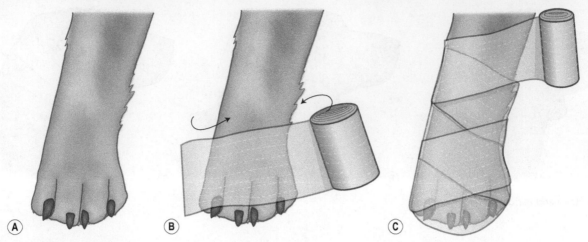

Fig. 20.15   Placement of a foot bandage

layer of conforming bandage commonly results in the slippage of the bandage, so the proximal end of the adhesive bandage should incorporate the patient's coat in order to anchor the dressing. Other techniques for tail dressings include the placement of a syringe case of a 10- or 20-ml syringe barrel with the tip removed, which may then be used to cover the tail tip and can be anchored to the tail using adhesive bandage; or pipe insulating material may be used to cover the tail, which again can be secured in place with adhesive bandage. This latter technique is useful as the pipe insulator is lightweight, therefore making it easier to secure the dressing in place.

FOOT BANDAGE

This is a commonly used dressing applied in an emergency to control haemorrhage and postoperatively to protect wounds and control swelling (Fig. 20.15).

Placement

Cotton wool or other padding material should be placed between the patient's toes and beneath the dewclaw. This padding helps to prevent pressure sores which may arise as a result of sweat from the glands of the foot and friction between the toes. It must be ensured that the pieces of padding are not too thick as this will make the overall dressing uncomfortable; at the same time strips must not be too thin.

Any wounds which may be present should be covered with a suitable dressing, then a padding layer should be applied over the whole of the carpus/tarsus; in foot bandages it is useful to extend the dressing as far proximally as the next joint, i.e. the carpal joint in the fore limb and hock joint in the hind limb. This technique has the advantage of preventing the dressing from slipping down; however, care must be taken, particularly in the hind limb, to prevent pressure points over the hock which may result in ischaemic areas. The padding layer can be either cotton wool or a synthetic padding material, e.g. Soffban or Cellona. It should be ensured that the padding is applied evenly. A layer of conforming bandage for the secondary layer should be used as this conforms well to the contours of the patient's limb and is generally easier to apply than other bandages, e.g. white open weave. A final layer should be added, using a cohesive bandage, e.g. Vetwrap, or adhesive bandage, e.g. Elastoplast. If adhesive bandage is used then it is useful to apply two shorter

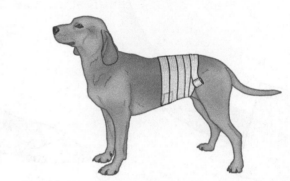

Fig. 20.16   Placement of an abdominal bandage

strips in a cranial to caudal, and then a lateral to medial direction; this will be useful to cover and protect the bottom of the bandage. The remainder of the adhesive bandage can then be unwound around the remainder of the foot, with the bandage being applied distally, working upwards around the limb. It is wise to unwrap both cohesive and adhesive dressings partially in order to prevent the bandage being applied too tightly.

If the bandage is being applied to control haemorrhage, the bandage can be observed to detect bleeding of the limb though the outer layers of the bandage. If this situation arises, then a further layer of padding material may be applied, covered with layers of conforming bandage and then another tertiary layer, again with the bandage being observed for further bleeding.

THORAX AND ABDOMINAL BANDAGES

Such dressings are often placed to cover wounds, surgical incisions, drains or as pressure bandages in cases of suspected abdominal bleeding. These bandages need to be applied firmly, but at the same time ensuring that there is no constriction of the chest or abdomen. When an abdominal pressure bandage is placed with the aim of controlling haemorrhage, the layers of the bandage should be applied firmly (Fig. 20.16). It may be useful when removing such a bandage to do this very slowly, starting at the cranial end and making a 1-inch incision into the bandage every hour until the dressing is removed; this is generally done when there is strong suspicion of abdominal bleeding.

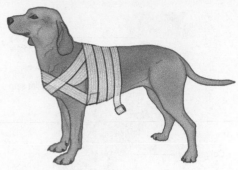

Fig. 20.17 Placement of a thoracic bandage

Placement

If a wound is present on the chest or abdomen, then this should be covered with a suitable dressing, or if a discharging drain is present then suitable absorbent material should be used in order to absorb any exudate, e.g. sterile laparotomy swab. Several layers of padding material should then be applied; this padding layer should overlap by approximately one-half to one-third; this should then be secured in place with a layer of conforming bandage, and then a tertiary layer of cohesive or adhesive bandage. The dressing can be prevented from slipping backwards or forwards by wrapping the intermediate and tertiary layers between the legs and over the shoulders (Fig. 20.17) or hips in a criss-cross fashion.

STOCKINETTE

One type of dressing which is incredibly useful and versatile in practice is stockinette (Surgifix). This dressing is available in several sizes but only two sizes need to be kept in stock to dress any animal from a kitten to a St Bernard. It is most useful for patients with thoracostomy tubes in place, as it allows easy access to the drain, but keeps all attachments associated with the drain in place, hopefully preventing accidental removal of the drain. I have also used this dressing incorporated into chest/body bandages where regular dressings may slip, or where wound dressings require to be retained in place before further dressing layers are applied.

Fractures

Fractures are breaks in the bone and are named according to the type of damage that has occurred (Fig. 20.18).

EMERGENCY TREATMENT

Emergency management of fractures can improve the systemic condition of the animal, and reduce complications when it comes to fixation. Adequate analgesia should be provided. Large amounts of blood can be lost from the circulation into the fracture site, especially in femoral, humeral and pelvic fractures. Cats with pelvic fractures will commonly be markedly anaemic a day or two after initial stabilisation. Further clinical monitoring of these cases along with PCV/TP serial measurement may be useful in documenting further haemorrhage.

Clinical signs such as deformity, swelling, crepitus, instability and pain will often be present. Important factors to assess are the position of the fracture, its relationship to critical structures

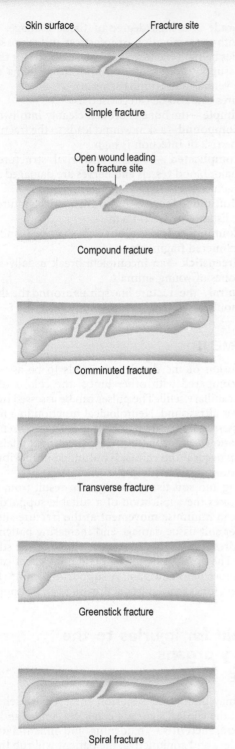

Fig. 20.18 Types of fracture

and whether it is open or closed. Open fractures are those where the skin has been broken. Open fractures should be covered with a sterile dressing, then clipped, lavaged and dressed again.

Open fractures are graded as follows:
- Grade 1: a bone fragment penetrates the skin ('inside out'). The fragment usually retracts in again, leaving a puncture wound.
- Grade 2: a penetrating external wound causes a fracture ('outside in'). The bone is not usually exposed.

- Grade 3: a high degree of tissue damage, commonly with contamination or infection and exposed bone.

Extremities below a fracture should be assessed for the presence of blood supply, pain sensation and any oedema (indicating impaired venous and lymphatic return).

Fractures can also be categorised as:

- **Simple** – the bone is broken cleanly into two pieces
- **Compound** – a skin wound leads to the fracture site and the risk of infection is high
- **Complicated** – organs and vital structures such as major blood vessels and nerves are damaged around the fracture site
- **Multiple** – there is more than one fracture site with a distance between them
- **Comminuted** – the bone is shattered and there are splintered fragments
- **Greenstick** – an incomplete break usually seen in the bones of young animals
- **Spiral** – the fracture line spirals around the shaft – commonly associated with the humerus.

ASSESSMENT

The perfusion of the distal limb needs to be assessed by its warmth compared with other limbs, the colour of pads/nail beds and capillary refill. The pulses can be assessed by palpation or Doppler ultrasound. Neurological function in a limb can be simply assessed by firmly pinching the digits. Absence of deep pain sensation carries a poor prognosis, although false-negative results can occur if the animal is obtunded or moribund due to systemic disorders.

Swelling and soft tissue damage can result from instability. In some cases the application of a suitable supportive padded dressing can minimise movement at the fracture site, preventing further soft tissue damage and increasing patient comfort. Support dressings applied above the elbow or the stifle are less effective. They often slip, and a pendulum effect causes more fracture movement and pain. A supporting splint (Fig. 20.19) or a Robert Jones-type support dressing can be applied.

First aid for injuries to the sensory organs

THE EYE

The eye may be injured either on the eyeball itself or on the eyelid but the clinical signs are generally similar and include:

- **Conjunctivitis** – reddening and inflammation of the sclera and conjunctiva; the patient will rub the eye with a paw or on the floor/furniture and thus cause further damage
- **Epiphora** – increased tear production
- **Photophobia** – avoiding bright light by closing the eye or burying the head
- **Blepharospasm** – scrunching up the eye to avoid the light.

Eyeball injuries

1. Corneal injury – care must be taken to avoid touching the cornea, as this may cause ulceration. The cornea may be injured by:

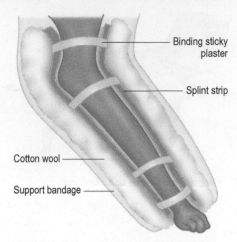

Fig. 20.19   Supporting a fracture – placing a splint

- Binding sticky plaster
- Splint strip
- Cotton wool
- Support bandage

- Penetrating wounds – during fights or road traffic accidents. These cause a loss of aqueous humour and subsequent intraocular pressure, and the cornea may take on a shrunken, wrinkled appearance. It is vital that the eye is disturbed as little as possible.
  - Non-penetrating wounds, e.g. ulcers, which may have been caused by foreign bodies, such as thorns or claw scratches.
2. Direct trauma to the eyeball, causing haemorrhage within the eye – known as hyphaema.
3. Fractures to the skull – can cause the eye to be bruised, which is often seen as a red blister on the sclera, or the eye may protrude slightly from the socket as a result of haemorrhage in the soft tissues behind the eyeball – retrobulbar haemorrhage.

General treatment of eyeball injuries – this includes the following:

- Flush with saline to clean the area.
- Place a sterile gauze swab over the eye and attach loosely in position with adhesive tape.
- Reduce any possibility of self-trauma by applying an Elizabethan collar.
- Place the patient in a darkened area to help with photophobia.
- Keep warm.
- Monitor for any changes or signs of shock.

4. Prolapse of the eyeball – the eye becomes dislodged from the socket and is exposed. This may result from fighting and is more likely in breeds with more protruding eyeballs, e.g. Pekinese. In this state the eyeball is unprotected and may dry out, causing the cornea to ulcerate, and damage to the optic nerve may also result.

Treatment includes the following:

- Although it is vital that the eye is replaced as soon as possible, this must not be attempted by anyone other than a veterinary surgeon.
- Lubricate the eye using false tears or contact lens fluid. If neither of these is available, boiled and cooled water can be used.
- Prevent self-trauma, e.g. use of an Elizabethan collar or cover the feet in socks or bandages.

Eyelid injuries

The eyelid may be injured by:

1. Foreign bodies – the most common are grass seeds, which become lodged either under the eyelids or beneath the third eyelid. They cause excruciating pain and the patient will keep the eye tightly shut, making an examination very difficult. They may also cause trauma to the eyeball by scratching it.

    Foreign bodies may be treated in a number of ways depending on their size. If they are large enough to be removed, then do so, taking care not to cause any further damage. Removal should not be undertaken, however, if the cornea is penetrated. If the foreign body is small it can be flushed out with warmed saline.

2. Wounds – due to trauma such as fights and road traffic accidents or as a result of self-trauma. Wounds should be cleaned to remove any contaminants by flushing with warmed saline.

3. Inflammatory or allergic reactions – cause oedema to the conjunctiva which can be seen as the conjunctiva bulging from under the eyelid – chemosis. The pain caused by all eyelid injuries can be reduced by applying ice packs to the eye, but take care to ensure that the ice is covered in a soft, non-abrasive material to reduce the possibility of damage to the cornea.

THE EAR

External injuries

The most common injuries are those to the ear pinna. They may be caused by scratches, bites and stings or self-trauma resulting in aural haematomata or blood blisters.

Clinical signs

- Haemorrhage – the pinna can bleed profusely, which can be very alarming to the owner.
- Shaking of the head – leads to wide distribution of blood droplets.
- Self-trauma – rubbing and scratching at the ear.
- Swelling – formation of a haematoma within the tissue of the pinna.

Treatment

1. Stop the haemorrhage – apply a pressure pad to the wound. The owner can use a folded handkerchief or similar bandage. In the surgery the pinna can be held back over the head with a bandage – care must be taken not to wrap the bandage too tightly under the head as this will cause asphyxia.
2. Pain may be reduced by the use of ice packs held against the ear pinna.
3. Treat insect stings according to their cause.
4. Aural haematoma – this must be treated surgically by the veterinary surgeon.

Internal injuries

Foreign bodies such as grass seeds are the most common cause of inner ear problems. Grass seeds are most often seen in the summer and are able to travel down the ear canal and become lodged deep in the ear, causing severe irritation and pain. A general anaesthetic is required to locate the foreign body and

remove it without causing further damage; owners should not try to remove the object themselves.

THE NOSE

As the nose is of the respiratory tract any injury may restrict the oxygen supply to the body and could be fatal. Any difficulty in breathing should always be investigated. Injuries to the nose may result in epistaxis or nose bleed, which may be unilateral or bilateral and can be caused by:

- Trauma, e.g. a direct blow – check for crepitus around the nose, indicating a possible fracture
- Presence of a foreign body, e.g. grass seed or blades of grass – also cause persistent sneezing and rubbing the nose on the ground or with the paw
- Infection – due to bacterial, viral or fungal infections
- Tumours in the nasal cavity – if these are very large the patient may show mouth breathing or snoring respiration.

Treatment

1. If the nose is injured, avoid muzzling the animal as this may cause further complications.
2. Cold compresses can be applied to the nose to alleviate haemorrhage. Pressure placed on the nose should be gentle, as it may make the situation worse and compromise the respiratory tract.
3. Place the patient in a quiet, darkened kennel – this will reduce the stress to the animal, allowing the heart rate and blood pressure to return to normal, which may assist with the haemorrhage.
4. Observe the patient. Watch out for signs of dyspnoea and vomiting, which may be caused by swallowing blood. Concussion may also be seen in cases where a serious blow or other trauma has occurred.

THE MOUTH

The mouth is often injured, as animals use it for investigating and in searching for food. Injuries include:

- Foreign bodies – these are a common problem, e.g. sticks caught in the back of the throat, fish hooks, various 'chews' and bones wedged across the hard palate
- Fractures – following direct blows, as seen in road traffic accidents
- Insect stings – most often on the lips but sometimes inside the mouth.

Clinical signs

- Pain and swelling of the affected area
- Pawing or rubbing at the face
- Salivation and drooling
- Dysphagia – difficulty in eating – the animal may go to the food and sniff it but walk away leaving it uneaten or the food may drop out of the mouth.

Treatment

- Foreign bodies must be removed quickly in order to reduce the distress caused to the animal. Retrieval in a conscious animal is not always a safe option, and can potentially cause more trauma. These cases should be brought to the surgery as soon as possible and anaesthetised by the veterinary surgeon so that the foreign body can be removed.

- Fractures are difficult to treat using first aid and should be treated under a general anaesthetic, once the animal is stabilised. In the majority of cases a feeding tube will be required as the jaw heals.
- Insect stings are treated as appropriate.

Seizures

Seizures can be caused by many different conditions. True epilepsy is caused by waves of disorganised electrical activity within the brain. The sight of their animal having a fit can be very distressing for owners. There are many causes of fits but very often they are idiopathic, i.e. there is no known cause.

Specific causes include:

- Brain damage caused by disease or trauma
- Poisoning
- Viral or bacterial infections
- Metabolic disease, such as chronic liver or kidney failure, hypoglycaemia in diabetics
- Cerebral anoxia, e.g. due to anaesthetic accidents.

CLINICAL SIGNS

Clinical signs of fitting can be divided into three phases:

a. **Pre-ictal phase** – the patient may become hyperexcited or overanxious and may have an 'aura' or an apparent awareness that something is about to happen.
b. **Ictal phase** – the patient becomes recumbent – usually laterally. The body is tense, with the limbs extended and sometimes the patient will 'paddle'. Eyes are fixed and staring. Drooling and frothing at the mouth can be seen. Bladder and rectal control may be lost. The patient is unaware of its surroundings.
c. **Post-ictal phase** – the patient is usually dazed, unsteady and appears to be exhausted. It may sleep for long periods after the event.

The timescale varies with the individual, but no animal should be allowed to seizure for more than 5 minutes. In some cases, the animal may have one fit after another – a condition known as **status epilepticus.**

TELEPHONE ADVICE

The most common situation will be that the owner of the animal will telephone the surgery for advice. The owner will be distressed and panicking and you must remain calm and patient. Very little can be done to the animal while it is having a fit. However, the following should be recommended:

- Ensure that only one person is left with the patient.
- Do not touch the patient.
- Remove any objects that could fall onto the animal and cause further harm.
- Reduce the light and noise levels.
- Once the fit has subsided, allow the patient to rest.
- Make a note of how long the fit lasted, what the symptoms were and any occurrences that might have stimulated the fit. When the fit has subsided the owner should arrange for the veterinary surgeon to check the animal. If the fit persists for longer than 5 minutes or has clusters of more than three in a 10-minute window, the

owner must bring the animal into the surgery as soon as possible.

Cardiopulmonary resuscitation – CPR

INTRODUCTION

The year 2011 marked the 50th anniversary of the first articles published about cardiopulmonary resuscitation (CPR) based on the work of Dr Guy Knickerbocker, at the Johns Hopkins Medical School in Baltimore, Maryland, USA.

Sadly, after more than 50 years, and despite impressive advances in technology, basic science and pharmacology, the rates of success have not improved dramatically, and still we do not have a clear understanding about which are the best interventions and what protocols we should adopt.

The published reports of success rates in veterinary medicine after cardiac arrest and CPR are around 13% in dogs and 15.4% in cats, and the rate of hospital discharge following successful CPR is less than 16%.

Cardiopulmonary resuscitation is a very complex and challenging situation, and because of that, periodic re-examination of the protocols and recommendations by experts, institutions, and senior leaders in that field occur, leading to changes that sometimes may be perceived as drastic. Even the name has been changed, and different denominations have been proposed. However, by the last consensus, it seems that the term **CPR** is more simple and easy to understand for everyone, even if it does not describe completely all the interventions and manoeuvres that will be attempted.

Every 5 years the American Heart Association (AHA) releases International Liaison Committee on Resuscitation (ILCOR)–based updates on CPR – this information is a review of the previous 5 years of research to determine if there is any new evidence that affects guidelines for CPR; the AHA guidelines are available free online through the *Circulation* journal. This information is primarily based on human research, and application in veterinary medicine may be inappropriate or simply wrong. However, the good news is that a group of very well-known and dedicated specialists and professionals put together the Reassessment Campaign on Veterinary Resuscitation (RECOVER) in order to publish the first evidence-based consensus CPR guidelines for veterinary medicine.

RECOVER identified five areas to be investigated:

- Preparedness/prevention
- Basic life support (BLS)
- Advanced life support (ALS)
- Monitoring
- Post-arrest care

PREPAREDNESS/PREVENTION

RECOVER recognised that training the team is critical for success, and expecting the unexpected is of the preparation. This training should include regular drills in the training refreshers.

CPR team

The ideal number of participants in a resuscitation attempt is three to five. In a small practice, when staffing is limited, it may be helpful to train the receptionists and kennel help to be a part of the CPR team. Each person can be taught to carry out a specific task.

The team leader is usually the veterinary surgeon; if the vet is not available, then the person with the most experience in performing CPR should lead the team. People will be needed to provide ventilation, do chest compressions, establish IV lines, administer drugs, attach monitoring equipment, record the resuscitation effort and monitor the effectiveness of the team's efforts. Practice a protocol for reception, intervention and monitoring **for all people in the hospital, including reception staff if necessary.**

Practice drills should be held monthly. A stuffed animal can be used as the patient during these drills. Each person should understand what his or her responsibilities would be during an arrest. After each practice session or true resuscitation, a self-evaluation should be performed.

Resuscitation area

One of the first decisions to be made is where the resuscitation attempt will take place. Some people prefer to perform CPR wherever the patient is located and bring the resuscitation equipment and supplies to the patient. Others prefer to designate an area in the clinic. When selecting an area, take into consideration the space available; is there enough room for a CPR team (three or more people) and equipment? An oxygen source should be readily available. Good lighting is a must; it facilitates endotracheal intubation and visualisation of veins, and, if open-chest massage is attempted, it will allow visualisation of internal structures. If CPR is to be performed on a table, then the height of the table should be adjustable. If a table is too tall for the person performing chest compressions, he or she may find it difficult to perform effectively. If the height of the table is not adjustable, then a footstool should be made available or CPR should be performed on the floor. Avoid grated surgical prep tables if at all possible. They have too much 'give,' which can be counterproductive when performing chest compressions. If you have no choice and must use a prep table, then put a board on or below the grate to provide extra support. The table must have a solid surface. If some form of crash cart is not used, then the drugs, ECG and defibrillator should be in close proximity. A shelf and a few drawers may be set aside for the emergency supplies.

Crash cart/kit

A crash cart/kit may be as simple as a plastic box or as elaborate as a mobile tool chest. Crash carts/kits help to make the resuscitation endeavour more efficient by having all the supplies readily available. If a cart is used, then in addition to the endotracheal tubes, drugs, catheters, syringes etc., equipment may be stored on the cart such as suction machine, ECG and defibrillator. The crash cart or kit should be checked at the beginning of each shift and restocked immediately after each use.

CPR protocol

Clinic staff can respond more efficiently if a protocol is established as to how cardiac arrest will be managed. The protocol can be organised either as a numerical list of steps or an algorithm (flowchart). It is also helpful to have a chart of drug dosages, which is based on the patient's body weight. If a computer is available, a program can be set up using a spreadsheet. By entering the patient's body weight, all the emergency drug doses can be calculated, printed, and placed in the patient's record. A drug dosage chart can also be based upon a small, medium, large or giant patient. The protocols should be reviewed periodically to ensure that they are up to date.

Recognition of cardiac arrest

The existence of cardiac arrest must be recognised early if we are to effectively resuscitate the patient. The ABCs (airway, breathing and circulation) should be rapidly checked in the apnoeic unresponsive patient. The absence of a palpable pulse, audible heart sound, or effective ventilation (agonal breaths should not be considered effective breaths) all support the assessment of cardiopulmonary arrest. Even under the best of circumstances it may be difficult to palpate a pulse; therefore, not much time should be spent trying to assess pulses. If there is any question that cardiac arrest has taken place the patient should be treated as such until proven otherwise. If in doubt, commence CPR – time should not be wasted checking for pulses, auscultating the thorax or looking for respirations. In patients under anaesthesia, aggressive CPR should be commenced as soon as possible – patients under anaesthesia have an increased chance of survival.

BASIC LIFE SUPPORT

Basic life support (BLS) should be initiated as quickly as possible following diagnosis of cardiac arrest using the circulation, airway, breathing (CAB) concept. Circulation should be addressed first, as ventilation will be ineffective if there is no cardiac output, and evidence suggests that outcome worsens as delay to the initiation of chest compressions increases.

Circulation: chest compressions

Patients with cardiac arrest have no forward blood flow out of the heart and no delivery of oxygen to the tissues. An immediate consequence is the exhaustion of cellular energy stores, cell depolarisation and thus loss of organ function. This quickly results in increasing severity of ischaemic organ injury and sets the stage for escalating reperfusion injury upon reinstitution of tissue blood flow. The initial goals of chest compressions are to provide (1) pulmonary blood flow for oxygen uptake and CO_2 elimination, and (2) tissue perfusion for oxygen delivery to restore cellular metabolic activity. Experimental evidence suggests that even well-executed external chest compressions produce at best 30% of normal cardiac output, making proper technique critical. Chest compressions should be started as soon as possible after diagnosis or suspicion of cardiac arrest. Delay in the start of high-quality chest compressions reduces the likelihood of return of spontaneous circulation (ROSC). Chest compressions should be done with the dog or cat in lateral recumbency with a compression depth of $\frac{1}{3}-\frac{1}{2}$ the width of the chest at a rate of 100–120 compressions per minute regardless of size or species. Use of aids to ensure correct compression rate, such as a metronome or a song with the correct tempo (e.g., 'Staying Alive') is recommended. Leaning on the chest between compressions must be avoided to allow full elastic recoil. Chest compressions should be delivered without interruption in cycles of 2 minutes, and a new compressor should take over after each cycle to reduce the effect of rescuer fatigue. Any interruption in compressions should be as short as possible, as it takes approximately 60 seconds of continuous chest compressions before coronary perfusion pressure (CPP) reaches its maximum. CPP in turn is a critical determinant of myocardial blood flow and the likelihood of ROSC.

The physiology of blood flow generation is fundamentally different during CPR compared to spontaneous circulation. Two distinct theories exist to explain how chest compressions lead to systemic blood flow. The cardiac pump theory is based on the concept that the left and right ventricles are directly compressed, increasing the pressure in the ventricles, opening the pulmonic and aortic valves and providing blood flow to the lungs and the tissues respectively. Recoil of the chest between compressions due to the elastic properties of the rib cage creates negative pressure within the chest, improving filling of the ventricles before the next compression. The thoracic pump theory is based on the concept that external chest compressions raise overall intrathoracic pressure, forcing blood from intrathoracic vessels into the systemic circulation, with the heart acting as a passive conduit. Given the chest wall stiffness in medium and large dogs, blood flow generated by the thoracic pump mechanism likely predominates in these patients. It is recommended therefore that the chest be compressed over the highest point on the lateral thoracic wall with the patient in lateral recumbency (i.e., the widest of the chest). In contrast, in very keel-chested dogs (e.g., sight hounds) it is reasonable to do chest compressions directly over the heart as the cardiac pump mechanism likely predominates. In markedly barrel-chested dogs (e.g., English Bulldogs), compressions over the sternum with the patient in dorsal recumbency may be more effective in eliciting the thoracic pump mechanism than lateral chest compressions. In these and other large dogs with low chest compliance, considerable compression force is necessary for CPR to be effective. The compressor should maintain locked elbows with one hand on top of the other, and the shoulders should be directly above the hands. This allows compressions to be done using the core muscles rather than the biceps and triceps, reducing fatigue and maintaining optimal compression force. If the patient is on a table and the elbows cannot be locked, a stool should be used or the patient should be placed on the floor.

Most cats and small dogs tend to have higher thoracic compliance and narrower chests than larger dogs, making the cardiac pump mechanism achievable in these patients; therefore, chest compressions should be done directly over the heart. Compressions may be performed using the same two-handed technique as described earlier for large dogs, or may be done using a single-handed technique where the compressing hand is wrapped around the sternum and compressions are achieved from both sides of the chest by squeezing. Circumferential compressions of the chest using both hands may also be considered.

Airway and breathing: ventilation

If an endotracheal tube and laryngoscope are available, the patient should be intubated as soon as possible. Both dogs and cats can be intubated in lateral recumbency, so chest compressions should continue during endotracheal tube placement. If an endotracheal tube is not readily available, mouth-to-snout ventilation will provide improved oxygenation and CO_2 removal. The patient's mouth should be held closed firmly with one hand. The neck is extended to align the snout with the spine, opening the airway as completely as possible. The rescuer makes a seal over the patient's nares with his or her mouth and blows firmly into the nares to inflate the chest. The chest should be visually inspected during the procedure and the

breath continued until a normal chest excursion is accomplished. An inspiratory time of approximately 1 second should be targeted.

In non-intubated patients ventilated using the mouth-to-snout technique, ventilation cannot be performed simultaneously with chest compressions: 30 chest compressions should be delivered, immediately followed by two breaths. Alternating compressions and ventilations should be continued for 2-minute cycles, and the rescuers rotated every cycle to prevent fatigue. Chest compressions and ventilations should be performed simultaneously in intubated patients because the inflated cuff of the endotracheal tube allows alveolar ventilation during chest compressions and interruptions in chest compressions are minimised. Intubated patients should be ventilated at a rate of 10 breaths per minute with an inspiratory time of approximately 1 second. If a spirometer is available, a tidal volume of approximately 10 ml/kg should be targeted. This low minute ventilation is adequate during CPR since pulmonary blood flow is reduced. Care should be taken not to hyperventilate the patient, as low arterial CO_2 tension leads to cerebral vasoconstriction, decreasing oxygen delivery to the brain.

ADVANCED LIFE SUPPORT

Once BLS procedures have been implemented, the CPR team should initiate advanced life support (ALS), which includes monitoring, drug therapy, and electrical defibrillation. Drug therapy is preferably administered by the IV or intraosseous route. Therefore, placement of a peripheral or central IV or intraosseous catheter is recommended, but should not interfere with continuation of BLS.

MONITORING

Many commonly employed monitoring devices are of limited use during CPR due to their susceptibility to motion artefact and the likelihood that decreased perfusion will compromise accurate readings. Low-yield monitoring devices include pulse oximeter and indirect blood pressure monitors, including Doppler and oscillometric devices. The two most useful monitoring devices during CPR are the electrocardiogram (ECG) and the end-tidal CO_2 (ETCO$_2$) monitor.

Electrocardiogram

Although the ECG is highly susceptible to motion artefact and is of limited use during ongoing chest compressions, an accurate rhythm diagnosis is essential to guide drug and defibrillation therapy. The goal of ECG monitoring during CPR is to diagnose which of the three most common arrest rhythms are present: (1) asystole, (2) pulseless electrical activity (PEA) or (3) ventricular fibrillation (VF). The ECG should be quickly evaluated while compressors are being rotated between 2-minute cycles of CPR, the rhythm diagnosis should be called out to the group by the team leader, and differing opinions on the diagnosis should be solicited. Discussion about the rhythm diagnosis should not prevent rapid resumption of chest compressions.

End-tidal CO$_2$ monitoring

ETCO$_2$ data can be used in multiple ways during CPR, and regardless of the technology used is highly resistant to motion artefact. The presence of measureable CO_2 by ETCO$_2$

monitoring is supportive of (but not definitive for) correct placement of the endotracheal (ET) tube. Because ETCO$_2$ is proportional to pulmonary blood flow, it can also be used as a measure of chest compression efficacy under conditions of constant quality of ventilation. Upon return of spontaneous circulation (ROSC), ETCO$_2$ dramatically increases due to the rapid increase in circulation, and therefore is a valuable early indicator of ROSC during CPR.

Drugs

Epinephrine (adrenaline) is a strong alpha-adrenergic. Alpha-adrenergic drugs work on alpha-receptors causing arterial vaso-constriction. Diastolic blood pressure is increased, which results in augmented coronary and cerebral blood flow. The drug also causes constriction of large veins, which would increase intrathoracic blood volume and thus 'cardiac output'. Initial doses of epinephrine should be 0.01 mg/kg (low dose). In the case of a prolonged arrest, a dose of 0.1 mg/kg (high dose) might be considered. Epinephrine should be re-administered every 3–5 minutes. To minimise underdosing and overdosing, epinephrine should be administered during every other BLS cycle.

Vasopressin is the naturally occurring antidiuretic hormone. In doses higher than required for the antidiuretic hormone effect, vasopressin acts as a direct peripheral smooth muscle vasoconstrictor. Vasopressin is an effective vasoconstrictor and may be used as an alternative to epinephrine in the treatment of cardiac arrest. The suggested dose is 0.08 U/kg IV. It may be used as a substitute or in combination with epinephrine every 3–5 minutes.

Atropine is indicated in the treatment of asystole. It plays the central role in the prevention and management of cardiac arrest associated with intensive vagal stimulation, which can occur during certain surgical procedures. The recommended dose is 0.04 mg/kg given once.

Crystalloid fluids are indicated only if the patient is hypovolemic. Lactated Ringer's or a lactated Ringer's–like solution is a reasonable choice. In one study, dextrose solutions were implicated in increased morbidity and mortality in association with cardiac arrest; therefore, dextrose should not be used. The dose of fluids in the dog is about 40 ml/kg and 20 ml/kg in the cat. The fluids should be given rapidly intravenously, in boluses sufficient to maintain effective circulating volume. When anaemia or hypoproteinaemia is present, whole blood or plasma or a synthetic colloid may be indicated.

Reversal agents such as naloxone, flumazenil, and atipamezole may be considered if an opioid, benzodiazepine or alpha-2-agonist respectively has been administered recently prior to the cardiac arrest.

Sodium bicarbonate (NaHCO$_3$) is used to correct metabolic acidosis, which is generated by anaerobic metabolism in hypoxic tissues. NaHCO$_3$ may be given empirically at a dose of 1 mEq/kg if the cardiac arrest is greater than 10–15 minutes.

Calcium is not currently recommended in the routine treatment of cardiac arrest. Calcium may be indicated when the patient is hyperkalaemic or hypocalcaemic. The dose of calcium is 0.1 ml/kg of 10% calcium chloride or 0.4 ml/kg of 10% calcium gluconate.

Route of drug administration

It appears that a central vein is the best route for drug administration. With this route drugs are administered close to the heart. Peripheral venous drug administration tends to deliver the drug to the heart in a lower blood concentration and at a slower rate as compared to the central venous route. Experimental studies in animals demonstrate that drug delivery after peripheral injection is enhanced by following the injection with 10–30-ml saline flushes and elevation of the extremity. The circulation time was shorter and the peak concentration was higher.

An alternative to the IV route is the intraosseous route. This route requires the placement of an intramedullary cannula inserted into the femur (through the greater trochanter), humerus (through the greater tubercle) and wing of the ilium or tibial crest. Medications and IV fluids can be injected into the medullary canal and rapid uptake is provided by the abundant endosteum-medullary blood supply.

The intratracheal route has been advocated for drug administration when venous access is not available. Some studies have indicated that drug uptake from the tracheal surface during resuscitation is sporadic, undependable and delayed. The drugs that may be administered by this route include epinephrine, atropine, and vasopressin. If this route is to be used, then the dose of the drug should be doubled and added to sterile saline or water for volume. The drugs are injected down the endotracheal tube via a long catheter that extends beyond the endotracheal tube and down to the level of the carina.

Intracardiac injections are not recommended because of the potential problems that can occur with this route. Problems include myocardial trauma, lacerated coronary arteries, pericardial effusion and refractory ventricular fibrillation when the heart muscle is injected with epinephrine. The American Heart Association recommends that this route be used when no other is available, and others feel that its use is indicated only during open-chest heart massage.

Defibrillation

Defibrillation is the treatment of choice for ventricular fibrillation (VF) and pulseless ventricular tachycardia (PVT). If the patient has VF or PVT and the duration is less than 4 minutes or if VF is diagnosed during a rhythm check between BLS cycles, the heart is defibrillated immediately. However, if the duration of VF or PVT has been suspected to be greater than 4 minutes, then a 2-minute cycle of BLS must be performed prior to defibrillation.

Following the application of a contact gel and the defibrillator charged to the desired energy level, BLS is stopped and the patient placed in dorsal recumbency. The defibrillator paddles are placed firmly over the heart on each side of the chest; the defibrillator is discharged after clearing the area around the patient of people. The energy necessary for defibrillation is 4–6 joules/kg and 2–4 joules/kg for monophasic and biphasic defibrillation, respectively. The monophasic and biphasic internal defibrillation energy level is 0.2–0.5 joules/kg. In the past, it was suggested to rapidly repeat defibrillation up to three times if the patient had a refractory VF or PVT. It is now suggested that a full 2-minute cycle of CPR be performed before re-evaluating the ECG and defibrillating again.

The precordial thump is a method of mechanical defibrillation where the patient is struck with the heel of the hand directly over the heart in the hopes of converting the patient. While there is minimal efficacy for this technique, it should be considered only if a defibrillator is not available.

POST-RESUSCITATION CARE

After the arrest the patient should be monitored closely. Special attention should be paid to the cardiovascular system, pulmonary system and CNS. It is helpful to monitor as many parameters as possible for each system; this gives you a clear overview of the patient's status.

BIBLIOGRAPHY

Aspinall, V., 2003. Clinical Procedures in Veterinary Nursing. Butterworth-Heinemann, Oxford.

O'Dwyer, L., 2007. Wound Management in Small Animals. Butterworth-Heinemann, Oxford.

RECOMMENDED READING

Aldridge, P., O'Dwyer, L., 2013. Practical Emergency and Critical Care Veterinary Nursing. Wiley Blackwell, Oxford.

    An excellent general overview of the practical application of emergency and critical care, written with the veterinary nurse in mind.

Burkitt Creedon, J.M., Davis, H., 2012. Advanced Monitoring and Procedures for Small Animal Emergency and Critical Care. Wiley Blackwell, Oxford.

    An excellent, in-depth, comprehensive textbook aimed at both veterinary surgeons and nurses.

King, L.G., Boag, A., 2007. BSAVA Manual of Canine and Feline Emergency and Critical Care, second ed. British Small Animal Veterinary Association, Gloucester.

    An excellent second edition to this essential textbook for those not only working in emergency and critical care environment, but also for those less familiar with some of the techniques and procedures.

21

Prevention of the Spread of Infectious Diseases

HELEN HARRIS | AMANDA ROCK

KEY POINTS

- Infectious diseases are caused by pathogenic microorganisms, including bacteria, viruses, fungi and protozoa.

- Pathogens are able to leave the body via any of the normal orifices and within any of the body secretions.

- To cause infection, a pathogen must be transmitted by a method that ensures that it reaches the susceptible animal as quickly as possible or ensures its survival in the environment before it enters the animal.

- Methods used to control the spread of disease are mainly aimed at preventing transmission of the pathogen.

- Once a pathogen enters the body, the immune system initiates a series of responses aimed at overcoming the pathogen and preventing the development of clinical signs.

- Immunity can be divided into innate factors, which produce the same response to every type of 'attack', and acquired factors, which produce a specific response to the individual pathogen.

- Vaccination is based on the acquired immune response and results in lifelong immunity to a disease without suffering the symptoms of the disease.

Introduction

An infectious disease is one that is caused by the invasion of harmful microorganisms or pathogens, which will establish and grow in the body tissues. The pathogens are then transmitted between individuals and the disease spreads. When dealing with infection, it is important to understand how the pathogen leaves the infected animal, how it transfers and how it enters the susceptible animal or new host. Each pathogen has its own pattern, evolved to achieve optimum pathogen survival and virulence. Through training and experience, the nurse will play an important role in the survival of the animal and elimination of the disease. Useful definitions relating to infectious diseases are included in Box 21.1.

Spread of infectious diseases

CAUSAL AGENTS

Microorganisms are living creatures seen only with the aid of a microscope or macroscopically when grown in colonies. They come in many forms and have varying forms of transmission and effects on the body. Not all microorganisms are pathogenic, i.e. capable of causing disease; some are normal inhabitants of the living body and live in harmony with the host without causing disease (see Chapter 30 for further details). Pathogenic microorganisms are categorised as follows:

Bacteria

Bacteria are single-celled organisms that range in size from 0.5 μm to 5 μm in length. They can replicate outside the living cell, ensuring their survival and making them difficult to eliminate. There are three basic shapes that are recognised:
- Bacilli (cylindrical or rod-shaped), e.g. *Salmonella* spp.
- Cocci (spherical), e.g. *Streptococcus* spp.
- Spirochaetes (spiral), e.g. *Leptospira* spp.

They are further divided into groups depending on whether or not they stain with Gram's stain (see Chapter 31). For example:
- Gram-negative *Salmonella* spp. live within the intestines.
- Gram-positive streptococci cause respiratory disease.
- Gram-variable *Leptospira canicola* causes leptospirosis.

Most bacteria reproduce most effectively at body temperature but are not always pathogenic. They may be:
- Commensals – live on or in the animal and do not normally cause disease
- Facultative pathogen – become pathogenic within immunosuppressed animals
- Obligate pathogens – will always cause disease.

In addition:
- Saprophytic bacteria will only replicate on dead tissue and are responsible for the decay of dead animals and plants.
- Symbionts or mutualistic bacteria are organisms that both provide a benefit to the host and derive a benefit for themselves – this process is known as symbiosis or mutualism.

Viruses

Viruses are extremely small, simple structures incapable of replicating outside the body cell. They are obligate intracellular parasites and are sometimes classified as non-living. Viruses vary in their stability and, with the exception of poxvirus, parvovirus and rotavirus, they do not survive well outside the host. They are difficult to treat once established, as they are protected within the host cells and the chosen methods of treatment are prophylactics, vaccination and good nursing. Examples of viruses include canine adenovirus (CAV-1), which causes canine infectious hepatitis, and feline parvovirus, which causes feline infectious enteritis.

BOX 21.1   USEFUL DEFINITIONS

- Infectious disease – a disease caused by microorganisms that can be spread between individuals.
- Non-infectious disease – a disease that is not caused by microorganisms but is usually due to a disturbance in the normal metabolism of the animal, e.g. diabetes mellitus, neoplasia, poisoning.
- Contagious disease – a disease that is able to spread from one animal to another via direct or indirect contact.
- Direct contact – physical contact between animals. Skin surfaces of animals will come together during licking, grooming, sleeping, fighting and, in rare circumstances, coitus. Microorganisms transmitted via this route need to live in or on an animal to survive. Pathogens spread in this way are frequently fragile and easily destroyed.
- Indirect contact – no physical contact between animals. Transmission occurs when the animal contaminates the environment with body fluids, e.g. urine or faeces. The microorganism is transported on fomites or by vectors and can survive in the environment for varying periods depending on the species.
- Fomite – a contaminated, inanimate (non-living) object, e.g. feeding bowls or litter trays.
- Vector – an animate object that carries the microorganisms. These can be further grouped into:
  - Biological vector – acts as intermediate host in the life cycle of some microorganisms or parasites. Some of the organism's development occurs within the intermediate host before it is eaten by the final/definitive host. For example, the cat flea is the vector for the larval form of the dog and cat tapeworm *Dipylidium caninum*.
  - Non-biological vector/mechanical vector – these play no role in development of the microorganism or parasite and simply transfer the disease from one animal to another. There are two types:
    - Transport host – will carry the infection to another animal without becoming affected by it at all. They maintain the viability of the microorganism; for example, the cat flea transports the virus that causes feline panleukopenia and the rickettsia *Haemobartonella felis*, which causes feline infectious anaemia.
    - Paratenic host – must be eaten by the final host to continue the life cycle and spread the infection. The microorganism lives within the paratenic host's tissue but there is no further development; for example, cats eating raw lamb from individuals infected with the protozoon *Toxoplasma gondii* will then become infected.

Chlamydias and rickettsias

This group have characteristics of both bacteria and viruses and cause such diseases as psittacosis in birds, chlamydiosis in cats and Q fever in a range of mammals, including humans.

Parasites

Parasites are defined as eukaryotic organisms that live off another organism to the advantage of the parasite (see Chapter 29). They may be:

- **Ectoparasites** – living on the outside of the body. They may cause discomfort and sometimes they act as vectors of disease, e.g. *Ctenocephalides* spp. and *Trichodectes canis* transmit the tapeworm *Dipylidium caninum*; *Ctenocephalides felis* transmits *Haemobartonella*, the causal agent of feline infectious anaemia; ticks carry *Borrelia burgdorferi*, the bacteria which causes Lyme disease.
- **Endoparasites** – living inside the body. Any detrimental effects on the animal's health will depend on the species.

Some may also be zoonotic, i.e. they can be transmitted from the animal to humans; for example, *Toxocara canis*, the roundworm of the dog, may cause visceral larva migrans and *Echinococcus granulosus*, a dog tapeworm, causes hydatidosis in humans.

Protozoa

Protozoa are single-celled organisms causing varying levels of disease within animals depending on the species. Some may also be zoonotic, e.g. *Toxoplasma gondii*, found in cats, may cause cysts within body tissues and abortion and birth defects in humans. Certain species of *Coccidia* live within the intestines of rabbits and poultry but can become pathogenic in intensively managed animals, causing coccidiosis, which may be fatal.

Fungi

Most fungi are non-pathogenic but some are able to invade healthy tissues and cause disease. They can be divided into yeasts, e.g. *Malassezia pachydermatis*, a common cause of skin disease in dogs, and dermatophytes, e.g. *Microsporum canis*, which is a cause of ringworm in many species.

ROUTES OF TRANSMISSION

In order to cause disease a pathogen must leave the host animal, be transmitted between the host and the susceptible animal and then enter the susceptible animal.

Pathogens are able to leave the host through any of the body orifices (Fig. 21.1) and within any of the body secretions – the choice depends on the species of pathogen (Table 21.1).

TABLE 21.1	Methods by which pathogens can leave the body	
Part of the body	**Secretion**	**Examples of disease**
Eyes	Ocular discharge	Cat flu Chlamydia Myxomatosis
Nose	Serous nasal discharge	Cat flu Kennel cough Distemper
Mouth	Oral discharge: saliva Vomit	Rabies Feline leukaemia virus Feline immunodeficiency virus Salmonella
Ear	Wax	*Otodectes cynotis*
Skin	Ectoparasites	*Ctenocephalides felis* *Linognathus setosus* *Trichodectes canis*
Mammary glands	Milk	*Toxocara canis* Feline leukaemia virus
Circulatory system	Blood	*Haemobartonella felis*
Gastrointestinal tract	Faeces	*Toxocara* spp. *T. gondii* *Salmonella* spp. *Campylobacter* spp.
Urinary	Urine	*Leptospira canicola* Canine infectious hepatitis
Reproductive	Vaginal discharge	*Brucella canis*

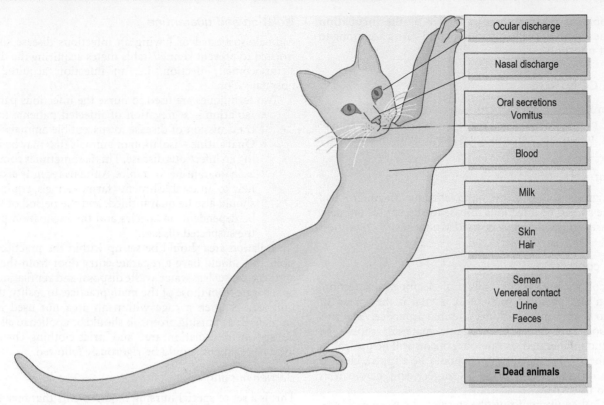

Fig. 21.1 Methods by which pathogens leave the infected animal

When the pathogen has left the body it must be transmitted to a susceptible animal. This may be almost instant, e.g. droplets transmitted by sneezing or coughing, or may take many weeks or even years, e.g. eggs of *Toxocara canis* may survive in grass for up to 2 years ready to be ingested by a susceptible dog. The following list shows the methods of transmission used by different groups of pathogens.

- **Direct contact** – the host animal touches the susceptible animal, e.g. during grooming, licking, etc., and the pathogen is transferred from one to the other. Commonly occurs in the transmission of ectoparasites
- **Indirect contact** – the host and the susceptible animal may be some distance apart and the pathogen requires a means of transport and a means of survival – often protection from drying out. The following are examples of indirect contact:
  1. **Aerosol droplets** – pathogens that cause respiratory diseases survive within the water droplets coughed or sneezed into the environment. The contaminated atmospheric air is inhaled and the pathogen will reach the nasal chambers and the pharynx.
  2. **Topical (inoculation)** – via bites or scratches. The skin is penetrated, allowing the pathogen to enter the body systems, e.g. *Staphylococcus* spp.; the hookworm *Uncinaria stenocephala* is able to burrow through the footpads of the dog; feline leukaemia virus is spread by bites and scratches during cat fights.
  3. **Faeces** – contains many pathogenic organisms, e.g. worm eggs and viruses such as parvovirus.
  4. **Vomit** – may carry parvovirus, salmonella or distemper virus.
  5. **Saliva** – may carry rhabdovirus, causing rabies, or feline leukaemia virus.
  6. **Blood** – may transmit feline immunodeficiency virus or *Haemobartonella felis*.
  7. **Oral** – a common route for the ingestion of pathogens that affect the digestive tract, e.g. roundworms, *T. gondii*, *Salmonella* spp., *Cryptosporidium* spp.
  8. **Venereal** – occurs during coitus, e.g. *Brucella canis* and transmissible venereal tumours.

Carriers

Some diseases may be transmitted by carriers. These are animals that secrete the pathogen at intervals and are a risk to contact animals. They may be classed as:

- **Convalescent carriers**, i.e. animals that have recovered from the disease, e.g. cat flu, canine infectious hepatitis, but secrete the pathogen, particularly when they are stressed
- **Healthy carriers**, i.e. animals that have apparently never had the disease and may be immune to it. Healthy carriers, e.g. of ringworm, are a particular risk, as there is no history of having had the disease.

Once the pathogen has entered the susceptible animal it must establish itself and replicate within the tissues. The most common site is in the lymph nodes local to the point of entry. When sufficient numbers of pathogens have been produced they are carried around the body by the blood or the lymph to their favoured site of action and symptoms will develop. The time lag between the entry of the pathogen into the body and the development of symptoms is known as the **incubation period**. The length of the incubation period varies according to the type of infection.

DISEASE CONTROL

The transmission of microorganisms can be minimised with the use of prophylactics, good nursing care and client education. The following are examples used within veterinary practice:

Treatment

Rapid diagnosis followed by rapid effective treatment will prevent the spread of infectious disease to susceptible animals. In some cases euthanasia may be used as a means of prevention of spread.

Infection control

Infection control involves all aspects of cleaning, disinfection, sterilisation and personal hygiene. It is vital if the spread of disease is to be prevented within a veterinary practice. All urine, faeces, blood and discharges (organic material) should be removed and incinerated, as microorganisms will be present in large numbers. The soiled animal should be clipped, cleaned and dried on admission, prior to surgery and before it is returned to its owner.

All surgical equipment must be sterilised between each use:

- Cleaning – reduces the number of pathogens and physically removes them by the use of water and detergents
- Disinfection – kills all pathogens with the exception of bacterial spores by the use of disinfectants
- Sterilisation – kills all pathogens and bacterial spores by the use of heat, ethylene oxide gas or radiation.

Disinfectants

When controlling microorganisms within the hospital environment, it is essential to clean and disinfect correctly to prevent the transmission of pathogens between animals. **Antiseptics** are disinfectants designed for use on skin and are used for scrubbing up prior to surgery and for preparation of the surgical site. Removal of organic matter, e.g. faeces, blood, dust and hair, will ensure that disinfectant agents are not inactivated before they reach the microorganisms. Most disinfectants are used at a lower strength for routine use and higher concentrations for specific disease-causing conditions, but it is important to read the manufacturer's instructions.

Each disinfectant will have different properties and may be classified as either bactericidal, i.e. it will destroy the microorganisms, or as bacteriostatic, i.e. it will inhibit their replication for a period of time.

As a guide:

- Most disinfectants are effective against Gram-positive bacteria, as they are easily destroyed.
- Gram-negative bacteria are more resistant, as are bacterial spores; the aldehyde and halogen groups are most effective against them.
- Halogens (hypochlorites) are used for viral infections.
- Fungi should be eradicated with a designated fungicide to ensure elimination of fungal spores.
- Pine oil disinfectants have no activity against the major microorganisms and should never be used, especially if fungi are present.

Isolation and quarantine

Animals suspected of having an infectious disease should be isolated to prevent kennel/stable mates acquiring the disease as a nosocomial infection, i.e. an infection acquired during hospitalisation.

Two techniques are used to nurse the infectious patient:

- **Isolation** – segregation of infected patients to reduce transmission of disease to susceptible animals
- **Quarantine** – isolation of animals that may be incubating an infectious disease. This is sometimes compulsory, as in quarantine for rabies. Animals recently acquired or new to an establishment (farm, kennels, equine yards) should also be quarantined, and the period of time will be dependent on species and the incubation period of the suspected disease.

An isolation area should be set up within the practice. If possible, this should have a separate entry door from the outside and services such as water, waste disposal and ventilation should be separate from those of the main practice. In reality, the isolation area is often a cage within an area not used by other animals. Basic nursing protocols should be applied to all patients housed in the isolation area and strict clothing changes and hygiene regimens should be rigorously followed.

Barrier nursing

This is a set of special nursing requirements that mean that an effective 'barrier' is created preventing the transmission of a pathogen by a fomite, e.g. clothing or cleaning equipment:

- Keep the animal in strict isolation.
- Use the same kennel, if possible, for the duration of the stay.
- Clean and treat the patient after all others; separate staff nursing the isolated patients, if possible.
- Keep separate equipment, e.g. cleaning and feeding equipment, for each patient.
- Disinfect all animal areas after use.
- Use disposable suits, gloves, apron and foot baths.

Parasiticides

Routine eradication of parasites will prevent their transmission to other animals, reduce the effects, such as anaemia, emaciation and failure to thrive, and improve the animal's immune system. It will also minimise the chances of the owner developing a parasitic zoonotic infection, e.g. visceral larva migrans.

Vaccination

Vaccines are given to stimulate antibody production, so preventing a specific disease. Hyperimmune serum contains ready-made antibodies and can be given to the animal where there is a high and immediate risk of contracting a disease. The level of immunity must be kept up by the use of regular booster vaccinations.

Balanced diet

An animal receiving the correct nutrients will develop a healthy immune response, which will enable the body to fight any disease with which it comes into contact.

Client education

Clients must be educated as to what is required when looking after an animal. This should include vaccination, parasite control and basic hygiene, all of which will help in the control of disease.

Zoonoses

A zoonosis is the term used to describe any disease transferable from animal to human, its opposite being an anthroponosis, which is a disease transferable from human to animal, e.g. gorillas may be infected by human measles. An increasing number of households now own a pet, so animal owners and veterinary personnel are at increased risk of contracting a zoonotic disease.

Unsuspecting owners may show moderate to severe illness, which may, on occasion, be fatal. Some examples of zoonotic diseases are shown in Table 21.2. They include:
- Leptospirosis – Weil's disease
- *Cheyletiella* spp. – mange
- *Sarcoptes scabiei* – scabies/mange
- Ringworm
- *Toxocara canis* – roundworm
- Toxoplasmosis
- Salmonellosis
- *Chlamydophila psittaci* – psittacosis.

TABLE 21.2	**Zoonotic diseases**					
Zoonosis	**Causal agent**	**Body system affected**	**Clinical symptoms**	**Incidence/ prevalence**	**Transmitted within**	**Symptoms found in humans**
Campylobacter	*Campylobacter jejuni*	Gastrointestinal (GI) tract	Tenesmus diarrhoea: • Mucoid • Watery • Bloody • Bile streaks Occasional fever Anorexia Intermittent vomiting	Dogs Higher in puppies Less commonly affects adult cats but kittens up to 6 months of age	Faeces Poorly sanitised kennels Asymptomatic carriers	Fever Abdominal pain Diarrhoea
Cat scratch fever	*Pasteurella*	n/a	(none, as *Pasteurella* is a commensal bacterium – unless immunosuppressed)	Cats	Bites Scratches	Inflammation at scratch/bite wound Cellulitis Occasional fever Regional lymphadenopathy
Cheyletiellosis	*Cheyletiella* spp.	Skin/exocrine	Pruritus Scaling	Animals within shelters Boarding and grooming establishments	Hair and dander	Pruritus Urticarial weals on trunk and arms
Chlamydiosis	*Chlamydophila psittaci*	Ophthalmic Respiratory GI tract Reproductive tract	Unilateral conjunctivitis leading to bilateral Nasal discharge	Adult cats Kittens between 2 and 6 months of age Birds	Ocular discharge	Mild conjunctivitis
Cryptosporidiosis	*Cryptosporidium* spp.	GI tract	Diarrhoea	Dogs (esp. > 6 months of age) Cats	Faeces	Vomiting Diarrhoea Headache Abdominal pain
Hydatidosis	German Shepherd dogs spp.	GI tract	Malnutrition	Dogs fed on raw meat	Faeces	Abdominal pain Jaundice Chest pain Cough
Leptospirosis	*Leptospira canicola* *Leptospira hardjo*	Primarily: • Renal • Hepatobiliary Can also affect: • Nervous • Respiratory • Cardiovascular • Reproductive • Ophthalmic	Pyrexia Jaundice Vomiting Diarrhoea	Unvaccinated dogs Rarely found in cats	Urine Contaminated bedding	Fever Vomiting Headache Muscle ache Jaundice Nephritis
Rabies	Rhabdovirus	Nervous system Salivary glands	Change in attitude and behaviour depending on dumb or furious Mandibular and laryngeal paralysis Dropped jaw Hypersalivation	Dogs Bats Foxes	Saliva	Fever Anxiety Headaches Dysphagia Hydrophobia Convulsions Death

Continued

TABLE 21.2	Zoonotic diseases—cont'd					
Zoonosis	Causal agent	Body system affected	Clinical symptoms	Incidence/ prevalence	Transmitted within	Symptoms found in humans
Ringworm	*Microsporum canis*	Skin/exocrine	Alopecia Crusty lesions Erythema Hyperpigmentation Pruritus	Dogs Cats – especially long-haired breeds	Skin and dander	Dermatitis Alopecia Erythema Ring-shaped crusty lesions
Roundworm	*Toxocara canis*	GI tract	Abdominal distension Cachexia Coughing Diarrhoea	Dogs, especially puppies	Faeces containing L2 larvae	Can cause blindness (temporary or permanent) in young children
Salmonellosis	Gram-negative bacteria	GI tract	Vomiting and diarrhoea Systemic disruption Organ infarction Anorexia Malaise	Dogs – young, pregnant Cats normally have a high resistance but stressed, hospitalised cats	Faeces Densely populated areas Pig ear treats Exposure to carrier animals Exposure to raw meat	Watery diarrhoea Dehydration Abdominal pain Fever
Sarcoptic mange	*Sarcoptes scabiei*	Skin/exocrine	Pruritus Scaly lesions Alopecia	Dogs	Skin lesions	Intense pruritus Red lesions at site of contamination or between fingers, under breasts or in groin region
Toxoplasmosis	*Toxoplasma gondii*	Reproductive	Normally asymptomatic	Cats	Faeces Infected hair	Fever Headache Lymphadenopathy Cough, although symptoms often ignored **Pregnant women:** Foetal changes, abortion

The main defence against zoonoses are education and basic but rigorous hygiene routines. The veterinary practice must devise its own rules and ensure that all staff are aware of them. Care must be taken when handling infected animals and their secretions. General guidelines to protect against contracting a zoonotic disease include:

- Owner education – make sure that they are aware that such diseases exist.
- Wear protective suits, aprons, gloves and, in some cases, eye protection and masks when dealing with infected patients.
- All faecal and urinary samples for testing should be treated with care and disposed of correctly without contaminating personnel.
- Always wash hands with chlorhexidine or povidone-iodine after handling animals or their products.
- Change infected clothing immediately after dealing with the animals.
- Keep kennel runs, gardens and children's sandpits free from faeces.

Infectious diseases

THE DOG

Canine parvovirus

Aetiology: Canine parvovirus 2 (CAV-2).

Very infectious disease. Virus mutated from feline parvovirus or panleukopenia in the 1970s. The virus is shed in the faeces during the incubation period and is very stable, surviving within the environment for up to 5 months. Barrier nursing and correct use of virucidal disinfectants are essential in controlling nosocomial infections within the hospital. The most critical stage of the disease for the animal is the first 3–4 days.

Transmission: via direct or indirect contact with faeces.

Incubation period: 4–7 days

Pathogenesis: Virus can only replicate in rapidly dividing cells such as lymph nodes, bone marrow, epithelial linings of lung, liver and intestines, which makes this disease very common in young, developing puppies. Rottweilers,

German Shepherd dogs and Dobermans have a greater susceptibility to this disease.

Clinical signs: Depression, vomiting, anorexia. Vomiting follows 48 hours after the onset of profuse, watery, haemorrhagic diarrhoea. Loss of body fluids leads to dehydration, which is the most common cause of death in these patients.

Diagnosis: History, clinical signs leading to enzyme-linked immunosorbent assay (ELISA) testing for CAV-2 antigen during early stages of infection, as this is when the virus will be shed. The antigen test can provide false negatives after the rapid decline in viral shedding that tends to occur within 10 days of infection.

Treatment: Isolation and barrier nursing. Rehydration and maintenance fluids to replace the fluid deficit. Antibiotics to treat secondary infections. Early enteral nutrition and the use of recombinant feline interferon has been shown to lessen clinical signs.

Prevention: Vaccination of dam before mating and puppy from 8 weeks of age using a live vaccine. In high-risk areas the dam can be given a killed vaccine during gestation and puppies can receive antiserum or start early vaccination at 6 weeks of age, followed by the usual primary vaccine course. A further vaccine at 16 weeks ensures that the maternally derived antibodies have not interfered with the vaccines response and is recommended in high risk areas. Puppies who survive the disease will develop very good immunity, which may last a number of years. Booster vaccinations should be given after 1 year and then every third year, dependent on the vaccination manufacture's guidelines.

Canine distemper

Aetiology: Canine distemper virus – a morbillivirus related to rinderpest and measles.

A multisystemic viral disease that can become chronic, affecting the dog several years after infection. The virus is labile and is easily destroyed by sunlight, heating and drying. Poor hygiene is normally to blame for disease outbreak.

Transmission: Via aerosol droplets and ingestion.

Incubation period: 7–21 days although an initial fever may occur after 3 days, accompanied by anorexia and leucopaenia which subsides and reoccurs several days later along with the rest of the clinical signs.

Pathogenesis: The virus replicates in the tonsils and lymph nodes, causing a viraemia. The next stage depends on the animal's immune response. In animals with poor immunity, further replication occurs within the epithelial cells of the respiratory and gastrointestinal cells. The skin can also become affected, leading to the 'hard pad' syndrome. In animals with more established immunity, mild signs may be observed but in each the virus will affect the nervous system.

Clinical signs: Pyrexia, nasal discharge, coughing, vomiting, diarrhoea, chorea (twitching) and hyperkeratosis of the pads. Fifty per cent of patients will be subclinical cases. Chronic signs include encephalitis and rheumatoid arthritis.

Diagnosis: Blood samples show red and white blood cell inclusions and lymphopaenia. Lymph nodes will harbour the virus and are normally viewed during post-mortem examination. Thoracic radiographs may show a pattern typical of viral pneumonia. Immunofluorescent assay or PCR of smears from conjunctiva or tracheal epithelium may aid diagnosis.

Treatment: Good nursing care and symptomatic treatment – fluid therapy, antibiotics, antiemetics, anticonvulsants, antitussives. Euthanasia may be considered in some cases.

Prevention: Vaccination. Immunity can last for 3 years following the first booster but annual vaccination may be needed in high-risk areas.

Canine leptospirosis

Aetiology: Bacteria – *Leptospira canicola* (affects the kidney) and *Leptospira icterohaemorrhagiae* (affects the liver). Other serovars may become more prevalent due to widespread vaccination programs.

It is a zoonotic bacterial disease contracted from contaminated water, especially stagnant woodland pools where rats drink and bathe.

Transmission: Direct or indirect contact with contaminated water or urine. Can also be spread via transplacental and venereal infection.

Incubation period: 4–12 days

Pathogenesis: Bacteria penetrate broken skin and mucous membranes and replicate in the liver and kidney, causing hepatitis, acute renal failure and intravascular coagulation. *Leptospira* can be excreted in the animal's urine for months or years after recovery.

Clinical signs: Pyrexia, vomiting, shock, interstitial nephritis and hepatitis. Signs dependent on animal's age, immunity and environmental factors.

Diagnosis: Blood samples show elevated urea and creatinine and elevated liver enzymes alanine aminotransferase (ALT) and alkaline phosphatase (ALKP). Serology is the most commonly used diagnostic test for dogs.

Treatment: Rehydration fluids, to include plasma or blood to correct the intravascular coagulation. Antibiotics, antiemetics and dietary management to assist with liver and kidney function.

Prevention: Vaccination at yearly intervals, especially in high-risk animals – working or outdoor dogs. Good hygiene procedures to prevent spread and development of a zoonosis.

Infectious canine hepatitis

Aetiology: Canine adenovirus (CAV-1).

Also known as Rubarth's disease.

Transmission: Direct or indirect contact with faeces, urine, saliva and fomites.

Incubation period: 5–9 days.

Pathogenesis: Virus enters the mouth and replicates in the tonsils and lymph nodes via the thoracic duct. Viraemia results and further replication occurs within the vascular endothelium, causing pericardial effusions, hepatitis and vasculitis.

Clinical signs: Anorexia, pyrexia, vomiting, diarrhoea, hepatomegaly, conjunctivitis, photophobia, petechiae and jaundice. Death can occur within 24 hours.

Diagnosis: Blood samples show increased liver enzymes ALKP and ALT and bile salts. ELISA, serologic and PCR testing are available.

Treatment: Supportive therapies – fluids, antibiotics for secondary infections, antiemetics, good nursing care. Plasma or whole blood may help with the coagulopathies.

Prevention: Vaccination. Live CAV-2 vaccine is used to protect against CAV-1 and CAV-2. Live CAV-1 will cause mild symptoms and 'blue eye'. Immunity lasts for 3 years after the booster.

Kennel cough

Aetiology: Numerous pathogens can be responsible, including *Bordetella bronchiseptica*, parainfluenza (pi) virus 2, CAV-2, reovirus, herpes virus and secondary bacterial infections.

Also known as canine infectious tracheobronchitis or canine contagious respiratory disease (CCRD).

Transmission: Aerosol droplets, via direct or indirect contact. This is a common disease found where several animals share the same air space, e.g. boarding kennels and hunt kennels.

Incubation period: 5–7 days.

Pathogenesis: Organisms replicate within the upper respiratory tract (parainfluenza virus is unable to replicate in macrophages). Secondary infection attacks the damaged tracheal epithelium. Ciliostasis (paralysis of the cilia on the mucous membranes) can occur, due to toxins that are produced in response to a *Bordetella* infection.

Clinical signs: Dry, hacking cough, with or without a terminal retch, which is precipitated by exercise, excitement or palpation of the trachea. Animals are not normally pyrexic unless a secondary infection is evident. A mucopurulent nasal and ocular discharge and bronchopneumonia can result from serious infection.

Diagnosis: Clinical signs and history. Further tests are of limited value.

Treatment: Antibiotics, antitussives, restricted exercise, rest. Most animals recover well and quickly.

Prevention: Vaccination – parenteral and intranasal.

Lyme disease

Aetiology: *Borrelia burgdorferi* – a bacterium.

Transmission: Via deer tick (*Ixodes scapularis*). This is now the most common arthropod-borne illness in man in the USA and is becoming more common in the UK, particularly in areas where ticks are found in large numbers, e.g. Exmoor, Dartmoor and parts of Scotland. May affect dogs walking in these areas.

Incubation period: Not known, as the bacteria may lie dormant for several months.

Clinical signs: This is a multisystem inflammatory disease that affects the skin and then spreads to the joints, nervous system and other organs in the later stages. Symptoms include lameness, pyrexia, lethargy, lymphadenopathy, cardiac arrhythmias.

Diagnosis: Serological testing is an adjunct to diagnosis.

Treatment: Removal of any ticks. Antibiotics and supportive therapies.

Prevention: Regular treatment with a recognised ectoparasiticide, especially before visiting wooded areas that the tick may inhabit. Transmission of *B. burgdorferi* does not begin until the tick has been attached for 36–48 hours, so after walking the dog it should be checked for the presence of ticks, which should be removed immediately.

THE DOG AND CAT

Rabies

Aetiology: Rhabdovirus belonging to the genus Lyssavirus. This notifiable zoonotic disease affecting all warm-blooded animals has been eradicated in the UK because of its strict quarantine regulations.

Transmission: Saliva within bite wounds.

Incubation period: Variable between 1 and 6 months – depends on the area bitten and its proximity to the central nervous system, the immune status of the animal and the strain of the virus.

Pathogenesis: Replication of virus in the injured muscle tissue before it enters the peripheral nervous system and central nervous system. Antibodies can attack the virus while in the muscle tissue but once the virus has entered the nervous system nothing can be done.

Clinical signs: There are two forms – furious and dumb. Both follow a prodromal period in which general character changes are seen within the animal before specific clinical signs develop. Some cases may be atypical:

- Furious form: Hyperexcitability, interspersed with periods of calm, pica, biting and 'snapping' – often at imaginary objects, ataxia, progressive facial paralysis, drooling, dysphagia, frothing of saliva. Death normally occurs after convulsions. This form is most likely to be seen in carnivores such as the dog and cat.
- Dumb form: Animals are timid, often affectionate, and have a generalised paresis leading to paralysis and ataxia. Death normally results from paralysis of the respiratory muscles. This form is most likely to be seen in herbivores such as the cow.

Diagnosis: Clinical history. Histopathological examination of the brain following death demonstrating the presence of Negri bodies, which are seen in 75% of cases.

Treatment: None. Supportive therapies are not used because of the zoonotic potential and disease prognosis. DEFRA and the police must be contacted by the veterinary surgeon as soon as a case of rabies is suspected. The animal must be kept in the practice until the Division Veterinary Officer (DVO) from DEFRA arrives; then it will be destroyed and taken away for tests.

Prevention: Animals in the UK are not routinely vaccinated against rabies unless they are to travel abroad under the Passports for Pets Scheme (PETS).

Salmonellosis

Aetiology: *Salmonella typhimurium* – a bacterium.

This zoonotic disease is caused by a facultative bacteria living within the intestines of the animal.

Transmission: Raw, uncooked meat. Immunosuppressed animals may precipitate their own illness. Enteritis often caused by faecal–oral route.

Incubation period: Impossible to specify, as the bacteria have permanent residency within the gut.

Clinical signs: Depending on the severity – acute or chronic gastroenteritis, drooling saliva, pyrexia, abdominal pain, slight icterus, breeding problems.

Diagnosis: Faecal or saliva sampling to isolate high numbers of the microorganism.

Treatment: Isolate and barrier-nurse. Rehydration and maintenance fluids. Rest and allow the animal to recover to encourage its own immunity to develop. Antibiotics are not normally used as they can destroy healthy bacteria living within the gut.

Prevention: Reduce the use of unnecessary antibiotics as this may lead to the development of antibiotic resistance. Ensure that all food offered to animals is fresh and cooked.

THE CAT

Feline upper respiratory tract disease (FURTD)

Aetiology: Feline calicivirus (FCV) and feline herpes virus (FHV). Also *Chlamydia felis*, *Mycoplasma felis* and reoviruses.

Also referred to as cat flu or feline influenza. Once recovered, cats can become carriers and reinfect themselves and other cats, especially at times of stress.

Transmission: Aerosol droplets via the oral, nasal and conjunctival route. Can be direct or indirect contact.

Incubation period: 2–12 days.

Pathogenesis: The virus will replicate in the tissues of entry into the body, e.g. mouth and nares (see Fig. 21.1).

Clinical signs: These are slightly different depending on the causal virus:

- FCV – sneezing, oral ulceration, chronic stomatitis, pyrexia and occasional intermittent lameness
- FHV – symptoms are more severe – sneezing, pyrexia, conjunctivitis, keratitis, corneal ulceration, anorexia, depression.

Secondary infections can cause damage to intranasal structures and chronic illness.

Diagnosis: PCR of nasal, pharyngeal or ocular secretions.

Treatment: Antibiotics, fluid therapy and good nursing to include ensuring that the animal's airways are patent. Encourage the animal to eat, using smelly foods such as sardines or by placement of a naso-oesophageal tube if anorexic. It is important to remember that cats will not eat if they cannot smell the food.

Recovered cases can become carriers and therefore a source of infection. Overt signs of sneezing may begin to show as a result of stress such as being put into boarding kennels or being taken into the veterinary surgery for procedures such as castration or spaying.

Prevention: Annual vaccination. Owners should ensure that the boarding cattery they use has strict procedures for vaccination and isolation. Sneezing cats should be isolated immediately or discharged if there is no secondary infection evident.

Chlamydiosis

Aetiology: *Chlamydophila psittaci*.

Also called feline pneumonitis. This disease is potentially zoonotic and the persistent conjunctivitis often gets overlooked. It often occurs as part of FURTD.

Transmission: Direct contact with ocular discharges.

Incubation period: 3–10 days.

Pathogenesis: The virus replicates within the point of entry, the eyes and mouth (see Fig. 21.1).

Clinical signs: Unilateral conjunctivitis, which can become bilateral. Mild rhinitis.

Diagnosis: Conjunctival scrapes/swabs. PCR tests.

Treatment: Topical and systemic antibiotics – to be given over a period of weeks. All in-contact cats should be treated to control further outbreaks. Chlamydia is sensitive to disinfectants, so kennels must be thoroughly cleaned.

Prevention: Vaccination of animals in contact with *Chlamydia* carriers.

Feline infectious peritonitis (FIP)

Aetiology: Feline coronavirus (FeCoV).

This disease predominantly affects young cats, causing the body cavities to fill up with effusions.

Transmission: Intrauterine.

Incubation period: Variable. Cats shed virus in faeces within 1 week of infection via the oronasal route.

Pathogenesis: Virus replicates within the lymph nodes of the gut and within macrophages, then transfers to endothelial layers of the body, to include pleura, peritoneum, meninges and the kidneys, eyes and blood vessels. It is a combination of viral genetics and host immunity that leads to the development of disease in some cats.

Clinical signs: There are two forms:

- Effusive (wet) – this is the acute form of the disease: signs include ascites, pleural effusions, dyspnoea, pyrexia, weight loss, jaundice
- Non-effusive (dry) – the more chronic form of the disease: weight loss, neurological signs, ocular lesions, hepatomegaly.

Diagnosis: Serology, haematology and biochemistry, analysis of ascitic/pleural fluid. Serum amylase A (an acute phase protein) increases 10 times in the serum of infected cats.

Treatment: None, although steroids may be used in the short term. Symptomatic nursing by the owner is beneficial.

Prevention: Isolate breeding queens before kittening.

Feline infectious anaemia (FIA)

Aetiology: *Haemobartonella felis*, now known as *Mycoplasma haemofelis* – a chlamydia.

Transmission: *Ctenocephalides felis*, the cat flea, ingests blood as it bites. It then passes on the organism at its next bite.

Incubation period: Unknown.

Pathogenesis: Severe anaemia can occur in immunosuppressed or debilitated animals. Parasitised red blood cells are phagocytosed by macrophages within the spleen.

Clinical signs: Sudden onset of weakness, lethargy and anorexia. Pale mucous membranes with associated tachycardia, tachypnoea and splenomegaly.

Diagnosis: Examination of a blood smear – blood to be collected within an EDTA coagulant as this will free the parasite from the red blood cells. PCR assay.

Treatment: Tetracycline antibiotics and steroids.

Prevention: Control of arthropod vectors.

Feline leukaemia virus (FeLV)

Aetiology: A retrovirus.

Most common in younger cats in multicat households, where direct contact occurs during social grooming.

Transmission: Vertically – via the placenta to the kittens; horizontally – in milk or saliva via bites and scratches.

Incubation period: Viraemia occurs 2–4 weeks after infection.

Pathogenesis: Virus replicates in the oropharynx and related lymph tissues, leading to viraemia. Some animals may recover but in others the virus will further replicate in the lymph nodes and bone marrow. Some cats have a latent infection; others will be persistently viraemic and continue to shed the virus in their saliva.

Clinical signs: Many remain asymptomatic for years before showing immunosuppressive signs and related disease conditions. Reproductive problems such as resorption, abortion or stillbirth can be apparent before diagnosis.

Diagnosis: ELISA tests detect the p27 protein. Immunofluorescent assay and PCR.

Treatment: There is no known cure. As infected cats shed the virus they are a continual threat to others and euthanasia may be the best option. Feline interferon omega may aid survival.

Prevention: Vaccination is available.

Feline immunodeficiency virus (FIV)

Aetiology: A retrovirus.

This disease is common in free-roaming, older male cats, with the highest incidence at the age of 5–9 years.

Transmission: Via bite wounds.

Incubation period: A few weeks to a few months.

Pathogenesis: The virus replicates at the site of the bite wound, causing viraemia which cannot be eliminated from the body. A permanent infection remains, leading to a further depletion of T lymphocytes and resultant immunodeficiency.

Clinical signs:
- Primary infection – pyrexia, neurological signs, weight loss, lymphadenopathy, lymphopenia, increased risk of neoplasia
- Secondary infection – chronic stomatitis, upper respiratory tract infections, skin changes, diarrhoea.

Diagnosis: ELISA tests can detect the viral antibodies, although early infections may not be very reliable.

Treatment: Nothing is effective, although low-dose steroids may be beneficial for a short time.

Prevention: Control breeding of infective cats by neutering. Keeping cats housed indoors will significantly reduce the risk. There is no vaccine available.

Toxoplasmosis

Aetiology: *Toxoplasma gondii* – a protozoon.

Transmission: After 3 days, infected cat faeces contain sporulated oocysts, which are ingested by a variety of intermediate hosts, e.g. cattle, horses, sheep, mice and humans. Within the intermediate host the parasite settles mainly in the musculature and causes few if any symptoms. If cats are fed raw meat from an infected animal, the disease is transmitted (see Chapter 29).

Incubation period: 2–5 weeks.

Pathogenesis: The end host for *T. gondii* is the cat, where it is found within the small intestine.

Clinical signs: Normally asymptomatic, although mild cases of diarrhoea, lethargy, jaundice may show if cysts are present.

Diagnosis: ELISA blood test to detect antibodies.

Treatment: Antibiotics.

Prevention: Cook meat before feeding, clean litter trays regularly before the faeces reach the infective stage. There is no vaccine available in the UK. This disease is zoonotic and pregnant women are at risk – infection may result in foetal deformities, although this is rare.

THE RABBIT

Respiratory disease

Aetiology: The most common bacterial cause is *Pasteurella multocida*; however, other organisms such as *Staphylococcus aureus*, *Enterobacter* spp. and *Pseudomonas aeruginosa* are not uncommon pathogens cultured from the respiratory tract. *Bordetella bronchiseptica* has also been isolated from some severe cases.

Often the only sign of respiratory disease is a small amount of discharge matted on the medial aspect of the forepaws where the rabbit has rubbed it nose with its paws. Infection may progress rapidly and cause abscesses in the rabbit's chest, significantly compromising the lung capacity.

Transmission: Both direct and indirect contact. Rabbits develop little effective immunity following infection and many are asymptomatic carriers, which perpetuates the infection in the community.

Pathogenesis: After initial replication in the upper respiratory tract, the organisms may spread to associated structures such as the nasolacrimal ducts or the middle ear. The condition may end in septicaemia, bronchial congestion, tracheitis, splenomegaly and subcutaneous haemorrhages. Pneumonia is a secondary and complicating factor, which causes pleuritis, pyometra and pericardial petechiae.

Clinical signs: Upper respiratory tract infection is usually characterised by a serous exudate from the eyes and nose, which later becomes a mucopurulent discharge. Infection may manifest as any of the following: rhinitis (snuffles), pneumonia, otitis media, conjunctivitis, abscesses, genital infections or septicaemia.

Diagnosis: Culture a sample of discharge taken from at least 2 cm into the nasal cavity. The retracted swab can be used in an indirect fluorescent antibody test or plated into a culture medium. There is an ELISA test for detecting antibodies against *Pasteurella multocida*. When culturing abscesses, the capsule wall should be sampled rather than the contents, which are often sterile.

Treatment: Therapeutic agents must be carefully considered, as severe dysbiosis (loss of intestinal flora responsible for digestive function) and life-threatening enteritis can occur if the wrong antibiotic is chosen. Safe antibiotics include the fluoroquinolones, enrofloxacin, chloramphenicol or trimethoprim/sulfadiazine (Tribrissen) given orally once daily for 10–14 days. Penicillin G is an effective treatment given every 3–4 days to reduce the gastrointestinal effects. Pasteurellosis is considered an essentially incurable infection, so the aim is to alleviate clinical signs. In cases where there is improvement, therapy may be indicated for several months. A useful adjunct to systemic therapy is the use of nebulisation. Antibiotics, a mucolytic agent, a bronchodilator and saline to moisten the turbinates can all be combined for this therapy. The nebulisation is usually well tolerated through a mask over the rabbit's nose.

Prevention: Isolation of new rabbits until testing has been performed. Detection and culling of carriers. Rabbits with exudative rhinitis should be isolated from others.

Myxomatosis

Aetiology: A pox virus.

Myxomatosis is a fatal disease of all breeds of domestic rabbits and the European wild rabbit.

Transmission: Biting by mosquitoes, biting flies and fleas, and by direct contact.

Pathogenesis: The virus replicates and does its damage in the dermis, and lesions are seen in the mucous membranes as well as fibrotic nodule formation over the nose, ears and forefeet. There are few other characteristic lesions found at necropsy, although the spleen is occasionally enlarged and is almost always devoid of lymphocytes when examined histologically.

Clinical signs: Conjunctivitis develops, rapidly becomes more marked and is accompanied by a milky ocular discharge. The animal is listless and anorexic and the temperature reaches over 42°C (107.6°F). In acute outbreaks some animals die within 48 hours while those that survive become progressively depressed and develop a rough coat. The eyelids, lips, ears and coat become oedematous and the vulva and scrotum swell. A purulent nasal discharge appears and breathing becomes laboured. Death occurs within 1–2 weeks of the appearance of clinical signs.

Diagnosis: The clinical appearance and the high mortality are of diagnostic significance. Large, eosinophilic, cytoplasmic inclusion bodies in the conjunctival epithelial cells are also helpful.

Treatment: Supportive therapy is often tried but, as the disease is invariably fatal, euthanasia is recommended.

Prevention: An attenuated vaccine is available. This should be given every 6 months using a 25 gauge needle. 10% of the vaccine should be deposited intradermally and the rest administered subcutaneously.

Viral haemorrhagic disease (VHD)

Aetiology: A calicivirus causing an acute, highly contagious infection first described in 1984.

Transmission: Aerosol transmission seems to be important, although all secretions and excretions are sources of infection. Mechanical transmission by fomites, rodents and other vermin, rabbit by-products and humans are all implicated in spread of the disease. Insects do not seem to be important vectors.

Pathogenesis: Replication is rapid, the incubation period being only 24–72 hours, and animals are found dead but in good condition. Gross lesions are subtle and generally restricted to congestion of the respiratory tract and liver. There is intense congestion of the lungs and trachea, which may be filled with froth. Haemorrhage in the thymus is common and there is congestion of the liver, spleen and kidneys. Histologically there is a massive, focal, coagulative hepatic necrosis.

Clinical signs: In protracted cases, dyspnoea, congestion of the eyelids, orthopnoea, abdominal respiration and tachycardia are seen. Before death there is violent cage activity, with rapid turns and flips that resemble convulsions or mania. Some cases show a blood-tinged nasal discharge.

Diagnosis: The peracute course of the disease is the most important feature. Symptoms of respiratory distress, high mortality and rapid spread are all significant. Fluorescent antibody techniques and immunostaining techniques can be used to identify the viral antigen. Liver, spleen and lung are the specimens of choice as they contain a high number of virus particles.

Treatment: The disease is always fatal and death often occurs before a diagnosis is made.

Prevention: There is a vaccine for use in countries where the disease is already widespread and eradication efforts are difficult to employ. Quarantine measures must be applied to rabbits entering from countries where VHD is present. Several vaccines are available, one of which also protects against myxomatosis.

Encephalitozoon cuniculi

Aetiology: A protozoan that affects many mammals. It can be zoonotic in immunodeficeint humans.

Transmission: Organisms are shed in the urine and spread by ingestion, inhalation or to the developing foetuses by the transplacental route.

Pathogenesis: Levels of serum antibodies rise 21 days post infection and peak at 63 days. Protozoal spores are shed in urine for 9 weeks. The target organs are the liver, kidney, lung, heart and brain.

Clinical signs: The infection may be latent and cause no clinical signs; however, a range of signs may be seen including those of renal disease, ataxia, weight loss, polyuria and polydipsia, torticollis, convulsions and death. Cataract formation may also occur.

Diagnosis: Serological tests are reported back as titre levels.

Treatment: Rarely successful in neurological cases. Fenbendazole given at 20 mg/kg for 4 weeks is suggested as effective treatment although evidence is anecdotal.

Prevention: The use of fenbendazole for 9 consecutive days 2–4 times a year is recommended as this disease is widespread and potentially zoonotic.

THE HORSE

Equine herpesvirus

Aetiology: There are four equine herpes viruses (EHV). EHV-1 is associated with respiratory disease and is the most commonly diagnosed infectious cause of abortion. EHV-2 does not seem to cause disease. EHV-3 causes genital problems and EHV-4 is primarily a respiratory pathogen.

These viruses are endemic worldwide. They result in abortion and respiratory disease, resulting in a significant financial loss to breeders, and are a major cause of loss of performance in racehorses.

Transmission: The virus is easily spread through respiratory tract secretions and morbidity may be 100%. Foetuses aborted are heavily contaminated with virus and serve as a source of infection to other in-contact horses.

Pathogenesis: After respiratory infection with virus, it travels transplacentally in pregnant mares by migrating leukocytes within which it can establish latent infection.

Clinical signs: Respiratory disease is characterised by a transient elevation of temperature to 40°C (104°F), inappetence, nasal discharge, pharyngitis, depression and sometimes limb oedema.

Diagnosis: Serological diagnosis can be made on the basis of a rising antibody titre (i.e. a fourfold rise in antibody levels over a 2-week period). Diagnosis of abortion is usually made on post-mortem examination of the foetus and on virus isolation.

Treatment: Symptomatic treatment, including antibiotics to prevent secondary bacterial infection. Minimising stress is also important.

Prevention: Both killed and live attenuated EHV-1 vaccines are available. There is also a vaccine containing inactivated EHV-4.

Equine influenza

Aetiology: Viruses of the orthomyxovirus group. They are subject to constant change, known as antigenic drift.

Transmission: Droplet infection and inhalation. The short incubation period of 1–5 days and the persistent coughing that releases large amounts of virus into the air contributes to the rapid spread of the disease.

Pathogenesis: The virus infects the ciliated respiratory epithelial cells, which lose their cilia and become oedematous. The impaired clearance mechanism results in susceptibility to secondary infection.

Clinical signs: Elevation in temperature to 41°C (105.8°F) followed by a deep cough. Serous nasal discharge, which soon becomes purulent, inappetence and enlarged mandibular lymph nodes. Occasionally there is oedema of the legs and scrotum.

Diagnosis: Isolation of the virus from nasopharyngeal swabs or serological examination. Antigen detection kits are available.

Treatment: One week of complete rest for every day of elevated temperature. Non-steroidal anti-inflammatories and antibiotics to prevent secondary infection.

Prevention: Inactivated vaccines. Safe live attenuated vaccines are difficult to manufacture as the virus is capable of rapid mutation.

Equine viral arteritis

Aetiology: An arterivirus (an RNA togavirus) that causes international concern because of its abortigenic potential.

Transmission: The virus is spread through respiratory and venereal routes and through indirect contact with fomites. Aborted foetuses are heavily contaminated with virus.

Pathogenesis: There is a predilection for the arterial walls, so the main lesions seen are necrotising arteritis.

Clinical signs: Variable range and most infections are subclinical. Fever, depression, inappetence, limb oedema, stiffness in gait, inflammation of the conjunctiva (pink eye) and ocular and nasal discharges.

Diagnosis: Virus isolation/PCR and/or serology (ELISA test for antibodies).

Treatment: Supportive therapy and rest. Most horses make a speedy and uneventful recovery.

Prevention: Restriction of movement of horses from infected premises and, where permissible, by vaccination with a modified live vaccine. It is a notifiable disease.

Tetanus

Aetiology: *Clostridium tetani* – a bacterium. This is a disease which can affect many warm-blooded species including man.

Transmission: Abundant in equine faeces and occurs in the gut of other herbivores and in the soil. The organism is anaerobic and is only able to multiply in damaged tissue where necrosis and lowered oxygen tension combine.

Pathogenesis: A toxin is released by the organism within deep wounds, which enters the local motor and sensory nerves. Free toxin may enter the capillaries and lymphatic channels.

Clinical signs: Incubation period varies from 1–3 weeks. Inability to retract the nictitating membrane and spasms in the facial muscles. The ears are pricked; there is stiffness, trembling, difficulty in eating and chewing. Muscular responses become exaggerated. Sweating is profuse and the heart rate is elevated. The mortality rate is about 80%; death occurs within 1 week of the start of clinical signs.

Diagnosis: Based on clinical signs. The bacteria can be readily grown in the laboratory.

Treatment: Large doses of antitoxin prevent the toxin from damaging further nervous tissue. Prognosis is poor.

Prevention: Immunoprophylaxis is essential in horses as the risk of tetanus following injury is so great. Vaccination with tetanus toxoid, regular boosters and the use of antitoxin when a horse is wounded are all essential.

African horse sickness (AHS)

Aetiology: An orbivirus which causes a highly fatal disease, last seen in Europe in the late 1980s.

Transmission: Climate change has sparked significant concern in the UK about AHS as it is transmitted by the same insect species as the recently problematic Bluetongue virus in cattle and sheep. The biting insects responsible are midges (*Culicoides* spp.).

Clinical signs: Respiratory and circulatory damage, fever, loss of appetite; 70–90% mortality rate.

Diagnosis: Based on clinical signs and virus identification.

Treatment: None as infected animals should be culled.

Prevention: Almost no horses have antibodies against foreign diseases, because they have never been exposed to them. This results in a large, highly susceptible population and an ideal scenario for a major outbreak. The AHS outbreak in Spain and Portugal was eradicated by slaughtering infected animals, movement restrictions, vector (insect) control, and horse vaccination. No vaccine for AHS is currently licensed in the EU. Use of a modified live vaccine for AHS carries a risk of vaccine virus reversion to wild type (i.e. the virus used in the vaccine can potentially undergo changes that mean it could actually infect vectors, and subsequently susceptible Equidae). Thus at the present time, the vaccine will not be considered for use in the UK other than in an emergency situation.

Immunity

Also called functional or protective immunity, this describes security against a particular pathogen, which makes the animal non-susceptible to certain specific diseases. It involves the introduction of a foreign body, usually a protein or antigen, into the body and the body responds by enabling the lymphocytes (white blood cells) to produce specific antibodies or immunoglobulins (Fig. 21.2) to fight against that antigen. Antibodies are Y-shaped proteins with specific binding sites on the tips of the 'Y' which are formulated to attach to a specific antigen and by a variety of methods they then inactivate the antigen.

Lymphocytes are the key constituents of the immune system which can produce antibodies against millions of invading foreign agents. All microorganisms carry on their surface or

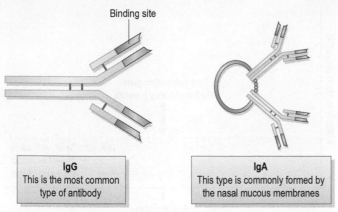

Fig. 21.2 Two types of antibody showing the binding sites on the tips of the Y-shaped proteins

secrete large protein molecules (the antigens), which initiate the immune response. B lymphocytes, cells originating in the bone marrow, have proteins on their surface that bind to the antigens. Binding, in turn, stimulates the B lymphocytes to mature into plasma cells and secrete antibodies at the rate of 2000 per second from each cell, which are then released into the blood circulation in response to the enemy invasion. These mature cells develop a memory of that particular invader and, if the antigen re-enters the body later in the animal's life, it will be recognised by the memory cells, specific antibodies will be produced and the antigen will be attacked and eliminated before clinical symptoms are observed. This is humoral immunity. Immature lymphocytes within the bone marrow are not competent to carry out their immune functions.

In addition, cells of another type, T lymphocytes, may bind to the antigen surface and assist with the immune response. T lymphocytes, which mature within the thymus gland, have proteins on their surface called T-cell receptors, which bind directly to the antigen. They are responsible for cell-mediated immunity. There are three types of T cell involved: the cytotoxic or killer T cells, which bind to and destroy other cells displaying antigens on their surface; the helper T cells, which assist B cells to stimulate antibody production; and suppressor T cells, which reduce B-cell activity, reducing the possibility of an autoimmune response.

Lymphoid organs, e.g. spleen and thymus gland, are responsible for filtering bacteria and other foreign substances into the lymph nodes and for producing lymphocytes to combat infection. The thymus gland, in the neck, contains macrophages and immature and mature T lymphocytes. The spleen, found in the cranial abdomen, acts as a defensive filter for blood and as a site of B- and T-cell function. Other areas of lymphoid tissue, such as the palatine, pharyngeal and lingual tonsils, are permanent sites of lymphocyte aggregation, meeting and fighting microorganisms that enter via the oral or nasal route.

Lymph nodes are found at portal sites throughout the body and act as a defensive filter for lymph and a site of B- and T-cell function. The cortex of each node is densely packed with B lymphocytes, the medulla consists of lymphocytes and plasma cells and the paracortex (junction of cortex and medulla) contains T cells.

TYPES OF IMMUNITY

There are two types of immunity:
- Innate immunity
- Acquired immunity.

Innate immunity

Innate immunity is hereditary and congenital, i.e. present at birth. There are many non-specific factors that affect the ability of the animal to resist invasion by pathogens. The response of these factors is always the same no matter what the injury or type of pathogen. They include the following:
- Genetic factors – may be due to the animal's species, breed or strain
- Physical barriers – external or mechanical defence of the body
- The inflammatory response – a non-specific response to tissue damage.

Genetic factors. Animals are automatically immune to certain diseases that affect some species but not others. For example, myxomatosis affects rabbits but not dogs or cats, while foot and mouth disease only affects cloven-hoofed animals. This may even be extended to certain strains or families of animals which may carry a predisposition to a particular disease while other strains are not. The colour of an animal may also be a genetic factor in its protection. White animals, e.g. horses, and the white ears of cats may be more susceptible to damage by the ultraviolet rays of the sun which may result in some types of tumour.

The physical barrier. Often referred to as the external or primary defence mechanism. Providing they are not damaged and the animal is healthy, the following will create an external and internal barrier to prevent 'invasion' of the body:
- Skin – the largest organ in the body provides protection as the external covering of the body. The sebaceous glands produce sebum, which creates an acid surface pH that prevents replication of pathogenic bacteria while creating an environment for the survival of normal commensal bacteria. Sweat glands release sweat, which contains lysozymes with antibacterial properties.
- Mucous membranes – produce secretions, which wash away any foreign material. The conjunctiva keeps itself clear by producing tears, the respiratory tract produces mucus and saliva contains more lysozymes.
- Hairs – microscopic hairs or cilia are found as part of epithelial tissues in selected areas of the body, in particular within the respiratory system. They are found in association with mucus-producing glands and are collectively termed 'ciliated mucous epithelia' (see Chapter 6). Their function is to trap bacteria or foreign particles within the mucus and the hairs then sweep them away from susceptible organs.
- Secretions – in addition to the above, semen contains antibacterial proteins and zinc; the vagina maintains an acidic environment that inhibits bacterial growth; and stomach acids provide an inhospitable environment for any pathogen that is swallowed.

The inflammatory response. When the body is damaged, e.g. by wounds or by infection, it responds by releasing histamine from mast cells within connective tissue. Histamine causes vasodilation of blood capillaries, increasing the blood supply to the area, and the area becomes reddened. It also changes the permeability of blood capillaries so that plasma proteins and tissue fluid leak out into the surrounding tissues, which then become swollen. Chemical mediators are transported by the tissue fluid to the site and attract white blood cells, in particular the polymorphonuclear leucocytes (PMNs), which are able to phagocytose dead and damaged tissue and bacteria to fight the infection. The inflammatory response is essential in the elimination of the initiating factor but it can lead to chronic problems if not controlled.

Acquired immunity

This form of immunity is acquired by the animal continuously throughout its life. It is also referred to as specific immunity, as it has a definite role to play in combating specific infectious diseases. Acquired immunity involves the development of specific antibodies in response to attack by specific antigens. For example, canine parvovirus antibodies will be produced by the lymphocytes in response to infection with canine parvovirus. It can be further classified as follows:

a. **Natural active immunity** – antibodies are produced in the body by lymphocytes in response to the animal actually having had, and survived, the disease. This type of immunity is more pertinent to viral disease conditions than to bacterial or protozoal infections and the antibodies produced following eradication of a pathogen give lifelong protection.

b. **Artificial active immunity** – this involves the introduction of an inactivated form of the disease into the animal's body to encourage the lymphocytes to produce specific immunoglobulins but without actually causing clinical symptoms. This is the basis of vaccination: a vaccine is an inactive form of a disease.

c. **Artificial passive immunity** – the animal acts as the recipient for antibodies via antiserum or hyperimmune serum, which have been already been produced within a donor animal. The transfer of this protection is vital for animals with a poor or undeveloped immune system. It gives them instant protection against diseases that they may be susceptible to because they are too young to form their own antibodies or because they have had no previous exposure in the form of the disease or through vaccination. This form of immunity lasts for only a few days because the antibodies themselves are foreign protein and are broken down by the body's defence system.

d. **Natural passive immunity** – neonatal animals have an inherent ability to respond immunologically to some antigens but the response is much slower and weaker than in an older animal that has been exposed to many pathogens during its life. This means that a neonate is at risk of contracting a disease until it develops the ability to produce its own antibodies. Maternally derived antibodies, supplied to the neonate in the colostrum or first milk, provide protection for the first 8–12 weeks of life (Fig. 21.3).

Neonates must consume the colostrum within hours of birth, as at this stage there is an absence of digestive enzymes and the large antibody protein molecules will be able to pass undigested through the intestinal wall into the blood stream. A small percentage of maternal antibodies also reach the foetus via the placenta. The dam can only supply the level of protection that she has accumulated over her life via regular vaccination and disease exposure. Her reaction to antigen identification and antibody formation rely on a healthy immune system and vaccination prior to coitus or during early gestation. Any neonate

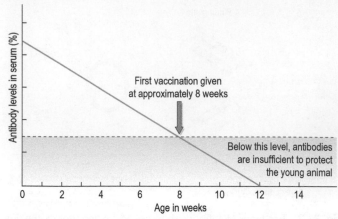

Fig. 21.3   Graph to show levels of maternal antibody in the young animal

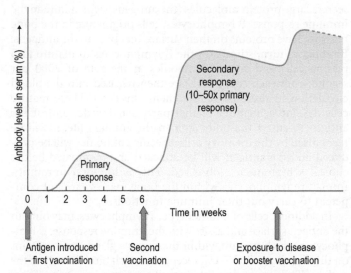

Fig. 21.4   Graph to show antibody response to the introduction of an antigen by natural exposure or vaccination

deficient in colostrum will be susceptible to illness until its own immune system has developed.

The timing of the administration of the first vaccine to the young animal is related to the levels of maternal antibodies remaining in the body. If the levels are too high they will destroy the antigen which is injected to stimulate the immunity of the animal; if the animal is not given its first vaccination until the levels of the maternal antibodies have becomes very low, then the animal is at risk of disease. The recommended time for the first vaccination is at about 8 weeks (see Fig. 21.3).

IMMUNE RESPONSE TIME

The first time that an animal encounters a specific pathogen, antibodies will be produced within 7–10 days – known as the primary response. By this time the animal may already have developed symptoms; however, if the animal meets the antigen later in its life the immune system, having retained the memory of the first response, is able to produce the antibodies within 24 hours, long before symptoms develop. This secondary response is 10–50 times greater than the primary response and is the principle behind the idea of regular booster vaccinations (Fig. 21.4).

Vaccination

Young animals have an insatiable curiosity and, as they investigate the world around them, will come into contact with infectious diseases. The purpose of vaccination is to provide immunity to the susceptible animal by introducing a disrupted and harmless version of the pathogen into the body. This stimulates the defence system to produce an immune response in the absence of clinical disease. Although it has not been proved that vaccination will completely protect the animal, it will protect the animal from expressing all clinical symptoms when naturally exposed to the disease. Vaccines are available against most of the common infectious diseases of companion animals and horses (Table 21.3). A list of useful definitions relating to vaccines is shown in Box 21.2.

TYPES OF VACCINE

There are two types of vaccine used within current veterinary practice and they both have advantages and disadvantages (Table 21.4):

- Live attenuated (modified) vaccine – contains live organisms that have been attenuated by culturing the pathogen in controlled conditions, e.g. canine parvovirus, feline infectious enteritis. These stimulate a good immune response but have the risk of causing the disease.

- Killed (inactivated) vaccine – contains dead organisms killed by ultraviolet, heat or sublethal chemicals such as formalin, e.g. leptospirosis. As the dead organisms cannot replicate within the body and are gradually removed by phagocytosis, several doses are required to produce sufficient antibody levels. Killed vaccines may be made more potent by the addition of an adjuvant such as oil or aluminium. This slows the release of the vaccine and delays its removal from the body by phagocytosis. Adjuvenated vaccines stimulate better immunity and in some cases remove the need for additional boosters.

VACCINE MANAGEMENT

A course of two or sometimes three vaccinations are given to provide protection to the vulnerable young animal whose

---

BOX 21.2 VACCINE TERMINOLOGY

- Vaccine – a preparation containing a small inactivated quantity of an organism that would normally cause disease.
- Toxoid – a chemically or heat-treated toxin that has a reduced pathogenicity but is still able to stimulate the production of antibodies.
- Hyperimmune serum/antiserum – serum containing antibodies to a particular disease. The antibodies are extracted from an animal that has produced high quantities as a result of vaccination. Used when an animal is in contact with the disease and requires instant protection, e.g. in a canine parvovirus outbreak.
- Autogenous vaccine – a vaccine made from the animal's own cells. A sample is taken and prepared by a laboratory before being injected back into the donor animal. Used in cases of skin infection where traditional therapies have not been successful.
- Adjuvant – a substance that is added to an inactivated vaccine to increase its efficacy and prolong its action.
- Attenuation – the virulence of an organism can be reduced (attenuated) to a point where it is able to replicate but is no longer pathogenic.
- Subunit vaccine – contains only a component of the microorganism, which is enough to produce an immune response but cannot cause the disease, e.g. FeLV vaccine.

TABLE 21.3 Vaccines available for the prevention of infectious diseases in the dog, cat, rabbit and horse

Species	Infectious disease	Form available	Route
Dog	Distemper	L or ML	Subcutaneous
	Hepatitis	L (CAV-2)	Subcutaneous
	Parvovirus	L or ML	Subcutaneous
	Leptospirosis	K	Subcutaneous
	Parainfluenza virus	L or ML	Subcutaneous
	Bordetella bronchiseptica	L	Intranasal
	Rabies	K	Subcutaneous
	Tetanus	K	Subcutaneous
Cat	Feline infectious enteritis	L, ML or K	Subcutaneous
	Feline influenza	ML or K	Subcutaneous
	Feline leukaemia	L (non-replicable) K or subunit	Subcutaneous
	Feline Chlamydia virus	K	Subcutaneous
	Rabies	K	Subcutaneous
	Tetanus	K	Subcutaneous
Rabbit	Viral haemorrhagic disease	K	Subcutaneous
	Myxomatosis	L	Subcutaneous
Horse	Influenza	K	Subcutaneous
	Herpes virus	Inactivated EHV-1	Subcutaneous
	Rotavirus	K	Subcutaneous
	Tetanus toxoid	K	Subcutaneous
	Rabies	K	Subcutaneous

Data taken from Mueller, P., 2004. Henston Companion Animal and Equine Veterinary Vade Mecum, twenty-second ed. Henston, Peterborough.
K, killed; L, live; ML, modified live.

TABLE 21.4 Comparison between live and killed vaccines

Modified live (attenuated)	Killed (inactivated)
One dose required	Two doses required
Allows controlled virus replication	No viral activity
Low antigen numbers required	High antigen numbers
Adjuvant not used	Adjuvant used – a reaction may be noted
Mild clinical signs may be observed	Killed so no risk of clinical signs
Contraindicated in immunocompromised animals	Safe in immunocompromised animals
Contraindications in pregnant animals – may affect the foetus	Safe to use in pregnant animals
Gives rapid and long-lasting protection	Shorter protection

immune system is underdeveloped. The first vaccination is given as the maternally derived antibody levels begin to fall (see Fig. 21.3), and antibodies will be formed within 7–10 days. A second dose is given 2–3 weeks later, stimulating the production of yet more antibodies with a quicker response time of 12–24 hours (see Fig. 21.4). This initial course provides antibodies for several months and should be reinforced 1 year later with a 'booster' vaccine to 'top-up' the acquired immunity. Failure to present the animal for the initial booster may result in a two-dose vaccine programme comparable to the primary course. In addition, the animal can gain natural active immunity when exposed to disease, creating further antibodies and protection.

The vaccines are administered by the following routes:

- **Subcutaneous route** – this is the most common route and is given in the scruff. The site of injection needs to be varied to prevent skin irritation if this route is to be used for a course of injections. Sterile equipment will be required but the use of a spirit swab is not advised, as it may precipitate a vaccine reaction.
- **Intranasal route** – drops placed into the external nares via a modified syringe create local antibody and cell-mediated immunity for respiratory diseases such as *Bordetella bronchiseptica*, a causative agent for kennel cough.
- **Oral route** – available for some European vaccines, e.g. rabies vaccine used in wild foxes.

Vaccines will only be effective if they are stored in a refrigerator at 2–4°C (35.6-39.2°F) and remain cold. Warmth will kill the microorganisms within a live vaccine. Stock control should be observed and those with the shortest expiry date should be used first. The veterinary surgeon or nurse should understand how to reconstitute vaccines and know which vaccines can be mixed to reduce the number of injections to be given. The veterinary nurse can prepare the vaccination certificate, but the veterinary surgeon is responsible for the document and must check all details and sign to authenticate it; veterinary nurses can sign records of vaccination cards, but not certificates of vaccination.

FAILURES IN VACCINATION

Vaccines may be ineffective for various reasons and owners must be aware that the veterinary surgeon may refuse to vaccinate their animal if an underlying illness or complications are suspected. Newly acquired puppies should not be brought to the surgery until they have had time to settle, as stress will have a negative effect on the immune system, causing vaccine failure. Older animals presented for vaccination without a current vaccine certificate will, depending on age and health, be given a full booster vaccination to ensure that the animal is truly protected against all infectious diseases (see Table 21.3).

Primary vaccine courses should be administered when the passive immunity received from the mother has decreased, as maternally derived antibody (MDA) interferes with the neonate's ability to respond to a vaccine (see Fig. 21.3). Delaying vaccination until MDA wanes may result in some puppies or kittens becoming infected and suffering the disease. Animals suffering systemic disease will suffer from immunosuppression and protective antibodies will not be produced in response to the antigen. A risk of clinical disease within patients suffering

from FeLV and FIV has resulted in an abandoned vaccine schedule.

Other causes of vaccine failure include:

- Animal has been exposed to the disease shortly after vaccinating – before the body has produced sufficient antibodies
- Animal was actually incubating the disease at the time of vaccination
- Vaccine has passed the expiry date
- Vaccine was not stored correctly
- Incorrect administration route
- Use of antibiotics or corticosteroids at the same time
- Incorrect timing of primary vaccine course
- Failure to boost the vaccine
- Animals may have a poor immune system
- Excessive use of alcohol or disinfectant on the skin.

ADVERSE REACTIONS

When introducing any foreign substance into the body there is a risk of an allergic reaction. Owners should be made aware of possible effects and asked to report to the veterinary surgeon if any are observed. Symptoms may range from mild lethargy to severe shock and may include:

- Swelling of injection site
- Urticaria
- Vomiting
- Diarrhoea
- Depression
- Ataxia
- Shivering
- Collapse.

Corticosteroids may be given as treatment and, if there are signs of shock, supportive therapy must be administered. The reaction should be recorded on the animal's treatment card and a different type of vaccine should be used for the next dose.

DIAGNOSTIC USE OF ANTIBODIES – ELISA TESTS

Enzyme-linked immunosorbent assay (ELISA) is based on the ability to produce monoclonal or polyclonal antibodies to a specific antigen or isolation and production of a specific antigen. In kits to detect antigens, antibodies specific for the antigen are bound to the wall of the test well, wand or membrane. The blood, serum or plasma sample is then added and any antigen present will bind to the antibody present. Washing of the test kit removes any unbound antibody. A second enzyme-labelled antibody is added, followed by a second washing. To finish, a substrate is added to develop a specific colour if the antigen is present.

At present there are commercial tests kits available to recognise the p27 protein found in FeLV and to test for antibodies in FIV cases. Fewer steps within the kits reduce the likelihood of human error and for further accuracy most tests contain a positive and negative control. These kits are of most use in cats showing suspected clinical symptoms, animals that have been in contact with a suspected case and as a precaution prior to breeding.

BIBLIOGRAPHY

American Lyme Disease Foundation. Available from: <www.aldf.com/lyme.shtml>.

Bowden, C., Master, J., 2003. Textbook of Veterinary Medical Nursing. Butterworth-Heinemann, Oxford.

Cooper, B., Mullineaux, E., Turner, L., 2011. BSAVA Textbook of Veterinary Nursing, fifth ed. BSAVA Publications.

Davol, P.A., 2002. Vaccines, Infectious Diseases and the Canine Immune System. Available from: <http://www.labbies.com/immun.htm>.

Fraser, C.M., 1991. The Merck Veterinary Manual, seventh ed. Merck & Co., Inc., Whitehouse Station, NJ.

Higgins, A.J., Wright, I.M., 1994. The Equine Manual. Baillière Tindall, London.

Kelleher, S., 2003. Respiratory disease in the rabbit. In: British Small Animal Veterinary Association Congress 2003 Scientific Proceedings. British Small Animal Veterinary Association.

Lightfoot, T.L., 2002. Hyaluronidase: Therapeutic applications including egg-yolk disease. In: Proceedings of the Association of Avian Veterinarians.

Mackean, D., Jones, B., 1985. Human and Social Biology. John Murray, London.

Mueller, P., 2004. Henston Companion Animal and Equine Veterinary Vade Mecum, twenty-second ed. Henston, Peterborough.

Pratt, P.W., 1998. Principles and Practice of Veterinary Technology. C V Mosby, St Louis, MO.

Tilley, L.P., Smith, F.W.K., 2004. The 5-minute Veterinary Consult: Canine and Feline, version 3. (Available as CD-ROM.). Lippincott Williams & Wilkins, Philadelphia, PA.

RECOMMENDED READING

Bowden, C., Master, J., 2003. Textbook of Veterinary Medical Nursing. Butterworth-Heinemann, Oxford.
Entire book dedicated to the subject designed for veterinary nurses and those taking more advanced courses.

Ramsey, I., Tennant, B., 2001. Manual of Canine and Feline Infectious Diseases. BSAVA, Quedgeley, Gloucester.
Written for the veterinary surgeon but information is comprehensive and approachable.

Access to all of the equine disease surveillance reports can be obtained from the Animal Health Trust website on www.aht.org.uk or from the DEFRA website www.defra.gov.uk or the BEVA website www.beva.org.uk.

22

Common Medical Conditions of the Body Systems

PAULA HOTSTON MOORE

Introduction

The common medical conditions covered in this chapter may be described as those which result from a problem within one or several body systems and are neither infectious nor require surgery to correct them. Many of these conditions elicit a *differential diagnosis* – a list of potential causes of the condition. A veterinary surgeon will work through the presenting clinical signs together with a history from the client and undertake various diagnostic tests that will eventually either confirm the diagnosis or reach a conclusion on how to treat the presenting clinical signs.

Respiratory system

ACUTE RESPIRATORY DISTRESS

Acute respiratory distress is a true respiratory emergency and has many possible causes which include:

- Airway obstruction (Fig. 22.1), e.g. by a foreign body such as a ball or stenotic nares
- Trauma, e.g. road traffic accident
- Laryngeal paralysis
- Poisoning
- Neoplasia
- Overdose of anaesthetic
- Pneumonia.

Treatment

1. A patent airway must be maintained in order that air can pass through the trachea to the lungs.

2. The use of suction will remove secretions such as haemorrhage or excess saliva.
3. Intubation will maintain an open and clear airway in the unconscious patient.
4. Placement of a tracheostomy tube is a semi-permanent solution to maintain a patent airway.
5. Oxygen therapy will ensure that air reaching the alveoli is rich in oxygen and thus aid oxygen exchange.

Oxygen may be administered in several ways – select the method that is readily available and is most easily tolerated by the patient (see also Chapter 17):

- A commercial oxygen cage is the ideal way to administer oxygen as this provides an enclosed environment that prevents the oxygen leaking away. Cage fronts can be purchased that can be fitted on to the front of an existing cage when oxygen therapy is required. As it is transparent, the oxygen cage allows observation of the patient and prevents the animal from feeling enclosed. An oxygen tube is fed into the cage via a hole in the cage front. This type of cage is not available in all practices and therefore alternative methods need to be employed.
- A Hall's anaesthetic mask is placed on or near the patient's nose and mouth to allow it to inspire oxygen-rich air (Fig. 22.2).
- An oxygen tent can be made from a large plastic bag, with the patient placed inside and an oxygen tube leading into it. A clear plastic bag allows the patient to see out and helps to prevent the animal from struggling. If only a coloured or black plastic bag is available, then cut a hole in the bag and reseal it with cling film to provide a 'viewing hole' for both observer and patient. Some animals, but not all, will tolerate this technique.
- An alternative is to place an Elizabethan collar on the patient and cover the front with cling film. An oxygen tube is placed through the neck opening of the collar. This creates an almost enclosed area in which to deliver oxygen therapy.
- Nasal prongs deliver oxygen to the patient and cause minimal stress.
- Respiratory stimulants such as doxapram hydrochloride may be given to patients that do not have respiratory obstruction.
- Bronchodilators may also help in cases of acute respiratory distress.
- Nasal cannulas, which ensure the highest oxygen saturation levels, cannot be used in cases of head trauma.

COUGHING

A cough is defined as 'a reflex action causing sudden expulsion of air from the respiratory tract'. Coughing is a common clinical

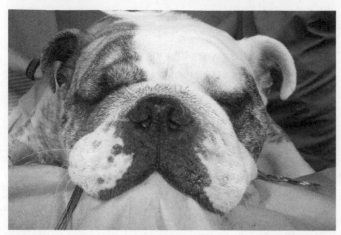

Fig. 22.1 Bulldog exhibiting respiratory obstruction caused by stenotic nares

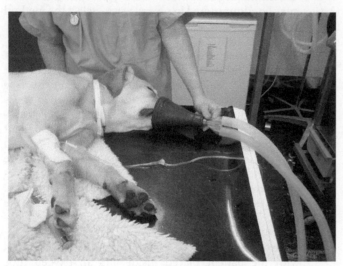

Fig. 22.2 Oxygen being administered via a mask

> ### BOX 22.1 POINTS TO CONSIDER WHEN TAKING THE HISTORY OF A COUGHING ANIMAL
>
> - Breed of animal (some breeds are predisposed to certain conditions)
> - Age of animal
> - Presence of exercise intolerance
> - Length of time the cough has been present
> - Type of cough – dry/hacking or moist and productive
> - History of any trauma
> - Presence of any other medical conditions
> - Exposure to possible infections
> - In contact animals showing similar clinical signs
> - Time of day when cough occurs or is worse

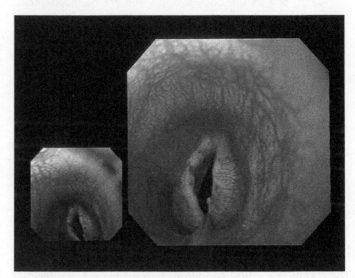

Fig. 22.3 Tracheal collapse shown on endoscopy

sign that occurs in several medical conditions, and it is important to determine whether the cough is dry and hacking or whether the cough is moist and productive because this will determine the differential diagnosis. Animals do not often expectorate but usually swallow the material instead. A comprehensive history from the client together with a thorough clinical examination will ascertain the type of cough. Box 22.1 shows points to be considered.

Coughing may be caused by:

- **Heart failure** – in left-sided congestive heart failure the patient may present with a moist cough caused by pulmonary oedema. Thoracic radiographs will show the severity of pulmonary congestion and help to decide the treatment regime. Thoracic radiographs should be taken with the patient in right lateral recumbency if possible. Alternatively, a dorsoventral thoracic radiograph will still be diagnostic and will also be more comfortable for the patient if severe coughing or respiratory distress is present. During radiography it is vital to cause a minimum of stress to the respiratory-challenged patient; consideration needs to be given regarding the drugs selected for sedation or anaesthesia of this patient.

Allowing the animal to adopt a near-natural position will help to prevent further respiratory distress.

- **Upper airway obstruction** – may be due to laryngeal paralysis or an inhaled foreign body. Laryngeal paralysis is paralysis of the vocal folds, usually bilateral, and is often a degenerative condition of the older dog. Laryngeal paralysis responds well to a surgical procedure known as a laryngeal tieback.
- **Viral or bacterial infection** – for example, kennel cough causes a dry hacking cough.
- **Feline asthma** – other terms are used interchangeably in the feline, such as chronic bronchitis, allergic airway disease and allergic bronchitis. Chronic disease of the bronchioles with unknown exact causes is often present. The feline patient presents with dyspnoea, coughing and noisy breathing/wheezing. Treatments include bronchodilators and identification of possible irritants.
- **Tracheal collapse** – most commonly a condition of toy and small breeds of dog. The tracheal rings collapse inwards and cause coughing on exercise, often accompanied by dyspnoea. Manual palpation of the trachea in the neck and the use of radiographs and endoscopy will confirm the diagnosis (Fig. 22.3). Most cases are managed medically by treatment of underlying causes, e.g. bronchitis.

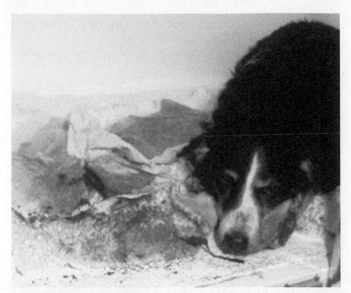

Fig. 22.4 Dog with epistaxis

- **Allergies** – allergies are more commonly seen in cats; see feline asthma.
- **Aspiration pneumonia** – may be linked to syringe feeding or feeding neonates via a dropper or syringe.
- **Bronchitis** – this condition can be acute or chronic and caused by allergens, infection or degenerative. The patient presents with coughing or dyspnoea. Treatments include antibiotics, steroids or bronchodilators.
- **Pulmonary oedema** – the commonest cause in both cats and dogs is cardiac failure. The patient presents with dyspnoea with a moist cough. The underlying cause is treated and supportive therapies administered.
- **Lungworm infection** – caused by *Aelurostrongylus abstrusus* in the cat. *Angiostrongylus vasorum* is the more common parasitic infestation in the dog, and slugs and snails act as the intermediate host. Dogs ingest larvae from eating the molluscs or from eating grass contaminated with slug trails, drinking from outside water bowls or playing with outside toys contaminated with larvae from slugs or snails. Larvae are coughed up and swallowed and are then passed out in faeces (see Chapter 29). Clinical signs in the dog include coughing, dyspnoea, tachypnoea, wheezing, blood clotting problems (coagulopathy), anaemia, anorexia and depression. Faecal tests and respiratory secretions tests are performed to confirm the diagnosis (see Chapter 29). Treatment includes parasiticides and possible steroid administration.
- **Respiratory neoplasia** – confirmed by radiography.
- **Inhalation of a foreign body** – patient will show severe distress.
- **Tuberculosis** – more common in cats than dogs and can be localised in the nose and feet, generalised or pulmonary. Tetanus is usually caused by an infection following exposure to wildlife.

Nursing care
- Allowing the patient to adopt a natural position in which they feel comfortable and do not struggle, often

sternal recumbency, will allow calm and efficient breathing between episodes of coughing.
- Antitussives suppress coughing and are useful if coughing is causing distress but must only be used in patients where suppressing the cough will not cause further harm. Alternative drugs are opiates, such as codeine or theophylline.
- Nebulisation is an effective way of hydrating the patient's respiratory tract and will increase the effectiveness of coupage (see Chapter 18). A commercially available nebuliser is used to deliver sterile water to the patient via a mask or with the patient restrained in a cage.
- The living conditions of the animal must be thoroughly investigated. Environmental factors should be examined and adjusted if necessary. Dusty or fluffy bedding material such as straw or old-type blankets must be exchanged for bedding materials that do not separate into particles. A dusty or damp atmosphere will worsen a cough.
- Owners should be advised that animals are susceptible to passive smoking, so a smoke-free home environment is essential.

DYSPNOEA

Dyspnoea is defined as 'laboured or difficult breathing'. This implies that oxygen supply is insufficient to meet the demands of the body. Dyspnoea can be seen on close observation of the animal or by auscultation of the thorax. It may be caused by:
- **Upper airway obstruction**, e.g. by a foreign body, will not allow sufficient air to pass into the trachea, causing the patient to become dyspnoeic.
- **Laryngeal paralysis** – this will present as inspiratory dyspnoea as the paralysed vocal folds obstruct the passage of air into the trachea.
- **Tracheal collapse.**
- **Feline asthma.**
- **Pulmonary oedema.**
- **Pulmonary neoplasia.**
- **Pneumonia.**
- **Brachycephalic obstructive airway syndrome (BOAS)** – commonly affected brachycephalic breeds include the bulldog, pug, Pekinese and Cavalier King Charles spaniel. The condition presents as dyspnoea due to problems such as an extended soft palate, stenotic nares and laryngeal deformities. These conditions interfere with the inflow and outflow of air into the upper respiratory system.
- **Heart failure.**
- **Smoke inhalation** following a house fire causes dyspnoea because there is little or no oxygen in the inhaled air during the fire. The smoke also irritates the respiratory system, causing inflammation and the release of inflammatory fluid into the alveoli. Fluid in the alveolar spaces prevents air entering the alveoli and interferes with gaseous exchange.
- **Poisoning**, e.g. from chemicals such as paraquat or chlorates (weed killers), paracetamol and carbon monoxide (exhaust fumes/poorly ventilated gas fires or boilers). Ingestion of paracetamol and chlorates causes haemoglobin to change into methaemoglobin, which is unable to transport oxygen around the body and leads to dyspnoea. In cases of carbon monoxide poisoning,

the haemoglobin combines with the carbon monoxide rather than with the oxygen, resulting in a much lower oxygen content of blood.

- **Pain** caused by compression of the thorax, e.g. during gastric dilation and volvulus. The abdominal contents press on the diaphragm and restrict the expansion of the thoracic cavity. Compression on the caudal vena cava also reduces venous return and compromises the cardiovascular system.
- **Thoracic wall injury**, e.g. diaphragmatic hernia or invasive foreign body – leads to dyspnoea, as air enters the pleural cavity and prevents the lungs from fully expanding.

Nursing care

- Keeping the animal free from distress and anxiety will avoid making the dyspnoea worse.
- Confine the animal to a small space where it can adopt a comfortable position and not become agitated or move excessively.
- Avoid handling the patient unless it is absolutely necessary, to avoid a possible struggle.
- Oxygen therapy, as described previously, may be helpful.
- Monitor and record the patient's vital signs, i.e. temperature, pulse and respiration.

EPISTAXIS

Epistaxis is defined as 'haemorrhage originating from the nose', i.e. a nosebleed (Fig. 22.4). The original source of the blood is not necessarily the nose but may be some other part of the respiratory system. Epistaxis is usually bilateral. Unilateral epistaxis may be caused by a foreign body, neoplasia or trauma.

Causes of epistaxis include:

- **Direct trauma**, e.g. road traffic accident
- **Nasal neoplasia** – often unilateral; confirm diagnosis by radiography of the affected area
- **Foreign body**, e.g. grass seeds, blades of grass, etc. – will cause trauma to the nasal lining
- **Ulceration of nasal epithelium** – may be due to fungal infection caused by *Aspergillus* spp. or diseases affecting the mucocutaneous function; a long-term condition such as cat flu may also cause ulceration of the nasal epithelium

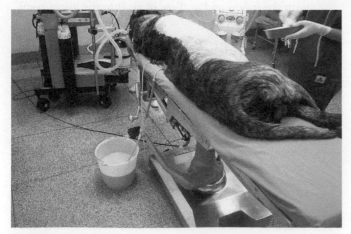

Fig. 22.5 Dog with chylothorax prepared for fluid drainage

- **Blood clotting problems** – haemophilia is the most common in small animals
- **Severe skull fractures** – rare but may cause epistaxis.

Nursing care

- Where dyspnoea accompanies epistaxis, treatment must be given for dyspnoea.
- If a foreign body is visible then it should be removed. In some more difficult cases it may be advisable to remove it when the animal is sedated or anaesthetised.
- A cold compress applied to the nose will alleviate pain and help arrest haemorrhage.
- Topical vasoconstrictor drugs may be squirted into the nose to prevent haemorrhage.

DISCHARGES

Discharges involving the respiratory system are usually nasal in origin. Serous discharges are clear in colour and often due to a viral infection. Mucopurulent discharges are thicker in consistency and often yellow or green in colour. These are often a result of a secondary bacterial infection following an initial viral infection.

FUNGAL INFECTIONS

The most frequent fungal infection of the respiratory system is due to *Aspergillus fumigatus*, which invades the nasal mucosa. It is more common in long-nosed (doliocephalic) breeds of dog and very rare in cats. Clinical signs are a mucopurulent nasal discharge, which may become blood stained, sneezing and pain. Diagnosis is confirmed by radiography, nasal culture, rhinoscopy and nasal biopsies. Surgical treatment is usually successful, using indwelling catheters placed in the frontal sinuses and then flushing the nasal chambers with fungicides.

Nursing care

- The administration of a fungicide via indwelling nasal catheters is often performed.
- Regularly monitor vital signs.
- Prevent patient interference of the nasal catheters, e.g. use of an Elizabethan collar.
- Clean the nostrils to maintain patient comfort.
- Tempt the patient to eat with warmed food or by hand feeding.
- Coupage (see Chapter 18) is used to loosen mucus in the lungs, which is then coughed up by the animal. Percussion of the chest is ideally performed with the animal in sternal recumbency or in a standing position. Cupped hands are placed on either sides of the lateral thorax, starting at the diaphragm. Maintaining cupped hands and loose wrists, the hands move along the length of the thorax, progressing cranially, percussing the chest along its length. Coupage should be performed for 10 minutes, three to four times a day. It is typically well tolerated by the patient. Using nebulisation prior to coupage can help loosen dehydrated mucus.

PLEURAL DISORDERS

These are summarised in Table 22.1.

TABLE 22.1	Conditions affecting the pleural cavity
Condition	**Definition**
Pneumothorax	Presence of air in the pleural cavity
Pyothorax	Accumulation of pus in the pleural cavity
Haemothorax	Accumulation of blood in the pleural cavity
Chylothorax (Fig. 22.5)	Accumulation of chyle in the pleural cavity
Hydrothorax	Accumulation of serous fluid in the pleural cavity

TABLE 22.2	Types of pneumothorax
Type of pneumothorax	**Definition**
Open pneumothorax	An opening into the thoracic cavity is present, e.g. from a penetrating wound. Air enters the thoracic cavity, thus destroying the negative pressure within the pleural cavity, leading to lung collapse
Closed pneumothorax	Lung tissue is torn or crushed, e.g. by a fractured rib, allowing air to escape into the pleural space and destroying the normal vacuum. The lungs are then unable to expand in the normal way and the animal becomes dyspnoeic
Tension pneumothorax	A type of closed pneumothorax in which the air pressure in the pleural space increases every time the animal breathes in, resulting in progressive lung collapse

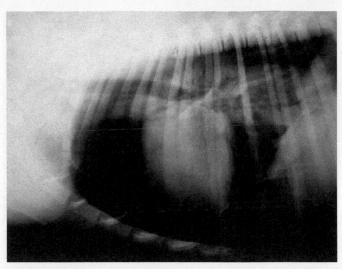

Fig. 22.6   Pneumothorax – lateral radiograph of a dog

Pneumothorax frequently occurs as a result of trauma, e.g. a road traffic accident, gunshot wound, bites to the chest wall or as a result of an impaling injury. A patient with pneumothorax will show signs of dyspnoea and, depending upon the severity of the case, asphyxiation and unconsciousness leading to death (Table 22.2).

Diagnosis may be confirmed by the use of radiography (Fig. 22.6). The removal of the air or fluid from the thoracic cavity by thoracocentesis is essential in both the diagnosis and treatment of these conditions.

Urinary system

RENAL DISEASE

Renal disease is only noticed clinically when 75% of the renal tubules are functionally impaired. Until this happens the kidney is able to compensate and function normally, so by the time clinical signs are evident the condition is already severe. All parts of the kidney work together, so if any part is diseased, kidney function as a whole will be affected.

Causes of renal disease include:

- **Poisoning**, e.g. mercury, ethylene glycol, sulphonamide
- **Nephritis** – to any inflammatory condition of the kidney

- **Glomerulonephritis** – often immune-mediated, affecting the renal glomerulus and thus renal filtration
- **Pyelonephritis** – infection of the renal pelvis, usually due to an ascending bacterial infection from the lower urinary tract
- **Interstitial nephritis** – affects the tissue between the nephrons but clinical signs are similar to those of any type of nephritis; associated with blood-borne infections, e.g. leptospirosis, canine adenovirus
- **Urinary calculi** – the formation of calculi or 'stones' within the bladder
- **Urinary obstruction** – if the calculi move along the urinary tract they may cause obstruction
- **Neoplasia**
- **Trauma.**

ACUTE RENAL FAILURE

May be due to severe dehydration, circulatory failure, poisoning, urinary tract obstruction or trauma. The patient shows signs of acute abdominal pain, anorexia, pyrexia, vomiting and oliguria, which may become polyuria at a later stage. Acute renal failure can usually be reversed. Treatment of the underlying cause, e.g. poisoning, obstruction, is essential. Correction of dehydration status by intravenous fluids is required, together with supportive therapies such as antibiotics and nursing care.

CHRONIC RENAL FAILURE

May be due to congenital problems, interstitial nephritis, glomerular nephritis, pyelonephritis or long-term urinary obstruction. Usually seen in older animals, where onset is gradual and the condition may not be diagnosed until the kidney fails to compensate. Presents as polydipsia and polyuria, anorexia and weight loss, anaemia, gingivitis, oral ulceration, halitosis and hypertension. Treat symptomatically but, once the condition is established, very little can be done.

URINARY OBSTRUCTION

Commonly caused by 'stones' (calculi or uroliths; Fig. 22.7). The formation of calculi, or urolithiasis, is complicated but is

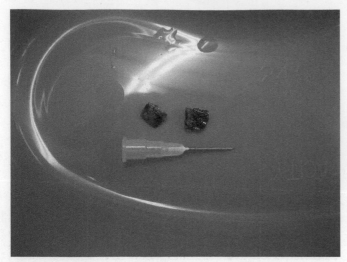

Fig. 22.7 Bladder stones from a cat

TABLE 22.3	Common types of urolith	
Type of urolith	**Found in acidic/ alkaline urine**	**Notes**
Struvite/triple phosphate	Alkaline	Often an incidental finding in dogs and cats. More common in bitches than male dogs. Bacterial infection often present in dogs. Most common in cats
Calcium carbonate	Alkaline	Less common in dogs and cats but common in herbivores, e.g. rabbits
Uric acid	Acidic	Common in Dalmatians
Ammonium urate/ Ammonium acid urate	Acidic	Common in Dalmatians. In other breeds often accompanies liver failure. Often poorly radiopaque so not always identified on plain radiographs
Calcium oxalate	Acidic	Sometimes an incidental finding in dog and cat urine
Cystine	Acidic	Less common urolith, almost always found in male dogs

considered to be due to high concentrations of salts in the body. In dogs and cats 50% of uroliths are struvite, composed of magnesium ammonium phosphate salts known as triple phosphate. Other calculi may be made of oxalate, urate, uric acid or cystine (Table 22.3).

The presence of urinary calculi may or may not cause clinical signs. Where clinical signs do occur, the patient will show varying signs of local pain and discomfort, haematuria, urinary tenesmus, dysuria or possibly anuria or urinary incontinence. Urinary calculi may obstruct the urethra, often at the ischial arch in male dogs, or they may cause irritation of the lining of the bladder.

A diagnosis is reached from interpretation of the clinical signs and the inability to pass a urinary catheter and it is confirmed by the use of radiography, particularly the use of contrast media (see Chapter 32).

Surgical removal of the calculi is often necessary, followed by prophylactic measures to avoid recurrence, e.g. control of urinary infection, increasing water intake, dietary changes and using urinary acidifiers. Encouraging the patient to pass urine frequently discourages re-formation of calculi. Renal function must also be checked in such cases by performing routine biochemistry. Chemical analysis of the removed urinary uroliths will help in the treatment and prevention of recurrence. Nutritional management of these cases is important, alongside environmental management in stress-related FLUTD cases (see Chapter 10).

OTHER URINARY PROBLEMS

Neoplasia

Uncommon. Surgical removal of the tumour is possible but this condition offers a poor prognosis. Diagnosis is confirmed by radiography.

Trauma

Trauma, e.g. a road traffic accident or a kick, may cause haematuria and anuria and the patient may show signs of acute renal failure. Diagnosis is confirmed by radiography and paracentesis – removal of fluid from the abdomen. A ruptured bladder will require surgical repair. Milder trauma will resolve with medical management, e.g. fluid therapy and supportive treatment.

Cystitis

Cystitis in cats is inflammation and is caused by stress rather than infections. Treatment in cats is based on the reduction of stress and pain management for the inflammation. In dogs, however, cystitis is normally due to a bacterial infection. It is more common in females than males because of the position of the opening of the tract in relation to the anus – often caused by faecal contamination. An infection is more likely if a urinary obstruction is present or where trauma to the urinary tract has occurred. The animal will pass smaller amounts of urine more frequently, often showing signs of tenesmus and haematuria. Treat with antibiotics following a urinary bacterial culture and sensitivity test.

Urinary incontinence

This is the involuntary passage of urine. Diagnosis is made from an extensive client history, radiography and urinary catheterisation. Causes include:
- Congenital anatomical malformation, e.g. ectopic ureter (Fig. 22.8) – can be corrected surgically
- Neoplasia
- Hormonal – in spayed bitches; treatment is with drug therapies
- Displacement of the bladder, e.g. after a road traffic accident
- Prostate disease
- Neurological disorders, e.g. spinal trauma or disease
- Senility
- Psychological, e.g. excitement or fear.

URINARY CATHETERISATION

Urinary catheterisation is performed for many reasons (see also Chapter 17).

An aseptic technique must be used to place the urinary catheter to avoid introducing infection into the bladder. Antibiotics should be avoided in cases of blockages in cats, though there is more likelihood of a urinary tract infection following catheterisation if the patient is immunosuppressed, if recurrent catheterisation is necessary or if there is already trauma to the urinary tract; the veterinary surgeon should culture any urine to see if there is a requirement for antibiotics. To avoid damaging the urethra the catheter should always be introduced with care and not forced into the urethra. In cases of urolithiasis in the urethra the catheter will not pass; an alternative means of treatment must be sought. If the catheter becomes blocked, flushing with sterile water or sterile saline may clear the blockage (hydropulsion).

Urinary catheters are purchased pre-sterilised (Table 22.4) and other than metal urinary catheters (which are no longer used), all urinary catheters are for single use only. Catheters should be stored flat and not allowed to curl, since this will hinder catheter placement. All urinary catheters must be lubricated and checked prior to use, maintaining the sterility of the catheter. The stylet, if present, is checked for ease of movement and the balloon in the Foley catheter is inflated prior to use to check for holes and then deflated for insertion. Where indwelling urinary catheters are in place, patient interference must be avoided. An Elizabethan collar is commonly used.

CYSTOCENTESIS

In some cases cystocentesis may be used as an alternative method of draining the bladder. An area of hair on the ventral abdomen, over the site of the bladder, is clipped and surgically prepared. Locate the bladder by palpation and firmly hold it in situ. A sterile needle with attached syringe is inserted through the abdominal wall into the bladder and urine is withdrawn. This procedure can be performed in a conscious animal in either lateral recumbency or in a standing position. Cystocentesis is well tolerated in most patients.

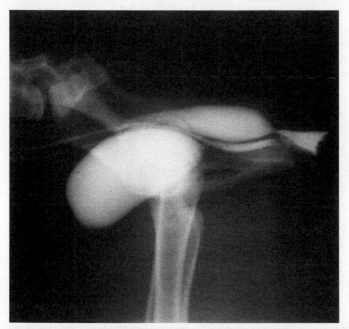

Fig. 22.8 Radiograph showing an ectopic ureter in a dog

Table 22.4	Types of urinary catheter	
Types of urinary catheter	**Dog/cat**	**Comments**
Jackson cat catheter	Cat Commonly used in male cats but can also be used in female cats	Can be used as an indwelling catheter, but can be very uncomfortable Has a Luer fitting Available in two sizes: 3 and 4 FG Has a stylet to aid insertion
Silicon cat catheter	Cat	Can be used as an indwelling catheter Has a stylet to aid insertion, but a Slippery Sam should be used to unblock first. Available in different sizes and lengths
Plastic plain urethral catheter	Dogs, bitches and female cats	Longer than the Jackson cat catheter Has no stylet Available in a variety of diameters and lengths Has a Luer fitting Can be used as an indwelling catheter
Foley catheter	Bitches	Can be used as an indwelling catheter Available in a variety of diameters and lengths Catheter does not come with a stylet but a separate stylet is often necessary to aid insertion Does not have a Luer fitting so a connector is required to attach the catheter to the urinary drainage system When used as an indwelling catheter the balloon is inflated with sterile water or sterile saline. The amount of fluid required to inflate the balloon is stated on the end of the catheter Care must be taken with lubricants and latex rubber – KY jelly is the lubricant of choice
Tiemann's catheter	Bitches	Not used as an indwelling catheter as impossible to suture in place effectively Curved tip aids insertion Has a Luer fitting Has no stylet

Cardiovascular system

HEART DISEASE

Heart disease may be:

- **Congenital** – present at birth but usually detected at the time of first vaccination. Congenital heart lesions represent about 5% of canine cardiac disease (Detweiler & Patterson 1965). They are commonly diagnosed when the heart is auscultated during the check-up prior to the first vaccination consultation. Table 22.5 describes the range of conditions and their treatment.
- **Acquired** – may develop as the animal ages. Acquired heart disease represents approximately 95% of canine cardiac diseases (Detweiler & Patterson 1965). Table 22.6 describes the range of conditions and their treatment.

ARRHYTHMIA

The term arrhythmia indicates an abnormality in the normal rhythm of the heart. Table 22.7 describes types of arrhythmia and their treatment.

HEART FAILURE

Heart failure is defined as 'an inability of the heart to provide sufficient output to maintain the blood circulation'. Heart failure is either acute, having a sudden onset, or chronic, having a gradual onset over a period of time. Numerous diseases or conditions affecting the heart lead to heart failure. The heart is able to compensate for many defects, so many heart conditions go unnoticed until the condition severely affects cardiac output.

The heart may compensate in the following ways:

- Peripheral vasoconstriction – increases circulating blood volume
- Tachycardia – increases cardiac output
- Enlargement of the heart chambers
- Myocardial hypertrophy
- Decreased renal perfusion, leading to:
  - Aldosterone release and an increase in plasma volume
  - Followed by angiotensin release, peripheral vasoconstriction and thus hypertension.

Many factors can affect the ability of the heart to compensate, including:

- Myocardial disease
- Heart valve disease
- Obesity
- Sudden excessive exercise or activity
- Excessive environmental temperature, leading to hyperthermia
- Pregnancy
- Respiratory disease
- Shock
- Haemorrhage
- Anaemia.

TABLE 22.5	Congenital heart conditions				
Congenital condition	**Clinical signs**	**Diagnosis**	**Comments**		**Treatment**
Pulmonic stenosis	Exercise intolerance Syncope	Radiography	This is a narrowing of the pulmonary semilunar valve Will lead to right-sided congestive heart failure		Surgical correction
Aortic stenosis	Syncope Exercise intolerance	Radiography	This is a narrowing of the aortic semilunar valve		Surgical correction
Patent ductus arteriosus (PDA)	Stunted growth Sudden death Exercise intolerance Coughing Dyspnoea Heart murmur	Radiography	Persistence of a small vessel which links the aorta to the pulmonary artery – normally closes over at birth Seen in young animals, commonly detected at vaccination consultation Breed predisposition – German Shepherd dogs, Irish setters and crossbreeds		Surgical ligation
Ventricular septal defect (VSD)	Exercise intolerance Signs of congestive heart failure	Radiography	Commonly known as 'hole in the heart' – this is a hole in the interventricular septum		Requires heart bypass – not generally available in the UK
Mitral or tricuspid valve dysplasia	Heart murmur	Clinical examination	A common congenital condition		Requires heart bypass – not generally available in the UK
Tetralogy of Fallot	Heart murmur Exercise intolerance Weight loss Cyanosis	Clinical examination	A combination of ventricular septal defect, pulmonary stenosis, a displaced aorta and hypertrophy of the right ventricular wall		Surgery possible but not often performed Very guarded prognosis
Persistent right aortic arch/vascular ring anomaly	Usually no cardiac signs are present Regurgitation Oesophageal diverticulum cranial to the stricture Possibly aspiration pneumonia	Radiography	Causes oesophageal constriction		Surgical ligation

TABLE 22.6	**Acquired heart disease**				
Acquired condition	**Clinical signs**	**Diagnosis**	**Comments**	**Treatment**
Endocardiosis	Left-sided heart failure leading to congestive heart failure Heart murmur	Clinical examination Client history	Valvular disease Valves leak when closed Common in small breeds of dog Mitral valve commonly affected and occasionally the tricuspid valve	No specific treatment Management of heart failure
Endocarditis	Weight loss Anorexia Lethargy Inflammation of other body parts, e.g. lameness, joint pain Pyrexia Bounding pulse	Electrocardiography (ECG) Clinical examination Haematology	An uncommon disease Associated with a bacterial infection present elsewhere in the body and having spread to the heart valves	Antibiotics Supportive therapy, e.g. rest, warmth, TLC Guarded prognosis
Myocarditis	Pyrexia	Clinical examination	Very rare Infection of heart muscle	No specific treatment but treat underlying cause – antibiotics and corticosteroids
Pericardial disease	Ascites Muffled heart sounds	Auscultation Clinical examination Radiography	Leads to right-sided heart failure Usually accompanied by pericardial effusion	Aspiration of fluid
Bradycardia	Incidental finding on clinical examination while investigating ECG underlying medical disease, e.g. Addison's disease	Auscultation	Usually defined as a heart rate <60 beats per minute	Treat the underlying disease
Tachycardia	Incidental finding on clinical examination while investigating underlying medical disease, e.g. feline hyperthyroidism or adrenal neoplasia	Auscultation	Usually defined as a heart rate of >150–200 beats per minute Commonly found in congestive heart failure Remember that environmental and physical factors, e.g. fear, pain, excitement, can cause tachycardia	Treat the underlying disease
Arrhythmias	Vary from none through syncope to sudden death	ECG	A deviation from the normal heart rhythm	Medical therapy, e.g. lidocaine

TABLE 22.7	**Types of arrhythmia**			
Type of arrhythmia	**Diagnosis**	**Comments**	**Treatments**
Sinus arrhythmia	Auscultation	Commonly found in normal dogs. Related to breathing: heart quickens on inspiration and slows on expiration	A normal finding in dogs
Premature beats/ missed or dropped beats	Auscultation Electrocardiography (ECG)	Caused by ventricles beating prematurely	Medical drug therapy, e.g. propranolol
Atrial fibrillation or 'flutter' (tumultuous heart)	Auscultation ECG	A random variation in heart rhythm More common in large and giant breeds In dogs, may develop as part of congestive heart failure Often accompanies cardiomyopathy	Medical drug therapy, e.g. propranolol
Heart block	Auscultation ECG	Conducting system of heart fails, producing slower and less forceful contractions Varies in severity, most important is third-degree block, resulting in severe bradycardia	Surgical implantation of a pacemaker

Heart failure may affect one particular side of the heart and is then referred to as right-sided heart failure or left-sided heart failure:

a. Left-sided heart failure – may be caused by:
- Aortic stenosis
- Mitral valve dysplasia
- Endocardiosis
- Cardiomyopathy
- Obstruction of aorta
- Dysrhythmias.

The clinical signs include pulmonary oedema and congestion, tachypnoea, dyspnoea, coughing, lethargy, tachycardia and pulmonary râles. All signs will become worse with exercise and in severe cases exercise must be limited to avoid precipitating cardiac arrest and death.

b. Right-sided heart failure – may be caused by:
- Pulmonic stenosis
- Tricuspid dysplasia
- Endocardiosis
- Congestive cardiomyopathy
- Pericardial effusions
- Neoplasia
- Myocarditis
- Following long-term left-sided heart failure.

The clinical signs include pooling of blood in the veins leading to oedema, hepatomegaly, splenomegaly, ascites, muffled heart sounds and dysrhythmias.

Congestive heart failure occurs when both the left and the right sides of the heart fail simultaneously. This can often happen following a one-sided heart failure.

Treatment

The main treatment of heart failure is by using drugs and Table 22.8 shows the main groups of drug that are commonly used. In addition to drugs, the following may also be used:

- **Diuresis** – in heart failure, fluid is retained and accumulates in the body tissues because the heart is unable to pump effectively. This results in pooling of fluid in the tissue spaces, leading to oedema, ascites and pulmonary congestion (Fig. 22.9). Diuretic drugs are used to overcome fluid retention (see Table 22.8).
- **Dietary management** – this plays an important role in the longer-term management. Sodium is the main cation of extracellular fluid and leads to the retention of fluid, which increases blood volume and increases the workload of the already failing heart. A low-sodium diet will reduce fluid retention and assist in treating heart

failure. Many proprietary diets have a high sodium content, so a specific cardiac diet with a low sodium content must be fed (see Chapter 10).
- **Weight control** – obesity puts unnecessary overload on the heart. If obese, the patient must lose weight and then maintain a constant weight.
- **Exercise** – should be regular and not excessive. Patients must maintain a constant exercise regimen in terms of both frequency and amount. It is important to avoid sudden bouts of exercise, as this will put an unexpected overload on the heart. Owners must be warned against 'weekend exercise' when they may take their dog for longer walks than on weekdays.

CARDIAC ARREST

A 'heart attack' is a failure in cardiac output and is uncommon in dogs and cats. It results mainly from a sudden increase in demand, such as sudden exercise, excitement or an underlying deterioration of an existing medical disease or condition.

Signs of cardiac arrest include:
- No heartbeat
- No peripheral pulse/weak or absent main pulse
- Cyanotic mucous membranes
- Dilated pupils
- Respiratory arrest or apnoea
- Prolonged capillary refill time.

Treatment

This is an emergency and first-aid rules apply (see Chapter 20). These include:
- Establish a patent airway, e.g. using an endotracheal tube, tracheostomy, extend the neck to lengthen airway, extend the tongue and check for anything blocking the pharynx and trachea
- Breathe for the animal – artificial respiration via endotracheal tube or tracheostomy tube or directly into the animal's mouth and nose
- Cardiac massage
- Administration of cardiostimulant drugs
- Electrical stimulation to restart the heart.

TABLE 22.8	Drugs used in the treatment of heart failure	
Drugs used in the treatment of heart failure	**Effect of drug**	**Example of drug**
Glycosides	Affect heart muscles, cause stronger contractions	Digitalis
Vasodilators/ angiotensin-converting enzyme (ACE) inhibitors	Increases the diameter of blood vessels, thus increasing the vascular space. ACE inhibitors are especially useful in the treatment of congestive heart failure. They work by blocking angiotensin-converting enzyme, which reduces fluid retention and thus blood pressure	Prazosin, enalapril
Diuretics	Increase urine output, thus removing excess fluid in ascites and oedema	Furosemide
Xanthine derivatives	Act on heart muscle to strengthen contractions	Theophylline
Inodilators	Used in the treatment of congestive heart failure, a vasodilator and acts on heart muscle	Pimobendan

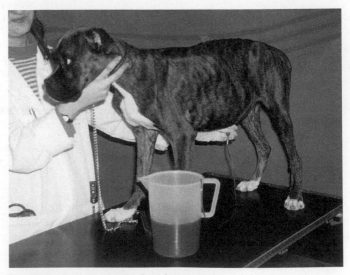

Fig. 22.9 Draining ascitic fluid from a dog

METHODS OF DIAGNOSIS OF HEART DISEASE

Auscultation

Auscultation of the thorax using a stethoscope will identify heart sounds, the heart rate and its rhythm. The optimum area for auscultation is between the third and sixth ribs on the mid-ventral thoracic wall usually on the left side:

- Heart sounds will be muffled if hydrothorax or neoplasia is present.
- The area for satisfactory auscultation will be displaced in cases of cardiac neoplasia.
- The rate and rhythm of the heart should be noted, as changes to this may indicate heart disease.
- A heart murmur is a vibration due to the turbulence of blood flow through the cavity of the heart. Heart murmurs are usually systolic and diastolic murmurs are uncommon. Heart murmurs are graded according to their intensity (Table 22.9).
- Other chest sounds are also heard on auscultation, e.g. respiratory noise, the presence of fluid.

Radiography

Radiography (see Chapter 32) is used to diagnose changes to heart size, heart chamber enlargement, congenital abnormalities, pleural effusions and dilated blood vessels. A plain radiograph is taken initially, centering over the heart, which is level with the caudal border of the scapula. A dorsoventral view will define the outline of the heart. A lateral view will enable an approximate measurement of the heart within the thoracic cavity to be made. The normal size of the heart should span 2.5–3.5 rib spaces; on a dorsoventral radiograph the heart should fill less than three-quarters of the depth of the thorax.

Introduction of an intravenous iodine-based contrast agent to perform an angiogram to assist in diagnosing congenital cardiac defects. Fluoroscopy with angiography is used to diagnose congenital cardiac defects and pleural effusions. (Fluoroscopy converts X-rays into light, multiplies the intensity of the light and then converts it to photoelectrons. A 'moving radiograph' is then seen.)

Ultrasound

Commonly referred to as echocardiography, this uses ultrasonic sound waves to produce an image. As the image is in 'real time' it can be used to visualise the heart as it beats. Doppler ultrasound or ultrasound in M mode is used to examine the movement of blood through the chambers of the heart.

Electrocardiography

Electrocardiography (ECG) is the technique of recording the electrical activity of the heart and is used to investigate the heart rate and rhythm. Electrodes are attached to the fore limbs, a hind limb and the thoracic wall and lead to an amplifier and recording apparatus. To ensure good electrode contact with the skin, the hair should be clipped and surgical spirit applied to the area prior to connecting the electrodes. The patient's coat must be dry and an insulated table will aid contact.

Electrical signals received by the machine are converted to tracings on a screen or a paper strip and provide a permanent record either on paper or as a digital recording. This ECG trace is then compared to that of a normal animal and is used to make a diagnosis. It must be remembered that an animal that is dying of heart failure will still have an ECG reading – an ECG does not measure cardiac output.

Laboratory tests

There are no specific laboratory tests used in the diagnosis of heart disease but some of the general tests will aid diagnosis (Table 22.10).

Haemopoietic system

ANAEMIA

Anaemia is a term describing an abnormally low number of circulating red blood cells, which affects the overall oxygen-carrying capacity of the blood. Anaemia is a clinical sign of an underlying disease rather than a disease itself.

Clinical signs

These are all related to the lack of oxygen reaching the tissues and include:

- Lethargy
- Exercise intolerance
- Pale mucous membranes
- Possible heart murmur
- Tachycardia
- Tachypnoea
- Reduced packed cell volume (PCV).

Causes

Anaemia may be caused by:

- Acute haemorrhage – sudden and excessive loss of red blood cells which may be internal or external, e.g.

TABLE 22.9	Gradation of heart murmurs
Heart murmur	**Definition**
Grade 1	Faint heart murmur that is not immediately heard on auscultation
Grade 2	Faint heart murmur heard within a few seconds
Grade 3	Murmur heard immediately and widespread
Grade 4	A loud heart murmur that is heard with the stethoscope not quite in full contact with the chest wall
Grade 5	Very loud murmur that is heard with the stethoscope slightly withdrawn from the chest wall

TABLE 22.10	Laboratory tests that may aid the diagnosis of cardiac disease	
Laboratory test		**Abnormality may indicate heart disease**
Leukocytosis		Congestive heart failure
Neutrophilia		Endocarditis
Urea		Congestive heart failure
High liver enzyme levels		Congestive and right-sided heart failure
Low globulin (and other plasma proteins)		Heart failure
High muscle enzymes		Myocardial disease

trauma, surgery, rupture of an organ, clotting disorder, haemangiosarcoma, haemorrhagic gastroenteritis or warfarin poisoning

- Chronic haemorrhage – gradual but extensive loss of red blood cells which may internal or external, e.g. haematuria, epistaxis, heavy ectoparasite or endoparasite burden, gastrointestinal bleeding
- Haemolysis – excessive destruction of red blood cells, e.g. immune-mediated haemolytic anaemia (IMHA), *Haemobartonella* infection
- Non-regenerative anaemia – insufficient production of replacement red blood cells, e.g. bone marrow hypoplasia, renal disease.

Laboratory tests

These are used to help confirm the diagnosis and to assess the degree of anaemia (see Chapter 31):

- Packed cell volume – measures the percentage of red blood cells within the blood. The normal parameters for the species and the time between onset of the condition and measurement of the PCV should be considered. PCV should always be measured alongside total protein/total solids, as this will aid to differentiate between acute and chronic loss of erythrocytes.
- Blood smear – examination of a smear will help to determine whether the anaemia is regenerative or non-regenerative:
  - Regenerative – presence of reticulocytes (immature red blood cells) which are produced to compensate for those being lost
  - Non-regenerative – little or no evidence of reticulocytes and there will be insufficient new red blood cells to compensate for the loss. Associated with bone marrow problems, chronic inflammation and renal disease.

Treatment

This should be aimed at the specific cause but very often the patient is treated symptomatically. The following are used:

- Corticosteroids – to reduce inflammatory processes
- Vitamin K_1 – involved in the formation of clotting factors in the liver
- Good-quality, high-protein diet – provides the nutrients for the formation of body tissues
- Dietary supplements, e.g. vitamin B and iron
- Intravenous fluid therapy – blood transfusion or colloids can be indicated in cases of acute and chronic conditions
- Stress-free environment and cage rest.

LYMPHOMA

Lymphoma is a neoplastic condition of the lymphocytes and is also known as lymphosarcoma. It is a relatively common disease in both dogs and cats. In cats lymphoma is associated with feline leukaemia virus (FeLV) infection; however, in dogs, lymphoma is a spontaneous condition. The most common form of the disease involves the infiltration of various organs (Table 22.11). Clinical signs relate to the system involved but may include enlargement of the affected organ, e.g. lymphadenopathy or enlargement of the lymph nodes (Fig. 22.10). In some cases the affected organ may fail, e.g. renal failure. Some

TABLE 22.11	Types of lymphoma
Affected organ	**Type of lymphoma**
Lymph nodes	Multicentric lymphoma
Gastrointestinal tract	Alimentary lymphoma (see Fig. 22.10)
Thymus	Thymic lymphoma
Kidneys	Renal lymphoma
Skin	Mycosis fungoides

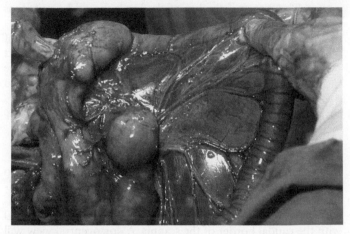

Fig. 22.10   Alimentary lymphoma

lymphomas secrete a parathormone-like hormone, which induces hypercalcaemia.

Diagnosis of lymphoma is confirmed by taking a biopsy of the affected tissue. Some cases respond well to chemotherapy, e.g. thymic and multicentric lymphoma. It is very unusual for cases of lymphoma to recover.

LEUKAEMIA

Leukaemia is a special form of lymphoma in which there is an abnormally high number of white blood cells, in particular lymphocytes, in the peripheral circulation. This is a result of bone marrow neoplasia. Leukaemia is rare in dogs and cats and may present as a chronic or an acute condition. Chronic lymphocytic leukaemia responds reasonably well to chemotherapy but the acute form has a poor prognosis. Leukaemia is diagnosed by haematology and confirmed by bone marrow biopsy.

BLOOD CLOTTING AND BLEEDING DISORDERS

- **Rodenticide poisoning** – most commonly due to warfarin and related agents, which cause a disruption in blood clotting. Warfarin poisoning is more common in dogs. Treat with vitamin K_1 and supportive therapy.
- **Thrombocytopenia** – this is a low platelet count due to an autoimmune destruction of platelets (immune-mediated thrombocytopenia [IMT]) or bone marrow suppression. Suppression of the bone marrow is caused by lymphoma or oestrogen toxicity, e.g. during the oestrus period in ferrets, Sertoli cell tumour and excessive oestrogen therapy.
- **Von Willebrand's disease** – this is an inherited bleeding disorder affecting both males and females. The affected animal lacks the von Willebrand factor, which is an

essential part of normal haemostasis. Some cases show spontaneous haemorrhage, while others have only abnormal bleeding following trauma or surgery. Treat by the administration of a blood transfusion (the blood product cryoprecipitate or fresh frozen plasma [FFP] is the product of choice in these cases – see Chapter 25) and supportive care. There is a breed disposition to von Willebrand's disease – Dobermans are commonly affected

- **Haemophilia** – this is a deficiency of factor VIII or factor IX in the clotting cascade. It is a sex-linked inherited disease seen in males and carried by the X chromosome. It is rare for females to be affected but they can carry the disease and pass it to their offspring. Unless the animal suffers trauma or requires surgery, haemophilia is unlikely to be identified until routine neutering is performed. Commonly affected breeds are German Shepherd dogs and Dobermans.

Tests for clotting and bleeding disorders

Diagnosis is by:

- **Buccal mucosal bleeding time (BMBT)** – a reliable method of measuring platelet number and function. A commercially available kit is used to make a small incision in the lip and the lost blood is then blotted with filter paper. The time is measured from making the incision to when bleeding stops. The normal buccal mucosal bleeding time for a dog is 1.7–4.2 minutes; in the cat normal bleeding time is 1.4–2.4 minutes. A longer than normal buccal mucosal bleeding time indicates von Willebrand's disease, low platelet numbers or other disorders of platelet function.
- **Activated clotting time (ACT)** – measured by collecting blood into an ACT tube, keeping at body temperature and after 60 seconds examining for clot formation. A clot should form within 90 seconds. A longer time than this indicates the possibility of a clotting disorder. Further clotting tests can be performed by commercial laboratories.
- **Measurement of platelet numbers** by routine haematology tests.
- **The von Willebrand antigen test** examines the genetic status of suspected individuals.

Nervous system

EPILEPSY

Epilepsy is a disorder in which an irritable focus within the brain causes disorganised electrical activity resulting in convulsions or fits and a sudden loss of consciousness. It is a condition affecting dogs, rather than cats (see also Chapter 20). Convulsions are violent and uncoordinated contractions of muscles that occur when the animal has lost consciousness. The animal has periods of alternating relaxation and heightened muscular activity, which raises the body temperature. Box 22.2 shows the advice to be given to the owner of a dog during its convulsions.

Epilepsy is more common in some breeds, e.g. poodles, German Shepherds, Cavalier King Charles spaniels. The cause is often unknown, i.e. idiopathic, but may be due to:
- Neoplasia of the brain
- Meningitis

BOX 22.2   ADVICE TO OWNERS DURING CONVULSIONS

- Make a note of the time convulsions begin.
- Monitor the animal and observe exactly what happens during the convulsion.
- Remove any harmful objects from the animal's reach.
- Maintain a darkened, quiet environment.
- Do not move or handle the animal during convulsions.
- Reassure the animal once convulsions cease.
- Make an appointment at the veterinary surgery for a clinical examination once convulsions have ceased.

- Hyperthermia
- Bacterial infection
- Viral infection
- Poisoning
- Renal disease
- Hypoglycaemia
- Hypocalcaemia
- Hydrocephalus.

Clinical signs

The convulsion is divided into three phases:
- **Pre-ictal phase** – the period of time just prior to the fit starting. Animals may be restless, anxious (described as an 'aura'), be asleep or appear normal with no noticeable signs.
- **Ictal phase** – the animal collapses, falls on to its side, loses consciousness and moves its legs in a 'paddling' motion. Often the animal will involuntarily urinate and defecate and may chomp its jaws. Convulsions are very distressing for the owners to witness.
- **Postictal phase** – the time immediately following the convulsion, when the animal may appear dazed or disorientated, gradually returning to its normal demeanour. The animal may appear to be exhausted and will sleep for several hours.

Status epilepticus is a series of repeated convulsions without the animal regaining consciousness, and is life-threatening. **Petit mal** is a short minor convulsion where slight muscle tremor is noticed but a full convulsion does not take place.

A convulsion is often witnessed by the owner and, since it only lasts for a few minutes, is rarely seen by veterinary staff. The advice given to owners while their dog is convulsing is shown in Box 22.2. The animal will appear perfectly normal on later clinical examination. It is important that a thorough and detailed history is taken from the owner and the person who saw the convulsion in order to be able to both determine the timing of the convulsion and its likely cause. To determine the exact cause of epilepsy, a number of tests may be performed, e.g. haematology, biochemistry, magnetic resonance imaging scan, urinalysis and cerebrospinal fluid tap.

Treatment

If it is known, removal of the underlying cause will prevent further attacks. In cases of idiopathic epilepsy, long-term anticonvulsive drug therapy is recommended if the frequency of seizures is high enough or the intensity severe enough. The animal will require a maintenance dose of an anticonvulsant. Oral anticonvulsants are not used during a convulsion, but intravenous or rectal anticonvulsants may be administered.

ATAXIA

Ataxia is defined as an irregular or unsteady gait caused by incoordination of the muscles. Causes of ataxia include muscle weakness, depression of the central nervous system, disease of the vestibular (balance) centre and spinal disease. A detailed clinical history will aid diagnosis. A detailed neurological examination must be carried out to determine the severity of ataxia and the presence of accompanying clinical signs.

Neurological examination

The patient will require a full neurological examination to assist in the diagnosis. Table 22.12 shows the neurological tests performed during a clinical examination.

PARALYSIS

Paralysis is the loss of voluntary muscle control resulting in either a partial or complete loss of movement in the affected body part (Fig. 22.11). Paralysis is due to nerve damage and is commonly a result of trauma to the brain or spinal cord. It may be further defined according to the extent of the paralysis:

- **Paraplegia** – paralysis of both hind limbs
- **Tetraplegia** or **quadriplegia** – paralysis of all four limbs
- **Hemiplegia** – paralysis of one side of the body.

Paresis is defined as muscular weakness and is often described as partial or incomplete paralysis.

A detailed neurological examination is performed to determine the extent of paresis or paralysis. The underlying cause must be treated or removed to gain long-term treatment.

Nursing care

- Patients with paralysis are unable to walk unaided, urinate and defecate, and must be walking-assisted by the use of a long towel (see Chapter 18) or walked with the aid of slings placed under the abdomen or hind

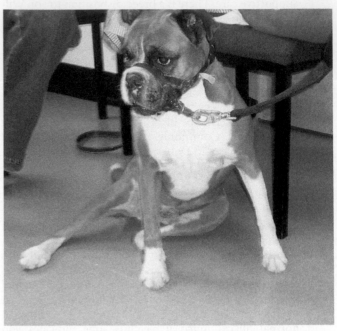

Fig. 22.11 A partially paralysed paralysed dog

TABLE 22.12	Neurological tests performed during a clinical examination
Body part	**Examination**
Consciousness	Fully conscious Depressed Stuporous Comatose
Posture	Presence of a head tilt Position of the head in relation to rest of the body Wheelbarrow reaction – hold animal's hind limbs and abdomen so all the weight is supported on the front limbs, 'walk' the animal forwards and backwards using a wheelbarrow motion – the normal animal is able to perform this
Spine	Visually examine the position of the spine for lordosis, scoliosis or kyphosis Spinal reflexes: • Patellar or quadriceps myotactic reflex, tested with a hammer • Flexor reflexes – skin between the toes is pinched, normal reflex is to withdraw the foot
Limbs	Increased or decreased muscle tone Limbs held in extension Normal stance or wide gait Presence of knuckling over of feet (proprioception) Proprioceptive positioning reaction – flex animal's foot until dorsal aspect is in contact with the floor – normal reaction is to replace foot correctly on floor Alternatively, place animal's foot on a piece of paper and withdraw the paper laterally in a sudden movement – normal reaction is to regain normal stance
Movement (examine standing still and during movement)	Presence of any involuntary movements Note the animal's gait Presence of muscular spasms Presence of muscular tremors
Skin	Panniculus reflex is tested by bilaterally pinching skin on flanks with a pair of forceps – normal reaction is a bilateral twitching of the panniculus muscle under the skin
Anus	Anal reflex is tested by stroking ring of anus with a solid object – winking of the anus should be seen

limbs to support the patient's weight. In cases where the animal is unable to support any of its weight an indwelling urinary catheter and collection bag avoids urine scalding and maintains constant bladder drainage.

- Soiled bedding must be changed immediately and any long hair around the perineum must be clipped to aid the passage of faeces and keep the anal area clean.
- Monitoring of urine and faecal output is important and should be recorded on the hospital chart.
- Soft bedding will alleviate decubitus ulcers on pressure points; for example, a plastic-covered deep foam mattress with a Vetbed covering will provide comfort and cushioning.
- Turning the patient every 2–4 hours will prevent hypostatic pneumonia.
- Provide support to position the animal in lateral or sternal recumbency, e.g. foam wedges and sand bags.
- Grooming the animal maintains patient interest and keeps the coat clean and free from matts.
- Ensure food and water is within the patient's reach. Use hand-feeding if necessary and syringe water into the mouth if the patient is unable to move the head and neck. Tube feeding will provide adequate nutrition in cases when the patient is unable to consume sufficient food (see Chapter 25).

- The paraplegic patient is not always able to maintain its body temperature because it is unable to move around. Monitoring and recording patient vital signs, including temperature, is important. Avoid hyperthermia by the use of fans.
- Physiotherapy of the limbs and the use of coupage are required to stimulate the patient and aid healing of affected tissue.

Endocrine system

There are several endocrine diseases that affect both dogs and cats. Table 22.13 shows their cause and effects.

DIABETES MELLITUS

This is a disease caused by the degeneration of the beta cells within the islets of Langerhans of the pancreas, which fail to secret the hormone insulin (see Table 22.13). Insulin lowers the

TABLE 22.13	Endocrine disorders			
Endocrine disease	**Comments**	**Clinical signs**	**Diagnostic tests**	**Treatment**
Diabetes insipidus (DI)	May be due to: 1) Pituitary gland fails to produce ADH (central diabetes insipidus) due to a pituitary tumour or trauma 2) Failure of kidneys to respond to ADH (nephrogenic diabetes insipidus)	Pronounced polydipsia and polyuria Production of very dilute urine	Urinalysis – low specific gravity Water deprivation test Slightly high PCV	Central diabetes insipidus – administer synthetic ADH, e.g. desmopressin in the form of nasal or eye drops Nephrogenic diabetes insipidus – guarded prognosis, drug therapy may reduce urine output but no long-term effective treatment is available
Hyperadrenocorticalism (Cushing's disease)	Common in dogs, rare in cats Excessive levels of cortisol are produced from the adrenal glands due to either: 1) An adrenal gland tumour or 2) A pituitary gland tumour – most common type – causes excess of adrenocorticotrophic hormone (ACTH), which stimulates adrenals to produce excess amounts of cortisol	Polyphagia Polydipsia Polyuria Bilateral alopecia on lateral flanks Muscle wastage 'Pot-bellied' appearance Possible change in coat colour Calcinosis cutis (calcium deposits in the skin)	ACTH stimulation test showing high post-stimulation cortisol levels Dexamethasone suppression test Increased blood alkaline phosphatase (ALP) Ultrasound to identify adrenal gland enlargement	If due to adrenal tumour – adrenalectomy (usually only one adrenal gland is affected so one remains intact) If due to pituitary tumour – drug therapy, e.g. oral mitotane or trilostane, suppresses adrenal function, maintenance dose for long-term use once condition is under control NB. Health and safety note – gloves must be worn when handling mitotane
Hypothyroidism (Fig. 22.12)	Rare in cats Common in dogs aged 6–10 years Usually associated with autoimmune disease or thyroid gland atrophy	Cold and clammy skin Lethargy Weight gain Poor appetite Muscle weakness Bilateral alopecia of flanks Loss of temporal facial muscle to give a 'drawn' facial expression	Thyroxine (T4) Thyroid stimulating hormone (TSH) test Raised liver enzymes High cholesterol levels	Oral thyroxine drug medication, long-term medication required NB. Regular monitoring of thyroid hormone levels is necessary

Continued

TABLE 22.13	Endocrine disorders—cont'd			
Endocrine disease	**Comments**	**Clinical signs**	**Diagnostic tests**	**Treatment**
Hyperthyroidism	Very rare in dogs Commonly seen in cats aged >10 years Most are due to benign thyroid tumours causing excess production of thyroid hormone NB. Most common endocrine disease in cats	Restlessness Aggression Polyphagia Tachycardia Weight loss Diarrhoea Poor coat Poor skin Mass palpable in thyroid gland (goitre)	T4 Clinical examination: enlarged thyroid gland is palpable	Thyroidectomy of affected gland (preferred treatment) Radiotherapy using iodine-131 Carbimazole drug therapy but difficult to stabilise in long-term management NB. Frequently, during surgical intervention, the parathyroid glands are damaged or removed inadvertently. This causes hypocalcaemia and the animal may show signs of muscle tremors and convulsions. Clinical signs indicate hypocalcaemia. Immediate treatment is necessary – calcium and vitamin D supplementation is essential. During the immediate postoperative period following thyroidectomy the patient is monitored for signs of low blood calcium levels. Calcium supplementation is sometimes only required for a few weeks postoperatively if the parathyroid glands are still intact and only disturbed during surgery
Diabetes mellitus (DM)	Commonly affects middle-aged entire bitches Also affects cats Due to a carbohydrate metabolism problem Blood sugar levels increase as cells do not take up glucose due to an insulin shortage. Glucose remains in the circulation and is eventually excreted in urine. NB. In the normal animal, insulin is secreted by beta cells in the pancreas when blood glucose naturally rises, e.g. following a meal. Insulin lowers the blood glucose level by increasing the uptake of glucose into the cells and by storing glucose	Polydipsia Polyuria Polyphagia Obesity As the condition worsens: Anorexia Vomiting Diarrhoea Dehydration Lethargy	High blood glucose levels	Establish a strict daily routine: 1) Follow a strict dietary regimen; exact amounts at same time each day 2) Daily injections of insulin – either once a day or twice daily 3) Neuter entire females to maintain hormone stability 4) Treat underlying medical conditions/diseases
Hypoadrenocorticism (Addison's disease)	Affects mainly dogs Caused by atrophy of the adrenal cortex, resulting in decreased amounts of cortisol and mineralocorticoid production and a severe sodium and potassium imbalance Often an autoimmune disease	Vomiting Diarrhoea Anorexia Lethargy Collapse Signs of dehydration Bradycardia NB. Clinical signs are often intermittent	Low blood sodium and high blood potassium levels ACTH stimulation test (showing low cortisol levels that do not rise following administration of ACTH)	Oral hormone replacement – synthetic mineralocorticoids, e.g. fludrocortisone, and glucocorticoids, e.g. prednisolone
Insulinoma	A tumour of the beta cells in the Islets of Langerhans of the pancreas that produce insulin. An excess of insulin is produced	Signs of hypoglycaemia Collapse Convulsions	Low blood glucose levels Ultrasound to identify insulinoma	Surgical intervention to remove the insulinoma although the tumour is highly likely to metastasise, so successful treatment is not possible. Drug therapy, e.g. diazoxide or prednisolone, will manage the clinical signs but not provide a permanent solution

blood glucose levels by enabling glucose to pass through the cell membranes into the cells, where it is used as source of energy and any excess glucose is stored in the liver as glycogen. Lack of insulin leads to hyperglycaemia, or raised blood glucose levels, and the clinical signs of diabetes mellitus are a result of this.

There are two types of diabetes mellitus:

- Insulin-resistant diabetes – most commonly seen in cats. Insulin is secreted but the tissues fail to respond
- Insulin-dependent diabetes – most common in dogs. The pancreas fails to produce insulin.

Clinical signs

Initially the patient is bright and shows polyuria, polydipsia and polyphagia. As the condition advances the patient may show anorexia, weakness, lethargy, vomiting and diarrhoea; some may develop cataracts. If left untreated, the body begins to utilise protein and fat as an energy source, resulting in metabolic acidosis and a build-up of ketones – ketoacidosis. This is an emergency and the patient will show signs of depression,

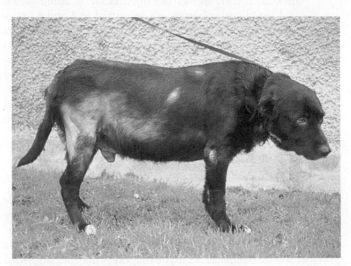

Fig. 22.12 Dog with hypothyroidism

inappetence, vomiting and later coma. Soluble insulin and intravenous fluid therapy are administered, alongside correction of electrolyte imbalances. Blood glucose levels are monitored hourly. Once ketoacidosis is reversed the patient will require initiation of therapy for diabetes mellitus; those animals already receiving therapy will require their medical protocol to be reviewed.

Laboratory tests

These are used to confirm the diagnosis. Urinalysis will show the presence of glucose in the urine and in advanced cases may also show ketonuria. Blood tests will show a raised fasting blood glucose level, as stress can also show hyperglycaemia. Fructosamine levels should also be evaluated. Blood ketone levels can be assessed using handheld meters.

Treatment

Treatment requires the owner to administer daily insulin injections balanced by a rigid regimen of regular amounts of exercise and a constant amount of food given at the same time every day. Table 22.14 provides the details of the management of the condition.

The standard treatment is to provide insulin in the form of regular injections. There are three main forms of insulin:

- Short-acting (soluble) insulin – this is given intravenously or intramuscularly. It has a rapid effect and does not last for long and is used in hyperglycaemic emergencies (ketoacidosis). It is not used for long-term treatments.
- Intermediate-acting (insoluble) insulin – may be given twice a day. This is currently the only veterinary licensed medicine of insulin in the UK, and the most commonly utilised.
- Long-acting (insoluble) insulin – the activity of the insulin is slowed down by the addition of zinc. There are several forms of long-acting insulin and the timing of peak activity is related to the size of the zinc insulin crystals.

TABLE 22.14	Management of diabetes mellitus
Treatment	**Details**
Monitoring	Can be achieved at home with species-specific glucometers, or in practice. Serial glucose testing should be taken into consideration alongside clinical signs (body condition, weight, water and food intake) and fructosamine levels
Diet	Food must be given in relation to insulin administration; see below under Administration of insulin for details. In dogs, a higher fibre diet (low in simple sugars) allows weight control, slows gastric emptying, slows glucose absorption from the small intestine and prolongs the time during which glucose is absorbed. In cats a diet high in protein and fat with low carbohydrate levels is indicated The same diet must be fed at the same time each day to maintain the stability of this condition. No titbits are fed
Administration of insulin	Insulin levels should be adjusted by a very small amount once every 7–10 days under direction of the veterinary surgeon after serial glucose testing. The insulin bottle is gently agitated to suspend the contents, an insulin syringe is used to withdraw the correct amount of insulin and is injected subcutaneously, alternatively an insulin injection pen can be used Insulin is either administered once or twice daily: • If administering once-daily insulin, one-third of the food is given with insulin and two-thirds of the food is given 8 h later • If administering twice-daily insulin, the food is divided into two equal meals, each meal given with the dose of insulin Insulin must be administered at the same time/s each day
Exercise	The same quantity and quality of exercise at the same time each day and for the same amount of time. A change to the animal's exercise regimen will increase the uptake of glucose and upset the stability of the animal's condition

At the start of treatment care is taken to identify three very important factors: that the insulin works in the patient by reducing blood glucose level, at what time the nadir occurs, and the length of action of the insulin. Cats may be difficult to stabilise as they tend to suffer with stress hyperglycaemia, which is exacerbated by such things as being in the hospital kennels and handling. Serial blood glucose testing may be used to assist in the initial stabilisation of the patient or in the later stages, to help identify the three factors listed previously. Regular blood glucose levels are plotted at hourly intervals on a graph. From these results it is possible to recognise peaks and troughs in the blood glucose levels related to the activity of the insulin in use. The feeding times and periods of exercise are also plotted on the graph and will help to indicate any reasons as to why the patient is not stabilising on the treatment. The plots on the graph should never be joined up, as on a conventional graph, as it gives a misinterpretation of what the blood glucose levels were doing at that specific time.

HYPOGLYCAEMIA

Defined as an abnormally low blood glucose level, this is a complication of the management of diabetes mellitus. It is often referred to as 'hypo'. The most likely cause of hypoglycaemia is cats going into remission or an overdose of insulin, either by injecting too much or because the animal has not eaten and the insulin has no glucose on which to act. An insulinoma (tumour of the pancreas) will also cause hypoglycaemia, as it secretes too much insulin (Fig. 22.13).

Clinical signs

Present at the time of the nadir of insulin injection, or in the cases of insulinomas after eating. The animal may shake and appear weak, lethargic, disorientated, ataxic, and may collapse and go into a coma.

Treatment

If the animal is conscious it should be offered sugary food, e.g. honey, jams, sugar or glucose solution; if unconscious the veterinary surgeon will instigate administration of intravenous dextrose, diluted to an appropriate concentration.

CUSHING'S DISEASE

This is also called hyperadrenocorticalism (HAC) and results from excessive levels of adrenal corticosteroids. Clinical signs of the condition are shown in Table 22.13. The diagnosis may be confirmed by the:

- **Adrenocorticotrophic hormone stimulation test** – this is used to aid the diagnosis of Cushing's disease (Fig. 22.14) or of Addison's disease, which is hypoadrenocorticalism. Adrenocorticotrophic hormone (ACTH) is normally secreted by the pituitary gland to stimulate the secretion of cortisol from the adrenal cortex. A blood sample is taken and cortisol levels are measured. A synthetic ACTH is then administered intravenously or subcutaneously and blood cortisol levels are measured again within 60–90 minutes of the injection; timing is dependent on how the synthetic ACTH is administered.
- **Dexamethasone suppression test** – a high or low-dose dexamethasone test is used to aid diagnosis of Cushing's disease. A blood sample is taken and cortisol levels are measured. Intravenous dexamethasone is administered and blood cortisol levels are measured at 3 and 8 hours following injection. In the normal animal, dexamethasone suppresses adrenal function and an absence of cortisol is found in blood following administration of dexamethasone. In the animal with suspected Cushing's disease, a low-dose dexamethasone test will show incomplete suppression of cortisol production. A high-dose dexamethasone suppression test is used to distinguish between adrenal- and pituitary-dependent Cushing's disease.

DIABETES INSIPIDUS

This results from the failure in production of antidiuretic hormone (ADH) from the posterior pituitary gland or a failure of the kidneys to respond to ADH. The clinical signs are polyuria, polydipsia and the production of urine with a low specific gravity (SG) (see Table 22.13). The diagnosis may be confirmed by performing the water deprivation test:

- The bladder is drained by catheterisation and the SG of the urine is measured.
- The animal's weight is recorded. Calculate 5% of the body weight.
- Place the animal in a cage and withhold food and water.

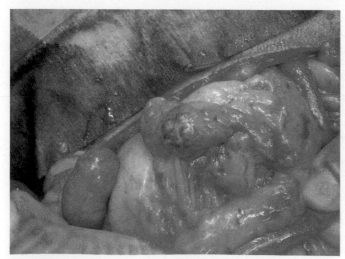

Fig. 22.13 Insulinoma in a dog

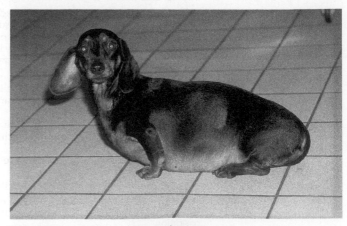

Fig. 22.14 Dog with Cushing's disease

- Collect a urine sample every 1–2 hours – catheterisation is often necessary.
- Measure the SG and weigh the animal.
- Repeat until 5% of body weight is lost. At this point a normal animal will have concentrated its urine and SG should exceed 1.030. Animals with diabetes insipidus are unable to concentrate the urine and the SG will remain the same.

The water deprivation test must not be used in patients that display signs of dehydration or in cases where alternative causes of polydipsia and polyuria have not been investigated fully. If the patient shows any signs of dehydration during the test, it must be abandoned immediately. Constant monitoring of the patient undergoing a water deprivation test is vital as it is potentially harmful if managed inappropriately.

Digestive system

REGURGITATION

Regurgitation is defined as the return of undigested material from the stomach via the mouth with no abdominal effort in the regurgitating; it occurs shortly after eating. It is vital that owners are able to distinguish whether their animal is vomiting or regurgitating. Causes include:

- Megaoesophagus (Fig. 22.15)
- Vascular ring anomaly/persistent right aortic arch
- Oesophageal stricture
- Oesophageal foreign body
- Oesophagitis.

VOMITING OR EMESIS

Vomiting is defined as the violent expulsion of stomach contents via the mouth. Forceful abdominal contractions are required to eject the vomitus and it occurs several hours after eating. The vomit may be partly digested food from the intestines, bile or water. Severe cases of vomiting will lead to dehydration and a loss of electrolytes. Causes include:

- Gastritis
- Distension of the stomach following intestinal obstruction

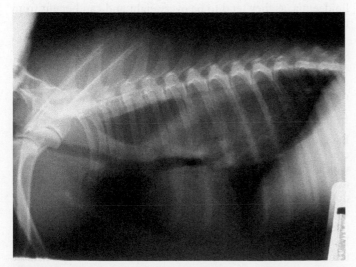

Fig. 22.15 Radiograph of a dog with megaoesophagus

- Gastric ulceration
- Gastric neoplasia
- Gastric foreign body
- Gastric dilatation
- Infection
- Systemic disease.

Blood tests may be used to monitor electrolyte levels and dehydration. Radiography will identify an obstruction or foreign body. Endoscopy will identify gastritis and gastric ulceration.

Treatment

Removal of the underlying cause of vomiting is essential. Intravenous fluid therapy is used to treat dehydration. Surgery is necessary to remove foreign bodies and repair gastric dilatation. Medical management of gastritis and ulceration may be needed, and antiemetics should be utilised if indicated. Nutritional support is still required in these cases (see Chapter 25).

DIARRHOEA

Diarrhoea is defined as abnormally frequent emptying of the bowel, usually producing soft and watery faeces. Fluid and electrolytes are lost in diarrhoea resulting in dehydration and leading to metabolic acidosis (Fig. 22.16). Causes, some of which may be life-threatening, include:

- Colitis
- Enteritis
- Bacterial infection
- Viral infection
- Heavy intestinal parasite burden
- Stress
- Secondary to systemic disease
- Neoplasia of the gastrointestinal tract
- Dietary hypersensitivity
- Sudden dietary change
- Intestinal foreign body
- Malabsorption conditions
- Inflammatory bowel disease.

A full clinical examination and client history will determine whether the diarrhoea is due to a problem in the gastrointestinal system or whether a systemic disease, e.g. Addison's or pancreatic disease, is present. Some patients with diarrhoea appear bright and alert while others are lethargic and non-responsive. Less severe cases respond well to simple dietary management while more severe cases require aggressive fluid therapy and supportive treatment. It is useful to determine whether the diarrhoea is from the large or small intestine (Table 22.15).

Diagnosis of the cause of the diarrhoea is based on a range of tests including radiography, haematology, biochemistry (including species specific pancreatic lipase tests), faecal tests, ultrasound, biopsies and endoscopy.

TABLE 22.15	Comparison between small intestinal and large intestinal diarrhoea	
Small intestinal diarrhoea	**Large intestinal diarrhoea**
Large volume of diarrhoea	Small volume of diarrhoea
Very soft/liquid faeces	Soft faeces; fresh blood or mucus may be present
Diarrhoea passed less frequently: 3–5 times daily	Diarrhoea passed more frequently: 8–12 times daily

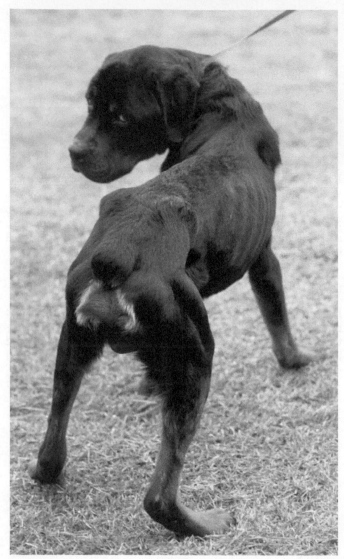

Fig. 22.16 A Rottweiler with emaciation caused by prolonged diarrhoea

Management

- Identify and treat the underlying disease
- Fluid therapy to correct fluid, electrolyte loss and metabolic acidosis
- Antibiotics if bacterial infection present
- Parasiticides if parasite burden present
- Surgery to remove neoplasia or an obstruction
- Dietary tests to establish hypersensitivity
- Dietary management
- Drug therapy, e.g. in cases of chronic diarrhoea.

CONSTIPATION

Constipation is the failure to pass faeces in either the normal amount or normal frequency. Constipation is more common in elderly patients that have reduced exercise. Causes include:

- Dehydration – producing excessively dry faeces
- Low-residue diet
- Neoplasia of the intestinal tract
- Foreign body in the intestinal tract
- Prostatic disease – obstructing the rectum
- Pelvic fracture
- Spinal paralysis
- Megacolon.

Constipation is often presented as faecal tenesmus, i.e. straining, and the animal will feel pain on defecation and will not be able to empty the rectum fully because of hard, impacted faeces. This is treated with an enema. Surgical removal of an obstruction such as a foreign body or neoplasia will relieve constipation. Prevention of constipation can include feeding a high-fibre diet and encouraging the animal to take regular exercise and to defecate at regular times during the day. In some cases a low-residue diet is indicated, e.g. in megacolon cases, alongside medical therapies such as cisapride.

PANCREATITIS

The exocrine pancreas is highly responsive to changes in nutritional substrates present within the diet. When the pancreas becomes inflamed, clinical signs such as depression, anorexia, vomiting, diarrhoea and displays of abdominal pain can present. Pancreatitis, whether in an acute or chronic form, is a common occurrence seen in veterinary practice. Pancreatitis is exceptionally painful and requires analgesia as its primary treatment. This is because the proteolytic enzymes are activated *in situ* resulting in autodigestion. Many factors can predispose to pancreatitis, including breed, age, gender, neuter status and body condition. In cats, nutrition is generally supplied by enteral means (gastrostomy feeding tube), in order to avoid hepatic lipidosis. There is no clinical evidence that this type of nutrition exacerbates the course of acute pancreatitis. There is also evidence that enteral support is superior to parenteral support as described previously. Oral intake in cats should only be restricted if persistent vomiting is occurring, and then for as short a time as possible.

Dietary long-term control of pancreatitis is vital, but initially confirmation of the presence of hyperlipidaemia needs to be obtained. Those dogs suffering from pancreatitis with associated hyperlipidaemia will need to be maintained on a different diet than those without. If the lipid levels in the bloodstream are within normal levels then a highly digestible low-fat diet can be used. If hyperlipidaemia is concurrent then a low-fat diet is required again, but these types of diets can have a corresponding high fibre content, thus reducing digestibility. This can be advantageous in the majority of dogs which suffer from hyperlipidaemia, as they tend to be overweight and can benefit from this type of diet.

Weight control is important in these cases, as a major predisposing factor is obesity and being fed high-fat treats. By altering the diet in order to reduce fat content, most animals will gradually lose weight, but this does need to be monitored regularly.

Exocrine pancreatic insufficiency

Exocrine pancreatic insufficiency (EPI) is a result of the pancreas producing insufficient amounts of pancreatic enzymes, which means that the animal is unable to digest fat. EPI often occurs in dogs of 1–2 years of age, commonly German Shepherd dogs. Affected animals initially develop well but then lose weight, have a ravenous appetite and produce pale, rancid faeces (steatorrhoea), with possible diarrhoea, and are coprophagic. Diagnosis is based on a serum trypsin-like immunoreactivity test (TLI). Treatment depends on the provision of pancreatic enzymes, usually given with each meal. Dietary management is also important and the dog should be given a low-fat but easily digestible diet.

LIVER DISEASE

The liver has a huge capacity for regeneration, and a substantial loss of hepatic tissue (around 70%) is present before any clinical signs of liver disease are seen. Clinical signs of liver disease are often non-specific because the liver is affected by many other metabolic diseases. Causes include:

- Infectious canine hepatitis
- Leptospirosis
- Poisons
- Drug overdose
- Hepatic trauma, e.g. following a road traffic accident
- Primary neoplasia of liver or bile ducts (less common than secondary neoplasia)
- Bile duct obstruction
- Secondary neoplasia
- Storage diseases/enzyme deficiencies, e.g. copper toxicosis in Bedlington terriers
- Secondary to cardiac disease, diabetes mellitus, hyperadrenocorticalism, hypothyroidism.

Confirmation of liver disease is by blood biochemistry tests, e.g. alanine transaminase (ALT), serum alkaline phosphatase (SAP/ALKP), bilirubin, plasma total proteins, haematology (see Chapter 31). Radiography of the liver is used to determine size and position, ultrasound, biopsy to confirm a diagnosis and exploratory laparotomy. Management of liver disease involves the use of supportive therapy until a definitive diagnosis is made, and nutritional support.

SPLENIC DISEASE

An enlarged spleen is usually palpable on clinical examination but it must be remembered that general anaesthesia with some barbiturates causes a temporary enlargement of the spleen. Causes of splenic disease include:

- Neoplasia, e.g. lymphoma or haemangiosarcoma
- Viral or bacterial infection
- Splenic torsion
- Idiopathic
- Anaemia.

Radiography and ultrasound are used to confirm the diagnosis. Surgical intervention, i.e. splenectomy, is often the preferred treatment.

JAUNDICE

Jaundice, also known as icterus, is defined as staining of the tissues by the yellow bile pigment bilirubin, produced in the liver as a result of haemoglobin breakdown. Diagnosis is confirmed by measuring plasma bilirubin, routine haematology, analysis of blood liver enzymes and the presence of pale faeces.

Jaundice is treated by identifying and treating the underlying cause, which includes:

- Obstruction of the bile duct, e.g. gallstones
- Haemolysis (jaundice often occurs when the liver is overloaded with bilirubin)
- Blood transfusion reaction
- Leptospirosis
- Leishmaniasis
- Haemobartonellosis
- Babesiasis
- Hepatic jaundice – accompanies liver disease.

PORTOSYSTEMIC SHUNT

This is a vascular abnormality where the hepatic portal vein empties directly into the caudal vena cava, thus bypassing the liver (Fig. 22.17). A portosystemic shunt may be either congenital (most common) or acquired. Diagnosis is confirmed by analysing blood liver enzymes, radiography and ultrasound. Typically, affected animals have a small liver. Treatment is by surgical correction, and medical management can be used to reduce clinical signs prior to surgery. This includes using a low-protein diet and lactulose.

Reproductive system

FEMALE

Many of the problems associated with the female reproductive tract are treated surgically; however, some, such as pyometra, may be managed medically to stabilise the bitch before an ovariohysterectomy is performed.

False pregnancy (pseudocyesis or pseudopregnancy)

This condition is commonly associated with the bitch, although it may occur in the queen as a result of a sterile mating. Signs in the queen are simply a failure to return to oestrus.

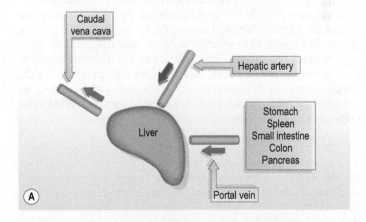

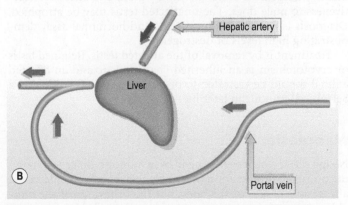

Fig. 22.17 (A) The normal portal circulation. (B) The abnormal portal circulation seen in cases of portosystemic shunt

False pregnancy may occur about 40–60 days after oestrus and is linked with high levels of circulating progesterone secreted by the corpus luteum. This is a normal part of the oestrous cycle but only a small percentage of bitches develop clinical signs. Those that show signs in one oestrous cycle are likely to show them during subsequent cycles.

Clinical signs include maternal behaviour, e.g. nursing soft toys or slippers, nest-making, aggression to anyone who tries to remove the toy, mammary development and lactation. Some bitches may be more seriously ill, with vomiting and loss of appetite.

Before treatment is instigated, check that the bitch is not actually pregnant. Hormones to suppress lactation can be given, e.g. oestradiol benzoate or methyl testosterone over several days and in a reducing dose. A bitch that has repeated false pregnancies should be spayed during anoestrus. The idea that a bitch should be allowed to have a litter in order to get the hormonal cycle to return to normal is largely an old wives' tale.

MALE

Prostatic disease

Enlargement or hypertrophy of the prostate gland is associated with older dogs and results from hormonal stimulation. The gland pushes upwards, causing pressure on the rectum and consequent faecal tenesmus. The gland may become infected by ascending infection from the urethra, which runs through the centre of the gland. The patient may show signs of cystitis and, in severe cases, pyrexia, anorexia and weight loss. Cysts and neoplasia may also develop inside the prostate gland. Diagnosis is confirmed by rectal palpation and the use of ultrasound.

Treatment usually includes castration, which will reduce the size of the gland. Chemical castration by the use of drugs may give an indication as to whether surgical castration will produce a permanent response. If infection is present it should respond to antibiotics, after culture and sensitivity of prostatic fluids. Surgical removal of tumours is difficult and rarely justified, as the tumour metastasises readily. Radiotherapy may relieve the clinical signs for a time.

Sertoli cell tumour

This tumour of the Sertoli cells, which line the seminiferous tubules within the testis and secrete oestrogen, is usually associated with a retained testis. Clinical signs often seen in dogs over 6 years old include bilateral symmetrical alopecia over the flanks, enlargement of the mammary tissue and onset of attractiveness to male dogs. The unaffected testis may be atrophied. Diagnosis is based on clinical signs and hormonal assay demonstrating high levels of oestrogen.

Treatment is by removal of the affected testis. Retained testis or cryptorchism is an inherited characteristic and an affected animal should be castrated to prevent the risk of developing a Sertoli cell tumour in later life.

Neoplasia

Neoplasia or the development of a tumour or cancer is an uncontrolled proliferation of a single type of cell. Neoplasia can affect most tissues of the body, but the behaviour of the individual types of tumour in terms of growth rate and the method, degree and site of spread (metastasis) depend on the cell type.

Tumours can be classed as:
- **Benign** – grows slowly and do not often spread to other sites. Their size may cause clinical signs by pressing on adjacent organs
- **Malignant** – locally invasive and metastasises to other organs by means of the blood or lymphatic systems. This type is more likely to cause clinical signs.

Chemotherapy, giving cytotoxic drugs, is used in the treatment of neoplasia in both cats and dogs (Fig. 22.18). These highly potent drugs either destroy rapidly dividing neoplastic cells or inhibit their growth. They have a very narrow dose range so that the drug kills the neoplastic cells but causes minimal damage to surrounding body cells (Table 22.16). The calculation of the dose rate is based on the patient's surface area rather than body weight. This is because the blood supply to the liver and kidneys is related to body surface area rather than body weight.

Cytotoxic drugs are excreted via the liver and kidneys and must be used with extreme care in animals with compromised renal or liver function, since their excretion may be impaired and toxicity could occur.

Side effects from cytotoxic drugs are common and include vomiting, diarrhoea and anorexia, but these may decline with prolonged use of the drug. The veterinary surgeon and owner will together decide on the best course of treatment and which clinical signs are to be tolerated in each individual patient.

Cytotoxic drugs are irritant and carcinogenic and extreme care must be taken in the handling of such drugs in veterinary

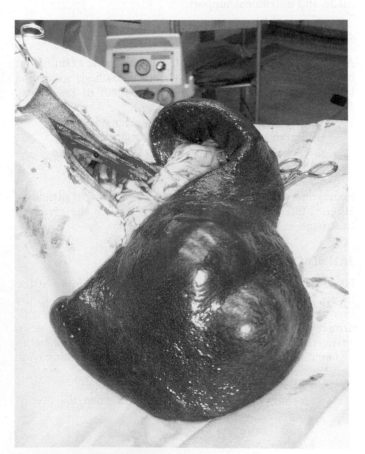

Fig. 22.18 Splenic lymphoma

TABLE 22.16	Drugs used in chemotherapy
Drug name	**Comments**
Cyclophosphamide	Used in treatment of lymphoma in dogs and cats. Available in tablet and injectable forms
Vincristine	Widely used in cats and dogs for treatment of leukaemias and lymphomas. Administered via intravenous route. Sometimes given in combination with other drugs. Perivascular injection causes sloughing, as drug is very irritant
Doxorubicin and epirubicin	Administered intravenously. Used in dogs for treatment of lymphoma
Cisplatin and carboplatin	Administered intravenously. Used in dogs for treatment of sarcoma, e.g. osteosarcoma following limb amputation

BOX 22.3   PRECAUTIONS TO BE TAKEN TO ENSURE SAFE HANDLING OF CYTOTOXIC DRUGS

- Tablets must not be broken or crushed.
- Disposable gloves must be worn when handling tablets.
- Cytotoxic drugs must be dispensed in child-proof containers.
- Cytotoxic drugs must be labelled with name of the drug and warnings regarding safe handling of the drug by owners.
- Keep all cytotoxic drugs out of children's reach.
- Wash hands after handling.
- Wear gloves when administering tablets to patient.
- Dispose of drugs by incineration.
- Cytotoxic drugs must not be handled by pregnant women.
- Wear protective personal equipment, e.g. gloves, long-sleeved gown, face mask, when reconstituting drugs.
- Have eye-wash station and water available when reconstituting the drugs.
- Do not inhale cytotoxic powders, e.g. when reconstituting drug.
- Employ a good technique when handling cytotoxic drugs, e.g. care with pressure in vial of drug.
- Label all cytotoxic drugs when in syringes.
- Transport with care.
- Administer via an intravenous catheter rather than a needle.
- Restrain patient adequately for administration of drug.
- Avoid skin contact with urine/faeces/vomit from patients undergoing cytotoxic drug therapy, since excreta will contain the drug.
- All soiled bedding from treated animals must be incinerated as it will be contaminated with cytotoxic drug.
- Dispose of used needles and syringes in the clinical waste.
- Wash hard surfaces, e.g. floors, table tops, with plenty of water following contact with patients after administration of cytoxic drugs.

practice. Local rules must be displayed in the practice area where cytotoxic drugs are used and all personnel must be made aware of the dangers (Box 22.3). Personnel are at risk during all stages of the procedure, i.e. when dispensing the drugs, when reconstituting (when injectable forms are in powder form and require mixing with a fluid) and administering them, when disposing of them and when caring for the patient following its treatment with cytotoxic drugs.

BIBLIOGRAPHY

Detweiler, D.K., Patterson, D.F., 1965. The prevalence and types of cardiovascular disease in dogs. Ann. N. Y. Acad. Sci. 127, 491.

RECOMMENDED READING

Aspinall, V., 2014. Clinical Procedures in Veterinary Nursing, third ed. Butterworth-Heinemann Elsevier, London.

Aspinall, R., Aspinall, V., 2013. Clinical Procedures in Small Animal Veterinary Practice. Saunders, Elsevier, London.

Bowden, C., Masters, J., 2003. Textbook of Veterinary Medical Nursing. Butterworth-Heinemann Elsevier, Oxford.

Hotston-Moore, A., Rudd, S., 2008. BSAVA Manual of Canine and Feline Advanced Veterinary Nursing, second ed. BSAVA, Gloucester.

Principles of Surgical Nursing

JULIE OUSTON

KEY POINTS

- Surgery always involves the creation and/or treatment of wounds.

- An understanding of the normal healing process is vital so that appropriate care can be given.

- Careful cleaning and debriding of wounds is essential to optimise the healing process.

- Wound dressings should be chosen carefully to match the type of wound and the stage of healing.

- All animals requiring surgery or wound management require holistic assessment and care for them to make the best recovery.

Wounds and wound management

CLASSIFICATION

A wound can be defined as an injury in which there is a forcible break in the continuity of the soft tissues. This includes both open wounds, in which the skin or mucous membrane surface is broken, and closed wounds, in which the damage is below the surface.

Wounds are divided into different groups based on their cause and the resulting type of damage (Table 23.1). Wounds may also be categorised on the basis of the degree of contamination (Table 23.2).

Operating order is always dictated by the cleanliness of the surgery. Clean surgery should be carried out first, followed by clean-contaminated conditions. Contaminated surgery should be carried out last. Dirty procedures should not be carried out in theatre but in another area of the practice.

WOUND HEALING

Wound healing occurs in three phases:

Haemorrhage, inflammation and primary wound contraction

Primary haemorrhage occurs at the time of injury. This then clots and forms a scab, which protects the wound from external contamination. Inflammation follows, encouraging white blood cells to the site. In the first few hours there is primary wound contraction as fibroblasts contract and the size of the wound decreases. This phase is also referred to as the **inflammatory phase**.

Proliferation

After 12 hours, epithelial proliferation starts. New cells are produced and slide over the surface of the wound. This occurs at a rate of up to 2 mm per day if the wound is kept moist. After 36 hours, fibroblasts and new capillaries are produced, forming granulation tissue. This is usually bright red and firm but is quite easily damaged.

Maturation

During epidermal growth new collagen is laid down and forms scar tissue. This is continually remodelled up to 2 years after the original incident. Once the wound cavity is filled, the wound undergoes secondary wound contraction and the size of the scar is reduced.

Open wounds can take weeks or even months to heal, depending on the severity of the initial injury. These wounds are described as healing by second intention. Wounds that are closed surgically with good apposition of the skin edges heal by first intention. This process is usually far quicker, as very little granulation tissue forms and the skin edges simply join together.

Whichever type of healing has taken place, whether by first or second intention, it is important to appreciate that healed wounds are never as strong as the original tissue, and only reach about 70–80% of the original strength.

INFLAMMATION

It is important to appreciate that inflammation is the reaction of normal tissue to injury and is part of the body's natural defence mechanisms. When cells are damaged, chemicals such as histamine and prostaglandins are released and these stimulate the inflammatory response. There is dilation of local vessels, and white blood cells and proteins are attracted to the site. This is all needed to start the healing process. Administration of anti-inflammatory drugs will reduce healing in the early phases, so generally should not be used. Protracted inflammation may cause problems, however, and this is where the use of drugs such as the non-steroidal anti-inflammatory drugs (NSAIDs) might be indicated.

FACTORS AFFECTING WOUND HEALING

Wound healing is a delicate process and many factors can delay the rate of healing. These include:

- Movement
- Infection
- Tension – e.g. sutures placed too tightly will produce cell death

427

TABLE 23.1	Wound classification	
Wound type	**Possible cause**	**Type of damage**
Incised	Sharp knife/scalpel Glass Tin	Clean cut with little damage to surrounding tissues Wound edges usually gape and bleed freely
Puncture	Nail Thorn Fish hooks Teeth (especially cats')	Small external wound but may be deep Little obvious sign on the surface Infection is a potential problem as bacteria or foreign material are carried deep into the tissues
Lacerated	Dog fight Road accident Barbed wire	Large irregular wound with considerable damage to the skin and superficial tissues The severity varies with the size and depth of the wound and the degree of damage to other tissues, such as muscles, nerves and blood vessels Infection is common and necrosis of the edges of the wound is likely
Abrasion	Friction	The epidermis is removed to expose the dermis. These are not full-thickness wounds and, although they are painful, are not usually serious
Avulsion	Dog fights	An avulsion wound occurs where there is forcible separation of a tissue from its attachments
Degloving	Road traffic accidents	Degloving injuries occur in a similar way to an avulsion wound or through damage to the blood supply such that an area of tissue dies and sloughs away over a period of time These are often heavily contaminated with dirt and bacteria
Shear	Road traffic accidents	These occur in the same way as degloving injuries, although as well as the removal of skin there is damage to the underlying bones and/or joints These are heavily contaminated and are often very serious
Contusion	Blunt trauma	Blood vessels rupture under the skin The blood seeps into the tissues and eventually clots Breakdown of the red blood cells and haemoglobin results in the discoloration of the skin that appears as the contusion heals
Haematoma	Blunt trauma Excessive head-shaking	Greater blood loss occurs than with a contusion and a pocket of blood develops under the skin The blood eventually clots and scar tissue is generated, which contracts with time Most usually associated with the ear

TABLE 23.2	Wounds classified by degree of contamination
Wound type	**Description**
Clean	There is no break in sterility An incision is made into a tissue that has been surgically prepared and no contaminated body systems are entered
Clean-contaminated	A contaminated area (such as the gastrointestinal, urogenital or respiratory tract) is entered but there is no spillage or spread of contamination
Contaminated	Wounds in which there is either spillage from a contaminated area or severe inflammation, but without infection Fresh, open wounds are also included in this category, but these can be converted to clean-contaminated wounds after thorough lavage and debridement
Dirty	Wounds in which there is leakage from a pus-filled organ or there is pus or infection present within the wound Dirty wounds also include traumatic wounds with devitalised tissue or those containing foreign bodies

- Interference with blood supply – e.g. bandages that are too tight, or heavily contused wounds
- Persistent irritation and self-trauma
- Tumour cells invading a wound
- Presence of foreign material or necrotic tissue.

These are all factors that relate specifically to the wound but there are also some general factors that will also influence the way in which wounds heal:

- Age – youngsters will heal faster than older animals.
- Region of the body – some areas of the body have better blood supply than others.
- Malnutrition or specific nutrient deficiency will delay healing.
- Concurrent treatment, e.g. with corticosteroids, can decrease wound healing.
- Other diseases will also affect the rate of wound healing.

Research into wound healing was carried out in 1962 by George Winter when he looked at whether allowing wounds to dry out was the best method, or whether maintaining a moist wound environment provided better healing. His results were quite clear – wounds left to heal in the open took twice as long to epithelialize as those that were covered with a polymer film, and this is now an important principle in the management of any wound.

MANAGEMENT OF WOUNDS

Wounds heal in a totally predictable way following the three stages described earlier. The key to good wound management is to ensure that conditions for healing are optimised which will give fastest recovery. Remember, though, that the healing process can never be accelerated; we can only prevent it being delayed.

Wound management can be summarised as follows:

1. First clean the wound thoroughly and remove any devitalised tissue.

2. The wound should then be repaired surgically or left as an open wound.
3. Dressings should be applied as indicated by the type of wound to encourage moist wound healing.
4. Follow-up checks should be carried out.

Cleaning and debridement

Wounds should always be cleaned carefully before any further management is undertaken. A heavily contaminated wound should be flushed thoroughly using a safe lavage solution that has been warmed. Sterile Hartmann's solution is currently thought to be best, but 0.9% saline can also be used. A large syringe (20–30 ml) and 18-gauge needle can be used to provide an appropriate pressure of approximately 8 psi. A dilute disinfectant solution such as 0.05% chlorhexidine may also be used, but this does have an effect on fibroblast activity, and will slow wound contraction. After lavage, any remaining dead or devitalised tissue needs to be removed. This can be achieved in a number of ways:

- **Surgical debridement** is the most effective, as all damaged tissue is simply excised leaving a clean wound which can then be allowed to heal.
- **Non-surgical debridement** techniques may be needed if surgical debridement is not possible. One of the simplest methods is the use of wet-to-dry dressings to mechanically debride wounds by applying dressings soaked in Hartmann's or saline to the wound, allowing them to dry out over 12–24 hours, and then gently peeling it away pulling with it debris and exudate when it is changed. Enzymes such as collagenase or chemical solutions are available and can be used to

debride wounds. Sterile medical grade maggots can also be used, though this is an expensive option.

Some dressing materials also assist in the debriding process, particularly those that are able to hydrate wounds, such as the hydrogels or hydrocolloids, as well as products containing honey, which has a number of beneficial properties (see Tables 23.3A and 23.3B).

Wound closure

Wounds usually heal more quickly if they can be closed surgically, so this is done wherever possible. Wounds can be closed using a number of methods:

- Suturing – commonly used and generally well tolerated. Most patients may require general anaesthesia for both restraint and analgesia.
- Staples – can be very quick and carried out in the conscious patient.
- Tissue adhesive – glues are available suitable for skin closure.

Wound closure can be carried out at different stages depending on the type of wound and the degree of contamination:

- **Primary closure:** the wound is closed immediately after presentation once cleaned and debrided.
- **Delayed primary closure:** this is carried out 3–5 days after the initial injury. The delay allows removal of contamination or any exudate that would compromise healing. At this stage granulation tissue has not yet started to form.
- **Secondary closure:** this is similar to delayed primary closure, except that it has taken longer to remove any infection and therefore some granulation tissue has

TABLE 23.3A	Dressing materials	
Dressing type	**Use**
ADHERENT CONTACT LAYER	
Wet-to-dry dressing	Sterile swabs soaked in Hartmann's solution or saline are placed close to the wound. The dressing dries out and, when removed, takes with it any exudate and debris. These dressings should be changed every 12–24 hr.
Dry-to-dry dressing	Dry swabs are directly applied to the wound so that debris and necrotic tissue adheres to the swabs and is pulled away when the dressing is changed. This is an effective but painful way of debriding wounds, so is not commonly used now.
NON-ADHERENT CONTACT LAYER	
Hydrocolloids, e.g. Granuflex	These help to rehydrate wounds and encourage debridement.
Perforated film dressing, e.g. Melolin, Rondopad, Primapore	Usually used for surgical wounds with little exudate. Provides a clean, dry environment for wound healing, so their main role is protective. Also available with adhesive to be simply stuck in place covering the surgical wound.
Foam dressing, e.g. Allevyn, Advazorb plus	Very good for absorbing fluid from wounds where there is likely to be heavy exudate, and also protects the wound from external contamination.
Alginates, e.g. Kaltostat, AlgiSite	These are derived from seaweed and are usually presented as a soft, woven dressing. They react with sodium ions in exudate, releasing calcium ions and the gel formed holds a considerable amount of fluid and ensures excellent moist wound-healing conditions. They should not be used on dry wounds as they can lead to desiccation of the wound.
Gauze impregnated with petroleum jelly, e.g. Jelonet, Grassolind	A non-adherent dressing that was used for many years, but has now been superseded by synthetic dressings which leave less residue within the wound.
Knitted viscose, e.g. N-A	This can be used to protect granulating wound beds.
Silicone mesh, e.g. Mepitel	Very good as a dressing over skin grafts as they do not adhere to the wound surface at all, but are expensive.
Semi-permeable film dressing, e.g. OpSite, Tegaderm, Bioclusive	These are used in situations with very little exudate since there is minimal absorption by these dressings. They do provide a good moist wound-healing environment.
Barrier sprays, e.g. Cavilon	These can be used to protect fragile tissues during the healing process.

TABLE 23.3B	Topical wound treatments	
Topical wound treatment	**Description**	
Hydrogels, e.g. IntraSite	Hydrogels are commonly used in practice and have the advantage of reducing bacterial contamination of wounds, as well as providing an excellent moist environment that promotes wound healing and some natural debridement.	
Maggots	Very effective at debriding wounds. Sterile stage 1 larvae must be purchased, and placed in contact with the wound. These can be purchased in a mesh bag so that they are contained at the required site. At this stage the larvae do not have chewing mouthparts and do not cause further damage. They must, however, be removed before they reach stage 2, which are able to chew.	
Silver, e.g. Acticoat, Aquacel AG	Silver has very good antimicrobial properties, and has been shown to have activity against bacteria such as methicillin-resistant *Staphylococcus aureus* (MRSA) and *Pseudomonas*. There are a number of creams and dressings that contain silver. Care must be taken to follow directions with these products, as they are quite specific in some cases.	
Honey, e.g. Manukacare 18+, Activon	This can be used as a debridement dressing. It draws fluid from the wound and lowers pH, so therefore should not be used on granulating tissue. Care must be taken that the mix is free from bacterial contamination, so sterile medical-grade honey must be used. There are also commercially available dressings which incorporate honey. To date Manuka honey has been found to have the highest antimicrobial activity, and is therefore the honey of choice.	

started to form. This usually is carried out after 5–7 days.

Dressings and bandages

Not all wounds are amenable to closure and some wounds are best left to heal by second intention. This is particularly the case where there is a large skin deficit, and these wounds will certainly require dressings and bandages to facilitate wound healing.

Bandages can help to:
- Protect a wound from bacterial contamination
- Debride a wound
- Provide comfort and pain relief
- Prevent patient interference
- Support an area with a wound and reduce movement of the skin edges
- Prevent desiccation of a wound
- Reduce the development of swelling and oedema
- Absorb any exudates
- Provide a cosmetic appearance for the owner.

Whenever bandages are used it is very important that clients are given clear instructions about when they should return to the surgery for a planned check-up and about any signs that could indicate a problem.

General guidance on bandage care is as follows:
- The animal should have restricted exercise – either cage rest, or lead walks only.

- The bandage must not be allowed to get wet, so it may need to be protected if the animal is taken outside. If it does get wet it will need to be changed.
- The animal must not be allowed to be interfere with the bandage. The use of Elizabethan collars, bitter-tasting bandages/sprays, additional protection or distraction techniques can all help. If the animal keeps worrying at the area it may also indicate that the bandage itself is causing the animal pain or discomfort.
- The owner must check the bandage regularly for any sign of slippage, damp or any smell or discharge.
- The owner should also monitor the animal's general demeanour and appetite. If the animal becomes depressed, lethargic or goes off its food, these are all signs that there could be an issue with the wound.
- The owner should be encouraged to contact the surgery if they have any concerns so that any problems can be managed as soon as possible.

A bandage should consist of three layers:
- **Primary or contact layer** – this touches the wound and must be sterile
- **Secondary or intermediate layer** – padding, usually added for comfort or absorption
- **Tertiary or protective layer** – applied over the other layers to hold them in place, prevent interference and minimise contamination from the environment.

There are several types of skin dressing available for the management of open wounds (Table 23.3A). The dressing materials chosen depend on the stage of wound healing and the degree of contamination or necrosis. Topical treatments may also be helpful (Table 23.3B).

Drains

In some wound cases, drains can be very valuable. A drain is a device that allows fluid or air to pass from a wound or body cavity to the surface. Several situations may benefit from the use of a drain, including the management of contaminated wounds, deep abscesses, and seromas where they are used to prevent the accumulation of fluid in dead space that may be created in surgical wounds.

Drains can be described as either active or passive:
- **Passive drains** – rely on pressure and gravity to allow the fluid to drain. In order to be effective they should be placed so that the opening is in a dependent position, i.e. below the level of the area from which the fluid is to be drained. The most common drain is a soft flexible tube known as the Penrose drain. Fluid follows the external surface of the drain. This type of drain should be left in place until such time as fluid production is minimal and the risk of dead space development has been removed. They can be made of either soft latex rubber or silicone. Other types of passive drain that are occasionally used are corrugated drains, tube drains and sump drains.
- **Active drains** – require some source of suction to work, and are the preferred choice of drain to use in surgical cases. Suction devices include small compressible plastic containers (grenades), syringes or evacuated blood tubes. For continuous, low-level suction these must be permanently attached to a drainage tube and bandaged in place. Alternatively, intermittent suction can be used, e.g. a syringe used in conjunction with a three-way tap

to ensure that air does not flow back into the area. Tube drains are usually used in these situations.

Monitoring – while in situ, any drain should be checked regularly to ensure that it is still in place and to assess the healing process. There should be no odour associated with the drain and the wound should appear clean, without excessive inflammation. Any fluid emerging should be almost clear, or possibly slightly blood-tinged, but not purulent.

Animals should not be allowed to interfere with drains. Drains are usually covered with bandage to protect against contamination and infection but passive drains may need to be left open to function. An Elizabethan collar or other preventative measures may be needed to prevent the patient worrying at the site.

Removal – when drains are removed, it is usually a simple matter of cutting the sutures that hold the drain in place and then withdrawing the tube. If the drain has been exposed at both ends, the proximal part should be trimmed first so that it is not pulled through the wound, potentially drawing bacteria with it. Check that the drain is intact and that no material has been left behind. This could act as a foreign body and induce a marked tissue reaction.

Thoracic drains are more specialised and consist of a fenestrated tube drain placed using a trocar. Insertion is carried out either under general anaesthesia, e.g. at the time of chest surgery, or under local anaesthesia. For drain placement in a closed thorax a skin incision is made between the 9th and 12th ribs and a subcutaneous tunnel made through to the level of the 8th intercostal spaces. Even those animals under general anaesthesia will require the administration of local anaesthesia at the site of skin incision, through the subcutaneous tunnel and down to the intercostal space that the drain will be inserted. The drain is pushed through the intercostal muscles at this site. Once in place the tube must be sealed to prevent air entering the thorax. This procedure must be carried out under aseptic conditions. Mechanical suction can then be used as necessary. Suction should always be applied via a one-way valve such as a Heimlich valve or water trap, which also prevents excessive suction being applied. Alternatively, a syringe can be used, either attached directly to the chest drain or via a three-way tap. With any thoracic drain it is essential that air is not allowed to enter the thoracic cavity as the drain is checked or the suction device is attached. A gate clamp can be placed on the chest drain as an additional safety feature. These must be opened before emptying the drain.

Reconstructive surgical techniques

Where there is extensive tissue loss, standard surgical closures may not be possible but the site may still be amenable to surgical techniques to replace the missing tissue. These include skin grafts and skin flaps.

If the skin of an animal is tented it is possible to see that there is considerable slack in some areas of the body while the skin is quite tight in other areas. This means that it is possible to remove skin from one of the 'slack' areas and still close the remaining hole. With skin grafts, the skin is usually totally removed from the donor area. With skin flaps, however, the skin is left partially attached to the original site so that its blood supply is maintained. The flap is then rotated or slid in order to cover the recipient site:

- **Skin flaps** are preferred to skin grafts as these conserve the natural blood supply to the tissue. There are many

different flaps possible, based on the position of major vessels, and careful planning is needed to ensure that the best site is used to get the desired result.
- **Skin grafts** can be defined as full or partial thickness, depending on the depth of skin taken. Full-thickness grafts include the epidermis and dermis, whereas split-thickness grafts only include the epidermis and part of the dermis. These are more fragile than full-thickness grafts but tend to take more easily. Hair growth is poor, they are more difficult to collect and the site they have been harvested from has to be managed as an open wound. Due to this, split-thickness grafts are less commonly used in small animal practice.

Skin grafts can also be described according to the amount of tissue used. Sheet grafts are designed to fully cover the deficit, whereas pinch grafts, punch grafts or strip grafts are designed to break up the deficit and provide a start point for epithelialization. Sheet grafts are preferred in small animal practice as often the other types of graft do not provide a good functional or cosmetic result. Before usage, the graft needs to be prepared by carefully removing any hypodermal tissue, and then making a number of small incisions through the graft which will allow drainage of the considerable amount of exudate which forms in the first few days after the graft has been applied.

As well as careful collection of the graft, the recipient site also needs to be well prepared. The site should be free of contamination, and a good layer of well-vascularised granulation tissue should be present so that the graft has a good chance of 'taking'. Alternatively, fresh surgical wounds or clean wounds that have been thoroughly debrided can be suitable sites. The grafts are then placed in situ. Sheet grafts are usually carefully sutured in place, whereas small pinch or punch grafts are simply embedded into the granulation tissue.

Postoperative care is essential in these cases and careful bandaging is required. The bandage should have a non-adherent dressing in contact with the graft such as silicone mesh, which is then covered by a second dressing, padding and an external protective layer. Splints may be used to prevent movement at the site. The bandage must be maintained carefully – it must not be allowed to get wet or to be interfered with by the patient. The graft should be checked every 24–48 hours and each time the dressing is changed great care should be taken to avoid disturbing the graft.

WOUND COMPLICATIONS

Wound dehiscence

Wound dehiscence is defined as the breakdown of a surgical wound. There are a number of reasons why this might occur:

- Insufficient debridement – such that the wound edges start to become necrotic
- Poor local blood supply
- Suture reaction – in some cases sutures act as a focus for a reaction
- Movement of wound edges.

The signs include redness, swelling, discharge, separation of the wound edges, irritation and the animal may start to appear unwell. Clinical signs seen can depend on the stage of dehiscence, whether it was noticed early or not.

To manage these cases, the underlying problem must first be identified so that steps can be taken to avoid repetition, then the wound should be cleaned and debrided again. Where possible, surgical closure should still be carried out, but occasionally it is necessary to keep the wound open and treat it as an open wound.

Wound infection

Wound infection is a major concern when dealing with any type of wound. If the wound has been lavaged thoroughly and debrided fully, the chances of infection are minimal. It is still very important that general hygiene is maintained so that the risk from environmental contamination is minimised, and, of course, animals with reduced immune function are more at risk.

If a wound becomes infected then the animal may show systemic changes, becoming anorexic, lethargic and/or pyrexic. The wound site will also show changes – the area will be red, swollen and uncomfortable and there may be an abnormal discharge.

Treatment is similar to that for wound dehiscence and the wound must be cleaned thoroughly and debrided again. If possible, it should then be managed as an open wound, as sutures may act as a focus for any residual infection. Swabs should also be taken and cultured so that appropriate antibiotics can be used. Systemic antibiotics must be used, but topical treatments may include the use of ointments or dressings containing antimicrobials such as silver. Topical antibiotics are not very useful as they tend to be absorbed by the dressing rather than going into the tissues.

Seroma formation

This is the accumulation of serous fluid under the skin. It usually forms where the surgery has involved the removal of subcutaneous tissue, or the skin is particularly loose or mobile, creating an empty or 'dead space'. In most cases seromas do not cause problems but may appear unsightly. Seromas may delay wound healing and are particularly worrying where skin grafts or flaps have been carried out. Most cases, however, do not actually require treatment as the fluid will be reabsorbed gradually over time. Pressure bandages may help if the site is amenable to bandaging. Some will require surgery, and the wound carefully cleaned, debrided and repaired once more. Where there is 'dead space' an active drain can be utilised to prevent further development of seromas.

Surgical conditions

In general practice much of our time is spent supporting animals requiring surgery. The cases range from relatively routine elective procedures to emergency life-saving operations. In all cases nursing staff carry out a vital role, ensuring that the animals are given the necessary care and support, and also helping owners to understand both the surgery and the aftercare required.

GENERAL CUTANEOUS CONDITIONS

Abscess

An abscess is a localised collection of pus. Pus is tissue debris, dead and degenerating neutrophils and is usually cream or green in colour. An abscess usually contains pyogenic (pusforming) organisms, but can be sterile. The wall of the abscess is lined with granulation and fibrous tissue. Note that abscesses can be found in any tissue, e.g. skin, muscle, bone, organs and brain.

Most abscesses will give rise to the signs of pain, local swelling and reduced function of the area. In time, the abscess is likely to come to a head and may rupture on to a surface. For subcutaneous abscesses this usually helps, because the pressure is reduced and drainage is established. Deep abscesses are more of a problem as, if these rupture, the pus will leak into the abdominal cavity and peritonitis may develop, which can be life threatening. It can also be serious if the pus enters the bloodstream – the animal will develop pyaemia and toxaemia.

Treatment of abscesses always involves the same basic principles no matter where the abscess is located:

- **Establish drainage** – superficial abscesses can be lanced and flushed with Hartmann's solution, sterile saline or weak disinfectant solutions, e.g. 0.05% chlorhexidine. Hydrogen peroxide should not be used as this is extremely tissue-toxic. Hydrogels may be used to pack the abscess site. Deep abscesses require surgery and drains are usually required in order to allow sufficient ongoing drainage.
- **Maintain drainage** – superficial wounds should be kept open through regular bathing and flushing with mild solutions. Deeper abscesses also require flushing via the drain.
- **Treat with appropriate antibiotics** – these are only of benefit if drainage has been established. Without drainage the abscess will reduce in size but it is unlikely that all the bacteria within it will be killed, and once antibiotics are stopped it is likely to recur.

In most cases the protocol described above will allow the abscess to settle down but, if there is insufficient drainage or if there is any foreign material within the abscess cavity, then further treatment will be needed.

There are some occasions where the type or location of the abscess makes it more amenable to complete surgical excision. Providing this is done without spillage it can result in complete removal of the problem. However, dead space will be created so drains are often placed to prevent the accumulation of any serum within the operation site. Excision is often the treatment of choice in rabbits, even for superficial abscesses, as the prognosis is considerably better than when using local drainage.

Ulcers

An ulcer is defined as the loss of the epithelial surface of a tissue, usually skin or mucous membrane, leaving a raw area, which is often slow to heal. Examples include oral ulceration, pressure sores (decubitus ulcers) and corneal ulcers.

Treatment involves the removal of the primary cause, keeping the surface clean and dressing the wound if possible. This will avoid further aggravation of the ulcer. Any secondary infection should be treated with antibiotics.

Fistula

This is a channel that passes from one mucous membrane to a second mucous membrane or the skin, i.e. it passes from one epithelial surface to another. The fistula itself is also lined with epithelium. In general, these should be repaired surgically but the specific treatment will vary with the location of the individual fistula:

- **Anal sac fistula** – an opening forms between the anal sac and the external skin, usually as a result of chronic infection. This will probably require surgical excision of the anal sacs and the overlying skin.

- **Rectovaginal fistula** – usually a congenital abnormality where an opening remains between the rectum and the vagina lying ventral to it. This is uncommon but may be corrected surgically. The condition is also likely to be inherited and affected animals should not be bred from.
- **Oronasal fistula** – may occur after extraction of the canine teeth, which have extremely long roots, which leave a channel between the oral and nasal chambers. The hole should be closed surgically or food will lodge in the site, which may lead to chronic nasal infection.

Sinus

This is an opening or canal running from deeper tissues to the skin or mucous membrane. It is not lined with epithelium and is blind-ending. It is often associated with infection:

- **Foreign body tract** – grass seeds commonly cause problems in animals by penetrating the skin and tracking through the subcutaneous tissues. Bacteria are carried deep into the tissues and there is marked tissue reaction to both the foreign body and the infection. Treatment involves careful surgical exploration of the site and removal of the foreign body.
- **Anal furunculosis (perianal fistulation)** – a deep pyoderma leading to many sinus tracts forming within the tissues. It can be very debilitating and painful and a number of treatment options are available, including radical surgical excision of the affected tissue and anal sacs, or the use of immunosuppressive drugs such as cyclosporine, prednisolone or topical tacrolimus.

HERNIAS AND RUPTURES

These are similar, since in both cases abdominal contents come to rest in an abnormal position through an opening in the muscular wall. The difference between them is that in a hernia, the opening in the abdominal wall is natural – such as the umbilicus or inguinal ring. In a rupture there is a tear in the muscle wall that allows the abdominal contents to migrate through.

In all cases, the contents of the hernia/rupture should be replaced in their normal position. This is sometimes quite simple and can be done through gentle manipulation. Such

hernias are described as **reducible**. The condition is likely to recur, so surgery is usually needed to close or reduce the size of the opening. With ruptures, adhesions may develop between the contents of the rupture and the wall, and they may then be **irreducible**.

In some cases the blood flow to the contents becomes compromised. Initially the venous flow is affected, as the vessels are relatively thin walled and more easily compressed, and blood is able to enter the area but not to leave it. Very quickly the tissues become engorged and then even the arterial vessels are affected. The hernia is then said to be **strangulated** and the tissue trapped in the sac will very quickly become devitalised. These cases are emergencies and require emergency surgery to prevent the animal's condition deteriorating. The surgery for each type of hernia is different in each case (Table 23.4).

Diaphragmatic rupture

Although often referred to as a hernia, this is usually a rupture caused by trauma forcing the diaphragm to tear. This allows abdominal contents to move through into the thorax and compromise respiratory function.

Affected patients need careful handling to prevent the situation deteriorating, and treatment of shock is the primary concern. Surgery should be attempted only after the animal has been stabilised. During this time the animal should be encouraged to remain in sternal recumbency with its head and thorax propped up such that they are higher than the abdomen. This allows the abdominal contents to slide back towards the abdomen under gravity rather than migrating forward into the thorax. Stabilisation can take a prolonged period of time depending on the presence of other injuries. Factors such as nutrition and pain control do need to be attended to during this period. Strict rest is essential as any activity increases the oxygen demand by the tissues, and the patient needs to be hospitalised in a quiet, calm area of the surgery to minimise stress. Additional oxygen can be helpful, providing this can be given without causing the animal any stress. Some cases may have no signs of any respiratory distress at the time of the trauma, and only diagnosed years later. These cases can prove to be exceptionally difficult surgical cases, due to the high levels of adhesions within the thorax and abdomen, and the issues surrounding postoperative re-expansion pulmonary oedema.

During surgery, the animal is usually placed in dorsal recumbency and the approach is via a cranial laparotomy incision. As

TABLE 23.4	Hernias – causes and treatments	
Type of hernia/rupture	Description	Treatment and prognosis
Umbilical hernia	Protrusion of abdominal contents through an enlarged umbilical opening	Surgical repair of the linea alba Rarely any complications
Inguinal hernia	Abdominal contents migrate through the inguinal canal to the groin region More common in bitches and rabbits	Surgery to draw abdominal contents back into the abdomen and to reduce the size of the hole in the abdominal muscle layers Can be serious if tissues have become devitalised, particularly if the bladder is involved
Perineal hernia	Muscle layers around the anal sphincter gradually break down and allow the rectal wall to stretch and form a diverticulum; this results in constipation and impaction Most common in intact male dogs	Muscle reconstruction of the perineal area is possible Castration is also recommended, since the condition is hormone-related Prognosis remains guarded because of possible long-term difficulty in passing faeces or incontinence There is a risk of the other side developing the same condition – particularly if the dog is left intact

the thoracic cavity is approached, the lungs tend to collapse, so there must be strict attention to the patient's respiration. Respiratory augmentation is often used to assist the animal. This can be achieved by gently squeezing the respiratory reservoir bag on the circuit at the same time as the animal's own respiratory movements. Thus the amount of air the animal takes in with each breath is increased and oxygenation is improved. Use of a ventilator is the preferred choice, alongside monitoring with a capnograph to ensure good ventilation (also see Chapter 27).

Postoperatively, a chest drain is usually placed, and as much trapped air as possible is withdrawn from the thoracic cavity to encourage the lungs to re-expand before the animal is allowed to recover, and the patient must be monitored closely to ensure that respiratory function is adequate. It may still be necessary to place the patient in an oxygen-rich environment during the recovery phase and to aspirate the drain every 1–4 hours. Once the patient's breathing has returned to normal and no more air is obtained from the drain, it can be removed. The prognosis for cases suffering a ruptured diaphragm does vary; patients who have been involved in this type of trauma may have other injuries that will influence the outcome.

TUMOURS

The words tumour and neoplasia are usually used to refer to any abnormal new growth occurring in the body. These growths are either benign, with no tendency to spread, or malignant, which infiltrate extensively into local tissues and can spread throughout the body. The suffix '-oma' denotes tumour or other abnormal growth, while the prefix normally denotes the tissue of origin.

Benign growths

These usually have well-developed fibrous capsules and remain in the one site. They include:

- **Lipoma** – tumour comprised of adipose tissue
- **Fibroma** – superficial tumour of the skin and occasionally the mouth, made up of fibrous or connective tissue
- **Adenoma** – benign tumour of glandular tissue, e.g. anal adenoma, adenoma of the thyroid gland; 'adeno-' means 'pertaining to a gland'
- **Papilloma** – 'warty' growths found on the skin and occasionally in the bladder arising from epithelial tissues; grow exophytically (outwardly projecting)
- **Melanoma** – tumour of the melanocytes in the skin; although named as if they are benign, such tumours are usually malignant.

Malignant growths

These are poorly differentiated tumours with indistinct edges. They tend to spread (metastasise) both into local tissues and systemically. They include:

- **Carcinoma** – produced from epithelium. Squamous cell carcinomas (often seen affecting the ear tips of white cats) and mammary tumours, which are usually adenocarcinomas, i.e. affecting glandular epithelium are all examples.
- **Sarcoma** – produced from mesodermal (connective) tissues; examples include osteosarcoma and fibrosarcoma.
- **Malignant melanoma** also come into this category. Strictly this should be called a melanocarcinoma, and therefore fits with other epithelial cell tumours.

Malignant tumours often show ulceration, local infiltration and metastasis, i.e. they spread to sites distant from the original tumour site.

Carcinomas tend to spread to local lymph nodes via the lymphatic system, whereas sarcomas tend to spread via the bloodstream and lodge in tissues where the blood passes through capillary networks, such as the lungs.

Haematological tumours – involve the lymphoid and myeloid tissues and can be solid or circulating: e.g. lymphosarcoma (solid) and leukaemia (circulating).

Common sites for tumours

Tumours can occur at any site in the body and in all species. The risk of developing some type of tumour increases as an animal gets older, since cellular repair mechanisms become less effective with age.

Complications of tumours

Tumours cause a number of problems within the body. Local effects include pain and ulceration leading to secondary infection. The physical presence of the tumour can also cause problems such as restriction of movement or prevention of the normal flow of ingesta through the intestines.

Metastases. These are secondary tumours that usually develop as small clumps of cells break away from the primary tumour and enter the circulation. When they encounter a mesh-like filter such as the capillaries in the spleen or lungs or the reticular structure within lymph nodes, they are caught (sometimes called 'seeded') and start to multiply or metastasise at that site.

Metastases can occur in almost any site, but the lymph nodes, lungs, liver and spleen are the most common. All metastases will produce loss of function at the affected site, which adds to the problems that may be developing at the primary site. The clinical signs will depend on the area affected.

Hormone production. Secretory tumours can overproduce normal hormones and affect the body's metabolism. Common endocrine tumours include thyroid adenomas, insulinomas, pituitary gland tumours and adrenal gland tumours.

Tumours affecting non-glandular tissues can also secrete substances that may behave like hormones: e.g. lymphomas and bone tumours can produce a substance that behaves like parathyroid hormone and causes hypercalcaemia; insulin-like hormones are produced by some tumours, leading to hypoglycaemia.

Haematological complications. These may also develop as a result of invasion of bone marrow by the tumour or changes in production of blood cells, platelets and clotting factors.

Causes of tumours

There is a considerable amount of research into why and how tumours develop and, although not all the answers are known, the following are thought to contribute:

- **Mutations** – random events leading to uncontrolled proliferation of mutated cells. There may be an inherited component as to why these occur in some breeds more than others.
- **Viruses** – including feline leukaemia virus and papillomaviruses.

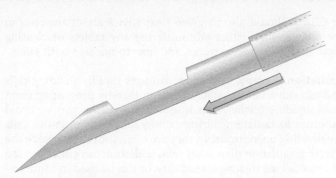

Fig. 23.1 Simplified diagram of a Tru-Cut needle

- **Carcinogens** – chemicals that induce mutations in the DNA such as those released through smoking, or solvents such as benzene.
- **Radiation** – is known to damage DNA and lead to changes.
- **Ultraviolet light** – sunlight has long been known to be involved in the development of some skin cancers.

Tumour diagnosis

Diagnosis of the actual tumour type is usually confirmed by means of a sample of tissue, which is examined histologically to determine both the cell type and the degree of malignancy. The results will give an indication of the prognosis and the most appropriate treatment. Diagnostic imaging such as radiography, ultrasonography, magnetic resonance imaging (MRI) and computed tomography (CT) will also detect the presence of a space-occupying mass (see later in the section).

Wedge biopsy. A section of the tumour is taken after surgical excision. This is often the best method as it provides cells from the centre and the edge of the tumour. The sample should then be fixed in formol-saline at a 10% concentration.

Tru-Cut needle biopsy. A specialised needle is used to take tiny samples from parenchymal tissues (Fig. 23.1). The needle has a small notch cut out of its barrel and a cover that is slid down so that a small quantity of tissue is caught between the notch and the cover. This can then be fixed and examined histologically.

A Tru-Cut needle can be used to obtain tissue from organs such as the liver and kidney. Biopsy of the kidney can even be performed percutaneously with ultrasound guidance. It is not as good as the wedge biopsy, as you only get a small sliver of tissue for analysis and could miss the area where the cancerous cells are located.

Grab or pinch biopsy. Samples from mucosal surfaces such as the intestine, respiratory tract or urogenital tract may be collected using small biopsy forceps which are often attached to endoscopes to allow visualisation of the tissues being collected. The main issues are that the samples collected are often very small and are only superficial, and may not fully represent the types of cells actually present.

Needle aspirate. This technique is commonly used for lymphomas and may also be used to differentiate between abscesses and other cutaneous swellings.

Method
1. Introduce a 1 inch × 23 G needle into the mass.
2. Move the needle to and fro within the mass, changing the direction.
3. Withdraw.
4. Connect an air-filled syringe.
5. Depress the plunger of the syringe sharply, and blow out the cells on to a slide.
6. Make a smear from the cells, stain and examine under the microscope, or fix before sending to an external laboratory.

It is also possible to obtain samples by suction, i.e. by having the syringe already attached and drawing back on the plunger to collect the cells. Lymphoma cells, however, are fragile, and if this is suspected, the needle-only method may give better results. Examination of the stained smear may give sufficient information to start treatment, though in some cases it may prove non-diagnostic.

Exfoliative cytology. Cells taken from the surface of the tumour are collected and analysed. This method is only used if other diagnostic techniques are not possible, as it is the least reliable. It can be carried out in several different ways, depending on the accessibility of the tumour:

- Tissue scraping – a scalpel blade is used to collect cells from the surface of a mass.
- Impression smears – a glass slide is touched onto the surface of the lesion, which has been cleaned prior to collecting the sample.
- Exudate is collected and then examined.
- Sterile saline is flushed over the surface of the suspect tissue and then collected. Any cellular matter is then examined. Flushes can be used to examine the nasal cavity, bronchi and trachea and prostate gland.

If tumour cells are found, then the technique is diagnostic; if none are identified, it might simply mean that the tumour cells were not collected.

Tumour imaging. Diagnostic imaging techniques may also be very important in the initial diagnosis of the tumour, checking for evidence of metastases and monitoring the progress of the patient. Several imaging techniques are now available, including radiography, ultrasonography, MRI, CT and scintigraphy (see Chapter 32). The choice of imaging technique depends on the nature of the particular tumour under investigation and location.

Treatment

Surgery. This is generally the treatment of choice as, by complete removal of the tumour, the animal may be cured of that particular cancer. Operations should be carried out as soon as possible to decrease the risk of further growth of the tumour and to minimise the risk of metastasis.

Care should be taken when preparing the site for surgery. Wide excisions are needed to ensure that all the tumour cells are removed, but different tumours require different margins based on both their type and their degree of malignancy, and therefore biopsies should be completed prior to excisional surgery. The area clipped and prepared for surgery must therefore be sufficient for the particular tumour. The site should also be cleaned quite gently; if the site is scrubbed too hard there is possibly an increased risk of the tumour metastasising.

Owners may need support and counselling preoperatively and postoperatively. Some radical resections will be life changing for the animal and a challenge for owners to deal with (e.g. surgery for an osteosarcoma may mean limb amputation, or a squamous cell carcinoma on the nose of a cat may require reconstructive surgery), so owners need to be prepared for this. It can be useful to provide pictures of other cases that have had similar treatment, or even getting support from other clients whose own animals have undergone the same procedure.

Postoperative care will vary depending on the amount of tissue that had to be removed, but pain relief and general wound management protocols will be needed.

In some cases it is not possible to remove the tumour completely and debulking surgery may be performed. This is indicated if it will either improve the animal's quality of life or reduce the amount of tumour sufficiently for follow-up treatments using radiation or chemotherapy to be more successful.

Chemotherapy. This is the treatment of tumours using cytotoxic drugs, and is most commonly used for tumours that have spread systemically or those affecting the bone marrow or lymphatic system. They can be used as the sole treatment method for some tumours, or may be used in combination with surgery or radiation treatments.

There are a number of different drugs available for use as chemotherapeutic agents and different protocols involving combinations of these products have been developed for different types of cancer. Most are given at intervals to provide maximum tumour cell death, while allowing time between treatments for the animal's healthy cells to recover. Newer protocols are being devised in which lower doses of drugs are used, but given continuously, rather than in higher doses less often. This type of treatment schedule is known as metronomic dosing and is undergoing trials at present.

These are obviously very potent drugs and care is required whenever they are handled. During preparation of the product, care must be taken to avoid any form of contact, whether on skin or via inhalation. The practice should have a standardised operating procedure (SOP) for the preparation and use of cytotoxic drugs, and all staff involved with their use made aware of the risks of working with these types of drugs and given training before they are expected to handle them.

There are good guidelines for the safety of staff provided by the European College of Veterinary Nursing Medicine of Companion Animals, and these should be checked and followed prior to any treatments. Drugs should be stored securely, and prepared in a biological safety cabinet. Protective clothing is essential; as a minimum two pairs of latex gloves, a full-length impervious gown, goggles and mask (not surgical) should be worn. A closed system should be used to administer the drugs wherever possible to prevent risk of spillage or accidental aerosol formation. If spillage does take place, there should be clear protocols as to how to deal with it.

It is not just during the preparation and administration of the products when care is needed, as body waste may also contain traces of the drugs, so gloves and protective aprons should be worn when handling faeces or urine from treated animals. Kennels containing patients being treated with cytotoxic drugs should be labelled clearly, and staff dealing with any waste must follow the correct practice protocol.

Clients should also be given clear advice about any risks to themselves when either administering any tablets or clearing their animals' urine or faeces, and how to manage both safely.

Radiation therapy. Radiation damages rapidly dividing cells and can cause chromosomal damage, thereby preventing them from dividing further. This is usually the reason why we avoid exposure to radiation during radiography. Since tumour cells are dividing uncontrollably, they are often more sensitive to the effects of radiation than other cells. Radiation can either be used as a standalone treatment modality, or can be used in combination with other treatments. Radiation can either be applied from an external source such as a linear accelerator which produces high-energy X-rays, or from an implanted source such as radioactive iodine or iridium wires (brachytherapy). If an external source is used, the total radiation dose required is usually split down into multiple small amounts given as often as daily – this is to avoid excessive damage to surrounding tissues.

Side effects, such as erythema of exposed skin and mucous membranes, alopecia, skin thickening and abnormal hair coloration, may occur. Owners must therefore be given careful advice before embarking on a treatment programme so that they are fully aware of the possible outcomes.

Surgical procedures by region of the body

The veterinary nurse has a number of very important roles to play in the management of surgical cases. This includes preoperative, intraoperative and postoperative care.

Preoperative procedures – on admission the necessary paperwork for the animal should have been completed fully and the client should have been made aware of what will happen during the surgery (informed consent). Discussion with the owner, or animal carer, to find relevant information on last feeding, what medications the pet is receiving (if any), is the animal in season, has the animal urinated or defecated etc. All animals should have access to water until the time that they are pre-medicated.

The animal should then be weighed and any premedication drug calculations completed. Medications should not be drawn up ready for administration as the plastic of the syringe can denature the drugs contained. The theatre should be prepared ready for the procedure and all the appropriate instruments should be made ready.

When the premedication is fully effective, anaesthesia should be induced (see Chapter 27). This should be done in the preparation area, and the animal should then be clipped up ready to be taken through into theatre. An initial skin preparation should also be done at this stage, and the proposed surgical site then covered before taking the animal through to theatre where the final skin preparation is applied.

Operative procedures – during the operation the veterinary nurse should provide assistance to the surgeon. This may mean that the nurse scrubs up and works alongside the surgeon, passing instruments, swabbing the site and cutting sutures as indicated. Alternatively, the nurse may remain non-sterile but be responsible for opening sterile packs for the surgeon, or monitoring the condition of the patient (also see Chapter 24). Note that the person monitoring the anaesthetic should not be involved in other aspects of the animal's surgery so that their full attention can be given to this important part of any procedure.

Postoperative procedures – the operation site should be gently cleaned before the animal starts to come round from the anaesthetic, and any dressings should be applied at this time. The patient should then be monitored carefully during recovery to ensure adequate respiration and return of the laryngeal reflexes. Patients should also be kept warm and the operation site should be checked regularly prior to discharge.

It is important that any nurse looking after a patient in the ward is fully aware of the procedures that have taken place, so that during recovery and in the immediate postoperative period all the relevant checks and treatments will be made. Owners may also wish to visit or call about the progress of their animal, and the nursing team should be able to respond to client questions about their animal.

Depending on the type of case, nurses may also be involved at discharge and need to be able to advise the client about the postoperative care for the animal, including details about any medication that needs to be given, when and what to feed, any special instructions relating to the operation, when to make the next appointment at the surgery and what possible problems to watch for.

THE EAR

Aural haematoma

Cause. Aural haematomas usually develop on the ear pinna as a result of self-trauma secondary to either an ear infection or a foreign body within the ear canal. More rarely it can be due to direct trauma. It is most commonly seen in dogs.

Clinical signs. The ear pinna is swollen, and on palpation the swelling is fluid-filled and warm to the touch. If there is otitis or a foreign body within the ear canal, the animal may resent examination of the ear, so care should be taken to ensure that no one is bitten.

Treatment. The ear should be examined carefully to determine the primary cause; this often needs to be carried out under general anaesthesia. If there is evidence of infection, the ear canal should be cleaned thoroughly using saline and the tympanic membrane checked prior to using any other solutions. If the tympanic membrane is damaged, then disinfectants or oto-lytic solutions should be avoided since these will cause problems within the middle ear.

There are a number of different options that can be used to manage aural haematomas. In some cases it may be possible just to drain the haematoma and then use an injection of long-acting steroids to reduce the inflammation and the likelihood of further bleeding under the skin. This method has the advantage of being less invasive, and does work in many cases. If the haematoma does recur then it may need to be followed with surgical treatment.

In all cases the pinna should be clipped and prepared for surgery. An incision is made on the inside of the ear to allow the blood to drain. The end of this incision is left open to allow continued drainage. Compression is then applied across the pinna to prevent the 'dead space' between the skin and cartilage from refilling with blood. This is usually achieved by using a number of mattress sutures, and the ear is then bandaged, either

in a downwards position or up over the head, which will prevent self-trauma, and also help absorb any seepage from the wound.

An alternative method is to use a device to continue to provide drainage or suction. A teat cannula or Penrose drain can be used to provide a route for passive drainage, or a small fenestrated drain can be created from a butterfly catheter, with the needle end inserted into a vacuum tube to provide continuous low-level suction. This must be bandaged to the patient's head or neck, so may not be tolerated by all patients.

Postoperative care. These cases require analgesia and antibiotics and will often need an Elizabethan collar to prevent self-trauma. It is usual to leave the sutures in place for slightly longer than a normal surgical wound just to make sure that the haematoma does not re-form immediately.

Lateral wall resection (Zepp's procedure)

This procedure is used in some cases of chronic ear infection in which the vertical canal has become chronically inflamed and narrowed. In this situation it is important that owners do not believe that this will provide a miracle cure for their animal – usually it just makes treatment of the underlying condition easier and allows air to circulate in the ear canal. Another indication for this surgery is an animal with polyps or a tumour affecting just the vertical canal. It is more commonly carried out in dogs than cats, particularly animals with 'floppy' ears where air circulation is reduced and infection more likely, e.g. Labradors and spaniels.

Preoperative preparation. The ear canal should be cleaned thoroughly and the area ventral to the external opening of the ear canal should be clipped and prepared for surgery. One of the most common reasons for wound breakdown postoperatively is infection, so it is helpful if the animal has already been on treatment for any otitis prior to the surgery, and any infection removed.

Procedure. The lateral wall of the vertical ear canal is resected and reflected such that when the operation is complete the medial wall of the vertical canal is exposed, as is the entrance to the horizontal canal.

Postoperative care. This is a painful procedure so analgesics are needed as well as antibiotics, due to the contaminated site. An Elizabethan collar is used to prevent the animal trying to scratch or rub the affected ear.

There is often a considerable discharge from the ear due to underlying infection so it is important that the operation site is kept clean in the postoperative period. Not all patients will tolerate this so it may be necessary for the dog to come back to the surgery for sedation, enabling the ear to be cleaned and checked.

Sutures should remain in place until the wound edges have obviously healed – this may take longer than most other surgical wounds and to avoid the need for suture removal some surgeons prefer to use absorbable sutures.

Total ear canal ablation (TECA)

If the infection or tumours within the ear are very severe, then a complete aural ablation may be necessary, in which the horizontal and vertical canals of the ear are excised. After this operation, the cosmetic result is actually better than after the lateral wall resection, since the skin is closed beneath the ear and a small hole is left that leads directly to the tympanic bulla.

Preoperative preparation. This is almost identical to the preparation required for the lateral wall resection.

Procedure. An incision is made overlying the vertical canal and the skin edges are reflected to expose the cartilage of the vertical canal. The canal is then carefully dissected away from the underlying tissues right down to the tympanic bulla.

A **bulla osteotomy** is also needed to prevent recurrent problems with infection. This involves opening the tympanic bulla in order to release any infection from within the middle ear. This does result in deafness in the affected ear, but in most cases requiring this type of surgery the animal is already unable to hear on that side.

Postoperative care. The basic care will be the same as for the lateral wall resection. The risk of complications is, however, far higher with this procedure, and damage to the facial nerve can result in a number of cases; this may be permanent. In addition other neurological complications can also arise due to the proximity of the tympanic bulla to many other structures, as well as the risks of wound dehiscence, chronic dermatitis or the development of a draining fistula from the site. This procedure is therefore not undertaken lightly, and owners need appropriate advice and guidance.

THE EYE

Prolapse of the eyeball (proptosis)

This is an emergency and is one of the few situations where an animal must be brought down to the surgery as soon as possible. It usually affects the brachycephalic breeds of dog such as Pugs and Pekinese but can also affect other species such as hamsters and guinea pigs, which also have protruding eyes. In cases of severe trauma, it can affect any breed or species.

Cause. The prolapse is usually caused by some type of trauma, e.g. road traffic accidents, in which case it may be accompanied by severe trauma to other parts of the body, and shock. Prolapse may also result from a fight or poor handling in the case of exotic species. It is therefore important that a full clinical examination is carried out so that any other injuries can also be assessed and treated.

Clinical signs. People often imagine that a prolapsed eye will be hanging from the socket but in reality this is not often the case unless there has been severe head trauma. The eye may simply appear more bulbous than usual and the conjunctiva is more apparent and quite congested. The prognosis for this condition is quite guarded, and the functionality of the eye should be assessed before surgery is considered. There are a number of long-term complications that may result, ranging from blindness to permanent damage to the eyelids or lacrimal gland, that can necessitate continued treatments. The alternative to replacement is enucleation, and while this seems drastic initially, it may be the better option for the patient.

First-aid treatment. The most important action is to prevent the eye from drying out. Saline, ophthalmic ointment or even a water-soluble jelly should be used to prevent this. The animal should also be stopped from traumatising the eye further by applying an Elizabethan collar. Any signs of shock should be assessed and treated as described earlier in this chapter.

Preparation. The fur around the eye should be clipped carefully and the area should be prepared using dilute povidone-iodine solution. The surface of the cornea should be protected with water-soluble jelly, which can then be rinsed off, taking with it any hair that might otherwise have become stuck to the surface of the eye. The surface of the eye should also be cleansed using a solution of povidone-iodine diluted with saline to produce a 1:50 solution.

Surgery. The eye should be replaced as soon as possible under general anaesthesia. A lateral canthotomy (making an incision at the lateral canthus) is required to allow the eyelids to be opened sufficiently to allow the eye to be replaced. To prevent immediate recurrence, the eyelids are often sutured together for a short while to allow the bruised and swollen conjunctiva to heal and the eye to settle back into its normal position.

Postoperative care. An Elizabethan collar may be needed for a few days postoperatively to prevent the animal from rubbing the eye. Once the eye has been in place for 1–2 weeks it should be safe to remove the sutures and collar. Topical antibiotics and atropine should be used as well as systemic antibiotics and anti-inflammatories. The animal will need quite a bit of care and reassurance during this time, so will need to be approached and handled gently to minimise stress.

Corneal damage

The most common type of corneal damage seen in general practice is a corneal ulcer.

Clinical signs. The eye is very painful and the animal usually holds the eyelids closed – described as **blepharospasm**. There is increased flow of lacrimal fluid due to the pain and irritation and this results in tear overflow or **epiphora**. Depending on the initial cause of the ulcer there may also be infection present, leading to a purulent ocular discharge.

Treatment. The eye should be examined carefully to see if the cause of the ulceration is still present. Small pieces of debris or bedding materials may be caught behind the third eyelid, which may have caused considerable damage to the corneal surface. Local anaesthetic drops such as proxymetacaine may be needed to aid the examination. Medical treatments are often tried first and topical antibiotics and pain relief may be sufficient in the majority of cases. The lack of direct blood supply to the cornea does mean, however, that the healing process is very slow compared with that of other tissues. To provide additional protection for the cornea, corneal bandages, similar to contact lenses, can be used.

Surgery. As the aetiology of corneal ulcers is complicated, for other cases a surgical approach may be preferred. The simplest surgery is the third eyelid flap, known as a **tarsorrhaphy**. In this procedure the third eyelid is sutured in the closed position so that it does not move across the surface of the ulcer and irritate it further.

Depending on the type and cause of the ulcer, it may need to be debrided using a dry cotton bud, and it may be necessary to excoriate the surface of the ulcer and perform a grid keratotomy. This involves the use of a 27-G needle to produce a grid pattern of superficial scratches on the surface of the cornea across the ulcer and extending into the healthy tissue around it. This may seem to be the exact opposite of what is required, but often stimulates healing in an area that had become quite dormant.

More refined surgery for deep ulcers involves the use of conjunctival grafts. Pedicles of conjunctiva are sutured to the cornea to cover the ulcer. Rather like the use of skin flaps, these still have their vascular supply intact to allow nutrients to reach the ulcerated site more easily. After a few weeks the flap is freed from its origin and trimmed to leave just a small area covering the defect. With time this remodels and becomes less obvious.

Tissue glue has also been used in the repair of small ulcers. After debriding the ulcer and allowing the surface of the cornea to dry, the glue is very carefully applied to the area where it is needed. This is then left in place until the ulcer is healed, and then either removed with forceps under local anaesthesia or allowed to slough away gradually.

Postoperative care. The most important thing is that the animal itself does not interfere with healing and aggravate the wound or injury still further, and it may be necessary for the animal to be fitted with an Elizabethan collar. Topical antibiotics and pain relief are continued even while the third eyelid flaps or conjunctival flaps are in place. The sutures holding the third eyelid flaps are usually removed after 2–3 weeks (depending on the severity of the ulcer) and the ulcer is checked carefully.

Enucleation

This is indicated if the eye is too damaged to save, which may be due to any of the following conditions:

- Gross trauma
- Panophthalmitis (massive inflammation of the whole eye)
- Neoplasia – of the eye or behind the eye (retrobulbar)
- Untreatable glaucoma, which has led to blindness in the affected eye
- Irreducible prolapse or recurrent prolapse
- Retrobulbar abscess
- Any other conditions leading to blindness and pain.

Preparation. Before surgery, owners are often very concerned about the procedure and the likely postoperative appearance of their animal. It may be helpful if the practice has some photographs of animals that have undergone enucleation so that worried owners can see that the cosmetic effect in small animals is often not as bad as they had feared. The animals themselves tolerate enucleation very well.

The skin around the eyelids should be clipped and prepared using a dilute povidone-iodine solution as described previously.

Surgery. If the eye itself is the only problem the eyeball is removed, but the muscles can be left in place so that the skin does not fall so far back into the socket. If, however, the surgical procedure is due to a retrobulbar tumour or chronic abscess in that region, more tissues will need to be removed; this procedure is referred to as an exenteration. It is possible for prostheses to be used to avoid the sunken appearance but these are not commonly used in general practice. The eye is carefully dissected from the surrounding tissues, the third eyelid is removed and a strip of tissue is removed from the edge of each eyelid so that these can be sutured together.

Postoperative care. Some veterinary surgeons bandage the site, which helps to prevent seroma formation within the orbit and is perhaps helpful for the owners in the initial postoperative period. This can be removed after 2–3 days and the wound can then be left open. To prevent the animal from rubbing the area an Elizabethan collar may be used.

Systemic antibiotics may be necessary for a few days postoperatively but should only be continued for any length of time in cases where there was gross infection within the orbit area prior to surgery. Analgesics should be prescribed on a case-by-case basis. Owners should always be warned that the animal can have a bloody nasal discharge on the same side of the removed eye, but this should resolve in 2–4 days.

Cataracts

A cataract is an increase in the opacity of the lens and in a true cataract is due to deposition of material within either the capsule, the cortex or the nucleus of the lens. The changes seen in the eyes of old dogs with increased lens opacity are not cataracts. The lens is continually growing and increases in density so that gradually less and less light is able to pass through; they appear greyish-blue. There is potential that they can interfere with vision (Lowe, 2014).

Many cataract cases seen in veterinary practice are those also suffering with diabetes mellitus – 75% of all dogs diagnosed with diabetes mellitus go on to develop cataracts and ultimately blindness.

Surgery. True cortical or capsular cataracts can be managed by eye specialists using surgical techniques. An incision is required at the edge of the cornea, and this allows access to the lens capsule. The most common technique is phacoemulsification, which breaks up the lens material inside the lens capsule through a combination of irrigation and ultrasound vibration. The lens material is then aspirated, and a synthetic replacement lens is then introduced.

The alternative is intracapsular lens extraction where the entire lens is removed. The animal will have some vision restored, in that light will reach the retina again, but it will have lost the ability to focus, and there is a risk of developing glaucoma.

Postoperative care. Patients must be monitored closely and regular checks made on the wound to ensure there is no leakage, and intraocular pressure will need to be checked regularly during the first 24 hours after surgery to ensure there is no hypertension. Diabetic animals will require additional checks, as in all postoperative situations. Topical treatments will be needed including antibiotics and mydriatics such as tropicamide or atropine, as well as non-steroidal anti-inflammatories. NSAIDs are used in the treatment of cystoid macular oedema (CMO) following **cataract surgery**. The animal may need to go home with an Elizabethan collar, and owners must be given clear advice about continuing topical medications, and when they should return for recheck appointments. A harness should

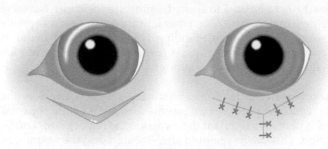

Fig. 23.2 V-Y plasty for ectropion management

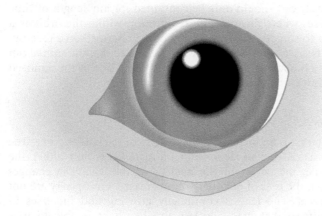

Fig. 23.3 Crescent-shaped sliver removal for entropion

be worn as a collar can press on the jugular veins and increase intracranial pressure and pressure within the eyes.

Entropion and ectropion

These are conditions of the eyelids. In entropion the eyelid rolls inwards, causing the eyelashes to irritate the cornea; in ectropion the eyelid bags open, exposing the conjunctiva. Occasionally, entropion and ectropion are found in the same eye. This is known as 'diamond eye' and a number of breeds, such as the St Bernard, are prediposed to this.

Clinical signs. Entropion leads to excess tear production and thus epiphora (tear overflow), which can be a cause of pain and irritation to the eye. The animal can show signs of blepharospasm (when there is sustained, forced, involuntary closing of the eyelid). Conjunctivitis is usually present, and without treatment corneal ulcers are a common consequence. Ectropion may also lead to conjunctivitis, as bacteria can easily gain access to the eye through the exposed area of conjunctiva.

Treatment. For both conditions this usually involves surgery of the eyelids. Small slivers of skin are removed to turn the eyelid out, or take up the slack of an oversized eyelid (Figs. 23.2 and 23.3).

It is essential that an assessment of the amount of tissue to be removed is made while the animal is conscious, and before the animal has had any premedication – the use of sedatives can make even a good eye appear like an ectropion.

Postoperative care. The main requirement is to ensure that the patient does not interfere with the wound, and particularly

in the case of animals that have had entropion surgery, it is likely that they will in fact be more comfortable postoperatively than they were before.

Distichiasis and ectopic cilia

Ectopic cilia are just one or two abnormally positioned eyelashes, whereas distichiasis involves a row of extra eyelashes inside the normal lashes.

Clinical signs. These are very similar to entropion – animals present with epiphora, conjunctivitis, blepharospasm and corneal ulcers.

Treatment. The extra eyelashes can be dealt with in a number of ways, of which the simplest is simply to pluck them. This only provides a temporary solution, since they will regrow. Electrolysis can also be used, which gives longer-lasting results, but is also not necessarily permanent. Surgery can be used to remove the roots of the lashes but this is very delicate surgery and requires specialised ophthalmic instruments. Cryotherapy is another alternative. Neither of these methods is commonly used in general practice.

Trichiasis

This occurs when hair growing normally rubs on the eye leading to problems similar to those described earlier. This occurs when normal hair, either from a prominent nasal fold or from the medial canthus, causes constant irritation to the eye. Surgery is required to correct this, and this can vary from a relatively simple procedure to full 'facelift' surgery.

GASTROINTESTINAL TRACT

Gastrotomy

The surgical technique involving the opening up of the stomach may be used as treatment for the following conditions:

Foreign bodies. These are very common and very varied in type. Throughout your time in practice you will undoubtedly see a number of items removed from the gastrointestinal tract of animals and will certainly gain experience in dealing with this type of case.

Clinical signs. These vary depending on the type of foreign body, whether solid or linear object, or if it causes a full or partial blockage. Sharp foreign bodies produce recurrent vomiting, often with blood, described as haematemesis, whereas others produce no obvious signs and might only be found when the animal is being investigated for something else.

Diagnosis. The most common method of confirming a diagnosis is radiography (see Chapter 32). Plain studies will be sufficient for some types but contrast studies may be needed to locate radiolucent objects such as plastic bags or pairs of tights.

Surgery. These patients usually require a laparotomy (celiotomy) and gastrotomy for removal of the object. If the problem has been present for some while, consideration will need to be given to the hydration status of the patient. All patients must be stabilised and be as physically well as possible prior to surgery. All surgical cases must be placed on intravenous fluids.

During the procedure it is important to minimise the risk of spillage of gastric contents into the abdomen; large laparotomy swabs should be used to pack off the stomach from the abdomen as it is exteriorised. If gastric contents do leak into the peritoneal cavity, it should be lavaged with copious amounts of warmed, sterile balanced electrolyte solution to remove bacteria and debris. This can range from 500 ml in a cat to several litres in large dog. All lavage fluids need to be removed from the cavity, as inadequate removal, via aspiration, can spread bacteria throughout the peritoneal cavity.

Postoperative care. Animals should be fed with a highly digestible diet postoperatively as soon as the pet can eat. The animal's normal food should then be reintroduced gradually over a period of days, if it was an appropriate diet. Antibiotics can be utilised if there was a break in contamination of the surgical field. Analgesics should be used to meet the animal's requirements, though NSAIDs should not be used due to their interference with the gastrointestinal tract (see Chapter 19). Careful monitoring is essential and any signs of vomiting, depression or pyrexia should be noted and the veterinary surgeon informed.

Gastric dilation and torsion (gastric dilation and volvulus [GDV]).

This condition can be seen in any dog, but most commonly affects deep-chested breeds, e.g. Greyhounds, Pointers and German Shepherds. The condition is multifactorial, and contributing factors include exercise after eating, reduced gastric motility, highly fermentable diets, age and breed. The dog becomes depressed and may start to salivate or attempt to vomit. Gradually the abdomen becomes distended and the animal may 'flank watch' as it tries to determine why it is feeling so uncomfortable. As time progresses the abdominal swelling becomes more obvious and the mucous membranes become a deep purple colour, as the distended abdomen presses on the vena cava, reducing venous return.

Pathogenesis. Initially the stomach dilates due to an accumulation of gas or fluid. The dilation may progress to torsion if the stomach starts to rotate about the oesophagus. The distal oesophagus and duodenum become twisted preventing ingesta leaving the stomach in either direction. The stomach continues to distend, which puts pressure on the hepatic portal vein and caudal vena cava and decreases venous return. This leads to hypovolaemic shock as blood is not returned to the heart and is not available to be re-oxygenated and delivered to the tissues. Without rapid treatment, this condition is fatal. In addition, the blood supply to the stomach is also compromised, leading to necrosis of the stomach wall. Toxins are able to leak into the bloodstream, which leads to endotoxaemia.

Management. **Gastric decompression** – the first thing to do is to decompress the stomach by attempting to pass a stomach tube to relieve the pressure in the stomach. In the majority of cases this will be unsuccessful as the distension is too high. A 16-G catheter can be placed and the stylet removed in order to release some of the gas and reduce the pressure on the torsed stomach.

- Introduce the needle into the right flank wall just behind the ribs. This will pierce the stomach and allow pent-up gas to escape. The stomach tube may then be passed and gastric lavage performed. The tube should be measured against the animal in order to determine the correct length and then gently passed through the oropharynx. If it will enter the stomach, then the stomach contents can be evacuated and the stomach can be flushed with warm water (gastric lavage).
- **Treat shock** – these patients are in shock, so intravenous fluids will be needed to restore the circulating blood pressure. This is the priority in these patients and the animal will require shock rate fluids before any gastric decompression is initiated. As these are normally large-breed dogs, two peripheral cannulas are usually required in order to gain the fluid rate requirements.

Surgery – in cases where dilation is the main symptom, passing the stomach tube may be sufficient initial treatment, after which the animal should be monitored. Cases involving a torsion will require surgery to relieve the torsion and reposition the organs. This should only be undertaken once the patient has been stabilised through gastric decompression and fluid therapy, and the symptoms of shock have been reduced. In some cases, when the stomach rotates, the spleen is taken with it and a **splenectomy** may also be needed, especially if the spleen has been caught in the twist for any length of time. In these cases the spleen must not be 'untwisted' prior to surgery, and simply removed. Resolving the twist to the spleen prior to removal releases micro-thrombi and toxins into the bloodstream. Surgery to create a **gastropexy** should be performed in all cases, but the timing can be delayed in cases that have been stabilised by decompression alone. In this procedure the stomach is sutured to the abdominal wall to prevent recurrence. Without this, there is a high chance of recurrence.

Postoperative care. Intravenous fluids and pain relief are needed initially, and patients are fed as soon as possible after surgery, with a highly digestible diet, little and often.

Close monitoring of these patients is essential, especially in the first 48 hours, as toxins trapped in the blood supply of the stomach are released into the circulation as the stomach is untwisted. It is possible for animals apparently doing well after surgery to suddenly relapse and die from endotoxic shock, so the prognosis should still be considered guarded. Blood pressure should be monitored throughout the postoperative period, alongside measurement of the dog's abdomen and thorax. This will help to gauge whether the dog is re-bloating.

Long-term management of these patients involves looking at their normal feeding and exercise regimens. Studies have found that patients have a reduced risk of dilation and torsion if they are fed three to four times a day rather than once a day. Owners should also exercise their animals before feeding, and avoid other stressors which have been implicated as a potential causal factor in GDV cases.

Enterotomy and enterectomy

- **Enterotomy** – a surgical technique involving the opening up of the intestine
- **Enterectomy** – the removal of a length of intestine.

These techniques may be used as treatment in the following conditions:

Foreign bodies. The clinical signs seen with intestinal foreign bodies vary but in most cases the animals vomit, have abdominal pain and become depressed and anorexic, leading to dehydration and shock. To treat these cases an enterotomy is usually carried out.

An incision is made in the wall of the intestine, the object is removed and the incision is closed immediately. Omentum or mesentery may be sutured over the point of entry to reduce the risk of leakage. If, however, the intestine is badly damaged, an enterectomy may be carried out. The damaged portion is removed and the two cut ends of the intestine are sutured together. This is referred to as an **end-to-end anastomosis**.

Intussusception. This describes the telescoping of a piece of intestine inside itself. It is most often seen in young animals, especially if they have had diarrhoea, as the peristaltic contractions are exaggerated compared with usual movements.

Clinically, the animals are subdued, with a depressed appetite. They may try to vomit or may pass small amounts of diarrhoea and on examination the intussusception may be palpable within the abdomen.

Management usually requires a laparotomy to reveal the extent of the problem. In mild cases, it may be possible for the intussusception to be reduced by simply teasing the intestine apart. If the blood supply has been severely compromised, an enterectomy will be needed.

Postoperative care. All animals undergoing intestinal surgery should be carefully monitored postoperatively, and analgesia provided – no NSAIDs. Water and food can be offered as soon as possible in these cases; an easily digestible diet, offered little and often, is favourable. Close monitoring of patient temperature is recommended as hypothermia is a concern in any small patient, and animals that have had long surgery with the abdomen open will also have potentially lost considerable amounts of body heat.

If the patient does not improve after the first couple of days, it should be checked thoroughly again, as the possibility of wound dehiscence cannot be ignored.

Rectum and anus

Surgery to the rectal and anal areas may be indicated for a number of reasons, including perineal hernias, as well as those detailed here:

Neoplasia and polyps. Growths within the colon are quite common and may cause problems with defecation. The owners may simply notice that the animal is having difficulty passing faeces (**dyschezia**) or is straining more than usual (**tenesmus**). There may also be fresh blood on the faeces.

To investigate problems in the terminal alimentary canal, proctoscopy is the most useful technique as it allows direct visualisation of the rectum. Digital palpation of the rectum can also be useful, and plain radiographs and contrast studies may also be used.

Some tumours and polyps are amenable to surgery and simple excision may be possible. Other cases require more radical surgery, in which the terminal part of the colon and rectum is removed. In all cases, postoperative care involves ensuring that the animal is able to pass faeces relatively comfortably, so the use of mild laxatives or hydrophilic compounds given orally may assist in keeping the faeces soft. Most importantly is using a diet that has a low residue, to reduce the volume of faeces that is being passed.

Anal furunculosis. A deep pyoderma develops in the perianal tissues and is characterised by the formation of deep sinus tracts. It is most often seen in German shepherd dogs, especially those with a low tail carriage. Anal furunculosis is a very painful condition and appropriate analgesia will be required.

Clinical signs. These animals are in considerable pain and consequently show dyschezia, faecal tenesmus and anal irritation.

Treatment. A number of different treatments have been tried. Medical treatments are usually used first, using immuno-suppressive drugs such as cyclosporin or topical tacrolimus, and some cases respond well to this. Others still require surgery during which the sinus tracts are fully debrided, leaving open wounds that are left to heal by second intention. If surgery is carried out, the anal sacs are normally removed at the same time.

Postoperative care. The wounds should be kept clean by gentle washing of the area with warmed saline or Hartmann's solution. Antibiotics are also needed to reduce the risk of further infection, and the patient must be closely monitored to ensure that it is able to defecate normally. Cases that require surgery carry a worse prognosis than those that can be managed by medical treatments alone, so clients will need appropriate advice about this.

Impaction and infection of the anal sacs. Impaction of the anal sacs is common, leading to anal irritation seen as bottom-rubbing, 'scooting' and biting at the rear end. Simple impaction can be managed by manual expression. If the impaction becomes frequent or abscesses develop, the sacs should be removed by surgical excision.

Treatment. Prior to surgery the anal area must be prepared. The anal sacs should be evacuated fully and then flushed or cleaned. The perianal area should be clipped up and prepared for surgery. Some surgeons may fill the sacs with anal sac gel or wax to aid their location during removal, but there is a very small risk that this material may leak into the surrounding tissues, leading to chronic reactions. Others may simply use a probe in the duct to help locate the sac. To prevent faecal contamination of the operation site, some veterinary surgeons use a purse-string suture around the anus, or a cotton wool plug. If this method is used, it should be noted, so that it can be removed at the end of the operation.

Postoperative care. Keep the area clean and ensure that the animal is able to pass faeces. Antibiotic cover is needed. Note that in some cases there is temporary faecal incontinence due to bruising of the anal sphincter tissues but this should settle down with time. A low-residue diet should be fed postoperatively for a period.

REPRODUCTIVE TRACT

The most common elective surgery carried out in practice is the neutering of pets. This surgery, while considered 'routine', is not risk free and it is always worth reminding owners of this when discussing the procedure. If appropriate care is taken then the risks are small, and we should encourage owners to be responsible and not breed animals indiscriminately.

Ovariohysterectomy (spay)

In most cases animals are spayed in order to control oestrous cycles and to prevent unwanted litters. In addition, an ovariohysterectomy may be carried out to prevent an animal developing mammary tumours, to treat a pyometra or to manage an animal that has recurrent false pregnancies.

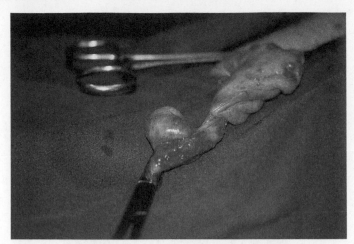

Fig. 23.4 Exteriorised ovary and uterine horn during a bitch spay

The timing of the surgery in the bitch is quite important and she can either be spayed prior to her first oestrus or during anoestrus – usually 2–4 months after the bitch has been in season or 6–8 weeks after giving birth.

The queen, during the breeding season, comes into oestrus every 3 weeks and it may be difficult to find a time when she is not in season. As a result, a veterinary surgeon will usually perform the operation any time after the onset of sexual maturity at around 5 months of age, though both cats and dogs can be neutered from 10 weeks of age, and some animal charities will neuter around this age.

Surgery. In the bitch, surgery is usually carried out via a midline linea alba incision, whereas in the queen it is more usually done through a sublumbar incision in the left flank. In both cases the ovaries, uterine horns and uterine body are removed (Fig. 23.4).

As the surgeon exteriorises the ovary, this can cause more pain, and the animal will breathe more erratically. Knowledge of the surgical procedure and when to plan for more painful elements of the procedure can ensure that the anaesthetic levels are maintained at an appropriate level to ensure that this does not occur.

More recently laparoscopic techniques are being used for a number of surgical procedures, including ovariectomy, where only the ovaries are removed providing that the uterus is healthy. This has been used in human surgery for quite a while, and is now becoming much more widespread in veterinary practice.

Postoperative care. The animal should be kept quiet for the first couple of days and, in the case of a bitch, restricted to lead exercise only until 10 days after surgery – this would have been when the sutures would have been removed, but it is now a rarity for veterinary surgeons to close with skin sutures that require removal; subcutaneous sutures are now the norm. Cats should be kept indoors until the wound has started to heal properly. If there is any interference with the sutures or any seepage from the wound, the animal should be brought back to the surgery for examination. Advice should be given about monitoring the patient's weight, as some animals will have a greater tendency to gain weight after ovariohysterectomy. With appropriate nutrition and exercise this should not be a problem.

Complications. These include the risk of haemorrhage from either the ovarian or uterine vessels. Internal haemorrhage may be recognised by pallor of the mucous membranes, rapid heart rate, increased respiratory rate and lethargy, possibly combined with abdominal swelling or leakage from the operation site. These animals should be checked carefully by a veterinary surgeon, as surgical intervention may be necessary in some cases. In others the use of a compression bandage to increase back-pressure may be sufficient.

Coat may change in texture and become coarser. This seems to be particularly true for certain breeds such as cocker spaniels and retrievers.

Hysterotomy (Caesarean section)

There are a number of reasons why a Caesarean section may be needed in a pregnant animal. These include:

- Primary or secondary uterine inertia
- Foetal oversize or a foetal monster
- Foetal malpresentation that cannot be reduced
- Obstructions of the birth canal such as pelvic deformities or vaginal polyps
- Neglected dystocias, especially if the foetal fluids have already been lost or a foetus has already died
- Elective reasons, particularly if the animal has had a history of problems previously, or is a breed that is prone to dystocia.

In all cases the aim of the surgery is to remove the young from the uterus to ensure that as many as possible survive, including the mother.

Preparation. Both the dam and her neonates must be considered, ensuring that suitable facilities are available to support all their needs. Additional nursing staff will be required and provisions must be made to attempt to call extra staff in, if on a shift where there are limited staffing numbers, particularly if a number of young are predicted and may require resuscitation. Towels should be at the ready and somewhere warm ready for the young to recover in – an incubator or a box containing a covered hot-water bottle may be suitable.

Surgery. The anaesthetic regimen should be chosen so that it has minimum effect on the respiration and cardiovascular function of the neonates. The mother needs to be pre-oxygenated, and this can occur while she is having an initial skin preparation. Rapidly acting induction agents such as propofol or alfaxolone are usually used without any premedicant. Once the neonates are removed, they should be stimulated to breathe by rubbing vigorously with a towel and clearing any mucus from the oral cavity. Doxapram may be necessary to stimulate respiration of any individuals that are reluctant to breathe.

Postoperative care. As soon as the dam has recovered from the anaesthetic, the young should be placed with her and watched closely to ensure that they are allowed to feed. It is essential that they receive the colostrum needed to provide them with both energy and antibodies. The dam may be reluctant to take the neonates initially but in most cases she can be persuaded to look after them. In very rare instances the young require hand-rearing or fostering because of maternal rejection.

Orchidectomy (castration)

Castration involves the surgical removal of both testes and ligation of the deferent duct on each side. It is often a more straightforward procedure than spaying, as the testes are more accessible. Retained testes should always be removed, and these can prove more difficult to find within the abdominal cavity. Some owners think that castration in animals is simply a vasectomy, in which the deferent duct is ligated and transected but the testes are left in place. This should be clarified with the owner before the surgery is carried out.

The indications for castration are varied. It may be to prevent breeding or roaming, or to prevent male behaviour traits such as spraying in tomcats that are driven by testosterone. Those behaviours that are not linked to hormones produced by the testes will not be affected, e.g. hyperactivity. It will also prevent the development of testicular tumours (particularly important if the testes are retained) and reduce the risk of prostate problems and anal adenomas.

Surgery. The procedure is slightly different in different species:

- Dogs – the incision is usually made just in front of the scrotum and the testes are each removed through this incision before it is closed.
- Cat – incisions are made through each scrotal sac to reach the testis on each side and these are usually left open.
- Rabbits – have particularly large inguinal rings and are able to retract their testes (often seen when clipping up the site in preparation for surgery). This also means that when the testes are removed, there is a greater chance of inguinal hernias, so many veterinary surgeons reduce the size of the inguinal ring or take other measures to reduce the risk of this occurring postoperatively.

Castration can be carried out using either a closed or an open technique. In **closed** castrations, the tunica vaginalis is not cut to expose the testes: the testes and covering are dissected away from the overlying skin and the whole spermatic cord is ligated and transected. **Open** castrations allow visualisation of the individual testicular vessels and these may then be ligated separately from the deferent duct. In both methods the tunica vaginalis is cut during the surgery. This tissue is simply an extension of the peritoneum, meaning that the procedure actually involves entry into a body cavity and should not be carried out by anyone other than a veterinary surgeon.

Postoperative care. The animal should be monitored for signs of haemorrhage or swelling at the operation site. Dogs and cats should be discouraged from licking, as this can cause complications, and it may be necessary to use an Elizabethan collar to prevent this. Since cats do not have any external sutures they may not need to return to the surgery, but most other species will require suture removal after about 10 days (though most practices now utilise subcutaneous sutures and tissue glue). A postoperative check should be recommended.

URINARY TRACT

Bladder

Cystotomy. Surgery on the bladder is quite common, e.g. to remove calculi (that cannot be medically managed), bladder tumours or to repair a ruptured bladder (Figs. 23.5–23.7).

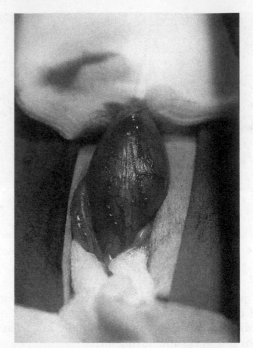

Fig. 23.5 Exteriorising the bladder and packing it off from the abdomen

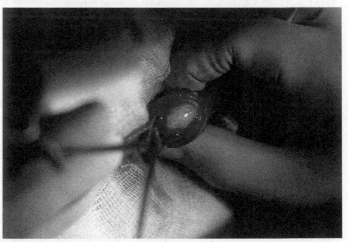

Fig. 23.6 Careful removal of urinary calculi from the bladder

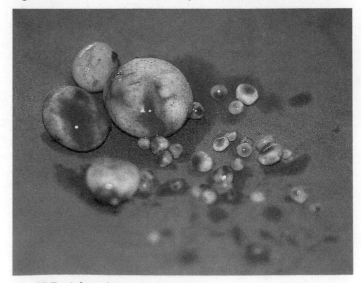

Fig. 23.7 A few of the calculi removed

Animals with calculi or tumours may not be particularly ill but may have shown signs of urinary tenesmus or haematuria that alerted their owners to the problem. Animals with ruptured bladders are more likely to have been involved in some kind of trauma and, unless the bladder is repaired quickly, the animal will rapidly become uraemic as the urea is reabsorbed via the peritoneum from the urine within the peritoneal cavity. It also will develop peritonitis unless the abdomen is lavaged thoroughly and quickly. Left untreated, both uraemia and peritonitis can be fatal.

Surgery. The bladder is usually approached via a ventral midline incision and should then be exteriorised and packed off from the rest of the abdomen with swabs to minimise the risk of contamination (see Fig. 23.5). If there is any spillage of urine or the bladder has already ruptured, the abdomen should be flushed thoroughly with a warmed sterile balanced electrolyte solution.

Postoperative care. Monitoring urine output is essential, and this can be easily achieved when a urinary catheter has been placed with a closed urine collection system. Trauma cases may need catheterisation initially; once the catheter is removed, observations need to be made on the ease of urination. All surgical cases require placement on intravenous fluids, but in these cases it is essential that fluids are maintained so that good urine output is achieved, and to help support renal function if there has been impairment.

Urinary catheters should be managed aseptically and connected to a closed collection system. The urine collected should be measured to ensure sufficient production and tested for evidence of infection; only culture of urine can give correct results for any urinary infection. Microscopic examination can provide false positives and false negatives. Antibiotics should be administered on evidence of culture growth and sensitivity results.

Urethra

Urethrotomy – creation of a temporary opening in the urethra

Urethrostomy – creation of a permanent opening in the urethra

Urethral obstruction. The most common surgical condition involving the urethra is urethral obstruction often caused by urinary calculi which have formed in the bladder, and then passed down the urethra where they have become stuck. This is seen predominantly in the male animal, where the urethra is much narrower than in the female. Signs of obstruction include urinary tenesmus, haematuria, lethargy and abdominal discomfort.

Treatment. Patients should be placed on intravenous fluids and anaesthetised to allow catheterisation of the urethra and flushing (hydropulsion) to dislodge the calculi. This is a painful procedure in most cases, so anaesthesia is required.

If the catheter cannot be passed, then decompression of the bladder can be achieved by means of a needle placed through the abdominal and bladder walls (cystocentesis). This will allow sampling of the urine, and it may then be possible to catheterise the patient after the pressure has been reduced.

If this has been successful, the animal is usually hospitalised and started on dietary management before returning home. Dietary dissolution is the treatment of choice in all cases. Radiography is required in all situations for all patients and must include the whole of the urinary tract, from kidneys through to the tip of the penis or vulva.

Surgery. If the condition recurs or the blockage cannot be removed, a urethrotomy or permanent urethrostomy is needed. The urethrotomy involves simply entering the urethra surgically, removing the obstruction and closing the wound. Postoperative strictures are quite common, so this procedure is not done very frequently and it is more usual for surgeons to decide to leave a permanent opening or urethrostomy.

In the dog, obstruction usually occurs at the base of the os penis, and a scrotal urethrostomy is the recommended procedure. For this technique castration and scrotal ablation are essential.

In the cat obstruction is usually higher and a high urethrostomy is needed where the incision is made in the perineal area. In the cat the distal penis is amputated at the same time.

Urethrostomy procedures are not undertaken lightly as there are risks of complications, so owners should be given careful advice about this.

Postoperative care. Most cases are hospitalised for several days after surgery to allow close monitoring, since it is essential that the animal is able to pass urine freely. An indwelling catheter is usually left in place during the early stages connected to a closed collection system. This allows urine to be passed easily and also ensures that the operation site does not contract down too much, preventing the urethrostomy site from working adequately. It is also important that the animal is given fluids or encouraged to drink in order to stimulate diuresis in the patient and prevent the recurrence of any calculi. An Elizabethan collar may be needed to prevent interference with the wound once the catheter is removed, particularly as the animal may feel urine dribbling from the site and wish to clean the area. It will take some training, particularly in dogs, for them to get used to the fact that urine emerges from a different site and owners may need to use protective barrier spray or cream around the area to prevent urine scald and keep the area clean.

With cats, shredded paper should be used instead of cat litter in the litter tray to avoid litter becoming stuck to the surgical wound and causing discomfort.

Any calculi removed should be sent for analysis, so that appropriate dietary management can be introduced to prevent recurrence. Any sutures that are placed within the urinary tract will act as a focal point or nidus for further calculi formation, which will occur more quickly as there is now a nidus to form around, thus making nutritional management even more important.

RESPIRATORY TRACT

Tracheostomy

This is the creation of an opening in the wall of the trachea. In most cases with respiratory distress an airway can be established using other techniques, but occasionally an emergency tracheotomy (creation of a temporary opening) or tracheostomy (creation of a permanent opening) has to be performed.

Technique. 1. The animal is restrained in dorsal recumbency with its neck extended over a sandbag, and the area clipped and prepared for surgical incision.

2. A small incision is made in the ventral midline of the neck. The best area is over the 5th and 6th tracheal rings since this is away from both the larynx and

the thoracic inlet and so there is least risk of the tracheostomy site being obstructed through normal neck movements.

3. Under the skin are paired longitudinal neck muscles that must be separated by blunt dissection, so that a cut can be made between the tracheal rings (about one-third of the way round the trachea).
4. Two stay sutures are placed in the rings adjacent to the tracheostomy site, in order to facilitate placement of the tube.
5. The tube should be measured at 50–60% of the tracheal circumference, then inserted and secured in place.

Care of the tracheostomy. The inner tube must be cleaned at least every 2 hours as it quickly becomes blocked with mucus. The best types of tubes have a separate inner sleeve that can be removed for cleaning. It should be cleaned just using warm water, dried and replaced.

Normally when patients breathe, the air is warmed and humidified as it passes through the nasal chambers and turbinates. The placement of a tracheostomy tube means that the air is cold and dry by comparison so this aggravates the inflammatory response already caused by the placement of the tube. Nebulisation is therefore needed, and transfer of the patient to a specialist facility may be required if the initial practice does not have these facilities or 24-hour nursing care.

It is also possible to use suction to help maintain the tube, but this may be stressful for the animal and cause it to panic, so should only be done when necessary. Pre- and post-oxygenation are required to avoid causing hypoxia.

Animals with tracheostomy tubes are critical care patients, and emergency equipment should be placed close to hand in case it is needed. These patients should be monitored regularly around the clock.

Pneumothorax

This is the presence of air within the pleural cavity. A pneumothorax may be due to a number of causes, including trauma or following surgery, e.g. for ruptured diaphragm. Whatever the cause, the aim of treatment is to encourage the correct inflation of the lung on the affected side so that full aeration of the lungs can take place again.

If the pneumothorax is small it may be managed conservatively. Air is gradually reabsorbed from the pleural cavity and the lung should eventually ventilate appropriately. This takes time and the animal's colour and respiratory function (including oxygen saturation) should be monitored closely during its recovery.

In more serious cases, it may be necessary for the air to be removed. This can be done with the patient conscious if it is suffering severe respiratory problems, but it is preferable for the animal to be under sedation, such as midazolam and ketamine combinations as these do not affect respiratory function (see Chapter 27), particularly if a drain is to be placed. Air can be removed in one of two ways:

- Butterfly needle or over-the-needle catheter and three-way tap attached to a syringe – this is the simplest technique and the air is removed by suction. The needle cannot be left in place and the technique is usually used when it is likely that the procedure will only be carried out once.
- Place a chest drain – between the ribs, usually at the level of the 7th or 8th intercostal space. The drain should actually emerge from the skin further caudally reducing the risk of air leakage around the drain. The drain should be connected to a gate clamp and three-way tap or a Heimlich valve so that air is unable to get back into the thoracic cavity. Air is removed by continuous or intermittent suction.

During treatment the animal will require supplementary oxygen. For small patients, oxygen can be pumped into incubators to provide an oxygen-rich environment, or a kennel may be adapted using plastic sheeting over the front. Other methods of oxygen administration include via a mask, though many patients do not tolerate this well, or via a nasal catheter. Close monitoring will be essential to check that the animal's colour, temperature, pulse and respiration all gradually return to normal as the lung regains its function.

Thoracotomy

This is entry into the chest via the thoracic wall and it may be required for several reasons, e.g. an oesophageal foreign body, repair of a cardiac condition such as patent ductus arteriosus or persistent right aortic arch, or lung surgery.

Thoracotomy is usually performed with the animal in lateral recumbency. The incision is made through an intercostal space and the ribs are then retracted using a self-retaining retractor (see Chapter 24). In some referral centres a median sternotomy ('sternal split') is carried out. For this procedure, the animal is positioned in dorsal recumbency and access to the thorax is via a midline incision through the middle of the sternum. With this technique the sternum must be repaired postoperatively using stainless steel wires, whereas with the other method no bones are actually cut or damaged. Splitting the sternum provides better access to the thoracic cavity for major surgery but is a very painful procedure, so pain management will be key in the perioperative period.

After completion, the thoracic cavity must be properly sealed and any air or fluid in the chest drawn off. This can either be done using a chest drain attached to a three-way tap and syringe, or other suction device. Postoperative monitoring is essential – not only basics such as checking temperature, pulse, respiration and colour regularly, but also due to the nature of the surgery oxygen saturation levels and blood pressure. Analgesics, including local anaesthetic blocks, will also be needed as well as appropriate antibiotic treatment depending on the type of procedure performed.

MUSCULOSKELETAL SYSTEM

Fractures

Fractures are a relatively common occurrence in small animal practice, and a good understanding of the types and management of different fractures is important when nursing trauma patients.

Types of fracture. Fractures can be classified in a number of different ways (Table 23.5).

Clinical signs of fractures. In most cases the clinical signs of a fracture are similar. The animal shows signs of pain, there may be swelling or deformity at the site and on palpation there may

TABLE 23.5	Fracture types	
Method of classification	**Type of fracture**	**Description**
Direction and location of the fracture line	Transverse	The fracture is at right angles to the long axis of the bone
	Longitudinal	The fracture is parallel to the long axis of the bone
	Oblique	The fracture is diagonal to the long axis of the bone
	Spiral	The fracture line spirals around the long axis of the bone
Extent of fracture damage	Complete	The bone is completely broken into two or more fragments
	Incomplete (greenstick)	The cortex is broken, but the periosteum remains intact on one side of the bone
	Fissure	There is a crack in the cortex, but no displacement of any fragments
Extent of soft-tissue damage	Closed	There is no wound over the surface of the fractured bone
	Open	There is a wound over the fracture site, such that the fracture is open to the environment
	Complicated	There is damage to other important tissues as well as the bone, such as nerves or major blood vessels
Number of fracture lines	Comminuted	There is one fracture site, but more than two fragments are produced
	Multiple	There is more than one fracture site and several fragments are produced
Position of the bone fragments	Depressed	The fracture fragments are pushed inwards to reduce the size of a cavity
	Over-riding	The two fracture fragments slide over each other to result in shortening of the area
	Impacted	The two fracture fragments are driven into each other to result in shortening of the area
	Distracted	The two fracture fragments are pulled apart by muscle activity
Position of the fracture	Avulsion	A fracture at the site of insertion of a tendon
	Physeal	A fracture through a growth plate
	Condylar	A fracture in which a condyle of a bone is separated from the rest of the bone
	Intercondylar	A Y-shaped fracture which involves two condyles being separated and fractured
Stability of the fracture	Stable	There is little tendency of the fracture fragments to move relative to each other
	Unstable	The fracture fragments are quite free to move relative to each other

also be crepitus (grating of the fracture fragments against each other). As a result, the animal will not be able to use the affected area normally.

First-aid treatment. It is rare that fractures are a priority in first-aid management; therefore basic checks should cover the whole animal and ensure that there is nothing life threatening that requires attention before the fracture itself is treated (see Chapter 20).

The following protocol should always be carried out:
- Check the animal's ABCs – airway, breathing and circulation.
- Control any haemorrhage and treat shock with intravenous fluids, oxygen and warmth.
- Analgesics and antibiotics should be given in accordance with the veterinary surgeon's instructions.

Only once the animal has been checked and supportive treatment given should the fracture be treated.

The aim of first-aid management of fractures is to minimise the movement of the fracture fragments so the bone should be handled as little as possible. In unconscious patients it may be appropriate to provide support for the fracture using either support bandages or splints. Most conscious patients protect fracture sites by holding them in the way that hurts the least. Attempting to bandage these might make the situation worse, particularly if the animal struggles.

Fracture repair. There are three basic principles that are often followed in fracture repair:
- Reduce the fracture – i.e. bring the fragments back together.
- Align the fragments – ensure that the contours of the bones fit.
- Immobilise the fragments.

Of these, the most important is that the fragments are immobilised. This will allow initial bone healing to occur more rapidly, and the patient is able to return to mobility sooner. This in turn promotes the gradual increase in strength of the healed fracture site.

There are different approaches to individual cases, and the type and location of the fracture can make a significant difference as to which method of repair or treatment is chosen.

Note that in all cases the patient is likely to take reduced exercise, so it is important that its diet is considered. The healing process requires the provision of a good-quality diet but enforced inactivity reduces the energy requirement.

Conservative treatment. This is the simplest option in which no actual surgery or fixation is carried out. The animal is confined so that movement of the affected area is restricted and bone healing will take place. This can be used for stable fractures where there is unlikely to be movement of the fracture fragments, e.g. some pelvic fractures, scapular fractures and impacted fractures. Careful rehabilitation may be needed after the cage rest period to allow the fracture site to strengthen, and this may mean that the total convalescent time is longer than if some type of surgical treatment had been carried out (see Chapter 18).

External fixation. Available methods include casts and splints. They provide a cheap method of fracture repair and have the advantage of being relatively easy to apply and do not run the risk of introducing infection into the fracture. These methods are only suitable for a limited number of fractures, i.e. only fractures that are stable and distal to the elbow or stifle. Note that this technique should not be used for fractures of the distal radius and ulna as evidence has shown that there is a high failure rate for fractures of this region using casts.

Casting materials are often based on polyurethane resin embedded on some type of bandage, are activated by

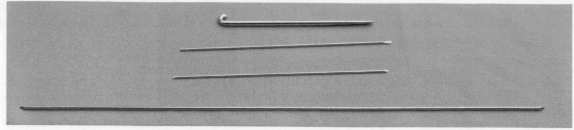

Fig. 23.8A Top to bottom: Rush pin, Kirschner wire, arthrodesis wire, Steinmann pin

immersion in warm or hot water, set within approximately 10 minutes and are fully weight bearing after about 30 minutes. They are radiolucent, so follow-up radiography can be carried out without actually removing the cast. The cast will require adequate padding as the casting material can be an irritant. Gloves must be worn during its application. Casts should be applied so that the pads and claws of the central digits can still be seen, as this helps both monitor the limb itself and helps patient tolerance of the cast. These casting materials can also be used to make bespoke splints for the limb, which can be reused at each dressing change. These are advantageous over general purpose splints as they will exactly fit the limb.

Aftercare of casts and splints is also important. Casts must not be allowed to get wet and must be regularly checked for sores. Cotton wool underneath casts may bunch up into hard lumps, whereas synthetic orthopaedic wool does not tend to do this and dries more easily should the animal start to sweat under the bandaging. The patient must be prevented from interfering with the cast and kept on minimal exercise (see previous section on bandage care).

There is a danger that the cast may loosen as the muscle atrophies through disuse, so regular check-ups must be made. Sometimes casts need to be replaced during the time the fracture is healing and sedation or anaesthesia will be required to replace them. As a result this treatment method can be more expensive than originally thought. 'Fracture disease' can also be a complication, in which tissues, including the bone, become weaker rather than stronger as a result of prolonged immobilisation. Used appropriately on the right kinds of fractures, casts and splints can work very well.

Internal fixation. A wider range of fractures can be treated using internal fixation techniques and, as the fixation is stable, normal activity can resume more quickly. The fixation device cannot be touched by the animal, so interference should be minimal. Aftercare is also reduced, providing that the surgery has been performed well.

There are some potential problems:

- In most cases open reduction is required, which increases the risk of infection and soft-tissue damage, particularly if the surgeon is inexperienced.
- The initial cost is higher and greater skill is required to perform the procedures well.
- It is possible that the implants may move after they are positioned.
- The animal may develop a reaction leading to hygroma formation (a fluid-filled 'blister' over the implant).

In most cases internal fixation provides good bone healing and can provide the equivalent of primary wound healing in soft tissues.

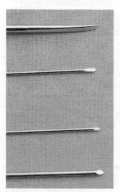

Fig. 23.8B The same pins as Fig. 23.8A – tips close up

TABLE 23.6	Orthopaedic pins
Type of pin	**Description**
Steinmann pin (see Fig. 23.8)	May have a trocar point on one or both ends
Kirschner drill wire (also referred to as K-wires; see Fig. 23.8)	Small, thin pins with a flattened spatulated end
Arthodesis wire (see Fig. 23.8)	Smaller versions of the Steinmann pin, designed to be used across joints
Rush pin (see Fig. 23.8)	The Rush pin has a pointed 'sledge-runner' tip at one end and a hook at the other; these can be used in pairs for physeal fractures, since they do not interfere with the growth of the long bone, but arthrodesis wires are now used more commonly

Types of orthopaedic implant. There are a number of different types of implant that can be used to repair fractures:

Intramedullary pins. These are metal rods inserted into the medullary cavity of a bone to immobilise a fracture (Fig. 23.8). Providing that it is the right type of fracture and the pin fits snugly in the medullary cavity, a pin can be very effective. A pin will cause problems if it is loose or used incorrectly. Several different types of pin are used in practice (Table 23.6).

Screws. These can be used as the sole method for fracture repair or can be used in conjunction with other techniques such as plates or wires. Used alone, they can be placed using a lag screw technique providing compression across the fracture site. Surgeons may also use some kind of splint or external support in these cases.

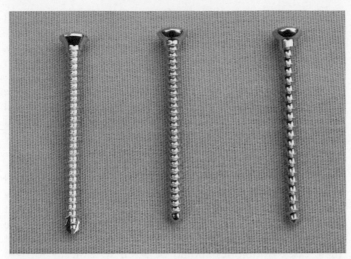

Fig. 23.9A Left to right: traditional screw, ASIF cortical screw, ASIF cancellous screw

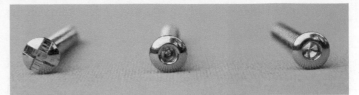

Fig. 23.9B Left to right: close-up of heads of traditional screw, ASIF cortical screw, ASIF cancellous screw

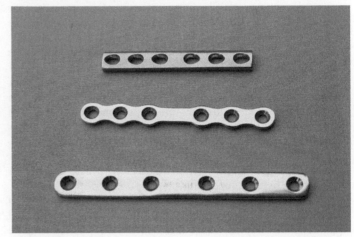

Fig. 23.10 Top to bottom: dynamic compression plate, Sherman plate, Venables plate

A number of different types of screw are currently used, and physically these can be classified in a number of ways:

- **Size** – This refers to the width of the screw including the thread.
- **Cancellous or cortical** – This describes the type of bone in which they are used. Cortical screws have a wider shaft and smaller thread pitch (the distance between each turn of the thread) than cancellous screws. The wider thread and deeper thread pitch of cancellous screws allows them to get a better hold in the loose structure of cancellous bone. Cortical screws are usually fully threaded, whereas cancellous screws may be fully or partially threaded.
- **Standard or locking** – Standard screws are simple screws where the shaft is the only part that is threaded. Locking screws have a thread on the head of the screw, and are designed to fit into a thread in the hole of a locking plate. These are being used extensively in human orthopaedics, and are now being used in veterinary practice for some specialist procedures. Locking screws have a star drive fitting, so use a different driver than other screws.
- **Self-tapping or non–self-tapping** – Self-tapping screws are designed so that they can be screwed directly into bone after a pilot hole has been drilled. As they are screwed in place they cut their own path. Non–self-tapping screws need the path to be cut first with the use of a separate instrument called a tap. Traditional self-tapping screws usually have a head that requires the use of a flat-bladed screwdriver, whereas the AO/ASIF (Arbeitsgemeinschaft fur Osteosynthesefragen; English – Association for the Study of Internal Fixation) screws have a hex fitting.
- **Cannulated or not** – Cannulated screws are similar in appearance to the standard AO/ASIF screws with a hex fitting, but have a hole through the centre of the screw, which allows it to be placed accurately over a guide wire.

Three of the common screws found in most general practices are shown in Figure 23.9.

All implants are available in a range of sizes and lengths, and it is important that a check is made prior to starting any surgical procedure to ensure that all the possible equipment the surgeon might require is available.

Orthopaedic wire. This is usually made of monofilament stainless steel. It is used around fracture fragments and the ends of the wire are then twisted together evenly, which brings the fragments closer together.

Bone plates. Bone plates are available in a number of different designs. Traditional plates are used with self-tapping screws. The two most commonly used are the Sherman plate and the Venables plate (Fig. 23.10).

More modern plates include the AO/ASIF plates (Fig. 23.10). The main plate in this system is the dynamic compression plate or DCP. This is available in several sizes and the holes are shaped such that the screws can be placed either in a neutral position or a loaded position. With appropriate placement of the screws, compression across the fracture site is achieved as the screws are tightened.

Postoperative care. The operation site should be checked regularly for any signs of swelling or discharge. Analgesics are usually needed in the initial postoperative period but as the animal starts to recover, review on a case-by-case basis needs to be made by the veterinary surgeon regarding requirement of analgesics. Limited exercise is essential for the first few weeks – for dogs lead exercise 2–3 times a day for 10–15 minutes each time is advocated, and for cats, restricting them to a large cage with occasional supervised excursions may be appropriate. Running and jumping in the early stages of healing should certainly be avoided, and stairs should certainly be out of bounds. Exercise can be gradually increased under the veterinary surgeon's direction as the patient improves. Generally, fractures take between 4 and 6 weeks to heal depending on the factors listed later.

External fixator (Kirschner-Ehmer device). The external fixator is useful in a number of situations where other methods of fracture fixation are not appropriate, e.g. open or infected fractures, since the pins can be placed away from the actual fracture site so that there is no implant device actually at the wound site. Access to the fracture site is also good and for infected sites this can aid treatment and recovery.

The device can also be used in cases of comminuted or unstable fractures, since the external bars of the fixator are able to take the animal's weight and hold the fracture fragments apart, preventing them from collapsing inwards. The fracture heals in the same way as a wound with tissue loss, i.e. by second intention. External fixation may also be used on a range of species. Avian fractures on both limbs and wings have been successfully managed this way and it also lends itself to use in other regions of the body such as pelvic fractures or mandibular fractures. In all cases it is essential that the surgeon has an accurate knowledge of the anatomy of the area so that the pins do not impinge on any vital structures. With care this repair method can be very successful.

The appearance of the device can be quite off-putting to start with but usually, with help from the practice, owners will appreciate the way in which the device works. There may be some discharge from the pin sites and these should be checked regularly to ensure that they are not becoming infected. Rods and clamps should be covered with protective bandage material to prevent any trauma from the metal, either to the animal or the owner.

Once bone healing is complete, the rods and pins are all removed under general anaesthesia. The pin entry wounds are left to heal by second intention and usually heal very quickly.

Fracture healing. Fracture healing, like wound healing, is affected by a number of different factors. These include factors specific to the injury, such as the stability of the fracture, the proximity of the fragment, the type of fracture and its location and blood supply. More general factors relating to the overall health of the animal, such as its age and species, also have an effect. Many exotic species, including birds, heal more quickly than cats and dogs, although with reptiles healing may take considerably longer.

Complications of fracture healing. Unfortunately, not all fractures heal smoothly, and it is important to be aware of the potential problems, so that the risks can be minimised or problems spotted early so that remedial action can be taken:

- Fracture disease – the bone weakens as the repair device takes the weight. Gradually muscle atrophy, osteoporosis, joint stiffness and tissue adhesions develop. It may even result in a non-union.
- Malunion – healing takes place but the alignment of the bones is altered from normal. Functionally this can have quite serious effects on the animal depending on the site of the fracture.
- Delayed union – the bone fails to heal within the expected normal time. This is usually due to the presence of a gap at the fracture site that takes longer to bridge. Occasionally the fracture does not heal at all, producing a non-union. In some cases bone chips, bone matrix, Nano-paste and bone granules can all be utilised to help with healing.
- Non-union – the bone fragments fail to heal properly. In some cases a fibrous connection may develop between the bones but in others there is no healing at all.
- Osteomyelitis – inflammation of the bone and bone marrow. It is usually the result of infection introduced at the time of surgery. It may be an uncontrolled virulent infection, or it may be more localised and controlled.

Treatment of osteomyelitis – first local drainage must be established, and all dead or necrotic tissue including soft tissue and bone should be debrided. Foreign materials, including any implants or sutures, must also be removed. This may mean that the original repair device has to be replaced with an alternative one. External fixators have been used with success in some of these cases. Antibiotics should be given systemically for 4–6 weeks based on culture and sensitivity tests on the bacteria found at the site.

Luxations and subluxations

- **Luxation or dislocation** – the persistent displacement of bones forming a joint
- **Subluxation or partial dislocation** – the bones are disturbed from their normal position but remain in contact.

Luxations can be divided into two types:

- Acquired luxations – caused by trauma. Hip and elbow joints are most commonly affected but the phalanges and the hocks may also be damaged
- Congenital luxations – due to anatomical abnormalities present from birth.

First-aid treatment. This follows the same basic pattern as for fractures as it is rare that a luxation is life-threatening:

1. Check A, B, C.
2. Treat shock and control haemorrhage.
3. In most cases, movement of the dislocated joint should be minimised to prevent further damage and pain. Pain management is an essential of first aid in these cases as it can exacerbate shock.

Treatment. The use of general anaesthesia is recommended for diagnostic imaging, and because it relaxes the muscles, which eases replacement. Radiography is essential to confirm the diagnosis, to ensure that there are no fractures and to make sure that the bones are replaced accurately. Many luxations can be reduced in a closed fashion, i.e. by manipulating the bones back into position. This is best done as soon as possible after the trauma, since blood clots and muscle contraction can lead to difficulties in replacing luxations left for some time.

If after relocation the joint is still very unstable, an open reduction is needed and surgical measures are needed to stabilise the joint, e.g. in luxation of the carpus where the collateral ligaments are disrupted.

Congenital dislocations are not uncommon and replacement of the bones is not usually sufficient. Surgical intervention is required to correct or modify the anatomical deformity. Patellar luxations can be repaired using one or more techniques depending on the severity of the anatomical deformity. Techniques include the use of a lateral imbrication, where the joint capsule overlying the patella is tightened; a trochleoplasty, which involves deepening the trochlear groove in the femur; and tibial tuberosity transposition, which is needed in some cases as the distortion of the limb is such that the tibial tuberosity has migrated medially.

Postoperative care. Avoid forces that could produce a recurrence of the luxation; for example, with hip luxations it may be necessary to use an Ehmer sling (figure-of-eight bandage) to prevent use of the limb for 5–7 days. This should be followed by restricted exercise for 3–4 weeks, in the same way as for a fracture.

Possible complications. Recurrence is the main complication, and this is true especially of luxations reduced by closed techniques. A recurrent luxation will require surgery to provide adequate stability, e.g. hip luxations may require surgery to the hip involving the creation of a synthetic round ligament.

Ruptured cranial cruciate ligament

The cranial cruciate ligament is a key component of the stifle joint, but unfortunately is quite easily damaged, especially in dogs. This can either be the result of some type of acute trauma, or can be due to a gradual weakening of the ligament due to chronic degenerative processes, which is more common in some breeds (e.g. Labradors, Rottweilers and Boxers).

Animals usually present with pain, causing lameness, and there is more joint laxity than normal due to the failure of the ligament. Veterinary surgeons can test for the laxity by checking for a cranial drawer movement (where the tibia can be moved relative to the femur when the animal is not weight bearing) or a cranial tibial thrust (where the tibial crest is pushed cranially when the hock is flexed in a standing, weight-bearing animal).

Cranial cruciate ligament rupture usually requires surgical management both to fully establish the extent of damage within the joint and manage this, and also to re-stabilise the joint.

There are a number of surgical options, and the choice used will depend on the size and weight of the animal, as well as the surgeon's experience and treatment preference.

Extra-capsular suture stabilisation (lateral fabellar suture stabilisation). In this technique a heavy-duty monofilament nylon stabilising suture is placed on the lateral aspect of the joint anchored to the tibia and around the back of the lateral fabella. This technique may be suitable for lighter dogs, but it is important that postoperative exercise is managed very carefully as the dogs need to be restricted for about 4 months.

Tibial plateau levelling osteotomy (TPLO). In this technique the cranial aspect of the tibia is cut using a circular cut, and rotated so that the top of the tibial plateau is roughly at 90° to the patella tendon. The tibia is then held in place using screws and bone plates designed specifically for this procedure. The result is that the stifle is more stable, and the cruciate ligament is no longer needed to hold the joint in place.

This is complex surgery and needs to be planned very carefully using good radiographs, so that measurements can be made to ensure initial osteotomy cuts are in the correct place and the bone is placed precisely once it has been rotated, using bones plates that are exactly the right size and shape for the individual animal.

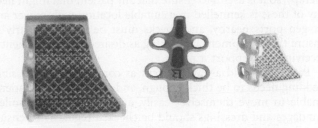

Fig. 23.11 Examples of different sized TTA cages

Tibial tuberosity advancement (TTA). This technique also involves an osteotomy, but this time the cranial aspect of the tibia (the tibial tuberosity or tibial crest) is cut away from the rest of the bone (but still left slightly attached), and a wedge-shaped spacer or other implant is used to push the front of the tibia away from the rest of the tibia (Fig 23.11). This results in a change in the position of the patellar tendon so that it is now about 90° to the tibial plateau. This is therefore a different way of achieving the same orientation as in the TPLO, and means that the joint is made more stable even without a functioning cranial cruciate ligament.

This too requires good planning, and skill to ensure that the placement of the tibial tuberosity is accurate.

All orthopaedic surgery is painful, but osteotomies are particularly so, and it is important that patients are given appropriate analgesia in the pre-, peri- and postoperative periods. Weight management will also be important as any excess weight will hinder recovery and could exacerbate any weakness in the cranial cruciate ligament of the other hind limb.

Pre- and postoperative physiotherapy is beneficial, but it is important that the exercises advised are followed carefully, and the dog is not allowed to do more than has been advised (see Chapter 18).

Nursing the surgical patient

All cases requiring surgery will remain in the practice for a period of time both before and after the procedure has been carried out. During that time, the care the patient receives can make a considerable contribution to its well-being and recovery time.

There are a number of aspects that should be considered for each patient:

TREATMENT PLAN

All staff involved with the care of a particular case need to know about the surgery that has or is about to take place, so that they are fully aware of the effect this will have on the patient and the specific care that will be needed. See Chapter 17 for nursing care plans.

Nursing and supportive care

All patients' vital signs should be checked regularly, and blood and urine samples may also need to be taken and assessed in order to monitor the animal's progress.

Patients may require supplemental oxygen, warmth or fluid therapy, so it is useful to ensure that any patient that might need any of these is kennelled in a suitable location with power and oxygen ports nearby, and checks must be made regularly to ensure that equipment is working as desired and the patient is receiving the support it needs.

Patients should always be kept as comfortable as possible. Bedding needs to be thick enough, and supportive for patients unable to move themselves easily, and changed when soiled. Bandages and dressings should be checked regularly to ensure that there are no problems, and if there is any chance of patient interference with any wound site, measures should be taken to prevent this.

Nutrition

All hospitalised patients should be monitored carefully during their stay to ensure that they are receiving adequate nutrition. The patient's weight should be recorded daily alongside body condition score (BCS) and its resting energy requirement (RER) calculated so that its intake can be assessed to see if additional nutritional support is required (see Chapter 10).

Nutrition also has an important role in the long-term management of surgical patients. In some cases, such as orthopaedic surgery, the animal needs to be on a restricted exercise regimen, whereas in others, such as neutering, its metabolism may be altered. In both cases the animal should not be allowed to gain weight, so the diet may need to be modified to prevent this.

Pain

Pain levels in surgical patients should always be assessed. There are a number of pain scoring systems that can be used for different species, and nursing staff should work together to ensure that these are used consistently so a meaningful assessment of the animal's progress can be made (see Chapter 27).

Different forms of pain occur at different stages during the animal's treatment, and these often require different types of pain management. A nurse's ability to recognise and report pain levels is an important part of helping any patient recover.

Stress management

For any animal, stress can have a very negative impact on its well-being and recovery. This is particularly true while it is hospitalised. This therefore needs to be recognised by the nursing team, and steps taken to reduce stress factors for the animal.

It is therefore helpful to learn a bit about the animal's normal behaviours and preferences from its owner, and to apply these where possible in the practice environment. For example, a dog that was nervous of other dogs would be best kennelled somewhere where it could not see other dogs, or one that was partially deaf would need to be approached in such a way that it was not startled.

For cats, the use of boxes in kennels can be very helpful, providing somewhere to hide and something to climb on, providing of course this is not contraindicated by the animal's condition. Another thing that can help is providing continuity of scent in the kennel. Cleaning the kennel regularly is obviously important, but using two beds, and removing and replacing just one each time (providing that it is not heavily soiled), will help.

For both dogs and cats the use of pheromones within the kennel areas is thought to help, though these cannot be relied on as a sole method of managing animal stress in practice.

Consideration of an animal's stress and anxiety should continue even once it has returned home. For example, active animals that are confined will need mental stimulation, and nervous animals may continue to need gentle reassurance from their owners during the recovery phase.

PHYSICAL THERAPIES

For some conditions, physical therapies such as physiotherapy, hydrotherapy or acupuncture will be an important part of the animal's recovery programme, and specific activities will be required in order to promote healing and its return to normality (see Chapter 18).

If these are to be used, it is important that the protocols are documented and followed exactly so that each time the procedure is done, it is carried out correctly and consistently. Similarly if owners are required to carry on with any form of rehabilitation, then they should be shown what to do as well as given clear, written instructions. Taking time to work with owners and ensuring that they fully understand what is required – and why it is required – will improve client compliance, and ultimately improve the chances of successful management of the animal's condition.

RECORD-KEEPING

Finally, hospitalisation charts, nursing plans, and all other records must be kept up to date throughout any patient's stay. This information will provide a complete record of the animal's treatments, nursing interventions and responses, so that its progress can be assessed as objectively as possible.

BIBLIOGRAPHY

Aspinall, V., 2014. Clinical Procedures in Veterinary Nursing, third ed. Elsevier, Oxford.

Baines, S., Lipscomb, V., Hutchinson, T. (Eds.), 2012. BSAVA Manual of Canine and Feline Surgical Principles: A Foundation Manual. British Small Animal Veterinary Association, Gloucester.

Brinker, P., Brinker, F., 1997. Handbook of Small Animal Orthopedics and Fracture Treatment, third ed. W B Saunders, Philadelphia, PA.

Brockman, D.J., Holt, D.E. (Eds.), 2005. BSAVA Manual of Canine and Feline Head, Neck and Thoracic Surgery. British Small Animal Veterinary Association, Cheltenham.

Capewell, L., 2012a. Get me a plate and some screws! Part 1. Equipment. Veterinary Nurs. J. 27 (6), 226–228.

Capewell, L., 2012b. Get me a plate and some screws! Part 2. Implants. Veterinary Nurs. J. 27 (7), 260–263.

Cooper, B., Mullineux, E., Turner, L. (Eds.), 2011. BSAVA Textbook of Veterinary Nursing, fifth ed. British Small Animal Veterinary Association, Gloucester.

Coughlan, A., Miller, A. (Eds.), 2006. BSAVA Manual of Small Animal Fracture Repair and Management. British Small Animal Veterinary Association, Gloucester.

Dobson, J.M., Lascelles, B.D.X. (Eds.), 2011. BSAVA Manual of Canine and Feline Oncology, third ed. British Small Animal Veterinary Association, Gloucester.

Gould, D., McLellan, G. (Eds.), 2014. BSAVA Manual of Canine and Feline Ophthalmology, third ed. British Small Animal Veterinary Association, Gloucester.

Harvey, A., Tasker, S. (Eds.), 2013. BSAVA Manual of Feline Practice: A Foundation Manual. British Small Animal Veterinary Association, Gloucester.

Hoad, J., 2006. Minor Veterinary Surgery. A Handbook for Veterinary Nurses. Elsevier, Oxford.

Hotston Moore, P., 2004. Fluid Therapy for Veterinary Nurses and Technicians. Butterworth-Heinemann, Oxford.

Houlton, J.E.F., Cook, J.L., Innes, J.F., et al. (Eds.), 2006. BSAVA Manual of Canine and Feline Musculoskeletal Disorders. British Small Animal Veterinary Association, Gloucester.

Lindley, S., Watson, P. (Eds.), 2010. BSAVA Manual of Canine and Feline Rehabilitation, Supportive and Palliative Care: Case Studies in Patient Management. British Small Animal Veterinary Association, Cheltenham.

Lowe, R., 2015. The Lens. In: BSAVA manual of canine and feline ophthalmology, third ed. BSAVA.

Mathews, K., Kronen, P.W., Lascelles, D., et al., 2014. WSAVA guidelines for recognition, assessment and treatment of pain. J. Small Anim. Pract. 55, E10–E68.

Tear, M., 2012. Small Animal Surgical Nursing Skills and Concepts, second ed. Elsevier, St Louis, MO.

Turner, S., 2005. Veterinary Ophthalmology. A Manual for Nurses and Technicians. Elsevier, Oxford.

Williams, J.M., Moores, A. (Eds.), 2009. BSAVA Manual of Canine and Feline Wound Management and Reconstruction, second ed. British Small Animal Veterinary Association, Cheltenham.

Williams, J.M., Niles, J.D. (Eds.), 2015. BSAVA Manual of Canine and Feline Abdominal Surgery, second ed. British Small Animal Veterinary Association, Cheltenham.

RECOMMENDED READING

Hoad, J., 2006. Minor Veterinary Surgery: A Handbook for Veterinary Nurses. Elsevier, Oxford.

An informative and detailed text covering all areas of surgery nurses may legally undertake as part of their role within the Veterinary Surgeons Act 1966 (Schedule 3 amendment).

Lindley, S., Watson, P. (Eds.), 2010. BSAVA Manual of Canine and Feline Rehabilitation, Supportive and Palliative Care: Case Studies in Patient Management. British Small Animal Veterinary Association, Cheltenham.

This book covers a range of cases highlighting the need for holistic care, and looks at the different things needed to optimise patients' recoveries from a range of conditions.

Roberts, L., 2013. Chemotherapy: toxins and barriers. Veterinary Nurse 4 (7), 372–381.

This is an excellent article covering the use of chemotherapeutic drugs and considering their safety both for the animal being treated and the staff involved with its care.

Tear, M., 2012. Small Animal Surgical Nursing Skills and Concepts, second ed. Elsevier, St Louis, MO.

This provides an excellent overview of all aspects of surgical nursing, with review questions at the end of each chapter.

White, R.A.S., Hollis, G., 2010. How to choose a wound dressing. Companion, July 2010, 12–20.

This is an excellent article for anyone wishing to familiarise themselves with the range of wound dressings available along with the rationale for their use

Williams, J.M., Moores, A. (Eds.), 2009. Manual of Canine and Feline Wound Management and Reconstruction, second ed. British Small Animal Veterinary Association, Cheltenham.

This is an excellent text for anyone wishing to develop their knowledge of wound management. There are very good chapters on graft techniques and reconstructive flaps.

24

Theatre Practice

EMMA BROOKS | SAM BELL

KEY POINTS

- Correct design and layout of the surgical unit is essential to provide an environment that is conducive to both effective surgical treatment and care of the patient and in which high standards of asepsis can be maintained.

- When preparing for surgical procedures the role of the veterinary nurse involves preparation of the operating theatre, instruments, other associated equipment and surgical gowns, gloves and drapes. The role may also include acting as a scrubbed or as a circulating nurse, both of which have their own specific roles in the procedure.

- A thorough understanding of the design, use and care of the standard surgical instruments is essential.

- The veterinary nurse should be able to understand how to care for the preoperative patient, intraoperative care of the patient for surgery, the basic principles behind the surgical procedure to be performed and then the postoperative care.

- Every veterinary practice should have a developed, rigid routine for the maintenance of asepsis at all stages of surgery. This includes disinfection and subsequent sterilisation of anything that comes into contact with the surgical site.

Introduction

The care and maintenance of the theatre suite, instruments and equipment is very important for the smooth running of any surgical procedure performed in the operating environment. Whatever type of surgical suite you have, there are fundamental rules that must be followed. This chapter will cover the preparation of the operating suite and the patient, and the care and maintenance of instruments and equipment. It will also cover the preoperative, intraoperative and postoperative care of the patient.

The surgical unit

It is unlikely that the layout and design of the surgical unit is the responsibility of the veterinary nurse. It is important, however, to have an idea of suitable requirements and features of a theatre suite, so that the best can be made of existing facilities. A model surgical unit should consist of:

- Operating theatre
- Anaesthetic preparation area (where the surgical site has its initial preparation)
- An area for washing and sterilising equipment

- Sterile equipment store
- Scrub area for personnel
- Changing rooms
- Recovery room.

OPERATING THEATRE

A majority of practices only have one operating theatre, which is used for all different types of surgical procedures. Some larger practices and hospitals have several theatres, which are used for particular types of surgery, e.g. orthopaedic surgery, general surgery and contaminated (dental) surgery. The size of a theatre will depend on the use for which it was intended. Orthopaedic theatres are fairly often large to accommodate the amount of equipment needed. If the theatre is too small, working conditions are compromised and it becomes difficult to maintain asepsis. Theatres do need to be large enough to accommodate the patient and table, the anaesthetic equipment, the surgical instruments and trolley, any other equipment and the surgical team.

There are several other requirements that are desirable, if not essential:

- The theatre should be an end room, not a thoroughfare to other rooms.
- Materials within the theatre should be easily cleaned. The walls and floors should be made of impervious material. Walls and ceilings should be painted with a light, waterproof paint. Drains should be avoided if possible.
- There should be as little shelving and furniture as possible, as this can harbour dust.
- Good lighting is essential. Natural light should be used if possible. Avoid clear glass windows to the outside, which can cause distraction. Windows must not open, as this will inhibit asepsis. Light fittings should be flush with the ceiling and walls and there should be an overhead theatre light to allow good visualisation of the surgical site.
- An adequate supply of waterproof electric sockets recessed into the wall should be available to enable theatre equipment to be used without the use of extension sockets, which can be hazardous.
- An ambient temperature of 15–20°C should be maintained, as anaesthetised animals struggle to regulate their body temperature. Panel heaters are ideal, but expensive. Fan heaters should be avoided as they cause air and dust to move and risk breaching asepsis.
- Air conditioning and ventilation is necessary under the Control of Substances Hazardous to Health (COSHH) regulations so there must be a scavenging system for waste anaesthetic gases.

- An air supply for power tools is desirable. Medical air should be piped in from cylinders outside the theatre. Anaesthetic gases should also be delivered in the same way.
- There should be an X-ray viewer or screen flush to the wall.
- There should be a clock to monitor the anaesthetic and time of surgery.
- There should be a dry wipe board for recording details such as number of swabs used, suture materials used, blood loss etc.
- There should be double swing doors that are kept closed.
- The operating table should be adjustable to suit the height of the surgeon and the position of the patient.
- All equipment should be able to be easily cleaned to ensure asepsis.

ANAESTHETIC PREPARATION AREA

The anaesthetic preparation area should be a separate area where induction and preoperative procedures take place. The area should lead directly to the theatre. Clippers, vacuum cleaner and other materials to enable surgical site preparation should be available in this area. It is sensible to have an anaesthetic emergency box located here.

AREA FOR WASHING AND STERILISING EQUIPMENT

Preparation of equipment should be within a specific room where any dirty equipment and instruments can be washed and sterilised in a controlled environment. The area should be close to the theatre but away from the sterile store area to prevent contamination. It should contain a washing machine if reusable drapes and gowns are used within practice, a tumble dryer, sterilisation equipment, autoclaves and an ultrasonic cleaner.

STERILE STORE AREA

Sterile packs should be stored in a closed cupboard near to or within the theatre. This room should be large enough to lay out instrument trolleys before surgery. It should have an entrance directly into the theatre. If this area is within the theatre, the cupboards should be clearly labelled with instrument location and cupboards should have doors.

SCRUB AREA

There should be a separate scrub area within the theatre suite but not in the theatre itself. It should lead into the sterile store area, then the theatre. Swing doors should separate the rooms. This is to prevent contamination of the surgical site prior to surgery from hand disinfection.

CHANGING ROOMS

These should be ideally situated at the entrance to the theatre. A line marked on the floor should delineate the sterile area of this room. Theatre footwear should be kept at the entrance to the theatre beyond the line. A one-way traffic system should be in place to maintain asepsis.

RECOVERY ROOM

This should be close to the theatre in case of an emergency. It should be quiet, warm and contain emergency equipment, e.g. oxygen, crash box etc.

Theatre maintenance

Routine cleaning of the theatre suite is essential if asepsis is to be kept at a high standard:

- **Daily damp dusting** – at the start of each day, all furniture, surfaces and equipment can be damp dusted with a disinfectant.
- **Between operative procedures** – the theatre suite should be cleaned as soon as the patient is removed from the operating theatre and before the next one arrives. All of the dirty instruments should be removed for cleaning and re-sterilisation. All surfaces should be wiped over with a suitable disinfectant. All waste should be removed and disposed of correctly. The floor should be cleaned if necessary, and then the instruments and equipment can be prepared for the next patient.
- **At the end of each day** – floors should be cleaned thoroughly to remove debris. They should be washed with disinfectant solution. All waste should be removed and disposed of correctly. All surfaces, including the scrub sink, should be washed with a disinfectant solution.
- **Deep cleaning** – once a week a thorough deep cleaning should be performed or when asepsis has been compromised due to a patient's clinical condition and procedure, e.g. clean-contaminated surgery. All equipment should be removed and walls and floors should be scrubbed. Any excess solution should be removed and then the surfaces should be allowed to dry, not rinsed off. This ensures a longer residual activity time for the disinfectant.

All cleaning equipment for the theatre should be kept separate from other cleaning equipment and should be rinsed and dried after each use. Where possible, mop heads should be laundered each day separately from other laundry. Any cleaning equipment must be stored away from the sterile store area.

Preparation for surgery

THE OPERATING LIST

This should be planned so that clean surgery, such as abdominal or orthopaedic surgery, is done first, followed by clean-contaminated surgery, such as closed pyometritis, oral and anal operations and then contaminated surgery such as contaminated wounds. An exotic surgery (reptiles and tortoises) should be completed at the end of the operating list.

PREPARATION OF DIATHERMY EQUIPMENT

There are two types of electrocautery equipment, also referred to as diathermy – monopolar and bipolar. If monopolar electrocautery is to be used, the patient must be 'earthed' by a contact plate placed in a suitable position between the patient and the table. Contact gel is applied to the plate. For bipolar electrocautery there is no contact plate.

PREPARATION OF OTHER EQUIPMENT

a. Turn on the anaesthetic monitoring equipment and check that all systems are fully operational. (See Chapter 27 for more details on setting up anaesthesia equipment.)

b. Connect the scavenging systems and anaesthetic circuit. Conduct pre-anaesthetic machine and circuit checks.

c. Ensure adequate scrub solutions or hand-disinfectants are available, brushes, sterile hand drying towels, gowns and gloves for the surgical team, including any additional scrub assistants if required.

d. Prepare skin preparation methods ready for the patient, e.g. chlorhexidine solutions, sterile irrigating fluids, swabs, iodine for eye surgery and reptiles and tortoises.

e. Establish that correct surgical instrumentation is selected for the procedure and place on or near instrument trolley, adding any spare instruments, drapes, sutures and swabs that may be required (Box 24.1).

SURGICAL ATTIRE

Suitable theatre clothing should be worn in the theatre. This usually consists of a two-piece scrub suit. A clean scrub suit should be worn every day and if necessary between every procedure if personnel become contaminated.

- **Footwear** – antistatic footwear, e.g. white clogs or wellingtons, is essential to prevent explosions caused by sparks when inflammable anaesthetic gases are used. They should be cleaned frequently and only worn in theatre.
- **Headwear** – a theatre cap should be worn; these are usually made of cloth or paper and ideally disposable.
- **Facemasks** – these are used to filter expired air from the nose and mouth; they are only effective for a short time and should be changed between operations.

SCRUBBING-UP PROCEDURE

As it is not possible to sterilise skin, the aim of scrubbing up is to destroy as many microorganisms as possible before putting on a sterile gown and gloves. There are many different scrub routines. Your practice should adopt a tried and tested routine and adhere to it (Box 24.2).

GOWNING PROCEDURE

The aim of a surgical gown is to provide a barrier preventing the transmission of microorganisms. There are two types of

gown available – those that tie at the back and those that wrap around and tie at the side:

a. Take the sterile gown from the pack and hold at the shoulders, allowing it to fall open without it touching any surfaces, including the floor.

b. Place a hand into each sleeve. Do not try to adjust the gown or pull it over your shoulders, as this can lead to contamination. An unscrubbed assistant will pull the gown over the shoulders by only touching the inside of the gown, and tie the ties at the back (Fig. 24.1).

c. Hands stay inside the sleeves and the waist ties are picked up and held out to the sides. The unscrubbed assistant takes the ties and secures them at the back. The back of the gown is now unsterile.

d. If disposable gowns are used, the process of tying gowns may be slightly different. Stage 1 is used, but stage 2 is altered by affixing a Velcro type fastening at the neck. Inside ties at the back of the gown are tied by an unscrubbed assistant. The gown's external ties are affixed normally with a cardboard holder. One tie is removed from the holder and the holder passed to the unscrubbed assistant. The tie is then passed around the waist of the scrubbed personnel, the second tie is removed from the holder and is tied sterilely.

GLOVING PROCEDURE

Gloves are worn as a barrier between the surgeon's hands and the tissues of the patient. They should fit snugly but not too tightly. Sterile gloves should be worn for all surgical procedures.

There are three methods for gloving up – closed, open and plunge methods.

Closed method

a. Hands stay inside the gown sleeves. This minimises contamination. The glove packet is opened and turned

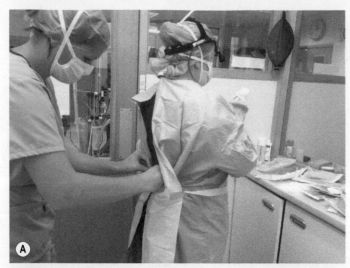

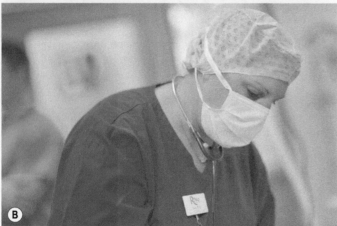

Fig. 24.1 (A) An unscrubbed nurse ties the ties of the sterile surgical gown. (B) Correct wear for an unscrubbed nurse

so that the fingers are pointing at the body. (The right glove will be on the left and vice versa.)

b. Pick up glove at the rim of the cuff of the glove.

c. Turn hand over so that the glove is on the palm surface with fingers pointing at the body.

d. Pick rim up with opposite hand and pull over finger and the dorsal surface of wrist.

e. The glove is pulled on as the fingers are pushed forwards.

Open method (Fig. 24.2)

a. The hands are out of the gown's sleeves in this technique. With the left hand, pick up the right glove by holding the inner surface of the turned-down cuff.

b. Pull on to right hand. Do not unfold the cuff.

c. Repeat steps 1 and 2 for left hand.

d. Put gloved finger under cuff of opposite hand and pull on firmly.

e. The rim of the glove is hooked over the thumb while the cuff of the gown is adjusted, then the cuff of the glove is pulled over the cuff of the gown using the opposite hand. Repeat for other hand.

Plunge method

A sterile glove is held open by a scrubbed assistant and the hand is inserted into the glove. This method is not used often, as there is a high risk of contamination.

Role of the theatre nurse

In veterinary practice the nurse may take one of two roles within the theatre – either a scrubbed nurse or a circulating nurse.

SCRUBBED NURSE

The scrubbed nurse is an important role as an understanding of the surgery to be performed is essential so that the needs of the veterinary surgeon can be anticipated:

- The instrument trolley should be prepared just before it is needed, i.e. just before the patient arrives in theatre. It is essential to know what and where the instruments are on the trolley at the start and during surgery.
- Swabs, needles and sutures should be counted at the beginning of the procedure and at the end before the incision is closed.
- The surgeon must be watched and listened to closely to anticipate his or her needs.
- Instruments should be passed so that they are ready to use and not upside down. They should be put back on the trolley in the same place so that you know their location. Do not leave instruments at the operation site or on the drapes in case they fall on the floor or into the surgical site.
- Instruments should be wiped over with a dry swab before replacing them on the trolley.
- Only one swab at a time should be given. There should be a constant check on the number of swabs. If any extra swab packets are opened, these should be counted carefully too.
- Swabs should be firmly applied to bleeding, without wiping, as this can destroy any clot formation.
- Handle tissues, especially viscera, carefully to avoid unnecessary trauma.
- Irrigation of tissues may be required with warm saline to prevent desiccation, especially during long operations or for flushing of cavities.
- At the end check that all instruments, needles and swabs are on the trolley and accounted for. Dispose of needles and blades in a sharps container.

CIRCULATING NURSE

The circulating nurse is there to assist with all non-sterile procedures:

- Help prepare the instrument trolley for surgery with packs and individual instruments.
- Open and tie surgical gowns, and open surgical gloves.
- Position the patient on the operating table in an appropriate position for the surgery required.
- Prepare the surgical site aseptically.
- Connect apparatus, e.g. suction, electrocautery, air tools, etc.

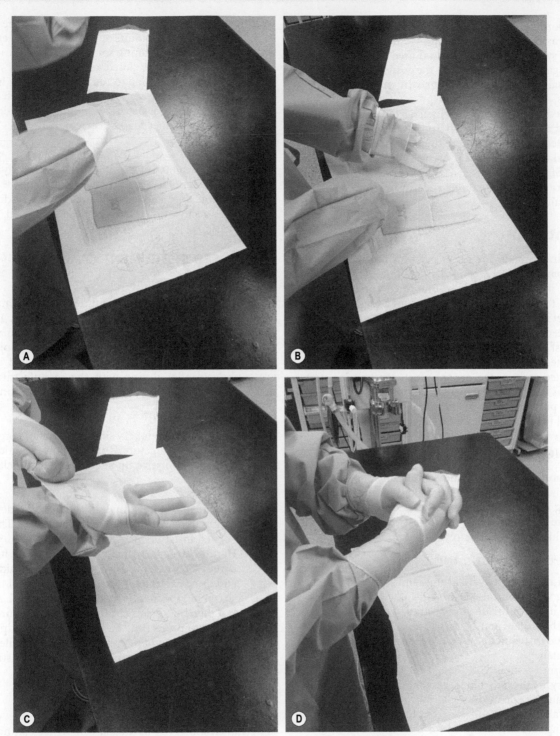

Fig. 24.2 A closed gloving method

- Open packs of swabs, suture material, etc.
- Count swabs with the scrub nurse and keep a running tally.
- Be in theatre when surgery is in progress.
- Assist the anaesthetist if required.
- Prepare postoperative dressings and post-surgical site cleaning.
- Clear theatre at the end of surgery.

Health and safety within the theatre

The COSHH regulations are designed to ensure safety at work, including in the operating theatre (see Chapter 5):

- **Equipment** – it is very important that all nursing staff are told how to use and maintain new equipment. All equipment should be serviced regularly and tested for electrical safety, and standard operating procedures are in place for guidance.

- **Pollution from gas** – all staff should be aware of the danger associated with inhaling anaesthetic gases. A scavenging system must be fitted and used at all times, with annual gas monitoring to check the possibility of any leaks.
- **Disposal of needles/sharp instruments** – all blades, needles, stylets etc. must be disposed of in commercially produced sharps containers. When full they must be sealed, labelled as contaminated sharps waste and removed by a licensed contractor, where they will be incinerated.
- **Clinical and pathological waste** – it is a requirement of COSHH that all veterinary waste is separated from ordinary refuse with colour-coded bags (see Chapter 5 for details).

Instrumentation

Good-quality instruments are expensive but they will have an extended lifespan if properly looked after. Stainless steel is the best choice as it combines high resistance to corrosion with great strength. Tungsten carbide is sometimes added to the tips of stainless steel instruments if used for cutting or gripping, e.g. scissors and needle holders. It is hard and resistant to wear but is an added cost. Instruments with tungsten carbide added are usually indicated by gold handles. Instruments made from chromium-plated carbon steel are the most common in veterinary practice as they are cheaper than stainless steel; however, they will rust, pit and blister when in contact with chemicals and saline, and tend to blunt more quickly.

MAINTENANCE OF INSTRUMENTS

Instruments should always be handled carefully. Do not drop onto trolleys and into sinks. Any sharp edges should be cared for. Sharpening may be required to enable continual use. New instruments are supplied without lubrication so you should wash, dry and lubricate them before use.

Cleaning instruments after use

COSHH states that protective clothing and gloves should be worn if dealing with surgical instruments:

a. Sharp items, i.e. blades and needles, should be removed from the trolley first.
b. Delicate instruments should be separated and cleaned separately.
c. Instruments should be cleaned as soon as possible after surgery to prevent blood and saline from drying on and causing corrosion.
d. Open all the joints and soak in cold water or a chemical cleaning solution designed for instruments.
e. Clean under warm running water with a scrubbing brush. Pay attention to ratchets, joints and serrations. Abrasive agents should not be used as they will damage the surface of the instrument. Ordinary soap causes an insoluble alkali film on the surface, trapping bacteria and protecting them from sterilisation.
f. After washing, rinse and dry carefully.

Ultrasonic cleaners

Bench-top cleaners are suitable for use in veterinary practice. They are effective at removing debris in areas inaccessible to brushes, e.g. box joints. Ultrasonic cleaners work by producing sinusoidal energy waves at a high frequency. After an initial soaking in cold water, place the instruments in the wire basket of the cleaner with their joints open. The unit is then filled with water and ultrasonic cleaning solution and the basket is placed in the solution. The lid is closed and the cleaner is switched on, and set to a cycle according to the manufacturer's instructions. When finished, remove the basket and rinse each instrument under warm running water. Dry carefully, as water trapped in areas such as joints may lead to corrosion.

Lubrication

This should be done on a regular basis, especially if using an ultrasonic cleaner. There are several antimicrobial water-soluble lubricants available. The instruments are usually dipped in the solution for a short time, then removed and dried. There is no need to rinse.

SPECIALISED-INSTRUMENT CARE

Compressed-air machines

These machines must never be immersed in water. All detachable parts should be cleaned in the normal way. Instruments should be detached from the air hose and then wiped with disinfectant. Pay attention to triggers and couplings. Rinse without immersing. The air hose can be cleaned in the same way. Lubricate after drying with the manufacturer's recommended lubricant before packaging for sterilisation.

Motorised equipment

Care of these machines is very similar to that of compressed-air machines. The manufacturer's instructions should always be followed, as they can seize up after repeated autoclaving.

Dental instruments

Dental instruments must be maintained to a high degree if good dental work is to be performed (see Chapter 26). There are two types of dental instrument:

- **Handheld** – these include scalers, picks, luxators and curettes. They have delicate tips and should be washed and dried carefully. These instruments will then require sharpening with an Arkansas stone and oil. Autoclaving can then be carried out in the normal manner, remembering to protect the delicate points and tips.
- **Mechanical** – these include ultrasonic scalers and polishers. Always follow the manufacturer's instructions for each piece of equipment.

Laparoscopic Equipment

This equipment is often very fragile and requires gentle handling and cleaning. Pay particular care with cleaning ports, trochars, biopsy forceps and camera equipment, and always follow the manufacturer's guidelines to ensure equipment is kept in good working order.

SURGICAL INSTRUMENTS

There are many different types of instrument available (Fig. 24.3). It is not necessary to know every single one, but a broad knowledge of the more common ones is essential (Table 24.1).

Orthopaedic instruments

Common types are described in Table 24.2 and Figure 24.4. Other instruments may be needed, depending on the technique

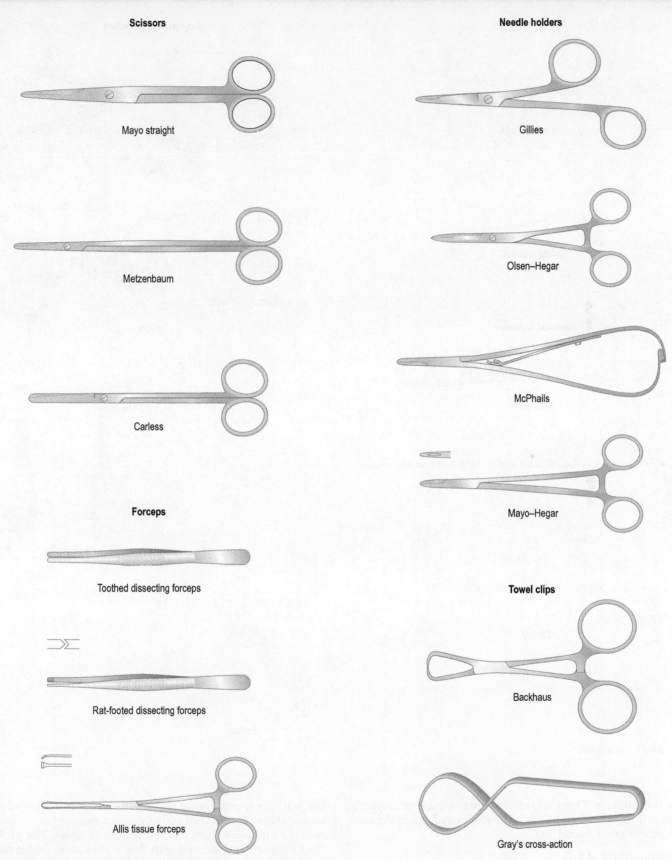

Scissors

Mayo straight

Metzenbaum

Carless

Forceps

Toothed dissecting forceps

Rat-footed dissecting forceps

Allis tissue forceps

Needle holders

Gillies

Olsen–Hegar

McPhails

Mayo–Hegar

Towel clips

Backhaus

Gray's cross-action

Fig. 24.3 A range of surgical instruments

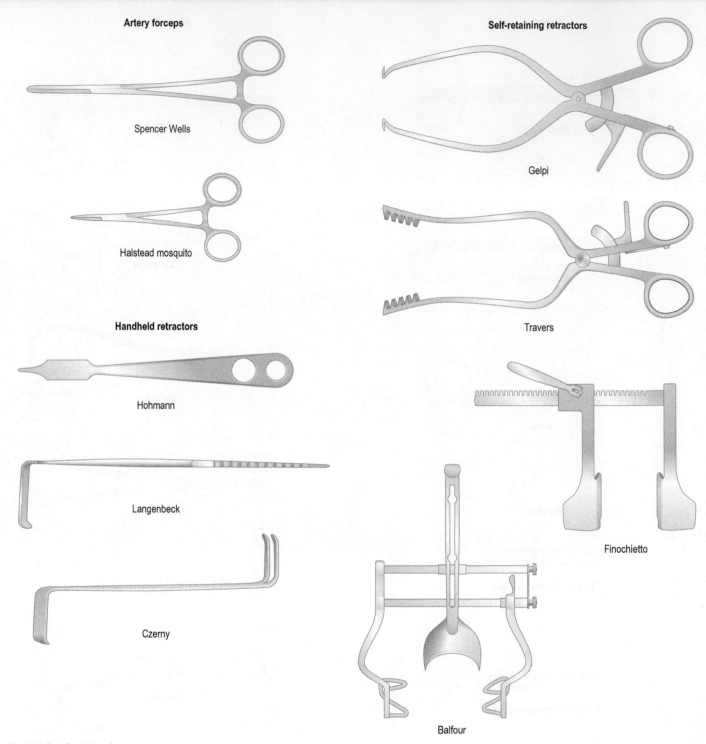

Fig. 24.3   Continued

and the surgeon. These include Steinmann pins, orthopaedic wire, arthrodesis wires, bone plates, screws and external fixator equipment (see Chapter 23).

Packing surgical kits

Instruments are often packed together with swabs, drapes, suction tubing, etc. The pack is usually wrapped so that the outer layers will cover the instrument trolley when unwrapped. Ideally, a metal or plastic tray is used and the instruments are laid out in a specific order (usually the order of use), and any swabs, drapes etc. are then added. A water-resistant drape is laid over the top followed by two layers of linen sheet. The pack is then wrapped and secured with Bowie Dick tape, and it must be labelled and dated before sterilisation.

Other methods of preparing surgical packs include wrapping the surgical kit in a concertina pattern for basic surgery, and using sturdy commercially available plastic or metal fenestrated boxes.

TABLE 24.1	General surgical instruments (see also Fig. 24.3)			
Name	Type	Use	Comment	
Scalpel		Divide tissues with minimal trauma	Size 3 handle used for small animal surgery. Use 10, 11, 12 and 15 blade Size 4 handle used for large animal work. Use 20, 21 or 22 blade A small (beaver) handle is available with a very small blade. Good for ophthalmic work	
Dissecting forceps (thumb forceps)	Plain Rat-toothed Debakeys	Holding tissue Plain ends hold delicate tissue Rat-toothed hold dense tissue Delicate tissue	Hold like a pencil	
Scissors	Mayo dissecting Metzenbaum Carless Paynes	Routine surgery Delicate surgery Suture cutting Removing sutures	Hold with ring finger and thumb inserted into ring of the scissors Index finger is placed on shaft to guide scissors	
Haemostatic artery forceps	Spencer Wells Dunhill Criles Cairns Kelly Halstead/mosquito	Clamping blood vessels to stop bleeding	Many different lengths and shapes. Most have transverse striations to help hold tissue. Mosquito forceps are the smallest and are used for fine blood vessels. Hold as for scissors	
Towel clips	Backhaus Gray's cross-action	Attach drapes to patients and instruments to operating site		
Needle holders	Gillies Olsen–Hegar Mayo–Hegar McPhail's	Hold suture needles during suturing and knot tying	Gillies – have scissor action for cutting suture ends. No ratchet so must hold needle tightly Olsen–Hegar – have cutting edge and ratchet to hold needle securely. Very easy to cut suture material Mayo–Hegar – like long-handled artery forceps. Have ratchet but no cutting edge McPhail's – usually have copper or tungsten carbide insert in tip. Have spring ratchet so that squeezing jaws together opens holder and releases needle	
Retractors	Handheld: Langenbeck Senn Czerny Self-retaining: Gelpi West's Travers Gusset Balfour Finochietto	Expose operating field	Can be handheld or self-retaining Gelpi, West's and Travers for muscle or joints Gusset and Balfour for abdominal surgery Finochietto for thoracic surgery	

TABLE 24.2	Orthopaedic instruments (see also Fig. 24.4)	
Name	Use	Comment
Osteotome	Cutting and shaping bone	Tapered on both sides
Chisel	Cutting and shaping bone	Tapered on one side only
Gouge	Cutting and shaping bone	U-shaped edge to remove larger pieces of bone or cartilage
Curette	Scoop surface of dense tissue to remove loose or degenerate tissue	The cup has a sharp cutting edge. Available in many sizes
Periosteal elevators	Lift periosteum and soft tissue from bone surface	Many sizes available
Bone-holding forceps	Grip bone fragments while reducing or aligning fractures	
Bone cutters	Cutting large pieces of bone	
Bone rasps	Remove sharp edges following arthroplasty	
Bone rongeurs	Cutting small pieces of dense tissue, bone or cartilage	
Drills	Hand drills are used around delicate structures where minimal drilling is required. Most surgery will require the use of a battery or air drill	Battery drills are slower and more cumbersome but less expensive than air drills
Saws and burrs	May be driven by air or electricity. Take care when connecting Do not switch on until all the couplings are assembled	
Wire forceps	Used to apply cerclage wire and when stabilising bones with wire	Various types available
Gigli wire and handles	Saw through bone with cheese wire effect	

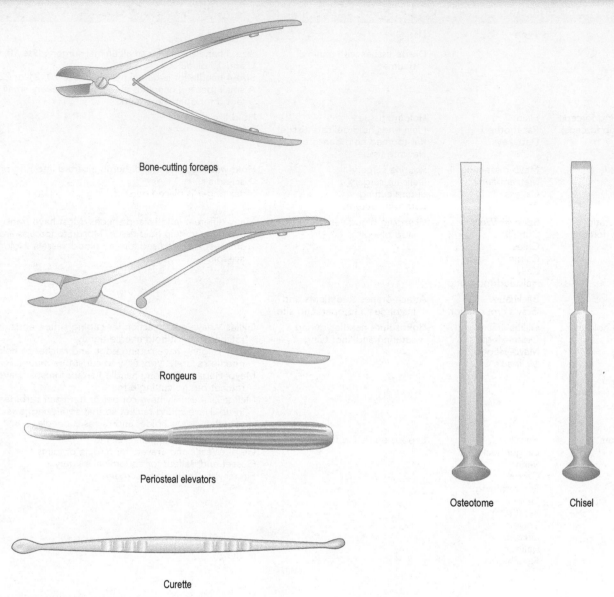

Bone-cutting forceps

Rongeurs

Periosteal elevators

Osteotome   Chisel

Curette

Fig. 24.4 Orthopaedic instruments

Instrument sets

These collections of specific instruments are made up to suit the technique and the needs of the individual practice. Some practices have sets for specific operations, e.g. bitch spay kit. Others have standard sets that are used for all operations but have extra instruments that can be added depending on the procedure. It is important that each standard kit contains the same number and type of instruments so that the surgical team know what is there and can check at the end of the procedure that all instruments are present. Personnel must all be aware of kit contents and how to repack to eliminate mistakes from occurring. Guidelines for types of kit are shown in Table 24.3.

Sutures

SUTURE MATERIALS

The choice of suture materials used within the veterinary practice depends on:

- Type of tissue to be repaired
- Risk of contamination

- Length of healing time, i.e. how long the suture material must remain effective within the tissue
- Personal preference.

There are two categories of suture material – non-absorbable and absorbable. Each category can be subdivided into:

- Natural or synthetic
- Monofilament or multifilament
- Coated or uncoated
- Antibacterial.

Tables 24.4 and 24.5 describe the most commonly used suture materials and their properties.

ALTERNATIVES TO SUTURES

Today there are an increasing number of alternatives to suture materials (see also Chapter 23). These include:

- **Staples** – there are several different types of metal staple available. The most common type is skin staples but specialised staples are available for intestinal anasto-

TABLE 24.3 Suggested contents of different types of surgical kit

Type of kit	Contents	Type of kit	Contents
General surgical kit	Scalpel handle no. 3 Dissecting forceps (plain and rat-toothed) Scissors (Mayo and Metzenbaum) Artery forceps ×8 Allis tissue forceps ×2 Retractors (Gelpi and Langenbeck) Backhaus towel clips ×4 Needle holders Suture scissors	Abdominal kit	General kit Self-retaining retractors Long-handled artery forceps ×6 Long dissecting forceps ×2 Bowel clamps ×4
		Thoracic kit	General kit + periosteal elevator Rib cutters Rib retractors Long-handled artery forceps ×6 Long dissecting forceps ×2 Lobectomy clamps
General eye kit	Eyelid speculum Small scalpel handle (beaver) Fine dissecting forceps Fine scissors Corneal scissors Capsular forceps Irrigating cannula Vectis Iris repository Castroviejo needle holders	Orthopaedic kit	General kit + periosteal elevator Osteotome Chisel Mallet Curette Hohmann retractor ×2 Rongeurs Bone-cutting forceps

TABLE 24.4 Non-absorbable suture materials

Suture material	Trade name	Mono- or multifilament	Synthetic or natural	Coated	Knot security	Duration	Comments
Polyamide (nylon)	Ethilon (Ethicon)	Monofilament	Synthetic	No	Fair	Permanent	Causes minimal tissue reaction and has little tissue drag
Polybutylester	Novafil (Covidien)	Monofilament	Synthetic	No	Fair	Permanent	Similar to polyamide with similar properties
Polypropylene	Prolene (Ethicon)	Monofilament	Synthetic	No	Fair – can produce bulky knots that untie easily	Permanent	Very inert. Produces minimal tissue reaction Very strong but very springy. Little tissue drag
Braided silk	Mersilk (Ethicon)	Multifilament	Natural	Wax coat	Excellent	May eventually fragment and break down	Good handling properties, but high tissue reactivity Do not use in infected sites
Braided polyamide	Supramid or Nuralon (Ethicon)	Multifilament	Synthetic	Encased in outer sheath	Good	Outer sheath can be broken	Better handling than monofilament polyamide Can be used in skin but not as a buried suture
Surgical stainless steel wire		Available as monofilament or multifilament	Synthetic	No	Excellent, although knots are difficult to untie	Permanent	Not commonly used now, but is useful in bones or tendon Difficult to handle

moses and vessel ligation. Staples are usually packed in a gun-type applicator.

- **Tissue glue** – used for skin closure. It is designed for rapid healing and is most commonly used on small superficial wounds.
- **Skin adhesive** – A flexible secure skin closure which can add strength and can inhibit bacteria, e.g. Dermabond Advanced®.
- **Adhesive tape** – mainly used in human skin closure. Mainly used in large animal abdominal closure, e.g. Dermabond Prineo®.

SUTURE NEEDLES

There are several types of suture needle and they are available with the suture material swaged onto them or with eyes through which the suture material is threaded. Choice is dependent on the type of wound to be sutured, the type of tissue and the characteristics of the needle.

The needle shape may be:

- **Curved** – the entire length of the needle is curved into an arc. Various degrees of curvature are available – half circle is most common.

TABLE 24.5 Absorbable suture materials

Suture material	Trade name	Mono- or multifilament	Synthetic or natural	Coated	Duration of strength	Absorption	Comments and uses
Polyglactin 910	Vicryl (Ethicon)	Multifilament	Synthetic	Yes – calcium stearate	Retains 50% of tensile strength at 14 days and 20% at 21 days	Absorbed by 60–90 days by hydrolysis	Dyed or undyed. Low tissue reactivity. Uses: in subcuticular layer, muscle, eyes and hollow viscera. Also available in an antibacterial form (Plus)
Polyglactin 910	Vicryl Rapide (Ethicon)	Multifilament	Synthetic	Yes – calcium stearate	Retains only 50% of tensile strength at 5 days. Provides wound support for 10 days	Absorption complete by about 42 days. Absorbed by hydrolysis	Although the same as Vicryl it is manufactured to make it loose tensile strength and be fully absorbed much faster. Also available in an antibacterial form (Plus)
Polydioxanone	PDS II (Ethicon)	Monofilament	Synthetic	No	Retains 70% tensile strength at 14 days and 14% at 56 days	Only minimal absorption by 90 days. Absorbed by 180 days, by hydrolysis	Good for infected sites as monofilament. Very strong but springy. Minimal tissue reaction. Uses: in subcuticular muscle, sometimes eyes. Also available in an antibacterial form (Plus)
Polyglycolic acid	Dexon (Covidien)	Multifilament	Synthetic	Can be coated with polymer	Retains 20% at 14 days	Complete absorption by 100–120 days. Absorbed by hydrolysis	Similar to polyglactin but has considerable tissue drag. Uses: as for polyglactin
Polyglecaprone 25	Monocryl (Ethicon)	Monofilament	Synthetic	No	Retains about 60% at 7 days, 30% at 14 days. Wound support maintained for 20 days	Complete absorption between 90 and 120 days. Absorbed by hydrolysis	Less springy than other monofilament absorbables with minimal tissue drag. Available dyed or undyed. Also available in an antibacterial form (Plus)
Polyglyconate	Maxon (Covidien)	Monofilament	Synthetic	No	Retains 70% at 14 days	Complete absorption by 60 days. Absorbed by hydrolysis	Similar to polydioxanone but easy to handle. Uses: similar to polydioxanone
Chromic catgut		Essentially monofilament	Natural (made from purified animal intestines)	Coated with chromium salts	Retains tensile strength for approximately 28 days	Absorbed by enzymatic degradation and phagocytosis	Always causes a moderate inflammatory response
Plain catgut		Essentially monofilament	Natural (made from purified animal intestines)	No	Retains tensile strength for approximately 14 days	Absorbed by enzymatic degradation and phagocytosis	Also causes a moderate inflammatory response and rapidly loses tensile strength

TABLE 24.6	Cross-sectional design of suture needles	
Cross-sectional design	**Features**	**Uses**
Cutting	Triangular in cross-section with apex on inside of curve Point and sides of needle have cutting edges, which are very sharp	Skin and other dense tissue
Reverse cutting	Triangular in cross-section with apex on outside of curve Point and sides of needle have cutting edges, which are very sharp	Skin and other dense tissue
Round-bodied	Round in cross-section No sharp edges	Delicate tissues, e.g. fat, viscera
Taper point	Becomes round-bodied as needle widens Similar to cutting needle at tip	Dense tissues other than skin, e.g. fascia, thick-walled viscera, mucous membranes

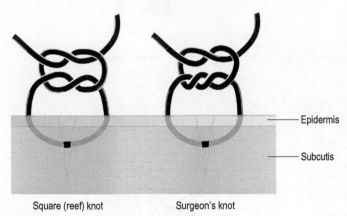

Square (reef) knot   Surgeon's knot

Fig. 24.5 Surgical knots

- **Half-curved** – the sharp end of needle is curved but the eye end is straight.
- **Straight** – the entire needle is straight.

The cross-sectional design may vary according to the tissue that is being sutured (Table 24.6).

COMMON SUTURE PATTERNS

As registered veterinary nurses are legally allowed to perform minor acts of surgery under the Veterinary Surgeons Act 1966 (Schedule 3 amendment), including suturing, it is important that you are familiar with basic suturing techniques. Remember always to seek practical instruction from a veterinary surgeon in charge of the case beforehand.

SURGICAL KNOTS

A surgical knot has three components:
- The loop – the part of suture material within the opposed or ligated tissue
- The knot – made from a number of throws or from a locking suture knot
- The ears – the cut end of the suture that prevents the knot from being untied.

Knots can be hand-tied or instrument-tied. The basic surgical knot is a reef knot, or square knot. A surgeon's knot has an initial double throw, not a single throw. This reduces the risk of the first throw loosening while the second throw is being placed (Fig. 24.5). Hand-tying will help prevent loosening and slippage of the first throw, as tension can be placed on both ends of the suture. It is, however, very wasteful of suture material.

The knots of skin sutures should be pulled to one side of the incision. The suture loop should be loose. Sutures that are placed tightly will compromise the vascular supply and delay healing. They will also cause irritation and cause the patient to interfere with the wound.

Interrupted sutures

Each suture is tied individually and cut distal to the knot (Fig. 24.6). The main advantage of interrupted sutures is the ability to maintain strength and tissue apposition if one part of the suture line fails. The disadvantages are the amount of suture material required and the length of time it takes to place the sutures.

Continuous sutures

A continuous line of sutures is placed and only knotted and cut at the beginning and end of the suture line (see Fig. 24.6). The advantages are the ease of application and removal and the fact that less suture material is used. The main disadvantage is that slippage of the knot at either end of the suture line will cause the entire suture line to break down.

Various patterns of sutures may be used depending on the site and the purpose of the suture line (see Fig. 24.6):
- Simple interrupted
- Simple continuous
- Ford interlocking
- Interrupted vertical mattress
- Interrupted horizontal mattress
- Cruciate mattress.

Sutures should be placed at least 5 mm from the wound edge and placed squarely across the wound. Atraumatic forceps should be used to handle the skin and the wound edges should be apposed or slightly everted, with no gaping or overlapping.

Patient care

PREOPERATIVE CARE

On admission all relevant details about the patient should be recorded:
- The reason for admission must be checked.
- Ensure that the owner understands what is to be done and the procedure explained.
- Check that the patient is in good general health or that the symptoms have not changed since last examined.
- Make sure a contact number is taken and the general anaesthetic consent form is signed.
- Check that the patient has been starved – usually food is withheld for a period of time prior to surgery to

Suture patterns

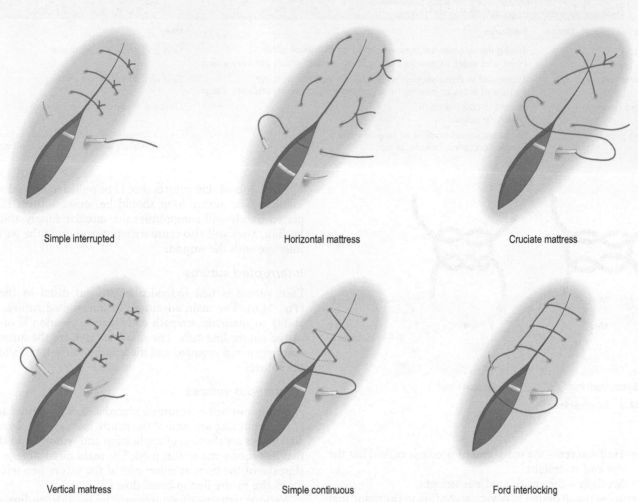

Simple interrupted Horizontal mattress Cruciate mattress

Vertical mattress Simple continuous Ford interlocking

Fig. 24.6 Common suture patterns

prevent regurgitation under anaesthesia, but length of time is an individual practice's decision and is dependent on species, age and procedure.

- Ideally, the patient should be bathed before surgery to minimise contamination of the surgical site.
- The patient should have been given the opportunity to urinate and defecate before surgery; in some cases an enema may be required.
- The patient should be weighed and any medication given, e.g. antibiotics, analgesia and premedication.

PREPARATION OF THE PATIENT FOR A SURGICAL PROCEDURE

Some form of premedication or sedation is given intramuscularly or subcutaneously 15–30 minutes before the induction of anaesthesia dependent on the drug choice. Antibiotics and analgesics are usually given at the same time or at induction.

Clipping

This is necessary for most surgical procedures. Clipping can be done before or under general anaesthesia. A large area should be clipped to allow an adequate area for the surgical procedure and for any extensions to the surgical site that may be required to prevent intraoperative clipping. Clips should be neat so as to be aesthetically pleasing to the owner. Before beginning a clip, ensure that the clipper blades are in good working order, as nicks in the skin will cause irritation and excessive licking postoperatively. All clipping should be done away from the theatre to minimise contamination.

Hair which has been clipped but is still in the surgical site can be removed by vacuuming and sticky rollers, especially in areas of sensitive tissue, before skin preparation can be started.

Skin preparation

As it is not possible to remove all bacteria from the skin, the aim is to significantly reduce the number of organisms without damaging the skin itself. Antiseptic and detergent properties are needed in a skin cleansing agent and surgical scrub preparations such as chlorhexidine or povidone-iodine are ideal. There are various methods of skin preparation; the one outlined as follows is commonly used:

a. Wear surgical gloves to prevent contamination of the patient's skin by the nurse's hands.
b. Use lint-free swabs to wash the site with the practice's preferred surgical scrub and a little water. Begin at

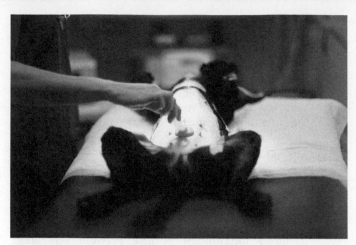

Fig. 24.7 Position and prepare the patient for surgery

the operating site and work out to the edges of the clipped area. At the edge of the clipped area discard the swab and use a new one. Continue until the skin is clean, i.e. no discoloration on swab.

c. A small amount of alcohol solution can be sprayed over the site to remove any remaining detergent. Do not use on mucous membranes or open wounds.

d. Move patient to theatre and position for surgery (Fig. 24.7).

The site will be contaminated now, so clean once again in the same fashion but using sterile swabs and gloves. Alternatively chlorhexidine gluconate combined with alcohol preparation can be used. These are used at the direct surgical site of 30 seconds, then moved outwards toward the peripheral clipped area, and left to air dry.

Preparation of eyes and mucous membranes

Most skin preparations are irritating to the eye and mucous membranes. Dilute solutions of povidone-iodine at a dilution of 1:50 sterile saline can be used to irrigate the eye and oral cavity. Alcohol solutions must not be used. The skin around the eye is very thin and sensitive, so minimal clipping is required. Oral preparation may require a commercially available veterinary oral rinse.

Preparation of the foot

Between the toes can be particularly sensitive and difficult to prep effectively. Once an initial scrub is complete, placing the foot in a glove filled with skin preparation and massaging the foot within the glove, which has been occluded at the glove rim, can help clean between the pads and metatarsals.

Draping the surgical site

This is done to maintain asepsis by preventing contamination of the surgical site by hair and the immediate environment. Drapes should be large enough to cover the entire patient and preferably the whole operating table, leaving only the surgical site exposed. Disposable drapes should be utilised in all circumstances, as they are more cost effective than reusable cloth drapes and are more impervious to strike-through.

Plain drapes. Four rectangular drapes are used to create a window for the surgical site (Fig. 24.8). The first drape is placed

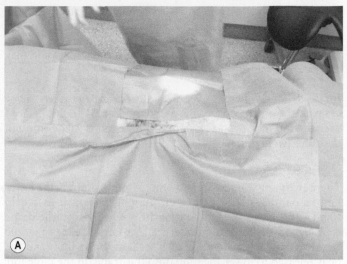

(A)

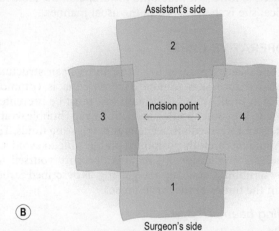

Assistant's side

Incision point

Surgeon's side

(B)

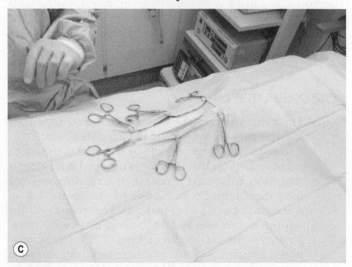

(C)

Fig. 24.8 Draping the patient. (A) Plain drapes placed on the patient ready for surgery. (B) Order of placing plain drapes on the patient. (C) Drapes secured in place with towel clips

between the surgeon and the nearest side of the patient. The second drape is placed on the opposite side of the patient. The remaining two drapes are placed at each end of the patient. They are then secured with towel clips and/or may have the benefit of a sticky strip if disposable.

Fenestrated drapes. These achieve the same effect as plain drapes but the 'window' is already formed within a single drape. The drape must be large enough to cover the entire patient. Such drapes are commonly used for cat and bitch spays and may also be disposable.

Incise drapes. These are sterile, adhesive plastic sheets. They are placed over the entire site. Standard drapes are then placed over the top in the usual fashion. An incision is made through the adhesive material.

Draping limbs

There are many ways to drape a limb. Most commonly the lower limb is bandaged and tied to an upright pole such as a drip stand – this keeps the limb out of the way while a sterile drape is placed on the table top underneath. A sterile drape or sterile cohesive bandage material is then secured to the limb and the tie is released to lower the limb onto the drape on the table top. The surgical site is then draped in the usual manner.

INTRAOPERATIVE CARE

Care must be taken to position towel to avoid delicate structures and to help reduce skin trauma. Hypothermia is common, particularly in small animals, and heat loss must be prevented. Use heat pads, hot-water bottles, insulating wrap (bubble wrap), foil blankets and warmed intravenous and irrigating fluids. The patient should be carefully positioned on the table to avoid any postoperative complications. If required, prepare yourself for surgery by scrubbing, gowning and gloving, as described earlier, to perform the duties of the scrub nurse.

Controlling haemorrhage

Haemorrhage can be controlled by using swabs, instruments (e.g. Spencer Wells or Halstead mosquito artery forceps; see Fig. 24.3), ligatures or electrocautery. If using swabs, blot the haemorrhaging area as opposed to wiping it, as wiping will disrupt any clot formation.

POSTOPERATIVE CARE

- The patient should not be left unattended until conscious, sitting up and able to maintain its airway.
- The endotracheal tube should be removed as the cough reflex returns (in cats the tube is removed just before it returns to reduce the incidence of laryngospasm) and the patient must be watched closely to ensure that an adequate airway is maintained. The colour of the mucous membranes and the presence or absence of respiratory noise are good indicators of effective ventilation. Monitoring should continue until the animal is completely recovered. Body temperature should be monitored and maintained.
- Heart rate and pulse rate should also be monitored and any changes noted.
- Dressings should be done before the patient regains consciousness. Any purse-string sutures and swabs should be removed.
- The patient should be placed in a warm, comfortable and quiet recovery kennel.
- Turn the patient regularly if it is unable to do this for itself.

- Administer any analgesic drugs prescribed by the veterinary surgeon. If you observe any signs of pain, inform the veterinary surgeon (see also Chapter 27).
- When fully recovered allow the patient to urinate and defecate.
- Provide food and water if appropriate for the case, especially to very old or young patients, and always ensure the patient has no specific dietary requirements.

INTUBATION

The advantages of intubation are:
- It provides a secure airway and protects it from saliva and other secretions such as water during dental procedures.
- It allows intermittent positive pressure ventilation (IPPV) (see Chapter 27).
- It reduces anatomical dead space.
- It allows the maintenance of anaesthesia and provides a means of supplying oxygen (see Chapter 27).
- It reduces pollution from waste anaesthetic gases.

Disadvantages include:
- The endotracheal tube may kink during positioning; however, armoured tubes are available to help prevent this. If tubes become damaged or become too flexible, they should be discarded.
- Overinflation of the cuff may occlude the tube and cause damage to the trachea.
- A tube that is too small may increase the resistance to breathing.
- Traumatic laryngitis may develop as a result of poor technique or oversized tubes, particularly in cats.

Method of intubation

Dogs

a. Place the anaesthetised patient in lateral recumbency.
b. The assistant holds the head up, supporting the base of the neck with the left hand and holding the maxilla and nose with the right hand. If there are any concerns regarding a cervical spine disease process, intubation should occur with the patient's head in lateral.
c. Gently ease the tongue out of the mouth and pull it down to lower the mandible. This enables the larynx to be viewed.
d. Using a correct-sized lubricated tube, insert it into the mouth towards the soft palate. The diameter of the tube to be placed roughly relates to the width of the nasal septum.
e. Insert the tube over the epiglottis and between the vocal folds.

Some people prefer the dog to be in sternal recumbency in order for intubation. Laryngoscopes can also be used for ease of placement.

Cats

a. Place the anaesthetised patient in lateral recumbency.
b. The assistant holds the head up, supporting the base of the neck with the left hand and holding the maxilla and nose with the right hand. Keep fingers out of the mouth. If there are any concern regarding a cervical spine disease process, intubation should occur with the patient's head in lateral.

c. Gently ease the tongue out of the mouth and pull it down to lower the mandible. This enables the larynx to be viewed.

d. If using a laryngoscope, hold the tongue with your thumb and forefinger and hold the laryngoscope with the same hand. Use the blade of the laryngoscope to push the tongue down, not the epiglottis, enabling the larynx to be viewed.

e. To prevent the occurrence of laryngeal spasm, spray the larynx with local anaesthetic to desensitise it. Wait 60–90 seconds.

f. Insert a correct-sized lubricated tube into the mouth and between the laryngeal folds during inspiration. The laryngeal folds can be seen moving in and out as the cat breathes.

Removing the endotracheal tube (extubation)

In dogs the tube should be removed when the swallowing/gag reflex returns; in cats it should be removed before the reflex returns. Leave the cuff inflated until ready for removal. On removal, deflate the cuff and carefully pull the tube out in a downward direction to avoid damage to the trachea and larynx.

IMMEDIATE/SHORT-TERM POSTOPERATIVE COMPLICATIONS

Haemorrhage

Control any external haemorrhage with digital pressure or pressure bandages. Internal haemorrhage is more complicated. Usually, the patient will have to be re-anaesthetised and the surgical site opened up to control the haemorrhage with instruments and ligatures.

Laryngospasm

Keep the endotracheal tube in place if you have not already removed it. Steroid treatment may help or, in severe cases, a tracheostomy may have to be performed.

Shock

Monitor all vital parameters, i.e. heart rate and pulse rate, mucous membrane colour, capillary refill time and respiration rate. Prepare warm intravenous fluids and administer according to the veterinary surgeon's instructions. Keep the patient warm using blankets or bubble wrap. Do not apply direct heat using heat pads. Administer antidote to the anaesthetic agent, if appropriate (see Chapter 27).

Hypothermia

Keep the patient warm using blankets, bubble wrap and heat mats. Maintain room temperature between 21°C and 23°C. Monitor rectal temperature every 10 minutes or more frequently if required. Administer warmed intravenous fluids.

Vomiting

Monitor the patient at all times. Hold the head and neck down, or hang over the side of the table with the body raised so that the head and neck are in a downwards position. Keep in this position until the patient regains consciousness. Administer any antiemetic drugs that the veterinary surgeon has prescribed.

Asepsis and sterilisation
PRINCIPLES OF STERILISATION

The saying 'prevention is better than cure' is very true. Infection of clean surgical wounds is always of great concern. Antibiotics should not be relied upon as a means of protection against infection because of poor aseptic technique. Every veterinary organisation should have a routine that is adhered to, from correct theatre attire and scrubbing-up techniques to the cleaning of instruments and the practice environment and when to use antibiosis. Box 24.3 provides some useful terminology.

SPREAD OF INFECTION

Contamination usually comes from four sources – the operating theatre and its environment, the equipment used, the personnel and the patient:

- **Operating theatre and its environment** – many microorganisms are airborne. Any movement within the theatre will cause them to disperse. Good ventilation is necessary, as hot humid conditions are also a threat to asepsis. Cleaner procedures should be done first, as organisms from the contaminated site will remain in the air. The operating room should be easily cleaned and contain little furniture. Aerosol disinfectants are often useful to ensure decontamination in the hard to reach places within theatres.
- **Equipment** – all equipment, e.g. instruments, must be sterile and a new set must be used for each operation.
- **Personnel** – There should be as few people in the theatre as possible, as the presence of unnecessary personnel increases the risk of infection. Correct theatre clothing should be worn (theatre scrubs, clogs, hats and masks) and those in the surgical team must prepare their hands aseptically. Sterile gowns and gloves should be worn.
- **Patient** – the patient is the greatest source of contamination. Microorganisms are either:
  - Endogenous – within the body of the patient, or
  - Exogenous – outside the body on the skin and coat of the patient.

Wounds may be classified as clean, clean-contaminated, contaminated or dirty, and a wound does not necessarily have to be obviously infected for microorganisms to be present. Other factors also need to be taken into account, such as the virulence of the organism, the resistance of the patient and the duration of the surgery. The infection rate doubles for every hour of surgery, and surgical techniques can also increase the risk of contamination, especially if there is excessive trauma and damage to the vascular supply. Impaired host resistance, the use

---

BOX 24.3 DEFINITIONS OF COMMON TERMS

- Sepsis – presence of pathogens in the blood or tissues, i.e. infection
- Asepsis – freedom from infection
- Antisepsis – prevention of sepsis by destruction of pathogens
- Sterilisation – destruction of all microorganisms, including bacterial spores
- Disinfection – destruction of all microorganisms except bacterial spores
- Disinfectant – a chemical agent that destroys microorganisms

of drugs, nutritional problems and underlying disease will contribute to wound contamination.

STERILISATION

All instruments and equipment must be sterilised before use. There are several methods of sterilisation available and the choice, which must be both safe and economical, depends on:
- Amount of equipment to be sterilised
- Type of equipment to be sterilised
- Cost
- Available space within the practice.

There are two types of sterilisation: cold sterilisation and heat sterilisation.

Cold sterilisation

Ethylene oxide. This is a highly penetrating and effective method of sterilisation; however, it is toxic, irritant to tissues and a flammable gas. Ethylene oxide works by inactivating the DNA of cells and stopping cell reproduction. It is effective against vegetative bacteria, fungi, viruses and spores. Several factors influence the ability of ethylene oxide to destroy microorganisms, including temperature, pressure concentration, humidity and time of exposure.

An ethylene oxide steriliser is a metal unit fitted with a ventilation system to prevent gas from entering the workplace. It must be used in a clean, well-ventilated area away from any work areas. The temperature of the room must be at least 20°C during the cycle. Items are placed in a specific polythene liner bag with a gas ampoule and the bag is sealed with a tie and placed in the sterilising unit. The top of the vial is snapped from outside the liner bag to release the gas. The steriliser door is then closed and locked, the ventilator is turned on and the items are left to sterilise. Cycles are either 12- or 24-hour processes depending on the equipment being sterilised. At the end of the period a pump is switched on to ventilate the container and the door may be opened 2 hours later. Items must be left for a further 24 hours to allow the ethylene oxide to dissipate.

Suitable items to be sterilised include anything that might be damaged by heat, e.g. fibre-optic equipment (endoscopes), laparoscopic equipment, plastic catheters, anaesthetic tubing, plastic syringes, optical equipment, high-speed drills, burrs and battery-operated drills. Most things can be sterilised but the limiting factors are the size of the container, the duration of the cycle and the toxicity. Equipment containing polyvinyl chloride (PVC) cannot be sterilised in this way, as PVC may react with the ethylene oxide gas.

All materials must be clean and dry. The presence of protein and grease slows sterilisation and reduces its effectiveness. Bungs, caps and stylets must be removed to allow the gas to penetrate freely. Items can be packaged, as ethylene oxide penetrates more easily than steam, but do not use nylon film bags. To monitor the effectiveness of the process, indicator tape can be used that has yellow stripes that turn red; however, this does not guarantee sterility as the stripes change colour after only a short exposure to the gas. Chemical indicators placed in the centre of the pack will change colour when exposed for the correct length of time. Spore strips can be added to the load. These can later be added to a culture medium and incubated for 72 hours. They are useful for checking the efficiency of the system but they are not an indicator of sterility.

Formaldehyde. This is used in a similar way to ethylene oxide, but COSHH regulations now restrict its use.

Chemical solutions. These are not very effective sterilants and are really only a means of disinfection. Some manufacturers guarantee sterilisation if immersed for a long time – usually 24 hours. This method is useful for equipment that cannot be sterilised by any other means, e.g. endoscopic equipment.

Chlorhexidine-based solutions. These can only be used as disinfectants as chlorhexidine has poor activity against spores, fungi and viruses.

Irradiation. Gamma irradiation can only be used in a controlled environment. Pre-packaged items such as needles and syringes are sterilised in this way.

Heat sterilisation

Dry heat – hot air oven. Dry heat will kill microorganisms by oxidative destruction of the bacterial protoplasm. Microorganisms are more resistant to this method than if heated with moisture, so higher temperatures are required – about 150–180°C. If the temperature is below 140°C then it will not destroy spores in less than 4–5 hours.

Hot air ovens are usually small and economical to run. The oven is heated by electrical elements. The door is usually fitted with a device to prevent opening before it is cool. Any items sterilised must have a long cooling period before they can be used. It is important not to overload the oven, to allow the free flow of air.

Spore strip tests and Browne's tubes can be used to test the sterility in the oven.

Items that can be sterilised by this method include glass syringes, cutting instruments, ophthalmic drill bits, powder and oils that cannot be sterilised with moisture. Fabric, rubber and plastic cannot be sterilised by hot air as they are destroyed by the high temperatures.

Hot air ovens are not recommended, for health and safety reasons.

Steam under pressure – autoclave. This is a common and efficient method of sterilisation. Instruments, drapes, gowns, swabs, most rubber products, glassware and some plastic can be sterilised in this way. Fibre optics, lenses and plastics, however, are usually heat sensitive and are thus easily damaged.

There are three types of autoclave:
- **Vertical pressure cooker** – this is the simplest of autoclaves. It works by boiling water in a closed container. There is an air vent at the top that is closed after the air is evacuated from the container, and the pressure is then allowed to build up to 15 psi. The biggest disadvantage of this system is that the air vent is at the top, so some air may remain trapped underneath the steam; the temperature in that area is lower and sterility cannot therefore be guaranteed. It is also manually operated, so there is room for human error.
- **Horizontal/vertical downward displacement autoclave** – this is a larger and completely automatic autoclave. It uses an electrically operated boiler that is also a source of steam. The air outlet is at the bottom, so the air is driven out more effectively by downward displacement. Usually there is a choice of programmes with

varying temperatures. This autoclave is designed for sterilisation of loose instruments rather than packs, as the drying cycle is insufficient. Damp packs will allow microorganisms to penetrate the pack during the storage period.

- **Vacuum-assisted autoclaves** – this autoclave works on the same principle as the other two, but there is a high-power vacuum pump to evacuate the air from the chamber at the beginning of the cycle. Steam penetration happens quickly and sterilisation is faster. A second vacuum cycle takes the moisture out after sterilisation and dries the load. There is a choice of cycles with different temperatures and pressures. It is suitable for all instruments, drapes and equipment and is fully automatic, with fail-safe mechanisms.

Use of the autoclave

Autoclaves differ but the principle remains the same. Water boils at 100°C and converts into steam, and the temperature of the water therefore remains the same however long the water is heated.

Many bacteria and bacterial spores are resistant to high temperatures no matter how long they are exposed; however, if the pressure is increased the temperature of the steam rises and the bacteria and spores will be killed. It is the increased temperature, not the increased pressure, that destroys the microorganisms, and the higher the temperature the shorter the time needed for sterilisation.

The central sterilising chamber of the autoclave is surrounded by a jacket of steam. When the pressure in the jacket is raised, steam enters the chamber, displacing the air downwards. When all the air is evacuated, the vents close and steam continues to enter the chamber until the desired pressure is reached. The steam condenses on the colder surfaces of the contents of the chamber, producing heat, which penetrates to the innermost layers of the pack – it is the moisture that increases the penetrability of the heat. After a specific time frame the steam is evacuated and the temperature and pressure drop to normal.

Effective sterilisation relies on loading the packs correctly. There must be adequate space to allow the steam to circulate freely. You must not overload the autoclave or block the inlet and exhaust valves. Instruments must also be free of grease and protein material to allow effective penetration of the steam. The autoclave itself should be regularly serviced by a qualified engineer to comply with health and safety regulations and to ensure that effective sterilisation takes place. Any faults should be dealt with immediately, and no further cycles run as equipment may not be sterile and pose risk if used.

Monitoring sterilisation

- **Chemical indicator strips** (TST strips) – these change colour when the correct temperature, pressure and time have been reached. The strips should be placed inside the pack. It is important that the appropriate strip is used for each different time/pressure/temperature cycle or a false result may occur.
- **Browne's tubes** – these change colour when the correct temperature, pressure and time have been reached. They are small glass tubes partly filled with an orange/brown liquid that changes to green when certain temperatures have been maintained for a set length of time. It is

essential that the correct tube is used for the selected cycle.

- **Bowie Dick tape** – this is usually used to seal an instrument or drape pack. It is beige-coloured tape impregnated with a chemical strip that turns dark brown when a temperature of 121°C has been reached. The tape is limited in value, as it does not ensure that the temperature has been maintained for the set time.
- **Spore tests** – these are strips of paper impregnated with dried spores. The paper is placed in a load and on completion of sterilisation it is placed in the culture medium provided and incubated at room temperature for 72 hours. If sterilisation is effective there will be no growth. These tests are more accurate than chemical indicator strips but the delay in results is a major disadvantage.
- **Thermocouples** – these are electrical leads with temperature-sensitive tips. They are placed in various parts of the sterilisation chamber with the leads passed out of an aperture to a recording device. The temperature of the chamber is constantly checked and recorded throughout the cycle.

PACKING SUPPLIES FOR STERILISATION

There are many packing materials and containers available, all with advantages and disadvantages (Table 24.7). Your choice will depend on several factors:

- Size of autoclave.
- Packing material must be resistant to damage.
- Steam or gas must be able to penetrate wrapping for sterilisation to occur and must easily exhaust when sterilisation is complete.
- Microorganisms must not be able to penetrate from the outside of the wrapping.
- Cost.
- Time taken to reach sterility.
- Personal preference.

EQUIPMENT CARE AND STERILISATION

Gowns and drapes

If non-disposable gowns and drapes are being used then they should be washed, dried and inspected for damage. They should be folded correctly (Figs. 24.9 and 24.10) to achieve flat packs and to allow penetration during sterilisation. The outside of the gown should be on the inside so that the surgeon can put it on aseptically. Drapes should be folded in a concertina pattern to allow free flow of steam during sterilisation.

Both gowns and drapes can also be sterilised with ethylene oxide but it is fairly uneconomical because the steriliser is small and the cycle is long. Autoclave sterilisation is much quicker and more efficient. A hot air oven cannot be used as it will burn the material. Gowns and drapes can be sterilised in bags or packs. Hand towels can be placed with the gowns and drapes in the instrument pack.

Swabs

These can be bought pre-sterilised and are fairly inexpensive. Non-sterile swabs are packed into bundles of 5 or 10 – the number of swabs is not important as long as it is consistent and all the staff are aware of the number, which should be written on each individual packet. Swabs may be incorporated into the

TABLE 24.7	Advantages and disadvantages of packing materials used for sterilisation of surgical equipment	
	Advantages	**Disadvantages**
Nylon film (usually sealed with Bowie Dick tape)	Variety of sizes available Reusable	Becomes brittle after repeated use and develops tiny holes, leading to contamination Difficult to remove sterile item without contaminating it on the edges of the bag
Seal and peel pack	Variety of sizes available Can be used with ethylene oxide or autoclave Risk of contamination is small	Paper backing tears easily
Paper	Elastic and conforming	Water-repellent therefore ideal as an outer layer
Textiles (usually linen)	Conforming Strong Reusable	Permeable to moisture
Metal drums	Last for years Use for instruments, gowns and drapes	Expensive Contamination risk every time lid is opened Rarely used now
Boxes/cartons	Inexpensive Reusable	Can only use in autoclave

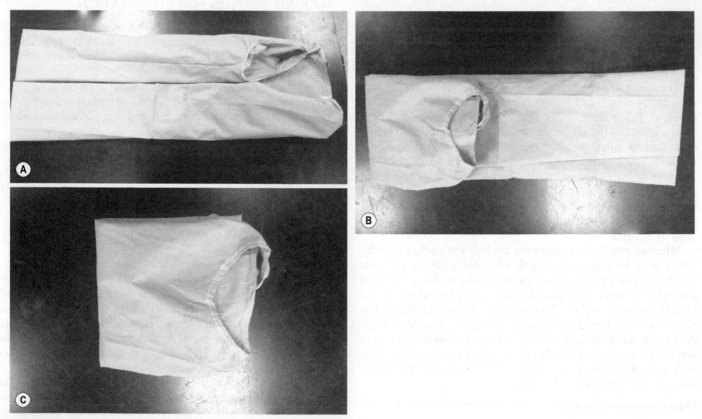

Fig. 24.9 Folding a gown. (A) The gown is laid out flat and the sides are folded into the middle (B). Then concertina it lengthways (C) to achieve a flat pack

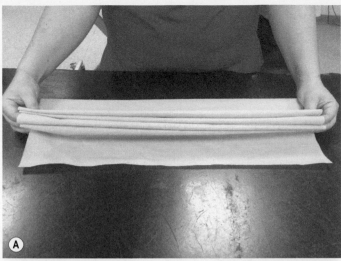

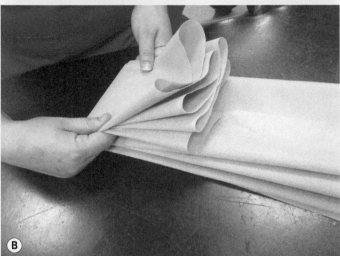

Fig. 24.10 Folding surgical drapes. **(A)** Concertina the cloth width-ways. **(B)** Then concertina lengthways to achieve a flat pack

instrument pack or packaged alone. They can be sterilised in boxes or bags.

Liquids

These are usually bought pre-sterilised but some of the more sophisticated autoclaves have a cycle for sterilising liquids. The risk of breakage is high and it is far more economical to buy commercially prepared fluids.

Power tools

Air drills, saws and mechanical burrs can be autoclaved, but follow the manufacturer's instructions. Autoclaving can cause motors to jam. Ethylene oxide can be used for all air-driven tools. Battery drills usually have a plastic casing that melts in the autoclave, but they can also be sterilised by ethylene oxide. Alternatively, an unsterile drill can be placed in a sterile sleeve with a sterile chuck attached, assembled once in the theatre.

STORAGE AFTER STERILISATION

There should be a separate dry, dust-free, well-ventilated area in the surgical unit for storing sterile packs. A closed cupboard is ideal. Handle the packs as little as possible to minimise damage, and pack loosely on the shelves so that the bags are not damaged. The length of time that sterile packs can be stored is debatable and all packs should carry the date of sterilisation. A sealed pack should remain sterile for a limitless period but it can become contaminated by handling, damage to the pack or moisture, and it is recommended that packs are repacked and sterilised every 6–8 weeks.

BIBLIOGRAPHY

Aspinall, V., 2014. Clinical Procedures in Veterinary Nursing, third ed. Butterworth-Heinemann Elsevier, Oxford.

College of Animal Welfare, 2000. Veterinary Surgical Instruments – An Illustrated Guide. Butterworth-Heinemann, Oxford.

Cooper, B., Mullineaux, E., Turner, L. (Eds.), 2012. BSAVA Textbook of Veterinary Nursing, fifth ed.

British Small Animal Veterinary Association, Gloucester.

Moore, M. (Ed.), 1999. Manual of Veterinary Nursing. British Small Animal Veterinary Association, Cheltenham.

Orpet, H., Welsh, P., 2011. Handbook of Veterinary Nursing, second ed. Wiley & Sons Ltd., Oxford.

Welsh, L. (Ed.), 2009. Anaesthesia for Veterinary Nurses, second ed. Wiley & Sons Ltd., Oxford.

RECOMMENDED READING

Aspinall, V., 2014. Clinical Procedures in Veterinary Nursing, third ed. Butterworth-Heinemann Elsevier, Oxford.
  All tasks performed in the preparation of the surgical environment are described in a step-by-step format with explanations as to why you do it.

Moore, M. (Ed.), 1999. Manual of Veterinary Nursing. British Small Animal Veterinary Association, Cheltenham.
  Includes several useful chapters on surgical procedures and theatre practice.

Orpet, H., Welsh, P., 2011. Handbook of Veterinary Nursing, second ed. Wiley & Sons Ltd., Oxford.
  Many step-by-step instructions for surgical procedures and theatre practice.

Fluid Therapy and Nutritional Support

SAMANTHA MCMILLAN | NICOLA ACKERMAN

KEY POINTS

- Fluid therapy is the mainstay of treatment for shock, with the exception of cardiogenic shock.

- Early recognition of the signs of shock and rapid restoration of the cardiovascular system to optimise tissue oxygen is essential.

- There are options for the administration of fluid therapy including type of fluid, volume needed, rate administered and route given, but these will ultimately all be prescribed by the veterinary surgeon in charge of the case.

- Hydration status of all animals needs to be assessed and addressed before any nutritional support is instigated.

Introduction

Fluid therapy is one of the most frequently administered treatments in veterinary medicine and something that many veterinary nurses will be involved with in some way on an almost daily basis. Many disease processes require differing fluid therapy strategies and fluids are not appropriate in all cases. Before administering fluid therapy a number of simple questions need to be answered:

- Does the animal require fluid therapy?
- What type or types of fluid should be given?
- Which route is most appropriate?
- How much should be given?
- Over what period of time should administration take place?

Each of these questions needs to be carefully considered before a fluid therapy plan can be formulated. It is important to remember that all fluid types do not suit every situation, every patient or every disease process. Some combinations may be completely contraindicated. Fluids can be considered as a drug therapy with dose ranges for different conditions and potential side effects. Before these questions can be answered an understanding of fluid dynamics in the body in the normal animal and in common disease processes is needed. This understanding is vital to know how best to treat each individual animal and its condition as inappropriate fluid therapy can cause more harm than good. Although the veterinary nurse will not often choose the type of fluid that is administered to a patient, it is essential to have a thorough understanding of why different fluids are administered and their potential side effects.

Shock

Shock is a syndrome characterised by a number of clinical signs and essentially caused by decreasing the effective circulating blood volume and poor perfusion to tissues. Shock is generally caused by loss of circulating intravascular volume (hypovolaemic shock), maldistribution of vascular volume (distributive shock) or failure of the cardiac pump (cardiogenic shock). Early recognition, through vigilant monitoring and nursing care, is essential to allow the veterinary surgeon to instigate care. Rapid therapy to restore the cardiovascular system and maintain adequate tissue oxygen delivery is needed to maximise the possibility for successful outcomes in these cases. The main component of treatment for all types of shock, with the exception of cardiogenic, is intravenous fluid therapy. Vascular access is essential in these cases but venous access can sometimes be difficult due to the lack of vascular volume or reduced cardiac output. The type of fluid therapy selected for shock cases will be dependent on the veterinary surgeon's clinical assessment but will often be initiated with lactated Ringer's solution (Hartmann's solution).

CLASSIFICATION OF SHOCK

- **Hypovolaemic shock** results from a reduction in the circulating intravascular volume – either through loss of volume from the intravascular space through haemorrhage or from the extravascular space via vomiting, diarrhoea, severe dehydration, third space losses, burns and neoplasia.
- **Cardiogenic shock** is due to the inability of the heart to pump effectively. This can be caused by valvular insufficiencies, some arrhythmias and cardiomyopathy.
- **Distributive shock** is due to excessive vasodilation. The vascular volume itself has not changed but the vessel size has increased meaning that blood pressure is not maintained resulting in lack of tissue perfusion or oxygen delivery to the tissues. This can occur with systemic inflammatory response syndrome (SIRS).

CLINICAL SIGNS

Hypovolaemia is the most commonly encountered type of shock and monitoring should include heart rate, pulse palpation to assess pulse quality, pulse deficits and rate, mucous membrane colour and capillary refill time. Electronic monitoring that may become essential in shock cases that are worsening includes electrocardiogram (ECG), blood pressure monitoring and pulse oximetry.

In hypovolaemic shock the body tries to compensate for the reduction in cardiac output by causing vasoconstriction, increasing cardiac contractility and increasing heart rate. Clinical signs may be subtle initially and continued monitoring is necessary to evaluate trends in these patients. As hypovolaemia progresses the following clinical signs may be identified in dogs and cats:

- Pale mucous membranes
- Increased capillary refill time (CRT)
- Tachycardia in dogs but either tachycardia or inappropriate bradycardia in cats
- Weak, thready pulse – peripheral pulses such as the dorsal pedal will become weaker before central pulses such as the femoral; in the early stages of hypovolaemia pulses may be easily palpable and be described as bounding; as the process progresses the dorsal pedal pulse is more difficult to palpate before diminishing completely and the femoral pulse becomes weaker
- Depression.

A drop in blood pressure does not normally occur until the hypovolaemia is somewhat advanced due to the compensatory mechanisms. Reduced organ perfusion will ultimately result in signs of organ failure, such as oliguria as a result of kidney failure and death.

Fluid therapy

BODY WATER DISTRIBUTION

In the average healthy patient the total volume of body water is approximately 60% of body weight. There are natural variations to this figure related to species, age, gender and body tissue composition (mainly fat content). Animals less than 6 months of age generally have a higher than average body water percentage at approximately 75% whereas older or obese patients have a reduced percentage of body water which can be as low at 50%.

The largest volume of water within the body is contained within the cells – the intracellular fluid (ICF). This volume comprises approximately 40% of the patient's body weight and two-thirds of total body water composition. Any fluid not contained within the cells is classed as extracellular fluid (ECF). This makes up 20% of body weight and one-third of total body water composition. The extracellular fluid can be further categorised into interstitial fluid, that found in the spaces between cells, at about 15% of body weight; fluid contained within the vascular compartment at about 5% of body weight, including blood vessels; and transcellular fluid at less than 1% of body weight, including cerebrospinal fluid, synovial fluid and bile. Sodium is the main cation in extracellular fluid with most of the body's sodium being contained within this compartment. The main anions in extracellular fluid are chloride and bicarbonate. Extracellular fluid also contains a small amount of the cation potassium. The intracellular compartment has potassium and magnesium as its main cations with most of the body's potassium being contained within cells. The main anions in intracellular fluid are organic phosphates and proteins. A small amount of the cation sodium is also contained within intracellular fluid.

FLUID BALANCE

There are two main homeostatic (balancing) mechanisms that maintain the osmolarity (osmotic concentration) and volume of extracellular fluid within the body; see Figure 6.5 in Chapter 6.

Antidiuretic hormone

When pure water is lost from the body an increase in plasma osmolarity occurs. This is detected by osmoreceptors in the hypothalamus. This stimulates thirst and the release of antidiuretic hormone (ADH) from the posterior pituitary gland. ADH acts upon the distal convoluted tubules of the kidney and increases water reabsorption thus increasing the concentration of urine. The increased water intake and reduction in urinary water loss reduces the osmolarity of ECF back towards normal. If osmolarity decreases due to excessive water intake then ADH secretion is reduced and water reabsorption in the kidneys is reduced increasing urinary water losses.

Renin-angiotensin-aldosterone system

Hypoperfusion of the kidney (decrease in renal blood flow due to low blood pressure) causes the release of renin from juxtaglomerular cells within the kidney. Renin activates angiotensinogen, which converts angiotensin I to angiotensin II. Angiotensin II increases water and sodium reabsorption in the proximal tubules of the kidney. Angiotensin II also mediates aldosterone release from the adrenal cortex. Aldosterone in turn causes increased sodium reabsorption in the distal tubules. This results in an increase in osmolality so also causes increased ADH secretion. This all acts to expand extracellular fluid volume in the face of hypovolaemia.

- The osmolarity (concentration) of extracellular fluid is controlled mainly via water balance.
- The volume of extracellular fluid is controlled by changes in both water and sodium balance.

MAINTENANCE OF BLOOD PRESSURE

Blood pressure is maintained by cardiac output (the amount of blood pumped by the heart in a given period) and by systemic vascular resistance (the tone of blood vessels, mainly arterioles).

Blood pressure = Cardiac output × Systemic vascular resistance

Cardiac output in turn depends on heart rate and stroke volume. Stroke volume is the amount of blood pumped by the heart in a single beat. Increasing heart rate and/or stroke volume will increase cardiac output to an optimal point. It should be noted that above this optimal level further increases in heart rate cause a decrease in stroke volume due to the ventricles not having time to fill in diastole.

The body has compensatory mechanisms in which to maintain blood flow to the vital organs (heart, lungs, brain and to a certain extent the kidneys) when faced with acute or severe reductions in circulating blood volume. In the face of hypovolaemia baroreceptor (pressure receptor) reflexes cause a discharge of the sympathetic nervous system, which increases heart rate and cardiac contractility (strength of heartbeat) thereby increasing cardiac output. Vasoconstriction also occurs to varying degrees. In mild hypovolaemia full compensation is possible and mean arterial blood pressure is maintained. As

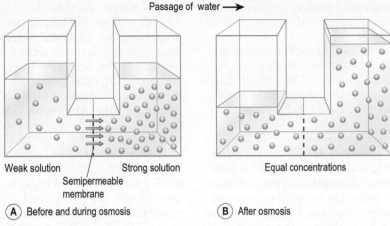

Passage of water ⟶

Weak solution   Strong solution

Semipermeable membrane

(A) Before and during osmosis

Equal concentrations

(B) After osmosis

Fig. 25.1   Processes that occur during osmosis

hypovolaemia becomes more severe the cardiac compensatory mechanisms are unable to increase cardiac output further, but vasoconstriction in the periphery and in the splanchnic circulation increases in an attempt to maintain blood pressure. Blood flow to the major organs is maintained but perfusion to organs such as the gastrointestinal tract is reduced. Once the cardiac and vasoconstrictive mechanisms are maximised progressive hypovolaemia leads to drops in arterial blood pressure and perfusion to the major organs.

FLUID MOVEMENT ACROSS CAPILLARY BEDS

Hydrostatic and colloid oncotic pressure

Fluid movement into and out of a capillary depends on the osmotic pressure of the substances dissolved within plasma and the hydrostatic pressure, as compared to interstitial fluid.

The capillary endothelium is readily permeable to ions and water. The pressure difference between plasma in the capillary and the interstitial fluid, the hydrostatic pressure, will cause movement of fluid and ions from the vessel into the interstitial space (Fig. 25.1).

The capillary endothelium is not readily permeable to larger molecules such as proteins. As smaller molecules tend to balance themselves across the capillary endothelium the osmotic pressure within the capillary is principally determined by plasma proteins. As a result the 'osmotic' pressure of blood is referred to as the colloid oncotic pressure (COP). Albumin generates about 70% of the oncotic pressure of plasma with the remainder made up by globulins.

- Hydrostatic pressure can be thought of as the power of the pressure within the capillary to cause fluid to leave the vessel.
- Colloid oncotic pressure can be thought of as the power of larger molecules (colloids) within plasma to hold/pull fluid within/into vessels.
- Across the capillary bed of a normal healthy animal these forces balance themselves out.

Alterations of hydrostatic pressure or COP can occur in many disease states.

Decreased colloid oncotic pressure in capillaries

Decreased COP in capillaries can occur due to hypoproteinaemia or damaged capillary endothelium.

Hypoproteinaemia, specifically hypoalbuminaemia, causes a drop in COP, which means that fluid has a tendency to leak from the capillaries. This leads to oedema (an increase in interstitial fluid).

Following damage to their endothelium capillaries can leak protein. This occurs in disease processes such as sepsis and SIRS, where runaway inflammation causes damage to the vessel wall. Loss of protein into the interstitial fluid causes a drop in COP and therefore fluid moves from the plasma. This leads to tissue oedema – an increase in interstitial fluid volume.

Decreased hydrostatic pressure in capillaries

If central blood pressure drops, hydrostatic pressure in the capillaries decreases. Reflex arteriolar vasoconstriction also occurs, which further reduces the pressure in the capillary. As a result fluid lost from plasma in the capillary bed is reduced. As the colloid oncotic pressure remains the same there is a net gain of fluid to the plasma across the capillary bed. This leads to an 'auto-transfusion' that helps to compensate for volume loss during hypovolaemia.

Increased hydrostatic pressure in capillaries

Increased hydrostatic pressures can occur due to increased venous pressure. Increased venous pressure in turn can be caused by heart failure or by fluid overload (overzealous fluid therapy).

In each of the above cases the increase of hydrostatic pressure within the capillary bed causes an increase in fluid loss and leads to the formation of oedema. Oedema can form in peripheral tissues or in the lungs. Alternatively if the increase in hydrostatic pressure occurs in the hepatic vasculature ascites can form.

BODY WATER LOSSES

In the healthy animal water is lost via urine and faeces and via respiratory and cutaneous evaporation. Although it can vary, about 20 ml/kg/day of water is lost through urine, 10 ml/kg/day is lost via faeces and a further 20 ml/kg/day is lost through respiratory and cutaneous evaporation. This gives a normal water loss of 50 ml/kg/day; therefore 50 ml/kg/day, or approximately 2 ml/kg/hr, is considered a maintenance fluid rate for adult cats and dogs.

It should be noted that neonates and paediatric patients (cats and dogs) have a higher maintenance fluid requirement of about 75–125 ml/kg/day.

Abnormal water losses can occur through vomiting and diarrhoea, polyuria, haemorrhage, increased evaporation due to pyrexia/hyperthermia or panting, wound exudation, third space losses into the pleural, peritoneal cavity or interstitial space (can also be removed from the body via chest/abdominal drains).

Fluid loss can be acute predominantly from the circulation/extravascular compartment (hypovolaemia), or chronic generalised loss from both the intracellular and extracellular compartments (dehydration). It is vital to understand the difference between hypovolaemia and dehydration in order to appropriately treat these animals. Whether the patient has hypovolaemia or dehydration (or both) can be established through clinical examination of the patient.

Hypovolaemia

Hypovolaemia means 'decreased circulating volume' and it directly affects the perfusion status of the patient. Acute loss of fluid from the circulation causes hypovolaemia. Haemorrhage, vomiting, diarrhoea, severe dehydration, third space losses and severe metabolic disease are the most common causes of hypovolaemia. Hypovolaemia leads to the compensatory mechanisms previously discussed. The degree of the response is proportional to the degree of hypovolaemia. The following clinical descriptions for varying degrees of hypovolaemia are for dogs.

In mild hypovolaemia increases in heart rate (130–150 beats/min), improved contractility and mild vasoconstriction occur. This leads to tall and narrow pulses, rapid capillary refill time (less than 1 second) and normal or slightly pinker mucous membranes.

In moderate hypovolaemia heart rate increases further (150–170 beats/min) and vasoconstriction continues. This leads to a moderate decrease in pulse height and duration, paler than normal mucous membranes and a slightly delayed capillary refill time.

In severe hypovolaemia heart rate increases to its optimal rate (170–220 beats/min) and vasoconstriction is maximised. This leads to severe decreases in pulse height and duration, extremely pale (white/grey/muddy) mucous membranes and a markedly delayed capillary refill time (over 2 seconds).

In cats assessment of hypovolaemia is more challenging than in dogs. Feline heart rates are normally around 170–200 beats/min, their mucous membranes are generally paler than dogs and their pulse profile is smaller and narrower. Hypovolaemia is often accompanied by marked hypothermia in cats. Cats are also prone to inappropriate bradycardia (130–150 beats/min) despite being in severe hypovolaemic or redistributive shock.

Heart rates above 220 beats/min in dogs should raise suspicions of a tachydysrhythmia rather than a compensatory tachycardia. Inappropriate bradycardia alongside other signs of hypovolaemic shock should raise suspicions of a bradydysrhythmia such as is caused by hyperkalaemia secondary to hypoadrenocorticism, acute renal failure or urinary tract obstruction.

Distributive hypovolaemia occurs secondary to runaway inflammation due to disease processes such as sepsis or SIRS. The intravascular space increases but the actual circulating volume remains the same. This leads to a relative hypovolaemia. Patients will be tachycardic with bounding pulses, mucous membranes are generally deep/brick red and capillary refill time is rapid (less than 1 second). Capillary endothelium often becomes 'leaky' and proteins are lost into the interstitium leading to peripheral oedema.

The fluid therapy approach to hypovolaemia is to rapidly replace the fluid lost from the circulation over a short period of time, i.e. at high fluid rates. Fluid therapy for hypovolaemic patients is generally thought of in terms of boluses, e.g. a 20-ml/kg bolus given over 20 minutes. As estimating fluid losses and responses to fluid therapy can be difficult it is often best to give smaller boluses of 10–20 ml/kg over a 10–15-minute period and then reassess the patient and repeat the boluses as necessary rather than to give each patient the 90-ml/kg dose that is often reported for shock. This means that the fluids given are tailored to the individual patient. The target should be to improve the patient's perfusion parameters, stabilising the cardiovascular system and aiming for a more normal heart rate with strong pulses, pink mucus membranes, and a normal 1.5-second capillary refill time – although this may not be possible in many patients without further intervention.

A guideline to the amount of isotonic crystalloid fluid that is required in different states of hypovolaemia over the first hour of therapy is given below. It should be noted that the fluid rate to be administered will always be prescribed by a veterinary surgeon.

- Severe hypovolaemia: dog, 60–90 ml/kg; cat, 30–60 ml/kg
- Moderate hypovolaemia: dog, 30–60 ml/kg; cat, 10–30 ml/kg
- Mild hypovolaemia: dog, 10–30 ml/kg; cat, 5–10 ml/kg

Where pre-existing cardiac, respiratory or brain disease is identified fluid therapy should be approached with caution and may be contraindicated. It is therefore vitally important to establish if diseases of these systems are contributing factors to the animal's condition as far as is possible during the clinical assessment of the patient as this may change the fluid plan.

Fluid therapy for the replacement of acute losses causing hypovolaemia must be replaced by the intravenous (or intraosseous) route. Multiple catheters can be placed to facilitate this in large animals. Remember, the gauge of the catheter is the most important factor determining the rate of fluid that can be administered.

Dehydration

As opposed to hypovolaemia (loss of circulating volume) dehydration is loss of water from the entire body. As circulating volume only makes up a twelfth of total body water, losses from the circulation are generally small until dehydration becomes severe.

Dehydration of under 5% tends not to cause any clinical signs. Dehydration of about 5% will cause dry mucous membranes only. Between 6% and 12% dehydration will lead to increasing severity of reduced skin turgor (skin tent), increased heart rate and reduced pulses. At 12–15% the fluid loss will be sufficient to start displaying worsening signs of hypovolaemic shock. By 15% dehydration the patient will be moribund and severely hypovolaemic.

Body weight can be used as a guide of dehydration in hospitalised patients. Dehydrated patients receiving fluid therapy should be weighed twice daily on accurate scales; this is an

BOX 25.1 MOVEMENT OF FLUID

Osmosis – the movement of water through a semipermeable membrane from an area of low concentration to an area of high concentration (see Fig. 25.1). The cell membrane is said to be semipermeable, permitting the passage of some substances but not of others. Osmosis will continue through it until the concentration is equal on either side. The pressure that must be applied to prevent this movement is called the osmotic pressure or potential

Isotonic – osmotic pressure is equal to that of the plasma and refers to solutions which cause no transfer of fluid either into or out of a cell

Hypertonic – solutions with an osmotic pressure higher than that of plasma

Hypotonic – solutions with an osmotic pressure lower than that of plasma

Diffusion – the movement of substances from an area of high concentration to one of low concentration. The substances are passing down a diffusion gradient

especially important element in the hydration status of exotic species.

For the animal that is dehydrated but not obviously hypovolaemic, fluid, electrolyte and acid/base deficits should be replaced over a 24–48-hour period. Fluid therapy tends to be thought of as multiplications of maintenance, for example, for an isotonic crystalloid solution 'twice maintenance' would be a rate of 4 ml/kg/hr (if maintenance is considered 2 ml/kg/hr). An estimate of the fluid deficit should be made. For every 1% dehydration there is a fluid deficit of 10 ml/kg and this should be added to the patient's maintenance requirement. This deficit should then be replaced over a 24–48-hour period. The general guideline is to replace half of the deficit over 6–12 hours and then reduce the rate to replace the remaining deficit over a longer period.

Pure water and hypotonic fluid loss

Pure water loss is rare in small animals and is generally seen in animals that produce large volumes of hyposthenuric urine, i.e. diabetes insipidus. This increases the osmolarity of the extracellular fluid. Fluid loss is distributed throughout the body and volume loss from the circulation is minimal. Animals do, however, commonly have a free water deficit due to water deprivation.

Hypotonic fluid loss is where water is lost in excess of sodium. This is seen in some animals with vomiting and diarrhoea and in animals with chronic renal failure. See Box 25.1 for definitions regarding the movement of fluid.

Isotonic fluid loss

Bleeding is an example of isotonic fluid losses. In these cases there is no change in osmolarity so no water movement occurs until compensatory mechanisms begin.

Hypertonic fluid loss

Hypertonic fluid can be lost in severe secretory diarrhoea such as parvovirus and haemorrhagic gastroenteritis. Loss of hypertonic fluid from the circulation causes hypovolaemia and also leads to extravascular fluid becoming hypotonic. This causes further movement of fluid from the extravascular space into the intravascular compartment worsening the hypovolaemia.

HYPERVOLAEMIA/FLUID OVERLOAD

Everyone involved in the administration of fluid therapy should be aware that it is not a benign treatment. In most healthy animals mild and often moderate increases in circulating volume can be dealt with relatively easily by the cardiovascular system, the lymphatics and the kidneys. However, in animals with cardiac insufficiency, respiratory disease, inflammatory disease, anuric/oliguric renal failure, or hypoalbuminaemia or in animals receiving massive overdoses of fluids, large increases in hydrostatic pressure can occur and lead to increased interstitial and third space fluid accumulation.

Initial signs of fluid overload are serous nasal discharge, tachycardia, polyuria, unexpected/unanticipated weight gain, jugular venous distension and potentially jugular pulsations. This can then develop into peripheral oedema ('pitting' oedema) generally best noted over the hock/Achilles tendon and bony prominences. Pulmonary oedema can also occur, which will clinically manifest itself as tachypnoea, dyspnoea and harsh lung sounds leading to pulmonary crackles. Fluid can also leak into the peritoneal and pleural cavities causing ascites and pleural effusion respectively. Ultrasound can be used to confirm the presence of free pleural or peritoneal fluid. Animals prone to ascites should be both weighed and have their abdominal girth measured regularly during hospitalisation. Generally (if infection is not involved) it is only worth performing large volume abdomino-centesis or thoraco-centesis if there is associated clinical signs of dyspnoea or discomfort as fluid can reform rapidly.

This potential is higher in cats who have a lower cardiovascular reserve and where the incidence of subclinical heart disease is high. A heart murmur or gallop is an indicator that fluid therapy needs to be monitored carefully. In some animals overaggressive fluid therapy can uncover previously asymptomatic cardiac insufficiency. Regular assessment of the major body systems (cardiovascular, respiratory and neurological) and of body weight should be carried out in all animals receiving fluid therapy to help avoid these problems.

Treatment should include immediate alteration of the fluid therapy regimen and diuretics may be necessary.

ELECTROLYTE AND ACID/BASE ABNORMALITIES

Electrolyte levels and pH are maintained within tight limits in the body in order to preserve normal cellular function. Fluid, electrolyte and acid/base balance are intrinsically linked and it is difficult to consider one without the others; however, it is beyond the scope of this chapter to discuss this in its entirety.

Alongside the treatments stated it is also vitally important to correctly treat the disease process causing the abnormality.

Acid/base

Via metabolic reactions the body continually produces CO_2, a volatile acid (from carbohydrates and fats), and H^+ ions (from proteins and phospholipids). CO_2 is excreted via the lungs and H^+ ions are excreted via the kidneys. The body uses buffering systems to facilitate handling of the acid load (to keep blood pH normal) and to a small extent this can help with pathological increases in acid load. Bicarbonate is the most important buffer in the body although haemoglobin and plasma proteins also play a role. Bicarbonate is continually regenerated by the kidneys and returned to the circulation.

Normal blood pH in dogs is 7.35–7.45. If pH is lower (more acidic) this is an acidaemia. If pH is higher (more alkaline) this is an alkalaemia. The processes that cause acidaemia and alkalaemia are termed acidosis and alkalosis. There are respiratory and metabolic causes of both acidosis and alkalosis. A respiratory cause of an acidosis/alkalosis is caused by alterations in CO_2. Increased CO_2 causes an acidosis and decreased CO_2 an alkalosis. A metabolic cause of an acidosis/alkalosis is caused by alterations in acid/alkali other than CO_2.

The body can compensate for a respiratory acidosis/alkalosis to a certain degree by altering renal acid excretion and bicarbonate reabsorption but this can take hours to days. The body can compensate for a metabolic acidosis/alkalosis by increasing or decreasing ventilation in the lungs, respectively, thus increasing or decreasing removal of CO_2 from the blood; this can take minutes. In most cases of acid/base disturbances the underlying cause and any electrolyte disturbances should be treated rather than trying to treat the acidaemia or alkalaemia directly.

Sodium abnormalities

As sodium balance is intrinsically linked with water balance and circulating volume disorders of sodium balance are generally thought of in terms of the patient's volume status.

Hypernatraemia can occur in hypo-, normo- or hypervolaemic patients. Hypovolaemic hypernatremia occurs when water is lost in excess of sodium. Some cases of vomiting, diarrhoea and renal failure are prime examples of this. Hypervolaemic hypernatraemia occurs due to salt toxicity or the overzealous administration of sodium-rich fluids, especially hypertonic saline.

Normovolaemic hypernatraemia is caused by pure water loss and can occur with water deprivation/hypodipsia, diabetes insipidus and hyperthermia.

Signs can vary from lethargy to severe depression and even coma and depend on the severity of hypernatraemia and the speed of onset. These neurological signs are due to cerebral dehydration as water moves from the brain into the blood via osmosis.

Treatment means altering the patient's fluid therapy plan to drop the sodium levels at a desired rate. In patients with chronic hypernatraemia the brain is able to adapt, meaning a sudden drop in sodium levels can cause cerebral oedema and therefore deterioration in clinical signs. In most patients with severe hypernatraemia the administration of 0.9% sodium chloride is appropriate as, although it is sodium rich, it will have lower sodium than the animal's serum and therefore will help dilute it. Alternatively, Hartmann's (lactated Ringer's or compound sodium lactate) or Ringer's solution can be used. In a chronically hypernatraemic patient the aim should be for an hourly decrease of 0.5 mmol/L/hr. Acutely hypernatraemic patients can have their sodium levels dropped more rapidly. Animals with pure water deficits can receive 0.45% sodium chloride or 5% dextrose administered over 24 hours. The deficit can be calculated by the following equation.

$$\text{Free water deficit (L)} = 0.6 \times \text{current body weight}$$
$$\times [(\text{Current sodium level}) - 1]/(\text{Normal sodium level})$$

Hyponatraemia can also occur in hypo-, normo- and hypervolaemic patients. Hypervolaemic hyponatraemia is caused by reduced water excretion and seen in congestive heart failure, hepatic disease and renal disease such as nephrotic syndrome.

Normovolaemic hyponatraemia can be caused by hypotonic fluid administration, psychogenic polydipsia or inappropriate ADH secretion. Hypovolaemic hyponatraemia occurs when there is sodium loss in excess of water loss; this occurs in disease processes such as hypoadrenocorticism and in some cases of vomiting and diarrhoea. Clinical signs are generally related to the rapidity of onset rather than the severity of the deficit. Again signs are neurological but this time in acute cases the low sodium in serum as compared to the brain promotes water movement into the brain by osmosis thus leading to cerebral oedema. Patients with hypervolaemic hyponatraemia may develop oedema or ascites. In chronic cases the brain has time to adapt to the change in tonicity so cerebral oedema does not generally occur.

Patients with hypovolaemic hyponatraemia should receive volume resuscitation with isotonic crystalloid solutions. It is vital to establish the cause of hyponatraemia prior to commencement of fluid therapy. Hypervolaemic hyponatraemic patients, especially those with congestive heart failure, cannot tolerate fluid therapy and may need diuretic therapy if oedema is present. This is especially important in animals with left-sided congestive failure when failure to diagnose pulmonary oedema can be rapidly fatal.

Chronically hyponatraemic patients should have their sodium levels returned to normal at a rate of 0.5 mmol/L/hr to avoid the formation of cerebral dehydration which may occur with more rapid replacement.

Potassium abnormalities

Hyperkalaemia is an acutely life-threatening condition as high potassium levels will effect cardiac cell conduction by affecting membrane potentials. This can cause severe bradycardia and eventually asystole. The most common causes of hyperkalaemia are decreased urinary excretion due to anuric or oliguric renal failure, uroabdomen, urethral obstruction or hypoadrenocorticism. Other less common causes include massive cell death due to reperfusion injury, for example following aortic thromboembolism, severe trauma or heat stroke. If the patient is hypovolaemic fluid therapy with isotonic crystalloids (either Hartmann's solution or 0.9% sodium chloride) will dilute the potassium levels. Either is suitable as, although Hartmann's solution contains low levels of potassium, it does not clinically affect the lowering of serum potassium levels. In fact as hyperkalaemic patients often have a metabolic acidosis, sodium chloride can prolong recovery as it is an acidic solution. For animals with electrocardiographic changes associated with hyperkalaemia calcium gluconate can be given intravenously; 0.5–1.5 ml of a 10% solution works rapidly and lasts for 15–30 minutes. Although this does not reduce the potassium it does act to stabilise myocardial membrane potentials. Another treatment option is to administer regular insulin and glucose. This lowers serum potassium levels as potassium is taken into cells alongside glucose due to the action of insulin. This takes 20–30 minutes to work and the patient requires prolonged glucose infusions to prevent hypoglycaemia. Bicarbonate can also be used to drive potassium into cells by changing blood pH but it is rarely necessary.

Hypokalaemia can be caused by three things:
1. Decreased intake, e.g. anorexia and inappetance (or long-term fluid therapy without potassium supplementation)

TABLE 25.1	Guidelines for potassium supplementation of intravenous fluids with potassium chloride	
Serum potassium	Potassium chloride (KCl) that should be added to 1 litre of fluid
3.5–5.0 mmol/l	20 mmol
3.0–3.5 mmol/l	30 mmol
2.5–3.0 mmol/l	40 mmol
2.0–2.5 mmol/l	60 mmol
<2.0 mmol/l	80 mmol

Adapted from Boag (2007).

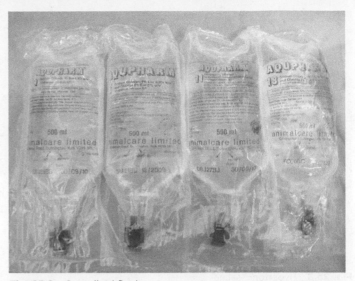

Fig. 25.2 Crystalloid fluids

2. Increased losses via the gastrointestinal tract (vomiting/diarrhoea) or via the urinary tract (chronic renal failure or diuresis, physiological or pharmacological)
3. Movement of potassium from the extracellular compartment into the intracellular compartment, i.e. with insulin therapy or alkalaemia.

Hypokalaemia generally causes non-specific signs of weakness, lethargy, anorexia and ileus. Severe muscle weakness manifesting itself as ventroflexion of the neck can be seen. Hypokalaemia should be treated by supplementation. Mild hypokalaemia with no overt clinical signs can be treated with oral supplementation (sometimes just the patient eating is needed). Intravenous supplementation should be administered in moderate to severe hypokalaemia where clinical signs are apparent. Supplementation should not be given at rates in excess of 0.5 mmol/kg/hr as myocardial conduction can be effected. Supplementation guidelines for different serum potassium levels are given in Table 25.1. Fluids containing potassium supplementation should be clearly marked and should not be bolused.

Chloride abnormalities

Hyperchloraemia commonly accompanies hypernatraemia. Normally treating the hypernatraemia is all that is required.

Hypochloraemia is caused by a loss of chloride-rich fluids such as occurs in gastric vomiting, when chloride is lost with hydrogen ions. This causes a metabolic alkalosis. Retention of sodium alongside bicarbonate in the hypovolaemic patient promotes this alkalaemia.

Treatment is through administration of chloride-rich fluid. Sodium chloride 0.9% is the treatment of choice. It should be given at rates to treat the hypovolaemia and then to counter ongoing losses.

Calcium abnormalities

Calcium is found in three forms in the body – ionised 55%, complexed 10% and bound to albumin 35%. Elevations and reductions in albumin levels especially can have a major action on total calcium levels but do not affect ionised calcium. Renal failure can increase total calcium by increasing complexed calcium levels. Ionised calcium is the biologically active form. Calcium homeostasis is controlled by the actions of parathyroid hormone, calcitonin and calcitriol. Calcium intake is via the gastrointestinal tract and excretion is controlled by the kidneys. Bone acts as a large store of calcium in the body.

Hypercalcaemia has many causes, including neoplasia, primary hyperparathyroidism, acute renal failure, hypoadrenocorticism, granulomatous infection (i.e. lungworm disease), vitamin D toxicosis (some rodenticides and psoriasis cream) and bone diseases. In cats idiopathic hypercalcaemia is possible.

Vague non-specific signs are associated with hypercalcaemia but polyuria/polydipsia is common alongside the signs of the underlying disease. Hypercalcaemia affects the kidney by impairing its ability to respond to ADH. This reduces the concentrating ability of the kidney forcing it to produce relatively dilute urine despite often having a prerenal azotaemia. Mineralisation of the kidney can lead to renal failure.

Although treatment depends on identifying and treating the underlying disease process, if clinical signs are apparent hypercalcaemia should be treated. Initial treatment should be in the form of diuresis with 0.9% sodium chloride. In addition to this furosemide can be given at 1–2 mg/kg 2–4 times daily. Glucocorticoids will also decrease calcium but may effect diagnostic tests so may make a diagnosis more difficult. Salmon calcitonin or drugs called bisphosphonates can also be administered.

Hypocalcaemia can be caused by hypoparathyroidism (primary, iatrogenic post-thyroidectomy or nutritional secondary), chronic renal failure, acute pancreatitis, intestinal malabsorption, hypovitaminosis D, massive transfusion of blood products and eclampsia. Clinical signs are related to hypocalcaemia causing increased excitation of skeletal muscle known as tetany. Facial pruritus is a common sign alongside muscle tremors, stiff muscles, panting, excitability and hyperthermia. Again treatment depends on identifying and treating the underlying disease. Patients with clinical signs should be treated with calcium gluconate; 0.5–1.5 ml of a 10% calcium gluconate solution can be administered intravenously slowly over 15–30 minutes (monitoring an electrocardiograph as arrhythmias are possible). Alternatively the dose can be diluted and given subcutaneously in several places. This is not ideal as it causes pain on injection and can cause tissue mineralisation and necrosis.

FLUID TYPES – CRYSTALLOIDS

Crystalloids are a group of solutions containing electrolyte, e.g. Na^+ and Cl^-, and non-electrolyte solutes, e.g. glucose, lactate and bicarbonate, all of which are capable of entering all body compartments (Fig. 25.2). They can be split into further groups

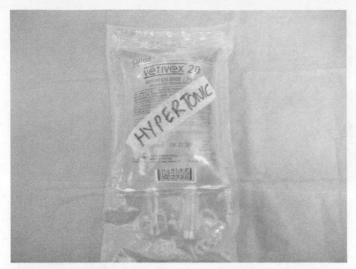

Fig. 25.3 Hypertonic saline

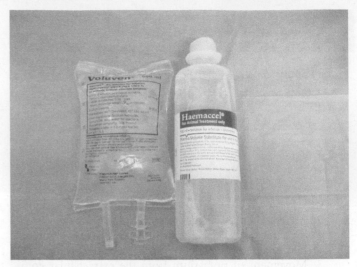

Fig. 25.4 Examples of colloids

according to their tonicity (the effective osmolality/concentration of a solution) compared to plasma, i.e. isotonic, hypertonic and hypotonic. Crystalloid solutions primarily exert their effects on the intracellular and interstitial compartments.

Isotonic

This is the most frequently used group of fluids in veterinary practice. They can be used to treat both hypovolaemia and dehydration and this group can be split further into replacement and maintenance isotonic crystalloids. Isotonic replacement crystalloids have an electrolyte composition that closely mimics that of the extracellular compartment with a reasonably high sodium concentration with little or no potassium. These fluids include Hartmann's solution (lactated Ringer's or compound sodium lactate), normal saline (0.9%) and Ringer's solution. When administered to the hypovolaemic patient these fluids do not constitute a change in concentration gradient between the intracellular and extracellular compartments and therefore do not cause water to move across the cell membrane. It should be noted that only approximately 20% of the infused crystalloid will remain in the vascular space 1 hour after intravenous administration. When replacement fluids are used for long-term fluid therapy the patient's serum potassium will become diluted causing the patient to become hypokalaemic and potassium supplementation should be considered. Serum sodium will often show a slight increase but this is generally not clinically significant.

Isotonic maintenance crystalloid solutions have an electrolyte composition that is designed to provide the electrolytes lost due to insensible losses. These fluids are not often used in veterinary practice with the primary one being Plasma-lyte M. They have a much higher potassium concentration than the replacement fluids with a conversely lower sodium concentration. This makes them only useful at maintenance rates, i.e. 2 ml/kg/hr.

Hypertonic saline

Hypertonic saline, NaCl 7.2%, has approximately 8 times the sodium concentration of plasma (Fig. 25.3). This means that when this solution is administered intravenously it creates a steep osmotic gradient causing water to be drawn rapidly and

in large quantity into the vascular space from the interstitial and intercellular compartments. This quickly increases intravascular volume with a small dose of solution, e.g. 4–7 ml/kg in the dog and 2–4 ml/kg in the cat given over approximately 5 minutes. The effects will, however, be short-lived as the sodium diffuses out of the vascular compartment within approximately 30 minutes of administration, similar to the duration achieved with isotonic crystalloids.

Hypertonic saline is useful where very rapid restoration of intravascular volume is required, i.e. severely hypovolaemic patients. It is contraindicated in patients who have severe dehydration, hypernatraemia, volume overload or uncontrolled haemorrhage. Serum sodium concentration should be closely monitored as hypernatraemia can be caused by administering more than one dose of this solution in quick succession. Hypertonic saline is also often used to treat raised intracranial pressure.

Hypotonic

Hypotonic crystalloid solutions include 0.45% NaCl, 0.18% NaCl with 4% glucose, and 5% glucose. There are very specific uses for these solutions, e.g. patients with pure water deficits, and they should be used with care. Infusion of hypotonic solutions can cause dilution of plasma electrolytes, especially sodium, and in extreme cases may result in acute cerebral oedema. Glucose-containing solutions can be considered as isotonic solutions while in the bag; however, once they are administered to the patient the glucose is metabolised by cells and only free water remains. Free water rapidly passes out of the vascular space and distributes across total body water. This means that these solutions are not suitable for vascular volume restoration in hypovolaemic patients and are really only the fluid of choice for patients suffering from pure water loss.

FLUID TYPES – COLLOIDS

The main reason for the use of artificial colloids is for volume expansion in the face of hypovolaemia and to provide colloid oncotic pressure (Fig. 25.4). Colloids are retained in the vascular space for longer than crystalloids. The length of time colloids remain within the vascular space generally relies on

TABLE 25.2	Colloids described according to type, molecular weight and COP			
Name of fluid	Type of fluid	Number molecular weight (kD)	Mean molecular weight (kD)	Colloid oncotic pressure (mm Hg)
Haemaccel®	Gelatine	–	35	26–29
Gelofusin®	Gelatine	23	30	33
Dextran 70	Dextran	39	70	40
Hetastarch 6%	Hydroxyethyl starch	69	450	30–35
Pentastarch 10%	Hydroxyethyl starch	12	264	30–40
Tetrastarch and Voluven®	Hydroxyethyl starch	–	130	≈30
Oxyglobin®	Polymerised haemoglobin	–	65–500 (≈200)	38

their molecular size (assuming microvascular permeability is normal). These solutions are described according to their number molecular weight (Mn), which is the total weight of all the molecules divided by the total number of molecules (Table 25.2). Artificial colloids contain a mixture of molecules of different molecular weights with the hydroxyethyl starches having a wider range of molecular weights than the gelatines or dextrans.

Gelatines

The two main gelatine-based solutions used are Haemaccel and Gelofusine. These solutions are created from the hydrolysis of bovine collagen. Gelatines have a shorter duration of action than the other colloids due to their smaller molecular size. The gelatines have been shown to be less antigenic and have minimal effects on coagulation compared to other synthetic colloids. Haemaccel also contains calcium and should not be administered alongside blood products. These are currently the only commercially available colloids in the UK.

Dextrans

Dextrans are prepared from macromolecular polysaccharides. They are supplied in both low- and high-molecular-weight forms, i.e. dextrans 40 and 70. Dextran is in part excreted unchanged by the kidneys, in the face of normal renal function, and the rest of the molecules are slowly metabolised to glucose by the liver. Dextrans can prolong bleeding times by interfering with fibrin clot formation, decreasing factor VIII and von Willebrand's factor, diluting clotting factors and affecting platelet function. These are not commercially available in the UK.

Hydroxyethyl starch

This group of colloids is derived from amylopectin, which is a form of plant starch. These solutions include Pentastarch, Hetastarch, Tetrastarch and Voluven. There has been some concern over the starch-based colloids and coagulopathy. It seems that the lower-molecular-weight hydroxyethyl starches have fewer effects on coagulation, e.g. Voluven, compared to the larger-molecular-weight starches, e.g. Hetastarch. Hydroxyethyl starch solutions usually increase plasma volume by at least the volume administered with the degree of expansion depending largely on the solution concentration. The hydroxyethyl starches have the longest duration of action of the three colloid groups. There is considerable controversy surrounding the use of starches. Recent human studies have demonstrated that the use of hydroxyethyl starch in sepsis resulted in the increased rates of acute kidney failure and increased morbidity and this has

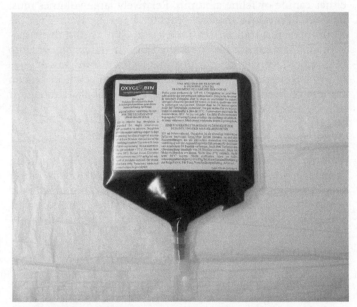

Fig. 25.5 Oxyglobin

resulted in the majority of these products not currently being available.

Polymerised haemoglobin

This solution contains polymerised bovine haemoglobin contained within a modified lactated Ringer's solution to provide oxygen-carrying capacity as well as colloidal support for patients where blood products are not available. Polymerised bovine haemoglobin is a powerful colloid. Oxyglobin is the product available for this purpose (Fig. 25.5). The dose listed for dogs is 10–30 ml/kg at a rate up to 10 ml/kg/hr; however, clinically much lower administration rates are often used. This product is licenced for intravenous use in dogs but not in cats in the UK. An off-label dose for cats is suggested as 10–15 ml/kg administered at 1 ml/kg/hr but this should only be administered with specific, informed consent from the owner and administered with caution.

Side effects include discolouration of the sclera, mucous membranes and urine. In dogs rates of administration over 10 ml/kg/hr are associated with increased central venous pressure, which can then lead to pulmonary oedema or other respiratory signs of fluid overload. In cats pleural effusion and pulmonary oedema have been found commonly in patients to whom polymerised haemoglobin has been administered.

Oxyglobin can alter results of serum chemistry tests depending on the dosage administered, the time since infusion and the analyser and reagents used. Plasma haemoglobin concentrations should be monitored using a haemoglobinometer. Urine dipstick analysis will be inaccurate while gross discolouration of the urine is present.

NATURAL COLLOIDS – ALBUMIN

Human serum albumin is available commercially and has been used in some institutions to treat small animals with hypoalbuminaemia. There is a risk of anaphylaxis when using human albumin in canine and feline patients as it is not identical to either canine or feline albumin. Relatively large volumes must be given to produce an effective increase in the patient's plasma albumin concentration. The increase in COP within the vascular compartment is transient as the albumin quickly moves into interstitial compartment, which may worsen third space losses in some conditions. Currently there are limited clinical data on the use of human albumin in veterinary patients, although it may be effective in certain situations.

Adverse effects of colloids

Volume overload. As previously discussed colloid solutions remain in the vascular compartment for considerably longer than crystalloids. This poses an increased risk if too much fluid is administered either accidentally or prescribed. Particular care should be taken in patients with pre-existing cardiac disease.

Renal failure. The kidneys are the major route of excretion for all synthetic colloids. They should be used with caution in patients with anuric or oliguric renal failure, especially low-molecular-weight dextrans, which have been reported to cause renal failure by blockage of the renal tubules and/or osmotic nephrosis.

Coagulopathy. Larger colloid molecules have a greater effect on coagulation than smaller molecules. The exact mechanism of coagulopathy caused by synthetic colloids is unknown but it would appear that it is directly related to the concentration of synthetic colloid within the intravascular compartment. Coagulation abnormalities will not occur in every case but the possibility should be considered as in a small number of cases it can result in significant bleeding. This side effect is generally only seen when doses greater than 20 ml/kg/day are administered of high-molecular-weight hydroxyethyl starch or dextrans.

Anaphylaxis. Anaphylactic reactions have been reported for all of the synthetic colloid groups. It should be noted, however, that the incidence of anaphylactic reaction to synthetic colloids is extremely low.

FLUID TYPES – BLOOD PRODUCTS

Blood types

Red blood cell types are classified according to antigens present on the surface on the cell. These antigens are inherited and species-specific.

Canine blood types. Canine blood types are described using the dog erythrocyte antigen (DEA) system. Seven canine blood groups have been described but typing sera are only available for six: DEA 1.1, 1.2, 1.3, 4, 5 and 7. For all of the DEA groups a dog may be determined as positive or negative for each. The relevance of each blood type is related to its potential to cause antigenic reactions. DEA 1.1 is the most antigenic blood type. DEA 1.1 is also the only group that can be easily tested 'in house' with testing kits and cards. As dogs have no naturally occurring alloantibodies to this type a transfusion reaction is unlikely from a transfusion with the first unit of incompatible DEA 1.1 blood; however, a DEA 1.1–negative dog that is transfused with DEA 1.1–positive blood will become sensitised and antibodies will be produced following exposure to the DEA 1.1 antigen. This means that if a further transfusion with DEA 1.1–positive blood is given during this patient's life then a transfusion reaction can result. Following sensitisation to an antigen it takes approximately 4 days for the antibodies to be produced after which time any further units being administered to the patient must be crossmatched. Transfusion reactions as well as being attributed to DEA 1.1 incompatibilities have also been shown to be significant in DEA 4–negative dogs given DEA 4–positive transfusions. DEA 7 is thought to be structurally related to an antigen in bacteria and a naturally occurring antibody against it has been found in some DEA 7–negative dogs. It could pose therefore some significance in transfusion reaction. It has been suggested that the ideal universal donor type should be negative for DEA 1.1, 1.2 and 7.

Feline blood types. There are currently three described feline blood types: A, B and AB. Unlike dogs, cats have naturally occurring alloantibodies against type A or type B cells. This means that typing all cats prior to transfusion is essential. Type B cats have strong antibodies against type A cells whereas type A cats have weaker antibodies against type B cells. This means that the risk of transfusion reaction is greatest when a type B cat is given type A blood. There is no universal donor type for cats and each cat should be blood typed and receive type-specific blood. Blood type AB is extremely rare and fortunately these patients do not require blood from an AB donor and can be given type A blood.

Crossmatching

Cross matching allows detection of antibodies in the plasma of the recipient or donor that may result in a transfusion reaction.

For canine recipients crossmatching is required if:

- The patient has received a previous transfusion more than 4 days ago
- The patient has a history of transfusion reaction
- The patient has previously been pregnant
- The patient has an incomplete medical history, e.g. a rescue dog where the owners cannot be sure if a previous transfusion has been given.

Feline recipients should be crossmatched if they require more than one transfusion.

The major crossmatch assesses the compatibility between the donor red blood cells and the recipient plasma or serum. The minor cross match assesses the compatibility between the donor plasma or serum and the recipient's red blood cells (Box 25.2).

1. Collect Ethylenediaminetetraacetic acid (EDTA) samples from both the recipient and donor.
2. Centrifuge both samples at 1000 × g for 5 minutes.
3. Using pipettes remove the plasma and transfer into separate tubes and label.
4. Wash the red blood cells with normal saline, centrifuge as step 2 and discard supernatant. Repeat 3 times.
5. Re-suspend the red blood cells with normal saline to make a 3–5% solution.
6. For each potential donor mix 1 drop of donor red cells with 2 drops of recipient plasma – major crossmatch.
7. For each potential donor mix 2 drops of donor plasma with 1 drop of recipient red cells – minor crossmatch
8. For the recipient control mix 2 drops of recipient plasma with 1 drop of recipient red cells.
9. Incubate all tubes at room temperature for 15 minutes.
10. Centrifuge tubes at 1000 × g for 15 seconds.
11. Observe tubes for signs of haemolysis.
12. Shake tubes gently to re-suspend cells.
13. Observe for signs of agglutination.

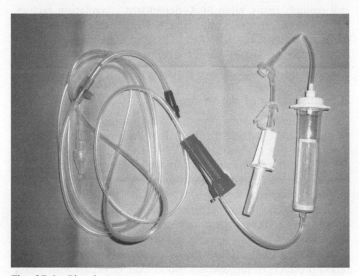

Fig. 25.6 Blood-giving set

Blood products

Changes in legislation over the last decade have seen the development of several commercial blood banks in the UK. This has meant that practices are no longer relying on finding a whole blood donor in an emergency. This has seen the promotion of the use of component therapy, which until several years ago was only available to the large university hospitals. The availability of blood components (i.e. packed red blood cells, fresh frozen plasma, stored frozen plasma, cryoprecipitate and cryo-poor plasma) means that transfusion therapy can now be specifically targeted to replace like with like and therefore lowers the likelihood of transfusion reactions. Unfortunately component therapy is not yet available for cats and most practices still rely on whole blood donors. All blood products should be administered through a specialised blood-giving set or in-line filter (Fig. 25.6).

Fresh frozen plasma. Fresh frozen plasma (FFP) is separated from the packed red blood cells and frozen within 8 hours of the unit being collected. The anticoagulant contained within the blood bag system is collected in the plasma fraction following separation. FFP provides clotting factors V and VIII as well as the other more stable clotting factors and plasma proteins. Plasma should ideally be placed in the freezer 6 hours after the unit has been collected to ensure thorough freezing prior to the 8-hour cut-off point. FFP can be stored for 1 year at −20°C. FFP may be indicated for coagulopathies, vitamin K deficiency, disseminated intravascular coagulation (DIC) (although this remains a topic of some debate) and patients with severe liver disease. FFP is also often utilised in hypoproteinaemic patients; however, it should be noted that large volumes and repeated transfusions may be required to achieve and maintain a clinically significant increase in the patient's plasma proteins. The dose of plasma is generally 10 ml/kg given over approximately 4 hours in the normovolaemic patient. Hypovolaemic patients will generally need to be given the plasma dose at a faster rate depending on the condition being treated.

Stored frozen plasma. Stored frozen plasma (SFP) is plasma that was not separated and frozen within the 8-hour window following collection. SFP can also be FFP that has been allowed to thaw and then been refrozen or FFP that has been stored for longer than 1 year. The more fragile coagulation factors V and VIII are lost. SFP may still be used to provide colloidal support and some vitamin K–dependant coagulation factors. Stored frozen plasma may be stored for five years at −20°C.

Fresh whole blood. Fresh whole blood (FWB) is collected aseptically and used within 8 hours of collection. It contains red blood cells, platelets, all coagulation factors and plasma proteins (Fig. 25.7). FWB not used within 8 hours of collection may be stored in a refrigerator at 1–6°C for up to 35 days depending on the anticoagulant used. FWB may be the only available source of blood products in some practices, although with the increase of blood banking component therapy has become increasing available. If components are available then FWB is generally only required for patients with anaemia in the face of other haemostatic complications. A general rule for administration of whole blood is that 2 ml/kg of whole blood will raise the packed cell volume (PCV) by 1%. A more accurate formula to calculate the required amount of whole blood for transfusion is as follows:

$$\text{Volume (ml)} = \text{Total blood volume}$$
$$\times [(\text{Desired PCV} - \text{Actual PCV})]/\text{Donor PCV}$$

Blood volume is about 90 ml/kg in the dog and about 60 ml/kg in the cat.

Packed red blood cells. Packed red blood cells (PRBCs) is the component remaining after the unit has been centrifuged and the plasma including the anticoagulant removed (Fig. 25.8). A 450-ml unit of whole blood will yield approximately 200 ml of PRBCs. This volume yield is obviously dependant on donor PCV. PRBCs should be stored upright in a refrigerator at 1–6°C. PRBCs may be stored for 20 days or up to 35 days if a red cell preservative such as Adsol is added to the red cells after the plasma is extracted. PRBCs are primarily used in anaemic patients. The initial dose for PRBCs is usually 6–10 ml/kg and will be continued until clinical signs improve.

Cryoprecipitate. This component is prepared by thawing FFP at 0–6°C. A precipitate forms which is removed from the plasma

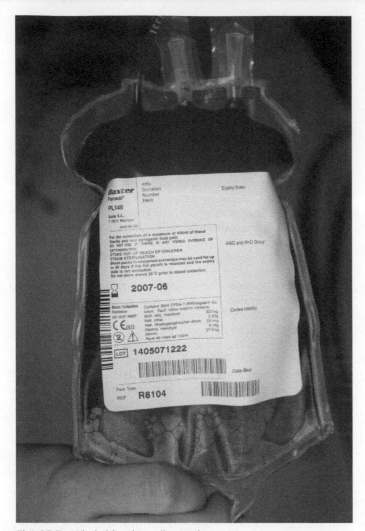

Fig. 25.7 Whole blood in collection bag

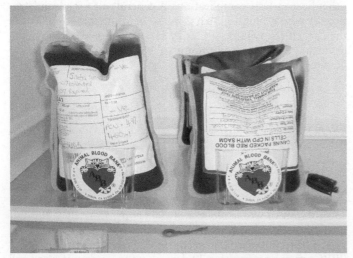

Fig. 25.8 Blood products

by centrifugation. The resulting components, cryoprecipitate and cryo-poor plasma, can then be refrozen. Cryoprecipitate contains a source of concentrated von Willebrand's factor, factors VIIIc and XIII and fibrinogen. Cryoprecipitate is the component therapy of choice for patients with von Willebrand's

disease. Cryoprecipitate can be prepared from a unit of FFP within 12 months from the date of collection. The cryoprecipitate and cryo-poor plasma (cryo supernatant) can then be stored for up to 1 year from the original date of collection of the unit. The administration of desmopressin (DDAVP) to the donor prior to collection of the unit will increase the yield of von Willebrand's factor in the resulting plasma or cryoprecipitate. In addition to its use in patients with von Willebrand's disease, cryoprecipitate may be administered to patients with bleeding due to a factor VIII (haemophilia A) or fibrinogen deficiency/disorder. The normal dose is 1–2 ml/kg given over 1 hour. Patients with severe deficiencies may need up to 5 ml/kg. Doses can be repeated every 30 minutes as necessary to provide coagulation factors.

Cryo-poor plasma/cryo supernatant. This is the plasma collected following centrifuging of FFP to produce cryoprecipitate. This can be refrozen and stored in the same way as cryoprecipitate. This component is plasma without the von Willebrand's factor, factors VIIIc and XIII and fibrinogen. It does however still contain many vitamin K–dependant coagulation factors, i.e. factors II, VII, IX and X, which makes it useful for the treatment of rodenticide toxicity. It may also be used for other coagulopathies that do not require the cryo components and hypoproteinaemia.

Administration of blood products

Examine the bag containing the blood product carefully prior to use. Is it the correct product? Is it the right blood type for the patient (for FWB and PRBC)? Is it within the expiry date? Also check that the bag is not damaged in any way and that the contents are of a normal colour and consistency.

Blood products should ideally be administered through a dedicated intravenous catheter, although they can be given through an intra-osseous catheter in an emergency where venous access is not possible. A specialised blood-giving set containing a filter should be used for administration of all blood products to remove any blood clots or debris which may cause an embolism. A specialised in-line filter can be utilised for cats where blood has been collected in syringes and is being administered via a syringe driver.

PRBCs and whole blood do not need to be warmed prior to administration unless they are being administered to very small patients or neonates where hypothermia is a consideration or if large volumes are to be administered. Plasma and cryoprecipitate require thawing prior to administration. The best way to do this is to use a water bath set at 37°C. It is important not to overheat the plasma as damage can easily be caused to the fragile plasma proteins and clotting factors.

Medication should never be administered through lines and catheters dedicated to blood products. Fluids containing calcium such as Hartmann's solution can cause coagulation if administered alongside blood through the same catheter as the calcium and can overcome the anticoagulant properties of the citrate. Fluids containing glucose can cause haemolysis of red cells. Consequently the only fluid that can be administered alongside blood products is normal saline 0.9%.

The rate of whole blood administration is often suggested at 0.25–1 ml/kg/hr for the first 15 minutes of the transfusion. If no signs of a transfusion reaction are encountered then the rate can be increased to deliver the remaining volume of whole blood over 4–6 hours. In patients with cardiac disease rates of 4 ml/kg/hr should not be exceeded.

Prior to transfusion the patient's PCV and total solids (TS) should be measured. PCV and TS should then be rechecked immediately following transfusion and then at 12 and 24 hours following transfusion.

Transfusion reactions

Careful observation of all patients receiving blood products is essential to quickly detect signs of a transfusion reaction. Heart rate, respiratory rate and temperature should be taken and recorded every 10 minutes for the first half hour of the transfusion and then every 15–30 minutes thereafter. Patients should be observed for signs of pyrexia, vomiting, diarrhoea, urticaria, tachypnoea, tachycardia, dyspnoea, haemoglobinaemia, and haemoglobinuria.

There are several types of transfusion reaction which may occur with the acute transfusion reactions occurring during the transfusion or within the first hour or so following the transfusion. Delayed transfusion reactions occur after the transfusion has been administered and may not be apparent for weeks to months after the transfusion.

Acute haemolytic immunological transfusion reaction. This type of transfusion reaction occurs because antibodies are present in the plasma of either the donor or the recipient that elicit an immune response. This is the type of reaction seen by a type B cat receiving type A blood or a DEA 1.1–negative dog that has been exposed to DEA 1.1–positive antigens and then exposed to them again through a second transfusion. Clinical signs may include pyrexia, vomiting, restlessness, salivation, lethargy, icterus, muscle tremors, collapse, haemoglobinaemia and haemoglobinuria. This type of reaction can quickly lead to shock, DIC and in some cases acute death. The transfusion should be stopped immediately if this type of transfusion reaction is suspected. Clinical signs should be treated and fluid therapy initiated. Antihistamines such as chlorphenamine and corticosteroids such as dexamethasone may be administered. These patients should continue to be closely monitored once the transfusion has ceased. This should include routine monitoring as well as arterial blood pressure, urine output (the kidneys are often damaged in this type of transfusion reaction) and thoracic auscultation. Central venous pressure monitoring may be warranted if the patient is critically ill following the reaction or if fluid overload is suspected.

Acute non-haemolytic immunological transfusion reactions. These are acute anaphylactic reactions. This is often a reaction to other cells and substances within the transfusion but not the red blood cells. Clinical signs include urticaria, dyspnoea, vomiting, oedema, erythema and pruritus. The transfusion should be immediately stopped. The anaphylaxis should be treated with chlorphenamine, corticosteroids and fluid therapy as necessary.

Delayed immunological transfusion reactions. This type of reaction typically occurs between 2 and 21 days following transfusion. These reactions can rarely be prevented by blood typing and crossmatching and are more likely to occur in patients that have been sensitised to red blood cell antigens through pregnancy or a previous transfusion. Compatible blood may have been given but the patient may have developed antibodies to any of the hundreds of red cell antigens present on the red cell surface. The owner may notice that the patient has become icteric and/or anorexic. Fever is the most common clinical sign on examination and PCV may have decreased.

Non-immunological transfusion reactions. This category encompasses reactions as a result of changes to blood during collection, storage or administration. Examples of this type of reaction include sepsis caused by transfusion of blood contaminated with bacteria, hyperkalaemia in patients receiving considerable volumes of stored blood (some cells haemolyse during storage, releasing potassium into the storage media), ionised hypocalcaemia due to the citrate contained within the anticoagulant, hypothermia in small patients receiving large volumes of refrigerated blood products, dilution of coagulation factors and volume overload.

Delayed non-immunological reactions include the transmission of an infection from donor to recipient via a transfusion. An example would be the transmission of feline immunodeficiency virus between cats and illustrates why a vigilant donor screening programme is imperative.

MONITORING FLUID THERAPY

Monitoring the patient undergoing fluid therapy is essential. While many of the observations and vital parameters recorded will be the same as for any patient under our care, there are some specific parameters and their interpretations that can help us to ensure the fluid therapy plan is accurately tailored to the patient.

The following parameters should be monitored:

- Pulse rate, rhythm and profile – the pulse profile represents the height/amplitude of the pulse as well as the width/duration of the pulse. It is essential to appreciate the pulse profile of resting, normovolaemic patients to enable recognition of abnormal pulse profiles.
- Heart rate and rhythm – this should include auscultation of the heart for any murmurs or abnormal rhythms.
- Respiratory rate, effort and pattern – this should include auscultation of lung fields to detect harsh lung sounds and crackles that could indicate fluid overload.
- Mucous membrane colour and capillary refill time.
- Skin turgor.
- Temperature.
- Body weight.
- General demeanour and mental status.
- Urine output.
- Central venous pressure if indicated.
- Arterial blood pressure if indicated.
- PCV/TS and electrolytes.

Body weight

This can be used as a monitoring tool for fluid resuscitation in dehydration. Dehydrated patients should gain weight following appropriate fluid therapy. Weighing the patient several times a day is necessary and will help estimation of fluid gain or fluid loss. If the patient's weight continues to decrease despite fluid therapy it can be assumed that on-going losses, e.g. high urine output (especially in cases of *E. coli* pyelonephritis and renal tubular disease), diarrhoea, vomiting, salivation or evaporative losses caused by pyrexia, hyperthermia or panting, are higher than the rate of fluid being administered and this should be addressed. Note that an increase in body weight in a patient that was not dehydrated to begin with may indicate that the patient is becoming fluid overloaded.

Urine output

Both hypovolaemia and dehydration can cause renal perfusion to become decreased. It is necessary to carefully monitor urine output to ensure adequate urine production is maintained by the fluid being administered. Normal urine production in the dog and cat is between 0.5 and 2 ml/kg/hr. The aim is to achieve 1–2 ml/kg/hr with a urine specific gravity of approximately 1.025 in the dog and 1.035 in the cat. In most cases this will be achieved with fluid therapy alone but in some conditions pharmacological intervention may be necessary.

The best way to monitor urine output is by placing an indwelling urinary catheter, which can either be connected to a urine collection system or drained via a bung at regular intervals. It may be possible to try and measure all the urine produced in ambulatory patients by catching the urine in receptacles and measuring it; however, this is time consuming and often not very accurate as some urine is invariably spilled. Another way often described is to weigh the urine-soaked bedding of recumbent patients but the author feels that from a nursing perspective this is unacceptable and will lead to the patient becoming urine-soaked and scalded when an indwelling catheter could be placed.

Urine should be drained from the bung or collection system on a regular basis, usually every 4 hours, in a strictly aseptic manner. The volume of urine drained should be recorded and the ml/kg/hr calculated and recorded with the veterinary surgeon being notified if the result is abnormal. The specific gravity of the urine should also be checked and recorded.

Central venous pressure

Monitoring central venous pressure (CVP) is a technique that can be utilised in critically ill patients undergoing fluid therapy. Individual CVP measurements will not give us an accurate picture of a patient's volume status but by monitoring trends we can build up a much more accurate picture when this is used alongside other monitoring techniques. CVP is the pressure measured in the patient's vena cava directly in front of the right atria. A central venous catheter must therefore be placed to facilitate CVP measurement. In addition to giving us information about the patient's intravascular volume, CVP can also be used to provide information on cardiac output.

The central venous catheter is placed aseptically into the right jugular vein. The brown port on the central catheter (if there is more than one port present) is connected to a manometer line filled with heparinised saline. This manometer line is then attached to a pressure transducer on an anaesthetic machine or intensive care unit monitor to produce a CVP trace and mean reading. Alternatively the measurement can be taken manually using a water manometer. These can be bought commercially or created using drip tubing, a three-way tap, a ruler and a syringe. The patient's central catheter in connected to one piece of drip tubing containing normal saline and connected at the other end to a three-way tap with drip tubing connected to each port. The second piece of drip tubing connected to the middle port of the three-way tap is placed vertically against a ruler and filled with saline to at least 20 cm via the third port on the three-way tap. The zero on the ruler should be level with the three-way tap, which in turn should be level with the

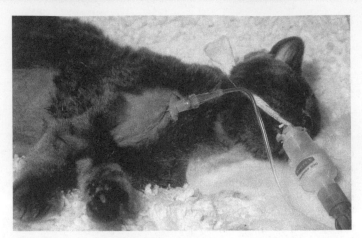

Fig. 25.9   Intra-osseous needle placement

patient's right atria. The three-way tap is turned to allow communication between the patient's central catheter and the vertical water column. Fluid will move backwards and forwards until it equilibrates with the patient's CVP, which can then be read manually on the ruler from the top of the meniscus on the water column.

Normal CVP is 0–5 cm H_2O. Low CVP can be indicative of decreased venous return whereas a high CVP may indicate volume overload, right-sided heart failure or increased intrathoracic pressure.

ROUTES OF FLUID ADMINISTRATION

The route of administration of fluid therapy will depend very much on hydration status, disease process and patient compliance.

Oral

This route is really reserved for patients whose disease process does not prevent them from eating and drinking normally, are not more than mildly dehydrated and do not have any degree of hypovolaemia. It can be used in addition to an intravenous fluid therapy plan and oral or feeding tube fluid intake should be taken into account when calculating a patient's fluid therapy plan.

Intravenous

This is the route of choice in hypovolaemic patients and those requiring blood component therapy. Intravenous access is essential in any critically ill patient.

Intra-osseous

This route can be an excellent choice in small patients or neonates where intravenous access is difficult especially if they are dehydrated or volume depleted (Fig. 25.9). This route is restricted to short-term access in emergency situations but provides good access to the vascular system via the medullary capillary beds until vascular access can be gained.

Intraperitoneal

This is a potentially hazardous route of administration and does not offer any advantage over other routes and is therefore generally redundant as a route of fluid administration.

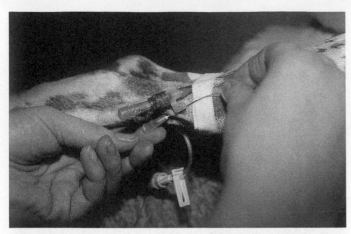

Fig. 25.10 A long catheter has been placed in the saphenous vein of a dog using the Seldinger technique. The catheter has been secured with tape and tissue glue, and sutures are being used to secure it further

Subcutaneous

This can be an inexpensive and convenient route for administering maintenance fluids in patients that do not need vascular access for ongoing fluid therapy or medication. The fluids used must be isotonic. This route is not indicated for fluid replacement. Complications associated with administering fluid via this route include pain, infection, inflammation, electrolyte imbalances, cellulitis and skin necrosis.

VASCULAR ACCESS

The type and insertion site of catheters will depend on the reason they are being placed, what they are to be used for, disease processes present (e.g. a jugular catheter may not be suitable for a coagulopathic patient), what will be administered through it, how long it needs to remain and place and the technical ability of the person placing it.

Peripheral catheters

Reasons to place peripheral catheters:
- Inexpensive and less technically challenging
- Well tolerated by most patients
- Easily accessible for quick catheterisation
- Generally minimal restraint required compared to central venous catheter placement
- Fewer significant complications compared to central venous catheters.

Sites for insertion include:
- Cephalic and accessory cephalic
- Medial and lateral saphenous
- Auricular – especially useful in rabbits and Bassett Hounds
- Dorsal common digital veins.

The lateral saphenous vein is larger than the medial saphenous vein in the dog and vice versa in the cat (Fig. 25.10).

Over-the-needle catheters are the most commonly used type for peripheral placement and can also be placed as a quick and easy method of central catheter placement in the cat. They are inexpensive, easy to place and are suitable for short- to medium-term use. Over-the-needle catheters can be left in place for 48–72 hours. There are also relatively few complications associated with placement of these catheters. They

comprise a needle with a closely fitting catheter over the needle and bonded to it. A wide variety of materials, lengths and gauges are available.

It should be noted that fluid flow through a catheter is related to the length and radius of a catheter. Catheter radius (r) has the greatest effect with flow related to r^4 therefore halving the diameter will result in a 16-fold decrease in flow.

Equipment required for the placement of a venous peripheral catheter (Box 25.3):
- Alcohol hand rub
- Non-sterile gloves
- Clippers
- 2% chlorhexidine gluconate solution
- Lint-free swabs
- Sterile applicator containing 2% chlorhexidine gluconate in 70% isopropyl alcohol
- Intravenous catheter the appropriate size for the patient
- T-connector or bung – if a T-connector is used this should be flushed with saline or heparinised saline in an aseptic manner prior to catheter placement
- Tape to secure the catheter
- Syringe and needle filled with saline or heparinised saline.

Central venous catheters

Central venous catheter placement is extremely useful in many situations:
- Administration of multiple drugs and fluids
- Administration of fluids with high osmolarity
- Administration of drugs by constant rate infusion known to cause phlebitis, e.g. mannitol, pentobarbital and diazepam
- Measurement of CVP
- Repeated blood sampling
- Total parenteral nutrition (TPN) – the high osmolarity of solutions used for TPN due to the lipid component not included in partial parenteral nutrition (PPN) make it essential for administration via a central catheter
- Long-term venous access – to reduce the repeated placement of peripheral catheters.

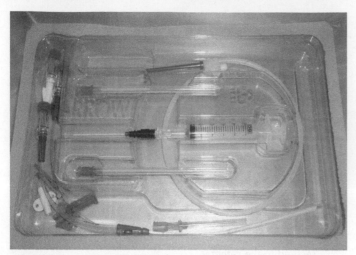

Fig. 25.11   Central venous line kit – Seldinger technique

Central venous catheter insertion sites include the jugular vein and the lateral and medial saphenous veins. In theory the cephalic vein could be used but catheters frequently will not pass the elbow and this is not a recommended site of insertion.

The placement of all central catheters should be done aseptically wearing sterile gloves. A large area over the vein should have been clipped and surgically prepared. A sterile drape is necessary when placing jugular catheters via a Seldinger technique or if the catheter is to be used for TPN.

Through-the-needle catheters

This type of catheter can be further categorised into those where the needle remains attached to the catheter outside of the vein in a protective guard and those placed using a 'peel-away' technique where the catheter is inserted through a plastic guide that can be peeled away and discarded. Through-the-needle catheters with attached needle guard are relatively inexpensive and technically quite easy to place (Fig. 25.11 and Box 25.4). The presence of the needle and needle guard makes these catheters bulky and more difficult to secure than those placed by the 'peel-away' or Seldinger techniques.

'Peel-away' catheter placement is similar to that used in the through-the-needle technique with the exception that it is surrounded by a peel-away sheath. The gauge of the catheter is limited to that of the peel-away sheath.

This method is very similar to the placement of the through-the-needle catheter. Steps 1–8 are performed as described in Box 25.4. Once the needle and sheath placement are confirmed by bleeding the needle is removed, leaving the sheath in place within the vein. The catheter is placed as above and once fully advanced the sheath is peeled apart by grabbing the tabs and pulling outwards and upwards. Once the sheath has been removed the catheter can be secured, flushed and bandaged as above.

Over-the-wire catheter – Seldinger technique

This technique uses a smaller introducing catheter or needle than other techniques and uses a guide wire to facilitate access to vessels or hollow organs. It can be used to place single- or multi-lumen catheters. It is also useful for replacing a catheter in the same location. The Seldinger technique for a multi-lumen catheter is described in Box 25.5.

BOX 25.4   PLACEMENT OF THROUGH-THE-NEEDLE CATHETERS WITH ATTACHED NEEDLE GUARD

1. Apply alcohol hand rub to hands using the WHO method.
2. Don non-sterile gloves.
3. Clip and aseptically prepare (2% chlorhexidine gluconate in a back-and-forth motion with lint-free swabs followed by sterile application of 2% chlorhexidine gluconate in 70% isopropyl alcohol) a large area of skin over the vein.
4. Pre-measure the catheter before beginning the procedure:
   a. For a jugular catheter the aim is for the tip of the catheter to lie in the cranial vena cava just cranial to the right atrium. This can be achieved by measuring the distance from insertion to the first rib.
   b. For peripherally inserted central catheters (PICCs) the distance from insertion to the vena cava is measured.
5. Reapply alcohol hand rub using the WHO method and then don sterile gloves using the open gloving technique.
6. Flush the central catheter with heparinised saline at this point to avoid air embolism.
7. All ports should be capped after flushing.
8. A sterile fenestrated drape should be used.
9. An assistant is asked to raise the vein without interfering with the surgical site.
10. The needle is aligned as close as possible to the longitudinal axis of the vein and the needle tip inserted into the vein. A flashback of blood should be seen.
11. Once the entire needle tip is within the vein the needle is stabilised and the catheter threaded into the vein.
12. Once the catheter is fully advanced into the vein pressure is applied over the venepuncture site and the needle backed out of the vein.
13. Once the bleeding has stopped the needle guard can be secured around the needle.
14. All ports should be aspirated (to avoid air embolism and check that blood flows freely), flushed with heparinised saline, capped and clamped (Fig. 25.12).
15. The catheter can then be sutured in place.
16. The catheter is then covered with a sterile dressing and bandaged appropriately.

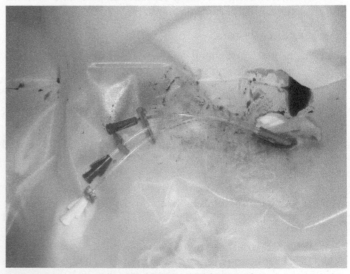

Fig. 25.12   Central lines flushed and clamped

Peripherally inserted central catheters

Peripherally inserted central catheters (PICCs) can be placed using either a through-the-needle or Seldinger technique. The catheter is inserted through a peripheral vein (usually a saphenous vein) and fed through so that it is lying within the vena cava

BOX 25.5 PLACEMENT OF OVER-THE-WIRE CATHETERS BY THE SELDINGER TECHNIQUE

1–4. Steps 1–4 are the same as for the through-the-needle techniques (see Box 25.4).

5. All ports should be capped after flushing with the exception of the distal port (usually the brown port), which is the one the guide wire will pass through.

6. A sterile fenestrated drape is placed over the vein.

7. An assistant is asked to raise the vein without interfering with the surgical site.

8. The vein is identified and a stab incision is made over the vein with a number 11 blade (the assistant should cease raising the vein while the stab incision is made).

9. The introducer needle or catheter is introduced through the incision and into the vein in a positive manner. A flashback of blood will be seen in the needle/catheter hub.

10. Once in the vein the guide wire will be introduced through the needle. The guide wire has a J tip to prevent damage to the vessel wire and it is normally necessary to wind this back so that it lies within the tip of the plastic wire introducer before inserting the wire into the needle. The ECG should be monitored during guide wire placement as arrhythmias will be seen if the guide wire is introduced too far and aggravates the myocardium. The guide wire should be introduced slowly to a pre-measured distance.

11. The needle can then be removed, leaving the guide wire in place. The guide wire should be held onto at all times to prevent embolism.

12. A vessel dilator is then fed over the wire and inserted into the vein using a twisting action to produce a larger hole in the skin and vessel wall for the catheter to pass through. Haemorrhage will occur when this is withdrawn as you have made a hole in the vessel larger than the guide wire. Pressure can be applied to minimise this as the dilator is removed.

13. The central catheter can then be fed onto the guide wire via the distal port until the proximal end of the guide wire protrudes from the hub of the catheter.

14. The catheter can then be fed into the vein and the guide wire removed.

15. All ports should be aspirated (to avoid air embolism and check that blood flows freely), flushed with heparinised saline, capped and clamped.

16. The catheter can then be sutured in place.

17. The catheter is then covered with a sterile dressing and bandaged appropriately.

BOX 25.6 CATHETER CARE AND MAINTENANCE

- All catheters should be checked at least twice daily. This should include unwrapping the bandaging and checking the site for oedema, erythema, discharge, unpleasant smell, contamination, pain and thickening.
- Central catheters and peripheral catheters used for PPN should be covered with a sterile dressing prior to bandaging.
- Care should be taken to ensure jugular bandages are not too tight as this may restrict breathing.
- Toes should be regularly checked for swelling.
- The area immediately above the bandage should be checked regularly for extravasation of fluid.
- When handling peripheral catheters gloves should be worn.
- When handling central catheters, peripheral catheters used for TPN or any vascular access sites in critically ill patients, sterile gloves *must* be worn.
- Catheters should be flushed regularly to check patency. If the catheter is not in continuous use this should be done every 4 hours. If the catheter is being used continuously then this should be done twice a day when unwrapping the bandaging. This should include the flushing of all ports on central catheters
- Swab injection ports with surgical spirit prior to injecting into them.
- Always check the catheter is patent before injecting medication into it.
- Prevent patient interference as necessary.
- Routine use of topical antimicrobial or antibiotic ointments is not recommended.
- Disconnection of fluid lines should be avoided and if necessary aseptic technique must be employed to reduce catheter contamination.
- Monitor the temperature of patients with vascular catheters and remove them if an unexplained temperature ensues.
- Catheters that are no longer required should be removed.
- Central catheters that no longer allow blood to be aspirated should be removed and/or replaced.
- It is recommended that all intravenous tubing and containers be changed every 48 hours or more often if contaminated.

(see Fig. 25.10). This requires pre-measurement of the catheter from the point of insertion to the vena cava.

Complications

Catheter care is exceptionally important, and catheters must be regularly checked for any complications (Box 25.6).

Catheter displacement. There is always a risk of displacement of any catheter. Needle catheters and stiff plastic catheters are more likely to cause perforation of the vein than polyurethane or silicone catheters. All catheters should be correctly secured and carefully monitored to prevent this. Flushing of catheters to check placement prior to administering drugs is essential. Extravasation of fluid may go unnoticed for several hours if the catheter has become dislodged. This is often indicated by oedema proximal to the catheter insertion site and pain on palpation of the area. If displacement of the catheter is suspected it should be immediately removed and a new catheter placed at a different site. The area can then be gently massaged at regular intervals to disperse the fluid and should be moni-

tored for signs of further complication. If irritant fluids or drugs have been administered perivascularly the consequences may be more severe and could cause necrosis and sloughing of the surrounding tissue. Displacement of central venous catheters may not become evident until much larger volumes of fluid have been displaced. This may lead to mediastinal or pleural effusions resulting in dyspnoea. Penetration of the right atrium is possible, although not common, with central catheters resulting in pericardial effusion from haemorrhage and cardiac tamponade.

Phlebitis. This is the inflammation of the vessel wall due to damage of the endothelial lining. Catheter sites should be checked regularly for pain, oedema and erythema, which may indicate phlebitis and potential secondary infection. Phlebitis can be caused by mechanical damage to the vessel (i.e. movement of the catheter within the vein), administration of highly osmolar fluids and infection. The presence of phlebitis will make the patient more susceptible to further complications such as endocarditis.

Thrombosis/thromboembolism. This is the formation of a thrombus on the catheter itself or on the vessel wall. These blood clots may occlude the catheter if they form within the lumen but those that form between the catheter and vessel wall are less obvious. Thrombi can become dislodged and form a thromboembolism. Diseases that predispose the patient to hypercoagulability will increase the risk of thrombosis (e.g. cardiac disease).

Catheter embolism. This is a rare but serious complication and occurs when a portion of the catheter breaks off and enters the circulation. This may occur due to a patient chewing the catheter or when cutting through the catheter bandage.

Infection. Catheter contamination and infection is usually caused by poor aseptic technique either on catheter placement or during subsequent management. Bacteria can easily track along the length of the catheter and into the vascular system. Pyrexia of unknown origin in critically ill patients should prompt replacement and culture of all vascular catheters.

Air embolism. This can occur with any indwelling venous catheter. The highest risk is with central venous catheters. The ports on these catheters should never be left open to the air. Clamps are present to allow closure of the catheter ports when the catheter hub is open, i.e. when aspirating blood, connecting fluid lines etc. It is also advisable to flush central catheters prior to placement. Air embolism is also possible if fluid-giving sets are not correctly run through before connection to the patient. In most cases small air emboli will remain in the pulmonary vasculature and have no adverse effect; however, large volumes of air will be rapidly fatal.

Exsanguination. This can occur whenever a catheter becomes disconnected from its bung, T-connector or fluid-giving set. The greatest risk is with arterial catheters as blood can be lost rapidly, which is especially problematic in small patients who can quickly lose a large proportion of their blood volume. Significant blood loss is not a common complication with venous catheters. All patients with intravenous catheters should be observed at regular intervals.

Intra-osseous catheter placement

This can be a useful technique where venous access is not possible, i.e. puppies, kittens and small mammals or animals in severe circulatory collapse. This is generally an emergency technique employed to administer large volumes of fluid therapy or emergency drugs into the marrow cavity where they can be quickly absorbed into the vasculature (see Fig. 25.9). This route can be utilised until vascular access is possible.

The following sites may be used:
- The wing of the ileum
- The medial aspect of the trochanteric fossa of the femur
- The proximal tibia
- The greater tubercle of the humerus.

The only contraindication is a fracture present in the bone to be used but care should be taken in young animals not to damage the growth plates.

Hypodermic needles or spinal needles can be utilised if intra-osseous catheters are not available. The area of insertion into the skin should be clipped and prepared in a sterile manner. The limb should be held firmly in one hand. The catheter can then be placed by aiming the needle's shaft down the bone parallel to the long axis. Resistance should be felt as bone is hit but this will reduce as the needle enters the marrow cavity. Once

in place the needle should feel secure in the bone and movement of the needle will move the limb. Saline should freely infuse into the marrow. These catheters are difficult to secure and will be displaced if the patient becomes active. This makes them really only suitable for short-term use.

The complication rate is low but complications may include osteomyelitis (especially if aseptic technique is poor), extravasation of fluid and pain.

The procedure for setting up a fluid infusion:
1. Remove the administration set from the packaging, and ensure the correct type of administration set is being used.
2. Turn off the flow regulator.
3. Check that the fluid bag is in date, fluid is clear (unless a blood product or Oxyglobin) with no deposits and the packaging is not damaged in any way.
4. Remove the fluid bag from the outer packaging and the drip stand.
5. Remove the protective tabs from the spike on the administration set and the insertion point on the bag of fluids.
6. Insert the administration set into the fluid bag using an aseptic technique – the spike of the administration set should not be touched during this process.
7. Squeeze the chamber on the administration set until it is one-third to one-half filled with fluid.
8. Slowly release the regulator to fill the drip line and then close the regulator when the fluid line is completely filled.
9. No significant air bubbles should remain within the line and there should not be any wastage of fluid if the regulator was turned on slowly and carefully.

Calculation of fluid administration rates. Things that need to be ascertained:
- The volume to be given, as directed by the veterinary surgeon – this may require calculating if given as ml/kg or ml/kg/hr
- How many hours the veterinary surgeon wishes for this to be delivered over
- The drip factor of the giving set

Drip factors for giving sets:
- Standard set: 20 drops/ml
- Paediatric set: 60 drops/ml
- Blood-giving set: 15 drops/ml

NB: This is provided as a guideline only and manufacturers' instructions should always be checked; for example some blood-giving sets are 20 drops/ml.

Calculations:

Total fluid required/Hours to be given over = ml/hr

Millilitres per hour/60 minutes = ml/min

Millilitres per minute × drip factor in drops/ml = drops/min

Examples:

A 25-kg dog requires 2 ml/kg/hr on a standard giving set

Millilitres per hour = 2 ml × 25 kg = 50 ml/hr

50 ml/hr ÷ 60 minutes = 0.83 ml/min

0.83 ml/min × 20 = 16.67 (17) drops per minute, i.e. 1 drop every 3.5 seconds

A 3.5-kg cat requires 105 ml over 3 hours using a paediatric giving set

TABLE 25.3	Clinical signs associated with dehydration
Water deficit (%)	**Associated clinical signs**
0–5	Concentrated urine, polydipsia, no clear clinical signs
5–7	Reduction in dermal elasticity (tenting), slightly sunken eyes, dry mucous membranes, increased capillary refill time, rapid weak pulse
7–10	Tented skin remains in place, sunken eyes, anuria, extremities, depression, weak pulse
10–12	Progression into shock phase, comatose, death usually inevitable

Millilitres per hour = 103 ml/3 hr = 35 ml/hr

35 ml/hr ÷ 60 minutes = 0.58 ml/min

0.58 ml/min × 60 = 34.8 or 35 drops per minute, i.e. 1 drop every 1.7 seconds

Fluid therapy can be a complex and often confusing area but this can be broken down by evaluating each patient and its fluid requirements individually and by considering a few simple questions. It is the 'gold standard' to replace like with like in terms of fluid loss so a range of fluid solutions should be considered, including crystalloids, colloids, polymerised bovine haemoglobin and blood component therapy. It will often be the decision of the veterinary surgeon in charge of the case as to which fluid the patient will be given but veterinary nurses should have a firm understanding of fluid types, administration rates, potential side effects and the monitoring required.

Assessing hydration status

There are various measurements and observations used to determine a patient's hydration status (Table 25.3), which include the following:

- Capillary refill time (CRT) – the gum is blanched by finger pressure and time taken for the gum to return to normal colour is recorded; in a dehydrated patient this may take a longer time than a healthy CRT.
- Dry mucous membranes are indicative of a dehydrated patient and can also be assessed while carrying out the CRT.
- Observing eye position within the socket – retraction of the eye back into its socket indicates that the patient is dehydrated.
- Dermal elasticity – this may be carried out by gently pinching or tenting the patient's skin. In a healthy patient the skin should resume its normal form almost immediately but in cases of dehydration there will be less elasticity within the skin and it will take longer to resume a normal position. This assessment is objective and depends on the age, condition and amount of subcutaneous fat in the patient.
- A packed cell volume (PCV) may be carried out if a blood sample is available. This test is normally used to measure the amount of red blood cells in a given volume of blood but the figure obtained can also be indicative of hydration status. The normal PCV for a cat or dog is 32–45%. A higher PCV (greater than 45%) would indicate dehydration, as the top layer of the plasma sample, the fluid component of the blood, is reduced

so that the relative proportion of red blood cells is greater. When assessing dehydration the rule is that a 1% increase in PCV is equivalent to a water loss of 10 ml/kg.

ARTERIAL CATHETERISATION

Arterial catheter placement

These are less commonly placed than venous catheters. They are more technically demanding but are very useful for monitoring direct arterial blood pressure and for taking serial blood gas samples. This is helpful during the anaesthesia of many cases, especially those with the potential to haemorrhage, develop hypotension and ventilatory complications and also for critically ill patients requiring intensive care.

The main sites for placement of arterial catheters are the dorsal pedal artery, palmar metacarpal artery, femoral artery, auricular artery and coccygeal artery.

The dorsal pedal artery is the most common of these sites used in cats and dogs. The patient should be placed in lateral recumbency with the designated leg placed closest to the table. The artery should be palpable just distal to the hock between the second and third metatarsal bones. The artery runs at approximately 30° to the long axis of the leg and runs from medial to lateral.

A 20–24-gauge catheter will be selected based on patient size and the artery selected.

The site should be gently clipped and prepared with a surgical scrub solution and surgical spirit. Overzealous scrubbing of the site may cause arterial spasm.

A small stab incision using a number-11 blade in the skin overlying the artery will facilitate placement by minimising damage to the catheter tip. Care should be taken not to penetrate the artery during this process.

The author prefers to flush the catheter with heparinised saline prior to placement as this facilitates a quicker flash to be seen in the needle hub.

Arteries, unlike veins, cannot normally be visualised so the catheter is introduced through the skin at a gentle angle while palpating the artery to guide the tip of the catheter to the correct position. Positive advancement is essential to penetrate the thick arterial wall once the catheter is orientated in the correct position. This is often indicated by a 'ticking' of the catheter. Once a flash of blood is seen in the catheter hub the catheter and stylet should be advanced slightly to ensure the catheter tip is through the thick arterial wall. The catheter can then be advanced. The catheter should be aligned parallel to the artery and as flat as possible after flashback and this will ease advancement. Once the stylet is removed pulsatile blood flow will be seen. A T-connector can be attached and the catheter secured and flushed with heparinised saline. The tape and T-connector should be clearly labelled to indicate that this is an arterial catheter. Arterial catheters should never be used for drug or fluid administration.

Management of arterial catheters is similar to that of venous catheters but includes regular flushing at least hourly. In small patients care should be taken to avoid excessive heparinisation.

Arterial catheters in cats should only be kept in place for 6 to 8 hours. This is due to poor collateral circulation in cats compared to dogs and they are prone to developing ischaemia due to vascular spasm and arterial occlusion. Arterial catheters are generally well tolerated in dogs but they can be easily dislodged due to excessive patient movement.

FLUID THERAPY FOR EXOTIC SPECIES

Fluid requirement for exotic species is as important as in companion animals. Each species has different requirements, and the route of administration will be based on species, equipment to hand and competency of staff. See Chapter 14 for administration methods.

FLUID THERAPY FOR RABBITS

Administering perioperative fluids will reduce the risk of the rabbit becoming dehydrated postoperatively and aid in the prevention of ileus. In healthy rabbits subcutaneous fluids are beneficial perioperatively; however, debilitated animals will require intravenous fluids, which offer greater support and aid recovery. Intravenous cannulation should be advocated in all animals requiring anaesthesia, and administration of fluids can utilise this access. Fluids which may be used include oral rehydration solutions such as lactated Ringer's (Hartmann's solution), a general purpose fluid useful for treatment of dehydration and for maintenance. It can be used in the treatment of metabolic acidosis, e.g. in individuals with chronic gastrointestinal problems. Protein amino acid/vitamin B supplements, e.g. Duphalyte at 1 ml/kg/day in malnourished individuals or those suffering from nephropathy, protein-losing enteropathy, hepatic disease or severe exudative disease. Colloidal fluids can be useful in the treatment of serious blood loss where an intravenous bolus will support central blood pressure. Where fluid deficits are large, rapid replacement risks overloading the patient's organ systems. Rabbits should be gradually rehydrated over 2–3 days or until the rabbit's body weight is stable.

A basic calculation of fluid requirements for rabbits is: Daily fluid maintenance (75–100 ml/kg of body weight per day) plus the correction of dehydration (10 ml/kg per 1% dehydration) with addition of any replacement of ongoing losses in the 24-hour window.

FLUID THERAPY IN BIRDS

Debilitated birds benefit from initial administration of warmed crystalloids at 30 ml/kg given intravenously, intra-osseously, or subcutaneously. When the bird appears stable, perform diagnostics including blood pressure monitoring and further treatment. One to three bolus infusions of crystalloids (10 ml/kg) and colloids (Hetastarch or Oxyglobin at 5 ml/kg) can be given in the same syringe intravenously or intra-osseously until blood pressure exceeds 90 mm Hg systolic.

A basic calculation of fluid requirements in birds is: Daily maintenance fluid requirements (2 ml/kg/hr or 48 ml/kg/day), plus any replacement fluid volume (ml) = estimated dehydration deficit (%) × body weight (kg) × 1000. Replace the total volume over 24 hours. Maintenance fluids will need to be provided until the bird is eating on its own. These fluids should be provided by dividing the bolus infusions over a 24-hour period.

FLUID THERAPY IN TORTOISES

Oral fluids can be administered using rubber, plastic or metal feeding tubes (Fig. 25.13). The tube should be placed to avoid

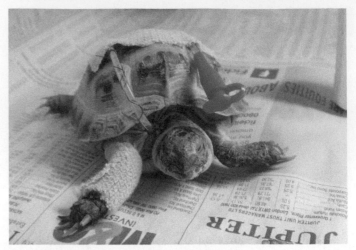

Fig. 25.13 Tube placement in a tortoise

the glottis to a position between the junction of the abdominal and humeral scutes of the plastron. Parenteral fluids can be administered via various methods including epicoelomic, intra-coelomic, intra-osseous or intravenous. Those fluids designed for use in mammalian species are appropriate (approximate osmolarity of 280–310 mOsm). All sites should be disinfected with an iodine-based scrub prior to injection; use of a toothbrush to prepare the site is ideal. The importance of warm water baths for tortoises should not be underestimated. Use tepid water at a depth that covers the entire plastron and a few centimetres of the carapace (this is dependent on the size of the tortoise). Tortoises will usually take the opportunity to void in the water, and take on fresh, therefore the water needs to be changed in order to encourage to take on fresh clean water. If any electrolyte solutions are added to the water, they must be rinsed off adequately.

A basic calculation of fluid requirements in tortoises is: A maintenance requirement of 30 ml/kg of body weight per day. Fluids can be given at the rate of 1% of body weight, up to 4 times daily, for rehydration. In severe cases, up to 6% of body weight may be given each day (typically by a combination of both oral and parenteral therapy). Fluids should be warmed prior to use.

FLUID THERAPY FOR REPTILES

Plasma osmolarity may be helpful in the selection of fluids that will be isotonic for an individual patient. Fluids may be administered orally for mild to moderate dehydration. Fluids can be administered intra-coelomically, intravenously, or intra-osseously for moderate to severe dehydration.

A basic calculation of fluid requirements in reptiles is: Maintenance requirements are estimated at 10–30 ml/kg/day, though different rates are quoted in different papers, ranging from 5–15 to 15–30 ml/kg/day.

Nutritional support

With all sick companion animals the nutritional goal is for the patient to eat the designated diet in its own environment. Unfortunately, in critically sick animals they will be in a hospital environment, where the added stress of this different environment can effect food consumption. Most animals will require or benefit from a veterinary therapeutic diet, but the initial goal is to ensure that the patient is receiving its daily calorific requirement. Analgesia should not be forgotten, as pain can reduce food intake in some animals. Hydration status must be maintained and corrected before any nutritional support can be initiated. The aim of critical care nutrition is dependent on the disease process and/or the individual's specific requirements. Each case must be considered on its own specific requirements once a full clinical examination and history have been achieved. This includes nutritional assessment and dietary history. The sole aim can be defined as to prevent and/or treat malnutrition when present. In order to define any nutritional aims in more depth, it is more beneficial to split the aims into short-term and long-term goals. The short-term aims are to:

- Provide for any ongoing nutritional requirements (both in terms of energy and nutrients)
- Prevent or correct any nutritional deficiencies or imbalances
- Minimise metabolic derangements
- Prevent further catabolism of lean body mass.

Long-term nutritional aims should include:

- Restoration of optimal body condition
- Provision of required nutrients to the animal within its own environment.

As disease processes change and the animal's physiological and metabolic responses alter the nature of the nutritional support, both the short-term and long-term nutritional aims may alter.

When assessing animals for the preferred method of critical care feeding the nutritional status of the animal needs to be evaluated. This should include body condition score (BCS), muscle condition score (MCS), hydration status, weight, hair coat quality, signs of inadequate wound healing, hypoalbuminaemia, lymphopaenia and coagulopathy (Chan, 2005). Thought should be given to 'fluid shifts' in these animals as they can severely affect haematological values and the animal's weight. Factors that should be identified include specific electrolyte imbalances, hyperglycaemia, hypertriglyceridaemia or hyperammonaemia, as they will have large consequences on the nutritional critical care plan. Adequate adjustments will be required to the feeding plan and possibly the formulation of any parenteral nutrition to be utilised.

The calorific intake required by the patient depends on:

- The rate of energy use for basal metabolism (resting)
- Nutrient assimilation
- Body temperature maintenance
- Activity levels.

Energy requirements during sickness are based on resting energy requirement (RER) values. This is due to the assumption that the patient is inactive and is often confined to a small area. Due to this calculated energy requirements, using an illness factor, are only a guideline. Daily weighing of the patient, assessing healing rates and assessing lean body mass are good indicators that the patient is receiving sufficient calories. In herbivores (horses and rabbits) vital parameters should also include gastrointestinal mobility and faecal volume, and appearance and frequency should be monitored. In the early phases of supportive feeding digital pulses in equines should be monitored. This is due to the potential to induce carbohydrate-induced laminitis.

As with all hospitalised patients, human and animal, malnutrition has been associated with increases in infectious morbidity, prolonged hospital stay and an increase in mortality.

The volume of liquid diets administered at each bolus feeding in dogs and cats should not exceed 50 ml/kg. This is only an estimate and each animal should be judged on an individual basis. Tolerance to liquid diets is best when small feeds are delivered frequently.

STARVATION AND ANOREXIA

Starvation can leave the animal severely emaciated, but also the gastrointestinal tract will become atrophied, due to the inadequate nutrient supply. Intestinal villi become atrophied and the epithelial layers become thin and fragile. Bacterial translocation will often occur in these cases. The gastrointestinal capacity to digest and absorb nutrients will become severely limited. The loss of lean body mass occurs from skeletal muscle and internal tissues. Nutritional support of these animals is vital and required immediately. Initially hydration, electrolytes and acid/base status of the patient need to be rectified. The diet chosen needs to be of a high digestibility, and primarily consisting of proteins and fats. This is due to the patient utilising these nutrients over carbohydrates. The patient will be suffering from protein energy malnutrition (PEM) and the quality (not just the quantity) of the protein feed is important. On initiating nutritional support to the patient small frequent meals are required, slowly building up over a period of time to the full daily nutrient and energy requirements. PEM has a potential to occur during times of illness and when increased demands of protein and energy are required (Buffington et al., 2004).

Transient diarrhoea is a common side effect in these cases due to maldigestion, and should resolve as the patient recovers. Inclusion of dietary fibre to the diet should be avoided as it will reduce the digestibility of the diet and bind nutrients up that are required.

RE-FEEDING SYNDROME

Re-feeding syndrome is seen in cats after periods of anorexia or starvation. Re-feeding syndrome is defined as the constellation of metabolic and physiological derangements associated with caloric depletion of the starved feline patient. Classically, re-feeding syndrome is characterised by the development of severe hypophosphatemia following the introduction of enteral or parenteral nutrition. Re-feeding syndromes in cats can also include hypokalaemia, hypomagnesaemia, vitamin deficiency, fluid intolerance and glucose intolerance. Typically re-feeding can occur 2 to 5 days after restarting feeding, but signs can be detected within hours of re-feeding or delayed for up to 10 days.

Many of these metabolic changes are believed to be due to a sudden release of insulin (stimulated by carbohydrate intake) in the presence of total body nutrient intake. Recommendations for reducing the risk of re-feeding syndrome in cats include the following (Chan, 2005):

- Supplementing phosphate, potassium and magnesium for the first 24 hours of therapy, providing that none of these electrolytes were above normal levels initially.
- Thiamine should be administered prior to therapy and then daily, until signs resolve.
- Nutritional support should start at 20% of RER on day 1, increasing slowly until 100% of RER is met over several days.

CLINICAL NUTRITION

Water (hydration levels)

The initial stage of nutritional support is correcting any dehydration, electrolyte replacement and normalisation of the acid/base status before starting assisted feeding. Initiating assisted feeding before the patient is haemodynamically stable can further compromise the patient. If oedema occurs or dehydration persists recalculation of flow rates is required. Monitoring of hydration level indicators is required during intravenous fluid therapy. Daily maintenance fluid requirements are approximately 50–60 ml/kg of body weight per day, or 2 ml/kg of body weight per hour. If persistent vomiting or diarrhoea is present these additional losses need to be factored in.

Where dogs and cats are able to consume fluids without vomiting, the use of an oral rehydration fluid should be advocated. Unless contraindicated placement of a bowl or bucket of water in the animal's kennel or stable should occur. If required, additional fluids can always be administered intravenously or via feeding tubes.

Protein

Nutritional support with adequate protein levels is vital, as patients in a catabolic state will utilise the skeletal muscle proteins. Sufficient calories need to be supplied to the patient from fats and carbohydrates. This will ensure that proteins are not used as a source of energy. The quality of the proteins provided is of importance as is the digestibility. Specific amino acids are supplemented to critical care diets. Glutamine is an important substrate for the increased levels of gluconeogenesis, used in rapidly dividing cells. Any deficiency in this amino acid has shown to lead to gut mucosal atrophy, and an increase in bacterial translocation, due to a compromise of the mucosal barrier. This can lead to the suggestion that glutamine may behave as a 'conditionally essential' amino acid during severe illness. The essential amino acid arginine has a positive effect on the immune system and can subsequently improve survival times of septic patients. Many enteral diets are supplemented with both glutamine and arginine. High doses of glutamine have a trophic effect on the gut mucosa.

The use of a novel protein source in these cases has been advocated. Due to atrophy of the gastrointestinal tract, protein antigens can cross through to the bloodstream and set up hypersensitivity processes.

Vitamins and minerals

The supplementation of vitamins and minerals for hospitalised patients will depend on the disease and its severity. Sodium, chloride, potassium, phosphate, calcium and magnesium should be used for short-term nutritional support. All animals that receive intravenous fluid therapy with or without parenteral support should have daily electrolyte levels monitored. If any polydipsia or polyuria is present, supplementation of the water-soluble vitamins is required. Zinc aids in promoting wound healing and plays a role in protein and nucleic acid metabolism. Supplementation of nutritional support diets with zinc has been recommended.

Carbohydrates

Carbohydrates within any critical care diet need to be of a very high digestibility. The quantities of fibre need to be kept to a minimum, as this will decrease digestibility and bind up impor-

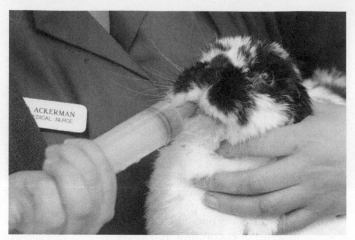

Fig. 25.14 Syringe feeding a rabbit

tant nutrients. The level of carbohydrate in the diet needs to be adequate to supply the required calories for recovery.

Fats

The quantity of fat in a critical care diet does need to be increased. A higher level of calories can be obtained from fat rather than via carbohydrates. The inclusion of omega-3 fatty acids can help decrease any inflammatory response.

RABBIT CRITICAL CARE NUTRITION

Rabbits need prompt treatment when anorexia presents, and this is especially important in obese rabbits and pregnant or lactating does. This is due to the greater risk of developing hepatic lipidosis and/or other clinical disorders.

Syringe feeding must be initiated in rabbits that have not eaten for more than 24 hours (Fig. 25.14). Nasogastric tubes are rarely utilised but are ideal, and can help in the reduction of bloat, as air can be drawn off. Rabbits do get stressed in unfamiliar environments; illness, anorexia and syringe feeding can exacerbate this. Several preparations are available on the market for critical care nutrition for rabbits, and it is important that they contain both soluble and insoluble fibre sources. Fresh grass and other foods should be made available to the rabbit at all times, even when not eating. The use of alfalfa to rabbits recovering from major surgery or severe illness is recommended. Alfalfa has a higher protein and calcium content compared to meadow or Timothy hay.

Analgesia should be routinely used, because pain will prevent the rabbit from eating and as a consequence reduced nutrient intake can occur. Gastrointestinal tract motility stimulants such as cisapride (0.5 mg/kg of body weight) and metoclopramide (0.5 mg/kg of body weight) can be used in order to aid in the prevention of gastrointestinal hypomotility in high-risk situations (e.g. after surgery).

SUPPORTIVE FEEDING METHODS

Supportive feeding methods should be considered when there is a history of greater than 10% weight loss; decreased food intake; anorexia; increased nutrient demands due to trauma or surgery; increased nutrient losses resulting from vomiting, diarrhoea, burns or scalds; acute exacerbation of chronic disease; or if specific areas of the alimentary canal need to be bypassed. The ideal diet to use in these cases should be highly palatable, highly digestible and have a high energy density. A relatively high percentage of energy should be achieved as protein and fat rather than carbohydrates. Table 25.4 gives suggested levels of critical care diets of nutrients in cats and dogs. Critical care diets for cats and dogs are available in three different forms: powdered, liquid and moist diets. Moist diets can have thixotropic consistencies, i.e. when mixed their viscosity decreases so they become thinner.

The use of assisted feeding methods does have great advantages, but care of the feeding tube is vital. The artificial opening through the abdomen into the gastrointestinal tract through which the tube is inserted is referred to as a stoma. The stoma must be treated as a surgical wound and cleaned daily with normal saline or cooled boiled water for the first 7–14 days, or until it is healed. Table 25.5 lists some problems that can arise with tube feeding. Deciding on which methods of tube feeding to be utilised depends on a number of different factors. Figure 25.15 shows a simple flow chart with deciding factors.

ENTERAL FEEDING

Whenever possible, it is preferable to use a method that makes use of the gastrointestinal tract, i.e. using the enteral route. It is very important to maintain the health of the intestinal mucosa and the function of peristalsis within the gastrointestinal tract to prevent destruction of the lining and malabsorption of food (Box 25.7).

There are several different types of feeding tube available that deliver food to the gastrointestinal tract when the patient is unable to ingest food normally (Table 25.6). The choice of tube will depend on the disease process or injury, the expected duration of assisted feeding, the food type to be used, and sometimes cost. Box 25.8 shows how to calculate the amount of diet required.

ENCOURAGING ANIMALS TO EAT

The process of encouraging animals to eat should never be forgotten. Voluntary intake can be established in a number of cases by taking time out to personally encourage the animal to eat. Grooming can actively encourage the animals (especially dogs and cats) to eat, removing any nasal discharge that is blocking their sense of smell, as can TLC, providing competition, hand feeding, providing a selection of different diets, taking the animal into a different environment and in some

TABLE 25.4	Macronutrient levels in critical care diets (as % energy content of diet)		
	Protein	Fat	Carbohydrate
Dog	20–25	50–55	25–26
Cat	25–37	41–50	22–25

BOX 25.7 ROLE OF MICROENTERAL NUTRITION IN FEEDING THE GASTROINTESTINAL TRACT

Microenteral nutrition is the delivery of very small amounts of water, electrolytes and easily absorbable nutrients directly into the gastrointestinal tract. This method is often underutilised in veterinary practices, but allows the nutritional requirements of the intestinal mucosal to be met. This helps to preserve the intestinal blood flow, the mucosal barrier and its immune function. Initial volumes of 0.05–0.2 ml/kg of body weight per hour are recommended, and will add exceptionally little to the volume of fluids normally produced by the stomach. Gradual increases can occur to 1–2 ml/kg of body weight per hour, over a 24–48-hour period. Enteral solutions that can be used include oral rehydrating solutions and those containing glutamine.

TABLE 25.5	Problems that can arise when utilising tube feeding		
Problem	Common causes	Signs and clinical symptoms	Treatment
Infection	Poor hygiene, contamination of the tube site by oral flora at the time of tube insertion.	Inflammation, malodour, pain, increased exudates.	Swab the site for culture and sensitivity, administer appropriate antibiotics. Apply dressings if indicated.
Leakage	Poorly designed tube, infection, and over-granulation.	Excessive movement of the tube or the tube cannot be moved, inflammation of the skin and/or excoriation.	Identify the cause of the problem. Use a barrier cream around the tube insertion site.
Over-granulation	Infection, incorrect positioning of the tube, excessive movement of the tube.	Inflamed, red raised tissue, bleeding, pain.	Treatment of any infection, correct any positioning problems.
Blocked tube	Inadequate flushing regimen, damaged tube, medication interaction.	Difficulty flushing tube, unable to administer water, feeds or medications.	Review flushing regimen, possibly medications. Flush with soda water or enzymatic solution. Preparations used in human medicine use commercially prepared enzymes e.g. Clog Zapper to remove blockages.
Feed-associated problems such as poor tolerance	Feed rate, technique, method, timing of feeds or medications, or type of nutrition used.	Bloating, nausea, vomiting, diarrhoea, constipation.	Eliminate other causes. Review all feeding and medication regimes. Use a diet with a slightly higher fibre content.
Aspiration	Incorrect positioning of the tube when feeding, feed rate/volume too high, poor gastric emptying.	Chest infection, aspiration pneumonia, coughing, regurgitation of the feed.	Review feed rate and administration method. Confirm that tube has been placed correctly, e.g. with radiography.

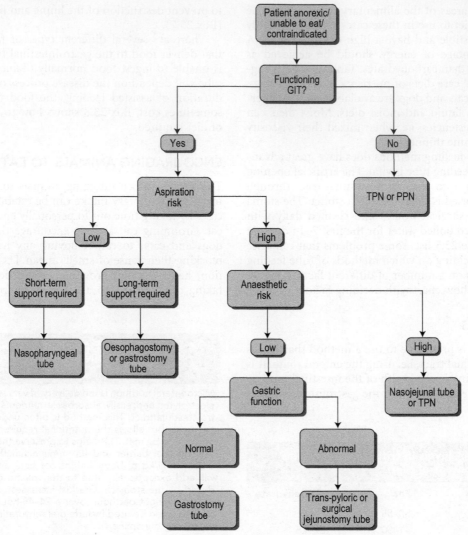

Fig. 25.15 Flow chart of feeding regimen

cases offering the animal some of the food that you are eating if it is suitable. This last method works especially well in dogs.

SYRINGE FEEDING

Many patients will tolerate syringe feeding well, as long as stress is limited during the process. Aversions can be initiated if the animal resents the process and the food is forcibly fed. Catheter-tipped syringes or Pasteur pipettes (cut down) are exceptionally useful in administering critical care diets (Fig. 25.16).

NASO-OESOPHAGEAL TUBES

Naso-oesophageal tubes (Fig. 25.17) are generally well tolerated by cats and dogs and are suitable for short-term nutritional support, usually 3–7 days, though longer periods have been documented. Contraindications for the use of these tubes include unconsciousness, vomiting, disease or dysfunction of the pharynx, larynx, and nares, swallowing reflex, oesophagus and stomach. The preferred placement of the naso-oesophageal tube is in the caudal oesophagus rather than the stomach as it reduces the risk of reflux oesophagitis.

Once the tube has been placed introduce a small amount of water injected slowly into the tube to see if a cough reflex is induced, indicating aspiration. Lateral radiographs can also identify that the tube has been correctly placed. Due to the narrow bore of the tube blockages may occur. Injection of 5–10 ml of water into the tube after introduction of the liquid diet should aid in prevention of any blockages. If blockages do occur small amounts of carbonated drinks, cranberry juice or solutions of pancreatic enzymes have been shown to aid in their removal. Pre-feeding administration of water is required to ensure that the tube is still positioned correctly.

OESOPHAGOSTOMY TUBES

Oesophagostomy tubes (Fig. 25.18) are commonly used in cats that have suffered facial trauma, usually after a road traffic accident. Oesophagostomy tubes are of use when bypassing of the nose and mouth is required in order to administer nutritional support. Animals that do not tolerate naso-oesophageal tubes well can have oesophagostomy tubes placed. Aseptic placement of the tube under general anaesthetic is required. Frequent cleaning and inspection of the tube is necessary under aseptic conditions. Complications can include

TABLE 25.6	**Types of tube used for enteral feeding**				
Tube type and use	Location	Duration of placement	Comments	Contraindications
Naso-oesophageal Short-term nutrition where upper gastrointestinal tract is functioning normally	Distal oesophagus via the nose	Short term, <7 days	Simple and non-invasive to place Reasonably well tolerated Inexpensive Can be maintained at home	Long-term nutritional support Trauma or disease to head, neck, nasal cavity, oesophagus Comatose and recumbent patients Abnormal gag reflex Vomiting; functional or mechanical gastrointestinal obstruction
Oesophagostomy Facial trauma, injury or disease involving the mouth and pharynx	Distal oesophagus via surgical placement into the cranial oesophagus through the skin	Short and long term (months)	Well tolerated Wide bore, so more selection of diets Can be maintained at home	Oesophageal disorder Vomiting Comatose or recumbent patients Following oesophageal surgery
Gastrostomy/PEG tube Injuries or surgery to oral cavity, larynx, pharynx or oesophagus	The stomach via surgical laparotomy or endoscopically through the ventrolateral abdominal wall (left side)	Mid to long term (months to years)	Well tolerated More invasive procedure to place Can be maintained at home Wide bore, so more selection of diets	Primary gastric disease (ulceration or neoplasia) Intractable vomiting Peritonitis
Enterostomy (duodenostomy or jejunostomy) When stomach or duodenum must be bypassed Pancreatic disease or surgery Biliary system disease	The small intestine via surgical laparotomy through the abdominal wall or endoscopically via gastric tube and through the pylorus	Long term (weeks to months) but term limited because of need for hospitalisation	Well tolerated Invasive procedure Not possible to maintain at home Very narrow bore	Patients must be stable enough for anaesthesia and surgery Dysfunction of the small intestine

PEG: percutaneous endoscopic gastrostomy

BOX 25.8 CALCULATION OF VOLUME OF FOOD TO BE ADMINISTERED

CALCULATIONS OF ENTERAL FEEDING AMOUNTS:

1. Calculate the RER of the animal:
   RER = 70 × (body weight [kg]) 0.75 for animals <2 kg or >45 kg, or 30 × (body weight [kg]) + 70
2. Add in the illnesses factor:
   RER × Illness factor = kcal/day
3. Choose the specific diet that is most beneficial for the patient and the method of feeding.
4. Divide the energy content of the diet (kcal/ml or gram) by the energy requirement of the animal (kcal/day) to achieve the daily amount of food required.
5. Divide the total amount to be given in 1 day by the total amount of feeding wished to be given, or by maximum volume of each feed.

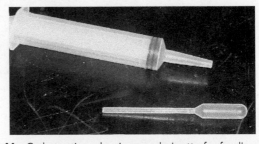

Fig. 25.16 Catheter-tipped syringe and pipette for feeding

airway obstruction, damage to the cervical nerves and blood vessels and infections.

PERCUTANEOUS ENDOSCOPIC GASTROSTOMY TUBES

Placement of percutaneous endoscopic gastrostomy (PEG) tubes (Fig. 25.19) is required under general anaesthetic, and the tube needs to be in place for at least 5 days prior to removal. PEG tubes are utilised when long-term nutritional support is required and when oesophageal problems are present.

Adhesions between the gastric serosa and the peritoneum can form within 48–72 hours. It should be noted that in malnourished patients these adhesions might take longer to form. Once the tube is placed, only a third of the calculated daily energy requirements should be administered; on day 2, two-thirds; and by the third day the full amount. Feeding through the PEG tube can commence 4 hours after its insertion. If patients are unable to take fluids orally, mouth care should be encouraged at least every 4 hours. This involves ensuring that the mucous membranes remain moist and that bacterial infections are prevented. This can be managed by the use of oral hygiene gels that contain chlorhexidine designed for dental care.

The procedure of removal of the gastrostomy tube in animals over 10 kg is to cut the catheter off flush with the skin after pulling it taught. The catheter tip is then passed in the faeces. The resulting gastrocutaneous fistula will rapidly heal if kept clean.

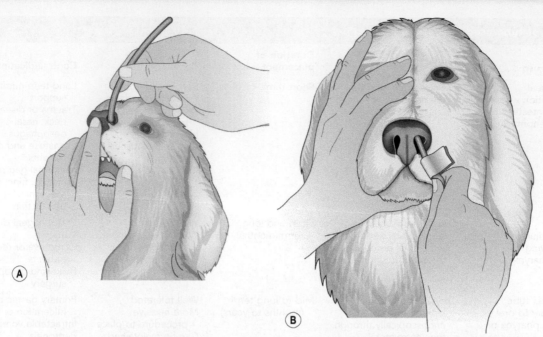

Fig. 25.17 (A) Placement of local anaesthetic into the nose is beneficial to the animal. Once working, the external nares are pushed dorsally and the tube is gently passed into the ventral nasal meatus. (B) The tube is fully inserted until the pen mark or adhesive tape tabs are reached. Glue or sutures are then used in order to secure the tube in position. It is useful to check correct placement of the tube prior to securing it in place.

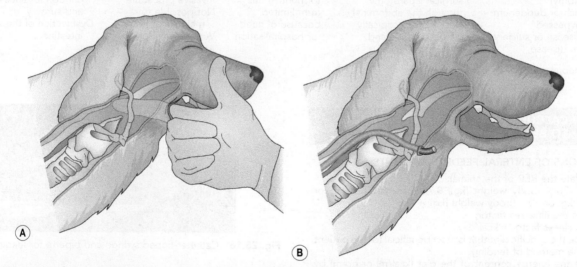

Fig. 25.18 Placement of pharyngostomy tube: (A) In order to correctly position a pharyngostomy tube, while anaesthetised a finger is used to palpate the hyoid apparatus. The tube exit needs to be as far caudally and dorsally along the pharyngeal wall as possible. Once an optimal site has been located a 1-cm skin incision is made over the bulging pharyngeal wall. Blunt dissection is advocated in order to tunnel caudally through the tissue from outside to inside. (B) Forceps are used to grasp one end of the tube, while the other end is passed down the oesophagus. The tube is secured in place with tape and sutures.

Maintenance of the feeding tube

When using nasogastric and oesophagostomy tubes it is necessary to check that the tube is still in the oesophagus before each feed as tubes can be dislodged through coughing. This may be done by placing 2 ml of sterile water down the tube beforehand and watching for any signs of coughing, which may suggest that the tube is lying in the trachea. A less common method is to check for a vacuum by attaching a 5-ml syringe to the end of the feeding tube, drawing back the plunger and releasing so that a vacuum is felt. This confirms that the tube is lying in the oesophagus. The feeding tubes must be flushed before and after each feed to prevent blockages. Fizzy drinks have been used, but these can cause nausea and vomiting in patients. Cranberry juice works just as well, with few unwanted side effects.

In most cases feeding tubes are used in conjunction with accessories such as stockinettes, abdominal bandages and buster collars to help keep them in place. They may require regular changing or altering and should be closely monitored for any signs of discomfort caused to the patient. The site of entry of a feeding tube should be treated as a surgical wound and will require daily cleaning and dressing to prevent any infection.

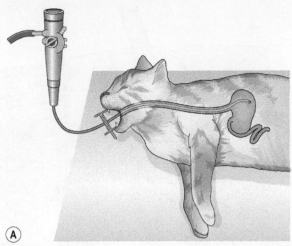

Fig. 25.19A Placement of a PEG tube required the animal to be placed in right lateral recumbency. The stomach is then insufflated with air introduced by the endoscope. The gastric wall will then come in contact with the body wall.

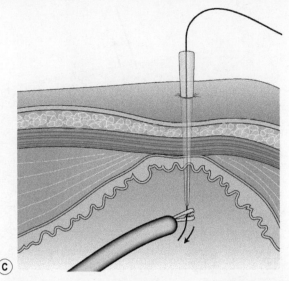

Fig. 25.19C A thick nylon suture is fed through the needle or catheter, and is grasped by the endoscope's retrieval forceps. As the endoscope is withdrawn, the nylon suture is pulled out through the mouth.

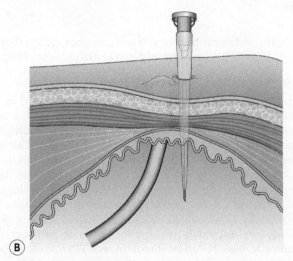

Fig. 25.19B The lighted tip of the endoscope can be seen when pressed against the abdominal wall. This area should be prepared and scrubbed aseptically. A large-bore needle or over-the-needle catheter is inserted into the stomach next to the endoscope tip.

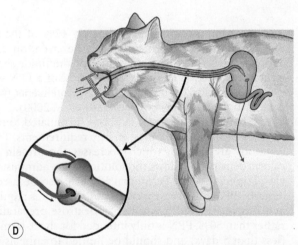

Fig. 25.19D The type of tube used will depend on the next stage. In order to allow the feeding tube to be pulled through the abdominal wall a catheter needs to be threaded onto the drawn-through nylon prior to the feeding tube being attached. Some commercial kits (e.g. Pezzer catheter assembly kits) already have a catheter guide in place. The lubricated catheter (with attached feeding tube) is drawn down the oesophagus into the stomach, by the suture, which is exiting the body wall.

The stomach capacity of a cat is 45 ml/kg and of a dog 90 ml/kg.

PARENTERAL NUTRITION

Parenteral nutrition (PN) is often fraught with complications, but should be considered in animals that are unable to tolerate enteral supportive feeding methods. This includes animals that are vomiting or regurgitating, or those unable to protect their airway. Complications such as hyperalimentation or overfeeding can be common and lead to metabolic complications, though these can be resolved easily by discontinuing and do respond fairly rapidly. Other complications can be more severe, and include localised infections, which can lead to septicaemia. The use of a central line (in TPN cases) for administering supportive nutritional methods requires careful attention to

aseptic techniques. The PN solution can also act as the perfect reservoir for bacterial growth.

Parenteral nutrition can be divided into two different categories:

1. TPN – where parenteral nutrition is formulated to meet 100% of the animal's energy requirements. In all animals receiving TPN hyperglycaemia and glucosuria can develop in some cases. This hyperglycaemic state can possibly reflect the decrease in peripheral glucose uptake resulting from mild insulin resistance. This can precipitate to laminitis in horses. As a general rule, intravenous dextrose solution should be used as the sole source of nutrition for no more than 2–3 days. An amino acid solution should be added to the dextrose solution, and then lipids. On day

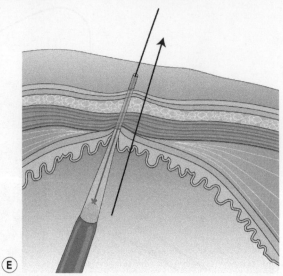

(E)

Fig. 25.19E When the lubricated catheter guide reaches the body wall resistance will be felt. Firm application of counter pressure to the body wall should allow the catheter tip to emerge through the skin. In order for the feeding tube to exit a very small incision (2–3 mm) may be required.

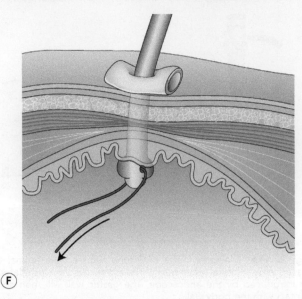

(F)

Fig. 25.19F As the feeding tube is pulled through, gentle traction will be required in order for the stomach and abdominal wall to come into close contact. A rubber flange is then slid down the tube and secured in place.

1 of the administration approximately 12% of the animal's total fluid requirement should be given, on day 2 approximately 24%. The remainder of the fluids should be administered via IV fluids. An example of a TPN solution will contain 32% lipid energy, 9% protein energy and 60% carbohydrate energy (Remillard et al., 2000).

2. Partial parenteral nutrition (PPN) – formulated to meet 40–70% of the animal's total energy requirements. These solutions are diluted, which decreases the protein and caloric density but allows the solution to be administered via peripheral veins. Peripheral PN can also be used to describe PPN. A lower osmolarity of solution is required, and this is achieved by using 5% dextrose preparations rather than 50%. PPN is only intended for short-term use (less than 5 days) and should be limited to animals that are not debilitated. It should be noted that purely dextrose solutions are not appropriate for the long-term treatment of hypoglycaemia. In critical care situations insulin resistance and glucose intolerance are exceptionally likely, and hence a fat source must be available. When using 5% dextrose infusions this will only provide less than 25% of the RER when administered at maintenance fluid rates.

Parenteral nutrition administration

Aseptic placement of a dedicated catheter is required in order to administer PN. When placing a catheter for TPN, a central venous (jugular) catheter is required. The use of multi-lumen catheters is advocated, as it can also be used for blood sampling, as well as the administration of fluids and intravenous medications, as a separate lumen is required for each purpose. As with enteral assisted feeding methods, TPN should be instituted gradually over a 3-day period. Flow rates of other fluids being concurrently administered should be adjusted accordingly.

Once the animal is consuming adequate nutrient intake voluntarily, the PN can be discontinued. TPN needs to be discontinued gradually over a 6–12-hour period. PPN can be discontinued abruptly. All animals receiving TPN and PPN should be closely monitored. Daily weighing of the animal must occur, alongside TPN throughout the day. The catheter site should also be monitored, and handled aseptically.

REFERENCES

Boag, A., 2007. Electrolyte and acid-base balance. In: King, L.G., Boag, A. (Eds.), BSAVA Manual of Canine and Feline Emergency and Critical Care, second ed. British Small Animal Veterinary Association, Gloucester, p. 49.

Buffington, T., Holloway, C., Abood, S., 2004. Manual of Veterinary Dietetics. Elsevier Saunders, St. Louis.

Chan, D., 2005. Parenteral nutritional support. In: Ettinger, S.J., Feldman, E.C. (Eds.), Textbook of Veterinary Internal Medicine, vol. 1, sixth ed. Elsevier Science, St. Louis, pp. 586–591.

Chan, D., 2015. Nutritional Management of Hospitalized Small Animals. John Wiley and Sons, Oxford.

Remillard, R.L., Armstrong, P.J., Davenport, D.J., 2000. Assisted feeding in hospitalised patients: Enteral and parenteral nutrition. In: Hand, M.S., Thatcher, C.D., Remillard, R.L., et al. (Eds.), Small Animal Clinical Nutrition, fourth ed. Mark Morris Institute, Missouri, pp. 351–399.

FURTHER READING

DiBartola, S., 2012. Fluid, Electrolyte and Acid-Base Disorders in Small Animal Practice, fourth ed. Elsevier Saunders, St. Louis.

Hopper, K., Silverstein, D., 2014. Small Animal Critical Care Medicine, second ed. Elsevier Saunders, St. Louis.

King, L., Boag, A., 2007. BSAVA Manual of Canine and Feline Emergency and Critical Care, second ed. British Small Animal Veterinary Association, Gloucester.

Pet Blood Bank UK: <www.petbloodbankuk.org>

26

Dentistry

CECILIA GORREL

KEY POINTS

- The veterinary nurse is an essential part of the primary dental care team and must be prepared to be both dental nurse and hygienist.

- Primary care dentistry requires the use of a range of specialised instruments.

- There are different degrees of cleanliness of equipment and instrumentation required for different oral/dental procedures ranging from visually clean to sterile.

- Suitable (clean, extremely clean, or sterile as required by the procedure) instruments should be available for each patient.

- Power equipment requires regular maintenance (daily, weekly) in the practice and regular servicing by the manufacturer.

- Oral examination and all dental procedures require general anaesthesia. Close attention must be given to preventing debris from entering the larynx and trachea and to the monitoring of the patient during the procedure and during the recovery period.

- All oral examinations and treatments should be recorded, and the use of specific dental record sheets is recommended.

- Professional periodontal therapy performed by the veterinary nurse includes supragingival and closed subgingival scaling and root planing.

- Home care carried out by the owner and based on regular tooth brushing is the most effective way to maintain oral hygiene. The veterinary nurse can play a major part in educating and training the owner in these techniques.

Introduction

In human dentistry the team that supplies primary oral care consists of the dentist, the dental nurse, the dental hygienist and the dental technician. Each of these individuals has a clearly defined role: i.e. the dentist is responsible for oral diagnosis and treatment; the dental nurse assists the dentist in these duties; the dental hygienist performs dental hygiene instruction and treatment as requested by the dentist; and the dental technician manufactures appliances as requested by the dentist. In addition to this primary care team, there are specialists in the various dental disciplines (periodontics, orthodontics, endodontics, oral surgery, prosthodontics, etc.). The specialists provide treatment that is outside the scope of the general dental practitioner.

The veterinary primary oral care team is not as easy to define. Despite the fact that oral conditions are common in our domestic pets, education in veterinary dentistry and oral surgery is not a big part of the undergraduate veterinary curriculum. Consequently, many veterinary surgeons are not comfortable with diagnosing oral conditions or with performing dental and oral surgery procedures. Moreover, dentistry is often not considered 'important' and is often delegated to nurses, who have even less knowledge of the discipline. In fact, oral health and disease is often not covered at all in the practical element of nursing training programmes. This is an unfortunate situation and does not benefit the oral health and general welfare of our domestic pets. There is today an urgent need to provide education in dentistry and oral surgery for veterinary surgeons as well as for nurses. Moreover, the legal role of the veterinary nurse in the dental care team needs to be clearly defined. In the UK, veterinary nurses may do the things specified in paragraphs 6 (applies to listed veterinary nurses) and 7 (applies to student veterinary nurses) of Schedule 3 to the Veterinary Surgeons Act 1966, as amended by the Veterinary Surgeons Act 1966 (Schedule 3 Amendment) Order 2002, SI 2002/1479, with effect from 10 June 2002.

Veterinary oral care should be structured similarly to human oral care – i.e. the veterinary surgeon is responsible for diagnosis and treatment; the veterinary nurse assists the veterinary surgeon in these duties, and also performs dental hygiene instruction and treatment as requested by the veterinary surgeon. In other words, the veterinary nurse takes on the duties of both 'dental nurse' and 'dental hygienist'.

The nurse can only perform these duties if specifically requested to do so by the veterinary surgeon and then only under their direct supervision. Moreover, the veterinary surgeon is accountable for the adequacy of any procedures performed by the veterinary nurse. In other words, the veterinary surgeon is ultimately responsible.

In addition to the veterinary surgeon in general practice, there are now veterinary surgeons who are specialists in dentistry. They provide treatment that is outside the scope of the general dental practitioner, e.g. complicated extractions and other surgical procedures, endodontics, prosthodontics, etc.

The veterinary nurse is an essential member of an effective oral care team. The trained veterinary nurse should be able to carry out the following procedures:
- Care for and maintain instrumentation and equipment.
- Perform an oral examination.
- Record findings on a dental record sheet.
- Take dental radiographs.
- Perform routine professional periodontal therapy.
- Perform oral/dental hygiene instruction.

General Considerations

Dentistry poses a health hazard for both operators and patients. There is the possibility of both indirect contagion (hands, nails, skin, clothes, instruments) as well as the dangers associated with the bacterial aerosol created by some procedures, e.g. scaling, but also by sneezing, coughing and by the water coolant and compressed air used. Consequently, dental procedures should be performed in a separate room which is carefully designed and maintained to minimise these hazards.

The room must have adequate light and ventilation. A bright light source is a mandatory requirement. A good dental light is expensive, but definitely worth the money. Some dental high-speed handpieces have lights built in.

Ergonomic considerations are of paramount importance in the layout of the dental operatory. All equipment and instruments should be within easy reach of the operator. Posture is important. Ideally, the operator should be seated.

It is essential to protect operator and staff. Designated operating clothes should be worn. Moreover, facemasks and appropriate eye wear (spectacles or face shield) to protect operators and assistants from the bacterial aerosol and other debris are essential. There is a risk of infection of skin wounds if the operator works in a dirty environment without gloves. The oral cavity is never a sterile site, so the use of surgical gloves is recommended. In addition, hand disinfection should be practised frequently.

Important patient considerations are as follows:
- General anaesthesia with endotracheal intubation is essential. This prevents inhalation of aerosolised bacteria (and other debris) and asphyxiation on irrigation and cooling fluid.
- The animal should be positioned on a surface that will allow drainage to prevent it becoming wet and hypothermic. This can be achieved by the use of a 'tub-tank' or placing the animal's head on a disposable 'nappy', which is frequently replaced.

Some important equipment and instrumentation considerations are as follows:
- Different degrees of cleanliness are required for different oral/dental procedures, ranging from visually clean to sterile.
- Some equipment and instruments need to be 'clean', i.e. units, lamps, tub tables etc., and need to be wiped clean with an all-purpose disinfectant.
- Any instrument that will be used inside the oral cavity but *without penetrating* the oral mucosa, e.g. examination instruments, burs, scalers, curettes, must be exceptionally clean as defined by European Standard (EN)/International Organization for Standardisation (ISO) document 15883. This degree of cleanliness is achieved by mechanical cleaning followed by heat or chemical treatment. This is best achieved using a disinfector, where both cleaning and disinfection occur automatically. Another alternative is placing the instruments in an ultrasound bath or ordinary dishwasher followed by disinfection in an autoclave. A third option is to use chemicals for cleaning and disinfection. The latter option is usually limited to equipment/instrumentation where heat disinfection is not suitable, e.g. instruments with plastic handles.
- Instruments that *penetrate* the oral mucosa or the pulp system of the tooth need to be sterile as defined by European Standard (EN) document 556. This entails packaging and sterilisation as detailed by EN/ISO document 14937.
- Suitable (clean, extremely clean, sterile as required by the procedure) instruments should be available for each patient. Ideally, several pre-packed kits with the required instruments for different procedures, e.g. examination, periodontal therapy, extraction, should be available.
- Power equipment requires regular maintenance (daily, weekly) in the practice and regular servicing by the supplier. Draw up checklists for these chores. Check maintenance and servicing requirements with the supplier.

Instrumentation and equipment for primary care dentistry

Primary care dentistry includes, but is not limited to:
- Oral examination and recording of findings
- Periodontal therapy
- Extraction
- Minor oral surgery.

Suitable (clean, extremely clean, sterile, as required by the procedure) instruments should be available for each patient. Ideally, several pre-packed kits containing the required instruments for the different procedures, e.g. examination, periodontal therapy and extraction, should be available.

Power equipment requires regular maintenance (daily and weekly) in the practice and regular servicing by the supplier. Checklists should be drawn up for these chores. Maintenance and servicing requirements need to be decided with the supplier.

INSTRUMENTATION FOR ORAL EXAMINATION

The details of how to perform an oral examination are covered later in this chapter.

The instrumentation required is shown in Figure 26.1.

The **periodontal probe** is a rounded, narrow or flat, blunt-ended, graduated instrument. Its blunt end can be inserted into the gingival sulcus without causing trauma. The periodontal probe is used to:
- Measure periodontal probing depth
- Determine degree of gingival inflammation
- Evaluate furcation lesions
- Evaluate extent of tooth mobility.

The **dental explorer**, a sharp-ended instrument, is used to:
- Determine the presence of caries
- Explore other enamel and dentine defects, e.g. fracture, resorptive lesions.

The explorer is also useful for tactile examination of the subgingival tooth surfaces. Subgingival calculus and resorptive lesions may be identified in this way. Dental explorers are either straight or curved. They are also either single-ended or double-ended, usually combined with a periodontal probe, i.e. one end is an explorer and the other end is a periodontal probe.

A **dental mirror** is a vital, but traditionally rarely used, tool in veterinary dentistry. It allows the operator to visualise palatal/lingual surfaces while maintaining posture. The dental mirror can also be used to reflect light on to areas of interest and to retract and protect soft tissue.

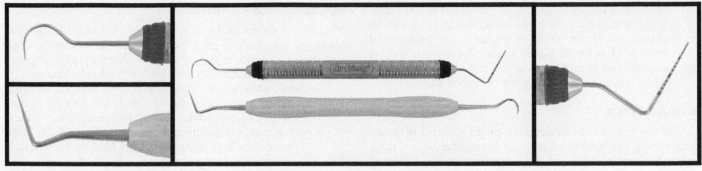

Fig. 26.1 Instrumentation for oral examination. Required instrumentation is a dental explorer and a periodontal probe. A dental mirror (not depicted) is also useful to reflect light on to areas of interest and to retract and protect soft tissue. The periodontal probe is a narrow rounded or flat, blunt-ended graduated instrument while a dental explorer is a sharp-ended instrument. Centre picture depicts double-ended instruments; top is a combined explorer and probe and lower (yellow handle) is a combined curved explorer and straight explorer. On the left are close-ups of a curved (top) and straight (bottom) explorer. On the right is a close-up of a periodontal probe

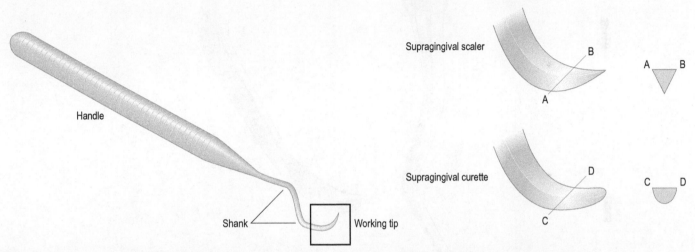

Fig. 26.2 Scaler and curette design. Each has a handle, a shank and a working tip. The working tip of a scaler is more robust than that of a curette. Also, the working tip of the scaler is pointed, while the curette has a rounded tip. A scaler is thus designed for supragingival work, while a curette can be used both supra- and subgingivally

EQUIPMENT AND INSTRUMENTATION FOR PROFESSIONAL PERIODONTAL THERAPY

Professional periodontal therapy includes scaling, root planing and crown polishing. The procedure is detailed later in this chapter.

Scaling describes the process whereby dental deposits, i.e. plaque, but mainly calculus, are removed from the supra- and subgingival surfaces of the teeth. Scaling may be performed using a combination of mechanical (powered) instruments, e.g. ultrasonic or sonic scalers, and hand instruments, i.e. scalers and curettes. Hand instruments should be used to remove large, bulky supragingival deposits before going on to powered scalers. Hand instruments are also required to adequately remove subgingival dental deposits.

Hand scaling instruments

Scalers and curettes are used to remove dental deposits from the tooth surfaces. Each has a handle, a shank and a working end or tip. They require frequent sharpening to maintain their cutting edges. The working end refers to that part of the instrument that is used to carry out the function of the instrument.

The working end of a sharpened instrument is called the blade. It is made up of the following components:
- Face
- Lateral surfaces
- Back
- Cutting edge(s).

The cutting edge is the line where the face and a lateral surface meet to form a sharp cutting edge. A blade designed with a pointed tip is called a scaler. A blade that ends with a rounded toe is classified as a curette. Figure 26.2 demonstrates the differences between a scaler and a curette:
- **Scalers** are used for the supragingival removal of calculus. As a scaler has a sharp, pointed tip it should only be used supragingivally. If a scaler is used subgingivally, the pointed tip will lacerate the gingival margin. A scaler should generally be pulled away from the gingiva towards the tip of the crown or the occlusal surface.
- **Curettes** are used for the subgingival removal of dental deposits and for root planing. They can also be used supragingivally. There are basically two types of curette, namely universal and area-specific, e.g. Gracey. The working end of a curette is more slender than that of a

scaler and the back and tip are rounded to minimise gingival trauma. A selection of scalers and curettes, as shown in Figure 26.3, is required for periodontal therapy. A separate scaler is not strictly required, as curettes can be used both above and below the gingiva while scalers are limited to supragingival use.

Calculus forceps

Calculus forceps have been designed to aid removal of heavy calculus from the surface of teeth. It is essential to use these forceps with extreme care and in the described manner, as inappropriate use will result in fractured teeth. These forceps must not be used to extract teeth.

Mechanical scaling instruments

Mechanical scalers enable fast and easy removal of calculus. However, they have a great potential for iatrogenic damage (overheating a tooth may cause irreversible pulp pathology) if used incorrectly. There are two types of mechanical scaler:

- **Sonic scalers** are driven by compressed air, so they require a compressed-air-driven dental unit for operation. The tip oscillates at a sonic frequency. Sonic scalers are generally less effective than ultrasonic scalers but generate less heat and are thus less likely to cause iatrogenic injuries and safer to use. Depending upon the design of the tip of the scaler, these instruments may be used for supra- and subgingival scaling. An insert with

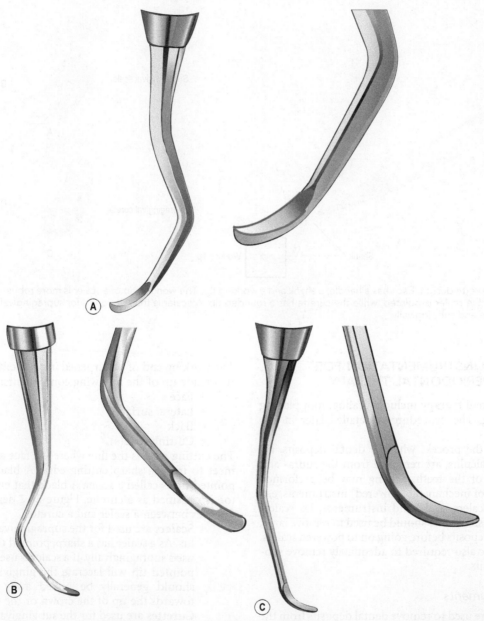

Fig. 26.3 A selection of hand instruments is required for periodontal therapy. (A) Sickle scaler. Due to its sharp pointed tip it would lacerate the gingiva if inserted subgingivally, so this instrument can only be used to remove dental deposits above the gingiva. Note the two cutting edges (highlighted red). (B) Universal curette. This instrument also has two cutting edges (highlighted red) but due to its rounded tip it can be used to remove subgingival deposits and restore the root surface to smoothness. It can also be used to remove supragingival dental deposits. (C) Gracey curette. This curette is considered an area specific curette and has only one cutting side (highlighted red)

a thin pointed tip, sometimes called a perio, sickle or universal insert, is recommended.

- **Ultrasonic scalers** are commonly used in veterinary practice. The tip oscillates at ultrasonic frequencies. They are driven by a micromotor rather than compressed air. The tip vibration is generated either by a magnetostrictive mechanism or a piezoelectric mechanism in the handpiece. The ultrasonic oscillation of the tip causes cavitation of the coolant, which aids in the disruption of the calculus on the tooth surface. Ultrasonic scalers are generally designed for supragingival use, but tips designed for subgingival scaling are available. A thin, pointed insert is recommended for supragingival use. Inserts specifically designed for subgingival use are recommended for subgingival scaling.

Polishing units

Polishing removes plaque and restores the scaled tooth surfaces to smoothness. A polished tooth surface is less plaque-retentive. Scaled teeth must be polished using either prophy paste in a prophy cup or in a brush in a slow-speed contra-angle handpiece, or by means of air polishing (particle blasting):

- **Prophy paste** in a cup or brush in a slow-speed contra-angle handpiece – the speed of rotation of the cup or brush can be regulated. To minimise the amount of heat generated, the prophy cup or brush should not rotate faster than 5000 revolutions per minute. Each patient should receive a new polishing cup or brush. Prophy paste is available in bulk containers and individual patient tubs. The latter are inexpensive and should be used to prevent contamination and iatrogenic transmission of pathogens.
- **Air polishing (particle blasting)** – this technique, based on the sandblasting principle, is used to polish the supragingival parts of the teeth. The particles used, e.g. bicarbonate of soda, will polish the tooth surface without causing damage to the enamel, if used properly. It is essential to protect the soft tissues, i.e. gingivae and oral mucosa, during air polishing.

A simple way of protecting the soft tissues is to cover them with a piece of gauze.

INSTRUMENTATION AND EQUIPMENT FOR EXTRACTION

Tooth extraction requires hand instruments and power equipment.

Hand instruments

Hand instruments required for tooth extraction include luxators, elevators, Extraktors, periosteal elevators, possibly extraction forceps and a small surgical kit including a scalpel blade, forceps, suturing instruments and suturing material.

Luxators, elevators and extraktors. A selection of dental luxators, elevators and extraktors of varying sizes is required. My preferred selection is shown in Figure 26.4.

These instruments are used to cut/break down the periodontal ligament, which holds the tooth in the alveolus. The different sizes are required so that an appropriate range for each size of root can be selected. Luxators have a very thin working end and are used to cut the ligament, but should not be used for leverage

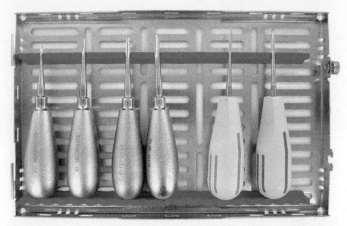

Fig. 26.4 Luxators and extraktors. My favourite extraction tools are depicted. On the left are extraktors and on the right are two luxators. Most extractions can be performed using the four different sizes (1.5, 3, 4 and 5) of extraktors

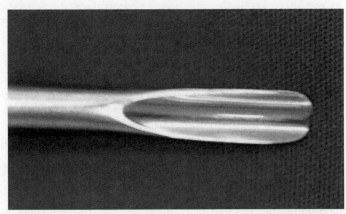

Fig. 26.5 The Extraktor. This newly developed instrument combines the advantages of both a luxator and an elevator. It is designed to conform to the shape of the root and can be used in an apical cutting motion as well as inserted horizontally between roots to apply leverage. It also has lateral cutting edges, unlike the luxator or elevator, which allow the instrument to slide around the circumference of the tooth

or they may break. Elevators have a more robust working end than luxators and are used to break down the periodontal ligament with a combination of apical pressure and leverage. The extraktor, shown in Figure 26.5, is a newly developed instrument (Accesia AB, Sweden) specifically designed for tooth extraction in the dog and cat. It combines the advantages of a luxator and an elevator into one instrument. They are shaped to adapt well to the shape of the root surface and can be used in an apical cutting motion as well as inserted horizontally between tooth roots to apply leverage. Moreover, they have sharp cutting edges on the lateral aspect, which allows them to slide around the circumference of the tooth. An extraction can be started with a luxator and completed with an elevator or it can be performed using different sizes of extraktors only.

Periosteal elevator. Periosteal elevators of different sizes, as shown in Figure 26.6, are required for open (surgical) extractions to expose the alveolar bone by raising a mucoperiosteal flap. However, even if a closed (nonsurgical) extraction technique has been used, the gingiva may be sutured over the

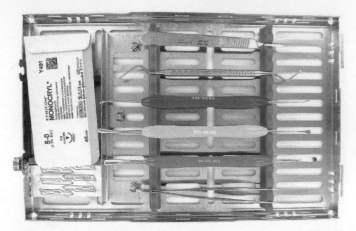

Fig. 26.6 Equipment for tooth extraction. A small surgical kit including my preferred periosteal elevators is shown. The size 15 blade shown (should always be used in a handle) is my preference

extraction socket. In this situation, a periosteal elevator is invaluable to free the gingiva, allowing suturing over of the extraction socket without tension.

Extraction forceps. Although forceps can be used to aid ligament breakdown by rotational force on the tooth, it is very easy to snap the crown off by using excessive force. There is some truth in the saying that the only extraction forceps required are your fingers. If the tooth cannot be lifted out with your fingers, then the periodontal ligament has not been adequately broken down. In short, dental forceps are not essential, but if they are to be used then a selection of sizes, to fit the root anatomy of the tooth being extracted, is required.

Scalpel blade. The use of a scalpel blade to free the gingival attachment to the tooth is recommended for both closed and open extraction technique. A size 15 or 11 blade, used in the handle, is ideal.

Suture kit and suture material. A suture kit with small ophthalmic instruments should be available. Monofilament, absorbable suture material with a swaged-on needle, should be used in the oral cavity. Monocryl® (polyglecaprone, Ethicon) is currently my suture material of choice.

Suction

Suction is invaluable. Excess water and debris can easily be removed, improving visibility for the operator and increasing safety for the patient (reduced risk of aspiration). In addition, blood loss can be estimated more accurately. Most compressed-air-driven units incorporate suction. A separate suction unit can also be deployed.

Power equipment

Power equipment is required to perform dentistry and oral surgery. Regular maintenance is essential to avoid problems with equipment failure.

Micromotor unit. A micromotor unit can be used for polishing teeth as well as for sectioning teeth, when the micromotor should be set at maximum speed. Micromotor units do not generally include water-cooling of the bur and an external

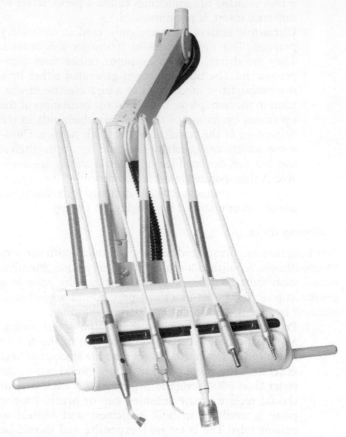

Fig. 26.7 A dental unit. The depicted unit has the following components from left to right: light gun (for transilluminating teeth and curing light-cure dental materials), an air–water syringe, an ultrasonic scaler (driven by a build in micromotor), slow-speed and high-speed outlet (will need separate compressor)

source, e.g. an assistant applying coolant continuously to the tissues, is required to prevent thermal damage to teeth and alveolar bone.

Compressed-air-driven unit. The basic compressed-air-driven unit consists of a high-speed outlet, which accepts a high-speed handpiece, a slow-speed outlet, which accepts a slow-speed handpiece, and a combination air/water syringe. The high-speed outlet is fitted with water cooling. The slow-speed outlet may be fitted with water cooling but often this feature is absent. Some compressed-air-driven units have suction, which is a real bonus. A typical dental unit is depicted in Figure 26.7. The different handpieces for dental units are depicted in Figure 26.8.

Burs. Dental burs are made of a variety of materials, including stainless steel, tungsten carbide steel and 'diamond'. A wide selection of burs are available to fit both slow- and high-speed handpieces (Fig. 26.9). The high-speed handpiece will only accept friction grip burs, while a slow-speed handpiece may accept either friction grip or latch key burs. A selection of round, pear-shaped, tapered fissure and straight fissure burs will be required for sectioning of teeth and removal of alveolar bone. 'Diamond' burs abrade rather than cut and may be safer for the inexperienced user. Blunted burs should be discarded.

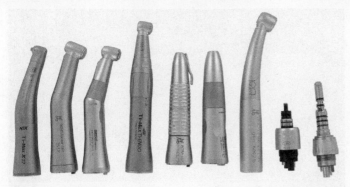

Fig. 26.8 The different handpieces for dental units. From the left are three slow-speed contra-angle handpieces, an endodontic handpiece, two straight handpieces; one with external water/saline and the other with internal, a high-speed (30,000 rpm or more) handpiece, a rotaquick connector (for motor and turbine or blaster) and a multiflex connector (for turbine or blaster). Slow-speed handpieces run at the speed of the micromotor, i.e. 20 to 40000 rpm unless geared up or geared down. A blue ring or no colour marking around the connecting end of the handpiece (third, fifth and sixth from left) means that the handpiece will run at the speed of the micromotor. A green ring around the connecting end of the handpiece (furthest left) means that the handpiece is geared down, i.e. runs slower than the micromotor. The degree of speed reduction is often engraved on the handpiece. The one depicted furthest left in the picture is 16:1, i.e. the handpiece will run 16 times slower than the micromotor. The handpiece depicted fourth from left is an endodontic handpiece with reduction gear 128:1. A red ring indicates that the handpiece is geared up, i.e. runs faster than the micromotor. The one depicted in the picture (second handpiece from left) is 1:5, i.e. runs 5 times faster than the micromotor

High-speed burs are used to section teeth and perform cavity preparation.

CARE AND MAINTENANCE OF INSTRUMENTATION AND EQUIPMENT

The care and maintenance of dental equipment and instrumentation is the responsibility of the veterinary nurse.

Sharpening of hand instruments

Instruments must be sharp if they are to work efficiently yet with minimal trauma to the gingival tissues. Scalers and curettes, luxators and elevators all require regular sharpening. The basic goals of sharpening are to conserve a sharp cutting edge and to preserve the original shape of the instrument. Sharpening is usually performed after cleaning and prior to sterilisation. Heat sterilisation will result in blunting, so a clean sharpening stone should be available for sharpening during the procedure. Alternatively, sharpening can be performed after cleaning and sterilisation.

In general, a fine grade stone, e.g. Arkansas, is recommended to avoid changing the basic shape of the instrument. A course grade stone removes too much metal and should not be used. Instruments that are very dull should be professionally reground or replaced with new ones that are maintained.

Scalers and curettes. Instruments must be sharp if scaling is to be completed efficiently with minimal trauma to the gingival tissues. When the blade of the instrument is maintained properly greater control of the working end occurs. Fewer repetitive strokes are required and there is thus less operator fatigue.

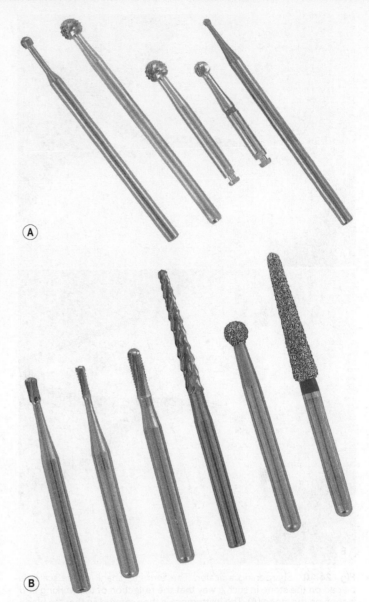

Fig. 26.9 Types of burs. (**A**) Slow-speed burs. The picture shows a selection of burs for slow-speed handpieces. The long burs with friction grip attachment are for use in a straight handpiece; while the shorter ones with latch-key attachment are for use in a contra-angle handpiece. Slow-speed burs can be used to section teeth but are predominantly used to safely remove alveolar bone during extraction. Water cooling is essential. (**B**) High-speed burs. The picture shows a selection of burs for high-speed handpieces. Note that all burs are friction grip. A latch-key attachment is not possible at speed in excess of 300000 rpm. High-speed burs are used to section teeth and for cavity preparation. To avoid thermal injury to tooth and bone and blunting of the bur the water should never be turned off when using high speed

Scalers and curettes should be sharpened before each use, i.e. after cleaning and disinfection. Sharpening of dirty instruments will contaminate the sharpening stone. Sharpening should be performed in a light room with a bright light, so that the cutting edge(s) of the blade are clearly visualised. Acrylic testing sticks are available to check the adequacy of the sharpening procedure.

Handheld sharpening stones are the best way to restore the cutting edge on a dull instrument while maintaining its original shape. Fine stones will maintain the cutting edge on

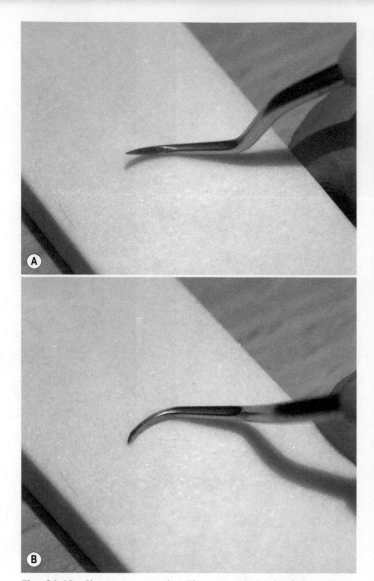

Fig. 26.10 Sharpening a scaler. The terminal shank of the scaler is placed on the stone in such a way that the reflection of the working end is seen on the stone (**A**). The instrument is then rotated so that the blade engages the stone and the shadow of the working end disappears (**B**)

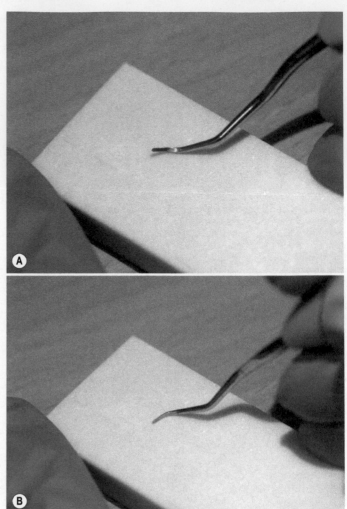

Fig. 26.11 Sharpening a curette. The terminal shank of the curette is placed on the stone in such a way that the reflection of the working end is seen on the stone (**A**). The instrument is then rotated so that the blade engages the stone and the shadow of the working end disappears (**B**)

instruments that are frequently sharpened, without removing an excessive amount of the blade. To prevent 'grooving', the whole surface of the stone should be used during sharpening.

Water (not oil) should be used on the stone. The care of stones requires wiping with a clean cloth to remove metal particles and then scrub or ultrasonically clean. Stones can be autoclaved safely.

There are several techniques for sharpening scalers and curettes detailed in the literature. A simple but effective technique is as follows:

1. The terminal shank of the scaler (Fig. 26.10A) or curette (Fig. 26.11A) is placed on the stone in such a way that the reflection of the working end is seen on the stone.
2. The instrument is placed so that the blade engages the stone and the reflection (shadow) of the working end disappears (Fig. 26.10B for scaler and 26.11B for curette).

3. The stone is held stationary and the engaged instrument is pulled towards you (Fig. 26.12).

Make sure that you are familiar with the component parts of the scaler and curette before attempting sharpening. It may be useful to have a sharp, unused scaler and curette available for comparison during the learning phase. Also, have an acrylic stick handy to test the cutting edge.

Luxators, elevators and extraktors. Luxators, elevators and extraktors also need to be sharpened regularly, usually after each use, i.e. after cleaning and disinfecting. If the working end has been damaged, they should be professionally reground.

Luxators and elevators are easily sharpened with a cylindrical Arkansas stone. I prefer to use a 'stationary stone, moving instrument technique' to sharpen these instruments. The technique is as follows:

- Place the cylindrical stone flat on the table.
- Place a few drops of water on the stone.
- Hold the handle of the luxator or elevator in the palm of the hand, with the index finger extended straight on the shank.

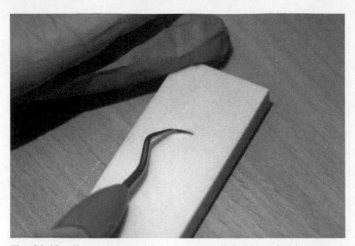

Fig. 26.12 Sharpening a scaler or curette. The stone is held stationary and the engaged scaler or curette is pulled towards you. Use a few drops of water (not oil) to lubricate the stone. Use the length of the stone and avoid using the same area every time to avoid grooving in the stone. Test the cutting edge with an acrylic stick and repeat until instrument is sharp, i.e. acrylic flakes are readily removed from the stick

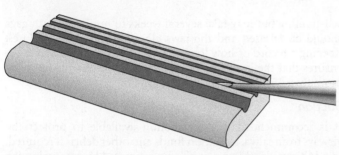

Fig. 26.13 Sharpening the extraktor. The extraktor is placed in the correct groove for its size with its convex side against the stone. The instrument is pushed forward while rotating it to maintain the unique lateral cutting edges

- Apply the working end of the luxator or elevator to the stone.
- Exert mild pressure and push or pull the luxator and elevator along the stone.
- Check sharpness on an acrylic stick.
- Repeat as necessary until instrument is sharp.

Extraktors can be sharpened using either a flat stone or ideally a specially designed stone (Fig. 26.13). If a flat stone is used, then place the extraktor with its convex side against the stone, angle around 20 degrees and push the instrument forward on the stone. For best results use the specially designed stone. Place the extraktor in the correct groove and push forward while rotating the instrument to maintain the lateral cutting edges.

Care and maintenance of power equipment

Power equipment also requires care and maintenance. The manufacturer and/or supplier of power equipment must supply you with detailed information on how to care for and maintain the unit you have purchased. An annual service contract should be part of the purchase agreement. There are similarities and differences in the care and maintenance of different units and you need to check with your supplier exactly how your unit should be looked after. The following is a general guideline.

TABLE 26.1	General maintenance of compressed-air-driven units			
Operation		Daily	Weekly	Annually
Drain air receiver		*		
Drain filter/regulator		*		
Check oil level			*	
Change oil				*
Change air intake filter				*
Change line filter				*
Check electrical connections and all pipe fittings				*

Cleaning and sterilising the ultrasonic scaler. The body of the ultrasonic scaler should not be cleaned in an ultrasonic bath. Instead, it can be cleaned using a cotton swab soaked in alcohol. Following cleaning, the handpiece should be sterilised (autoclave at 134°C at 2 bar [200 kPa] for 20 minutes). The procedure is as follows:

1. Separate the handpiece from the cord and remove the scaler tip.
2. Put the handpiece in the sterilisable cloth or bag if required.
3. Take the handpiece out of the autoclave as soon at the sterilisation is complete.
4. Carefully dry the electrical contacts and the cord connector before use.

Cleaning and sterilising handpieces. Handpieces need to be lubricated before and after sterilisation or the bearings will fail.

After removing the bur, a brush is used to remove foreign particles from the handpiece. It is then wiped clean with a moist cloth. For the high-speed handpiece, a fine wire is provided for cleaning the water spray hole. Instructions should come with each unit as to how to dismantle handpieces.

Lubricate the handpiece. This can be achieved by inserting two or three drops of oil lubricant via a lubricant nozzle into the air supply tube. If a spray lubricant is used, it should be activated for 3 seconds. Operate the handpiece with a bur installed for 15–20 seconds. Remove the bur from the handpiece and disconnect the handpiece from the unit. The handpiece is now ready for autoclaving. Follow manufacturer's directions. After autoclaving is complete, and the handpiece has returned to room temperature, it needs to be lubricated again prior to use.

Precautions:
- Never autoclave handpiece with a bur in place.
- Never operate handpiece without a bur inserted.
- Do not forget 'before and after sterilisation' lubrication procedures.
- Dry heat sterilisation is not allowed under any circumstances.

General maintenance. Table 26.1 indicates general maintenance, which must be carried out by the user. The high-speed handpiece requires clean air, and water that accumulates in the compressor must be removed daily. Refer to the handbook for details of how to empty the compressor.

Anaesthesia for dental procedures

GENERAL CONSIDERATIONS

Oral examination and all oral/dental procedures require general anaesthesia. The procedures are often lengthy and close attention to life support is needed. Some general principles of anaesthesia for the patient undergoing dental or oral surgery are as follows:

Airway security

During dental surgery, the airway must be secured by endotracheal intubation to prevent aspiration pneumonia, which may occur if debris such as irrigation fluid and blood from the oral cavity enters unprotected airways.

Endotracheal tubes

Endotracheal tubes must be checked for defective cuffs and obstructed lumens before use. Any defective tubes should be discarded. Lightweight circuits are recommended.

To reduce apparatus dead space and the risk of endobronchial intubation, the tubing should be cut to fit the patient from mid neck to the level of the incisor teeth. Excessively long tubes that protrude from the oral cavity are prone to kinking, which may lead to pulmonary oedema as the patient inspires against an obstructed airway. The use of guarded endotracheal tubes should be considered for patients at high risk of tube kinking. Moreover, excessively long tubes are difficult to secure to the jaw with gauze bandage, which increases the risk of accidental extubation, and increases the dead space. Knots should be tied around the adaptor and not around the endotracheal tube itself. The cuff should be carefully inflated to a point where there is no air leaking around it. Be careful not to inflate the cuff excessively, as this can cause tracheal injury. The status of the endotracheal tube and integrity of the cuff should be monitored continuously. The operator will usually change the animal's position during surgery or while taking radiographs and this may cause tube displacement and/or kinking.

Pharyngeal packing

Pharyngeal packing should be used for greater airway security. Commonly used pharyngeal packs include surgical swabs, sponges (Fig. 26.14) and gauze bandage. A simple way to pack the pharynx is to insert a length of damp gauze bandage around the endotracheal tube, with the free end left visible for easy removal. It is important not to pack too tightly, as this impedes venous return and results in swelling of the tongue. Packs will become saturated with liquid during procedures and will then no longer offer adequate protection and should be replaced as required. It is imperative to remove any packing prior to extubation. It is good practice to note on the anaesthetic monitoring sheet that the pack has been inserted and then removed, the same as a swab count in abdominal surgery.

Eye protection

The eyes should be protected from desiccation by applying a lubricant eye ointment as required during the procedure.

Mouth gags

Mouth gags should be used with caution. Keeping the jaws wide open for prolonged periods may result in neuropraxia and inability to close the jaws (Robins 1976). The condition is

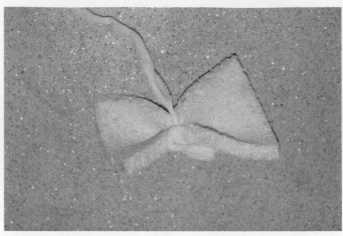

Fig. 26.14 Pharyngeal pack. Pharyngeal packing should be used for greater airway security. Commonly used packs include sponge, surgical swabs, gauze bandage. Packs will become saturated with liquid during procedures and will then no longer offer adequate protection and should be replaced as required. It is imperative to remove any packing prior to extubation

self-limiting but may take several weeks to resolve. Mouth gags should be released and the jaws closed every 10–15 minutes. Keeping a record of how long the mouth gag has been in place ensures that the jaws are not inadvertently kept wide open for more than 15 minutes.

Suction

It is recommended to have suction available to protect the airways from saliva, irrigation fluids and other debris if required. In addition, blood loss can also be estimated by measuring the volume of blood in the suction jar.

Hypothermia

Hypothermia is a complication of lengthy anaesthesia and the use of cool irrigation fluids. Body temperature should be monitored regularly, e.g. every 5–10 minutes, and the development of hypothermia should be prevented by supplying external heat by blankets and warmed intravenous and irrigation fluids. Patients should be insulated with towels or bubble pack to prevent thermal injuries due to 'hot spots', which may occur with electrical heating mats. Circulating warm water mats may be safer.

Hyperthermia

Hyperthermia can occasionally occur in large, heavy-coated dogs connected to rebreathing circuits for long periods. By monitoring body temperature every 5–10 minutes, the development of hyperthermia can be identified and active cooling by fans, cooling pads, etc., can be initiated before damage occurs to vital organs.

Haemorrhage

Periodontal and other dental treatment rarely results in extensive haemorrhage unless the patient has an underlying disorder, e.g. coagulopathy, septicaemia.

A full haematological examination and clotting profile should be performed prior to any potentially haemorrhagic procedure, e.g. major oral surgery such as a maxillectomy. The patient should also be cross-matched with a healthy donor prior to any such procedure. An alternative to cross-matching is autologous transfusion.

During the procedure, blood loss should be estimated either by weighing blood-soaked swabs or by measuring the amount of blood collected in a suction jar. As a rough guide a saturated 7.5×7.5 cm swab contains 7 ml of blood and a saturated 10×10 cm swab contains 10 ml of blood.

PATIENT MONITORING

All patients should be monitored continuously. Careful monitoring should enable the detection of problems before they become severe, so that they can be treated appropriately and crises can be avoided. Continuous anaesthetic monitoring is associated with reduced mortality (Dyson et al. 1998). It is impossible to both monitor anaesthesia and perform the procedure. Moreover, with some procedures a surgical assistant is required. The surgical assistant needs to be a different person from the one monitoring the anaesthesia.

Routine anaesthetic monitoring includes:
- Inspecting respiratory function
- Assessing the colour of the mucous membranes
- Checking capillary refill time
- Listening to the sound of breathing
- Palpating the peripheral pulse.

All findings should be recorded on an anaesthetic chart at regular intervals, e.g. every 5 minutes, for the duration of anaesthesia. Also record current oxygen, nitrous oxide (if used) and volatile agent level at each check. Any changes in the anaesthetic regimen, e.g. altering flow rate or concentration of volatile agent, should be recorded on the chart.

This basic monitoring can be augmented with mechanical aids, which give additional information and allow a more precise picture of the patient's status. This allows closer control over the course of the anaesthetic. The disadvantage of mechanical monitoring devices is that they in turn must be monitored to ensure that the information they are giving is accurate. Unexpected readings should be verified by examination of the patient before they are acted on, i.e. monitor the patient, not the equipment.

ANAESTHETIC RECOVERY

Anaesthesia should be lightened towards the end of the procedure. The oral cavity must be cleaned out, the pharyngeal pack removed and the cuff of the endotracheal tube deflated before recovery is allowed to proceed. Use of the three-way syringe (air–water spray) on the dental unit is recommended for removing debris from the tongue and gums. A dry swab can be used to remove any large blood clots. Ensure that there is no debris in the oropharynx before removing the pharyngeal pack and deflating the cuff of the endotracheal tube. The coat around the mouth and head should be cleaned and dried using a towel or hairdryer. The endotracheal tube is usually not removed until the animal has a swallowing reflex.

Anaesthetic recovery should be monitored closely and recorded. It should always occur in a warm environment. Animals that have had surgical procedures using flap techniques and suturing, e.g. open or surgical extractions or oronasal fistula repair, must be prevented from pawing at their mouths or rubbing their faces. In some animals, an Elizabethan collar may be used. If the surgical procedure has resulted in blood in the nasal cavity, e.g. oronasal fistula repair, it is wise to recover these patients in sternal recumbency with the head placed lower than the rest of the body to encourage drainage. Sneezing fits commonly occur in these patients on recovery.

IMMEDIATE POSTOPERATIVE CARE

Optimal immediate postoperative management involves appropriate analgesia and nursing. Sound nursing measures also have a profound impact on reducing the level of postoperative discomfort and pain. Giving the animal attention at regular intervals helps reduce the distress associated with pain and the unfamiliar environment, otherwise a cycle of pain/distress/sleeplessness can develop.

The provision of a comfortable bed in a warm, but not too hot, environment is beneficial. Food and water should be offered as early as possible in the postoperative period. Pain and inflammation increase the basic metabolic rate and a high level of nutrition is required to promote healing. Offering food as early as possible not only speeds recovery but can also have a soothing effect.

Oral examination and recording

Oral examination in a conscious animal will only give limited information. Definitive oral examination can only be performed under general anaesthesia. All detected abnormalities should be recorded. It saves time if one person performs the examination and another individual takes the notes and enters the findings on the dental record.

CONSCIOUS EXAMINATION

Oral examination of a conscious animal is limited to visual inspection and some digital palpation. Gentle technique is essential. Examination involves assessing not only the oral cavity but also palpation of:
- Face – facial bones and zygomatic arch
- Temporomandibular joint
- Salivary glands – mandibular/sublingual; the parotids are usually only palpable if enlarged
- Lymph nodes – mandibular, cervical chain
- Having looked at the entire face, the mouth is first examined by gently holding the jaws closed and retracting the lips (do not pull on the fur to retract lips) to look at the soft tissues and buccal aspects of the teeth. This is the optimal time to evaluate occlusion.

After evaluating the occlusion the animal is encouraged to open its mouth. One method of achieving this in the dog is to place a thumb and finger on the margin of the alveolar bone caudal to the canine teeth of the upper and lower jaw on one side and with gentle pressure encouraging the animal to open its jaws. Another method, useful for both dogs and cats, is to approach the animal from the side, place one hand over the muzzle and press the lips gently into the oral cavity while tilting the head slightly upwards. A finger from the other hand is placed on the lower incisors and gentle pressure is exerted. Do not use the fur under the mandible to try to pull the jaw down. Most animals allow at least a cursory inspection of the oral cavity once the jaws have been opened. The mucous membranes of the oral cavity should be examined as well as the teeth. Apart from colour and texture of the mucous membranes, look for evidence of a potential bleeding problem, e.g. petechiation, purpura, ecchymoses. In addition, look for vesicle formation, ulceration, which could indicate a vesiculo-bullous disorder, e.g. pemphigus, pemphigoid. Obvious pathology, e.g. tooth fracture, gingival recession, advanced furcation exposure relating to the teeth, can be identified. Assess the oropharynx (soft palate, palatoglossal arch, tonsillary crypts, tonsils and fauces) if possible. It is useful to identify any potential problems that may occur with endotracheal intubation prior to inducing anaesthesia.

EXAMINATION UNDER GENERAL ANAESTHESIA

The oropharynx (soft palate, palatoglossal arch, tonsillary crypts, tonsils and fauces) should be examined prior to endotracheal intubation. Normal anatomical features of the oral cavity should be identified and inspected. Refreshing your memory on these features from an anatomy textbook is highly recommended. It is only with knowledge of the normal that abnormalities can be identified.

Once the animal is intubated and anaesthesia stable, the full oral examination can commence. The periodontium of each tooth needs to be assessed. Examination of the periodontium is not routinely performed in veterinary practice. It is essential to perform a thorough periodontal examination in order to identify disease and plan treatment. The following indices and criteria should be evaluated for each tooth:

1. Gingivitis and gingival index
2. Periodontal probing depth (PPD)
3. Gingival recession
4. Furcation involvement
5. Mobility
6. Periodontal (clinical) attachment level.

In animals with large accumulations of dental deposits (plaque and calculus) on the teeth, it may be necessary to remove these to assess periodontal status accurately.

The purpose of the meticulous periodontal examination is to:

- Identify the presence of periodontal disease, i.e. gingivitis and periodontitis
- Differentiate between gingivitis – inflammation of the gingiva – and periodontitis – inflammation of the periodontal tissues, resulting in loss of attachment and eventually tooth loss
- Identify the precise location of disease processes
- Assess the extent of tissue destruction where there is periodontitis.

Periodontal probing depth, gingival recession, furcation involvement and mobility quantify the tissue destruction in periodontitis. Radiography to visualise the extent and type of alveolar bone destruction is mandatory if clinical evidence of periodontitis is found. In many cases, measuring or calculating the periodontal or clinical attachment level (PAL/CAL) is also useful.

1. Gingivitis and gingival index

The presence and degree of gingivitis (Fig. 26.15) is assessed based on a combination of redness and swelling, as well as presence or absence of bleeding on gentle probing of the gingival sulcus. Various indices can be used to give a numerical value to the degree of gingival inflammation present. In the clinical situation, a simple bleeding index is the most useful. Using this method, a periodontal probe is gently inserted into the gingival sulcus at several locations around the whole circumference of

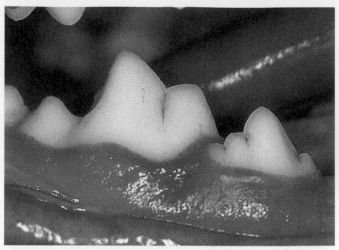

Fig. 26.15 Gingivitis is inflammation of the gingiva, which manifests as reddening, swelling and often bleeding of the gingival margin

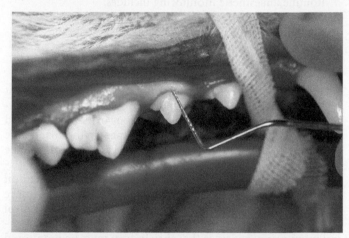

Fig. 26.16 Periodontal probing depth

each tooth; and the tooth is given a score of 0 if there is no bleeding and a score of 1 if the probing elicits bleeding.

2. Periodontal probing depth

The depth of the sulcus can be assessed by gently inserting a graduated periodontal probe until resistance is encountered at the base of the sulcus. The depth from the free gingival margin to the base of the sulcus is measured in millimetres at several locations around the whole circumference of the tooth (Fig. 26.16). The probe is moved gently horizontally, walking along the floor of the sulcus. The gingival sulcus is 1–3 mm deep in the dog and 0.5–1 mm in the cat. Measurements in excess of these values usually indicate the presence of periodontitis: the periodontal ligament has been destroyed and alveolar bone resorbed, thus allowing the probe to be inserted to a greater depth. The term used to describe this situation is periodontal pocketing. All sites with periodontal pocketing should be accurately recorded. Gingival inflammation resulting in swelling or hyperplasia of the free gingiva (Fig. 26.17) will, of course, also result in sulcus depths in excess of normal values. In these situations, the term pseudo-pocketing is used, as the periodontal ligament and bone are intact, i.e. there is no evidence of periodontitis and the increase in PPD is due to swelling or hyperplasia of the gingiva.

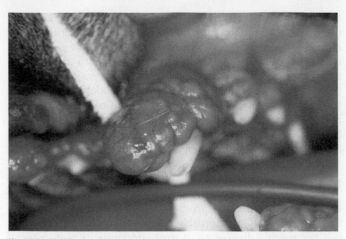

Fig. 26.17 Gingival hyperplasia

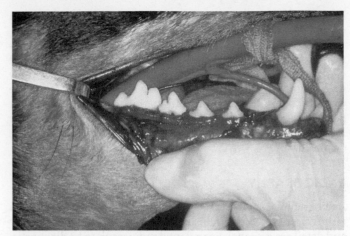

Fig. 26.19 Furcation involvement. The left maxillary second and third premolars have grade 2 furcation involvement and the fourth premolar has a grade 1 lesion

TABLE 26.2	Grading of furcation involvement
Grade 0	No furcation involvement
Grade 1	The furcation can be felt with the probe but horizontal tissue destruction is less than one-third of the horizontal width of the furcation
Grade 2	It is possible to explore the furcation but the probe cannot be passed through it from buccal to palatal/lingual. Horizontal tissue destruction is more than one-third of the horizontal width of the furcation
Grade 3	The probe can be passed through the furcation from buccal to palatal/lingual

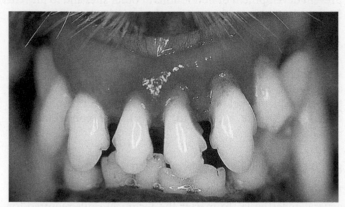

Fig. 26.18 Gingival recession is measured from the cemento-enamel junction to the free gingival margin using a periodontal probe. In this photograph of the upper incisors, the right second incisor has a normal gingival contour, while the right first incisor and the left first and second incisor all have gingival recession of varying degrees

TABLE 26.3	Grading of tooth mobility
Grade 0	No mobility
Grade 1	Horizontal movement of 1 mm or less
Grade 2	Horizontal movement of more than 1 mm*
Grade 3	Vertical as well as horizontal movement is possible

*Note that multirooted teeth are scored more severely and a horizontal mobility in excess of 1 mm is usually considered a grade 3 even in the absence of vertical movement.

3. Gingival recession

Gingival recession is also measured using a periodontal probe (Fig. 26.18). It is the distance (in millimetres) from the cemento-enamel junction to the free gingival margin. At sites with gingival recession, PPD may be within normal values despite loss of alveolar bone due to periodontitis.

4. Furcation involvement

Furcation involvement refers to the situation where the bone between the roots of multirooted teeth is destroyed by periodontitis (Fig. 26.19). The furcation sites of multirooted teeth should be examined with a periodontal probe. The grading of furcation involvement is listed in Table 26.2.

5. Tooth mobility

The extent of tooth mobility should be assessed using a suitable instrument, e.g. the blunt end of the handle of a dental mirror or probe. It should not be assessed using fingers directly, since the yield of the soft tissues of the fingers will mask the extent of tooth mobility. The grading of mobility is listed in Table 26.3.

6. Periodontal/clinical attachment level

Periodontal probing depth is not necessarily correlated with severity of attachment loss. As mentioned, gingival hyperplasia may contribute to a deep pocket or a pseudo-pocket if there is no attachment loss, while gingival recession may result in the absence of a pocket but also minimal remaining attachment. Periodontal attachment level records the distance from the cemento-enamel junction or from a fixed point on the tooth to the base or apical extension of the pathological pocket. It is thus a more accurate assessment of tissue loss in periodontitis. PAL is either directly measured with a periodontal probe or it is calculated, e.g. PPD + gingival recession.

RECORDING FINDINGS

The information resulting from the examination and any treatment performed must be recorded. A basic dental record consists of written notes and a completed dental chart. Additional diagnostic tests and radiographs are included as indicated.

A dental chart is a diagrammatic representation of the dentition, where information (findings and treatment) can be entered in a pictorial and/or notational form. A dental chart needs to be supplemented by clinical notes, radiographs, etc., to make a complete dental record.

A copy of dog and cat dental record sheets used in our practice is depicted in Figure 26.20. The front is used to record clinical findings and the back is used to enter diagnosis, draw up a treatment plan and record treatment performed. The nurse who performs the clinical examination completes the front page. The veterinary surgeon checks the clinical findings and interprets any radiographs taken, and then fills in the back page of the chart.

RADIOGRAPHY

Radiography is a vital tool in veterinary dentistry. Pathological radiographic changes are usually discrete and therefore clarity and detail are essential. For a dental radiograph to be diagnostic, it should be an accurate representation of the size and shape of the tooth without superimposition of adjacent structures. Intraoral radiographic techniques are therefore required; a parallel technique for the mandibular premolars and molars, and a bisecting angle technique for all other teeth. (For intraoral radiographic techniques see Chapter 32.) Attending a practical course is strongly recommended. While a trained nurse can take radiographs, the interpretation of the films is the remit of the veterinary surgeon.

Periodontal therapy

The management of periodontal disease is aimed at controlling the cause of the inflammation, i.e. dental plaque. Conservative or cause-related periodontal therapy consists of removal of plaque and calculus, and any other remedial procedures required, under general anaesthesia, in combination with daily maintenance of oral hygiene. In other words, the treatment of periodontal disease has two components:

- Professional periodontal therapy
- Maintenance of oral hygiene.

Professional periodontal therapy is performed under general anaesthesia and includes:

- Supra- and subgingival scaling
- Root planing
- Tooth crown polishing
- Subgingival lavage.

Maintenance of oral hygiene is performed by the owner and is often called home care. Its effectiveness depends on the motivation and technical ability of the owner and the cooperation of the animal. If no home care is instituted, then plaque will rapidly reform after a professional periodontal therapy procedure and the disease will progress. Before any treatment is instituted, the owner must be made aware that home care is the most essential component in both preventing and treating periodontal disease. Whenever possible, it is useful to institute a home-care programme before any professional periodontal therapy is performed. The veterinary nurse has an important role to play in instituting and maintaining home care.

The aim of treatment differs whether the patient has gingivitis only or if there is also periodontitis.

GINGIVITIS

Gingivitis is by definition reversible (see Fig. 26.15). Removal or adequate reduction of plaque will restore inflamed gingivae

to health. Once clinically healthy gingivae have been achieved these can be maintained by daily removal or reduction of the accumulation of plaque. In short, the treatment of gingivitis is to restore the inflamed tissues to clinical health and then to maintain clinically healthy gingivae, thus preventing periodontitis (Fig. 26.21). The purpose of the professional periodontal therapy in the gingivitis patient is removal of dental deposits, mainly calculus (which is not removed by tooth-brushing). Once the teeth have been cleaned, it remains up to the owner to remove the plaque that reaccumulates on a daily basis.

PERIODONTITIS

Untreated gingivitis may progress to periodontitis. Periodontitis is irreversible. It is important to remember that periodontitis is a site-specific disease, i.e. it may affect one or more sites of one or several teeth (Fig. 26.22). The aim of treatment is to prevent development of new lesions at other sites and to prevent further tissue destruction at sites that are already affected.

Professional periodontal therapy removes dental deposits above and below the gingival margin. It then rests with the owner to ensure that plaque does not reaccumulate. Meticulous supragingival plaque control, by means of daily tooth-brushing and adjunctive antiseptics when indicated, will prevent migration of the plaque below the gingival margin. If the subgingival tooth surfaces are kept clean, the sulcular epithelium will reattach.

PROFESSIONAL PERIODONTAL THERAPY

Professional periodontal therapy must be performed under general anaesthesia. To master the technical skills required for dentistry and oral surgery, attending practical courses is recommended.

Supragingival scaling

This is the removal of plaque and calculus above the gingival margin. It can be performed using hand instruments alone or a combination of hand instruments and mechanical scalers.

The recommended procedure is as follows:

1. Remove gross dental deposits – plaque-covered calculus – using rongeurs, extraction forceps or calculus-removing forceps (Fig. 26.23).
2. Remove residual supragingival dental deposits with sharp hand instruments, either a sickle-shaped scaler or a curette, as shown in Figure 26.24.
3. A mechanical scaler, either ultrasonic or sonic, is then used to remove residual dental deposits (Fig. 26.25).

Mechanical scalers generate heat and have the potential to cause iatrogenic damage if not used properly. Overheating a tooth will cause desiccation of the dentine and consequent damage to the underlying pulp tissue. Pulp damage may be a reversible pulpitis but it can become severe enough to cause pulp necrosis, which would necessitate extraction or endodontic treatment of the affected tooth.

An ultrasonic or sonic scaler should be used by gently stroking the tooth with the side of the tip and with continuous movement over the tooth surface. A plentiful supply of water is essential to cool the oscillating tip and flush away debris. Using the tip of the instrument or applying excessive pressure will cause gouging of the tooth surface as well as generating

Text continued on p. 524

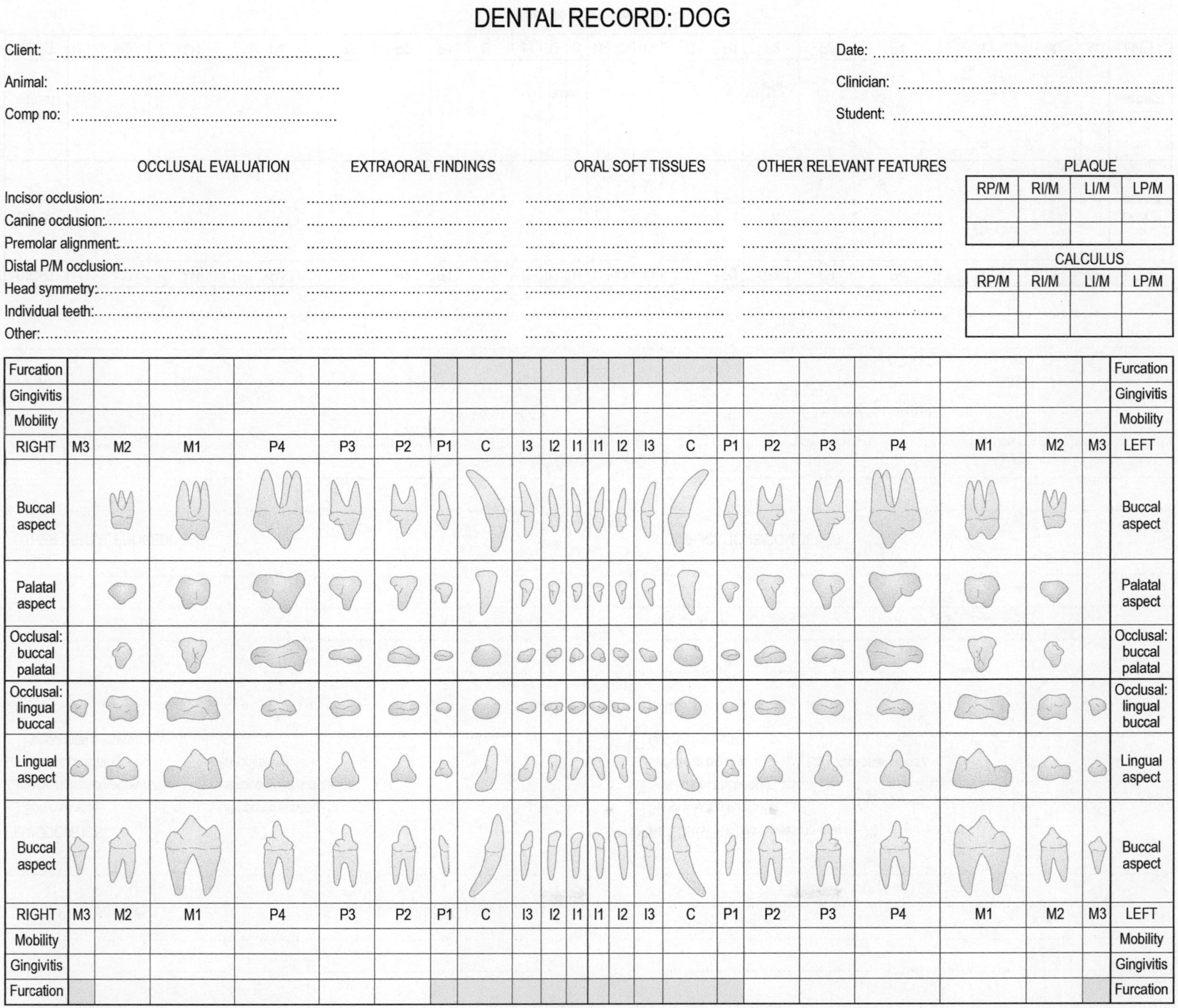

DENTAL RECORD: DOG

Client: ....

Animal: ....

Comp no: ....

Date: ....

Clinician: ....

Student: ....

OCCLUSAL EVALUATION

EXTRAORAL FINDINGS

ORAL SOFT TISSUES

OTHER RELEVANT FEATURES

Incisor occlusion: ....

Canine occlusion: ....

Premolar alignment: ....

Distal P/M occlusion: ....

Head symmetry: ....

Individual teeth: ....

Other: ....

PLAQUE	RP/M	RI/M	LI/M	LP/M

CALCULUS	RP/M	RI/M	LI/M	LP/M

Fig. 26.20A Dog dental record sheet – the front is used to record clinical findings and the back is used to enter diagnosis, draw up treatment plan and record treatment performed

Continued

ORAL PROBLEM LIST

THERAPEUTIC PLAN

PERIODONTICS

☐ Sonic scaling ☐ Ultrasonic scaling
☐ Subgingival curettage ☐ Periodontal debridement
☐ Pumice-polishing ☐ Air-polishing
☐ Periodontal surgery..............

ORAL SURGERY (Note sites on graph - X)
☐ Simple extraction(s):...............
☐ Surgical extraction(s):..............
☐ Incisional biopsy ☐ Excisional biopsy
☐ Other/comments.............

OTHER DENTAL PROCEDURES

COMPLICATIONS/COMMENTS

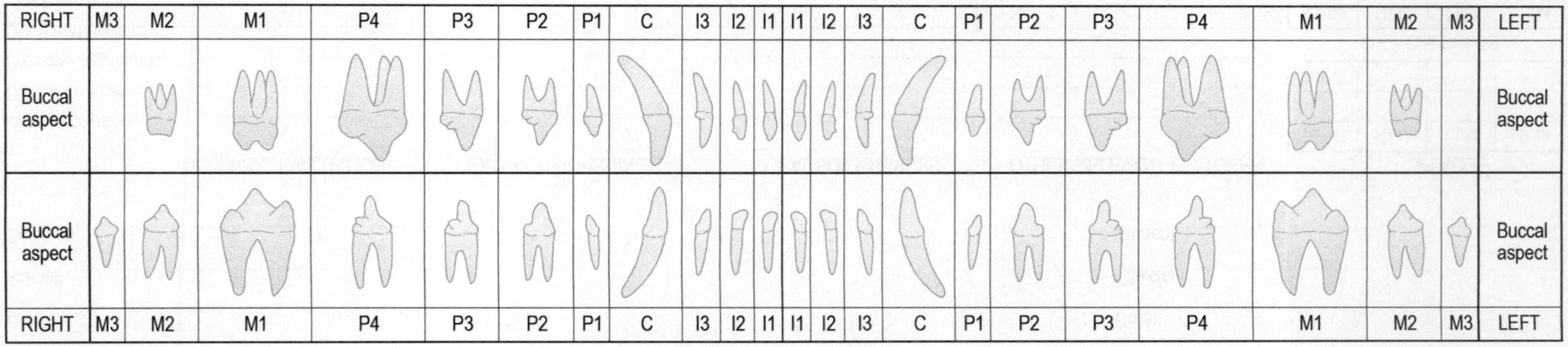

RIGHT	M3	M2	M1	P4	P3	P2	P1	C	I3	I2	I1	I1	I2	I3	C	P1	P2	P3	P4	M1	M2	M3	LEFT
Buccal aspect																							Buccal aspect
Buccal aspect																							Buccal aspect
RIGHT	M3	M2	M1	P4	P3	P2	P1	C	I3	I2	I1	I1	I2	I3	C	P1	P2	P3	P4	M1	M2	M3	LEFT

Fig. 26.20A, cont'd

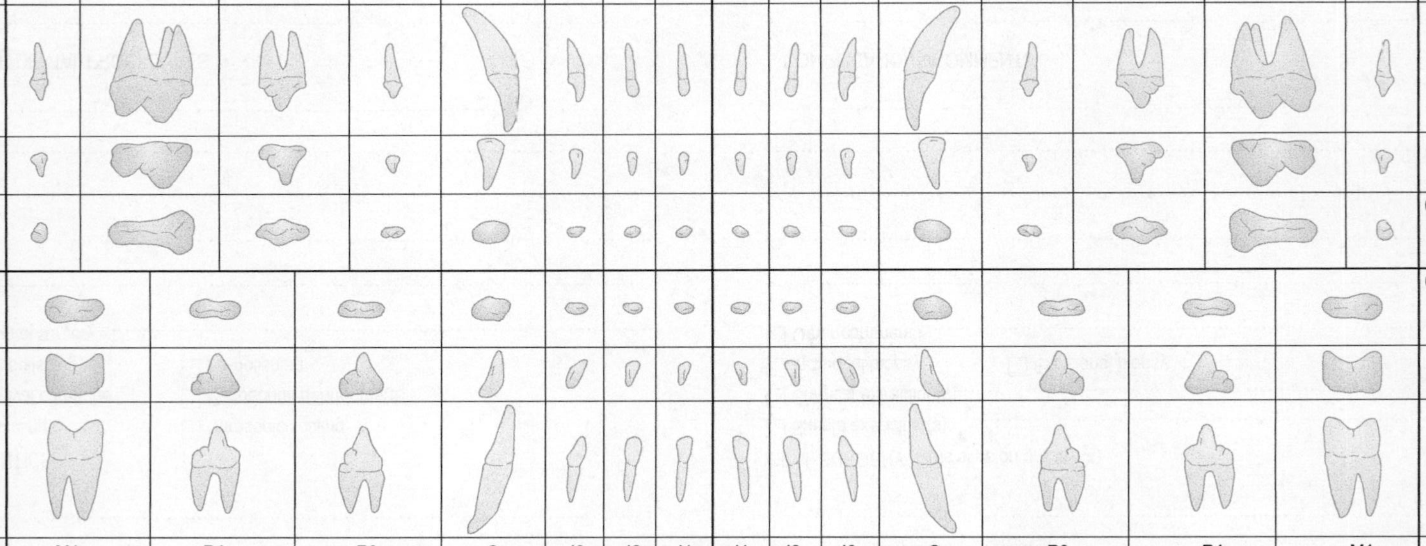

DENTAL RECORD: CAT

Client: .... Date: ....

Animal: .... Clinician: ....

Comp no: .... Student: ....

	OCCLUSAL EVALUATION	EXTRAORAL FINDINGS	ORAL SOFT TISSUES	OTHER RELEVANT FEATURES
Incisor occlusion:				
Canine occlusion:				
Premolar alignment:				
Distal P/M occlusion:				
Head symmetry:				
Individual teeth:				
Other:				

PLAQUE

RP/M	RI/M	LI/M	LP/M

CALCULUS

RP/M	RI/M	LI/M	LP/M

F.O.R.L.																	F.O.R.L.
Furcation																	Furcation
Gingivitis																	Gingivitis
Mobility																	Mobility
RIGHT	M1	P4	P3	P2	C	I3	I2	I1	I1	I2	I3	C	P2	P3	P4	M1	LEFT
Buccal aspect																	Buccal aspect
Palatal aspect																	Palatal aspect
Occlusal: buccal palatal																	Occlusal: buccal palatal

Occlusal: lingual buccal															Occlusal: lingual buccal
Lingual aspect															Lingual aspect
Buccal aspect															Buccal aspect
RIGHT	M1	P4	P3	C	I3	I2	I1	I1	I2	I3	C	P3	P4	M1	LEFT
Mobility															Mobility
Gingivitis															Gingivitis
Furcation															Furcation
F.O.R.L.															F.O.R.L.

Fig. 26.20B Cat dental record sheet

Continued

ORAL PROBLEM LIST

THERAPEUTIC PLAN

PERIODONTICS

☐ Sonic scaling   ☐ Ultrasonic scaling
☐ Subgingival curettage   ☐ Periodontal debridement
☐ Pumice-polishing   ☐ Air-polishing
☐ Periodontal surgery

ORAL SURGERY (Note sites on graph - X)
☐ Simple extraction(s):
☐ Surgical extraction(s):
☐ Incisional biopsy   ☐ Excisional biopsy
☐ Other/comments

OTHER DENTAL PROCEDURES

COMPLICATIONS/COMMENTS

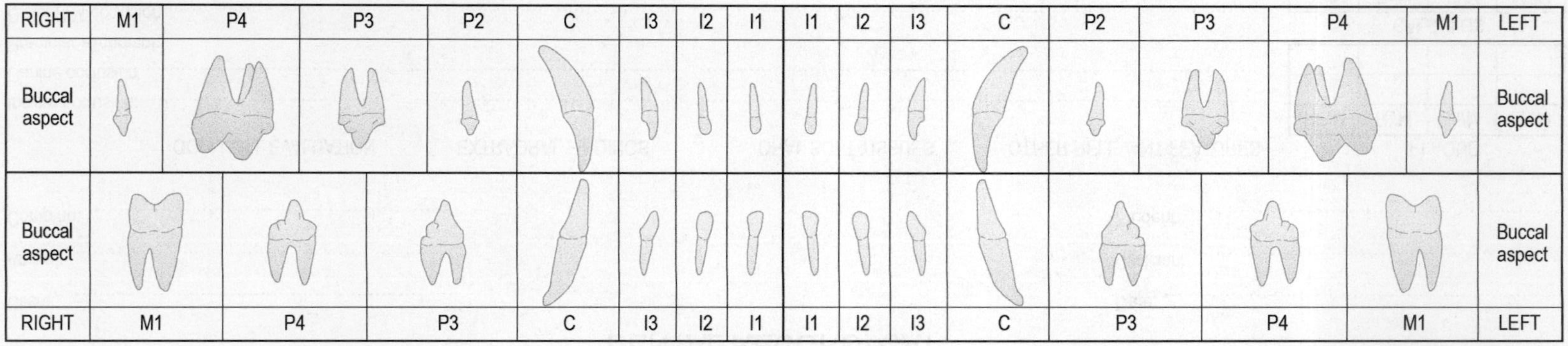

Fig. 26.20B, cont'd

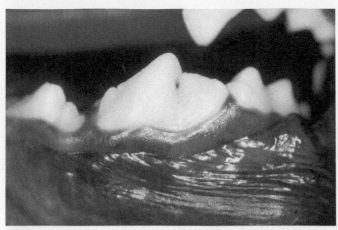

Fig. 26.21 Clinically healthy gingivae. This is the term used to describe gingiva that shows no clinical evidence of inflammation. There is no reddening, swelling or bleeding. The gingival margin is firmly adapted to the tooth surface

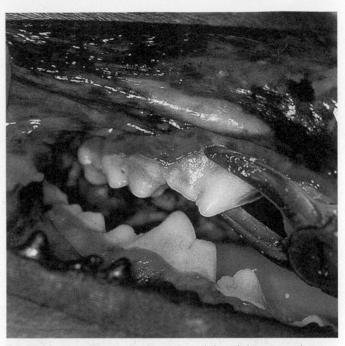

Fig. 26.23 Removing gross supragingival dental deposits with extraction forceps. Avoid traumatising the gingival margin with the forceps

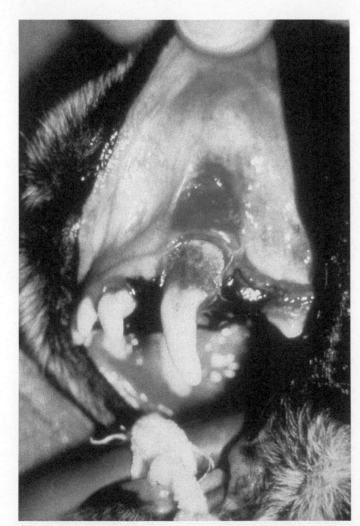

Fig. 26.22 Periodontitis. It is important to remember that periodontitis is a site-specific disease. Depicted is a lower first molar with periodontitis (destruction of periodontal ligament, bone loss and gingival recession) affecting the buccal surface of the distal root. The rest of the tooth shows no evidence of periodontitis (normal PPD and no gingival recession)

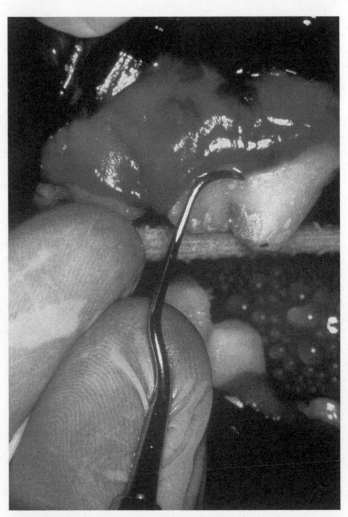

Fig. 26.24 Removing residual dental deposits with hand instruments. Here a universal scaler is being used to remove calculus

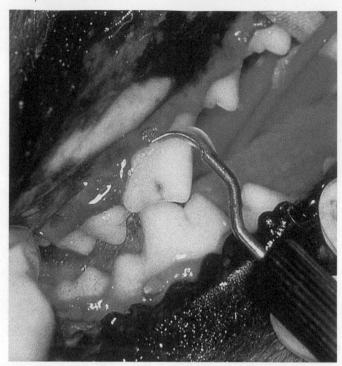

Fig. 26.25 Removing supragingival calculus with an ultrasonic scaler

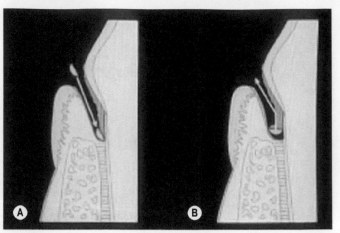

Fig. 26.26 Procedure for closed subgingival debridement. (A) The curette is inserted to the bottom of the gingival sulcus or pocket. (B) The cutting edges of the curette are engaged by turning the handle of the instrument, against the root surface and pulling out of the sulcus or pocket in this position. The instrument is worked in this way around the whole circumference of the tooth, using overlapping strokes. Mainly vertical, but also oblique and horizontal strokes are used

excessive heat. As an arbitrary rule, it is suggested that no more than 15 seconds of continuous scaling should be performed on any one tooth. If the tooth is not clean in that period of time, then return to it after scaling a few other teeth. This will allow the original tooth time to cool down.

Both sonic and ultrasonic scalers should be used with an insert that has a thin, pointed tip, sometimes called a perio, sickle or universal insert. An insert with a large (wide) tip is not recommended. A fine tip will remove dental deposits more accurately, with less likelihood of damage to the tooth enamel.

Subgingival scaling and root planing

This is the removal of plaque, calculus and other debris from the tooth surface below the gingival margin, i.e. within the gingival sulcus or periodontal pocket. There is no need to perform extensive subgingival scaling if there is no calculus below the gingival margin. However, the presence of subgingival deposits should always be investigated with a dental explorer and if any are identified they should be removed.

Root planing is the removal of the superficial layer of toxin-laden cementum from the root surfaces. Root planing produces a smooth root surface that is less likely to accumulate plaque and more likely to permit epithelial reattachment. Excessive root planing may damage the root surface (expose root dentine to the periodontal ligament) and predispose to further periodontal destruction. So, while a clean and smooth root surface should be obtained, overzealous root planing should be avoided.

Scaling and planing are achieved simultaneously using a curette. The procedure can be performed using either a closed (without raising an access flap) or open (raising an access flap) technique. An open technique is recommended for pockets deeper than 4 mm as it is difficult even for a skilled operator to ensure that all subgingival deposits have been removed without raising a gingival flap for direct access and visualisation. However, an open technique is only indicated in patients with

proven sufficient home care, i.e. it is not first-line treatment. The open technique is not a routine hygiene procedure. It is classified as periodontal surgery and should be performed by a veterinary surgeon with expertise in veterinary dentistry.

Ultrasonic and sonic scalers are designed for supragingival work. Once inserted into the gingival sulcus or pathological pocket, the water will no longer reach to cool the tip. The result is thermal damage of both hard and soft tissues. Quick subgingival excursions are permissible only if the gingiva is oedematous, or held mechanically out of the way to allow the water to reach the tip. Scalers with specially designed working tips where the water exits at the very end are safer to use under the gingival margin, but the removal of established subgingival deposits can only be adequately performed with meticulous use of sharp curettes.

The procedure for closed subgingival debridement is shown in Figure 26.26. It is often a lengthy procedure. It must be emphasised that removing subgingival plaque, calculus and debris as well as the superficial layer of toxin-laden cementum and restoring the root surfaces to smoothness is a most important step. Removing only the supragingival debris at a periodontitis site does not have any therapeutic benefit.

It will not prevent disease progression, as the cause of the disease – subgingival plaque – is still present.

Polishing

Scaling, even when done correctly, will cause minor scratches of the tooth. A rough surface will facilitate plaque retention. Polishing smoothes this roughness and helps remove any remaining plaque and stained pellicle.

Polishing is performed by applying a mildly abrasive prophylaxis paste to the tooth surface with a prophylaxis cup/brush mounted in a slowly rotating slow-speed handpiece (Fig. 26.27). The handpiece should be running at less than 5000 rpm to avoid generating excessive heat by friction. The amount of heat that can easily result from incorrect polishing can cause severe pulpal pathology. A surplus of paste is applied to the tooth surface, using light force. If a rubber cup is used, the force

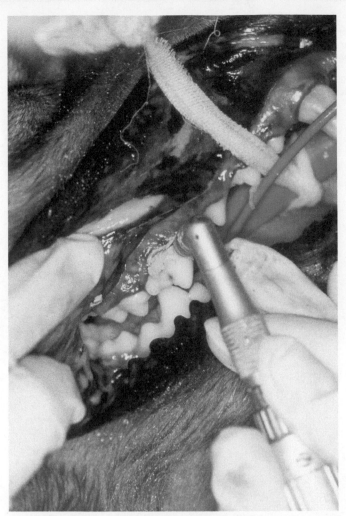

Fig. 26.27 Tooth crown polishing with a prophylaxis cup in a slow-speed handpiece

should be just enough to cause the cup to flare out on the tooth surface. The prophylaxis cup is kept moving over the entire tooth surface for a few seconds per tooth. The flared edge of the prophylaxis cup can be used to polish slightly subgingivally, taking care to avoid causing any further gingival damage. It is useful to check that all tooth surfaces are clean by using a plaque-disclosing solution after polishing. Any residual plaque is thus visualised and can be removed with further polishing.

Sulcular lavage

This involves gently flushing the gingival sulcus and pathological pockets with saline or dilute chlorhexidine to remove any free-floating debris. This step is particularly important in a deep pathological pocket as free-floating debris may occlude the orifice of the pocket and lead to the formation of a lateral periodontal abscess.

MAINTENANCE OF ORAL HYGIENE (HOME CARE)

The benefit of any professional periodontal therapy is short-lived unless maintained by effective home care. In fact, if no home care is instituted after professional periodontal therapy, then plaque will rapidly reform and disease will progress. It has been shown that 3 months after periodontal therapy, gingivitis scores are equivalent to those recorded prior to therapy if no home care is instituted (Gorrel & Bierer 1999).

The cause (dental plaque) and effects (discomfort, pain, chronic focus of infection, loss of teeth and possibility of systemic complications) of periodontal disease must be thoroughly explained to the pet owner. The owner must be made aware that home care is the most essential component in both preventing and treating periodontal disease. The responsibility of maintaining oral hygiene, i.e. keeping plaque accumulation to a level compatible with periodontal health, rests with the owner of the pet. Once instituted, home care regimens need continuous monitoring and reinforcement.

The veterinary nurse can play a vital role in educating clients, checking compliance and reinforcing the need for home care. It is strongly recommended that the trained veterinary nurse takes on the responsibility of educating and training pet owners to perform optimal home care by setting up preventive care clinics.

Tooth-brushing is known to be the single most effective means of removing plaque – studies have shown that in dogs with both experimentally induced gingivitis (Tromp et al. 1986) and naturally occurring gingivitis (Gorrel & Rawlings 1996), daily tooth-brushing is effective in returning the gingivae to health. In a 4-year study using the Beagle dog (Lindhe et al. 1975) it was shown that with no oral hygiene plaque accumulated rapidly along the gingival margin, with gingivitis developing within a few weeks. Dogs that were fed an identical diet under identical conditions but were subjected to daily tooth-brushing developed no clinical signs of gingivitis. In the group that were not receiving daily tooth-brushing, gingivitis progressed to periodontitis in most individuals.

Tooth-brushing is the gold standard for plaque control – every effort should be made to get every pet owner to commit to brushing their pet's teeth on a daily basis. The success of tooth-brushing depends on pet cooperation and owner motivation and technical ability. Tooth-brushing should be introduced gradually and as early in the animal's life as possible. Adult cats are generally less amenable to the introduction of tooth-brushing than adult dogs, but with patience and persistence, many will accept some degree of home care. In contrast, kittens often accept tooth-brushing more readily than puppies.

REFERENCES

Dyson, D.H., Maxie, M.G., Schnurr, D., 1998. Morbidity and mortality associated with anaesthetic management in small animal veterinary practice in Ontario. J. Am. Anim. Hosp. Assoc. 34, 461–471.

Gorrel, C., Bierer, T., 1999. Long-term effects of a dental hygiene chew on the periodontal health of dogs. J. Vet. Dent. 16, 109–113.

Gorrel, C., Rawlings, J.M., 1996. The role of tooth brushing and diet in the maintenance of periodontal health in dogs. J. Vet. Dent. 13, 139–143.

Lindhe, J., Hamp, S.-E., Löe, H., 1975. Plaque induced periodontal disease in Beagle dogs. A 4-year clinical, roentgenographical and histometrical study. J. Periodontal Res. 10, 243–255.

Robins, G.N., 1976. Dropped jaw – mandibular neurapraxia in the dog. J. Small Anim. Pract. 17, 753.

Tromp, J.A., van Rijn, L.J., Jansen, J., 1986. Experimental gingivitis and frequency of tooth-brushing in the Beagle dog model. Clinical findings. J. Clin. Periodontol. 13, 190–194.

RECOMMENDED READING

Aspinall, V., 2014. Clinical Procedures in Veterinary Nursing, third ed. Butterworth-Heinemann, Oxford.

Within the chapter on Surgical Nursing Procedures there is a step-by-step guide to scaling and polishing teeth.

Gorrel, C., 2013. Veterinary Dentistry for the General Practitioner, second ed. W B Saunders, Edinburgh.

Gorrel, C., Derbyshire, S., 2005. Veterinary Dentistry for the Nurse and Technician. Butterworth-Heinemann, Edinburgh.

Holmstrom, S.E., 1999. Veterinary Dentistry for the Technician and Office Staff. W B Saunders, Philadelphia, PA.

27 Principles of Anaesthesia and Analgesia

SAMANTHA MCMILLAN

KEY POINTS

- The role of the veterinary nurse in anaesthesia should prioritise the safety and comfort of the patient.

- Anaesthetic adverse events and fatalities are generally preventable.

- The majority of small animal fatalities occur in the maintenance and recovery period.

- A holistic approach to analgesia and pain management planning requires consideration of how agents affect the pain pathway, pain assessment and providing comfort through nursing care.

- Communication and vigilance in monitoring the anaesthetised patient are essential.

Introduction

General anaesthesia underpins what happens every day in veterinary practice as it facilitates many diagnostic, surgical and medical procedures, allowing them to be performed in a more humane manner than would otherwise be possible. Anaesthesia is a subject concerned with keeping animals safe and maintaining an animal's welfare during veterinary interventions. This can be achieved by identifying, minimising and managing the risk of adverse events and by ensuring pain is recognised and treated in an appropriate fashion. Anaesthesia is a complex process and one that is often performed in a suboptimal manner in general and even specialist practice. This is perhaps because it is considered by many as a 'means to an end' to facilitate diagnostic and surgical procedures rather than a complex procedure in its own right. This chapter is designed to allow the reader to become familiar not only with the drugs and equipment involved in anaesthesia but also the process of anaesthetising a patient.

Anaesthesia

WHAT IS ANAESTHESIA?

The word **anaesthesia** is coined from two Greek words: 'an-' meaning 'without' and '-aesthesis' meaning 'sensation'.

'Anaesthesia is a state of unconsciousness produced by a process of controlled, reversible drug induced intoxication of the central nervous system in which the patient neither perceives nor recalls noxious (harmful) stimuli.'
— C. Prys-Roberts (1987)

The term **balanced anaesthesia** is often used and, although this has many definitions, it can be generalised to mean the use of multiple drugs to achieve:
- Unconsciousness
- Amnesia
- Analgesia – inhibition of the neural pathways that lead to pain
- Suppression of reflexes – inhibition of movement
- Muscle relaxation.

The **triad of anaesthesia** is a simpler adaptation of this consisting of:
- Analgesia
- Unconsciousness
- Muscle relaxation.

Each of these elements will vary in their necessity depending on the procedure being facilitated. For example anaesthesia for exploratory laparotomy will depend on good levels of analgesia, unconsciousness and some degree of muscle relaxation to allow good surgical access to the abdominal cavity, whereas anaesthesia for radiography (e.g. for British Veterinary Association (BVA) hip scoring) should not be painful and will require minimal analgesia but a good level of unconsciousness with reasonable muscle relaxation to facilitate positioning for the radiographs.

RESPONSIBILITY FOR THE PATIENT UNDER ANAESTHESIA AND THE ROLE OF THE REGISTERED VETERINARY NURSE

Under the Veterinary Surgeons' Act 1966 and the RCVS Code of Professional Conduct and Supporting Guidance, anaesthesia is ultimately the responsibility of the veterinary surgeon. It is clearly stated in this legislation and set of professional guidelines that while registered veterinary nurses (RVNs) can administer a specific quantity of medication under direction of a veterinary surgeon to induce anaesthesia, they cannot administer medication incrementally or to effect. The responsibility for monitoring and maintaining the patient's anaesthesia also lies with the veterinary surgeon. The role of the RVN and student veterinary nurse has become critical in recent years in providing knowledgeable assessment of patients during the perioperative process. This is required in order to communicate changes in the patient's status to the veterinary surgeon while he or she is concentrating on performing the animal's procedure(s). In essence, RVNs and student veterinary nurses become an extension of a veterinary surgeon during the anaesthetic process by providing eyes, ears and hands to facilitate monitoring, pain assessment and drug administration. Critical to this role is the knowledge of when to alert the veterinary surgeon to a potential adverse event.

TABLE 27.1	Risk of anaesthetic fatality in dogs and cats listed by ASA status	
Species	Health status	Risk of anaesthetic-related death
Dog	Healthy ASA 1-2	0.05% (≈1 in 2000)
	Sick ASA 3-5	1.33% (≈1 in 75)
Cat	Healthy ASA 1-2	0.11% (≈1 in 1000)
	Sick ASA 3-5	1.40% (≈1 in 70)

TABLE 27.2	The percentage of anaesthetic fatalities in dogs, cats and rabbits by time point		
Anaesthetic time point	Dogs	Cats	Rabbits
After pre-medication	1%	1%	0%
Induction	6%	8%	6%
Maintenance	46%	30%	30%
Postoperative	47%	61%	64%

Royal College of Veterinary Surgeons (RCVS) day-one competencies of the registered veterinary nurse for anaesthesia include:

- Assist in administering and maintaining anaesthetics to patients – to include maintaining and monitoring of anaesthesia under the direction of a veterinary surgeon
- Assess pain and alert the veterinary surgeon.

It is therefore imperative that veterinary nurses entering the RCVS register:

- Be competent in the processes of anaesthesia, i.e. they understand how balanced anaesthesia and multimodal analgesia are achieved and they appreciate the concepts of anaesthetic safety (including the use of checklists)
- Have knowledge of the key anaesthetic drugs including their effects and side effects
- Be competent to assess and communicate regarding adverse events that may be likely to occur in a given procedure
- Be competent to monitor patients under anaesthesia and know when to alert the veterinary surgeon to changes in parameters
- Understand what to do if adverse events occur
- Be knowledgeable regarding how the equipment works, how it should be checked and how it is set up and used
- Recognise potential risk and intervene to prevent, where possible, complications occurring.

RVNs should have patient safety and comfort as their top priority when considering anaesthesia in any species, breed or individual. The aim of this chapter is to help RVNs and student veterinary nurses become safe practitioners in the area of anaesthesia by helping knowledge development and adoption of the tools required to develop safe systems of work.

FATALITIES AND RISK IN VETERINARY ANAESTHESIA

It is important to remember that almost all of the drugs that are used for sedation, analgesia and anaesthesia cause some degree of alteration to a patient's normal physiological homeostasis. Among other things, anaesthesia may affect cardiac output, blood pressure, respiratory rate, tidal volume and body temperature regulation. Given this, it is perhaps surprising that adverse events under anaesthesia do not cause fatalities more often.

The Confidential Enquiry into Perioperative Small Animal Fatalities (CEPSAF) evaluated anaesthesia-related fatalities in a mixture of general and referral practices in order to assess the fatality rate in small animal patients and whether this rate was improving (Table 27.1). It also evaluated a number of different factors and their effect on anaesthesia-related death.

The overall anaesthesia-related mortality rates found in the study were:

- 0.17% in dogs (≈1 in 600)
- 0.24% in cats (≈1 in 400)
- 1.39% in rabbits (≈1 in 70).

This indicates that the fatality rates in veterinary medicine are significantly higher than that of human anaesthesia. CEPSAF demonstrated that the majority of deaths occurred postoperatively in dogs, cats and rabbits with the second largest proportion occurring during the maintenance phase (Table 27.2). But why is this? After all, the anaesthetic is turned off and the procedure is over.

The answer to this, unfortunately, is that recovery is often the time when monitoring ceases and thoughts turn to the next anaesthetic despite the patient still being compromised by the anaesthetic. As a consequence complications can and do still occur in this period at an alarming frequency but often pass unnoticed. This study confirms that planning for recovery and any potential complications should be done as vigilantly as the preparation for the anaesthetic itself. Awareness of the risk during recovery must increase to enable a reduction in anaesthetic mortality rate.

Risk factors in veterinary anaesthesia from the CEPSAF study:

- Increased patient age, increased American Society of Anesthesiologists (ASA) status and decreased patient weight all increased the risk of fatality.
- Endotracheal intubation in cats undergoing short procedures increased the risk of fatality.
- Total inhalational anaesthesia in dogs increased the fatality risk.
- Intravenous fluid therapy increased the risk of fatality in cats.
- Continuous pulse monitoring (including pulse oximetry) decreased the risk of fatality.
- Procedural factors such as complexity, duration and urgency of anaesthesia were more important risk factors for fatality than the drugs used. This implies that more care should perhaps be taken when planning and preparing for anaesthesia in non-elective and more complex cases.

Death of course is not the only bad outcome of anaesthesia. Morbidity, such as organ damage, which does not lead to death is also possible. Alongside potentially long-term damage to a patient's health, morbidity can lead to increased hospitalisation, additional treatments and interventions and consequently costs. Unfortunately information on the frequency of anaesthetic-related morbidity is not currently available but it is likely that it occurs far more regularly than fatality.

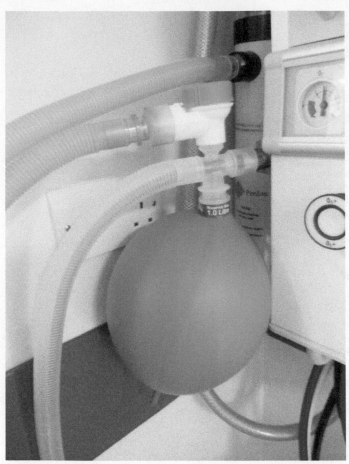

Fig. 27.1 APL valve should always be checked

BOX 27.1 POSSIBLE HUMAN ERRORS IN ANAESTHESIA

- Miscommunication
- Miscalculation of doses/administration error
- Incomplete clinical assessment
- Lack of knowledge of drugs and equipment
- Inadequate monitoring/failure to act
- Equipment not correctly set up/failure not recognised
- Failure to provide prophylactic treatment
- Misdiagnosis
- Airway mismanagement
- Fluid mismanagement
- Burns
- Corneal abrasions

An error may not harm the patient; however, consquences of medical error can sometimes be catastrophic. The worst thing about medical errors is that they are completely avoidable.

SAFETY IN ANAESTHESIA

Safe and effective anaesthesia should aim to minimise error and can be practiced at almost any veterinary practice regardless of the monitoring equipment and drugs available. The principles of safe anaesthesia encompass:

- Following a structured and organised approach centred around preparation of the patient, equipment and the 'anaesthesia team' (this could just be the veterinarian and nurse)
- Recognising and minimising the risks to the patient
- Vigilance: closely observing and examining the patient during the peri-operative period (before, during and after anaesthesia)
- Reacting appropriately when a problem is identified
- Utilisation of checklists
- Recording and reflecting on adverse events (especially those that occur frequently or those that result in fatality or significant morbidity) in order to develop measures to prevent them from recurring and to better manage them when they do.

Checklists

Checklists and procedural guides are proven to strengthen our cognitive processes and strengthen weaknesses in human factors, thereby greatly reducing error, adverse events and fatality. They simplify complex, long processes into lists of essential tasks or a 'step-by-step' guide to ensure that steps are not missed and that all staff approach processes in a standardised fashion. Checklists and procedural guides have been widely incorporated into human anaesthesia and surgery and have been shown to greatly reduce error, adverse events and fatality. This is an idea taken from aviation – the pilot runs through a checklist to ensure the plane is safe and ready to fly prior to take-off. The integration of simple anaesthetic checklists into a general practice situation and following simple recommended procedures when setting up for an anaesthetic can ensure that all anaesthetics are prepared for in the same manner and that important details are not left out.

The Association of Veterinary Anaesthetists have recently published an anaesthetic safety checklist and associated

More is known about anaesthetic complications and adverse events which if not managed appropriately can result in either morbidity or potentially fatality. It appears that adverse events (such as hypotension, hypoventilation, drug overdose, hypothermia, breakthrough nociception and patient's becoming too 'light' and moving) occur regularly under anaesthesia. Despite this in most practices adverse events are often not recorded or reflected upon.

MEDICAL ERROR

Medical error has been found to be a major cause of morbidity and mortality in human anaesthesia and it is likely that this is mirrored in the veterinary sector. Clarke and Hall (1990) documented errors of patient management in over 75% of deaths in healthy dogs and cats.

Errors can be made by anyone, however experienced, and they can be as simple as forgetting a vital piece of equipment, leaving an adjustable pressure-limiting (APL) valve closed (Fig. 27.1), not checking the spare oxygen cylinder, miscalculating a drug dose, misdiagnosing a problem or ignoring an alarm. Probably the most common errors seen in veterinary medicine include inadequate clinical examination and monitoring of the patient either before, during or after anaesthesia (Box 27.1). Another classic example is struggling to induce a stressed patient whose pre-medication has not worked as required.

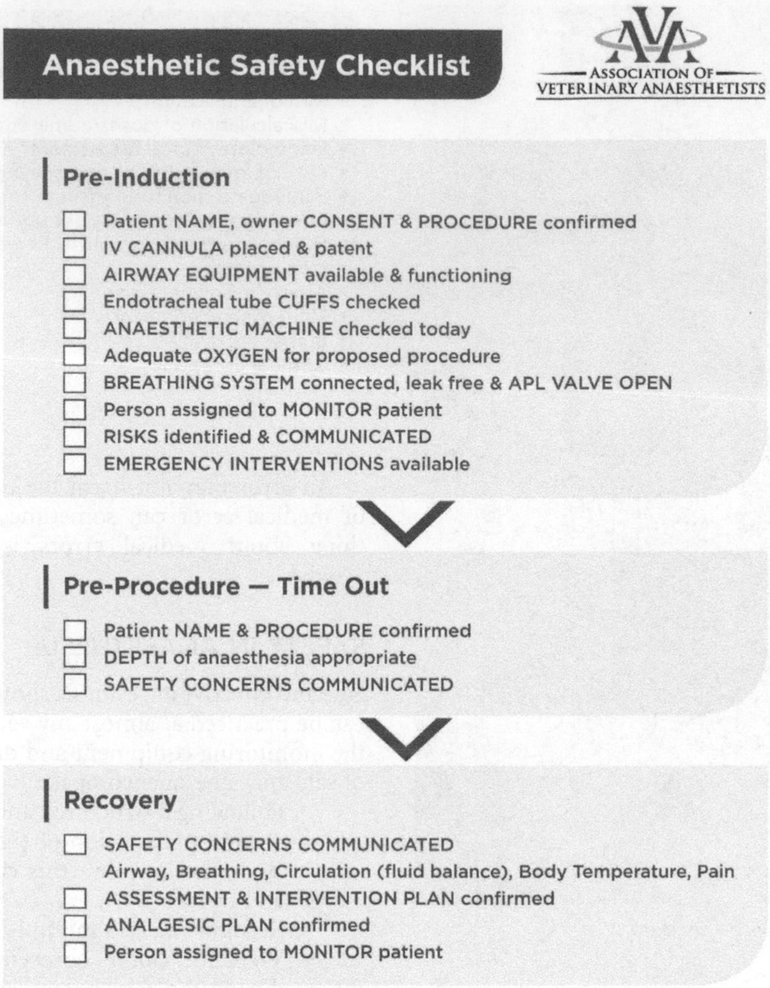

Anaesthetic Safety Checklist

ASSOCIATION OF
VETERINARY ANAESTHETISTS

Pre-Induction

☐ Patient NAME, owner CONSENT & PROCEDURE confirmed
☐ IV CANNULA placed & patent
☐ AIRWAY EQUIPMENT available & functioning
☐ Endotracheal tube CUFFS checked
☐ ANAESTHETIC MACHINE checked today
☐ Adequate OXYGEN for proposed procedure
☐ BREATHING SYSTEM connected, leak free & APL VALVE OPEN
☐ Person assigned to MONITOR patient
☐ RISKS identified & COMMUNICATED
☐ EMERGENCY INTERVENTIONS available

Pre-Procedure — Time Out

☐ Patient NAME & PROCEDURE confirmed
☐ DEPTH of anaesthesia appropriate
☐ SAFETY CONCERNS COMMUNICATED

Recovery

☐ SAFETY CONCERNS COMMUNICATED
Airway, Breathing, Circulation (fluid balance), Body Temperature, Pain
☐ ASSESSMENT & INTERVENTION PLAN confirmed
☐ ANALGESIC PLAN confirmed
☐ Person assigned to MONITOR patient

Fig. 27.2 AVA anaesthesia safety checklist

procedural guide (Figs. 27.2 and 27.3) modelled on the World Health Organization Surgical Safety Checklist but with more emphasis on anaesthesia (see http://www.ava.eu.com/resources/checklists/). It contains safety tasks that should be completed at key stages in the anaesthetic process:

1. Pre-induction
2. Pre-procedure
3. Pre-recovery.

It also incorporates a machine checklist and pre-anaesthetic patient assessment questions.

Such recommended procedures, checklists and equipment inventories can be printed and laminated and put next to each anaesthetic machine in a practice. During the setup and assessment period and prior to anaesthesia of each case, student and registered nurses or veterinary surgeons can check off the items as they prepare with a whiteboard marker. At the end of the case the checklist can be wiped clean ready for the next case.

It may seem like a waste of time (these are tasks done multiple times a day) but it has been found to reduce proper preparation time (time it takes to fully prepare without forgetting anything) for even the most experienced anaesthetists (it can decimate it for inexperienced staff) and can go a long way to reduce error due to factors such as inexperience, time constraints and fatigue.

Preparation for anaesthesia

Every anaesthetic has the potential to cause harm. This is more likely if the anaesthetic is not adequately prepared for and then carefully monitored. It is the proper preparation of the patient, drugs, anaesthetic equipment and the anaesthesia and surgery teams that helps prevent problems from occurring and allows for them to be rapidly and effectively managed if they do occur. The following AVA suggestions may be useful:

- Has anything significant been identified in the history and/or clinical examination?
- Do any abnormalities warrant further investigation?
- Can any abnormalities be stabilised prior to anaesthesia?
- What complications are anticipated during anaesthesia?
- How can these complications be managed?
- Would the patient benefit from pre-medication?
- How will any pain associated with the procedure be managed?
- How will anaesthesia be induced and maintained?
- How will the patient be monitored?
- How will the patient's body temperature be maintained?
- How will the patient be managed in the post-anaesthetic period?

Recommended Procedures

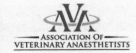
ASSOCIATION OF VETERINARY ANAESTHETISTS

Pre-Anaesthesia

★ Has anything significant been identified in the history and/or clinical examination?

★ Do any abnormalities warrant further investigation?

★ Can any abnormalities be stabilised prior to anaesthesia?

★ What complications are anticipated during anaesthesia?

★ How can these complications be managed?

★ Would the patient benefit from premedication?

★ How will any pain associated with the procedure be managed?

★ How will anaesthesia be induced & maintained?

★ How will the patient be monitored?

★ How will the patient's body temperature be maintained?

★ How will the patient be managed in the post-anaesthetic period?

★ Are the required facilities, personnel & drugs available?

Anaesthetic Machine

☐ PRIMARY OXYGEN source checked
☐ BACK-UP OXYGEN available
☐ OXYGEN ALARM working (if present)
☐ FLOWMETERS working
☐ VAPORISER attached and full
☐ Anaesthetic machine passes LEAK TEST
☐ SCAVENGING checked
☐ Available MONITORING equipment functioning
☐ EMERGENCY equipment and drugs checked

Drugs / Equipment

• Endotracheal tubes (cuffs checked)
• Airway aids (e.g. laryngoscope, urinary catheter, lidocaine spray, suction, guide-wire/stylet)
• Self-inflating bag (or demand valve for equine anaesthetics)
• Epinephrine/adrenaline
• Atropine
• Antagonists (e.g. atipamezole, naloxone/butorphanol)
• Intravenous cannulae
• Isotonic crystalloid solution
• Fluid administration set

Drug charts & CPR algorithm (http://www.acvecc-recover.org/)

Fig. 27.3 AVA procedural guide

• Are the required facilities, personnel and drugs available?

Clinical examination and history

All patients admitted for anaesthesia should be thoroughly assessed by a veterinary surgeon. This should include a full medical history (including any current drug therapies) alongside a thorough clinical examination. Previous anaesthetics should also be evaluated and any adverse events noted should be discussed with the team. The patient should also be weighed to ensure an accurate body weight for anaesthetic drug dosing.

As the RVN or student veterinary nurse involved in the case it is important to evaluate the patient's history, pre-existing conditions and risk factors prior to anaesthesia. This allows discussion of problems with the veterinary surgeon and helps to ensure that preparations have been made for the most probable eventualities. Examples of potentially significant problems may include brachycephalic obstructive airway syndrome, heart murmurs, electrolyte imbalance, endocrine diseases and neuromuscular diseases. Knowing that the patient is receiving drug therapy is also important. This will alert both the veterinary nurse and veterinary surgeon to the possible effects of that drug on the anaesthetised patient, avoiding problems such as the potential for drug interactions and overdoses. It is also prudent

to pay attention to the results of any diagnostic tests that have been performed (e.g. blood tests, ultrasound and radiographs) which might highlight problems that are not immediately obvious from the patient's presenting history. Whether blood screening is necessary will depend on the individual. Routine screening often constitutes haematology, biochemistry, packed cell volume, total protein, electrolytes, blood glucose and potentially coagulation profiles. Pre-operative blood screening is probably not justified in healthy patients under the age of about 8 years as results rarely change anaesthetic plans based on thorough clinical examination and historical assessment (Alef et al. 2008). Blood screening may be more useful in older geriatric patients even if they appear to be healthy due to an increased incidence of underlying disease.

During the appraisal of the patient's clinical notes it is also important to ascertain that signed informed consent has been obtained for anaesthesia, the clinical procedure to be performed and any additional techniques required such as local blocks.

It is a good idea for the RVN or student veterinary nurse to do a brief clinical examination of any patient that they will be helping to anaesthetise. This should be done prior to premedication of the patient and should include:

• Assessment of the patient's demeanour, temperament and behaviour

TABLE 27.3	Common breed-specific anaesthetic considerations and recommendations for their management	
Breed	**Considerations**	**Preparation**
Brachycephalic group including pugs, English and French bulldogs, Boston terriers, Pekinese	Hypoplastic tracheas, overlong soft palates, stenotic nares, everted ventricles in the larynx and this should prompt consideration that intubation may be challenging	Laryngoscopes, guide wires, a range of endotracheal tubes and aids to provide oxygen (Fig. 27.4) in the event of unsuccessful intubation should be considered Consider pre-oxygenation Late extubation and oxygenation in recovery may be necessary Careful monitoring after pre-medication and in recovery for airway occlusion
Dobermann pinschers	A breed with a high incidence of abnormally low von Willebrand factor concentrations	Screening or at the least a buccal mucosal bleeding time should be considered in all cases Dogs that are shown to be deficient in von Willebrand factor will require treatment usually with desmopressin and/or cryoprecipitate.
Boxers	Appear to have a genetic disposition to acepromazine (ACP) sensitivity	ACP doses should be reduced or the drug avoided altogether
Greyhounds and sighthounds	Metabolism of some drugs are reduced due to a deficiency in the P450 enzyme They also have problems with overactive fibrinolysis (clot breakdown) that can lead to rebleeding (heavy bruising and SC haemorrhage).	Some drug dosages will need to be reduced and recovery may be prolonged with some agents (e.g. acepromazine and propofol)
Collies	ABCB1 (formerly MDR1) mutations	The gene mutation results in drug accumulation in body fluids such as CSF and acepromazine and opioids in particular butorphanol are affected – doses should be decreased.

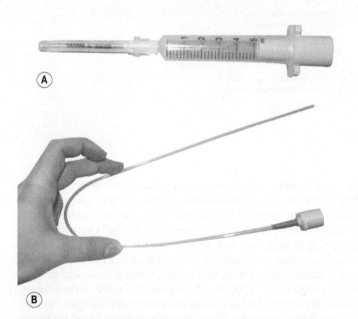

Fig. 27.4 Range of different endotracheal tubes in case of problematic intubation

- Palpation of peripheral pulses
- Observation of respiratory rate, effort and chest wall movement
- Auscultation of the heart and lungs
- Assessment of capillary refill time and mucous membrane colour.

This major body systems assessment should only take a couple of minutes but will give an objective baseline with which to compare monitoring assessments once the patient is anaesthetised – it is difficult to identify a change in a patient's mucous membranes or pulses if there is no pre-anaesthesia baseline to compare this to. It may feel 'weak', but is this the same as it was before the drugs were administered or is it vastly different? Obesity for example is a common cause of 'weak' peripheral pulses as normal pulses are damped by excessive subcutaneous fat.

Breed considerations

There are a large number of breed-specific anaesthetic considerations that should be considered prior to anaesthesia. A number of these are outlined in Table 27.3.

American Society of Anesthesiologists (ASA) physical status category, the 'ASA scale'

An American Society of Anesthesiologists (ASA) physical status category can be assigned to the patient. This is a scale from 1 to 5 (Table 27.4) with 1 being a healthy patient and 5 being moribund and unlikely to survive 24 hours without surgery. The ASA scale has been shown to be predictive of anaesthetic morbidity and mortality in humans. By giving each of the cases a category it will help to assign relative anaesthetic risk to each patient based on health status and allow the alteration of anaesthetic protocols accordingly. An 'E' can be added to any of the five categories to denote that the anaesthesia was for an emergency procedure.

If problems or abnormalities are identified then these should be stabilised prior to anaesthesia. Consider whether patients with newly diagnosed diseases would benefit from further stabilisation and work-up.

Fasting

Consider and discuss with the veterinary surgeon how long the patient has been/should be fasted for. A patient that has not been fasted will present a vomiting/regurgitation risk while a paediatric patient is at risk of hypoglycaemia if fasted excessively. It has been shown that prolonged fasting may increase

TABLE 27.4	American Society of Anaesthesiologists (ASA) scale of classification	
ASA scale	Physical description	Examples (use as a guide only as grading can be controversial)
1	A normal healthy patient	Ovariohysterectomy, castration Hip radiographs
2	A patient with mild systemic disease	Controlled diabetes mellitus, compensated cardiac disease, localised infection, obesity
3	Patients with severe systemic disease	Poorly controlled diabetes mellitus, anaemia, fever, heart disease resulting in exercise intolerance
4	Patients with severe systemic disease that is a constant threat to life	Uncompensated cardiac disease causing severe cardiovascular compromise, severe dehydration and hypovolaemia, sepsis
5	Moribund patient not expected to survive without the operation	Severe trauma, multiple organ failure

Adapted from the American Society of Anaesthesiologists (ASA) scale of classification.

TABLE 27.5	Approximate fasting times for companion species
Species	Approximate fasting times
Dogs, cats, ferrets	At least 4–6 hours prior to induction. No longer than 3 hours in paediatric patients (less than 12 weeks).
Rabbits, rats, mice	Do not regurgitate or vomit – fasting not required, however removing food 30 minutes prior to anaesthesia can ensure residual food debris does not remain in the oral cavity.
Guinea pigs	2 hours to prevent retention of food in the pharynx. Do NOT starve for longer.

gastric reflux and gastric acidity therefore prolonged fasting (over 8 hours) should be avoided where possible. In human medicine the fasting guidelines are 4–6 hours and this can be considered the minimum time to withhold food in dogs, cats and ferrets prior to induction of anaesthesia (Table 27.5). Paediatrics (less than 12 weeks of age) should be fasted for no longer than 3 hours and should be observed carefully for signs of hypoglycaemia.

Water should not be withheld for long periods to prevent dehydration but it is advisable to remove this when the patient's pre-medication is administered to prevent them drowning following profound sedation.

Other considerations

Type of surgery – this will assist will the evaluation of factors that may affect anaesthesia such as:
- Degree of pain – adequate analgesia
- Risk of haemorrhage – additional fluids and blood products may be necessary

- Length of anaesthesia – this has been shown to increase the likelihood of morbidity and mortality
- Possibility of hypothermia or hyperthermia occurring – e.g. where a thoracic cavity such as the abdomen is exposed to the environment or the patient is small with a large body surface area
- Ventilation – e.g. hypoventilation will be expected when pressure is being exerted on the diaphragm by a gravid uterus, surgical pressure in the cranial abdomen
- Whether neuromuscular blockade is required – therefore a ventilator (or an additional person for intermittent positive pressure ventilation [IPPV]) will be required.

PREPARATION OF THE TEAM

Proper preparation of the team involves planning and communication. Evaluation of patient, surgical and equipment consideration allows a plan to be made by the veterinary team as to the equipment and drugs that may be required for the anaesthesia, what adverse events may occur and what needs to happen in the face of those adverse events and may include:
- Identifying potentially useful drugs, and having their doses and infusion rates calculated and prepared for use. This may include drugs for cardiopulmonary resuscitation if the patient is particularly critical.
- Calculation of the patient's circulating blood volume and what a 10%, 20% and 30% blood loss would be in millilitres. Have scales available to weigh blood-soaked swabs.
- Appropriate intravenous fluids to be prepared and the rates discussed and calculated.
- The stock of other fluids such as glucose saline, colloids and blood products checked and kept close at hand; e.g. glucose saline may be required for a patient with diabetes mellitus and colloids or blood products if the patient is expected to haemorrhage profusely such as a splenectomy.
- Bair huggers™, Hot Dogs™ and other heating devices can be utilised to maintain appropriate temperature in patients at risk of hypothermia, e.g. the small Jack Russell terrier being anaesthetised for an exploratory laparotomy.
- Non-rebreathing anaesthetic systems or using higher fresh gas flow rates in a circle system and non-heating bacterial filters can be utilised for patients evaluated as at risk of hyperthermia, e.g. the Newfoundland that is being operated on for cruciate repair on a hot summer's day in the theatre with no air conditioning.
- Analgesic techniques such as local blocks or epidural can be discussed and prepared and strategies for breakthrough nociception prepared for. The doses of lidocaine or bupivacaine, for example, can be calculated for dental blocks.
- Equipment such as the glucometer for the diabetic patient, the ventilator for the thoracotomy, the syringe driver for the constant rate infusion or the suction machine for the mega-oesophagus patient at risk of oesophageal reflux can be checked and prepared ready for use.

This may seem like a long list of things to consider, but each case must be considered holistically and individually by listing the potential patient and surgical complications, considering anaesthetic protocols, discussing and planning for solutions to potential adverse events and gathering and checking equipment to ensure everything that is required is present and functioning properly. It is often not necessary to write an anaesthetic plan but the use of a checklist can help prompt patient evaluation and in more complex cases it is helpful to list the possible adverse events and what may need to be done or made available to either prevent or manage them. Indeed it is often easier and more time effective to put a plan down on paper than to try and recall it from memory in a stressful situation. As an example the brachycephalic patient (e.g. a pug or bulldog) may be more difficult to intubate and therefore will likely benefit from pre-oxygenation and a selection of different-sized endotracheal tubes being available. Alternatively, the patient admitted with a known history of diabetes mellitus will require regular blood glucose checks during anaesthesia and a patient with mega-oesophagus should be considered a regurgitation risk and therefore have suction available and be maintained in sternal recumbency with its head raised until an endotracheal tube is placed and cuffed.

These plans will increase efficiency during anaesthesia, create a more balanced anaesthetic for the patient, improve patient safety and ultimately reduce the number of adverse events and improve patient outcome in veterinary anaesthesia.

EQUIPMENT CONSIDERATIONS

Attention to detail is paramount when considering our anaesthetic equipment (this includes the anaesthetic machine and breathing system). By adequately checking and preparing equipment in advance we can minimise the risk posed by human error and consequent equipment failure. In addition to checking for faults we should make sure that we have all the required equipment ready before proceeding.

THE ANAESTHETIC MACHINE

The anaesthetic machine (Fig. 27.5) in combination with the vaporiser and breathing system is what fundamentally delivers oxygen, other carrier gases and volatile agents to veterinary patients undergoing anaesthesia. It is therefore vital that this equipment is understood and thoroughly checked prior to each use to maximise patient safety and minimise equipment failure and other potential adverse events resulting from human error.

The average veterinary anaesthetic machine will comprise:

- An oxygen supply (Fig. 27.6) – this could be from cylinders, a piped supply, a combination of both or from an oxygen concentrator
- Other carrier gases supplied via pipeline or cylinder, e.g. medical air and nitrous oxide
- Pressure gauge (Fig. 27.7)
- Pressure-reducing valves
- Flowmeters (Fig. 27.8)
- Back bar
- Oxygen flush
- Fresh gas outlet.

Cylinders and pipelines

Cylinder sizes are available in C to J and generally have a pin index system up to size E and then a bull nose or handwheel in sizes above this (oxygen has a pin index again at size J). The

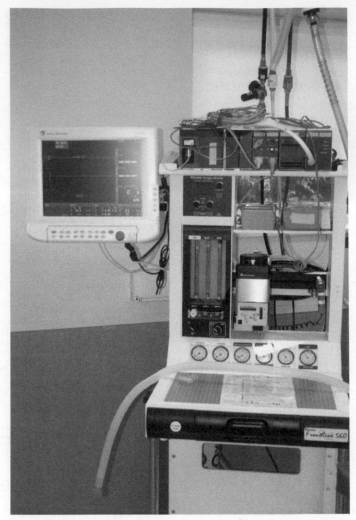

Fig. 27.5 Anaesthetic machine

smaller size cylinders are generally mounted directly onto anaesthetic machines while the larger cylinders support pipeline supplies. The pin index system means that the position of holes on the valve block of the cylinder are set in a unique position depending on the medical gas it represents. This will only fit onto the correct corresponding pins on the cylinder yoke of anaesthetic machine. This is a safety feature in addition to colour coding (Table 27.6) to prevent gases such as nitrous oxide being mounted in the place of oxygen. Anaesthetic machines that have medical gas cylinders mounted directly to them have a **Bodok seal** placed between the cylinder yoke on the anaesthetic machine and the valve block of the cylinder. This is a circular seal made from neoprene with a metal surround to promote a gas-tight seal.

Pipeline supplies generally have a Schrader probe on the end of a flexible hose from the anaesthetic machine that will connect with the corresponding socket in the wall (Fig. 27.9) or ceiling for the medical gas required. The flexible hoses and the sockets are colour coded (see Table 27.6) for safety, and the collar on the Schrader probe and its corresponding socket connection is unique to each medical gas to ensure the flexible hose cannot be connected to the incorrect socket (e.g. the oxygen hose on the anaesthetic machine cannot be connected to the sockets for nitrous oxide or medical air).

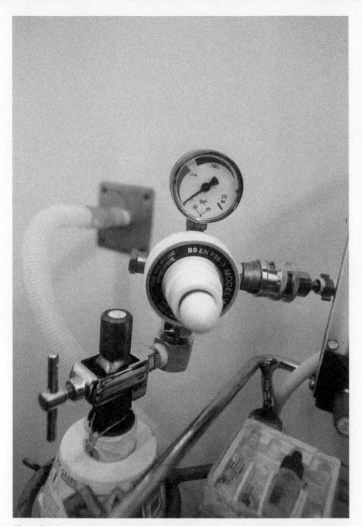

Fig. 27.6 Oxygen supply, with Pillar valve, regulator and pressure valve

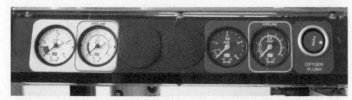

Fig. 27.7 Pressure gauge

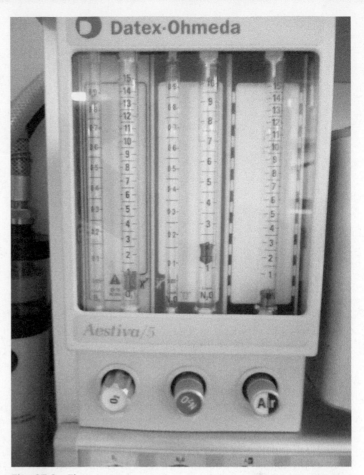

Fig. 27.8 Flowmeters

TABLE 27.6	UK colour code for common anaesthetic carrier gases and state of cylinder contents		
Medical gas	Cylinder colour in UK	Pipeline colour in UK	State of cylinder contents
Oxygen	White shoulders with a black body or may be all white	White	Compressed gas
Nitrous oxide	French blue shoulders and body	French blue	Saturated vapour above liquid
Medical air	Black and white shoulder with a grey body	Black	Compressed gas

Pressure regulating valves

The pressure of the medical gases in the cylinders is far higher than is appropriate to administer directly into a patient's airway. These valves regulate the pressure to a safer constant level, ensuring that gas pressure does not fluctuate especially as cylinder content declines. Each cylinder will have a pressure regulator and the piped supply will be regulated at its source (i.e. the cylinder supplying it).

Pressure gauges

These measure the pressure of the gas in either the cylinder or pipeline to allow monitoring of the level of gas remaining in the cylinder. Oxygen and medical air will show a corresponding decrease on the pressure gauge as the amount of gas in the

cylinder decreases. Nitrous oxide differs because it contains liquid with saturated vapour above it. The gauge measures the saturated vapour pressure and will remain constant until all the liquid evaporates after which the pressure gauge will decrease rapidly. The nitrous oxide pressure gauge is therefore not indicative of contents in the cylinder and instead the cylinders need to be weighed to accurately assess remaining contents.

Pressure relief valves

These are located in the back bar of the anaesthetic machine as a safety feature and open at high pressures to protect the

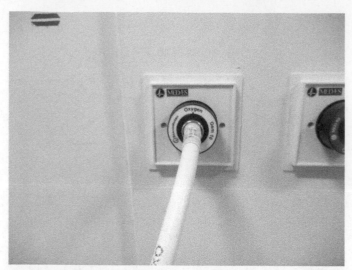

Fig. 27.9 Piped oxygen outlet

flowmeters and vaporiser in the event that the pressure regulating valves were to fail, or if downstream obstruction occurs.

Flowmeters

These consist of tubes of transparent glass or plastic tapered to be wider at the top than the bottom. A ball or bobbin is held within the tube to indicate the flow of a specific medical gas. If a ball indicator is present then the flow is read from the middle of the ball but if a bobbin is present then the flow should be read at the top of the bobbin. The level of gas is controlled by a knob at the bottom of the flowmeter which operates a needle valve. Each flowmeter is specifically calibrated for the gas it contains due to differences in laminar and turbulent flow between the medical gases. Flowmeters should be regularly inspected for cracks which could render them inaccurate.

Back bar

This is where the flowmeter block is supported and the vaporisers are mounted. The back bar has a double pin locking system for each vaporiser to ensure a seal and enable the vaporiser to function. Each anaesthetic machine will normally accommodate one to two vaporisers and in the UK the locking system is most commonly an Ohmeda 'Selectatec' system.

Fresh gas outlet

This is also sometimes called the common gas outlet and is where anaesthetic gases exit the anaesthetic machine and the point of connection for the breathing system.

Oxygen flush

The emergency oxygen flush receives oxygen directly from the cylinder or pipeline without it passing through the pressure regulating valve. The pressure of the oxygen delivered far exceeds that which is safe for the patient's airway and therefore the oxygen flush should not be utilised while a patient is connected to the breathing system to avoid barotrauma (pressure damage to the patient's lungs).

Vaporisers

These are temperature-compensated devices that are calibrated to deliver accurate concentration of volatile agents as

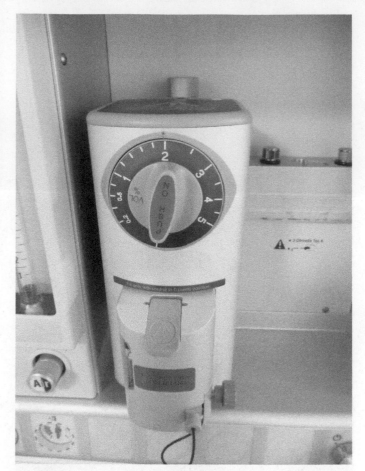

Fig. 27.10 Colour-coded purple isoflurane vaporiser

anaesthetic vapour. Vaporisers are calibrated for specific agents and are colour-coded purple for isoflurane (Fig. 27.10) and yellow for sevoflurane.

Most modern vaporisers are filled using a key fill system (Fig. 27.11). These systems minimise environmental contamination and therefore exposure to personnel and ensure that the vaporiser can only be filled with the correct agent.

Vaporisers have two channels: one that passes through the vaporising chamber and becomes saturated with anaesthetic gas and another that bypasses the vaporising chamber (Fig. 27.12). The two channels then combine before exiting the vaporiser. When concentration of anaesthetic gas required is set on the vaporiser, the amount of gas that is split off is adjusted to achieve the required concentration.

SAFETY FEATURES OF ANAESTHETIC MACHINES

In addition to some of the pressure reducing and relieving features outlined it is advisable to have an anaesthetic machine that incorporates the following:

Hypoxic guard – this device couples the oxygen and nitrous oxide flowmeters to ensure that when the nitrous oxide is turned on oxygen is also delivered in a minimum concentration. This prevents a hypoxic mixture of gas being delivered. Either the oxygen is automatically turned on or up as nitrous oxide is turned

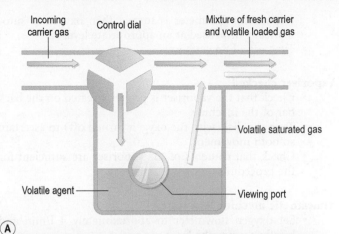

(A)

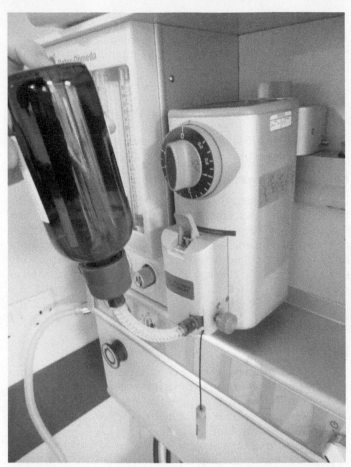

Fig. 27.11 Key fill system

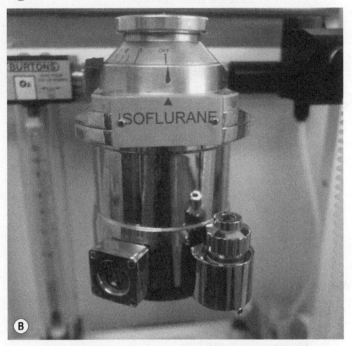

(B)

Fig. 27.12 Plenum vaporiser. (A) Schematic diagram. (B) Vaporiser attached to anaesthetic machine

on, or the nitrous oxide will only be able to reach a safe flow (up to twice that of the oxygen flow).

Low oxygen or oxygen failure alarm – when the oxygen pressure in the anaesthetic machine drops an audible alarm (most commonly a whistle) will sound to alert the user that the cylinder or pipeline pressure has dropped below a calibrated pressure. These are often combined with a nitrous oxide cut-off which stops nitrous oxide being delivered when oxygen reaches a low pressure and the alarm is sounding.

PRE-ANAESTHETIC EQUIPMENT CHECKS

Checking the anaesthetic machine

Primary oxygen source checked. If using cylinders:
- Check that there is adequate oxygen for the procedure by turning on the cylinder and reading the contents on the pressure gauge. This cylinder should be left on ready for use and marked with an 'in use' label. Full cylinder = 137 + 100 kPa.
- Check the backup cylinder is present and full by turning on and observing the pressure gauge. This cylinder should be turned off until needed to ensure it is not inadvertently used.

If using pipeline:
- Check the source of piped gas if no audible alarm system is installed to ascertain that there is enough oxygen in the source cylinder.

- Connect piped supplies on the anaesthetic machine to the gas pipeline and confirm security of Schrader probe and connecter with a tug test.

Oxygen alarm working
- Turn off all oxygen cylinders or disconnect the pipeline.
- Press the emergency oxygen flush to empty the system of oxygen.
- The oxygen alarm should sound to indicate low oxygen pressure in the system.
- Turn on the 'in use' cylinder ready for use.

Flowmeters working
- Turn the knob on the oxygen flowmeter an ensure that it moves freely and that the ball or bobbin moves freely throughout the range of the flowmeter.
- If using nitrous oxide ensure that the hypoxic guard is working so that if the nitrous oxide knob on the cor-

responding flowmeter is turned then oxygen is automatically dispensed at an appropriate level.
- Turn off all flowmeters.

Vaporiser checked
- Check that the vaporiser is properly seated on the back bar of the machine.
- Turn the dial (with the oxygen turned off) to ascertain smooth movement.
- Check that contents of the vaporiser are sufficient for the procedure.

Anaesthetic machine leak tested
- Set oxygen flowmeter to approximately 4 l/min and briefly occlude the fresh gas outlet.
- The ball or bobbin in the flowmeter should drop with the increased back pressure – if there were a leak then this pressure would be contained and the ball or bobbin would not drop.
- Turn off the fresh gas flow.

Scavenging system checked
- Charcoal canisters should be weighed to ensure that they have not reached capacity (the weight is normally listed on the outside of the canister).
- If using active scavenging then ensure that the system is switched on and that the air brake is working correctly – in most systems a disk in the air brake can be seen to visibly lift when the scavenging is working correctly.
- Ensure that the scavenging tubing is correctly connected to both the breathing system and the scavenging source, e.g. the charcoal canister or air brake.

Anaesthetic breathing system checked
- Visibly inspect the breathing system for contamination, cracks to the tubing and holes in the reservoir bag.
- Connect the breathing system to the fresh gas outlet of the anaesthetic machine.
- Fully close the APL valve.
- Turn on the oxygen flowmeter to approximately 4 l/min and allow the reservoir bag to inflate (this can also be done by pressing the oxygen flush button).
- Occlude the patient end of the breathing system and observe the reservoir bag fully inflate while listening for leaks.
- Once the bag is fully distended apply digital pressure and observe for obvious leaks – note that squeezing the bag hard will purge gas out of the APL valve on all systems except the Mini-Lack. This is normal and an integrated safety feature of these systems and testing this safety valve is also an important part of this procedure.
- Open the APL valve and leave the breathing system attached to the anaesthetic machine and ready for use.
- On the circle system inspect the unilateral valves.
- On the Bain occlude the inner tube with oxygen flowing at 4 l/min (there is a correct tool available for this but a biro will also fit). Observe the ball or bobbin on the flowmeter – it should dip as for the anaesthetic machine leak test if there are no leaks in the inner tubing of this system.

Monitoring equipment check
Any available monitoring equipment should be turned on and thoroughly checked/prepared for use. Examples of this may include:
- Ensuring the correct blood pressure cuff for the patient is selected and prepared
- Switching on the capnograph to allow calibration with room air
- Checking the pulse oximeter on a finger to ascertain that it is correctly detecting a pulse rate.

Emergency drugs and equipment checked
If it has been ascertained by assessment and planning for the anaesthetic that emergency equipment is required then this should be prepared ready for use. Otherwise the location and the contents of the crash box or trolley containing drugs for cardiopulmonary resuscitation and critical incidents should be regularly checked and restocked as necessary (also see Chapter 20).

ANAESTHETIC BREATHING SYSTEMS

Definitions
- **Tidal volume** – volume of air breathed in one breath
- **Functional residual capacity** – volume of air left in lungs following normal expiration
- **Residual volume** – volume of air left in lungs after forced expiration
- **Total lung capacity** – total amount of air breathed in with maximum inspiration
- **Vital capacity** – total volume of air in the respiratory tract that can be used during respiration
- **Mechanical dead space** – the volume within the system that may contain exhaled patient gas which will be rebreathed with the subsequent inspiratory breath
- **Anatomical dead space** – the volume of gas inhaled by the patient and residing in the respiratory tract which does not undergo gaseous exchange; this includes gas contained within the trachea, main-stem bronchi and bronchioles as gaseous exchange only takes place in the alveoli
- **Fresh gas flow** – the gases delivered to the patient via the fresh gas outlet on the anaesthetic machine. This is measured in litres per minute and depends on the amount of gas the flowmeters are set to deliver.

Anaesthetic breathing systems are used for three main functions:
- Delivering anaesthetic gases and oxygen to patient
- Removing CO_2 from exhaled gases
- Providing a means of manually supporting ventilation.

Components of breathing systems:
Unidirectional valves – discs of material enclosed within a gas-tight chamber. Gas enters the chamber, raises the disc and is able to pass. The inspiratory valve ensures that gas flow is maintained in the direction of the patient. The expiratory valve prevents rebreathing of exhaled gases and directs them to the absorbent canister.

Y connector – connects the endotracheal tube with inspiratory and expiratory limbs of system. The Y piece contributes to the system's mechanical dead space but in

TABLE 27.7	Non-rebreathing anaesthetic systems			
Non-rebreathing system	Patient size	Breathing system/ circuit factor	Suitable for IPPV?	Considerations
Ayres T-piece	Less than 10 kg	2.5–3 × Vm	Yes	
Bain	10 kg upwards	2.5–3 (1.5–2) × Vm	Yes	
Lack	10 kg upwards	1–1.5 × Vm	No	
Mini-Lack	2–10 kg	1–1.5 × Vm	No	No safety feature on valve

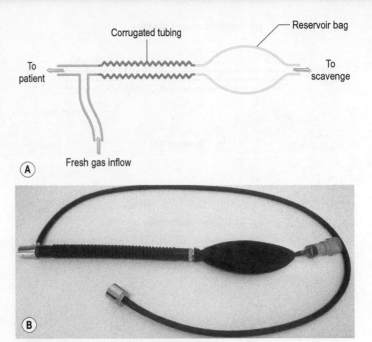

Fig. 27.13 Jackson-Rees modified Ayres T-piece

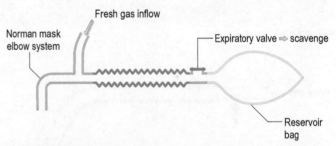

Fig. 27.14 Modified Ayres T-piece with variation in the scavenging valve, which provides greater assistance with expiration and can therefore be used in animals of 5–10 kg

paediatric systems a septum may be present to divide inspiratory and expiratory gas flow and reduce this dead space.

Adjustable pressure-limiting (APL) valve ('pop-off' valve) – vents gases to the scavenger system to prevent the build-up of excess pressure within the system.
- Open position – actuated by pressures of less than 0.1 kPa (1 cm H_2O).
- Closed position – pressure relief mechanism, actuated at 6 kPa (60 cm H_2O), but this safety feature is not present in the Mini-Lack.

Absorbent canister – contains CO_2 absorbent in rebreathing systems at a volume of approximately 50% with inter-granular space comprising the other 50%. Canister should be large enough to contain an air space between the granules that is equal to or greater than the patient's tidal volume.

Breathing tubes – corrugation helps prevent obstruction if the tubes are bent. These should preferably be on the outside of the tubing only leaving the internal walls smooth to minimise the generation of turbulent flow.

Reservoir bags – should practically contain at least twice the patient's tidal volume when the bag is in a neutral position but ideally 5 times the tidal volume or 50 ml/kg, which is equivalent to vital capacity.

Fresh gas flow rate calculations for non-rebreathing systems

Tidal volume (Vt) = 10–15 ml/kg
- Generally use 15 ml/kg for the tidal volume of small dogs and cats and 10 ml/kg for medium dogs upwards.

Minute volume (Vm) = Vt × Respiratory rate (RR)
- This takes the volume of air breathed in one breath and multiplies it by the number of breaths in 1 minute to give the total volume of air required for the patient to breathe for 1 minute.

Fresh gas flow = Vm × Circuit factor
- Quick fix – Vm = 200 ml/kg/min

Non-rebreathing systems

The non-rebreathing systems routinely used in veterinary practices are (Table 27.7):
- Ayres T-piece (Figs. 27.13 and 27.14)
- Bain (Figs. 27.15 and 27.16)
- Lack (Figs. 27.17 and 27.18)
- Mini-Lack (Fig. 27.19)
- Humphrey ADE in A mode.

Ayres T-piece
- Many modifications – most commonly has the Jackson Rees modification (open-ended bag) or a bag and an APL valve
- Patients less than 10 kg
- Lower resistance than other systems
- Minimal mechanical dead space
- The reservoir bag is on the expiratory limb
- On expiration the expired gases are exhaled into the expiratory limb and high fresh gas flow rates are therefore required to purge the alveolar gas that has undergone gaseous exchange from the system. This unfortunately means that gas that was residing in the anatomical dead space and had not undergone gaseous exchange is also lost as it is breathed out first and has to also be purged to remove the alveolar gas following it
- High fresh gas flow (FGF) rates required to prevent rebreathing of alveolar gas, i.e. 2.5–3 × Vm
- Suitable for long-term IPPV.

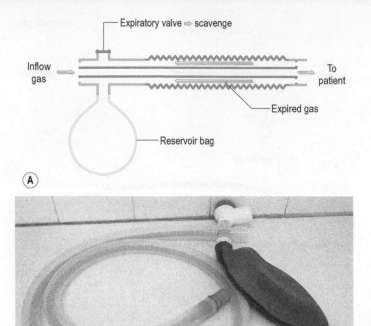

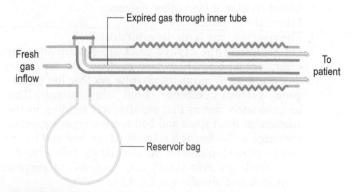

Fig. 27.15 The Bain circuit

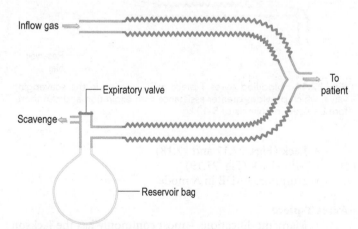

Fig. 27.16 The modified Bain circuit

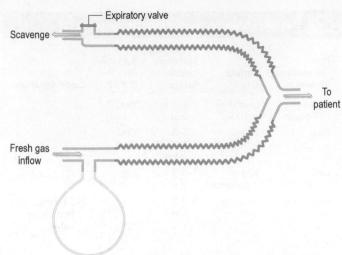

Fig. 27.18 The parallel Lack circuit

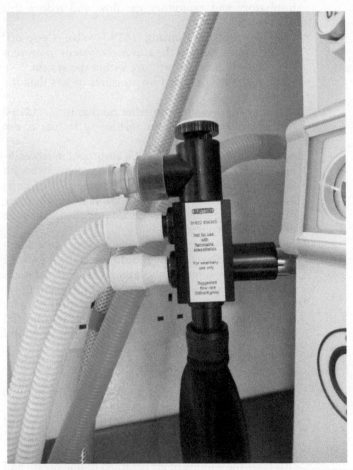

Figure 27.19 Mini-Lack

Fig. 27.17 The Lack circuit

Bain

- Very similar in the way it works to T-piece but higher resistance
- Patients 10 kg upwards although becomes uneconomical in larger patients
- Co-axial system – fresh gas delivered through the inner tube which allows warming of the inspired gas
- Minimal mechanical dead space
- The reservoir bag is on the expiratory limb

- High FGF required – a range of fresh gas flows have been suggested. Traditionally in veterinary nursing a fresh gas flow of 2.5–3 × Vm has been recommended to give a wider safety margin; however, 1.5–2 × Vm has been accepted as being appropriate in most situations
- Suitable for long-term IPPV.

Lack

- More economical than Bain and T-piece as it utilises anatomical dead space gas
- Patients 10 kg and upwards
- When the patient exhales the first portion of gas released has not undergone gaseous exchange but has been held within the anatomical dead space. This portion of gas enters the inspiratory limb while the alveolar gas which has undergone gaseous exchange exits through the scavenging via the expiratory limb. The 'dead space' gas is then inhaled with fresh gas as the patient inspires
- The reservoir bag is situated on the inspiratory limb
- Parallel Lack most common but coaxial versions available
- FGF 1–1.5 × Vm
- Not suitable for assisted ventilation over long periods as rebreathing will occur.

Mini-Lack

- Alternative to the modified Ayres T-piece for spontaneously breathing patients
- Expiratory valve should be fully open at all times
- Patients 2–10 kg
- Main advantage – economy of much lower fresh gas flows compared to Ayres T-piece
- Minimum FGF 200 ml/kg/min to prevent rebreathing of CO_2 – 1–1.5 × Vm
- Minimum flow rate of 1 l/min in patients weighing 2–5 kg if capnography unavailable
- Not suitable for assisted ventilation over long periods
- No safety device on expiratory valve – use with care

Calculating the patient's fresh gas flow for a non-rebreathing system

Minute volume × Breathing system factor
- So: a 25-kg dog has a tidal volume of 10 ml/kg and an observed respiratory rate of 15 breaths per minute

Tidal volume = 25 kg × 10 ml/kg = 250 ml
Minute volume = 250 ml × 15 breaths per minute = 3750 ml/min
For a Lack the breathing system factor is 1–1.5 so:
- Minute volume × Breathing system factor = 3750 ml/min × 1 = 3750 ml/min

Or
= 3750 ml/min × 1.5
= 5625 ml/min
To convert to litres simply divide by 1000, e.g. 3750/1000 = 3.75 L/min.

Humphrey ADE and circle system

- Developed for use in human anaesthesia to maximise efficiency and reduce FGF rates (Table 27.8)
- Includes detachable soda lime canister which allows it to function as a non-rebreathing or rebreathing system

TABLE 27.8	Recommended FGF rates following the normal induction process	
Fresh gas flow (after induction)	**Minimum 300 ml/min**
Cats – all weights	70–100 ml/kg/min – semi-closed – without absorber
Dogs under 10 kg	70–100 ml/kg/min – semi-closed – without absorber
Dogs over 10 kg	30 ml/kg/min induction – recycling with soda canister 10 ml/kg/min maintenance

- Patients 1–100 kg
- Bag on the inspiratory limb to help maximise efficiency
- Also employs a unique exhaust valve which saves as much dead space gas as possible

The valve is designed to open and close in four distinct phases:

Phase 1: Valve seat lifts with expiration. Valve lifts into the chimney but valve remains effectively closed.

Phase 2: Seat reaches the top of the chimney and the valve is now open. This effectively means that during the first phase of expiration, i.e. before the seat reaches the top of the chimney, all gas must flow into the inspiratory limb. The first section of this is 'dead space gas' which is then available for the next breath.

Phase 3: As expiration ends the valve drops back into the seat preventing the last few millimetres of gas from escaping. This has the effect of providing positive end-expiratory pressure.

Phase 4: Valve seat closes preventing gas from flowing back to the patient along the expiratory limb during inspiration and ensuring that the patient only receives gas from the inspiratory limb containing the 'dead space gas' and fresh gas from the anaesthetic machine.

The valve is designed so that the opening of the valve seat in phase 2 is increased at higher flow rates, i.e. the higher the flow rate the more the valve seat is lifted up and the more gas can escape. This ensures as little resistance as possible from the valve, and the system has been used safely in patients down to 1 kg.

Rebreathing systems

Rebreathing systems allow recycling of exhaled gases by removing CO_2 using an absorbent. The FGF must provide oxygen at least equivalent to the patient's metabolic oxygen demand. The two main systems are the circle system (Fig. 27.20) and the Humphrey ADE with the soda lime canister attached (Fig. 27.21).

Circle system

- Use from 10 kg (can go lower with modern circles if low-resistance tubing used)
- Recycles expired gases through carbon dioxide absorbent
- One-way valves ensure that gases more in the correct direction around the system
- High resistance due to the carbon dioxide canister, valves and tubing

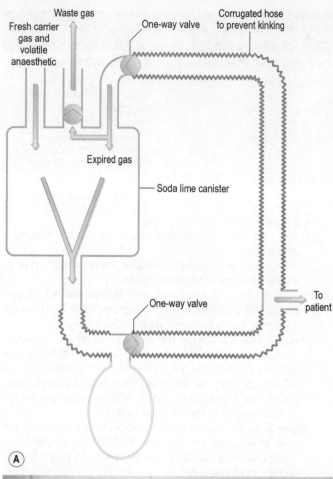

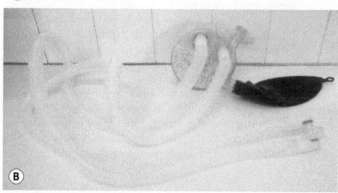

Fig. 27.20 The circle system

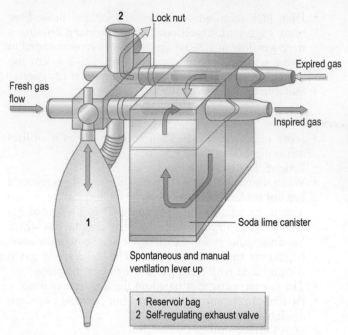

Fig. 27.21 Diagram to show set-up for the Humphrey ADE system

Carbon dioxide absorbent – can be caustic so gloves should be worn when handling it. The absorption of carbon dioxide will cause a colour change, e.g. from white to purple or pink to cream (this varies depending on the type of absorbent purchased) when the absorbent has become exhausted. Once the absorbent is exhausted it should be changed in accordance with manufacturer's instructions.

Chemical reaction:
$$CO_2 + H_2O \rightarrow H_2CO_3$$
$$H_2CO_3 + 2NaOH \rightarrow Na_2CO_3 + 2H_2O + heat$$
$$Na_2CO_3 + Ca(OH)_2 \rightarrow CaCO_3(chalk) + 2NaOH$$

Low-flow anaesthesia. Low-flow, closed and semi-closed are terms used to denote FGF rates for rebreathing systems

compared to the patient's metabolic oxygen demand. They do not describe any structural differences between the rebreathing systems nor do they indicate the position of the APL valve.

Metabolic oxygen demand. This is the amount of oxygen required by the patient for cellular metabolism. Factors affecting this include:

- Body weight
- Surface area
- Temperature
- Level of consciousness
- Age
- Type of anaesthetic drugs (e.g. ketamine)
- Disease process.

Estimates for metabolic oxygen requirements in anaesthetised cats and dogs vary between 3 and 8 ml/kg/min. A more accurate figure can be calculated using the equation $10 \times$ body weight$^{0.75}$. A safe baseline is often considered 10 ml/kg/min.

- **Closed system:** This occurs at low FGF rates when the oxygen entering the system approximates the patient's metabolic oxygen consumption. This does not indicate the position of the pop-off valve, which may be open or closed in this instance. Very little if any gas is vented into the scavenging. If valve is open the pop-off valve often leaks gas so ultra-low flow is not possible.
- **Low-flow anaesthesia:** For small animals this has been defined as an oxygen flow rate which exceeds that of the patient's oxygen demand but less than 22 ml/kg/min.
- **Semi-closed system:** Where the fresh gas flow exceeds the uptake of oxygen and anaesthetic by the patient. The patient's metabolic oxygen consumption times 3 is an appropriate guideline for flow rates. Significant amounts of gas are purged through the APL valve into the scavenging – less economical than closed and low flow systems.

Advantages of low-flow anaesthesia
- Economy – both oxygen and inhalant anaesthetics
- Reduction of waste gas – less exposure of personnel and harm to the environment
- Some retention of heat and moisture – helps to prevent hypothermia
- Suitable for IPPV

Points to consider with circle systems and low flow rates:
- **Initial outlay of the breathing system** – circle and Humphrey ADE systems tend to be more expensive than the non-rebreathing systems.
- **Vaporiser performance** – some vaporisers may not be accurately calibrated for flow rates less than 500 ml/min. Inspired and expired agent monitoring can be used to assess this.
- **Denitrogenation** – when a patient is initially connected to the rebreathing system the air that is breathed out will contain nitrogen (remember that room air is 78% nitrogen) as the patient was breathing room air prior to connection to the breathing system. The FGF rate must be relatively high initially (10–15 minutes) to purge the nitrogen from the system via the APL valve. As nitrogen is not absorbed by the carbon dioxide absorbent, if it were not purged then a hypoxic mixture could occur in the breathing system.
- **Nitrous oxide** – exhaled gases are being recycled but the carbon dioxide absorbent does not absorb nitrous oxide. The oxygen gets diluted by the nitrous oxide and this can mean that the oxygen level no longer meets metabolic demand and hypoxic levels occur. **Ratio of N_2O to O_2 should be no more than 1 : 1.**
- **Dust from CO_2 absorbent** – this can increase resistance and may also stop the unidirectional valves performing correctly.
- **Resistance** – the canister, lengths of tubing, valves and carbon dioxide absorbent all add resistance to the system making it unsuitable for smaller patients.
- **Overheating** – the carbon dioxide absorbent produces heat and moisture as part of a chemical reaction and this can be a factor in cases which are evaluated as having the potential to become hyperthermic.
- **Dilution factor** – the average circle system can accommodate over 4 l of gas. The fresh gas flow contributing to this is very small and exhaled gases contain proportionally less inhalational agent than fresh gas. This means that the % volatile agent in the fresh gas is diluted by the exhaled and recycled gases and the patient receives a lower % of the volatile agent than set on the vaporiser dial.

The larger the patient and the lower the FGF, the larger the discrepancy. Maintain the vaporiser setting until happy with the depth of anaesthesia and remember that any rapid changes to anaesthetic depth that are required will require an increase in FGF rate.

The time to change 97% of the gas in a circle system = (Volume of the breathing system/FGF) × 3

For example: A circle system with a 2-l reservoir bag accommodates a volume of approximately 6000 ml. So: 25-kg dog receiving 10 ml/kg/min has FGF rate = 250 ml.

6000 ml/250 ml = 24 minutes

24 minutes × 3 = 72 minutes to change 97% of the gas in the circle system.

By increasing the FGF to 1 l/min:

6000 ml/1000 ml = 6 minutes

6 × 3 = 18 minutes to change 97% of the gas in the circle system.

By increasing the FGF to 4 l/min:

6000 ml/4000 ml = 1.5 minutes

1.5 × 3 = 4.5 minutes to change 97% of the gas in the circle system.

Guidelines for low-flow anaesthesia using the circle system in practice
- Use a higher FGF initially for the first 10–15 minutes to ensure denitrogenation and adequate depth of anaesthesia.
- Maintain initial vaporiser setting until the desired depth of anaesthesia has been achieved.
- Decrease FGF after this initial period to approximately 10–20 ml/kg/min. Flow rates less than 10 ml/kg require capnography, gas monitoring and pulse oximetry to accurately assess the patient.
- The minimum FGF to ensure accuracy of most vaporisers is 300–500 ml/min. Do not reduce below this unless agent monitoring is available.
- Once the FGF has been reduced a higher vaporiser setting may be required compared to using a semi-closed system due to dilution.
- If using nitrous oxide use at a ratio of 1 : 1 with oxygen and ensure the FGF is at least 20 ml/kg/min. As with any breathing system, switch off the nitrous oxide 10–15 minutes prior to the end of anaesthesia.
- Routine monitoring should ensure that there is gas in the reservoir bag at all times. If there is not enough in the bag then the flow is too low and FGF should be increased. If there is too much in the bag then the FGF is too high and should be decreased.
- If you need to change the depth of anaesthesia rapidly increase the FGF until the desirable depth is achieved and then return to low flow.
- When the vaporiser is switched off at the end of anaesthesia FGF should again be increased and the contents of the reservoir bag dumped into the scavenging.

Calculating fresh gas flow for patients on a circle system
10–20 ml/kg/min

For example, a 30-kg dog requiring 10–20 ml/kg/min:

= 30 kg × 10 ml/kg/min = 300 ml/min

= 30 kg × 20 ml/kg/min = 600 ml/min

So the dog requires 300–600 ml/min and bear in mind that 500 ml/min is a recommended minimum to ensure vaporiser accuracy.

Heat and moisture exchangers. These devices can be utilised to warm inspired gases and prevent the loss of moisture from expired gases (Fig. 27.22). They are fitted between the endotracheal tube and the breathing system and often contain a bacterial filter which reduces the risk of contamination of the breathing system tubing. Some also have an attachment for the capnograph.

Scavenging. It is necessary to scavenge waste anaesthetic gases to minimise personnel to the exposure of vapour (for potential hazards and side effects see the section on maintenance/volatile agents).

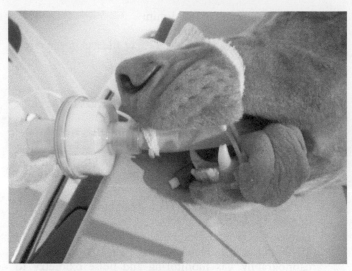

Fig. 27.22 Heat and moisture exchangers

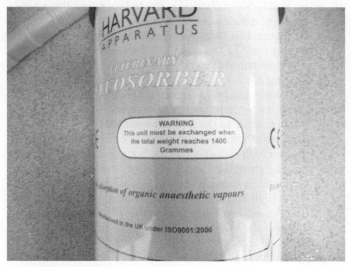

Fig. 27.23 Charcoal canisters

The recommended maximum accepted exposure concentrations in the UK are:
- 100 particles per million (ppm) for nitrous oxide
- 60 ppm for sevoflurane
- 50 ppm for isoflurane

All areas where inhalation anaesthesia is carried out should have a scavenging system. Excess gas escapes from the breathing system via an adjustable pressure-limiting (APL or pop-off) valve that can be connected to the following scavenging systems:

Charcoal canisters. A canister containing activated charcoal is connected to the outlet of the breathing system. The nature of halogenated anaesthetics (isoflurane, sevoflurane) allows them to be trapped by the charcoal by van der Waals forces as the gases filter through the canister. They are able to scavenge a fixed amount of anaesthetic. Once they have reached a certain weight they need to be disposed of in clinical/pharmaceutical waste (Fig. 27.23).

Advantages:
- No set-up cost – just pay for the canisters
- Mobile – moves with the machine

Disadvantages:
- Continuing cost of replacement
- Need to be weighed regularly to ensure that the charcoal has not been used up
- Does not remove nitrous oxide
- Heating the canister causes the release of the inhalational agents – keep them away from radiators

Passive scavenging. Consists of a tube connected to the breathing system valve by a shroud. The waste gases can be removed via:
- An open window
- A pipe passing through an outside wall
- An extractor fan vented to the outside air (*not* into the building's air-conditioning system)

Advantages:
- Inexpensive to set up
- Simple to operate

Disadvantages:
- May be impractical in some buildings
- Increased chance of leaks as compared to active systems

Active scavenging. These systems connect the exhaust of the breathing system to a hospital vacuum system. The vacuum is not directly attached to the exhaust hose of the breathing system but rather the waste gas is sucked into the vacuum via the Venturi effect using an 'air brake'. The vacuum system usually vents to the outside environment.

Advantages:
- Extremely efficient
- Low running cost once set up
- Convenient in large hospitals, where many machines are in use in different locations
- Allows the use of nitrous oxide

Disadvantages:
- Vacuum system and pipe work is a major expense, needs regular maintenance

INTERMITTENT POSITIVE PRESSURE VENTILATION

Intermittent positive pressure ventilation (IPPV; mechanical ventilation or controlled ventilation) is the act of applying a positive pressure into a breathing system in order to produce a pressure gradient into the chest (Fig. 27.24). As the pressure in the breathing system becomes greater than that in the chest, gas flows into the chest and the lungs expand. When this pressure is ceased expiration occurs in the normal manner. Pressure in a breathing system can be elevated in a number of ways:
- Closing the expiratory APL valve and squeezing the rebreathing bag (manual ventilation)
- Intermittently occluding the exhaust from circuit allowing the pressure of fresh gas flow to inflate the lungs. Known as artificial or mechanical thumbs (Vetronic services ventilator [SAV-03], Penlon Nuffield or Pneupac Ventipac with paediatric or Newton valve)
- Increasing the pressure within an airtight canister that contains a gas-filled bellows. The bellows is attached to the breathing system and when the pressure in the canister is increased the bellows empty – in effect this is squeezing the bag hence the name 'bag squeezers' (Hallowell)

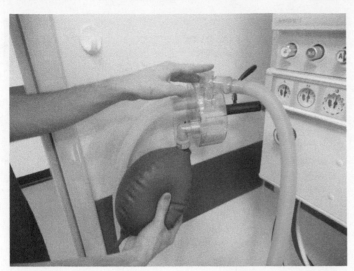

Fig. 27.24 IPPV

- Providing a flow of gas into the expiratory limb of the circuit (Penlon Nuffield or Pneupac Ventipac with patient valve)
- Taking a volume of gas from the anaesthetic machine and driving or squeezing it into the patient (minute volume dividers such as Manley ventilators or electronic ventilators such as the Vetronic MERLIN)

IPPV is not a benign act. Increasing intra-thoracic pressure during inspiration can decrease venous return to the heart and therefore have detrimental effects on cardiac output. It is not unusual to detect a transient decrease in pulse profile amplitude immediately after inspiration. This can be often be detected audibly on a Doppler flow detector or visually on a pulse oximeter's plethysmograph (pulse trace) or on a direct arterial blood pressure trace. Within the range of pressures and inspiratory times generally used for IPPV, changes are often small but the effects may become clinically significant the higher the pressure and the longer the inspiratory time. The cardiovascular effects of IPPV can be exaggerated by hypovolaemia or in animals with cardiac disease. Consequently the pressure which IPPV exerts should be carefully controlled.

In addition to this, overinflation of the lungs during IPPV can:

- Cause bradycardia secondary to a reflex mediated by pulmonary stretch receptors and the vagus nerve
- Lead to barotrauma, volutrauma and atelectrauma of the alveoli and airways; the resulting lung injury can lead to pulmonary oedema and other adverse pulmonary events
- Cause uneven ventilation in the lungs, which can affect pulmonary function especially in animals with pre-existing pulmonary disease
- Hyperventilate patients if not monitoring end-tidal carbon dioxide ($ETCO_2$).

IPPV is indicated when the patient's spontaneous ventilation is inadequate to maintain normocapnia or if there is ineffective gas exchange in the lungs. There are a number of patient and anaesthetic factors for which IPPV is always required and some where IPPV is recommended or advisable.

Absolute indications for IPPV:

- Diaphragmatic rupture
- Open chest
- Neuromuscular blockade
- Raised intracranial pressure
- Respiratory arrest

Relative indications for IPPV:

- Increased pressure on diaphragm secondary to abdominal enlargement (obesity, gastric dilation volvulus (GDV), insufflation of abdomen during laparoscopy, ascites and abdominal effusions, horses and other large animals in dorsal recumbency)
- Debilitated animals (muscle weakness)
- Long-duration anaesthesia
- When using potent respiratory depressants, e.g. fentanyl
- Animals breathing erratically
- Hypoventilation

Other advantages of IPPV:

- More accurate control of respiratory variables
- Constant arterial gas tensions create stable plasma pH and potassium concentrations
- Regular rhythm depresses ventilation, augments narcosis and improves operating conditions
- Mechanical ventilator frees anaesthetist (or nurse) for other duties

Generally IPPV will be performed at a tidal volume of between 10 and 15 ml/kg, a pressure of 10–20 cm H_2O and a respiratory rate that maintains partial pressure of carbon dioxide in the blood ($PaCO_2$) at a set level ($ETCO_2$ is often used as a surrogate for $PaCO_2$). This level is normally within the normal range or within the range of permissive hypercapnia that the anaesthetist has set. In patients with brain disease, especially if raised intracranial pressure is suspected, patients can benefit from being ventilated more than this. This is because increasing $PaCO_2$ levels increases cerebral blood flow and therefore can further increase intracranial pressure. In these circumstances the current recommendations are to ventilate the patient to a $PaCO_2$ (or $ETCO_2$) level of 35 mm Hg. Short-term hyperventilation can be used to further decrease intracranial pressure in the emergency situation but long-term hyperventilation is not advisable as it reduces cerebral perfusion to a level that can lead to cerebral hypoxia.

Hand ventilation

The simplest way of achieving positive pressure ventilation is by intermittent, controlled squeezing of the reservoir bag against a closed or semi-closed APL valve. This is labour intensive and it is difficult to keep consistent inspiratory pressures and volumes for long periods. Only certain breathing systems are suited to performing long-term IPPV: the T-piece, the Bain, and the circle (those with the bag on the expiratory limb). Other breathing systems such as the Magill and the Lack can be used in the short term with increased fresh gas flow but should be changed for a more suitable circuit for longer-term IPPV. The reason for this is that these breathing systems (those with the reservoir bag on the inspiratory limb) tend to cause rebreathing of expired gases.

Mechanical ventilation

As already discussed, in order for a ventilator to cause inspiration and then allow expiration it must intermittently force air into the lungs down a positive pressure gradient. Different types of ventilator perform this task in different ways; this helps classify the different types of ventilator.

- The first way of classification is by describing how the flow of gas is delivered. Most ventilators are volume controlled or pressure controlled. Volume-controlled ventilators provide a constant flow of gas during inspiration. Pressure-controlled ventilators provide a constant pressure of gas during inspiration.
- The second way of classifying ventilators is by how the ventilator switches from providing gas in inspiration to not providing gas in expiration. Ventilators can be time cycled, pressure cycled, or volume cycled. Time-cycled ventilators switch from inspiration to expiration after a set time. Pressure-cycled ventilators switch from inspiration to expiration once a set pressure is met. Volume-cycled ventilators change from inspiration to expiration once a set volume is met.

PRE-MEDICATION (AND SEDATION)

Pre-medication or pre-anaesthetic drugs are by definition given prior to induction of anaesthesia. Pre-medications are administered to decrease stress and/or anxiety (and the behaviours and physiological consequences of them), provide analgesia, cause sedation or muscle relaxation or a combination of these effects. The exact combination of drugs chosen by the veterinary surgeon will depend on the patient's medical history, concurrent underlying conditions, the procedure to be performed, the patient's temperament and the desired effect of the pre-medication. The importance of appropriate pre-medication cannot be overemphasised and administration of these drugs should aid a balanced approach to anaesthesia by meeting the following objectives:

- Reduce anxiety and limit stress at induction thereby reducing the excitement phase and the release of circulating catecholamines
- Provide pre-emptive analgesia and reduce the possibility of central sensitisation
- Provide analgesia and where possible reverse peripheral and central sensitisation in patients that are already in pain
- Facilitate a calm and comfortable recovery period
- Reduce doses of induction and maintenance anaesthetic agents thus limiting the effects of the cardiovascular and respiratory effects of these agents
- Pre-emptively counteract adverse effects of other anaesthetic drugs or due to the patient's pre-existing condition

The timing of the pre-medication should be thought about carefully. It is necessary to understand the onset time and duration of action of the drugs in order to appreciate that if the drugs are administered too early then they will be wearing off during the procedure and will need to be topped up and if they are administered too close to induction then they may not have reached peak effect. As previously discussed, none of the drugs that we administer during anaesthesia are inert and many have a set of often unwanted side effects as well as producing their desired effect in the patient. Patients should be carefully observed following pre-medication to enable rapid identification of any adverse events.

Classes of drugs included in this category include:

- Anticholinergics – atropine and glycopyrolate
- Phenothiazines – acepromazine
- Alpha-2 agonists – medetomidine and dexmedetomidine

TABLE 27.9	Comparison of the anticholinergics atropine and glycopyrolate	
Atropine	**Glycopyrolate**
Licensed	Not licensed in any animal species
Shorter duration of action	Longer duration of action
Rapid onset of action	'Gentler' less rapid onset of action
Greater lipid solubility	Less lipid soluble
Crosses the blood-brain barrier and placenta. Linked with cognitive impairment and delirium post-anaesthesia in humans	Does not cross the blood-brain barrier
Effects on the eye – mydriasis and possible rise in intraocular pressure	No effects on the eye

- Benzodiazepines – diazepam and midazolam
- Dissociative drugs – ketamine
- Opioids – pethidine, methadone, fentanyl, buprenorphine, butorphanol.

Definitions

Agonist – binds to and activates the receptor

Antagonist – may combine at the same site as an agonist but causes no effects and will block the effect of agonists at that receptor

Anticholinergics (muscarinic receptor antagonists) – these were historically popular as part of pre-medication protocols as they counteracted the side effects commonly seen with the inhalational agent ether (e.g. increased airway secretions). They are also still popularly administered in the USA to counter drug-induced bradycardia where higher doses of opioids are commonly utilised. They are generally regarded only for use now in the UK if the patient has a pre-existing condition or an anaesthetic history that requires a pre-emptive approach to counter bradycardia. It is more advisable in cases without these indications that these drugs only be used in response to observed bradycardia. They are also called **parasympatholytic** agents and are competitive antagonists whose chemical structures resemble that of acetylcholine (Ach) and block acetylcholine, which is the main neurotransmitter in the parasympathetic nervous system. They can be administered intravenously (IV), intramuscularly (IM) or subcutaneously (SC). See Table 27.9 for comparison between atropine and glycopyrolate.

Main effects:

- Inhibition of secretion – salivary, lacrimal, bronchial glands
- Effects on heart rate – tachycardia through block of cardiac muscarinic acetylcholine receptors; at low doses a paradoxical bradycardia can be seen prior to an increase in heart rate
- Effects on the gastrointestinal (GI) tract – inhibits GI motility
- Effects on other smooth muscle – relaxes bronchial, biliary and urinary tract smooth muscle. Bronchodilation except where bronchoconstriction is caused by local mediators, e.g. histamine and leukotrienes.

These agents are also used during anaesthesia where bradycardia is encountered. They should not be used to counter bradycardia induced by alpha-2 agonists.

Phenothiazines

These agents are generally administered to reduce anxiety and provide sedation. They are also considered as antipsychotic drugs and thus are called neuroleptics. In combination with an opioid they synergise the effects of both drugs to produce an increased level of sedation – neuroleptanaesthesia.

Acepromazine

Following intramuscular injection, sedation will generally occur within approximately 15 minutes with peak effect at 30–45 minutes. The duration of action depends on the dose (increasing dose increases duration and hypotension but not sedation) but is generally from 2–3 hours for good sedation and 4–8 hours for mild sedation and vasodilation. Sedation effects are often variable and not as reliable as the alpha-2 agonists but may be improved if the patient is kept calm and quiet. Works via SC/IM/IV routes (by half an hour there is no noticeable difference between routes). Oral administration also works but large first-pass metabolism reduces potency. Giant-breed dogs are more susceptible to the effects and the veterinary surgeon may consider reducing the dose in these cases. Some Boxer dogs have an increased sensitivity to acepromazine which may result in profound hypotension, vasovagal syncope or even death. The veterinary surgeon may elect to reduce the dose in Boxers, but this may not produce the required sedation in some individuals and alpha-2 agonists may provide an alternative choice depending on the health status of the individual. DO NOT USE in patients in shock or with pre-existing cardiovascular disease due to the risk of cardiovascular collapse.

Advantages:
- Sedation and management of stress-related behaviours
- Anti-arrhythmic properties – antagonist at alpha-1 adrenoreceptors in the heart; increased dose of adrenaline required to initiate arrhythmias (protects heart against catecholamine induced arrhythmias)
- Little effect on respiratory function
- Decreases the mean alveolar concentration of the inhalational anaesthetics
- Anti-emetic

Disadvantages
- Resets thermoregulatory mechanisms and causes vasodilation therefore may predispose to hypothermia
- Peripheral vasodilation and consequent hypotension – antagonist at alpha-1 receptors
- Liver metabolised forming conjugated and unconjugated metabolites which are renally excreted
- Can decrease stroke volume, cardiac output and mean arterial pressure by up to 25–30%
- Can decreases packed cell volume and total protein by 20–30%
- May increase the risk of gastro-oesophageal reflux as decreases gastric emptying and reduces gastrointestinal motility
- Decreases platelet aggregation but appears to cause no real haemostatic impairment
- May cause paradoxical excitement

BOX 27.2 CASES WHERE THE USE OF ALPHA-2 AGONISTS IS CONTROVERSIAL OR CONTRAINDICATED

- Diabetes mellitus
- Animals with immature cardiovascular and hepatic systems (under 10–12 weeks of age)
- Heart disease (especially dilated cardiomyopathy and mitral valve disease)
- Liver failure
- Raised intracranial or intraocular pressure

- Disinhibition, extrapyramidal excitement possible in highly strung animals or if 'interrupted' during early stages of sedation
- Profound hypotension can be seen in hypovolaemic or vasodilated animals due to the withdrawal of adrenergic tone
- Increases the vasodilatory effect of isoflurane
- Not reversible

Alpha-2 adrenergic agonists

This group has become one of the most widespread sedative/analgesic groups used in veterinary medicine. They act synergistically with the opioids and this will allow a lower dose of the alpha-2 agonist to be administered. Alpha-2 agonists interact with alpha-2 adrenergic receptors in the peripheral and central nervous systems. They invariably have some sort of alpha-1 activity and also interact with central imidazole receptors. Some alpha-2 agonists such as medetomidine and dexmedetomidine have been shown to have local anaesthetic–like qualities. They can be given systemically or via extradural or perineural routes. Due to the cardiovascular effects these drugs they may not be suitable for some patients with pre-existing cardiac conditions, e.g. significant mitral or tricuspid valve disease or dilated cardiomyopathy (Box 27.2). These drugs, however, are increasingly being chosen in low doses for use in some cardiac patients in place of acepromazine where some degree of sedation is required, and vasoconstriction is perhaps more preferable to vasodilation (e.g. aortic stenosis or hypertrophic cardiomyopathy).

Uses:
- Profound sedation and management of stress
- Neuroprotection and potentially anticonvulsant
- Analgesia – central and spinally mediated which contributes to a balanced, multimodal approach to patient analgesia
- Muscle relaxation assists the triad of anaesthesia and the balanced approach
- Cardiovascular stability due to sympathetic suppression
- Potent suppressors of the stress response
- Profound drug-sparing effect thus reducing the amount of induction and maintenance agents required

Drug effects:
- Systemic vascular resistance changes – initial direct vasoconstriction resulting in increased blood pressure followed by a central impairment of sympathetic tone and vasodilation resulting in a more 'normal' blood pressure

- Bradycardia initially reflex due to the hypertension then through central suppression of sympathetic tone (imidazole related)
- Reduced cardiac output
- Reduces respiratory rate but tidal volume may increase to compensate
- May cause some bronchodilation
- Thermoregulation changes – due to thalamic effects the thermoregulatory centres are depressed but peripheral vasoconstriction prevents heat loss and patients may become less hypothermic than those given acepromazine
- Emesis (perhaps serotonin mediated and more profound in cats) – do not use in patient where vomiting is contraindicated, e.g. head trauma, fragile eyes with raised intraocular pressure, gastric dilatation and volvulus or linear GI foreign body
- Reduces gut motility and perfusion – may predispose to gastric reflux
- Increase uterine activity and impair perfusion
- Cause hyperglycaemia (block β-cell insulin production)
- Diuresis (reduces antidiuretic hormone [ADH] secretion and antagonises ADH in collecting ducts and perhaps glucosuria; dogs) – this needs to be taken into account if measuring urine output
- Hepatic blood flow is reduced and the rate of metabolism of other drugs in the liver is reduced
- Reduce intraocular pressure (perhaps secondary to muscle relaxation – beware vomiting in small animals, especially cats), mydriasis in most species but meiosis in dogs
- Can be reversed with atipamezole, a highly selective alpha-2 antagonist that is licensed (in cats and dogs) so the drug of choice to reverse alpha-2 agonists.

Medetomidine and dexmedetomidine

Dexmedetomidine is the active isomer present in medetomidine. In chemical terms, medetomidine contains equal amounts of two mirror image enantiomers (dextro and levo isomers); the dextro-enantiomer possesses the sedative and analgesic properties while the levo-enantiomer does not. In dexmedetomidine, the inactive levomedetomidine enantiomer is eliminated.

These cases will need careful considered by the veterinary surgeon before an alpha-2 agonist is administered. It should, however, be recognised that sometimes it is necessary to use drugs for sedation in cases where most drugs would be contraindicated but that the effects of stress could be more detrimental than the side effects of these drugs. It is therefore down to the veterinary surgeon to do a risk-benefit analysis for the individual case.

Alpha-2 adrenergic antagonists

Atipamezole is the licensed reversal agent for medetomidine and dexmedetomidine and is an alpha-2 adrenergic receptor antagonist.

Benzodiazepines

- No benzodiazepines are licensed for veterinary use.
- Midazolam and diazepam have been used in veterinary species.

- Midazolam is a schedule 3 controlled drug and all schedule 3 drugs are advised to be kept locked in a secure cabinet by the RCVS.
- Diazepam is a schedule 4 part 1 drug and therefore has no safe custody requirements or advice.
- Limited sedative qualities in healthy animals (may actually cause paradoxical excitement – preferential inhibition of inhibitory transmission especially at lower doses) but may be useful in the old, young and very sick patients.
- Limited as pre-medication agents.
- Provide muscle relaxation.
- May have more of a role as a co-induction agent although the dose-sparing properties have been varied (midazolam is more effective than diazepam).
- Often considered to have a benign cardiovascular and respiratory profile.
- Have minimal cardiovascular effects although can cause a little vasodilation.
- Can have profound hypoventilatory effects in susceptible patients or if administered under general anaesthesia.
- Diazepam is considered the first-line antiepileptic drug during seizure management.

Opiates and opioids

Opiates are drugs derived from the poppies *Papaveretum somniferum* (morphine, codeine) or *Papavertum bracteatum* (thebaine). Opioids are drugs that act on opioid receptors and can include semisynthetic or synthetic versions of opiates. Structurally opioids are benzylisoquinoline alkaloids which act on the opioid receptors (OP) of which there are four main types: mu (MOP or OP3), kappa (KOP or OP2), delta (DOP or OP1) and nociceptin (NOP or OP4). Originally there was a sigma but this has been reclassified as it cannot be antagonised by naloxone.

Desired effects

- Analgesia with central, spinal and peripheral effects
- Sedation
- Anaesthetic/sedative sparing
- Reduce neuroendocrine stress response to anaesthesia and surgery (although ADH and cortisol can increase in response to opioid administration in some species)
- Depressed airway reflexes

Possible adverse effects

- Dysphoria/euphoria
- Nausea and vomiting (morphine)
- Ileus (via Mu MOP receptor activation in GI tract, reduces secretions, peristalsis and sphincter tone)
- Hypoventilation – not generally clinically significant except with highly potent agents such as fentanyl
- Decrease thermoregulatory thresholds in the thalamus
- Reduce central sympathetic outflow
- Vagal excitation (except pethidine, which has mild vagolytic/antimuscarinic effects)
- Histamine release (morphine and pethidine especially) direct non-opioid receptor effects on mast cells
- Depressed airway reflexes
- Reduced urine output through ADH stimulation (though effects are unclear)

- Urinary retention (extradural/spinal especially seems to increase sphincter tone)

Morphine

See under 'Pain assessment, patient comfort and analgesia' later in this chapter.

Methadone

- Methadone is a synthetic diphenylheptane
- It is made of two enantiomers: D-methadone and L-methadone
- Methadone is licensed in the UK (Comfortan; Dechra Pharmaceuticals) for analgesia in dogs and cats
- Schedule II controlled drug – needs to be kept in a controlled drugs cupboard and its use and wastage recorded in a controlled drug record
- IM, IV, SC – not routinely given by constant rate infusion or epidurally
- Methadone is a mu (MOP) receptor agonist
- NMDA receptor antagonist
- Duration of action is approximately 4 hours in dogs and 6 hours in cats
- May inhibit its own metabolism and accumulate after multiple dosing so individually tailored analgesia is important

Pethidine (meperidine)

- Synthetic, phenylpiperidine derivative opioid
- Pethidine is licensed in the UK for the use in the dog and cat for analgesia
- Schedule II controlled drug – needs to be kept in a controlled drugs cupboard and its use and wastage recorded in a controlled drug record
- Causes profound histamine release IV
- IM or SC only
- Mu (MOP) receptor agonist
- Sodium channel blocker
- ACh antagonist (antimuscarinic) – does not cause bradycardia as it has an atropine-like structure
- Duration of action is 45–60 minutes in the dog and 90–120 minutes in the cat

Fentanyl

See under 'Pain assessment, patient comfort and analgesia' later in this chapter.

Buprenorphine

- Buprenorphine is a long acting, semi-synthetic thebaine derivative
- Buprenorphine is licensed as an analgesic in dogs, cats (multiple forms with and without preservative)
- Schedule III controlled drug – keep it in a locked cupboard but does not need to be recorded
- Buprenorphine can be administered IV, IM and transmucosally (cats only)
- Buprenorphine is classically described as a partial mu (MOP) agonist.
- Buprenorphine binds avidly (but slowly) to mu (MOP) receptors and dissociates slowly
- Duration of action 6–12 hours

Butorphanol

Description

- Butorphanol is a morphinian type, synthetic opioid agonist-antagonist
- It is licensed for sedation and analgesia in dogs and cats
- Systemically IV, IM or SC
- Oral form used as antitussive
- Agonist at kappa (KOP)
- Antagonist at mu (MOP)
- Good sedative but poor analgesic in dogs and cats
- Not appropriate as a sole analgesic for surgical procedures in dogs and cats
- Good analgesic in birds
- Duration of action 45–90 minutes
- Not subject to controlled drug regulations

Antagonism of opioid agents

The effects of pure mu opioid agonists can be reversed with a mu opioid antagonist naloxone.

Naloxone

- Mu opioid antagonist
- Rapid onset 1–2 minutes
- Duration of action 30–60 minutes
- Can be used to reverse the mu agonists
- Has a higher affinity for the mu and kappa receptors than these drugs
- May not be as effective at reversing buprenorphine due to its high receptor affinity
- Administer slowly in intravenous increments until the desired effect is reached
- Not subject to controlled drugs regulations
- Complete reversal occurs so no analgesic effects remain and alternative provision for patient comfort should be made
- May need repeat dosing as it is shorter acting than many common opioids

Intravenous catheter placement

Following pre-medication of the patient and allowing sufficient time for this to work the next step in the anaesthetic process is to place a peripheral intravenous catheter. This is considered best practice and will allow:

- Administration of intravenous induction agents
- Rapid intravascular access in the case of an adverse event
- Administration of intravenous fluid therapy.

Sites for insertion include cephalic and accessory cephalic, medial and lateral saphenous, auricular and dorsal common digital veins. The lateral saphenous vein is larger than the medial saphenous vein in the dog and vice versa in the cat.

Over-the-needle catheters are the most commonly used type for peripheral placement and can also be placed as a quick and easy method of central catheter placement in the cat. They are inexpensive, easy to place and are suitable for short- to medium-term. Most over-the-needle catheters can be left in place for 48 to 72 hours, but should be checked regularly for any phlebitis, inflammation or misplacement.

It should be noted that fluid flow through a catheter is related to the length and radius of a catheter. Catheter radius (r) has the greatest effect with flow related to r^4; therefore halving the diameter will result in a 16-fold decrease in flow.

TABLE 27.10	Approximate sizes of endotracheal tube according to lean body weight	
Approximate lean body weight	Species	Sizes – internal diameter in mm
2.5 kg	Cat	3.0 cuffed or uncuffed
5.0 kg	Cat	4.5 or 5.0 cuffed or uncuffed
5.0 kg	Dog	6.0 cuffed
10 kg	Dog	8.0 cuffed
15 kg	Dog	9.0 cuffed
20 kg	Dog	10.0 cuffed
25 kg	Dog	11.0 cuffed
35 kg	Dog	12.0 cuffed
>40 kg	Dog	14.0 or 16.0 cuffed

Note: This table is intended as a guide only.

FLUID THERAPY UNDER ANAESTHESIA

It is considered best practice to provide intravenous fluid therapy to patients undergoing anaesthesia. This is normally lactated ringers (Hartmann's) solution but other preparations may be prescribed by the veterinary surgeon for different conditions. For example head trauma cases are often put on normal saline (0.7% sodium chloride) and diabetic patients may require glucose to be added to the intravenous fluids depending on glucometer readings.

The rate of fluids to be given under anaesthesia is the topic of much debate but should generally be considered as twice maintenance (4 ml/kg/hr) plus the ml/ml replacement of any fluids lost. Patients with congestive heart failure, for example, may be prescribed more cautious fluid rates and hypovolaemic patients may require higher rates but this is at the discretion of the veterinary surgeon in charge of the case.

PREPARING FOR INDUCTION

It is best practice to place an airway device in the majority of small animal patients unless the veterinary surgeon perceives that the risks of placement outweigh the risks of not having a secure airway. Airway devices for dogs, cats and rabbits include endotracheal tubes and for cats and rabbits supraglottic airway devices (V-gel™).

Once the anaesthetic machine, monitoring equipment and other checks have been made according to the checklist it is important to assess the patient to ascertain what size endotracheal tube or supraglottic airway device will be required.

When using endotracheal tubes: The length of the endotracheal tube will need to be measured from the patient's incisors to the thoracic inlet or the point of the shoulder when the neck is flexed. It may be necessary to cut the tube to the correct length and then reposition the connector. This is important because endotracheal tubes that are too long will contribute to mechanical dead space if protruding too far from the incisors or could cause endobronchial intubation if the long endotracheal tube is advanced beyond the tracheal bifurcation and into one of the main-stem bronchi. The widest tube that can easily be passed down the trachea will be selected so it is best practice to have a range of three sizes available to whomever is going to intubate the patient (Table 27.10).

Types of endotracheal tube include:
Red rubber
- Available in sizes 2–16 mm with some sizes being available in both cuffed and uncuffed versions
- Reusable but may perish over time (especially when exposed to sunlight)
- Autoclavable
- Less expensive than silicone
- Easy to intubate as pre-formed into a curve
- No Murphy eye – 'Murphy eye' is the eponymous name for a hole on the side of most endotracheal tubes that functions as a vent and prevents the complete obstruction of the patient's airway, should the primary distal opening of the tube become occluded
- Cannot be repaired
- Low volume high pressure cuff – superior protection of the airway due to a better seal but much higher risk of tracheal damage
- Pivot balloon does not self-seal and may come undone
- Blockages are not visible
- Irritant to airways
- Does not withstand kinking

Polyvinyl chloride (PVC)
- Available in sizes 2–11 mm with some sizes available as uncuffed versions
- Inexpensive
- Cannot be repaired
- Disposable
- Not autoclavable
- Non-irritant
- Easy to intubate due to pre-formed curve
- High pressure – low volume and low pressure high volume cuff versions available
- Blockages may be visible
- Withstands kinking better than red rubber tubes
- Self-sealing pivot balloon for cuff inflation

Silicone
- Available in a wide range of sizes 2–16 mm
- Expensive
- Can be repaired
- Autoclavable
- Non-irritant
- Re-usable
- More kink resistant than red rubber tubes but occlude earlier than PVC tubes
- May be more difficult to intubate – a stylet may be needed to stiffen and bend the tube
- Self-sealing pivot balloon for cuff inflation
- Low volume – high pressure cuff
- May be possible to see blockages

Armoured endotracheal tubes are available for surgeries where the risk of kinking and obstructing the endotracheal tube is high such as cerebrospinal fluid (CSF) taps, ophthalmic, oral or facial surgery. Other specialist tubes are available, e.g. for laser surgery.

Endotracheal tubes should be assessed for patency either by looking through the tube or by passing a stylet through. They should never be blown through as this poses an infection control risk. Endotracheal tubes should also be visually assessed for contamination and damage. Cuffs on the endotracheal tubes should be inflated for 5–10 minutes to check for leaks and then the air withdrawn to leave them ready for use. The connector should also be checked to ensure that it is securely seated in the endotracheal tube – this will minimise the risk of leaks.

Using cuffed endotracheal tubes in cats is the subject of much debate. The advantages of inflating the cuff mean that a good tracheal seal is achieved and may be necessary if ventilation is required or if there is a risk of aspiration of foreign material, e.g. during regurgitation or dental procedures. Red rubber tubes should never be cuffed in cats due to the low volume, high pressure cuff which can easily damage or tear the fragile trachea.

Equipment required for the induction of anaesthesia:
- Saline or heparinised saline in a syringe to flush the intravenous catheter
- Intravenous induction agent
- Anaesthetic machine with breathing system attached – both checked and ready for use
- Lidocaine spray for the larynx in cats
- A range of endotracheal tubes – checked for patency and cuff inflation or a range of supraglottic airway devices (cats only)
- Laryngoscope
- Woven bandage to tie the tube in

Process for the induction of anaesthesia and endotracheal intubation in the dog and cat:

1. An assistant restrains the patient usually in sternal recumbency – lateral recumbency may be chosen in individuals with spinal disease.
2. Flush the intravenous catheter with saline/heparinised saline to ensure it is in the vein and patent.
3. Pre-oxygenate the patient using flow-by oxygen technique (or well-fitting mask if tolerated).
4. Inject the intravenous induction agent over 60 seconds to effect – this will be done by a veterinary surgeon.
5. Assess depth of anaesthesia by assessing jaw tone and palpebral reflex (see monitoring) – do not attempt to intubate unless the patient is considered to be at a surgical plane of anaesthesia
6. The assistant will extend the neck and hold the upper jaw by the holding the mucous membranes under the lips or by using gauze bandage around the upper jaw behind the canines and holding both ends – care should be taken not to place fingers in the patient's mouth.
7. The tongue is extruded utilising the laryngoscope and then pulled forward and held against the base of the laryngoscope using the first finger on the non-dominant hand.
8. The base of the tongue is depressed, rostral to the epiglottis, using the laryngoscope blade to visualise the larynx (Figs. 27.25 and 27.26) – the laryngoscope blade should never be used directly on the epiglottis as this may cause damage and subsequent swelling may occlude the airway on extubation.
9. In cats the larynx is sprayed with lidocaine and then a period of 30–90 seconds should elapse to allow the lidocaine to work before attempting intubation – this is to desensitise the larynx and reduce the risk of laryngospasm. Pre-oxygenation and further incremental doses of induction agent can be continued during this period as required.
10. The endotracheal tube is passed over the epiglottis and between the arytenoid cartilages and vocal folds into the trachea (Fig. 27.27).

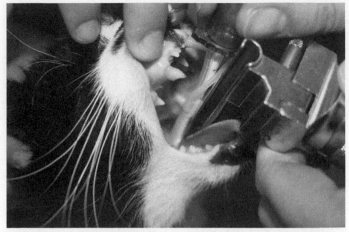

Fig. 27.25 Using the laryngoscope blade to visualise the larynx

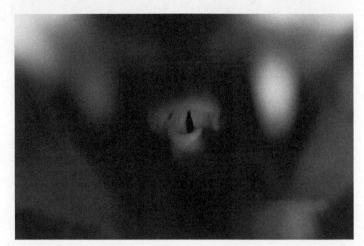

Fig. 27.26 The larynx

11. If the arytenoid cartilages are not open in cats then intubation should not be forced and it is necessary to wait for these to open before intubating to avoid laryngospasm and laryngeal oedema on extubation.
12. Once placed the endotracheal tube should be secured with the connector external to the incisors and with gauze bandage tied around the tube connector and then secured to the upper or lower jaw or around the patient's head.
13. The oxygen should be turned on and the breathing system connected to the endotracheal tube with a 'push and twist' action to avoid disconnection.
14. Placement of the endotracheal tube can be assessed using capnography, by visualisation of the simultaneous movement of the patient's chest wall and the reservoir bag if a capnograph is not available or by administering a positive pressure breath.
15. If the cuff is to be inflated this should be done while listening to air leaks from the mouth while an assistant administers a positive pressure breath – the cuff should not be inflated further when no more leaks are heard. If a large volume of air is required then consideration should be made as to whether a larger endotracheal tube may be warranted.

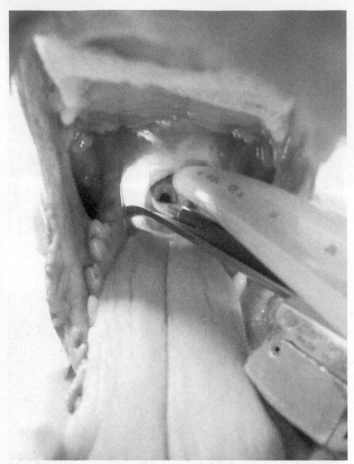

Fig. 27.27 The endotracheal tube is passed over the epiglottis and between the arytenoid cartilages and vocal folds into the trachea

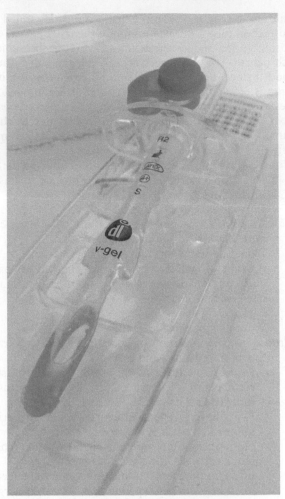

Fig. 27.28 The V-gel™ supraglottic airway device

ALWAYS disconnect the breathing system from the endotracheal tube when turning the patient to prevent tracheal damage. This has been a major factor in tracheal rupture of cats with cuffed endotracheal tubes.

Supraglottic airway devices

Supraglottic airway devices were originally introduced in human anaesthesia, due to the difficulty in intubating people, as a simple and effective alternative to the endotracheal tube. The V-gel™ supraglottic airway device (Fig. 27.28) has been developed as an alternative to endotracheal tubes in rabbits and cats. Both cats and rabbits were indicated by the CEPSAF as being higher anaesthetic risks than dogs and it is possible that this is in part attributable to airway complications in both species. Rabbits can be notoriously difficult to intubate due to difficulties in directly visualising the larynx. While some practitioners may be well practiced at blind intubation in this species, the majority are not and securing an airway is often either not attempted (resulting in masked anaesthesia) or intubation takes a prolonged period of time. Cats are also often not appropriately intubated and laryngospasm and laryngeal oedema are known to present as adverse events in the perianaesthetic period. This, combined with the continued use of red rubber tubes in cats (which can damage tracheal mucosa and cause necrosis complete tracheal rupture if the cuffs are used inappropriately), may make the use of supraglottic airway devices a useful and potentially safer alternative for short procedures where a capnograph is available.

The device size is selected by consulting the body weight guidelines provided by the manufacturer and also by measuring it against the patient. The airway opening should be placed adjacent to larynx (this can be felt) on the patient's neck (without touching the fur and contaminating the device) and the connector should reach just past the incisors if correct size of device has been selected.

Considerations:

- Ease of placement in both species
- Allows rapid airway security
- Allows IPPV
- Avoids airway trauma and prevents laryngeal spasm
- Well tolerated in recovery and does not need to be removed as early as an endotracheal tube
- Reusable and autoclavable
- Latex free and non-irritant
- The device does not sit in the trachea therefore the diameter of the trachea is not reduced
- Perceived as an expensive initial purchase – in reality the cost is only a few pounds per use
- Can twist and become dislodged even if well tied in so requires a capnograph to ensure correct placement and assess displacement during anaesthesia

- Has not been clinically evaluated for protecting the airway from regurgitated gastric contents
- Anatomically designed to be species specific

Procedure for induction of anaesthesia and placement of a supraglottic airway device:

- Steps 1 through 6 as for endotracheal intubation.
- The mouth should be examined for debris and the tongue pulled forward.
- Lidocaine spray should be administered onto the laryngeal area and a period of 30–90 seconds waited prior to placing the supraglottic device.
- The V-gel™ cuff should be lubricated with a water-soluble lubricant.
- The capnograph is connected to the port prior to insertion.
- The V-gel™ is then inserted into the pharynx with gentle finger-push pressure – if it cannot be inserted with this gentle pressure then a smaller size should be selected.
- The V-gel™ will guide itself into place with the tip of the device securing a seal to the upper oesophagus.
- The V-gel™ should continue to be inserted over the base of the tongue until the shoulders of the device come into contact with the pharyngeal arches and a positive stop will be felt when the device achieves the correct position.
- Placement is observed by observing the capnograph.
- The device is secured with gauze bandage around the patient's head to the loops on either side of the device.
- The oxygen should be turned on and the breathing system connected to the device with a 'push and twist' action.
- The breathing system should then be supported with a stand to ensure it is kept in line with the mouth and does not twist and displace the device.
- The cuff can be inflated to improve the seal of the supraglottic airway device if necessary.
- The device should be assessed for displacement throughout anaesthesia using capnography.

Cleaning endotracheal tubes and supraglottic airway devices:

- Some endotracheal tubes are designed to be disposable and therefore may not withstand cleaning and reuse.
- Endotracheal tubes and supraglottic airway devices should be cleaned with water and a soft bottle brush.
- Once all gross contamination has been removed endotracheal tubes and supraglottic devices should be soaked in an enzymatic cleaner for the appropriate contact time.
- During soaking a soft bottle brush should be used to clean the airway channels.
- Where endotracheal tubes are not going to be sterilised by autoclave they should then be soaked in a cold sterilising solution for the appropriate contact time.
- The tubes and devices should be rinsed thoroughly with water (ideally filtered sterile water) and left to dry.
- Red rubber and silicone endotracheal tubes can be autoclaved as necessary.
- Supraglottic airway devices should then be placed in their cradle into an autoclave pouch and autoclaved on a 121°C cycle.

INDUCTION AGENTS

There are only two induction agents currently licensed in small animals – propofol and alfaxalone. Propofol is currently available in two formulations – one with preservative and one without.

Propofol

- A substituted phenol with no preservative so it should be immediately discarded after vial breach
- The solution is a white, milky lipid solution containing soyabean oil, glycerol and egg lecithin
- Administered to effects over 10–40 seconds
- Duration of action up to 5 minutes
- Induction quality is generally smooth but may cause stage II excitation if given too slowly and apnoea if given too quickly
- May cause pain on injection, apnoea, stage II excitation, dose-dependent hypotension and bradycardia
- Impairs baroreceptor reflex so heart rate does not increase in response to hypotension
- Terminal plasma half-life approximately 90+ minutes in dogs and 480+ minutes in cats
- Intravenous use only
- Suitable for constant rate infusion for total intravenous anaesthesia (TIVA) but caution with cats due to accumulation and oxidative damage to the red blood cells
- Licensed in cats and dogs
- Repeated anaesthesia with propofol in cats may cause oxidative injury to red blood cells and Heinz body production. Recovery may also become prolonged. Limiting repeated anaesthesia to intervals of more than 48 hours will reduce the likelihood
- Propofol is metabolised by various P450 pathways with glucuronidation being the major pathway for phase II. As such the metabolism of propofol by cats is impaired. In dogs P450 may vary between different breeds of dog accounting for the longer duration of action in breeds such as greyhounds. Clearance of propofol is greater than hepatic blood flow suggesting that extrahepatic metabolism is significant – one suggested site is the lungs and propofol metabolites can be measured in expired breath
- Propofol infusion syndrome can be seen in patients receiving propofol for more than 24 hours and is characterised by the presence of metabolic acidosis, rhabdomyolysis or myoglobinuria, acute renal failure, sudden onset of bradycardia resistant to treatment, myocardial failure, and lipaemic plasma

Propofol with benzyl alcohol preservative

- Drug characteristics as propofol except that as it has benzyl alcohol as a preservative and can be kept for 28 days from vial breach
- Benzyl alcohol toxicity may lead to prolonged recovery and hyperkinesia in cats, and neurological signs such as tremors in dogs and fatalities in both species
- Not licensed in caesarean section and in humans parenterally administered benzyl alcohol has been associated with a fatal toxic syndrome in preterm neonates

- Not suitable for constant rate infusion. Licensed for up to half an hour but contraindicated for prolonged infusion due to benzyl alcohol
- MUST NOT exceed total dose of 2.4 ml/kg.

Alfaxalone

- A neuroactive steroid carried in a clear solution of the inert carrier agent 2-hydroxypropyl-beta cyclodextrin
- No preservative so should be discarded on vial breach but does not seem to promote bacterial growth in the same way as propofol
- Administer slowly to effect over at least 60 seconds
- Duration of action: 10 minutes (dog), 25 minutes (cat)
- Smooth induction evoking a sleep-like quality with no excitation generally seen
- Smooth recovery provided the patient has been appropriately pre-medicated
- Less apnoea than propofol as able to give more slowly to effect due to the absence of stage II excitation
- Causes vasodilation but does not impair baroreceptor reflexes so there is normally a reflex transient increase in heart rate – cardiac output normally increases although blood pressure may decrease slightly
- Appears to have a very wide safety margin when compared with propofol
- Has minimal effects on neonates when administered as an induction agent for Caesarean section and recently shown to provide better vigour in puppies than propofol
- Terminal plasma half-life is shorter than that of propofol: 25 minutes (dogs), 45 minutes (cats)
- Licensed in cats and dogs
- Suitable for constant rate infusion as not cumulative and causes no oxidative damage in cats
- While not currently licensed as it causes no tissue damage or irritation, it has been widely used for intramuscular sedation prior to anaesthesia.

DISSOCIATIVE ANAESTHETICS

These agents do not provide classical anaesthesia (generalised central and spinal cord depression) and as such are not classed individually as induction agents but may be used for co-induction or as part of an intramuscular combination. They interrupt ascending transmission to the brain and interfere with transmission between parts of the brain responsible for conscious and unconscious functions. These agents facilitate immobilisation through cataleptic anaesthesia, which gives a 'trance-like' state and 'superficial sleep'. They also offer profound analgesia.

Ketamine

- Phencyclidine derivative
- Aqueous solution, pH 3.5–5.5
- Can be administered IV and IM but stings on IM injection due to the pH
- Can be administered as a constant rate infusion as part of a partial intravenous anaesthesia (PIVA) protocol and for postoperative analgesia
- Contains preservative and can be kept for 28 days from vial broach
- Currently classified as a Schedule 4 controlled drug (CD) and therefore by law its use does not need to be recorded, nor does it need to be kept in the CD cabinet. Ketamine has recently been reclassified as a Class B drug by the home office but its schedule remains unchanged. The RCVS advises: Record the use of ketamine in an informal register. Store ketamine in a controlled drugs cabinet. Destroy ketamine in the presence of an authorised witness
- In other words, ketamine should be treated as though it is a Schedule 2 drug.
- Relatively rapid onset of action, approximately 2 minutes
- Antagonist at NMDA receptor
- Analgesia – somatic over visceral analgesia
- Muscle rigidity, convulsions, hyperexcitability can be seen but reduced by the co-administration of alpha-2 agonists or benzodiazepines
- Hypersensitivity to noise
- Recovery via redistribution from central nervous system
- Metabolised via the liver in most species
- Elimination in cats depends more on renal excretion than metabolism – care in cats with compromised renal function
- Indirect cardiovascular stimulation – acts directly as a myocardial depressant but sympathetic effects generally outweigh this; subsequent increase in myocardial work due to increased cardiac output and afterload
- Respiratory – does not depress the respiratory response to hypoxaemia. Respiratory rate and minute volume drop initially but normally return to baseline. Apneustic (prolonged inspiration/inspiratory hold) may occur as well as other abnormal breathing patterns
- May not obliterate cranial nerve reflexes so may still gag and have active palpebral reflexes
- Increased intracranial pressure seen (but generally associated with an increase in $PaCO_2$)
- Increases cerebral metabolic oxygen demand
- May offer neuroprotective effects
- May increase intraocular pressure (effect lost with benzodiazepines in dogs)
- Reduces gut motility
- May increase uterine tone

TRANSITION

Anaesthetic transition is the period between injecting an intravenous agent to induce anaesthesia and maintaining anaesthesia with an inhalational agent. The smoothness of this period will depend on:

- The duration of action of the induction agent chosen – if this is too rapid then the patient will often become 'light' and require a top up of intravenous induction agent or there is a tendency to increase the percentage on the vaporiser beyond what would normally be required
- The ease and speed of intubation of the patient
- Whether the patient is spontaneously breathing – if apnoea (if too much induction agent has been administered) or breath holding (the patient is not adequately anaesthetised prior to intubation) has occurred then the patient will not be spontaneously breathing and this should be addressed to prevent further adverse events.

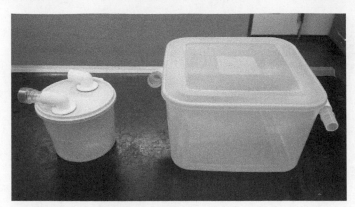

Fig. 27.29 Anaesthetic gas chamber

MASK AND CHAMBER INDUCTION FOR ANAESTHESIA

The use of inhalational agents for induction has been superseded in dogs and cats and is not considered best practice as there is an inability to rapidly control the airway. Mask induction was previously used in rabbits; however, they have a tendency to breath hold when exposed to inhalational agents when conscious, and the introduction of supraglottic airway devices and newer induction agents means that this is no longer necessary.

Small mammals such as rats and mice are often best anaesthetised using a chamber due to the inability for appropriate restraint and easy intravenous access in these species. A see-through chamber means that the patient can be clearly visualised (Fig. 27.29).

Procedure for chamber induction of rats and mice:
1. Fill the chamber with oxygen.
2. Place the patient in the chamber and allow acclimatisation.
3. Turn on the vaporiser.
4. Watch the patient continuously and when unconsciousness is reached – the righting reflex is lost – flush the chamber with oxygen to scavenge anaesthetic gases and remove the patient quickly before resealing the chamber.
5. Take care to minimise exposure of anaesthetic gases to personnel.
6. The patient is then maintained by delivering inhalational agent via a properly fitting face mask.

MAINTENANCE OF ANAESTHESIA

Maintenance of anaesthesia can be achieved in a number of ways:
- By continued use of the intravenous induction drug either by bolus or constant rate infusion –this is termed total intravenous anaesthesia (TIVA)
- By inhalational agent
- Using a combination of inhalational anaesthesia (e.g. isoflurane) but utilising constant rate infusions of other agents to reduce the inhalational requirements (such as ketamine, fentanyl and lidocaine) is termed partial intravenous anaesthesia (PIVA)
- Injectable agents given intramuscularly, e.g. the triple combination of ketamine, medetomidine and butor-phanol sometimes administered to cats for short procedures

INHALATIONAL OR VOLATILE AGENTS

These agents are by far the most common maintenance agents used in anaesthesia today although the use of TIVA is becoming more widespread. There are two main types of volatile agents:

Halogenated hydrocarbons

Halothane – no longer licensed for use in veterinary medicine

Fluorinated ethers

Isoflurane – licensed for horses, dogs, cats, ornamental birds, reptiles, rats, mice, hamsters, chinchillas, gerbils, guinea pigs and ferrets

Sevoflurane – licensed for dogs

Desflurane – not licensed for use in veterinary medicine

Mode of action

The exact mode of action of volatile anaesthetics is poorly understood. Much of the current understanding of volatile agent mode of action revolves around interactions with the $GABA_A$ receptor (the major inhibitory receptor in the central nervous system). Anaesthetics must work both in the brain to deliver unconsciousness and the spinal cord to block spontaneous and reflex movement. Generally unconsciousness occurs at lower concentrations of volatile agent than the inhibition of spinal cord function.

Differences between the volatile agents

What differs between these agents is their blood/gas solubility, potency and side effects. These will define the situations where each of the agents is most useful.

Blood/gas solubility

Blood/gas solubility is a ratio that defines the amount of agent dissolved in blood as compared to that in gaseous form at equilibrium. For example, a blood/gas solubility of 1 would give 1 part dissolved in blood to 1 part in gaseous form; a blood/gas solubility of 0.5 would give 1 part dissolved in blood to 2 parts in gaseous form (or 0.5 to 1) and a blood/gas solubility of 2 would give 2 parts dissolved in blood to 1 part in gaseous form.

Blood/gas solubility gives us an idea of how that vapour will behave in an animal's alveoli and helps define speed of onset and offset of anaesthesia. The more soluble an agent is in the blood then the slower the patient goes to sleep and recovers. Changes in vaporiser setting are slower to take effect the more soluble in blood the agent is. Sevoflurane is less soluble in blood (0.65) than isoflurane (1.4) and therefore induction, recovery and changes in vaporiser settings are more rapid.

Other factors influencing the onset of volatile anaesthesia

It is important to remember that other factors influence volatile anaesthetic onset:

Delivery phase
- Vaporiser setting
- Fresh gas flow for rebreathing systems

Pulmonary phase
- Alveolar ventilation
- Pressure of volatile agent in the pulmonary artery (decreases concentration gradient)
- Pulmonary blood flow (increasing perfusion, increases uptake and decreases speed of onset)
- Ventilation/perfusion mismatching – this is where areas of alveoli are well ventilated but poorly perfused or alternatively well perfused but poorly ventilated
- Concentration and second gas effects

Circulatory phase
- Cardiac output
- Cerebral blood flow
- Distribution to other tissues

Minimum alveolar concentration

Minimum alveolar concentration (MAC) is a means of comparing the potency of different agents as mg/kg doses are meaningless when looking at inhaled drugs (Table 27.11). MAC or MAC_{50} of an agent can be defined as the alveolar concentration of agent required to stop 'gross purposeful movement' (reflex movement such as withdrawal or tail twitch) following a 'noxious stimulus' (normally a clamp to an extremity but sometimes electrical stimulation) in 50% of a population.

This assumes that the volatile agent was used on its own with no analgesics or additional sedatives/anaesthetics.

MAC values are drug and species dependent but by definition animals within a population may fall above or below the population median.

Care: MAC is merely a method to compare volatile anaesthetic potency and care should be taken when interpreting MAC in clinical settings.

Factors affecting MAC:
- Species
- Analgesics/sedatives and other anaesthetic agents
- Hypothermia
- Hypotension
- Concurrent underlying disease – hyperthyroidism, pregnancy, electrolyte abnormalities
- Age
- Hypoxaemia – low blood oxygen levels
- Hypercarbia – high levels of carbon dioxide in the blood

VOLATILE AGENTS

All of the volatile agents have the following effects:
- Dose-dependent respiratory depression
- Dose-dependent depression of the cardiovascular system – systemic vascular resistance is reduced causing vasodilation and therefore hypotension
- Depression of the central nervous system
- No analgesic effects
- Very little liver metabolism as excreted by the lungs

Isoflurane
- Licensed for horses, dogs, cats, ornamental birds, reptiles, rats, mice, hamsters, chinchillas, gerbils, guinea pigs and ferrets in the UK
- More potent than sevoflurane – lower vaporiser settings are required
- More soluble in blood than sevoflurane so slower induction (when using inhalational anaesthesia), recovery and changes in depth.

TABLE 27.11	Illustrating blood/gas coefficient and MAC for dogs and cats for the volatile agents and nitrous oxide		
Volatile agent	Blood/gas solubility	MAC$_{50}$ % dogs	MAC$_{50}$ % cats
Nitrous	0.47	222 (least potent)	255
Desflurane	0.45	7.2	9.8
Sevoflurane	0.65	2.3	2.6
Isoflurane	1.4	1.3	1.6
Halothane	2.4	0.9 (most potent)	1.1

Note that halothane and desflurane are not licensed in veterinary species but are shown for illustrative purposes.

- Strong, pungent odour – makes it difficult to use for inhalational induction
- Irritant to airways

Sevoflurane
- Only licensed for dogs in the UK
- Less potent than isoflurane so higher vaporiser settings are required
- Less soluble in blood than isoflurane so faster induction (when using inhalational anaesthesia), recovery and changes in depth.
- Odourless – better choice for masked induction
- Less respiratory irritation than isoflurane
- Maintains metabolic flow coupling in the brain and potentially maintains cerebral autoregulation so is preferred by some anaesthetists to isoflurane in suspected brain space occupying lesions and head injuries
- May not impair hypoxic pulmonary vasoconstriction to the same degree as isoflurane therefore may be chosen in some respiratory cases
- A reaction with moist soda lime is known to produce compound A, which has been shown to be nephrotoxic (in laboratory rats) at very high concentrations. Not clinically significant.

Nitrous oxide

Nitrous oxide is a poor anaesthetic agent and requires a MAC of over 100%. It is therefore not potent enough to be used alone but is used in some practices as a carrier gas. Its main use in veterinary anaesthesia is an analgesic adjunct. It is a liquid at room temperature and is supplied in blue cylinders. Unlike with oxygen the dial on a nitrous oxide cylinder will read full until the cylinder is almost empty and then drop dramatically. Nitrous oxide cylinders should be weighed to accurately appraise how much is left in the cylinder.

Nitrous oxide can be utilised with oxygen at a ratio of no more than 2 parts nitrous oxide to one part oxygen (2:1) in non-rebreathing systems and in equal parts (1:1) with oxygen in rebreathing systems.

Pharmacology
- Poor anaesthetic agent – MAC_{50} greater than 100%
- NMDA antagonistic effects – provides analgesia
- Opioid receptor effects – possibly increasing endogenous opioid secretion
- Sympathomimetic causing an increase in systemic and pulmonary vascular resistance

- MAC sparing so can improve the hypotensive effects of isoflurane/sevoflurane by reducing the amount of these agents required
- Mild direct cardio-depressant effects
- Low blood/gas solubility – 0.47
- Diffuses into gas filled viscous when the gas has a lower solubility co-efficient – so methane (0.04) and nitrogen (0.015) filled spaces (pneumothorax, intestines, stomach etc.) but **not** capnoperitoneum (CO_2 blood/gas solubility is 0.48). Will double intestinal size in 2 hours of anaesthesia (which will affect visualisation during laparoscopy)
- **DO NOT use for patients with pneumothorax, GDV, bowel obstruction or for any surgeries or procedures where air is insufflated, e.g. gastroscopy or intraocular surgery.**

Nitrous oxide was previously utilised for its second gas effect when halothane was still available. Due to the low solubility of nitrous oxide it has a rapid onset time and when used as a carrier gas could be used to augment the uptake of the volatile agent (the second gas) thereby increasing the speed of the volatile agent attaining the required brain concentration to maintain the required depth of anaesthesia. There is little clinical benefit of the second gas effect when using isoflurane and sevoflurane.

Diffusion hypoxia. At the end of anaesthesia, when nitrous oxide is turned off the nitrous oxide rapidly leaves the blood and floods the alveoli. If the patient is not on supplemented O_2 but is rather moved straight to room air hypoxia will develop due to the dilution of O_2 in the alveoli with the nitrous oxide. This will lead to hypoxia – a decreased PaO_2. Due to this it is recommended that nitrous oxide be turned off 10 minutes prior to the end of anaesthesia and 100% O_2 administered.

Health and safety concerns of volatile agents and nitrous oxide. N_2O oxidises the cobalt ion in cyanocobalamin (vitamin B_{12}). N_2O therefore indirectly inhibits the production of methionine, thymidine, tetrahydrofolate and DNA. This mainly causes effects on the bone marrow resulting in anaemia but has to potential to cause degeneration of spinal cord and peripheral neuropathy as methionine is required for myelination. N_2O has also been shown to be teratogenic in rats – this has never been investigated in man but is often avoided in the first trimester of pregnancy; 50 ppm is the limit set in the UK for environmental exposure.

There is little evidence regarding the effects of exposure of sevoflurane and isoflurane but they have been reported to cause nausea, headaches, respiratory depression, bradycardia and hypotension. Exposure to these agents must be monitored according to legislation in the UK at least every 6 months and adequate scavenging facilities provided. Monitoring can be done easily using exposure badges. It is advisable to minimise exposure to these agents especially for pregnant individuals.

Minimising exposure to anaesthetic gases:
- Check the anaesthetic machine and breathing system for leaks before use
- Use vaporisers with key fill systems
- Avoid using masked or chamber inhalational induction procedures
- Do not turn vaporisers on until the patient is attached to the breathing system and the cuff on the endotracheal tube has been checked
- Fill vaporisers in a well-ventilated area at the end of the working day
- Recovery areas should be well ventilated
- Allow patients to breathe 100% oxygen for several minutes at the end of anaesthesia and empty the reservoir bag to scavenge waste gases
- Pregnant personnel should avoid being involved in marked inductions, recovery from anaesthesia and any procedures where the patient is maintained on inhalational anaesthesia and there are frequent disconnections of the breathing system from the airway device (e.g. where the patient requires turning frequently).

ENVIRONMENTAL EFFECTS

The estimated effect of anaesthesia as a whole on global warming over 1 year is thought to be that of 1 million cars/1 coal-fuelled power station. Other sources claim it to be 0.05–1% of the total greenhouse emissions. N_2O is a potent greenhouse gas (300 times the effect of CO_2 over 100 years). The Kyoto agreement suggested restricting N_2O emissions (but Copenhagen suggested that all fluorinated agents should be banned by 2030).

MONITORING THE ANAESTHETISED PATIENT

Monitoring of anaesthesia is key in ensuring that the patient is kept safe during anaesthesia. RVNs and student veterinary nurses play a critical role in patient monitoring and they should take responsibility to:
- Recognise and minimise the risks to the patient
- Maintain vigilance: closely observing and examining during the peri-operative period
- React appropriately when a problem is identified and alert the veterinary surgeon.

The continuous close monitoring of a patient undergoing anaesthesia or sedation has been demonstrated to reduce the likelihood of adverse accidents and incidents during the peri-operative period. The overall risk of the anaesthetic can be reduced by early observations of deterioration in the patient's condition and by detection of the consequences of any errors that have been made (Association of Anaesthetists of Great Britain and Northern Ireland [AAGBI], 2007).

Monitoring the patient begins with the RVN or student veterinary nurse who will be involved in the anaesthetic process performing a brief clinical examination prior to the administration of pre-medication drug. It is difficult to appraise and compare these parameters during anaesthesia if there has been no assessment made of what they felt like/looked like or sounded like prior to the administration of anaesthetic drugs.

It is important to remember that almost all of the drugs used during the anaesthetic process exert some degree of effect on cardiac output, blood pressure, respiratory rate, tidal volume, thermoregulation, neurological and metabolic function. Once the patient has been pre-medicated a continual assessment process to monitoring should be adopted with readings being recorded a minimum of every 5 minutes. It is strongly advised that the same standard of monitoring should apply to both general anaesthesia and sedation in human medicine (AAGBI, 2007) and this should be mirrored in veterinary medicine.

Anaesthetic monitoring records form part of the patient's medico-legal records and should be filled out in a timely and accurate manner to give a true account of the anaesthetic

TABLE 27.12	Utilising the senses to monitor patients	
Assessment method	What can we assess?	Parameters recorded
Observation/ see	Reservoir bag, chest wall movement, respiratory rate and effort, mucous membrane colour, eye position, patient movement, surgical site	Respiratory rate, effort and pattern Mucous membrane colour Depth of anaesthesia
Palpation/ touch	Pulse rate, strength and quality, capillary refill time, palpebral and pedal reflexes, jaw tone, muscle relaxation	Pulse rate, strength and quality Capillary refill time Depth of anaesthesia
Auscultation/ hear	Heart rate and rhythm, abnormal heart sounds, lung sounds, leaks in the breathing system, incomplete endotracheal tube seal, leaks in the anaesthetic machine	Heart rate and rhythm Abnormal heart and lung sounds Equipment failure

period. A graph format (Fig. 27.30) is more useful for monitoring trends in parameters and often allows problems to be identified in a timelier manner.

Our main concerns in the anaesthetised patient are:
- Anaesthetic depth
- Cardiac output
- Blood pressure
- Tissue oxygen delivery
- Volume status
- Ventilation
- Temperature.

Effective monitoring of the anaesthetised patient by RVNs or student veterinary nurses will depend on them having the knowledge to rapidly identify adverse events by evaluating changes in patient parameters and then reporting these to the veterinary surgeon. This must begin with the utilisation of the nurse's senses. This can be achieved utilising a 'hands on' approach to continually monitor the patient using observation, palpation and auscultation – see Table 27.12. Minimal equipment is required for baseline monitoring techniques to be performed well with the exception of a stethoscope or oesophageal stethoscope, a thermometer and some kitchen scales. Ensuring continuous accurate monitoring even without electronic monitoring equipment will improve patient safety by quickly identifying adverse events and preventing fatalities.

The addition of electronic anaesthetic monitoring equipment will often be advantageous but is merely an adjunct to the veterinary nurse. It is the knowledge and ability of the suitably qualified individual to interpret and act on the individual values and trends displayed by the monitors that is essential.

Routine monitoring should include:
- Respiratory rate, effort, chest wall movement and evaluation of the reservoir bag movement, lung sounds
- Colour of mucous membranes and capillary refill time
- Heart rate and some assessment of rhythm may be possible through auscultation
- Peripheral pulse strength, quality and rate
- Depth of anaesthesia via the assessment of cranial reflexes – eye position and jaw tone

- Temperature
- Monitoring for haemorrhage – calculating circulating blood volume and weighing blood-soaked swabs to assess blood loss.

Further electronic monitoring equipment may then give the possibility to monitor:
- Blood pressure – non-invasive (indirect) via Doppler or oscillometric equipment or invasively (direct) via an arterial catheter, manometer and multiparameter monitor
- Oxygen saturation of blood haemoglobin – pulse oximetry
- End-tidal carbon dioxide, ventilation status, respiratory rate, patency of airway, capnography
- Electrical activity in the heart – electrocardiogram (ECG)
- Central venous pressure via a central venous catheter (either a jugular catheter or peripherally inserted central catheter) and both manometer line and multiparameter monitor or water column.
- Blood/gas analysis to measure the partial pressure of oxygen (PaO_2) and carbon dioxide dissolved in arterial blood – requires a blood/gas analyser and the ability to take an arterial blood sample.

Anaesthetic depth

Anaesthetic depth is one of the key factors in adverse events under anaesthesia. Patients that are at an inadequate level of anaesthesia (too 'light') may exhibit the following signs:
- Hypertension – high blood pressure
- Tachycardia – fast heart rate
- Hyperventilation
- Regurgitation
- Movement

Patients that are at an excessive depth of anaesthesia (too 'deep') or have received an overdose may exhibit the following signs:
- Apnoea
- Hypoventilation
- Hypotension
- Bradycardia

These adverse events can be prevented by assessing the patient's depth of anaesthesia frequently. It should be noted that where one adverse event occurs then this can quickly give rise to others if it is not quickly identified and rectified.

Monitoring anaesthetic depth. In combination with the physiological parameters such as heart rate, respiratory rate and blood pressure there are also a number of cranial nerve reflexes that should be evaluated:

Eye position – the problem with eye position is that it will be up and central both when the patient is too light and when the patient is too deep. This means that this parameter needs to be assessed alongside the cranial reflexes such as palpebral reflex and jaw tone. At an adequate level of anaesthesia (surgical plane of anaesthesia) the eye will be rotated ventrally (down) (Fig. 27.31). Dissociative agents (e.g. ketamine) and neuromuscular blocking agents (NMBA) will affect eye position and it cannot be relied upon as an indicator of anaesthetic depth when these drugs are being used.

Palpebral reflex – this reflex is elicited by gently applying fingertip pressure to the medial canthus of the eye or by gently stroking the eyelid. This reflex diminishes with increasing depth

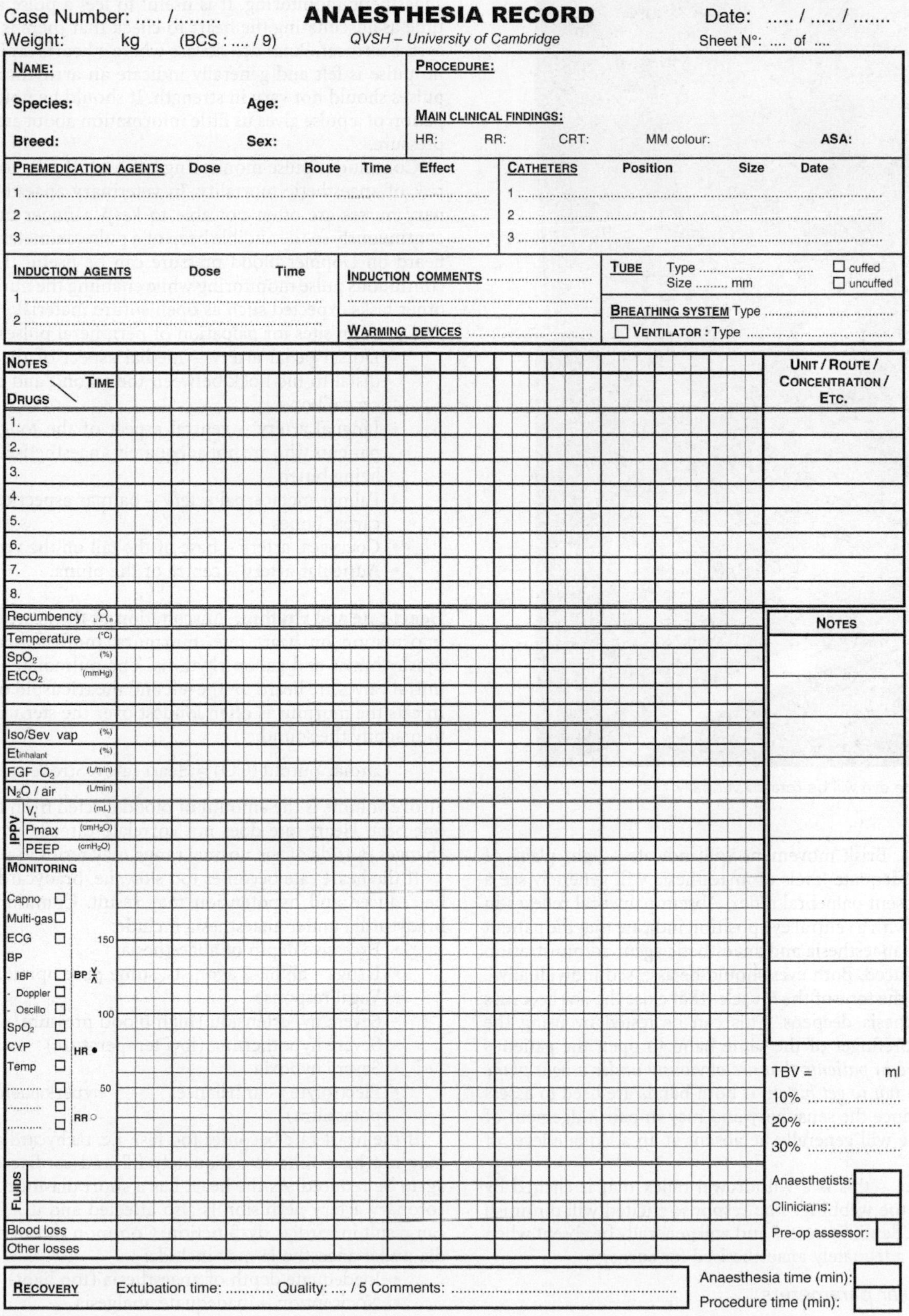

ANAESTHESIA RECORD
QVSH – University of Cambridge

Case Number: ..... /.........　Date: ..... / ..... / ....

Weight:　kg　(BCS : .... / 9)　Sheet N°: .... of ....

NAME:

Species:　**Age:**

Breed:　**Sex:**

PROCEDURE:

MAIN CLINICAL FINDINGS:

HR:　RR:　CRT:　MM colour:　**ASA:**

PREMEDICATION AGENTS	Dose	Route	Time	Effect
1				
2				
3				

CATHETERS	Position	Size	Date
1			
2			
3			

INDUCTION AGENTS	Dose	Time
1		
2		

INDUCTION COMMENTS ....

WARMING DEVICES ....

TUBE Type ....　☐ cuffed
Size .... mm　☐ uncuffed

BREATHING SYSTEM Type ....

☐ **VENTILATOR :** Type ....

NOTES

TIME

DRUGS
1.
2.
3.
4.
5.
6.
7.
8.

Recumbency
Temperature (°C)
SpO$_2$ (%)
EtCO$_2$ (mmHg)

Iso/Sev vap (%)
Et$_{inhalant}$ (%)
FGF O$_2$ (L/min)
N$_2$O / air (L/min)

IPPV
V$_t$ (mL)
Pmax (cmH$_2$O)
PEEP (cmH$_2$O)

MONITORING

Capno ☐
Multi-gas ☐
ECG ☐　150
BP
- IBP ☐　BP ˅ ˄
- Doppler ☐
- Oscillo ☐　100
SpO$_2$ ☐
CVP ☐　HR ●
Temp ☐
.... ☐　50
.... ☐
.... ☐　RR ○

FLUIDS

Blood loss
Other losses

UNIT / ROUTE / CONCENTRATION / ETC.

NOTES

TBV =　ml
10% ....
20% ....
30% ....

Anaesthetists: ☐
Clinicians: ☐
Pre-op assessor: ☐

RECOVERY　Extubation time: .... Quality: .... / 5 Comments: ....

Anaesthesia time (min): ☐
Procedure time (min): ☐

Fig. 27.30 Anaesthetic monitoring chart

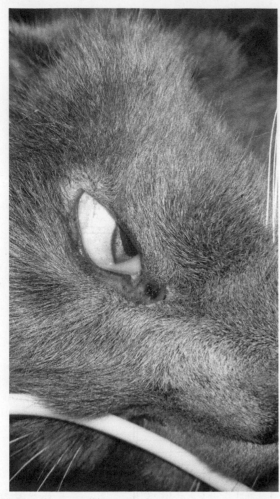

Fig. 27.31 The eye will be rotated ventrally

of anaesthesia. Brisk movement will indicate a light plane of anaesthesia. Adequate levels of anaesthesia will generally see a sluggish or absent palpebral reflex. Absent palpebral reflexes in combination with a central eye position indicate that the patient is under deep anaesthesia and anaesthetic agent administration should be reduced. Both eyes should be assessed individually.

Jaw tone – the tone of the muscles that close the jaw becomes less as anaesthesia deepens. This can be tested by using the thumb and forefinger of the same hand to open the patient's jaw – *take care in patients that are obviously under a light plane of anaesthesia not to get bitten.* If both hands are used to assess this it will reduce the sensitivity and may impair judgement of tone. Jaw tone will generally be absent at an adequate level of anaesthesia.

Pedal reflex – this is a withdrawal reflex that is elicited by pinching the toe webbing. The response elicited will diminish as anaesthetic depth increases and will generally be absent when the patient is adequately anaesthetised for surgery.

Cardiovascular parameters

Pulse. Pulse quality reflects stroke volume – the amount of blood ejected from the ventricle during contraction of the heart and therefore represents the difference between systolic and diastolic pressures. Peripheral pulses feel 'weak' and are lost much quicker than the central pulses in poorly perfused patients and it is recommended that peripheral pulses are utilised for

anaesthetic monitoring. It is useful to feel a pulse at the same time as auscultating the heart to check that there is a pulse for each heartbeat. Pulse deficits are where a heartbeat is heard but no pulse is felt and generally indicate an arrhythmia. Normal pulses should not vary in strength. It should be noted that palpation of a pulse gives us little information about arterial blood pressure.

Continuous pulse monitoring has been shown to reduce the risk of anaesthetic mortality. In veterinary anaesthesia veterinary nurses are often not able to keep a finger on the pulse continuously so the audible beep of a pulse oximeter or the flow heard on Doppler blood pressure can be useful. This enables continuous pulse monitoring while enabling the nurse to do the other tasks expected such as open suture material.

Common sites for palpation of peripheral pulses are:
- Dorsal pedal artery – medial aspect of the hind limb distal to the hock between the second and third metacarpal bones
- Lingual artery – ventral aspect of the tongue; care in patients who are not adequately anaesthetised to prevent being bitten
- Palmar metacarpal artery – palmar aspect of the metacarpal bones
- Coccygeal artery – base of the tail on the ventral aspect
- Auricular artery – centre of the pinna.

Heart rate and rhythm. Auscultation of the heart gives useful information on heart rate, murmurs, muffled heart sounds, dysrhythmias and gallop rhythms. The pulmonary, aortic and mitral valves are heard on the left and the tricuspid on the right. In cats the murmur is often loudest over the sternum as it acts to magnify the sound.

$$\text{Cardiac output (CO)} = \text{Heart rate} \times \text{Stroke volume}$$

Stroke volume is the amount of blood ejected from the heart in one beat. Heart rate does not correlate directly with CO and changes outside of the normal range may result in reduced CO.

If the heart rate becomes too slow, i.e. bradycardia, CO can be reduced and hypotension may result. Common causes of bradycardia under anaesthesia include:
- Excessive depth of anaesthesia
- Drugs – alpha-2 agonists, some pure opioids
- Vagal response
- Severe hypertension (high blood pressure)
- Severe hypothermia (low temperature)
- Severe hypoxia
- Electrolyte imbalances – hyperkalaemia (high potassium).

If the heart rate becomes too fast, i.e. tachycardia, the heart may not have time to adequately fill and cardiac output can again be reduced. As the heart has a short diastolic filling time coronary artery perfusion is also affected and if left untreated can result in cardiac dysfunction. Common causes of tachycardia under anaesthesia may include:
- Inadequate depth of anaesthesia (too light)
- Nociception – inadequate analgesia
- Hypotension – low blood pressure
- Hypovolaemia – lack of circulating volume in the vascular space
- Hypoxaemia – low levels of oxygen in the blood
- Hypercapnia – high levels of carbon dioxide in the blood

- Hyperthermia – high temperature
- Drugs – anticholinergics (atropine).

When evaluating heart rate it is important to consider whether it is having an effect on blood pressure, what the patient's pre-anaesthetic heart rate was, whether the heart rate has suddenly increased or decreased or if the change has been gradual. The veterinary surgeon should be alerted as soon as concerning changes occur.

Mucous membrane colour and capillary refill time

Comparisons with the pre-anaesthetic mucous membrane parameters are important – e.g. are the mucous membranes the same colour pink as they were previously and is the capillary refill time the same? Consistently writing down 'pink' for mucous membrane colour and 'less than 2 seconds' for capillary refill time does not give an accurate appraisal of the patient's clinical status; it is the monitoring of trends in conjunction with other parameters that is important. It should be noted that mucous membrane colour and capillary time may not be reliable indicators of peripheral perfusion under anaesthesia and can be altered by drugs such as alpha-2 agonists.

Normal mucous membranes should be pink with a capillary time of around 1.5 seconds. Prolonged capillary refill times can be indicative of poor tissue perfusion and may be caused by hypovolaemia, hypotension, reduced cardiac output and hypothermia. Shortened capillary refill times may indicate congestion and vasodilation and are often accompanied by red progressing to brick-red mucous membranes and can be indicative of hypercapnia, systemic inflammatory response or sepsis.

Vasoconstriction may lead to pale mucous membranes and can be caused by lack of analgesia (nociception), reduced tissue perfusion, drugs such as alpha-2 agonists and anaemia.

Hypoxia can lead to cyanosis (blue-tinged mucous membranes); however, this should not be the first sign of hypoxia that is observed when monitoring the anaesthetised patient as it generally occurs at SpO_2 below 80%.

Arterial blood pressure

Mean arterial pressure = Cardiac output × Systemic vascular resistance + Central venous pressure. Normal values will vary depending on the patient's pathology but a rough guide in the anaesthetised patient is:

- Systolic: 90–120 mm Hg
- Mean: 60–90 mm Hg
- Diastolic: 55–75 mm Hg

A mean of less than 60 mm Hg is the point at which perfusion to the major organs (most specifically the kidneys) begins to become compromised. This will result in the accumulation of lactic acid and increased oxygen demand and ultimately result in organ damage such as kidney failure.

- Systolic pressure is the pressure generated when the left ventricle of the heart is fully contracted.
- Diastolic pressure is the pressure within the left ventricle of the fully relaxed heart.
- Mean arterial blood pressure (MAP) is the mean of pressures generated throughout the cardiac cycle and can be estimated as:
  - MAP = Diastolic pressure + ⅓ (Systolic pressure − Diastolic pressure)
  - MAP gives an idea of the overall driving (perfusion) pressure to the tissues.

The body will generally try to maintain blood pressure as much as possible and can do this by:

- Increasing CO, e.g. by increasing heart rate
- By causing vasoconstriction of the peripheral circulation
- By trying to retain fluid at the level of the kidneys.

For these reasons the blood pressure may not drop initially on the monitors when haemorrhage occurs.

Blood pressure cannot be assessed by palpation of peripheral pulses as this will simply give an indication of systolic-diastolic pressure difference, which is difficult to evaluate. Peripheral pulse palpation should be monitored as a trend alongside blood pressure monitoring wherever possible.

There are several different ways of monitoring blood pressure. The most accurate method is direct arterial blood pressure monitoring, which requires the placement of an arterial catheter. The arterial catheter is connected via a manometer line to a pressure transducer, which turns the pressure signal into an electrical signal and then transmits the waveform to the patient monitor. This method provides systolic, mean and diastolic readings in a beat-by-beat fashion. It is, however, more technically challenging to place an arterial catheter as it requires specific equipment and monitors and therefore is often reserved for critical cases which require on-going, accurate blood pressure monitoring.

Indirect blood pressure monitoring can be done using either the Doppler or oscillometric techniques. Both methods rely on a pressurised cuff occluding blood flow and then depressurising in a steady and measurable fashion so blood flow then returns beneath the cuff. For either method the correct cuff size should be chosen. The width of the cuff should be approximately 40% of the circumference of the site where the cuff will be placed. The cuff should be long enough so that the bladder of the cuff fully encircles the site where the cuff is to be placed. A cuff that is too wide or too tight will give measurements that are falsely low whereas a cuff that is too narrow or too loose will give falsely high readings. *If the Velcro of a cuff meets perfectly it is likely that the cuff chosen is of the appropriate size.*

Doppler ultrasound – an array of piezoelectric crystals is placed over an area (that may need to be shaved) with the transducer perpendicular to the artery. Coupling gel is used ensure a good signal. The transducer is taped in place where the sound of the flow is detected. Changes in flow as seen with arterial pulsations cause a frequency change 'Doppler shift' in sound waves which is detected by the piezoelectric crystal and converted to sound. An inflatable cuff is placed proximal to the transducer and connected to a sphygmomanometer. The cuff is inflated to a pressure above the expected systolic pressure which occludes the artery. No flow is heard from the Doppler. The cuff is slowly deflated until the sound of flow is detected. This method should measure systolic blood pressure; however, this is a topic of some debate, especially in cats. It is likely, in fact, to measure somewhere between mean and systolic. This method is less accurate than direct arterial blood pressure monitoring but has the benefit of providing a source of continuous pulse monitoring and provides excellent information on changes and trends in blood pressure.

Oscillometric – This technique uses the cuff to occlude the artery and detects oscillations of the underlying artery while it is partly occluded. The cuff is snugly placed over the artery chosen and attached to the control unit that senses arterial oscillations and inflates the cuff to occlude the artery and then

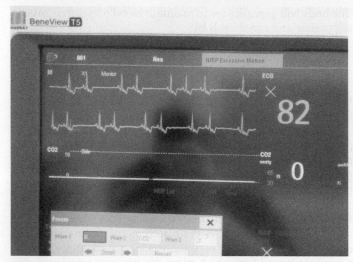

Fig. 27.32 ECGs give a trace of the electrical activity of the heart

automatically slowly deflates it. Systolic blood pressure is measured following the point that the first oscillation is detected. The largest oscillation detected gives us the mean pressure and oscillations disappear at diastolic pressure. This technique is less accurate than direct arterial blood pressure monitoring.

Hypertension – higher than normal blood pressure under anaesthesia can be commonly caused by:

- Insufficient depth of anaesthesia (too light)
- Inadequate analgesia – nociception
- Drug effects – alpha-2 agonists
- Hypercarbia – high levels of carbon dioxide in the blood
- Hypoxia – lack of oxygen perfusion to tissues
- Hyperthermia – high temperature.

Hypotension – lower than normal blood pressure under anaesthesia can be commonly caused by:

- Vasodilation caused by:
  - Inappropriate depth of anaesthesia (too deep) – the inhalational agents cause vasodilation resulting in an often significant drop in blood pressure
  - Sepsis or systemic inflammatory response syndrome
  - Other vasodilatory drugs – e.g. acepromazine.
- Hypovolaemia – pre-existing or due to haemorrhage
- Inappropriate tachycardia or bradycardia
- Myocardial dysfunction.

Blood pressure in combination with pulse oximetry and capnography has been shown to detect over 93% of perioperative adverse events.

Electrocardiography

Electrocardiograms (ECGs) give a trace of the electrical activity of the heart (Fig. 27.32). An ECG trace does not indicate that there is contractility, cardiac output or perfusion but can be helpful to monitor dysrhythmias and response to treatment. They are useful in patients where dysrhythmias may be expected, e.g. in cases of splenic torsion/neoplasia or gastric dilatation and volvulus. It also provides a value for the patient's heart rate.

If there is an ECG available in the practice then it is important to become familiar with what a normal ECG looks like. It is not necessary to be able to name an abnormal rhythm but learning what normal looks like will allow recognition of what is abnormal and allow the veterinary surgeon to be alerted to

this potentially abnormal rhythm. Be aware that electrical interference can occur from sources such as the diathermy and clippers and that this interference may look like an arrhythmia but will normally disappear when the interference is removed.

ECG electrode placement:

- Red: Right fore
- Yellow: Left fore
- Green: Left hind
- Black: Right hind

Where a three-electrode ECG is available the hind limb chosen is usually the left.

Where arrhythmias are identified the veterinary surgeon will often evaluate their effect on the patient's cardiovascular status by evaluating blood pressure readings and what the pulses feel like on palpation before deciding whether to treat the arrhythmia.

Central venous pressure

Monitoring central venous pressure (CVP) is a technique that can be utilised in anaesthetised and conscious intensive care patients. Individual CVP measurements do not give an accurate assessment so trends should be monitored. CVP is the pressure measured in the patient's cranial vena cava directly in front of the right atria and closely corresponds with the pressure in the right atrium. CVP affects the end diastolic volume of the right ventricle and therefore influences stroke volume and cardiac output. A central venous catheter must be placed aseptically in the right jugular vein to facilitate measurement and is generally reserved for critical cases. CVP is often utilised to guide fluid therapy, though it should be noted that evidence for this technique is poor.

Normal CVP is 0–5 cm H_2O (1 mm Hg = 1.4 cm H_2O). Low CVP can be indicative of decreased venous return whereas a high CVP may indicate volume overload, right-sided heart failure or increased intra-thoracic pressure.

Haemorrhage

The circulating blood volume of the dog and cat can be calculated as follows:

Dog = 90 ml/kg

Cat = 60 ml/kg

The veterinary nurse monitoring the anaesthetic is often in a better position than the veterinary surgeon to monitor the haemorrhage from the surgical site. It is good practice to work out the circulating blood volume of the patient prior to the surgery beginning, especially when haemorrhage has been identified during planning as a potential adverse event. This can be written on the anaesthetic record and the volumes for 10%, 20% and 30% of that patient's blood volume calculated and recorded. It is then very easy to compare these values to the actual blood loss and this gives the veterinary surgeon much more information to make a decision on what should be done.

For example:

A 25-kg dog has a circulating blood volume of 90 ml/kg.

Blood volume = 25 kg × 90 ml/kg = 2250 ml

10% = (2250/100) × 10 = 225 ml

20% = (2250/100) × 20 = 450 ml

30% = (2250/100) × 30 = 675 ml

A 3.5-kg cat has a circulating blood volume of 60 ml/kg.

Blood volume = 3.6kg × 60ml/kg = 210 ml

10% = (210/100) × 10 = 21 ml

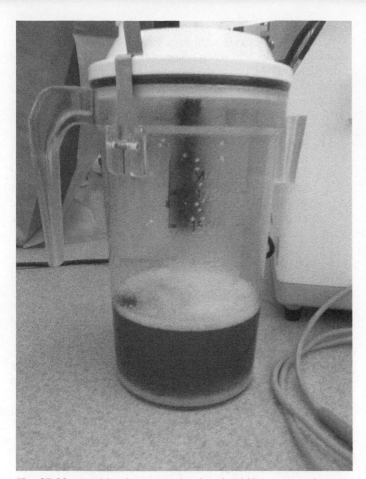

Fig. 27.33 Any blood in suction bottles should be measured

$$20\% = (210/100) \times 20 = 42 \text{ ml}$$
$$30\% = (210/100) \times 30 = 63 \text{ ml}$$

The weight of one dry swab can be recorded on the white board in theatre (or laminated and stuck to the wall). Blood-soaked swabs can then be weighed using electronic kitchen scales (in grams). The total dry weight of the number of swabs weighed should be deducted and the resulting weight in grams gives an approximation to the number of millilitres of blood lost. Any blood in suction bottles should be measured (Fig. 27.33) (remember to deduct any fluid given to the veterinary surgeon to lavage as this will also be in the suction bottle) and blood on the floor and the drapes should be estimated. The total blood loss estimated can then be compared against the patient's blood volume and percentage calculations to see how much this equates to as a percentage of the patient's circulating blood volume.

Urine output

This is often measured in critical patients under anaesthesia and in intensive care and can be monitored by placing a urinary catheter and urine collection system. This allows continual assessment and allows fluid therapy to be tapered accordingly.

Normal urine output = 1–2 ml/kg/hr

Parameters of oxygenation, ventilation and respiration

Respiratory rate, effort and pattern. This should be observed by watching the reservoir bag and the patient's chest wall movement simultaneously. It should be noted that this is an extremely subjective assessment and although it gives a rough idea of a patient's ventilation a capnograph is required to perform a proper assessment.

Auscultation of the lungs. Auscultation of the lungs for wheezes, crackles and inspiratory stridor should be performed whenever a respiratory complication such as hypoxaemia (low SpO_2) or hypoventilation is encountered. If the patient is apnoeic then auscultation should be performed while administering a positive pressure breath.

Airway gas analysers. These are incorporated into some multi-parameter monitors and enable the inspired and expired levels of nitrous oxide and the volatile agent to be monitoring as well as oxygen and carbon dioxide.

Pulse oximetry. This can be used to determine the arterial haemoglobin saturation with oxygen (SpO_2) – the amount of oxygen bound to the haemoglobin of the patient's red blood cells. In a healthy patient the haemoglobin should be greater than 95% saturated with oxygen when breathing room air. The anaesthetised patient breathing 100% oxygen should have a SpO_2 reading close to 100%. It is a monitor that mainly becomes useful when patients are apnoeic at induction, in the recovery stages of anaesthesia and later in intensive care.

Pulse oximeters are often considered to give spurious results – to see if the monitor is likely to be accurate think 'pulse before O_2'. If the pulse rate is correct to what has been palpated and the trace is clear then it is more likely that the oximeter reading can be believed.

The relationship between PaO_2 and SpO_2 forms a sigmoid curve meaning that below 93% SpO_2 a small decrease in SPO_2 will result in a large decrease in PaO_2. Pulse oximeter readings of 93% or higher are acceptable in non-anaemic critically ill patients. As 90% SpO_2 correlates to a partial pressure of arterial oxygen (PaO_2) of 60–70 mm Hg (severe hypoxaemia), oxygen should be supplemented where readings on the pulse oximeter are less than 93%. As a rule of thumb below 90% SpO_2 PaO_2 is approximately SpO_2 minus 30. If the pulse trace is not good try moving the probe to another location before assuming hypoxaemia as the place where the probe is located may merely be poorly perfused.

Pulse oximetry uses a simple principle that oxygenated blood is a different colour to blood that is not well oxygenated. Light is passed through a pulsating arterial vascular bed and the pulse oximeter can detect the oxygen saturation within that artery. It disregards absorption from tissues that are not pulsating, i.e. venous blood, skin and muscle. Oxyhaemoglobin and deoxyhaemoglobin absorb light differently at different wavelengths, which allows the microprocessor to detect the saturation. Most pulse oximeters cannot distinguish dysfunctional haemoglobin such as methaemoglobin (produced with paracetamol toxicity in cats) or carboxyhaemoglobin (from carbon monoxide/smoke inhalation). This means that they may continue to read greater than 90% in these instances even when the patient is severely hypoxaemic.

The probe can be placed on various sites including the tongue, pinna, lip, toe web and tail, but is sometimes not well tolerated in conscious patients. It is, however, minimally invasive, and where arterial blood gases are not available it can be a useful tool in monitoring trends and disease progression in

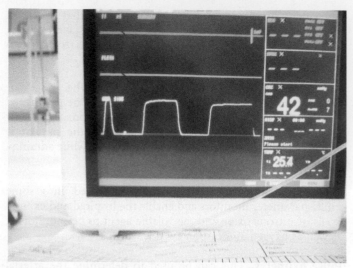

Fig. 27.34 Capnography

hypoxaemic patients and for tailoring oxygen therapy after anaesthesia.

The major limiting factor of pulse oximetry is tissue perfusion. Conditions such as shock and hypotension which reduce peripheral blood flow will prevent the pulse oximeter from accurately reading haemoglobin saturation.

It should be noted that fluorescent lighting, pigmentation, compressed tissue (from leaving the probe in one place for too long), cold extremities and patient movement can all interfere with pulse oximeter readings.

It should also be noted that the pulse oximeter gives no indication of the oxygen content of the blood, the amount of oxygen dissolved in the blood (PaO_2), ventilation, cardiac output or blood pressure; it does, however, allow evaluation of peripheral pulse profiles.

Pulse oximetry alone has been shown to detect 40–82% of perioperative adverse events and its use in veterinary anaesthesia as a form of continuous pulse monitoring is valuable.

Capnography. As carbon dioxide (CO_2) diffuses so rapidly from the blood into the alveoli it can be used as a measure of the adequacy of alveolar ventilation. To get a true indication of how well an animal is ventilating an arterial blood gas is required for the measurement of the partial pressure of arterial CO_2 ($PaCO_2$). Arterial CO_2 levels, however, are approximately equal to alveolar CO_2 levels, which can be more easily measured. Alveolar gases are the last gases to be expelled during expiration and therefore end-tidal CO_2 ($ETCO_2$) monitoring via capnography will give a breath-to-breath approximation of $PaCO_2$ and therefore the adequacy of ventilation (Fig. 27.34).

Capnography can also give an indication regarding respiratory rate, cardiac output, metabolism, rebreathing of alveolar gases (carbon dioxide), exhaustion of soda lime, airway obstruction, leaks around the endotracheal tube, displacement of supraglottic airway devices and return of spontaneous ventilation in apnoeic cases.

Normal values are 35–45 mm Hg. An $ETCO_2$ greater than 60 mm Hg is suggestive of excessive respiratory acidosis and these patients should be ventilated.

Hypoventilation is usually caused by a reduction in minute volume due to a decrease in respiratory rate and/or tidal volume.

It is defined as an $ETCO_2$ greater than 45 mm Hg. This leads to hypercarbia and can simultaneously cause hypoxaemia. Carbon dioxide forms an acid when retained in the blood – respiratory acidosis – and will cause the blood pH to decrease – respiratory acidaemia.

Common causes of hypoventilation in anaesthetised patients:
- Excessive depth of anaesthesia (too deep) – this depresses the respiratory centres in the brain
- Accidental endobronchial intubation – placing an endotracheal tube that is too long
- Abdominal distension – pressure on the diaphragm from the abdominal contents, e.g. Caesarean section or gastric dilatation and volvulus patients; this 'splints' the diaphragm preventing it from expanding and therefore reduces tidal volume
- Hypotension
- Hypothermia

Other less common causes include pleural space disease (pleural effusion), pulmonary disease (pulmonary oedema), diaphragmatic hernia or rupture and central nervous system disease.

Hyperventilation is usually caused by an increase in minute volume due to an increase in respiratory rate and/or tidal volume. It can be defined as an $ETCO_2$ of less than 35 mm Hg. This leads to too much carbon dioxide being removed from the body. Essentially, too much acid is lost – respiratory alkalosis – and the blood pH may rise and become alkalaemic.

Common causes of hyperventilation in the anaesthetised patient:
- Inadequate anaesthetic depth (too light)
- Inadequate analgesia – nociception
- Iatrogenic hyperventilation – overzealous IPPV
- Hypertension
- Hyperthermia

Combining capnography and pulse oximetry has been shown to detect 88–93% of perioperative adverse events.

Arterial blood gas analysis

Measurement of partial pressure of oxygen (PaO_2) and carbon dioxide ($PaCO_2$) in arterial blood is the gold standard for determining lung function as it gives information about oxygenation as well as ventilation.

Animals with normal lung function should have a PaO_2 greater than 85 mm Hg when breathing 21% oxygen (room air). A PaO_2 less than 80 mm Hg can be considered hypoxaemia and is usually treated by oxygen supplementation and addressing the underlying cause. Values less than 55 mm Hg are imminently life threatening and require immediate action. Increases in fraction of inspired oxygen (FiO_2) lead to increases in PaO_2 with a general rule of thumb being that PaO_2 should equal roughly 5 times FiO_2, e.g. a patient receiving 100% oxygen via an endotracheal tube should have a PaO_2 of approximately 500 mm Hg.

$PaCO_2$ gives a picture of how well the patient's alveoli are being ventilated. Normal $PaCO_2$ is 35–45 mm Hg. In simple terms, if the $PaCO_2$ is greater then there is either reduced ventilation of the perfused alveoli or there is an increase in CO_2 production. Conversely, if there is a decrease in $PaCO_2$ then either alveolar ventilation is increased or there is a decrease in CO_2 production.

There are several sites for arterial sampling: dorsal pedal artery, digital artery, auricular artery, lingual artery and femoral artery. The dorsal pedal artery is most commonly used for arterial sampling. If serial sampling is required an arterial catheter can be placed (see the section on vascular access). Pre-heparinised syringes should be used for arterial sampling. The area over the dorsal pedal artery is clipped and gently prepped. The artery is palpated so the pulsations can be felt while guiding the needle at a 60° angle towards the artery. When the needle penetrates the artery a flash of blood will be seen in the needle hub and the sample can be collected. All bubbles should be removed immediately, the sample tightly capped and run immediately if possible.

Temperature

Temperature should be regularly recorded in the anaesthetised patient to ensure that the patient is not becoming hypothermic or hyperthermic. Many practices routinely warm the patients undergoing anaesthesia but neglect to assess whether this is effective or if they have become too warm. Most patients will be susceptible to hypothermia under anaesthesia but this risk is increased in small patients, lean patients and those where body cavities are exposed to the ambient environment (e.g. laparotomy and thoracotomy).

Core temperature can be measured with an oesophageal temperature probe but a rectal thermometer will suffice where this method of temperature monitoring is not readily available.

Hypothermia can be relatively easy to prevent using fluid warmers and circulating warm air blankets; however, if these are not available then 'hot' hands, heat pads can be utilised. It is easier to attempt to avoid it than it is to treat. Care should be taken to avoid direct contact between the heat source and an anaesthetised patient as thermal burns may occur. Additional precautions should include:

- Warming fluid used to lavage body cavities
- Avoiding over-wetting the patient when performing skin preparation of the surgical site
- Using heat and moisture exchangers attached to airway devices
- Using rebreathing systems where appropriate
- Maintaining a reasonable ambient temperature in the preparation area, theatre and recovery
- Wrapping extremities with insulating materials.

Hypothermia reduces metabolic rate, which in turn decreases MAC and therefore the amount of inhalant anaesthetic agent required, which can lead to inadvertent overdose and will significantly slow recovery. Uncorrected hypothermia can also cause bradycardia, arrhythmias and coagulation problems. If a patient is hypothermic on recovery from anaesthesia they may shiver, which will increase metabolic oxygen demand.

Hyperthermia

Other monitoring that may be required:

Blood electrolytes – patients where electrolyte abnormalities have been diagnosed, e.g. hyperkalaemia (high potassium) in blocked cats

Blood glucose – monitoring of blood glucose throughout anaesthesia is warranted in patients with diabetes mellitus, paediatric patients (less than 12 weeks) and those with liver insufficiency

Haemoglobin – this may be a useful parameter to monitor if available in the face of acute haemorrhage as it is marginally more responsive than measuring packed cell volume

Total protein – in critical patients who are hypoproteinaemic this may be useful. This may also be an earlier indicator of haemorrhage than haemoglobin measurement.

RECOVERY FROM ANAESTHESIA

The recovery period is of utmost importance; 50–60% of small animal anaesthetic fatalities occur during the postoperative period with 50% of these being within the first 3 hours following cessation of anaesthesia.

Important factors to consider in recovery include:

- Pre-existing disease/patient health status – these should have been highlighted in the pre-anaesthetic assessment and ways that recovery may be affected already anticipated.
- Complications encountered during anaesthetic – these should be communicated clearly to the individuals recovering the patient.
- Planning ahead – preparation and planning for recovery is key to ensuring that the correct equipment is available and that there is someone available to closely monitor the patient. The AVA checklist includes a recovery section to help with this.
- Communication – this is a common cause of error and veterinary patients are normally transferred from the theatre to kennel team without a formalised handover. This does not need to take a lot of time but should be in a structured and repeatable format such as the SBAR technique – situation, background, assessment, recommendation. For example, 'Fluffy has had a general anaesthetic for ovariohysterectomy. She has been very stable. She is a little cold – 36.8°C. Can we monitor that every 30 minutes until it is normal please? Otherwise we have no concerns. Sally, can you watch her until she is awake and lying in sternal without assistance? Assess for pain and she is due some more buprenorphine prior to discharge'.
- Monitoring – patients should be continually monitored until they are fully awake and maintaining sternal recumbency.
- Hypothermia – one of the most common anaesthetic adverse events and will prolong recovery and may lead to further adverse events, yet only 11–14% of cases had temperature monitored in recovery in CEPSAF. Active warming should be provided in recovery for hypothermic patients and temperature monitored approximately every 30 minutes until normal.
- Patient stimulation – this should be minimised. Patients should be moved to their allotted recovery area prior to awakening. Temperature should be taken prior to cessation of anaesthesia. Shaking, turning or otherwise stimulating patients to try and make them 'wake up faster' is unacceptable – consider how a person would react. This will ultimately often lead to a more 'stormy' or excitable recovery. Noise should be minimised and some breeds such as greyhounds appear to be more noise sensitive in recovery.
- Comfort – analgesia should be evaluated. The dose of opioid administered in the pre-medication protocol may have worn off and should be topped up as necessary. Additional analgesia should be considered for the

event of 'break-through' pain and well communicated to the recovery team. Patients should be provided with comfortable padded bedding. Pain scoring should be utilised.

- Anxiety– if the sedation provided in the pre-medication protocol was not sufficient then it is unlikely the patient will have a stress-free recovery. With anaesthetic agents such as alfaxalone and isoflurane giving no residual effects in the recovery period it is down to the pre-medication to manage the patient's stress and comfort in recovery. Particular attention should be paid to the timing of the pre-medication and agents such as medetomidine repeated as necessary albeit in smaller doses than in pre-medication.
- Recovery environment – the ideal recovery environment would have a warm ambient temperature, be well ventilated (to remove waste anaesthetic gases) and be calm, comfortable and quiet. This is not always possible in a busy veterinary practice but the best should be made of what is available.

In veterinary medicine staff and time constraints coupled with a lack of appreciation of the adverse events that can occur in this period mean that many patients are not accurately monitored during this period. Only 33–34% of cases were continually monitored in recovery according to CEPSAF with 69% checked every 5 minutes.

Recovery begins when the anaesthetic agent is switched off. The anaesthetic agent should not be turned off until the veterinary surgeon has finished the procedure and all cleaning and bandaging procedures have been conducted. The anaesthetic drugs used are so rapidly eliminated that if the anaesthetic agent is turned off prior to this point then it is likely that the patient will awaken and need extubating during transfer to the recovery kennel or kennel area. Stimulation at this point can cause a 'stormy' or more 'excitable' recovery, especially if the pre-medication protocol was not adequate or the sedative and analgesic drugs have worn off.

Following cessation of the anaesthetic agent the reservoir bag should be emptied (the flow rate increased for rebreathing systems) and the patient should remain on 100% oxygen for a few minutes (where inhalational agents have been used) to scavenge the waste gases and minimise exposure to personnel. Once disconnected from the breathing system the patient should be quickly transferred from the theatre table to the area prepared for recovery. Brachycephalic patients and critical cases may need to be recovered in the theatre environment and close to the oxygen source and monitoring if these facilities are not available in a kennel or recovery area. In routine patients most of the monitoring will be removed at this point; however, this is the point where the pulse oximeter is most useful in detecting oxygen desaturation. In more critical patients the monitoring equipment may need to remain but oesophageal devices such as temperature probe and oesophageal stethoscope must be removed prior to extubation to prevent gagging and chewing of the devices.

Extubation with endotracheal tubes should be removed as the gag reflex returns in the dog and prior to return of the gag reflex (to protect the fragile laryngeal cartilages from laryngospasm) in the cat. This needs to be estimated by the return of the cranial reflexes. In rabbits extubation should occur once the swallowing reflex is observed. Supraglottic airway devices can be removed later in both rabbits and cats and do not seem to

cause laryngospasm in cats. These are usually removed in cats once the patient becomes intolerant of the device.

Intravenous catheters should not be removed until the patient is fully recovered from anaesthesia unless the patient's temperament dictates it would be safer to do so earlier (in terms of stress to the patient or risk of injury to patient or staff). This is important as it allows the administration of intravenous drugs in response to an adverse event or crash situation. For more critical patients it may be necessary to leave these in for longer periods to facilitate fluid therapy and drug administration.

Pain assessment, patient comfort and analgesia

WHAT IS PAIN?

Pain can be defined as an unpleasant sensory and emotional experience associated with actual or potential tissue damage, or described in terms of such damage (Merskey and Bogduk 1994).

The inability to communicate does not negate the possibility that an individual is experiencing pain and is in need of pain-relieving treatment. This is incredibly important to remember in veterinary patients. One of the most important roles in pain management for veterinary nurses is the assessment and recognition of pain in species that cannot verbalise their pain and ask for help. In effect this is one element where the veterinary nurse truly becomes the patient advocate and can make a huge difference to treatment, patient welfare and patient well-being.

Analgesia is the absence of pain in response to a stimulus that would normally elicit pain (Merskey and Bogduk 1994). While there are many pharmacological analgesic agents available in the veterinary toolkit the veterinary nurse's role in analgesia is about so much more than the individual drugs. It is important, however, to have an understanding of the properties of these agents, their actions on the pain pathway and their side effects (Table 27.13).

TABLE 27.13	The pain pathway and the role of pharmacological agents at various stages	
Point in the pain pathway	How	Pharmacological agent
Transduction	Prevent nociceptor activation	NSAIDs Local anaesthetics Opioids Alpha-2 agonists
Transmission	Inhibit nerve conduction	Local anaesthetics, alpha-2 agonists
Modulation	Reduces onward transmission from the spinal cord and enhancement/ amplification	Opioids Alpha-2 agonists NMDA receptor antagonists NSAIDs Tricyclic antidepressants Anticonvulsants
Perception	Alter sensory or emotional conscious processing	Inhalational anaesthetics Induction agents Opioids Alpha-2 agonists Benzodiazepines Phenothiazines

THE PAIN PATHWAY

The pain signal first undergoes a process caused **transduction** whereby the noxious stimulus is converted into a chemical signal at the nociceptor.

The signal is then **transmitted** along the nerve fibre to the dorsal horn of the spinal cord and through the spinal cord to the brain.

Modulation occurs at various sites in the spinal cord and brain with signals either being enhanced (sensitisation) or inhibited (hypoalgesia).

Perception is the conscious organisation of the information that has been transmitted and modulated.

PAIN PERCEPTION IN THE UNCONSCIOUS PATIENT

Nociception is the neural process of encoding noxious stimulation and denotes the response of the central nervous system to actual or potential tissue damage (**noxious stimulus**). This process encompasses the transduction, transmission and modulation of the noxious stimulus but does not include perception.

To perceive or feel pain an animal must be consciously able to process the sensory and emotional component of the noxious stimulus. When an animal is rendered unconscious through general anaesthesia the emotional and sensory component cannot be perceived but the automatic nociceptive pathways are not inhibited. If adequate analgesia is not provided then transduction, transmission and modulation still occurs resulting in physiological changes even in the adequately anaesthetised animal. This normally presents as tachycardia, hypertension and hyperventilation despite the depth of anaesthesia indicating that the patient is suitably anaesthetised for surgery. This often causes veterinary surgeons to instruct that the anaesthetic agent be increased but this can cause anaesthetic overdose and the resultant adverse events such as hypotension and hypoventilation. Repeated activation of the nociceptive pathways under general anaesthesia may also make the patient more sensitive to pain on recovery.

Hyperalgesia is an increased sensitivity to a noxious (painful) stimulus.

Allodynia is pain evoked by a stimulus that would not normally be painful, e.g. touch.

Multimodal analgesia – this involves utilising analgesic agents in combination to target the nociceptive pathway at different points to provide a more effective pain management plan than with a single agent.

Pre-emptive or preventative analgesia is where analgesic agents are given prior to an anticipated noxious (painful) stimulus. Where analgesics, for example, are given as part of the pre-medication protocol and allowed adequate onset time prior to a surgical incision. This should be a primary goal in all patients undergoing potentially painful diagnostic and/or surgical interventions.

Once tissue damage has occurred neuronal cells become activated leading to **peripheral sensitisation** and **hyperalgesia** meaning that greater doses of analgesic agents are required to provide relief to the same level of noxious stimuli than if the analgesics were given pre-emptively.

Central sensitisation occurs through repeated transmission of noxious stimulation to the dorsal horn of the spinal cord. *N*-methyl-D-aspartate receptors (NMDA) become activated and amplify the signal to the brain. This can result in enhanced neuronal response to pain (**hyperalgesia**) and the interpretation of innocuous stimuli as painful (**allodynia**). Once these signals have become amplified and the neuronal response enhanced it can be difficult to prevent stimulation without a pharmacological intervention.

CONSIDERATIONS IN PAIN

Tissue handling – the abilities of the surgeon can be a major factor in how much pain the patient is in after the procedure. If the tissue handling is gentle then peripheral and central sensitisation will be minimised.

Nursing care – ensure that the patient is comfortable with padded bedding and mattresses if necessary. Turning recumbent patients, evaluating bladder size, preventing urine scalding, facilitating movement, talking ambulatory patients outside to void and TLC are all major contributing factors in patient comfort.

Reduce fear and anxiety – the patient should be assessed for signs of fear or anxiety which could be mistaken for pain symptoms or possible mask them. Sedative or stress relieving drugs may need to be administered in conjunction with analgesics in trauma patients or in anaesthetic recovery to maximise patient comfort.

Adjunct therapies – acupuncture, physiotherapy and hydrotherapy can all be useful adjuncts to improving patient comfort.

PAIN ASSESSMENT

Pain assessment in small animals has many challenges and to date there is no universal, validated way of assessing pain for all veterinary species for both acute and chronic pain states. In human medicine it is still challenging to ascertain an accurate evaluation of pain but in most cases the patients can be asked about their pain, e.g. their level of discomfort, quality and intensity of the pain. Veterinary medicine faces the further challenge of not being able to discuss pain with the patient verbally and therefore must rely on other cues, such as behavioural change, which can be affected by the individual experience and subjectivity of the assessor.

It is now widely acknowledged that dogs and cats have similar neural pathways for the development, conduction and modulation of pain to humans and as such it is highly likely that they experience pain in a similar way. Due to better education in the veterinary sector and acknowledgement of pain in animals the majority of surgical, trauma and chronic pain cases will be provided with analgesia.

Many surgical cases follow a standard practice protocol for analgesia set without considering the individual patient or procedure. This often results in postoperative pain relief being administered as a rigid protocol at predetermined times, e.g. methadone every 4 hours or buprenorphine every 6–8 hours regardless of patient assessment. This ignores the fact that some analgesics may not suit some patients and that side effects may be more profound in certain individuals. Regular assessment of the patient allows a more fluid and individually tailored pain management plan to give analgesia when needed and may often result in less analgesia being administered and fewer side effects being observed. Consider the complexity of the pain pathway and then whether administering one analgesic agent on a regular schedule actually constitutes adequate pain relief.

Chronic pain cases often follow a similar pattern with patients being put on non-steroidal anti-inflammatory drugs (NSAIDs) at increasing doses as the chronic pain worsens rather than considering other pharmacological and non-pharmacological solutions alongside owner assessment of the patient's condition.

The question should not whether analgesics are provided or not but rather whether adequate pain relief is being provided to the patient and whether this is being adequately assessed. Answering these questions ensures that patients are provided with individually tailored pain management which contains not only analgesics but also non-pharmacological solutions to relieve pain.

Veterinary nurses play a key role in pain recognition and assessment due to the amount of time they spend with patients, which allows them to quickly learn how to recognise signs individual to each patient. Ideally pain should be assessed by the same person each time but this is often not practical and the introduction of a pain scoring or assessment system can be useful to standardise pain assessment within the practice. For chronic pain patients it is also helpful for the same person to assess the patient's pain each time and build up a rapport with the client to encourage their participation in the patient's pain assessment. This can often form a valuable part of nurse consultations or pain clinics.

It is an essential part of a veterinary nurse's role to help provide a balanced and multimodal approach to pain relief. Try writing down all the possible pain relief options for a patient including analgesic agents and non-pharmacological options including any pros and cons and any known drug interactions. This will then provide the basis for discussion with the veterinary surgeon to provide an individual analgesic plan for the patient and will often encourage a more holistic approach to pain relief. True evaluation of the patient history including previous analgesic treatment, the procedure being performed/trauma encountered or in the case of chronic pain the nature of the problem and type of pain (e.g. neuropathic pain) is essential.

Most attempts to assess clinical pain are based on behavioural observations but many factors can influence behavioural change:

- Strange environment
  - May alter normal behaviour and mask signs of pain.
  - Apprehension, excitement and nervousness alter clinical parameters and may be perceived as pain.
  - Prey animals are adapted to disguise signs of pain.
  - The presence or absence of the owner may dramatically influence behaviour.
  - The presence of other species may alter patient behaviour.
- Species difference
  - Behavioural effects of pain cannot be extrapolated from one species to another.
  - Care with anthropomorphosis.
- Within-species variation
  - Different breeds and individual animals may react to pain differently.
  - Some cats may hiss and vocalise with pain while others prefer to hide in a corner.

TABLE 27.14	Typical signs of pain in cats, dogs and rabbits		
Cats	**Dogs**	**Rabbits**	
Hunched in sternal recumbency	Reduced appetites/anorexia	Reduced appetite	
Aggression	Unusual aggression/resents touch	Hunched position	
Reduced appetite/anorexia	Attention seeking	Teeth grinding	
Decreased grooming	Over grooming/self-mutilation	Exaggerated responses to handling	
Vocalising/hissing	Restlessness	Immobility – unwilling to move	
Increased heart rate, respiratory rate and blood pressure	Unwilling to lie down/get up and move around	Increased respiratory rate and/or effort	
Squinting eyes with ears rotates and flattened	Trembling/shivering	Lack of grooming	
Self-mutilation/biting at the affected area	Whining/barking/growling	More of a tendency to hide than normal or may face back of kennel	
Immobility	Guarding the injury site	Squinting	
Hiding	Increased heart rate, respiratory rate and blood pressure	Excessive scratching or licking	

- A normally 'dominant' dog may show aggression when in pain.
- Drug effects
  - Many analgesic drugs have sedative properties.
  - Opioids can cause abnormal changes in behaviour.

Signs of pain

Clinical parameters such as temperature, heart rate and respiratory rate are notoriously difficult to interpret as they may be altered by things other than pain such as fear, anxiety, infection and dysphoria (Table 27.14). They are therefore not reliable parameters for pain assessment and should only be considered alongside behaviour and reaction to palpation around wounds. Behavioural signs can also be altered by other factors, e.g. dysphoria can lead to vocalisation, a stressful hospital environment may cause withdrawal, depression and inappetence, and drugs can affect many observations traditionally used to monitor pain (e.g. mentation and urination).

Composite pain scoring is a more comprehensive way to establish a pain score for each patient and evaluate the analgesia plan.

The following signs of pain may be exhibited by some patients and several of the signs being exhibited should make us consider whether the patient is receiving adequate analgesia.

Clinical signs associated with acute pain include:

- Increased respiratory rate
- Increased heart rate

- Increased blood pressure
- Increased temperature
- Dilated pupils
- Salivation.

Behavioural signs of acute pain may include:

- Agitation or restlessness
- Reluctance to lie down or sleep
- Depression
- Inactivity
- Resentment to handling
- Abnormal posture
- Alteration in gait
- Increased or decreased urination.

Assessing acute clinical pain

There are numerous methods of assessing and scoring pain in both humans and animals.

- Visual Analogue Scale (VAS) – this consists of a 100-mm line with no pain at one end and the worst pain imaginable at the other end. The person assessing the animal makes a mark on the line according to their assessment of the amount of pain they believe the patient to be in. It has the advantage that it avoids the use of descriptive terms and the need to assign a number to the pain. If used by an experienced observer this method can be a useful tool in mapping pain. Its disadvantages include variability in observer interpretation of worst pain imaginable and its sensitivity depends on observer training and experience. VAS scores have also been shown to significantly correlate with increases in vocalisation and respiratory rate not necessarily due to pain, i.e. due to dysphoria or anxiety. For these reasons it is often used in combination with other pain assessment tools.
- Numerical rating system (NRS) – this is much like the VAS but a number, e.g. 1–10 or 1–5, is assigned to the patient's pain rather than a mark on a line. One disadvantage is that it is an ordinal measurement and assumes that a change from 1 to 2 is equivalent in degree to a change from 2 to 3. Categories are assigned equal weighting and assigned equal importance to the overall pain score. This uneven weighting results in inconsistencies. There is again significant inter-observer variability seen with this scale.
- Simple descriptive scale (SDS) – consists of four or five expressions used to describe various levels of pain intensity (no pain, mild pain, moderate pain, severe pain). Each expression is assigned an index value which becomes the patient's pain score.
- Composite pain scoring systems – these scoring systems use multiple assessments of behavioural or physiological variables and combine them to give a more complete impression of the patient's pain. The Glasgow Composite Pain Scale (GCPS) is a pain scoring system questionnaire which evaluates not only intensity but also sensory and affective qualities of pain. The GCPS has been evaluated and validated for use in dogs with acute pain. Dogs are observed from a distance and then their responses to interaction and wound palpation are evaluated. This questionnaire is available in a short form that is less time consuming. For cats the UNESP-Botucatu Multidimensional Composite Pain Scale for assessing postoperative pain in cats has recently been validated and a GCPS for cats has also recently been developed.

Other pain assessment tools that have been used to evaluate pain include looking at 'pain faces' in mice, rats and cats.

Assessment of chronic pain

This relies heavily on structured pain questionnaires based on those used in human medicine for chronic pain patients. Owner input is essential to form an accurate picture of chronic pain as the owner is the person who is often most aware of what is 'normal' behaviour for the animal.

PHARMACOLOGICAL AGENTS

The general protocol for analgesia in small animal surgical patients would be:

- Opioid – included alongside the anxiolytic/sedative as part of the pre-medication protocol. Opioids may be administered on their own for this purpose in some cases such as critical ill patients and Caesarean sections.
- NSAID – if clinically appropriate (if does not have kidney, gastrointestinal or liver disease) and administered before, during or after anaesthesia depending on the veterinary surgeon's assessment and consideration of factors such as blood pressure and volume status.
- Local analgesic blocks – many surgeries and most dental extractions would benefit from blockade of the nociceptors involved in transmission and transduction of noxious stimulation (Table 27.15).
- NMDA receptor antagonist – trauma patients where peripheral and central sensation are present and as an adjunct for major surgeries.

Other agents where necessary, e.g. paracetamol, may be utilised where NSAIDs are not appropriate and gabapentin and tricyclic antidepressants may be included in on-going postoperative pain to alter modulation of pain.

Administration of analgesia peri-operatively:

- Oral/transmucosal – NSAIDs, gabapentin, tramadol, buprenorphine, paracetamol

TABLE 27.15	Characteristics for the local analgesic agents, lidocaine and bupivacaine	
Characteristic	**Lidocaine**	**Bupivacaine**
Onset of action	Shorter	Longer
Duration of action	Approximately 60–120 minutes	Approximately 4–6 hours
Indications	Topical – larynx, skin, nose, splash blocks Local infiltration Peripheral and central blockade	Local infiltration Peripheral and central blockade
Comments	Can be formulated with adrenaline (a vasoconstrictor) to prolong the duration of action for local infiltration Potential for localised ischaemia due to vasoconstriction	More cardiotoxic, contraindicated for intravenous infusion and intravenous regional anaesthesia (IVRA)

- Injectable bolus – IV, IM, SC, via chest drain/wound soaker catheter/continuous nerve block catheter, epidural catheter – NSAIDs, opioids, ketamine, local analgesic agents, paracetamol, alpha-2 agonists
- Constant rate infusion – IV, e.g. fentanyl, ketamine, lidocaine, alpha-2 agonists or via wound soaker catheter – lidocaine, bupivacaine
- Transdermal – fentanyl
- Local anaesthesia (LA) techniques – lidocaine, bupivacaine

Constant rate infusion versus bolus injection:

- Bolus injections cause peaks and troughs in drug plasma concentration
- Constant rate infusion will give constant plasma levels
- Eliminates waning analgesic effect
- Dose can be more accurately titrated

BUT

- Requires close patient monitoring
- Way of accurately giving drugs – equipment

Opioids

These agents work at many different points on the pain pathway and can affect transduction, modulation and perception of pain. The selection of opioids for analgesia generally begins with the one selected for pre-medication and then this will be 'topped up' during the procedure after the anticipated duration of action or as the result of pain assessment if the patient has recovered from anaesthesia. The most commonly used opioids are methadone and buprenorphine. Other opioids may be selected for epidural administration such as morphine or to provide additional analgesia at the mu receptors in addition to the buprenorphine or methadone administered. Opioids selected to provide additional analgesia during the procedure are often administered by intravenous constant rate infusion (although some can be given as a bolus dose) and include fentanyl, remifentanil and alfentanil.

See pre-medication for methadone, pethidine, buprenorphine and butorphanol.

Morphine

- Prototypical opioid agent against which all other opioids are compared
- Previously widely used and studied
- Schedule II controlled drug
- Available with preservative for systemic administration and preservative free for the epidural route
- Really only used in its preservative-free form epidurally now since methadone was licensed in dogs
- Shown to be effective systemically, via extradural and intrathecal routes and peripherally (intra-articularly)
- Pure opioid agonist at mu (MOP), kappa (KOP), delta (DOP) and NOP
- Can cause vomiting when used systemically
- Prolonged duration of action when administered extradurally and spinally (up to 24 hours) due to its hydrophilic nature meaning it has greater persistence in CSF compared to other opioids. This also means it has a greater area of spread up the cord.

Fentanyl

Description

- A short-acting, synthetic opioid
- Licensed intravenous version for dogs (Fentadon)
- Licensed transcutaneous liquid preparation (a 'patchless patch') for perioperative analgesia in the dog (Recuvyra)
- Schedule II controlled drug
- Systemically IV as a bolus or a constant rate infusion
- Transcutaneously as very lipid soluble – the 'patchless' system is formulated as a highly concentrated solution with a lipid-soluble carrier (octyl salicylate) and isopropyl alcohol; when absorbed this forms a depot of fentanyl in the stratum corneum which provide analgesia for 96 hours
- Mu (MOP) agonist
- Rapid speed of onset within 5 minutes when administered IV
- Duration of action 15–30 minutes (generally about 20 minutes) after a single bolus due to rapid redistribution to fat and muscle
- After 2 hours of constant rate infusion peripheral sites become saturated and elimination relies more on hepatic metabolism and renal excretion so half-life increases; care if using for longer procedures
- Metabolised in the liver and renally excreted
- Can cause profound respiratory depression so limited to anaesthetised patients
- May cause bradycardia
- Can be reversed with naloxone

Non-steroidal anti-inflammatory drugs

NSAIDs are analgesic and anti-inflammatory drugs commonly used in veterinary medicine for both acute and chronic pain and are effective at transduction and modulation points on the pain pathway. Despite differences in chemical structures and other potential mechanisms of action, these compounds share the effect of inhibiting the cyclooxygenase enzyme system and preventing prostaglandin production. Side-effect profiles may vary and this can often be an important factor in the veterinary surgeon's selection of one of these drugs in preference to another. There are many licensed NSAIDs for chronic pain but only three are currently licensed in an injectable preparation for perioperative use in dogs and cats: carprofen, meloxicam and robenocoxib.

Cyclooxygenase (COX)

- Cyclooxygenase is present in most tissues within the body and two primary forms of COX have been identified, COX-1 and COX-2.
- COX-1 produces prostaglandins that are responsible for numerous physiological responses including vasodilation, sensitisation of nociceptors enhancing both peripheral and central sensitisation, and a number of effects in the GI tract including increased mucus production, decreased gastric acid secretion, increased secretion of bicarbonate in the duodenum, increased turnover of mucosal cells and platelet aggregation.
- COX-2 produces prostaglandins that have some of the same physiological effects as COX-1 but also inhibition of platelet aggregation, alteration of renal physiology by increasing sodium excretion, inhibiting sodium reabsorption, and altering chloride transport and stimulating renin release and profoundly altering total renal blood flow and regional blood flow within the kidneys.

- COX-2 is also associated with both central and peripheral sensitisation.

Selectivity

- The COX-1/COX-2 inhibitory ratio is often referenced as a measure of NSAID safety. The higher the ratio above 1 the more COX-2 specific the NSAID is.
- Such statements must be interpreted cautiously due to numerous limitations.
- The COX selectivity or COX sparing concept only applies to the potential decrease in the frequency of GI adverse effects in healthy GI tissues, and has no association with renal or hepatic adverse effects, effects on diseased or injured gastrointestinal tracts, nor to efficacy.
- The renal adverse effects of NSAIDs may be more related to COX-2 inhibition and all commercially available NSAIDs inhibit COX-2.
- Hepatic adverse effects may be related to production of reactive metabolites and be independent of COX inhibition.
- Drugs which maintain some activity of COX-1 (i.e. COX-2 selective or COX-2 preferential inhibitors) have decreased frequencies of gastrointestinal adverse effects and subsequently a better GI adverse effect profile than NSAIDs which inhibit both COX isoforms.

Side effects and consideration of using NSAIDs

- GI effects can be the result of mucosal irritation due to the weakly acidic nature of the drugs or due to prostaglandin suppression.
- Prostaglandins have important gastroprotective effects including increased mucosal blood flow, increased mucus production, increased bicarbonate production, decreased acid secretion and increased turnover of GI epithelial cells.
- Both COX-1 and COX-2 are constitutively expressed in the canine GI tract and the inhibition of these enzymes can lead to GI adverse effects including gastritis, enteritis, ulceration and perforation.
- Newer more selective NSAIDs appear to exhibit decreased incidence of adverse GI effects and these side effects are more likely to be seen in long-term administration for chronic pain.
- COX-1 and COX-2 are involved in renal blood flow regulation and tubular function, therefore it cannot be assumed that COX-1-sparing NSAIDs infer greater safety in the kidney. This is particularly important in the anaesthetised patient where hypotension may be evident so there is further risk of renal compromise.
- Avoid in hypotension or if renal compromise is already apparent.
- Avoid in patients with hepatic compromise.
- Cats do not metabolise NSAIDs in the same way as dogs and therefore dosing intervals and duration of licensed use are generally considerably different.
- DO NOT use in patients receiving corticosteroids.

NMDA receptor antagonists

These drugs help to reduce central sensitisation as the activation of the NMDA receptor is central to these processes. Drugs that actively block the NMDA receptor are useful in trauma patients where these receptors are already activated and major surgery where these receptors could be activated on recovery if analgesia is not adequate. The most commonly used NMDA receptor agonists are methadone and ketamine. Methadone (see pre-medication) is generally administered as bolus doses and included in the pre-medication protocol for these cases. Ketamine can also be utilised as a bolus dose in conjunction with other agents (it should not be used on its own; see induction agents) and administered peri-operatively as a constant rate infusion. Nitrous oxide also has NMDA antagonist actions.

Alpha-2 agonists (see pre-medication)

As well as their use as a sedative from a pre-medication perspective these drugs can provide excellent short-term, visceral analgesia. This is due alpha-2 receptors in the periphery and the dorsal horn of the spinal cord that play a role in transduction, transmission and modulation of nociceptive signals. Incorporation of drugs such as medetomidine and dexmedetomidine into pre-medication protocols (in suitable patients) gives additional analgesia and can be topped up or administered as a constant rate infusion as necessary.

Other agents

Paracetamol (acetaminophen)

- A non-opioid antipyretic analgesic agent that can be administered concurrently with NSAIDs or corticosteroids
- Few anti-inflammatory effects
- Exhibits a central analgesic and antipyretic effect
- May block COX-1 variant COX-3
- May stimulate serotonin receptors
- DO NOT USE IN CATS – can result in methaemoglobinaemia due to their inability to metabolise it via glucuronidation
- Relatively safe in dogs
- Can be used intravenously and orally

Gabapentin. Gabapentin was originally used as an anticonvulsant drug in human medicine but has been found to provide analgesia for neuropathic pain in humans and small animals. The mechanism of action is currently unknown but it may be caused by the blockage of calcium channels. In acute pain gabapentin should be combined with other analgesics. It is only available in oral form. It does not undergo significant hepatic metabolism but is excreted by the kidneys so patients should have normal renal function. The major side effect of gabapentin is sedation although this may wear off with prolonged use.

Tramadol. Tramadol is categorised as an atypical, centrally acting opioid analgesic. Central analgesic effects are produced through activity of the parent drug and its active metabolites at mu receptors. Tramadol also inhibits serotonin and noradrenaline uptake, which may contribute to a reduction in nociceptive transmission in the spinal cord. Tramadol is a schedule 3 controlled drug (CD No Register POM) and is exempt from Safe Custody Regulations in the UK (see Chapter 19 for details on storage of controlled drugs). It is available in oral and parenteral forms. Side effects are rare but may include sedation and vomiting.

Local anaesthesia/analgesia. Local anaesthetic/analgesic agents can be utilised to block nociceptive transmission and transduction and can contribute significantly to multimodal analgesia (see Table 27.15). Local anaesthetics work by the blockade of sodium channels within the neuron's cell membrane. This prevents the action potential being propagated because the membrane is prevented from depolarising.

Sensory, motor and sympathetic neurons are blocked by local anaesthetic techniques and this results not only in the loss of nociceptive signal transmission but also a loss of motor function and vascular tone in the area that has been blocked. Depending on the duration of the agent administered this loss of motor function may be an unwanted side effect, e.g. the inability to stand following epidural administration. Ideally the administration of these drugs would only block the sensory pathway but this is rarely clinically possible.

Lidocaine. Lidocaine can also be administered intravenously as a constant rate infusion and while most commonly thought of as an antiarrhythmic it can actually be effective as a perioperative analgesic when administered systemically in this way. Lidocaine is neurotoxic and cardiotoxic if overdosed. A maximum safe dose should be calculated and not exceeded – care should be taken because more than one dose of lidocaine spray to a cat's larynx in a small patient could potentiate toxicity. Signs of toxicity include nausea, depression/sedation, muscle twitching and seizures followed by cardiovascular signs such as arrhythmias.

Bupivacaine. More cardiotoxic than lidocaine – do NOT administer intravenously.

Local analgesic techniques. These are relatively easy to perform as long as anatomical landmarks are familiar. These procedures require inexpensive drugs and little equipment yet can make a vast difference to the patient's overall perioperative comfort. All injection sites should be prepared aseptically as if they were surgical sites and the person administering the block should wear sterile gloves and maintain aseptic technique throughout.

For all the techniques described the maximum dose should be carefully calculated and not exceeded to prevent toxicity. For injectable techniques the plunger on the syringe should always be drawn back prior to injection to ensure the needle is not in a vessel (with the exception of intravenous regional analgesia where this is the intention).

- **Topical application** – this is utilised most commonly to desensitise the larynx prior to intubation in cats and to desensitise skin for venepuncture and intravenous catheter placement. Local analgesics can also be used topically to desensitise the cornea.
- **Splash blocks** – local analgesics can de directly applied to the tissues in a surgical site before closure.
- **Local infiltration** – the injection of local analgesic agents intradermally or subcutaneously to desensitise the tissues for minor surgical procedures.
- **Epidural** – indicated for hind limb, perineal and abdominal surgery. Local analgesic agents and preservative-free

opioids such as morphine can be administered into the epidural space at the lumbosacral junction via a spinal needle. The patient is positioned in sternal or lateral recumbency with the hind limbs drawn forwards to increase the lumbosacral space. Side effects include hypotension, hind limb ataxia and weakness post procedure until the local agent wears off, urinary retention and delayed hair growth at the clipped site. Epidural morphine may even provide analgesia for thoracotomy.

- **Spinal/intrathecal** – injection into the subarachnoid space instead of the epidural space. Duration of action is generally shorter but better consistency of analgesia may be observed and drug doses should be reduced when compared with epidural administration.
- **Brachial plexus block** – blockade of the nerves in the brachial plexus. A nerve stimulator is often utilised to guide placement for these blocks. Additionally blocks the axillary nerve as well as those blocked by the RUMM block. Useful for surgery in the fore limb from mid antebrachium (just above the elbow) distally. Side effects include pneumothorax.
- **Radial, ulnar, median and musculoskeletal (RUMM block)** – an alternative to the brachial plexus block for surgery to the fore limb (below the elbow).
- **Femoral/sciatic nerve block** – this is useful for hind limb surgery and blocks distal to the stifle. A nerve stimulator is often utilised for these blocks.
- **Intra-articular/intrasynovial block** – local analgesic agents and/or morphine can be utilised directly into the joint prior to closure during orthopaedic surgery.
- **Intravenous regional anaesthesia (Bier block)** – this is used to provide analgesia of the distal limb and may be indicated for digit amputation in dogs. Lidocaine is administered intravenously distal to a tourniquet (normally an Esmarch bandage). Analgesia persists until the tourniquet is removed.
- **Dental blocks** – these include:
  Maxillary block – blocks the maxillary nerve as it enters the infraorbital canal and provides sensory blockade to the caudal maxilla including the upper dental arcade and hard palate.
  Infraorbital block – blocks the infraorbital nerve at the infraorbital canal and provides sensory blockade to the rostral maxilla.
  Mental nerve – blocked as it exits the mental foramen and provides sensory blockade to the cranial aspect of the lower dental arcade and chin.
  Inferior alveolar nerve – blocked as it enters the mandibular foramen to provide sensory blockade to the lower dental arcade, tongue and chin.
- **Intraperitoneal instillation** – local analgesic agents can be instilled into the peritoneal cavity during abdominal surgery (often performed at the end). They have been shown to provide analgesia following ovariohysterectomy in the bitch.
- **Intrapleural block** – introduction of a local analgesic agent into the pleural cavity via a thoracic drain to

provide analgesia post-thoracotomy or following thoracic drain placement.

- **Intercostal block** – the intercostal nerves can be blocked at the caudal edge of each rib. This may be indicated for thoracic drain placement.
- **Wound catheters** – wound soaker catheters can be placed simply and inexpensively during surgery and allow repeated or continuous dosing of the surgical wound with local analgesia agents. These are especially effective for soft tissue surgeries such as limb amputation and mastectomy. Side effects may include movement of the catheter and sepsis. Should not be left in place for more than 72 hours.

Muscle relaxants

Muscle relaxation is a fundamental corner of the triad of anaesthesia. Most general anaesthetics and indeed sedatives, with the exception of dissociative agents such as ketamine, provide some spinally mediated muscle relaxation. Clinically this is often enough; however, in some circumstances further relaxation is required.

Neuromuscular blocking agents

The neuromuscular junction is where motor neurons synapse with skeletal muscle fibres. The neurotransmitter responsible for transmission at the neuromuscular junction is acetylcholine (ACh). Acetylcholine receptors are responsible for precipitating muscular depolarisation and contraction and are situated both on the pre- and post-synaptic membrane of the neuromuscular junction. Neuromuscular blocking agents act at the neuromuscular junction to prevent the action of Ach and therefore they cause relaxation of skeletal muscle. They do not affect smooth muscle or the myocardium but will cause complete paralysis of skeletal muscle including blockade of the muscles of respiration meaning that the patient will need to be manually or mechanically ventilated.

Possible indications for the use of neuromuscular blocking agents include:

- Ophthalmic procedures where the eye is required to be central, e.g. cataract removal
- For relaxation of the abdominal wall in deep abdominal surgery
- To facilitate IPPV – where the patient is 'fighting' the ventilator and control of lung inflation is necessary, e.g. with some thoracic surgeries.

These agents are rarely used in general practice. Neuromuscular blocking agents are quaternary ammonia compounds which are able to mimic the quaternary nitrogen radical of acetylcholine. They can be further classified as to their mode of action into those that cause depolarisation and those that do not.

Depolarising NMBA

- Succinylcholine or suxamethonium, which is basically two ACh molecules back to back.
- Depolarising NMBA are agonists at the neuromuscular junction (NMJ). They open the central acetylcholine receptor ion channel allowing muscle depolarisation

and initial muscle contraction but they are slow to dissociate therefore further depolarisations cannot occur until the drug concentration at the NMJ is reduced.
- Fast onset with a short duration of action.
- Succinylcholine has classically been administered to allow rapid tracheal intubation in human anaesthesia.
- This type of muscle relaxant does not have a reversal agent.

Non-depolarising NMBA

- Examples includes vecuronium, atracurium and rocuronium.
- These neuromuscular blocking agents are antagonists at the acetylcholine receptor. They compete with acetylcholine at the neuromuscular junction and bind to the acetylcholine receptor but do not elicit a change in the ion channel and therefore no depolarisation takes place.
- Over 75% of acetylcholine receptors must be occupied to cause neuromuscular blockade.
- More often used in veterinary medicine.
- Can be reversed using edrophonium or neostigmine. These agents must be combined with an anticholinergic such as atropine or glycopyrolate.

MONITORING NEUROMUSCULAR BLOCKADE

Monitoring depth of anaesthesia becomes difficult because the normal cranial reflexes are paralysed so the eye is central, the jaw relaxed and the palpebral reflex absent regardless of anaesthetic depth.

Physiological parameters must therefore be closely monitored to ensure the patient does not become 'light' despite being unable to move. Indicators that the patient is not adequately anaesthetised may include:

- Tachycardia
- Hypertension
- Increased salivation and lacrimation – difficult to assess under drapes during surgical procedures and often subjective.

The blockade itself must also be monitored and this is most effectively done with a train of four device to electrically stimulate a superficial peripheral nerve, e.g. the facial or ulnar nerve.

ANAESTHETIC ADVERSE EVENTS

Common anaesthetic adverse events have been discussed throughout the chapter but some of the common ones are summarised in Table 27.16. It should be noted that the veterinary surgeon should always be informed if an adverse event is suspected.

Cardiopulmonary resuscitation (CPR) is discussed in the emergency and critical care chapter and for anaesthetised patients care should be taken to turn off intravenous or inhalational maintenance anaesthetic agents as well as administering basic life support. Considerations should also be made as to whether anaesthetic and analgesic drugs could have contributed to the cardiopulmonary arrest and whether these agents can be reversed.

TABLE 27.16	Common anaesthetic adverse events under anaesthesia	
Common adverse events	**Common causes under anaesthesia**	**Troubleshooting**
Tachypnoea – increased respiratory rate	Inadequate depth of anaesthesia Nociception (pain)	Check depth of anaesthesia Discuss analgesic options if appropriate Increase anaesthetic agent
Bradypnoea – reduced respiratory rate	Overdose of anaesthetic agent Administration of potent opioids	Check depth of anaesthesia Consider ETCO2 – IPPV if necessary
Hyperventilation – end-tidal carbon dioxide less than 35 mm Hg (hypocapnia)	Increased minute volume – increased respiratory rate and/or tidal volume Inadequate anaesthetic depth Nociception (pain) Surgical stimulation Overzealous ventilation (iatrogenic) Hypoxia Hypotension Pyrexia Hyperthermia	Check anaesthetic depth Adjust anaesthetic agent as directed Discuss analgesia if appropriate Identify underlying cause
Hypoventilation – end-tidal carbon dioxide over 45 mm Hg (hypercapnia)	Decreased minute volume – increased respiratory rate and/or tidal volume Excessive depth of anaesthesia Pleural space disease, e.g. pleural effusion Pulmonary disease, e.g. pulmonary oedema, pneumonia Accidental endobronchial intubation Abdominal distension increasing pressure on the diaphragm Diaphragmatic hernia/rupture Severe hypotension leading to decreased cerebral perfusion	Check anaesthetic depth and adjust as directed Identify underlying cause IPPV
Apnoea/respiratory arrest	Overdose of anaesthetic agent Brainstem injury in head trauma patients Hypoxia Severe pulmonary disease Cardiac arrest Iatrogenic hyperventilation Neuromuscular blockade Neuromuscular diseases Equipment failure	Distinguish from breath holding (i.e. patient too 'light' when intubated) Check anaesthetic depth Check pulse oximetry reading IPPV Identify the underlying cause
Hypoxaemia – low oxygen content in arterial blood	Decreased partial pressure of oxygen – low inspired oxygen concentration (equipment failure), hypoventilation, diffusion barrier Decreased oxygen saturation – decreased partial pressure of oxygen or formation of carboxy- or methaemoglobinaemia Decreased haemoglobin caused by anaemia	Increase inspired oxygen concentration Evaluate ventilation Identify underlying cause IPPV Treatment of underlying disease, i.e. anaemia
Hypoxia – impaired oxygen delivery to tissues	Hypoxaemia Decreased cardiac output Decreased tissue perfusion Increased oxygen extraction from the tissues – pain, fear, shivering	As for hypoxaemia
Tachycardia – increased heart rate	Inadequate anaesthetic depth Nociception (pain) Hypovolaemia Hypotension Hyperthermia Hypoxaemia Hypercapnia	Check anaesthetic depth Discuss analgesia Assess other parameters to determine the underlying cause
Bradycardia – decreased heart rate	Excessive anaesthetic depth Drugs – alpha-2 agonists Vagal reflex Atrioventricular block Hyperkalaemia Severe hypothermia Terminal hypoxia Increased CSF pressure	Check anaesthetic depth Consider reversal of drugs contributing, i.e. alpha-2 agonists Assess other parameters to determine the underlying cause Anticholinergics may be administered (not with alpha-2 agonists)
Hypertension – increased arterial blood pressure	Inadequate depth of anaesthesia Nociception (pain) Hypercarbia Hypoxia Fever Metabolic acidosis Drug effects (adrenaline, ketamine) Secondary to raises in intracranial pressure (Cushing reflex)	Check depth of anaesthesia – adjust as directed Discuss analgesia if appropriate Identify underlying cause and treatment as directed for example IPPV if necessary

TABLE 27.16	Common anaesthetic adverse events under anaesthesia—cont'd	
Common adverse events	**Common causes under anaesthesia**	**Troubleshooting**
Hypotension – mean arterial blood pressure less than 60 mm Hg	Excessive anaesthetic depth Relative or absolute hypovolaemia Drug effects – isoflurane, sevoflurane, acepromazine Haemorrhage Vasodilation due to disease process – sepsis, systemic inflammatory response syndrome	Check depth of anaesthesia and adjust accordingly Identify underlying cause and treat as directed
Haemorrhage	Blood loss from surgical site	Weigh blood-soaked swabs Measure blood lost into suction bottle Estimate percentage blood loss Appropriate fluid therapy
Arrhythmias	Hypoxia Hypercapnia Sepsis Acid-base disturbances Electrolyte imbalances – e.g. hyperkalaemia Drugs – e.g. adrenaline, alpha-2 agonists GDV Splenic, hepatic or atrial haemoangiosarcoma	Assess the impact on the animal and assess pulse deficits and blood pressure Establish the underlying cause
Hyperthermia	Iatrogenic overwarming High ambient temperature	Active cooling of patient Increase FGF Remove heat and moisture exchange (HME) Change to non-rebreathing system if appropriate
Hypothermia	Inadequate monitoring of patient temperature Loss of heat from open abdominal cavity Over-wetting when preparing the surgical site Large body surface area	Active rewarming of the patient – heat pads, warm air blankets, warmed intravenous fluids, warm water to lavage body catheter Lavage bladder with warm water Warm water enema
Regurgitation/aspiration Clinical signs: airway obstruction, dyspnoea, tachypnoea, cough, pyrexia and increased lung sounds	Drugs – volatile agents, anticholinergics, opioids Fear Nociception (pain) Shock Inadequate depth of anaesthesia Abdominal pressure Prolonged fasting	Secure the airway Flush, lavage and suction oral cavity

REFERENCES

Association of Anaesthetists of Great Britain and Northern Ireland (AAGBI), 2007. Recommendations of Standards of Monitoring during Anaesthesia and Recovery, fourth ed. AAGBI, London.

Alef, M., von Praun, F., Oechtering, G., 2008. Is routine pre-anaesthetic haematological and biochemical screening justified in dogs? Vet. Anaesth. Analg. 35 (2), 132–140.

Clarke, K.W., Hall, L.W., 1990. A survey of anaesthesia in small animal practice. J. Vet. Anaesth. 17, (1) 4–10.

Prys-Roberts, C., 1987. Anaesthesia: A practical or impractical construct? Br. J. Anaesth. 59 (11), 1341–1345.

FURTHER READING

Dugdale, A., 2010. Veterinary Anaesthesia; Principles to Practice. Wiley-Blackwell, Oxford.

Bryant, S., 2010. Anesthesia for Veterinary Technicians. Wiley-Blackwell, Iowa.

Merskey, H., Bogduk, N., 1994. Classification of Chronic Pain, second ed. IASP Press, Seattle.

28

Equine Anaesthesia

ANJA WALKER | CATHERINE LANE

KEY POINTS

- The basic procedures performed in equine anaesthesia are very similar to those described for small animal anaesthesia.

- The major differences result from the fact that the horse is much larger and horses are 'flight' creatures and can react unpredictably to drugs, becoming anxious and excited during the induction and recovery period.

- Equine anaesthesia may routinely be carried out in a field and the choice of drugs and equipment must be suited to those conditions, which may be very different from those in an equine theatre.

- General anaesthesia is normally maintained by the use of rebreathing circuits, i.e. circle and to-and-fro, because the use of non-rebreathing circuits would be impracticable and costly in such a large animal.

- Local anaesthesia is a useful technique in the horse, allowing 'standing' surgery to be performed and thus avoiding the problems associated with general anaesthesia. It is also used for the diagnosis of lameness.

Introduction

Anaesthesia in equids incorporates general anaesthesia, standing sedation and local anaesthetic techniques and is carried out to perform painful or difficult procedures, to position the animal in dorsal or lateral recumbency, as a method of restraint for fractious or unhandled animals and as a diagnostic tool. General anaesthesia or standing chemical restraint of horses allows maintenance of a clean or sterile operating area, calm handling of large or difficult animals and a concomitant increase in safety for both patient and attendants. Modern sedative drugs available for use in equine practice, often combined with local anaesthetic techniques, allow many procedures to be performed standing that might previously have required a general anaesthetic, e.g. cheek tooth removal, and dorsal spinous processes surgery. Local anaesthesia, e.g. perineural and intra-articular anaesthesia (nerve or joint 'blocks'), has a major role to play in diagnosis, particularly of lameness. Local anaesthetics can also be used preoperatively to encourage a smoother anaesthesia.

Preoperative care

CLIENT INSTRUCTIONS FOR PRESENTATION OF ANIMAL FOR ANAESTHESIA

Clients should be aware of the procedure to be performed when making an appointment for anaesthesia of their horse.

Anaesthetics, either field- or clinic-based, should not be booked in at short notice, so that all parties can be adequately prepared.

On admission to the hospital (and increasingly in cases of field anaesthesia), it is essential that the client be asked to sign for informed anaesthetic consent. This is to safeguard the practice in a legal situation and gives the veterinary nurse the opportunity to inform the client of the risks of anaesthesia and to answer or redirect any questions or concerns before anaesthesia is performed. Box 28.1 provides a pre-anaesthetic checklist.

PATIENT PREPARATION

The patient's shoes should be removed prior to general anaesthesia, as shoes may cause trauma to the horse or the personnel during induction and may lead to damage to the induction room floor. When shoes cannot be removed, the horse's hooves should be wrapped with bandage material or tape. It is preferable for elective procedures to admit the horse to the clinic the night before a general anaesthetic, to minimise the stresses associated with travelling and immediate introduction to a new environment.

A jugular venous catheter should be placed using aseptic technique, side dependent on the position during surgery (left jugular for right lateral recumbency and vice versa). Intravenous catheters are necessary to prevent repeated venous trauma and thrombus formation, perivascular injection and necrosis, and also allow intraoperative fluid therapy and instant intravenous access in case of an emergency. Intravenous catheterisation of the horse is usually via the jugular vein. Cephalic and lateral thoracic veins can be used in cases where one or both jugular veins are occluded. Whether the catheter is placed with or against the direction of blood flow depends on the preference of the personnel involved. If large volumes of fluid are to be infused it is preferable to place the catheter with the blood flow; care must be taken as this position increases the possibility of air being drawn through the catheter and even a very small quantity of air in the circulation can cause a horse to collapse. Choice of catheter size depends on the size of the patient and the catheter's intended use.

Catheters for anaesthetic induction are usually designed for 'short-stay' and should be removed after recovery (Table 28.1). Catheters for use over several days are 'long-stay' and designed to be less irritant and more compliant to the lumen of the vessel, reducing the risk of thrombus formation within the vein. Preparation of the skin for 'long-stay' catheters is important and the site should be sterile to avoid the introduction of infection and the development of thrombophlebitis.

This risk is even greater when treating an animal in a state of septicaemia.

Preoperative starving of patients has been questioned recently and some clinicians are concerned that fasting may increase the risk of postoperative ileus. However, there has been no data to support or refute this, thus reduction of normal food rations overnight will reduce the pressure imposed by the weight of a full abdomen compromising diaphragmatic movements and thus leading to hypoventilation when the patient is positioned in dorsal recumbency. Water does not need to be restricted prior to general anaesthesia as water is rapidly absorbed from the stomach. Preoperative grooming and tail bandaging will reduce the level of contamination from the environment into the theatre suite, thus reducing the likelihood of surgical site infections. The patient should also have its mouth washed out before anaesthesia to prevent food debris from being pushed down the trachea during intubation. To reduce anaesthetic time, the patient should be preoperatively clipped and scrubbed prior to induction.

BOX 28.1 CHECKLIST FOR EQUINE ANAESTHESIA

- Owner is aware of procedure being performed
- Shoes to be removed
- Horse to be admitted the night before elective procedures
- If not being admitted, then starve overnight at home but allow water
- Owner must sign anaesthetic consent form

PATIENT ASSESSMENT AND RECORDING OF ANIMAL DETAILS

Pre-anaesthetic records and assessment of patients for elective procedures should at least consist of the following:

- Patient name, age, sex, breed, colour, and microchip number. All horses admitted to the hospital must be labelled with their name and owner's name, especially if several similar horses are present in the hospital at the same time to prevent confusion between patients.
- Owner name, address and telephone number, including number for contact during or after surgery.
- Record of any drug allergies known, tetanus vaccination status, feed requirements and any other relevant history; record what equipment is left with the horse.
- Quotes or estimates for the surgery may or may not be recorded in writing on the admission form.
- Anaesthetic consent forms should contain a written statement of the risks of anaesthesia and must be read, understood and signed. If a responsible party cannot attend, the form may be completed over the phone and faxed for signing.
- Record a full pre-anaesthetic clinical examination, including temperature, heart rate and rhythm, respiratory rate and auscultation of lung sounds, mucous membrane colour and capillary refill time.
- Weight should be measured as accurately as possible, using calibrated scales or a weigh tape which will ensure correct drug dosages are administered.

TABLE 28.1	Insertion of 'short-stay' and 'long-stay' catheters	
Short-stay	**Long-stay**
A small area over vein is clipped over the cranial two-thirds of the jugular vein and then aseptically prepared. NB. The catheter should not be placed into the distal one-third of the jugular vein, as there is a higher risk of puncturing the carotid in this region.	As for short stay but a larger area if clipped, to minimise contamination.
A subcutaneous 'bleb' of 2 ml local anaesthetic is injected over the vein. A stab incision is made through the skin over the vein in the localised skin area, using a scalpel blade.	As for short-stay.
The vein is raised by applying digital pressure and the catheter is inserted with gloved hands (sterile or unsterile due to practice preference), taking normal intravenous injection precautions.	The vein is raised as for short-stay and the catheter is inserted in a fully sterile manner using sterile gloving. The catheter should be primed with heparin saline (10 IU/ml) before insertion.
Placement with or against blood flow. Catheters placed against the direction of the blood (retrograde or up the vein) minimises the risk of air embolism, if the catheter become disconnected. Or catheters placed with the blood flow (antegrade or down the vein) may result in decreased turbulence of blood flow thus decreasing irritation of the endothelium of the vein.	Placement with blood flow.
The catheter should be advanced through the skin into the vein at around a 70° angle until blood wells up into the hub of the catheter. Once blood has been observed the angle of advancement should be reduced to between 20° and 30° and the stylet should be withdrawn as the catheter is advanced to reach the level of the skin.	As for short-stay.
A three-way tap or injection cap is applied to the hub of the catheter and a small amount of heparin saline is injected to prevent clotting.	A short length of purpose-made extension tubing with a valve or injection port is attached to the hub. All subsequent handling should be clean or preferably sterile.
The catheter and port are secured in place by pre-placed skin sutures, or skin glue.	The catheter with the extension is sutured in place as appropriate for its design.
Short-stay catheters are normally over-the-needle design and less than 15 cm in length.	Long-stay catheters can be over-the-needle or over a guide wire. They are longer and less thrombogenic than short-stay catheters.

- Any previously obtained relevant laboratory results. (At present, routine pre-anaesthetic blood sampling is only performed if abnormalities are detected during the clinical examination in elective equine surgery; however, it is more frequently used prior to emergency exploratory laparotomy surgeries, where there is a high risk of hypovolaemia or toxaemia.)

In addition to the above, especially in the case of emergency procedures, further information such as history of circumstances leading up to surgery and other diagnostic procedures used, e.g. joint or peritoneal fluid analysis, packed cell volume and total protein or radiographs, should be included in the records of the case.

CLASSES OF RISK ACCORDING TO PHYSICAL STATUS

Statistics show that routine general anaesthesia in horses carries an inherently higher risk than in other companion animals. This increased risk is related to their large size and temperament as well as to their anatomy. Awareness and careful assessment of these risks and the laying down of routine protocols to be carried out before, during and after all general anaesthetics are therefore of great importance.

The Confidential Enquiry into Perioperative Equine Fatalities (CEPEF) study (Johnston et al. 2002) identified risk factors in equine anaesthesia and found that animals could be categorised according to several factors. Emergency exploratory laparotomy surgery carries the highest risk of intra- or perioperative death, with mares in the last trimester of pregnancy and foals less than 1 month of age also in the high-risk category. Surgical conditions, such as dorsal recumbency, surgery performed out of normal work hours and anaesthesia administered without premedication, all carry a higher risk of perioperative death. The study concluded that the rate of perioperative death in equine anaesthesia is 1 in every 100.

Pre-anaesthetic assessment of risk for each individual should include the clinical parameters summarised earlier, as well as a careful evaluation of the type, age, reason for anaesthesia and physiological condition, e.g. pregnant, shocked, exhausted or frightened. These findings must be taken into account when preparing the animal for and performing general anaesthesia.

FACTORS DETERMINING CHOICE OF ANAESTHETIC AGENT

Drug choice in equine anaesthesia is usually determined by:

- **Type and duration of operation** – these have a bearing on drug choice; for example, muscle relaxants may be avoided in orthopaedic and short-duration surgery, as ataxia during recovery would increase the risk of injury.
- **Type and condition of patient** – pre-anaesthetic protocol may alter in a fractious or unhandled animal to improve induction conditions for the animal and the handlers. Drugs may be altered in anaesthetising a horse in a state of hypovolaemic shock in order to minimise the depressive effects of anaesthesia.
- **Normal facilities used for surgery** – surgery routinely performed in an operating theatre on a table will usually have gaseous methods of anaesthetic maintenance, whereas for field anaesthesia and anaesthesia performed on a cushioned floor, total intravenous anaesthesia may be more practical.
- **Anaesthetist familiarity** – frequent use of certain drug combinations will improve anaesthetic technique as the anaesthetist becomes familiar with the reactions of a variety of patients to a known drug protocol.
- **Cost** – this is a factor in most establishments and may restrict, for example, the acquisition of more than one vaporiser, restricting use of more than one type of volatile agent. Newer generations of anaesthetic gases are usually more expensive than the older drugs.

Premedication

Premedication is the use of a drug or combination of drugs given prior to or concurrently with administration of the drugs to induce general anaesthesia (Table 28.2). Premedication is used, as in other species, to create a relaxed and sleepy patient and in order to reduce stress and anxiety during the anaesthetic procedure for both the patient and its attendants. Lack of anxiety lowers the risk of complications that may occur as a result of epinephrine (adrenaline) release, e.g. cardiac arrhythmia. Judicious choice of drug combinations given prior to anaesthesia can allow a 50–75% reduction of the dosage of anaesthetic agents required to both induce and maintain anaesthesia, helping to minimise the depressant effects that these drugs have on circulatory and respiratory functions. In the horse, the use of premedication often aids or enables the control of unhandled, fractious or temperamental animals. Drugs may be included in premedication protocols for their physiologically beneficial effects, e.g. analgesia and myocardial protection.

PREPARATION OF DRUGS

The dosage of anaesthetic and premedicant drugs should be calculated as accurately as possible by accurate assessment of the weight of the animal. Once the premedication and anaesthetic protocol have been decided upon, dosages of the required drugs should be calculated and the drugs should be prepared and clearly labelled for use during premedication and induction of anaesthesia. Drugs should be ready for use either in syringes with needles appropriate for the route of administration, in drip bags or bottles with the required giving set available, or in a suitable presentation for other routes of administration. Diazepam should not be drawn into plastic syringes until immediately prior to injection.

Analgesia

Analgesia is a state of insensitivity to pain even though the subject is fully conscious. It involves the abolition of pain alone while normal sensation is maintained; anaesthesia removes both pain and normal sensation and, in the case of general anaesthesia, removes consciousness.

THE IMPORTANCE AND BENEFITS OF ANALGESIA

Non-steroidal anti-inflammatory drugs (NSAIDs) are routinely given intravenously an hour before surgery starts to ensure analgesia before induction and prevent wind-up and thus a smoother anaesthetic recovery. Analgesia in the equine patient

TABLE 28.2	Drugs used in premedication				
Group	**Drug**	**Classification**	**Form**	**Route/effect**	**Pharmacology**
Alpha-2 agonists (sedatives)	Romifidine	POM-V	Injection, 10 mg/ml	Intravenous (IV), quick predictable action	Combination with opioids increases depth and reliability of sedation
	Detomidine	POM-V	Injection, 10 mg/ml	Maximum effect 5 min after intramuscular (IM) injection, slow onset, less reliable, higher doses required	Side effect of hyperglycaemia and polyuria; possible hypotension Sedative potency: detomidine > romifidine > xylazine Analgesic potency: detomidine > xylazine > romifidine All are muscle relaxants Romifidine produces least ataxia and is a common premedication
	Xylazine	POM-V	Injection, 20 mg/ml or 100 mg/ml	Detomidine can be given by sublingual route in extreme cases; very slow onset of action	Horses can still kick! Sedivet (romifidine) has a 6-day meat withdrawal Xylazine and detomidine not for use in horses for human consumption
Phenothiazines (neuroleptics)	Acepromazine	POM-V	Injection, 10 mg/ml Paste, various concentrations Tablets, 10 mg or 25 mg	IV or IM most reliable route Oral, more reliable than tablets Slow onset of action Oral, unpredictable sedation Slow onset	Mild – moderate sedation with no analgesic properties Good anxiolytic (useful for shoeing, travelling, premedication) Given IV, peak effect is in about 5 min, duration of action 4–24 hr Orally, onset takes approximately 1 hr, duration of action 4–24 hr Contraindicated in hypotensive animals Not for use in breeding stallions/pregnant mares Not for use in horses intended for human consumption
Benzodiazepines (sedative)	Diazepam	Human drug not licensed for veterinary use	Injection 5 mg/ml in 2 ml Tablets 2 mg, 5 mg or 10 mg	Slow IV (do not give alone to adult horses)	Highly effective anxiolytics, low toxicity, short duration of action Useful for control of seizures in foals and pre-myelography Possible excitation in normal healthy animals if given IV Ataxia and panic in conscious horses due to muscle-relaxing effect Not for use in horses intended for human consumption
Opioids (opioid analgesics)	Butorphanol	POM-V	Injection, 10 mg/ml	IV	Extremely potent analgesia (far greater than NSAIDs)
	Morphine	CD (S2) Human drug	Injection, 10 mg/ml or 60 mg/ml, vials	IM, IV, epidural or intra-articular	Deepens and prolongs sedation when used in combination with alpha-2 agonists
	Pethidine	CD (S2)	Injection	IM	Morphine may cause excitement and box walking in pain-free horses Butorphanol (Tobugesic) has a meat withdrawal of 0 days Pethidine is not for use in horses intended for human consumption
Sedative-hypnotic	Chloral hydrate	POM-V	Crystalline powder	IV or oral	No longer in wide use May be useful to sedate untouchable horses by adding to water (nasty taste)

CD, controlled drug; NSAID, non-steroidal anti-inflammatory drug; POM-V prescription-only medicine – veterinarian; S2, Schedule 2 controlled drug.

is important not only on humane grounds to reduce suffering but also to reduce the undesirable effects of pain, e.g. violent rolling and self-trauma associated with colic or overload strain on a limb when resting the contralateral limb. Control of pain may improve temperament and aid handling. Perioperative pain control can reduce the amount of anaesthetic agent required and, by reducing the stimulus of pain, improve the quality of recovery.

Pain can be recognised in horses in many forms (also see Chapter 13):

- Subdued attitude
- Loss of appetite
- Increased (or decreased) respiratory rate and effort
- Increased (or decreased) pulse rate
- Alteration in pupil diameter
- 'Flehmen' or curling of the upper lip

- Teeth-grinding
- Reluctance to move or 'guarding' of painful area
- Limb-resting and lameness
- Recumbency
- Posturing to urinate without passing urine
- Rolling
- Flank-watching
- Objection to palpation of painful area.

General anaesthesia

General anaesthesia can be considered to take place in two stages:

- Induction – in which the animal becomes unconscious
- Maintenance – in which the animal is administered a continuous level of anaesthetic drug in order to keep it in a state of unconsciousness.

INDUCTION

Anaesthesia should be induced in an environment that is safe for both the horse and handlers and one that is quiet and conducive to relaxation on the part of the patient. Field anaesthesia in a fenced, clean field is a common place to perform anaesthesia outside an operating theatre. Account must be taken of the temperament and 'handle-ability' of the patient, and frightened or unhandled patients should be sedated prior to being taken into an open space. It may be necessary to compromise, and a hay barn with a clean, soft floor and bales to protect the horse from colliding with hard or sharp obstacles may mean not losing the patient.

Induction boxes designed for equine anaesthesia should have padded floor and walls and, if possible, should not have any corners, e.g. hexagonal in shape. Doors should have padding that is thick enough to ensure that they are flush with the walls on either side. Viewing hatches are desirable but mirrors placed so that the horse can be observed during recovery also work quite well. Boxes should be large enough to induce a large horse safely but small enough to prevent the patient from building up any speed during recovery.

Techniques for induction vary between practices. For all techniques an adequate number of trained personnel should be available to avoid mishaps and to deal with unexpected reactions on the part of the horse.

1. 'Free-fall' induction

The horse is positioned with the hindquarters in a corner and a handler on either side of the head to encourage the horse to drop its head and sink to the ground. This method does not require large numbers of personnel or special adaptations of the induction area.

2. 'Gate' technique

A padded gate is hung on one wall of the induction box and is used to restrain the horse against the parallel wall. One handler holds the head and another handler holds a rope that closes the gate by running the rope through a ring on the parallel wall in front of the horse, thereby controlling the fall and preventing the horse from moving forward. The alternative to this uses several handlers to replace the gate to push the horse against the wall as anaesthesia is induced; the effectiveness of this method is greatly improved if the handlers refrain from pushing

---

> **BOX 28.2   SUGGESTED CHECKLIST FOR FIELD ANAESTHESIA, E.G. CASTRATION**
>
> - Oxygen cylinder with tubing or demand valve
> - Choice of two suitable (different)-sized endotracheal tubes
> - Pulse oximeter (if available)
> - Clippers
> - Scrub bowl, cotton wool and scrub solutions
> - Spare buckets for rubbish and for retaining the emasculators
> - Surgical/stitch kit
> - Emasculators
> - Short-stay venous catheter, three-way tap and suture material to suture catheter in place
> - Needles and syringes, scalpel blades
> - Sterile swabs
> - Local anaesthetic, analgesics, antibiotics, tetanus antitoxin
> - Sedative/premedicant drugs, e.g. romifidine
> - Induction drugs, e.g. ketamine and diazepam
> - Maintenance drugs, e.g. sufficient ketamine for multiple top-ups or triple drip
> - Epinephrine (Adrenaline)
> - Atropine
> - Antibiotics
> - Tetanus antitoxin

against the horse until it starts to lose consciousness. If this does not happen the horse is likely to push against the handlers and increase the risk of injuring somebody or falling awkwardly.

3. Tilting operating table

The table is tilted to a vertical position and the sedated horse is restrained with straps against it, with a handler controlling the head. As consciousness is lost, the straps take the weight of the horse and the table is rotated into the horizontal position, the horse now being in lateral recumbency. Lifting may be necessary to alter the position or to place padding under the horse. Recovery may involve transfer to a recovery box or a reversal of the induction procedure.

FACILITIES REQUIRED FOR ANAESTHESIA

Field anaesthesia

Facilities required are as for induction but the area then becomes the operating site and positioning of the horse is facilitated by using bales, sandbags or similar.

The equipment required (Box 28.2) is similar to that for a theatre environment with some obvious changes. Intravenous catheterisation is desirable to allow easy 'top-up' of the anaesthetic drugs, and equipment to resuscitate the patient in an emergency is advisable. This includes a suitable endotracheal (ET) tube with an inflatable cuff and an oxygen supply with a demand valve or suitable tubing, and drugs to treat cardiac arrest. A pulse oximeter may be useful if available, as it is the most easily carried and quickly attached (non-invasive) piece of monitoring equipment.

Theatre anaesthesia

Anaesthesia in an induction box can be carried out as in the field, if it is to be carried out without lifting the horse, for short uncomplicated procedures. It is preferable to have facilities for gaseous maintenance as the anaesthetic machine doubles up as a means of ventilating the animal in an emergency situation.

For normal theatre anaesthesia, a machine for gaseous maintenance is necessary. A variety of sizes of ET tubes, mouth gags and K-Y jelly to aid intubation, syringes to inflate ET tube cuffs etc. should be available; a suitable scavenging system for the safe removal of waste gases from the area must be used. Spare oxygen canisters should be easily accessible if required during an anaesthetic procedure.

Various table designs are available, including tables that sink into the induction box floor to conventional tables in an operating area separate from induction, onto which the horse must be lifted. An electronic or manual hoist is usually necessary for lifting and positioning and if so it is necessary to have either a generator or a manual backup hoist, in case of power failure. Hoisting the patients by their legs can cause ventroflexion of the thoracolumbar spine and thoracic compression, thus a bar is attached to the hook of the hoist which attaches to the hobbled limbs as this will reduce the possibility of complications. Hobbles are used for lifting and these should be frequently checked for wear and tear.

Positioning of the horse and adequate padding are vital in a theatre, especially as the duration of the anaesthetic increases. Postoperative myopathies are distressing when a procedure has otherwise gone well. Horses may be positioned on purpose-made inflatable cushions or large foam rubber mats with waterproof covering. The induction box floor may be too hard for longer procedures and a cushion should be placed under the horse if surgery is to be carried out in that area. Attention must be paid to ensuring that there are no pressure points, particularly on the dependent muscles. In lateral recumbency, supports must be available to raise the legs slightly, so that upper and lower limbs are parallel with the ground, in order to reduce the pressure on the lower muscles and maximise venous return of blood from the limbs. Secure props or suspension from overhead supports can achieve this.

Facilities to measure electrocardiograph (ECG) and blood pressure should be available and acquisition of equipment in addition to this may depend on practice finances. A 'crash box' should be available. All personnel should be trained so that, in the case of an emergency, reaction can be quick.

INTRAVENOUS INDUCTION AGENTS

The most commonly used intravenous anaesthetic combinations are as follows:

Ketamine and diazepam

This combination is usually used after suitable sedation with an alpha-2 adrenoceptor agonist (see Table 28.2). Ketamine alone can potentially cause excitement and induction quality is greatly improved by combination with a benzodiazepine. Benzodiazepines cause profound ataxia, which might cause distress. For that reason they are typically given with ketamine. Ketamine (2 mg/kg) and diazepam (0.01–0.2 mg/kg) can be combined in the same syringe (diazepam deactivates in contact with plastic and therefore should be drawn up immediately before administration); the combination is given as an intravenous bolus 5 minutes after the alpha-2 adrenoceptor agonist has been given. There may be a moment of ataxia before the horse sinks smoothly into sternal and then lateral recumbency; the horse should not be handled and no noise made until full relaxation is achieved, which may take up to 30 seconds. Voluntary eye movement and brisk reflexes usually remain initially, making accurate assessment of anaesthetic depth difficult. Ketamine gives minimal depression of cardiac and respiratory functions

and is a good analgesic. Incremental top-up doses of ketamine can be used to prolong anaesthesia without significantly prolonging recovery time.

Ketamine/diazepam or thiopentone (thiopental) with glyceryl guaiacolate ether (GGE)

Thiopentone (thiopental) is becoming less available and hence its use in equine practice is becoming limited to 'top-ups' during anaesthesia. Ketamine/diazepam can be used as an induction agent with GGE and should be combined with alpha-2 adrenoceptor agonist sedation. GGE is given by rapid intravenous bolus to effect (50–100 mg/kg). As the horse becomes ataxic, GGE infusion is stopped and ketamine/diazepam as above or thiopentone (5–6 mg/kg) is given by intravenous bolus. The horse should be adequately restrained to avoid panic as ataxia develops. GGE should never be given without an anaesthetic agent as inhumane conscious paralysis will result. Thiopentone is strongly irritant if injected perivascularly and should always be administered via a catheter at the lowest practical concentration – in larger horses a 10% solution is required to make the dose required a practical volume. Thiopentone produces transient depression of respiration and blood pressure and has no analgesic properties. Anaesthesia can be prolonged for short periods with thiopentone and GGE top-ups but, at higher total doses, this will prolong recovery and increase ataxia.

Propofol

The use of propofol for the induction of anaesthesia in foals is increasing, although the volumes required and concurrent cost prevent its use in adult horses in most commercial settings. Propofol is administered intravenously to effect to induce anaesthesia.

Total intravenous anaesthesia (TIVA)

This is a method of anaesthetic maintenance that is useful in a field situation but can also be used in a theatre in place of gaseous methods. Anaesthesia is induced with an alpha-2 adrenoceptor agonist/ketamine/diazepam protocol; GGE induction should be avoided to reduce the risk of GGE overdose. TIVA combinations can be made with xylazine or detomidine (romifidine is cheaper but requires higher drip rates, increasing the chance of GGE overdose), ketamine and GGE, e.g.:

- 1 g ketamine
- 10 mg detomidine or 500 mg xylazine
- Added to 500 ml ready-made 10% solution of GGE.

Infusion is usually at a rate of about 1 ml/kg/hr. This method should not be used for procedures longer than 90–120 minutes as the accumulated dose of GGE and ketamine will increase the risk of a prolonged and ataxic recovery. Intubation and oxygen supplementation is recommended for procedures lasting more than 20–30 minutes.

HEALTH AND SAFETY ISSUES

Accidental self-administration of injectable drugs used for premedication and induction is dangerous, and can occur by absorption through skin and mucous membranes:

- Spills onto skin during drawing-up and administration should immediately be washed off with large amounts of water.
- Contamination of the atmosphere by volatile agents occurs during vaporiser filling and use. Vaporisers

should be filled with purpose-made attachments and outside the operating area when possible. Volatile agent monitoring should be carried out at annually to detect possible problems.

- Circuits should be regularly checked for leaks and scavenging systems should be used.
- Emptying of the rebreathing bag should be done through the scavenging system by fully opening the pressure release valve, rather than by detachment of the bag from the cylinder.
- Toxic effects on theatre personnel at the levels encountered during normal veterinary use have not been proved but COSHH and Health and Safety Executive regulations relating to the substances should be adhered to. Advice should be sought during pregnancy.

Storage

Anaesthetic drugs should be stored as other prescription-only medicines in an environment described by the Veterinary Medicines Regulations. See Chapter 19 for details on drug storage including controlled drugs. Compressed gas cylinders should be kept away from extremes of temperature or open flames and should be stored, according to fire regulations, outside the building, away from entrances and secured in a lockable metal cage where they cannot fall over or be damaged.

Withdrawal periods

Horses are considered to be 'food-producing animals' under European medicines legislation and should now have a signed passport declaration to say that the horse will not be used for human consumption before an anaesthetic is administered. If it is possible that the horse may enter the human food chain, products should be chosen that are licensed for use in food-producing animals (consult the Veterinary Medicines Directorate for lists of licensed products). Drugs and their withdrawal periods should be recorded on the passports of animals that may enter the human food chain. Use of any product 'off-licence' should be carefully considered and should be justifiable on the 'cascade' system (see Chapter 19). Consequences of the use of drugs in this way are, first, that the manufacturer is unlikely to take responsibility for any adverse reaction and, second, that in the event of an adverse reaction, a successful legal prosecution might be mounted against the practitioner. The owner's informed consent should be obtained in cases where it is necessary to go 'off-licence'.

MAINTENANCE OF ANAESTHESIA

In the horse, general anaesthesia may be maintained either by the inhalation of gases, or of liquids with sufficient vapour pressure to produce a gas, or by total intravenous anaesthesia, i.e. both induction and maintenance produced by intravenous agents. The advantages and disadvantages of both systems are shown in Table 28.3.

INHALATION OF ANAESTHETIC AGENTS

Volatile agents typically used in equine practice are isoflurane and sevoflurane. Isoflurane is commonly used in practice, as it has lower blood solubility than halothane, thus allowing a more rapid recovery from anaesthesia; also isoflurane is not metabolised in the liver. Sevoflurane has a lower blood solubility than isoflurane, thus patients recover quicker from anaesthesia when sevoflurane is used as an inhalation agent. Sevoflurane, like isoflurane, is not metabolised in the liver.

Oxygen is an anaesthetic gas commonly used in equine practice; carbon dioxide is rarely used in equine anaesthesia and nitrous oxide is less widely used in equine than in small animal practice. For moderate caseloads oxygen is usually obtained in 'G'-sized cylinders for ease of use and most large animal anaesthetic machines have the facility for two cylinders to be attached at a time (see Chapter 27). Larger hospitals may have banks of large gas cylinders (O_2 and N_2O) stored outside the building and piped into the operating theatre via colour-coded pipes to which the anaesthetic machine can be attached. The properties of these volatile agents and gases have been described in Chapter 27.

ANAESTHETIC EQUIPMENT

Once the animal is unconscious, gaseous agents are administered via ET tubes, nasotracheal intubation and facemasks attached to the appropriate type of anaesthetic circuit.

Endotracheal intubation

A range of sizes of ET tubes is required:
- 8-mm/10-mm diameter tube is suitable for a mini foal
- 12–16-mm diameter tube is suitable for a thoroughbred foal (or smaller for a pony foal)
- 18 mm is suitable for an older foal or small nasal tube
- 20 mm is suitable for Shetland or nasal tube
- 22 mm is suitable for a pony
- 24 mm is suitable for large pony
- 26–30 mm diameter for a 500-kg adult
- 34 mm or larger for adult heavy horse breeds.

The tube should be long enough to reach the middle to lower third of the cervical trachea.

Endotracheal intubation is used to maintain the airway and, by inflation of the cuff, to deliver a controlled mixture of gases to the lungs. Control of the airway is essential in anaesthetic emergencies so that oxygen supply can be artificially maintained. Intubation is usually via the mouth and a gag is inserted between the upper and lower incisors to aid insertion and to prevent the horse from biting on to the tube. In cases when oral surgery is to be carried out, the tube may be inserted into the trachea via the nose. Nasotracheal intubation is achieved by the use of a smaller-diameter ET tube than that used for tubing via the mouth; for example, a 20-mm diameter tube would be suitable for the average thoroughbred. Intubation of the airway increases its resistance by reducing its diameter and, in the case of nasotracheal intubation, this increase is exacerbated by the use of a small tube.

Once intubation has been achieved, correct placement can be checked by connecting to the anaesthetic machine and squeezing the rebreathing bag to check that the chest rises, rather than compressing the chest to check for breath coming out of the tube. Care must be taken in inflation of the cuff, as overinflation can cause damage to the tracheal lining and can compress the tube, causing increased resistance or complete obstruction; underinflation leads to leakage of gases and uncontrolled anaesthesia.

TABLE 28.3	The main pharmacological properties of each of the commonly used analgesics					

Group	Drug	Classification	Form	Route	Pharmacology (peculiar to individual drugs)
Non-steroidal anti-inflammatory drugs (NSAIDs)	Phenylbutazone (Equipalazone)	POM-V	Powder (1 g sachets) Paste (1 g per unit/6 g per tube)	Oral	Very commonly used because of low cost and convenient preparation Very irritant if injected outside the vein Greater analgesia achieved by the intravenous route
			Injectable solution (200 mg/ml)	IV	
	Flunixin (Finadyne)	POM-V	Powder (250 mg sachets) Paste (500 mg tube)	Oral	Commonly used NSAID licensed for use in horses intended for human consumption Meat withdrawal is 7 days from the last dose given
			Injectable solution (50 mg/ml)	IV	
	Ketoprofen (Ketofen)	POM-V	Injectable solution (10 mg/ml)	IV	
	Carprofen (Rimadyl)	POM-V	Injectable solution (50 mg/ml)	IV	The least damaging to gastrointestinal mucosa and hence the drug of choice for use in foals if the use of NSAIDs is unavoidable
			Granules (210 mg sachets)	Oral	
	Aspirin	Off licence therefore POM-V	Tablets (various formulations)	Oral	Not licensed for use in horses Occasionally indicated for treatment of thromboembolic disorders
	Meloxicam (Metacam)	POM-V	Injectable solution 20 mg/ml Oral suspension 15 mg/ml	IV	Licensed for use in horses intended for human consumption; 5-day meat withdrawal May be useful in foals
	Suxibuzone (Danilon Equidos)	POM-V	Granules (1.5 g sachets)	Oral	
Pharmacology pertaining to all of above			Effective in the relief of pain and swelling Act by inhibiting cyclo-oxygenase (COX), which acts to generate inflammatory mediators Highly bound to plasma protein; acute inflammation causes exudates rich in plasma protein, thus carrying high levels of the drug to the site Adverse side effects include gastrointestinal ulceration and nephrotoxicity Foals are particularly prone to gastric ulceration and NSAIDs should be used judiciously in the very young (see carprofen, above) Use of anti-inflammatory drugs is prohibited in competition, including racing: stop use at least 8 days prior to a race or competition With the exception of flunixin and meloxicam the use of NSAIDs is not licensed in horses intended for human consumption			

Opioid analgesics, see Table 28.2.

Facemasks

Gas induction via a facemask is restricted to use in foals and is rarely used in equine practice. The mask should be adequate to fit over the muzzle to form a seal around the nose without obstructing the nostrils. The advantages of this method are that it removes the need for repeated injections as well as reducing the number of anaesthetic drugs and their potential side effects, which is especially pertinent in the anaesthesia of sick foals. Disadvantages are that strong and healthy foals may struggle to resist the pungent smell of the gas and become stressed, and a transition has to be made to endotracheal intubation once induction has been achieved. The stress can be reduced by gradually increasing the volatile agent content of inspired gas.

Anaesthetic circuits

Circle and to-and-fro circuits are almost exclusively used in equine anaesthesia (Figs. 28.1 and 28.2). These are both rebreathing systems, i.e. the expired gas is reused after being passed through soda lime to remove CO_2 (see Chapter 27). Non-rebreathing systems, where the expired gases are pushed

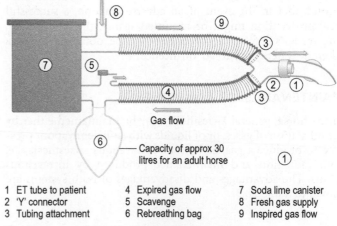

Gas flow

Capacity of approx 30 litres for an adult horse

1 ET tube to patient	4 Expired gas flow	7 Soda lime canister
2 'Y' connector	5 Scavenge	8 Fresh gas supply
3 Tubing attachment	6 Rebreathing bag	9 Inspired gas flow

Fig. 28.1 Large animal circle rebreathing circuit

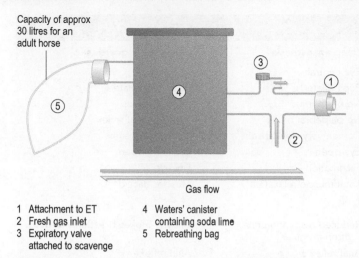

Capacity of approx
30 litres for an
adult horse

Gas flow

1   Attachment to ET
2   Fresh gas inlet
3   Expiratory valve
    attached to scavenge
4   Waters' canister
    containing soda lime
5   Rebreathing bag

Fig. 28.2   Large animal to-and-fro circuit or Waters' canister

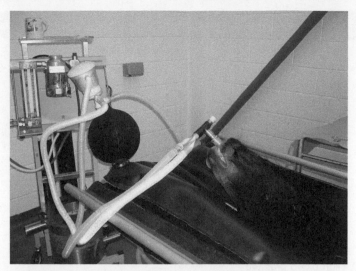

Fig. 28.3   Foal maintained on an adult human circle system

out of the circuit by providing a high flow of replacement gases to displace them, would be impractical and costly in large animal anaesthesia. The rebreathing circuit has advantages in its conservation of the warmth and humidity of the expired air, as well as its low gas-flow requirements, low volatile agent usage and hence low waste/pollution.

The disadvantages of such systems are the initial expense, high resistance to breathing, size and relatively slow changes that are possible in levels of anaesthesia. Rebreathing circuits rely on soda lime to remove CO_2 from the circulating gas and this must be checked regularly and changed as soon as it becomes exhausted. Soda lime is manufactured with a colour indicator; some change from pink to white and some from white to lilac when exhausted. (This depends on the manufacturer, so make sure you know which you are using and never mix them.) Active soda lime will become hot during use which is another indicator that it is working. Soda lime status should be checked immediately after use, as it will regain its active colour to some extent when not in use, but may not become chemically active again.

Rebreathing circuits can be used as 'open', 'low-flow' and 'closed' systems:

- **Low-flow system** – most easily operated and requires the flow of oxygen to slightly exceed the requirements of the horse, allowing the excess gas to escape via the pressure release valve, which is left partly open.
- **Open system** – one in which the pressure relief valve is left fully open, which would greatly reduce the efficiency of the circuit.
- **Closed system** – one in which the gas flow replaces, without exceeding, the anaesthetic and oxygen used by the horse. The closed system is the most efficient but is more difficult to operate than a low-flow.

Nitrous oxide (N_2O) should not be used in rebreathing circuits in horses as it is used at a different rate from oxygen and may result in the gas mixture becoming relatively low in oxygen.

The to-and-fro system must be attached close to the horse to reduce the amount of dead space from the extra tubing. The fresh gas inflow is situated near the ET tube and the air is exhaled through the canister containing soda lime into the rebreathing bag and inhaled in the opposite direction via the same path; hence 'to-and-fro'. Care must be taken to avoid soda lime dust being inhaled. The advantages are that the system is simple and relatively portable for use in field conditions if necessary.

Foal anaesthesia. The major consideration in choosing a circuit for foal anaesthesia is the resistance of the circuit. The immature chest cavity of a foal is not able to generate sufficient pressure to overcome a circuit with high resistance. The most convenient system available for foals up to approximately 100 kg is an adult human circle, with a rebreathing bag of approximately 6 l capacity (Fig. 28.3). Magill or Lack circuits can be used for gaseous induction in foals as they allow greater control than induction with a circle system (see Chapter 27).

Premedication in very young and debilitated foals should be avoided where possible; the foal has an immature hepatic detoxifying system, rendering it less able to cope with drugs than adults. If necessary, small foals can be restrained with diazepam; older healthy foals tolerate the use of alpha-2 adrenoceptor agonists such as xylazine quite well.

When anaesthetising foals it is important to keep them with the dam until the foal is unconscious and allow the foal to suck for as long as possible until induction. Sedation of the mare prior to handling the foal greatly reduces the stress in both animals. Romifidine is a good sedative in this case as the mare will be minimally ataxic when led back to the stable once the foal is fully anaesthetised. The mare can be returned before or after the foal is standing, depending on the system employed. The presence of the mare will stimulate the foal to stand but care must be taken to prevent the mare from stepping on it. The foal should be allowed to suckle up to and straight after anaesthesia. Because of their small size, foals are at risk of hypothermia during anaesthesia and steps should be taken from the outset to preserve body heat and to warm the foal if necessary. These steps could include covering the foal with bubble wrap, bandaging legs, applying a rug and regular monitoring of temperature.

Use of artificial ventilators

Intermittent positive pressure ventilation (IPPV) in its simplest form can be achieved by compression of the rebreathing bag having closed the pressure relief valve. This is a cumbersome

TABLE 28.4	Signs of anaesthetic depth for inhalation anaesthesia		
Light anaesthesia	**Medium anaesthesia**	**Deep anaesthesia**	**Anaesthetic overdose**
Eye central (or caudal)	Eye medially rotated	Eye central	Eye central
Pupil moderate dilated	Pupil dilation slight	Pupil dilated	Pupil very dilated
Nystagmus brisk	Nystagmus slow/absent	No nystagmus	No nystagmus
Brisk palpebral reflex	Sluggish palpebral reflex	No palpebral reflex	No palpebral reflex
Brisk corneal reflex	Sluggish corneal reflex	Cornea very slow/absent	No corneal reflex
Eye wide open	Eye closing	Eye open	Eye wide open
Lacrimation ++	Lacrimation +	Lacrimation −	Dry eye
Head and limb movement possible (tension in tendon of m. sternocephalicus)*	Muscle relaxation (tendon of m. sternocephalicus relaxes)*	Total muscle relaxation*	Muscles flaccid*
Breath-holding or rapid breathing	Regular breathing pattern	Reduced respiration rate, often irregular	Cheyne-Stokes breathing or gasps
Anal reflex +++	Anal reflex ++	Anal reflex ±	Anal reflex −
High blood pressure		Low blood pressure	Very low blood pressure
Mucous membranes pink, CRT < 2 sec	Mucous membranes pink, CRT < 2 sec	Mucous membranes pale/blue, CRT ↑	Mucous membranes grey/blue
Pulse easily palpable	Pulse good to moderate	Weak pulse	Pulse not palpable

CRT, capillary refill time.
*Muscle relaxants (glyceryl guaiacolate ether) will increase muscle relaxation further; horses can often vary from the 'normal' in their responses to anaesthesia.

procedure and is usually restricted to emergencies or for short periods.

Most modern equine anaesthetic machines incorporate a ventilator to allow automatic IPPV in horses that are hypoventilating, as indicated by hypercapnia. Ideally, blood gases, especially CO_2, should be monitored during IPPV to enable 'fine-tuning' of the tidal volume and ventilation rate according to the requirements of the patient. Most horses ventilate quite adequately by spontaneous respiration during anaesthesia. Cases in which IPPV may be used include those in which the respiratory rate falls below four breaths per minute, in which case the horse may be inspiring inadequate volatile agent to maintain a level plane of anaesthesia, and cases where abdominal distension restricts normal respiration. IPPV is always required for intrathoracic surgery.

Monitoring anaesthesia

Anaesthetic drugs (Table 28.4) have a depressive effect on the cardiac and respiratory functions of the patient. This depressive effect can be life-threatening if careful and ongoing assessment of these functions is not performed and the appropriate actions taken.

Anaesthetic monitoring should be continuous and should be carried out by one dedicated anaesthetist throughout a procedure; this varies from small animal anaesthetics and only a veterinary surgeon can perform anaesthesia in horses. Monitoring methods will depend on the conditions in which anaesthesia is being carried out – field conditions do not lend themselves to use of electrical monitors, which may take some time to set up and may prolong anaesthetic time for limited benefits. Whether in field or theatre conditions, the primary tool of anaesthesia should be observation by the anaesthetist and electrical equipment should only be used to

---

BOX 28.3 PATIENT MONITORING ROUTINE

- Clinical examination of horse at rest in the stable, record vital signs
- Observation of response to premedication
- Check vital signs after induction before lifting or positioning
- Intraoperative monitoring using manual checks and monitors as appropriate
- Periodic intraoperative checks on equipment
- Manual monitoring should continue after the horse is placed in recovery and observation at a distance maintained until it stands up

---

enhance careful monitoring. It is good practice to complete anaesthetic record charts, but this should not be done at the expense of careful patient monitoring. Familiarity with monitors should be gained through training during low-risk procedures. It can be argued that it is only useful to monitor things that you have the ability to alter. For example, it may not be useful to monitor blood oxygen without the facility for positive pressure ventilation.

Anaesthetic monitoring is most effective when a routine is established to reduce the likelihood that any areas are overlooked (Box 28.3). Equipment that should be checked prior to an operation includes:

- Oxygen cylinders, turned on and levels within the cylinders
- Adequate supplies of anaesthetic drugs required
- Leak check on endotracheal tube cuff, circuit and bag
- Mouth gag
- Soda lime
- Mats, etc., to position horse on floor or table
- Anaesthetic machine, including vaporiser fluid level
- Electrical monitor check
- Fill in patient information on anaesthetic chart.

TABLE 28.5	Advantages and disadvantages of inhalational and total intravenous anaesthesia	
Advantages	**Disadvantages**	
INHALATIONAL ANAESTHESIA		
Effective, controllable and normally predictable maintenance of anaesthesia	High cost of initial set-up	
Low running costs	Varying degrees of cardiovascular and respiratory depression	
Concurrent oxygen delivery	Required gases are potentially flammable/explosive	
Activity does not rely on metabolism by the body	Possible risk to personnel as a result of exposure to volatile agents	
Duration of anaesthesia can be safely increased within a certain range		
The airway patency is maintained		
TOTAL INTRAVENOUS ANAESTHESIA		
Minimal equipment required, convenient for field conditions	Drugs required are expensive	
Endotracheal intubation may not be required	Drugs have a cumulative effect and rely on clearance by the animals' metabolism. This may lead to prolonged recovery	
No reliance on respiratory function to deepen anaesthesia	Depth of anaesthesia can be easily increased but not decreased	
No flammable or explosive gases or cylinders are required	Causes respiratory depression and oxygen may be needed	

MONITORING DEPTH OF ANAESTHESIA

The eye

- The palpebral reflex is elicited by gently running a finger along the free margin of the upper eyelid; this is retained during anaesthesia.
- Lacrimation and rapid nystagmus are associated with a light plane of anaesthesia.
- Corneal reflex is not used routinely to assess the depth of anaesthesia.

Anaesthetists should interpret eye reflexes alongside their knowledge of the anaesthetic agent administered, e.g. when using inhalation agents the palpebral reflex is usually reduced and the eye rotates medially and ventrally.

Muscle tone

Inadequate depth of anaesthesia can cause changes in muscle tone, e.g. tightening of the muscles in the neck.

MONITORING EQUIPMENT – USES AND LIMITATIONS

Short routine procedures undertaken in a field or clinic environment are often monitored purely by observation, pulse palpation and use of a stethoscope (Table 28.5). All equine clinics undertaking surgery in a theatre on a regular basis should have, as a minimum, facilities for electrocardiography and blood pressure monitoring.

Stethoscope

Essential to auscultate heart and lungs, the stethoscope is a very portable, familiar piece of monitoring equipment. There is a limitation in auscultation of the heart in the unconscious horse

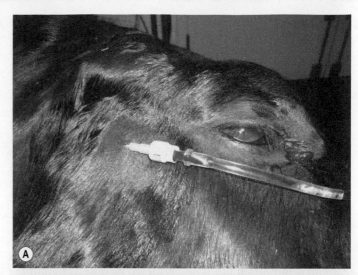

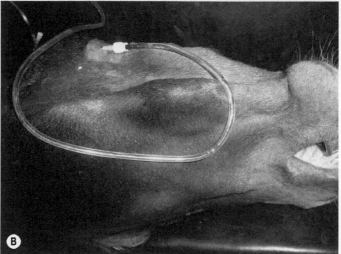

Fig. 28.4 Position of the arteries used for direct blood pressure monitoring

as it can fall away from the body wall, leading to a false diagnosis of cardiac arrest.

Electrocardiography

ECG monitors show the heart rate and the pattern of activity in the heart. They are easily and quickly applied and provide easily visible, reassuring monitoring of cardiac activity. Heart rate is displayed on the screen and an alarm will sound on most machines if this drops. The displayed heart rate should be periodically checked manually, because, as monitors are adapted for human use, they occasionally count more than one beat for each 'PQRS' complex. It is sometimes possible to correct this by altering the lead position. ECG in the horse is limited to giving information on rate and rhythm. Other electrical equipment and physical movement or vibration, e.g. by clippers, affect the monitor display.

Blood pressure

This is most reliably measured by direct methods, i.e. arterial catheter placement. Arteries used for this procedure are the facial, transverse facial and dorsal metatarsal arteries (Fig. 28.4). The blood pressure monitor is often combined with the ECG monitor. A direct blood pressure trace will give information on cardiac output, and blood pressure values are an important guide to depth of anaesthesia, i.e. higher for 'light' planes of anaesthesia and lower as the patient becomes 'deeper'. It also indicates peripheral perfusion, which is important in the horse because of the association of poor perfusion of muscles with postoperative myopathies. Mean arterial blood pressure should be maintained above 65 mm Hg to decrease the risk of myopathy. Desirable mean arterial blood pressure in anaesthetised horses is 65–85 mm Hg.

The main limitation of direct blood pressure monitoring is that some skill must be learned in the placement of arterial catheters and use of the machine. Indirect methods involving pneumatic cuffs applied around the leg or tail are available but are unreliable in horses.

Respiration monitors

Monitoring of respiratory rate, depth, rhythm and pattern is extremely important but is best achieved by observation of the chest wall movement, excursion of the bag and sound of the valves during respiration. Breathing should be rhythmical and deep, with a normal rate of 6–10 breaths per minute in the horse. Shallow breathing may lead to poor lung ventilation; mucous membrane colour and capillary refill time should be monitored to check this.

Respiratory monitors are usually limited to measuring rate of respiration and do not indicate tidal volume or lung perfusion. The expense of acquiring a machine is unlikely to be justified.

Pulse oximeters

Non-invasive monitoring of the haemoglobin oxygen saturation of the blood (SaO_2) can be achieved by a clip attached to the tongue or the nasal septum. These machines usually measure pulse rate as well as oxygen saturation and will bleep with each heartbeat. Pulse oximeters may be useful in field conditions because they are easily portable, quickly connected and the audible pulse signal may be useful.

Pulse oximetry is poor at predicting problems and tends to indicate when a problem has occurred. Correcting low oxygen haemoglobin saturation in the horse, without means of positive pressure ventilation, is extremely difficult, and the value of these monitors without the availability of an artificial ventilator is doubtful.

Capnograph

Monitors are very useful and relatively inexpensive; they measure the CO_2 in expired air ($PaCO_2$). Elevated $PaCO_2$ can be addressed by increasing ventilation by compression of the rebreathing bag manually with the pressure relief valve closed. Capnography may be more useful in showing trends in $PaCO_2$ than in giving absolute values.

Blood gas machines

These are expensive pieces of equipment that require the ability to take arterial blood samples for immediate analysis in order to obtain accurate results. Correct sample handling is vital if accurate results are to be obtained. A blood gas machine will measure $PaCO_2$, PaO_2 and pH, which are of great benefit if severely compromised patients are routinely being anaesthetised and acid-base monitoring becomes increasingly important, e.g. colic surgery (see Chapter 27). Portable blood gas analysers are exceptionally useful in equine practice, and can be used in the field. These can measure electrolytes alongside blood gases and lactate.

Recovery from anaesthesia

An ideal recovery involves the horse remaining calmly in lateral and then sternal recumbency until the effects of the anaesthetic drugs have worn off and it can stand without ataxia. Recovery time should be as short as possible within those limits.

A horse positioned in lateral recumbency during surgery should be placed on the same side in recovery; if the horse has been in dorsal recumbency it should be placed on its left side in recovery.

Turning a horse over from one side to the other from surgery to recovery will allow reperfusion of the formerly dependent muscles but results in atelectasis (partial collapse) of the newly dependent lung lobes. This can result in respiratory embarrassment as the lung lobes that have been dependent during surgery will already be in a state of atelectasis, which will not resolve quickly enough to allow adequate ventilation. Extubation can be carried out before the swallow reflex returns if the airway is clear. If a nasotracheal tube is to be placed for the full recovery, it should be secured in place to prevent it being pushed up the nose. (Wrapping adhesive bandage around the nasal end to form a 'ball' is quite effective.)

In some cases the horse can recover with the ET tube left in the mouth but this carries the inherent risk that the horse will obstruct its own airway by biting the tube, and a secure, safe mouth gag is needed.

To prevent the patient from standing too quickly, ensure that the horse has been administered adequate analgesia to reduce pain. The horse's bladder should be catheterised during surgery to prevent a distended bladder, and sedation should be administered; e.g. xylazine 0.1 mg/kg, administered intravenously, can be used to prolong recovery time and keep patients calm during the recovery period.

Recovery boxes should be designed to achieve a good, safe recovery (Fig. 28.5). The recovery room should be square with curved corners – horses use a fifth point of support when they stand with their head supported in a corner. The box should be of a size that allows free movement but is too small for the

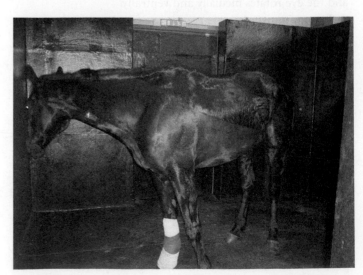

Fig. 28.5 Horse recovering from anaesthesia in a recovery box

recovering patient to gather speed. The walls and floor should be padded without protruding edges and the floor should provide good grip, even when wet. It should be possible to dim the lights and keep the area quiet while a horse is recovering to reduce patient stimulation during the recovery period to prevent horses getting to their feet too quickly, consequently increasing their risk of injury. A heat lamp can be used to minimise the risk of postoperative hypothermia.

Assistance during recovery may be required for foals to prevent injury and for adults in some cases of orthopaedic surgery. Assistance during recovery should only be given to adults by experienced teams and preferably with a method of restraint, such as ropes attached to the head collar and tail running through rings on the wall to provide a secure anchor. Slings are poorly tolerated unless the horse has previously become acclimatised to them.

The quality of recovery should be scored and recorded. A simple descriptive scale has been devised:

Score 5: no ataxia, no struggling, stood up at first attempt as if fully conscious

Score 4: slight ataxia, no struggling, stood up at first attempt as if fully conscious

Score 3: some staggering and ataxia, a few unsuccessful attempts to stand, ataxia immediately after standing up

Score 2: excitement, paddling when recumbent, several attempts to stand, severe ataxia once standing, may fall, danger of self-inflicted injury

Score 1: excitement when recumbent, persistent unsuccessful attempts to stand, aimless walking, high risk of self-inflicted injury

Score 0: very violent ('wall of death'), self-inflicted injury, prolonged struggling or unable to stand 2 hours after end of anaesthesia.

Complications and emergencies

EQUIPMENT AND DRUGS REQUIRED FOR EMERGENCY RESUSCITATION

The larger pieces of equipment used for routine anaesthesia are also used for resuscitation and are therefore readily to hand in an emergency. A 'crash box' containing a selection of needles, syringes, fluid-giving sets, intravenous cannulas and a stethoscope should be kept together with the drugs listed below.

Equipment required:
- ET tube to maintain airway.
- Tracheostomy/laryngotomy tube.
- Means for IPPV – anaesthetic circuit/ventilator/(Hudson) demand valve.
- Drugs for emergency resuscitation should be drawn up into capped syringes and labelled with the name of the drug and the appropriate weight of the horse.

Drugs required:
- Epinephrine (adrenaline) (1 mg/ml), which is a cardiovascular stimulant, which initiates or increases heart rate
- Atropine (0.6 mg/ml), which is an antiarrhythmic agent, which increases heart rate
- Lidocaine (lignocaine) (20 mg/ml), which is an antiarrhythmic agent, which treats ventricular arrhythmias

- Doxapram (20 mg/ ml), which is a respiratory stimulant, which initiates or increases breathing.

RESPIRATORY OBSTRUCTION

Causes include:
- Kinking of the ET tube – do not overflex the neck; check the tube inside and outside the mouth where it may be prone to kinking during movement
- Overinflation of the cuff leading to compression of the tube or inflation of the cuff over the end of the tube – become familiar with the amount of air usually required to inflate the cuff and measure this by using a normal syringe
- Foreign material in the airway, e.g. blood – if it is suspected that blood or gastric reflux may enter the airway, leave the ET tube in position with the cuff inflated until the patient is able to swallow to clear the airway
- Oedema of the nasal passages when the head has been in a position that is lower than the body during anaesthesia – leave a suitable design of nasotracheal tube in place for the duration of recovery; treatment includes topical administration of 5 ml 0.15% phenylephrine into each nostril 10–15 minutes before termination of anaesthesia
- Dislocation of the soft palate – stimulate the larynx to make the horse swallow or pass an ET tube gently to open the airway
- Laryngeal spasm – place a tracheostomy tube in a laryngotomy wound prior to recovery and leave in place overnight after surgery.

Complete airway obstruction during anaesthesia is shown by the presence of chest and abdominal movements without excursion of the rebreathing bag. Partial airway obstruction is often audible, as air will be forced through a narrowed airway, e.g. snoring when the nasal passages are narrowed by oedema of the nasal lining. Signs of hypoxia (inadequate oxygen supply to tissues) or anoxia (total lack of oxygen supply) include grey or blue mucous membrane colour and reduced blood O_2 and elevated blood CO_2 observed if blood gas analysis or capnography are available.

Emergency treatment

- Aim is to restore oxygen supply to the tissues.
- Establish cause of obstruction and remove or correct it if possible; if this is not possible, regain airway patency by passing a nasotracheal or ET tube or in the extreme case open the airway by tracheostomy.
- Ventilate manually, making sure no further anaesthetic gas is given.
- Monitor pulse and mucous membrane colour to check efficacy of ventilation.

Respiratory arrest

This is the cessation of breathing that results in apnoea. This frequently occurs transiently during induction, especially after placement of the ET tube. More serious causes of apnoea include respiratory obstruction, excessive resistance in the breathing circuit, central nervous depression during anaesthetic overdose and cardiac arrest.

Breathing after induction can often be restarted by stimulation of the larynx or other reflexes, or a sharp compression of the chest wall. These methods, as well as surgical stimulation, may also be effective during anaesthesia. If breathing still does not begin, e.g. because of drug effects or other conditions causing central nervous depression, then IPPV should be initiated and should continue until spontaneous breathing resumes. Doxapram (0.5–1 mg/kg) may be used in severe circumstances but its efficacy relies on an effective circulation.

Cardiac arrest

Cardiac arrest occurs when the heart no longer has any output and cardiopulmonary function fails to provide oxygen and metabolic substrate to central nervous and cardiac tissues. Clinical signs include loss of palpable peripheral pulse, loss of heart sounds (may also occur without cardiac arrest), cyanosis or pale mucous membranes, apnoea or terminal gasping ventilation, central eye position, pupillary dilation, and absent palpebral and corneal reflexes.

Cardiac arrest usually results from the occurrence of several factors simultaneously, e.g. inhalation agent overdose, hypoxia and hypercapnia (elevated blood CO_2). Vagal stimulation during head and neck surgery may cause cardiac arrest in horses with very little warning.

Emergency treatment

This involves the use of cardiopulmonary resuscitation (CPR). CPR has three main objectives:

1. Maintain oxygen delivery to vital tissues.
2. Prevent development of metabolic changes that cause irreversible tissue damage.
3. Restore normal myocardial activity.

CPR is a team effort, and each member of the team should know his or her role. The principles and technique of equine CPR are similar to those for small animals and humans. The ABCD steps should be followed:

- **Airway** – ensure it is clear; intubate if necessary.
- **Breathing** – initiate IPPV or manual compression of rebreathing bag – use pure O_2 if possible, thus switch off vaporiser.
- **Circulation** – cardiac massage is difficult in the horse. If possible, place horse on a hard surface and give a sharp blow to the precordial chest region to attempt to stimulate heart contraction. If this fails, attempt external massage by exerting strong force over the chest with the knees or foot (about 30 compressions per minute). If all else fails, surgical exposure of the heart and internal massage can be performed.
- **Drug treatment** should only be initiated when cardiac massage results in blood flow. IPPV and cardiac massage should be continued:
  - Epinephrine (adrenaline) given intravenously (0.3 ml per 100 kg) – if this is not possible, give directly into left ventricle of heart or into bronchial tree via ET tube.
  - Atropine intravenously (1.6 ml per 100 kg of 0.6 mg/ml solution = 0.01 mg/kg).
  - Repeat epinephrine (0.5 ml per 100 kg).
  - For ventricular fibrillation use lignocaine (2.5 ml per 100 kg of 20 mg/l = 0.5 mg/kg).

Normal mucous membrane colour and a palpable pulse (when cardiac massage is not occurring) show that the circulation is returning to normal.

Other anaesthetic complications

- **Hypoxaemia** – reduced arterial oxygen concentration; causes include lung atelectasis (lung collapse), anaesthetic equipment failure leading to low inspired oxygen concentration, respiratory depression caused by anaesthetic agents leading to hypoventilation, ventilation/perfusion mismatch (more commonly seen in horses in dorsal recumbency). Treatment includes inhalation of pure oxygen, check for respiratory obstructions, IPPV, maximise cardiac output with IVFT and administration of positive inotropes, and minimise respiratory depression caused by anaesthetic agents.
- **Hypercapnia** – increased arterial CO_2 concentration; caused by reduced ventilation or circulation. This can be treated by IPPV and ensuring that the anaesthetic machine is functioning correctly.
- **Hypotension** – low blood pressure, caused due to deepening of anaesthetic plane, loss of circulating volume, dilation of peripheral vasculature or reduced cardiac output. Hypotension is strongly correlated with myopathies. Treatment should include decreasing the inhalation anaesthetic agent, administering dobutamine (which increases blood pressure), administering ephedrine (which increases blood pressure more than dobutamine) and correcting volume deficits.
- **Cardiac arrhythmias** – loss of normal heart rhythm; occur as a result of drug administration. Arrhythmias that have a significant effect on circulation are rare. Treatment includes addressing underlying causes, e.g. electrolyte imbalances, and administration of lidocaine if the patient is suffering a ventricular arrhythmia.
- **Musculoskeletal injury** – usually long-bone fractures and head trauma; usually occur during unaided recovery as a result of attempts to stand before the drug's effects have worn off or as a result of previous injury or pain.
- **Post-anaesthetic myopathy** – ischaemic muscle damage, as a result of failure of blood supply to the muscle during anaesthesia; caused by poor positioning, lying on firm surfaces, prolonged anaesthesia, prolonged periods of hypotension. Clinical signs include difficult or prolonged recovery, lameness, hot swollen muscles, pain, sweating, muscle fasciculations and myoglobinuria. Treatment includes assistance to stand, padding and nursing if recumbent, Intravenous fluid therapy (IVFT) to maintain perfusion and hydration, administration of analgesia, acepromazine (ACP), vitamin E and selenium, dimethyl sulfoxide, mannitol and massage and hot compress of swollen muscles.
- **Post-anaesthetic neuropathy** – nerve damage as a result of trauma, pressure, stretching and failure of blood supply; caused by pressure of head collar on facial nerve during induction, stretching of limbs for the duration of surgery, e.g. positioning for arthroscopy, or focal pressure causing blood flow to be occluded. Patients that suffer post-anaesthetic neuropathies are not usually in pain, but do require supportive care.

Local anaesthesia

Local anaesthetic is used to desensitise a restricted area to allow painful surgical procedures or paradoxically to abolish existing pain to prove its existence, e.g. diagnosis of some types of lameness. Local anaesthetic techniques usually aim to abolish pain and sensation, leaving motor functions intact, but occasionally are directed at motor nerves to abolish movement as in the auriculo-palpebral nerve block to stop blinking during eye examination. Local anaesthesia can be combined with sedation to allow surgery to be performed 'standing' or it can be used during general anaesthesia to reduce pain and the amount of maintenance drugs required.

TYPES OF LOCAL ANAESTHESIA

Topical anaesthesia

Topical anaesthesia can be achieved using creams designed for skin absorption. For example, creams containing lignocaine (lidocaine) are available for treatment of minor but painful skin abrasions; local anaesthetic eye drops, e.g. amethocaine, are used to desensitise the cornea to aid examination or minor surgery. Absorption through intact skin is slow and the use of topical anaesthesia prior to injection has limited use.

Regional anaesthesia

Regional anaesthesia involves desensitisation of a specified area and includes several methods of administration:
- **Perineural infiltration of local anaesthetic**, i.e. infusion around a nerve whose precise position is known. This effectively prevents the transmission of impulses from beyond that point back to the brain and renders the structures supplied by that nerve insensitive. This is the principle used in lameness diagnosis.
- **Infiltration of local anaesthetic into a wide area**, often of skin, blocks the nerves that supply the area, which is then desensitised. This technique is commonly used in suturing wounds.
- **Intravenous anaesthesia** is useful for the desensitisation of the distal limb. As the technique requires the occlusion of blood flow from the area, a tourniquet is applied proximal to the area to be 'blocked' and local anaesthetic is injected distally into a prominent vein. This produces good anaesthesia in the area below the tourniquet while it is in position. This technique is rarely used in horses, and in large animal practice is mainly restricted to bovine digit surgery.
- **Epidural anaesthesia** is achieved by injection of local anaesthetic around a specific part of the spinal cord, blocking conduction in the spinal nerves of that area and sometimes the spinal cord itself. The structures supplied by the spinal nerves are then desensitised. A caudal block is the most commonly used in horses to allow surgery in the perineal region, e.g. to replace a rectal prolapse and prevent further straining. More cranial blocks carry the risk of desensitising the hind limbs and inducing collapse. Xylazine and xylazine/local anaesthetic combinations are useful in the horse to provide anaesthesia without ataxia.

Intrasynovial anaesthesia

Intrasynovial anaesthesia is used in equine practice and, like perineural anaesthesia, is primarily for lameness diagnosis. Local anaesthetic is injected directly into joints and tendon sheaths and produces anaesthesia of a known, specific structure.

A positive result is a good indication for medication or further investigation of the sheath or joint.

APPLICATION

Topical anaesthesia

- Place appropriate preparation on a dressing directly on to the skin for 1 hour.
- Apply appropriate drops on to cornea or into conjunctival sac.

Perineural infiltration and infiltration into a wide area

- Clipping hair is optional.
- Skin should be cleaned with spirit swab or chlorhexidine wash according to the level of dirt.
- Smallest possible needle is used to minimise patient reaction.
- Agent is injected into target site.

Intrasynovial and epidural anaesthesia

- Strict aseptic technique must be employed, i.e. clip hair, scrub, sterile gloving.
- Place an intradermal skin bleb of local anaesthetic.
- A suitable drug, volume and needle size are chosen.
- Adequate restraint of the horse will be necessary, e.g. sedation or twitch.
- Inject local anaesthetic through the bleb.

DRUGS USED FOR LOCAL ANAESTHESIA

Local anaesthetic drugs are variably lipid-soluble; those that have good lipid solubility diffuse quickly through tissues and nerve trunks and have a quicker speed of onset of activity (Table 28.6). Other factors affecting speed of onset include the accuracy of the injection and the concentration rather than the volume of agent used.

Duration of action is affected by the volume and type of drug chosen and whether a vasoconstrictor, i.e. epinephrine (adrenaline), has been combined in the preparation. Vasoconstriction slows the diffusion of drug out of the target area by reducing blood flow. Preparations containing epinephrine (adrenaline) should be confined to perineural and infusion techniques. Care must be taken to avoid significant systemic uptake.

Humane destruction of Equidae

INDICATIONS FOR EUTHANASIA

Euthanasia is usually carried out on grounds of welfare. This can range from severe inoperable injury resulting in intractable pain to ill or elderly animals that no longer have a 'good quality of life'. Euthanasia should be performed humanely and in the best interests of the animal. The British Equine Veterinary Association (BEVA) has issued guidelines for the decisions involved in the destruction of horses, with particular regard to insurance implications.

TABLE 28.6	Local anaesthetics used in equine practice		
Local anaesthetic drug	Applications	Speed of onset	Duration of action
Lidocaine (Lignol)	Topical Infiltration Perineural Epidural (without epinephrine)	<5 min	30–40 min (doubled by adding epinephrine)
Prilocaine (Citanest)	Infusion Perineural Intrasynovial Epidural Intravenous	5–15 min	Approx. 1 hour
Mepivacaine (Intra-Epicaine)	Infusion Perineural Intrasynovial Epidural	10–20 min	Up to 2 hour
Bupivacaine (Marcaine)	Infiltration Perineural Intrasynovial	15–20 min	Up to 8 hour
Amethocaine	Mucous membrane (topical) Corneal (topical)	<1 min	10–15 min
Proxymetacaine (Ophthaine)	Corneal (topical)	<1 min	15 min

CURRENT METHODS

The handling of the euthanasia of a horse is very important throughout the practice, and lack of sympathy or failure to act correctly can greatly affect clients. Informed consent must be obtained from the owner or keeper of the horse to be euthanised. If the animal is insured, then permission should be sought from the insurance company, if it is humanely possible to delay destruction of the animal. A euthanasia consent form should be signed prior to humane destruction of an animal and a description of the animal should be kept if necessary for insurance or other purposes. It may be necessary to perform a post-mortem examination and the whole carcass or the relevant part should be retained. It may be a good idea, if appropriate, to ask if the owner would like the shoes returned or a piece of mane or tail saved.

Methods available for the humane destruction of horses are as follows:

Gun

This is usually a single-shot 0.32 calibre free-bullet humane killer (weapons smaller than 0.32 calibre are not suitable and neither are captive bolt weapons considered appropriate for destruction of horses outside an abattoir situation, as death is induced by pithing, a process not aesthetically acceptable to the majority of horse owners).

Sedation is often used and assistance is required in the handling of the horse. It is vital that nurses/assistants are aware of people around the area. All humans and other animals should be removed from the area if possible, or at the least they should stand behind the person using the gun – including the assistant, even if the assistant continues to hold the animal.

Lethal injection

This uses a high dose of pentobarbital (pentobarbitone) or Somulose.

Somulose (cinchocaine and quinalbarbitone)
- Preload correct dose (10 ml per 100 kg) into a single syringe.
- A 14-G intravenous catheter is placed.
- The assistant restrains the horse, pulling its head down to encourage the horse to sink backwards.
- The full amount of Somulose is injected over about 15 seconds.
- Collapse will occur 35–45 seconds after the start of injection, death within 2 minutes.

Pentobarbital (pentabarbitone)
- Pentobarbital is preloaded into as many 50-ml syringes as required (dose 200 mg/kg).
- A 14-G intravenous catheter is placed.
- Sedative may be used if required, usually an alpha-2 agonist at full sedative dose.
- The assistant restrains the horse, being aware that sudden or violent movements may occur.
- The full volume of pentobarbital is injected as quickly as possible.
- Collapse should occur 35–40 seconds and death 1.5–2.5 minutes after injection; gasping may occur.

DISPOSAL OF THE CARCASS

Disposal of the animal should preferably be arranged prior to euthanasia and the preferred method of disposal discussed with the owner. Even though this may be difficult at the time, it may have a bearing on the method of euthanasia.

Common routes of disposal are:

Cremation/incineration:
- Expensive
- Method of euthanasia unimportant
- Ashes can often be returned if requested.

Carcass used for animal consumption by a hunt kennel or abattoir:

- Depends on personal wishes or opinions and may be distasteful to many horse owners
- Less expensive than incineration
- Horse cannot be euthanised with Somulose or pentobarbital.

Carcass used for human consumption:

- May retrieve 'meat' value of the animal, which gives some financial return

- Animal must be euthanised by gun
- Animal must not contain residues of any controlled drugs or substances and all medication must have been recorded in the passport under the passport scheme
- Horse will have to be transported alive to a registered abattoir.

BIBLIOGRAPHY

Bishop, Y. (Ed.), 1996. The Veterinary Formulary, third ed. Royal Pharmaceutical Society of Great Britain/Pharmaceutical Press, London.

British Small Animal Veterinary Association, 2015. Controlled drugs. Available from: <https://www.bsava.com/Resources/BSAVAMedicinesGuide/ControlledDrugs.aspx>.

Corley, K., Stephen, J., 2008. The Equine Hospital Manual. Blackwell, Oxford.

Coumbe, K. (Ed.), 2012. Equine Veterinary Nursing Manual. Wiley-Blackwell, Oxford.

Doherty, T., Valverde, A., 2006. Manual of Equine Anaesthesia and Analgesia. Blackwell, Oxford.

Hall, L.W., Clarke, K.W., Trim, C.M., 2001. Veterinary Anaesthesia, tenth ed. Butterworth-Heinemann, Oxford.

Johnston, G.M., Eastment, J.K., Wood, J.L.N., et al., 2002. The Confidential Enquiry into Perioperative Equine Fatalities (CEPEF): mortality results of phases 1 and 2. Vet. Anaesth. Analg. 29, 159–170.

Knottenbelt, D.C. (Ed.), 1997. Formulary of Equine Medicine. Liverpool University Press, Liverpool.

Taylor, P.M., Clarke, K.W., 1999. Handbook of Equine Anaesthesia. W B Saunders, Philadelphia, PA.

RECOMMENDED READING

Taylor, P.M., Clarke, K.W., 1999. Handbook of Equine Anaesthesia. W B Saunders, Philadelphia, PA.

This book is written for veterinary surgeons but provides useful information for the veterinary nurse.

Parasitology

MAGGIE FISHER

KEY POINTS

- Parasites can be divided into the ectoparasites and the endoparasites.

- Most ectoparasites are arthropods belonging either to the insect or to the acari groups but certain species of fungi are also ectoparasites.

- Endoparasites of companion animals or horses fall into four main groups – the nematodes or roundworms, cestodes or tapeworms, trematodes or flukes and protozoa.

- Each species of parasite has its own life cycle, which is its means of survival and spread between host animals.

- An understanding of the life cycle is the key to treatment and control of the parasite.

- The effect of a parasite on the host animal may be insignificant and treatment is only necessary to prevent an increase in parasite numbers in or on the host or in the environment and to prevent the spread of zoonotic disease.

- Parasites such as the lungworm *Angiostrongylus vasorum* and the heartworm *Dirofilaria immitis* can cause severe disease in their host, while other parasites can cause disease if present in sufficiently high numbers.

- There are many antiparasitic drugs, each with their own specific mode of action. Some may act against several parasite groups, which necessitates giving only a single treatment to the patient.

Definitions

- **Parasite** – a eukaryotic organism that lives off another (the host) to the advantage of the parasite.
- **Endoparasite** – a parasite that lives inside the host, e.g. a roundworm.
- **Ectoparasite** – a parasite that lives on or in the skin of the host, e.g. a flea.
- **Permanent parasite** – a parasite that lives for its entire life cycle on the host, e.g. a louse.
- **Temporary parasite** – a parasite that lives for only part of its life on a host, e.g. a flea – the adult stage is entirely parasitic but the immature stages live in the environment. A mosquito is still more temporary – only the adult females are parasitic as they take a blood meal from a human or animal.
- **Zoonoses** – animal infections that can infect humans.

- **Host specificity** – refers to the range of hosts that a particular parasite can utilise; e.g. lice are very host-specific as each species will only infect one specific host. Thus *Bovicola equi*, formerly *Damalinia equi*, the horse louse, will not infect dogs and *Linognathus setosus*, the sucking louse of dogs, will only survive on dogs. In contrast *Ctenocephalides felis*, the cat flea, has been recorded living successfully on cats, dogs, rabbits, ferrets, sheep, goats and calves.
- **Final host** – only occurs in a life cycle involving more than one host. It refers mainly to the host in which sexual reproduction of the parasite occurs, e.g. *Echinococcus granulosus* – this tapeworm occurs in dogs but the hydatid cyst, the immature stage, occurs in sheep, which are the **intermediate hosts**. These include:
  - *Paratenic* hosts – act as host for a parasite but little or no development of the parasite occurs within them; e.g. infective *Toxocara canis* eggs eaten by a mouse hatch and the larvae migrate into the mouse's tissue (the paratenic host), where it remains without further development until the mouse is eaten by a dog.
  - *Transport host* – simply carries the parasite from one host to another.
- **Vector** – an arthropod responsible for the transmission of a parasite among vertebrate hosts. The arthropod may act as an intermediate host, a paratenic host or a transport host.
- **Prepatent period** – the time between the ingestion of the infective stage, e.g. egg, and the production of eggs by the adults. A parasitic infection is said to be **patent** when e.g. eggs are found in the faeces.
- **Infective stage** – may be larvae or other stage that is capable of infecting the next host in the cycle.
- **Direct life cycle** (refers to nematodes) – a life cycle which does not involve an intermediate host. Larvae may be directly transmitted from host to host or be free-living in the environment, e.g. on pasture.
- **Indirect life cycle** – a life cycle in which the larval stages pass through an intermediate host.
- **Facultative parasites** – they can, but do not have to, infest living animals.
- **Obligate parasites** – cannot complete their life cycle without an animal host.

NOMENCLATURE OF PARASITES

It is normal to refer to a parasite by its genus and then species name, e.g. the canine worm, *Toxocara canis*: the genus is *Toxocara* and the species *canis*. After the first use the genus name can be abbreviated to its initial, in this case becoming *T. canis*.

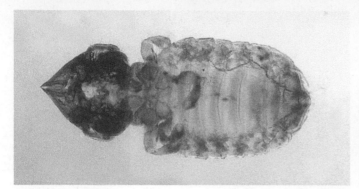

Fig. 29.1 *Felicola subrostratus*, the biting louse of the cat. Adult is 1–1.5 mm in length

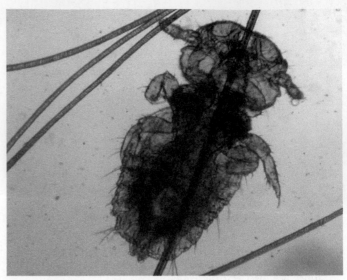

Fig. 29.2 *Trichodectes canis*, a biting louse of dogs. Adult is 1–2 mm in length

Ectoparasites

Ectoparasites include the arthropod species and certain species of fungi.

Most ectoparasitic arthropods belong either to the insect group, i.e. lice, fleas, mosquitoes, sand flies and *Culicoides* midges or the acari, a subgroup of the arachnids, i.e. mites and ticks. Adult arthropods have an exoskeleton (as opposed to the mammalian endoskeleton) and reproduce by laying eggs. The immature stages may be similar to the adult but smaller, e.g. lice or mites, or may be maggot-like and change to the adult form, e.g. flies and fleas during pupation.

Infection with ectoparasites may be termed 'infestation'.

INSECTS

Lice

Lice are small, wingless, permanently parasitic insects. They are dorsoventrally flattened and possess claws for clasping hairs or feathers. They are host-specific and there are many species of louse. Rather than focusing on identifying the species, it is usually more important to identify whether lice are present and whether they are sucking or biting lice. 'Sucking' or 'biting' (also known as chewing) refers to the method of feeding: biting lice have mouthparts adapted to chewing the surface of the skin and sucking lice have narrow mouthparts for piercing skin and sucking blood. A heavy burden of the latter can result in anaemia. Cats have just one species of louse, the biting louse *Felicola subrostratus* (Fig. 29.1). Dogs in temperate climates have one species of biting louse, *Trichodectes canis* (Fig. 29.2), and one species of sucking louse, *Linognathus setosus* (Fig. 29.3). On horses, *Haematopinus asini* is the sucking louse and *Bovicola equi*, formerly known as *Damalinia equi*, is the biting louse.

Life cycle: Female lice lay their eggs or nits on the host attached to hairs (Fig. 29.4) and these can give lousy animals a speckled appearance, depending on their hair colour. Immature lice emerge from the eggs and progress through a series of moults to become adults. The entire life cycle takes about 4–6 weeks.

Animals with clinical lousiness or pediculosis will rub and scratch themselves. A heavy burden may cause debility, particularly if sucking lice are present. Infection is most common in young, old or debilitated animals. Infection is seen relatively rarely in cats and dogs in the UK but more often in horses. Louse burdens can build up on horses during the winter when

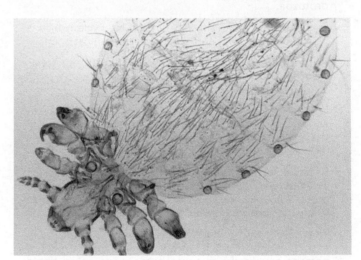

Fig. 29.3 *Linognathus setosus*, the sucking louse of dogs. Adult is approx. 2 mm in length

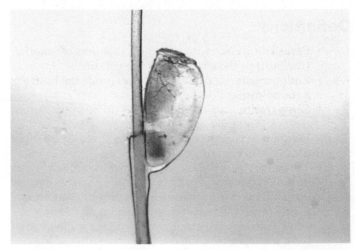

Fig. 29.4 Louse egg or nit on a hair shaft. Egg approx. 0.7 mm long

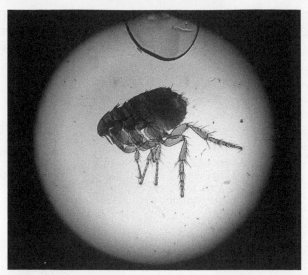

Fig. 29.5 Lateral view of an adult 'cat' flea, *Ctenocephalides felis*. Adult measures 1–2.5 mm in length

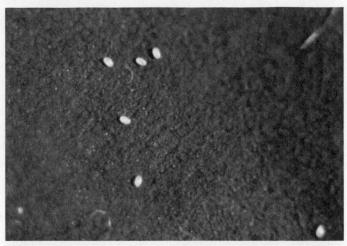

Fig. 29.6 Cat flea eggs are smooth and are laid by the adult female on the host but drop off into the environment. Egg is approx. 0.5 mm in length

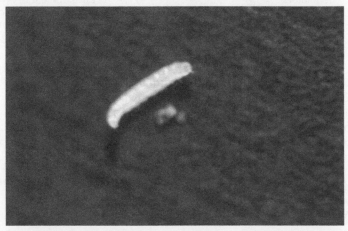

Fig. 29.7 Flea larvae go through two moults before pupating. Larvae measure approx. 0.5 cm

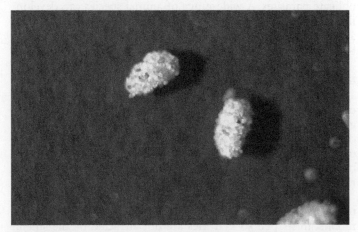

Fig. 29.8 Pupae are covered in sticky cocoons, which become coated in debris from the environment

they are stabled, with louse populations diminishing during the summer at pasture.

Infected animals can be treated with a suitable insecticide. Few insecticides penetrate the eggs, so unless a residual insecticide such as fipronil, selamectin or imidacloprid is used a repeat treatment may be necessary approximately 10 days after the first.

Fleas

Fleas (Fig. 29.5) are wingless, laterally flattened, dark brown insects capable of moving rapidly through a coat or jumping with their specialised legs. Their mouthparts are adapted for piercing skin and sucking blood. The details of the head, such as the presence of combs, are often characteristic of the species of flea and can be used for identification. One species, *Ctenocephalides felis*, more commonly referred to as *C. felis* or the cat flea, is the predominant species on cats and dogs in the UK and may also be found on ferrets and rabbits. The dog flea, *Ctenocephalides canis*, is more host-specific, is found on some dogs in the UK and is the most common flea on dogs in Ireland. Other species of fleas parasitize small mammals and birds.

Life cycle: Adult *C. felis* emerge from their pupal case in the environment and begin to seek a host. Once they have found a suitable host they begin to feed within 5 minutes. Female fleas begin to lay eggs approximately 24–48 hours after they begin to feed. The eggs (Fig. 29.6) are smooth and fall off into the environment, typically in the area where the animal rests. In ideal conditions the eggs hatch after about 2 days, although development is slower in cool conditions (Dryden and Rust 1994). Eggs and larvae require warmth and humidity to remain alive and develop – dry conditions and heat over about 35°C will kill them. Maggot-like larvae (Fig. 29.7) hatched from the eggs undergo two moults before pupating. The pupal case is sticky, so typically becomes camouflaged with environmental debris (Fig. 29.8). The life cycle can be completed in about 12 days in ideal conditions. Other species of flea, such as the bird flea *Ceratophyllus gallinae*, are nest-dwelling fleas, where the adults remain in the environment except when they find a host to feed.

Fleas suck blood and a moderately heavy burden can cause severe anaemia, particularly in small animals such as kittens. As fleas feed, saliva is injected, which contains antigens that provoke the development of an allergic response in some individuals. In cats and dogs this often manifests as a pruritic dermatitis or 'flea allergic dermatitis'. Fleas can transmit diseases and also act as the intermediate host for the tapeworm *Dipylidium caninum*.

TABLE 29.1	Flea control agents			
Chemical group	**Examples**	**Mode of action**	**Application to**	**Formulation**
Organochlorides	Lindane	Acts on the neuromuscular junction	Animal (broadly phased out now)	Topical
Organophosphates	Fenthion	Acts on the neuromuscular junction	Animal (broadly phased out now)	Topical
Carbamates	Carbaryl	Acts on the neuromuscular junction	Animal, particularly collars	Topical
Phenylpyrazole	Fipronil	Neurotransmitter inhibition	Animal	Topical
Semicarbazone	Metaflumizone	Neuronal sodium channel blocker	Animal	Topical
Oxadiazine	Indoxacarb	Neuronal sodium channel blocker	Animal	Topical
Pyrethrins and pyrethroids	Natural pyrethrin Permethrin Deltamethrin	Acts on the nervous system	Animal and environmental formulations available (NB. Cats are susceptible to pyrethroid toxicity)	Topical
Neonicotinoids	Imidacloprid Nitenpyram	Blocks nicotinic acetylcholine receptors	Animal	Topical Oral
Spinosins	Spinosad	Blocks nicotinic acetylcholine receptors	Animal	Oral
Macrocyclic lactones	Selamectin	Neurotransmitter inhibition	Animal	Topical
Insect growth regulators	Lufenuron	Chitin synthesis inhibitor (prevents development of immature stages)	Animal	Orally or by injection
	Methoprene	Juvenile hormone and analogues (prevents development of immature stages)	Animal or the environment	Topical
	Pyriproxyfen			Topical

C. felis is zoonotic and will bite, although not live on, humans. Control of an existing problem can be achieved by treatment of affected dogs or cats with an insecticide that is active for just a few hours, or with sustained activity. Depending on the severity of the infestation, elimination may be accelerated by concomitant treatment of immature flea stages in the environment by insecticide and/or by insect growth regulators that prevent maturation of eggs and larvae (Table 29.1). Fleas can be prevented by prophylactic use of insecticide or insect growth regulators.

Flies

Some fly larvae are facultative parasites, while some others are obligate parasites. A wide range of animal species can develop fly strike and the condition is seen occasionally in dogs and cats and more frequently in rabbits and sheep, particularly during the summer months.

Life cycle: Adult flies lay their eggs in moist conditions on the animal to which they have been attracted by odours, such as those of faeces. The larvae hatch rapidly and begin to feed on the surface of the animal and invade deeper tissues as they grow and moult (Fig. 29.9). Once fully developed the larvae drop to the ground and pupate. Proteolytic enzymes, secreted onto the animal to assist in tissue breakdown together with the breakdown products, have toxic effects on the host, which can rapidly become depressed and anorexic.

Careful husbandry is important during the summer months to prevent a build-up of faeces on the animal or, in the case of rabbits, in its pen so that flies are not attracted by the smell. Careful observation is needed so that if fly strike does occur it can be dealt with rapidly. Development of larvae on rabbits can be prevented by application of the larval growth inhibitor cyromazine. When an animal becomes fly-blown the wound must be cleaned and the larvae removed. Prognosis is good if the infection is caught early but reduces as the larvae burrow deeper into tissues and enter body cavities. Supportive nursing and adjunctive therapy may also be necessary.

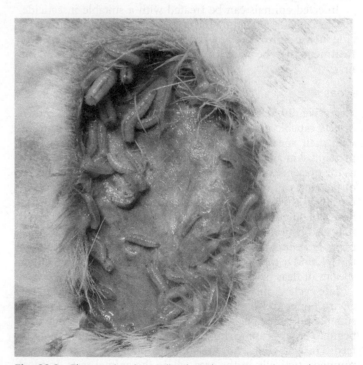

Fig. 29.9 Fly eggs hatch rapidly, then the maggots begin damaging the skin, which is often penetrated by the time the infestation is noticed. (Courtesy of Steve Warren). Each maggot measures approx. 0.9 mm

Various species of flies bite horses and feed off secretions around horses' eyes (Fig. 29.10). The flies can transmit infections, including the nematode *Habronema* spp. Horses may become hypersensitive to fly bites, and hypersensitivity to the small biting midge *Culicoides* spp. (Fig. 29.11) can result in a severe pruritic dermatitis, known as sweet itch, during the summer months. The tail, head and mane are often the most affected areas (Fig. 29.12). Horses can be protected from flies and midges in a number of ways, including keeping them

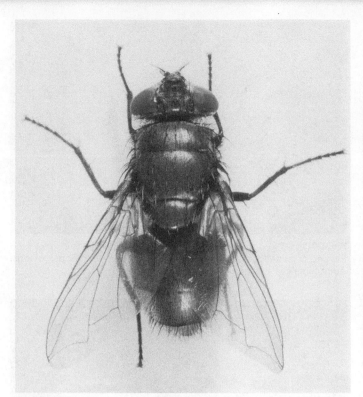

Fig. 29.10 Horses are worried in the summer by a number of species of flies that feed off eye secretions, etc. *(Courtesy of John McGarry.)*

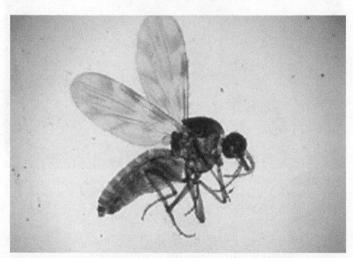

Fig. 29.11 Culicoides are also known as 'no-see-ums' because of their very small size *(Courtesy of John McGarry, © Liverpool School of Tropical Medicine).* Flies measure 1–4 mm

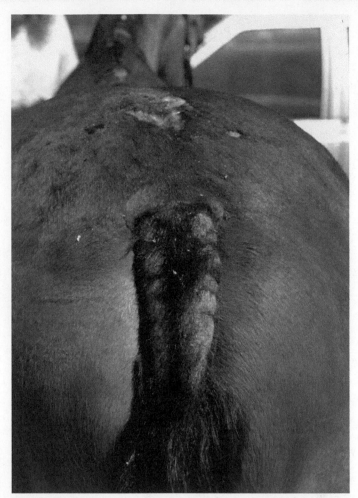

Fig. 29.12 'Sweet itch' is caused by *Culicoides* bites activating an inflammatory allergic response that is very pruritic, so the affected horse rubs affected areas, primarily the mane and tail *(Courtesy of Mark Craig)*

indoors and using proprietary insect repellents or head nets. Female mosquitoes and sand flies are temporary parasites, requiring a blood meal prior to egg laying. Mosquitoes are the vectors of heartworm caused by *Dirofilaria immitis* and sand flies are responsible for the transmission of *Leishmania* spp.

ACARI

Ticks and mites appear as a single sac without the definition of head, thorax and abdomen that is seen in the insects. The mouthparts protrude anteriorly and nymphal and adult stages possess four pairs of legs.

Mites

Mites can be roughly grouped into surface dwellers (Table 29.2), which have long legs, and subsurface dwellers, which typically have short, stumpy legs. The entire life cycle of most parasitic mites occurs on the host, with transfer from host to host occurring through close contact or occasionally by acquisition of mites from the environment, since some mites can survive in the environment for some time in some of their life cycle stages. Other species of mites are temporary parasites, e.g. *Dermanyssus gallinae*, opportunistic parasites or, in the case of *Trombicula autumnalis*, parasites only during their larval stage. Treatment of mite infections involves using an appropriate acaricide on single or repeated occasions. Symptoms of mite infection are collectively referred to as 'mange'.

Surface mites
- *Otodectes cynotis*, the ear mite – normally inhabits the external ear canal, although it is occasionally found elsewhere on the host. Cats, dogs and, occasionally, ferrets can be infected. The mites have bell-shaped suckers on the end of unjointed stalks (legs) or pedicels (Fig. 29.13). The mites are off-white and can be clearly seen against the brown of ear wax when magnified with an aurascope. The entire life cycle occurs on the host and begins

TABLE 29.2	Summary of mite species			
	Host species			
Mite species	Cat	Dog	Horse	Other pets
SURFACE MITES				
Otodectes cynotis	Yes	Yes	–	Ferrets
Chorioptes equi	–	–	Yes	–
Psoroptes spp.	–	–	*Psoroptes equi*	*Psoroptes cuniculi* in rabbits
Cheyletiella spp.	Yes	Yes	–	Rabbits
Trombicula autumnalis	Yes	Yes	Yes	–
SUBSURFACE MITES				
Sarcoptes scabiei and related species	*Sarcoptes scabiei* rarely *Notoedres cati*	*Sarcoptes scabiei* var. *canis*	*Sarcoptes scabiei* rarely in the UK	*Sarcoptes* spp. can infect rabbits and hamsters *Notoedres* spp. in rats *Trixacarus caviae* in guinea pigs
Demodex spp.	Yes, rarely	Yes	Yes, rarely	Hamsters

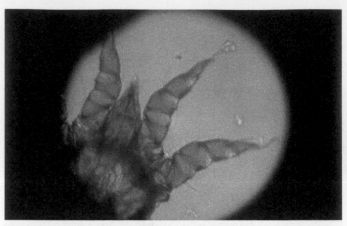

Fig. 29.14 *Psoroptes* spp. mites can be identified by the suckers on the end of jointed stalks or pedicels at the ends of the front pair of legs. Adult female is approx. 750 µm

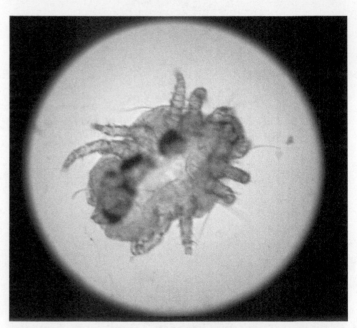

Fig. 29.15 *Cheyletiella* spp. mites are large surface mites with long legs. They have a characteristic waist, large palps at the anterior end each carrying a heavy claw and 'combs' on the ends of their legs

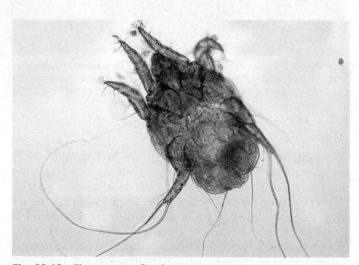

Fig. 29.13 The ear mite *Otodectes cynotis* can be recognised by the unjointed stalks or pedicels with suckers on the end that occur on the front two pairs of legs in all developmental stages. Adult mite approx. 300 µm

with the female mite laying eggs. Immature stages appear similar to those of adult mites and the life cycle is completed in about 3 weeks. Transfer from animal to animal probably occurs through close contact. Some animals tolerate the presence of ear mites without apparent discomfort, although the external ear canal may produce excessive wax, which appears like brown coffee grounds. Others, particularly dogs, will show pruritus and inflammation. Affected animals can be treated with an acaricidal product applied down the ear canal,

or with a systemic product such as selamectin or imidacloprid/moxidectin (Curtis 2004).

- *Chorioptes equi* – similar in appearance to *O. cynotis* but has cup-shaped suckers on the end of unjointed pedicels. It is found on the surface of horses' skin, particularly on the feathered lower legs of heavy horses.
- *Psoroptes cuniculi* (Fig. 29.14) – has trumpet-shaped suckers on the end of jointed pedicels or stalks and causes 'ear canker' in rabbits.
- *Psoroptes equi* – identical in appearance to *P. cuniculi* and causes an itchy dermatitis in horses.
- *Cheyletiella* spp. – are parasites of cats, dogs and rabbits, each host having its own species, although the individual species may not be entirely host-specific. The mites are large (about 0.5 mm in length) so can just about be seen with the naked eye. They possess large claws on their palps and comb-like appendages on the ends of their legs (Fig. 29.15). They typically cause a

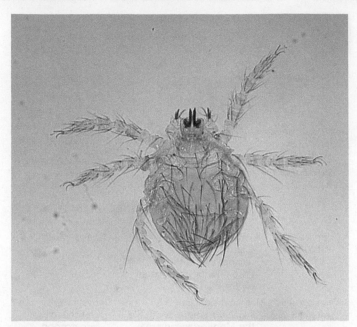

Fig. 29.16 The larvae of *Neotrombicula* or *Trombicula autumnalis* mites are hairy and have six legs. Measures approx. 200 μm

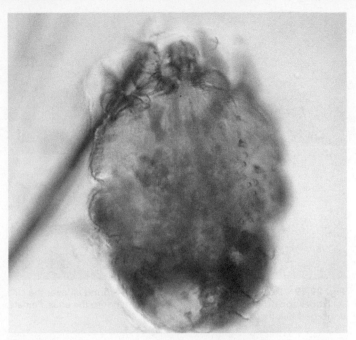

Fig. 29.17 *Sarcoptes* spp. mites are rotund with short legs. The back is covered in pegs and spines and the anus is terminal. Measures approx. 360 μm

scurfy dermatitis, sometimes with erythema, and the condition is often referred to as 'walking dandruff'. There is evidence that mites are capable of surviving for some days in the environment, so cleaning of the environment is recommended, alongside acaricidal treatment of affected animals.

- *Trombicula* or *Neotrombicula autumnalis* larvae (Fig. 29.16) parasitize animals for a short time in high summer. The mites are hairy and bright orange and can be seen as small orange spots formed by a cluster of larvae. Once they have fed, the larvae drop off into the environment and complete their life cycle. The larvae can cause pruritus and dermatitis.

Subsurface mites

- *Sarcoptes scabiei* (Fig. 29.17) – a parasite of foxes and dogs and occasionally horses, cats and rabbits. There appear to be different strains, referred to as, for example, *Sarcoptes scabiei* var. *canis*, relating to the host species. The mite has pegs and spines on its dorsal surface. Female mites burrow into the stratum corneum of the skin and lay eggs within the burrows. Immature mites hatch from the eggs, develop, then move to create burrows of their own. The infection typically begins in the pinna, elbow or hock area causing an erythematous, alopecic dermatitis that is extremely pruritic. Untreated, crusting lesions develop that can spread to cover much of the animal. A similar parasite of cats is *Notoedres cati*, which has a dorsal anus and concentric rings on its dorsum. It does not occur in the UK but is found in several European countries, as well as in other warmer parts of the world. Infection by *Notoedres* spp. also occurs in rats, where it can be associated with dermatitis. *Trixacarus caviae* is the burrowing mite that commonly occurs in guinea pigs and is similar in appearance to *S. scabiei*.

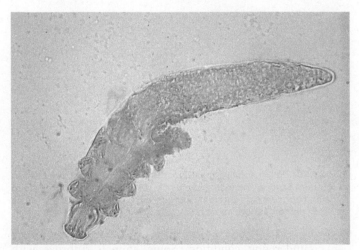

Fig. 29.18 *Demodex* spp. mites are often described as cigar-shaped. The legs are arranged in pairs at the front of the body. Measures approx. 0.2 mm

- *Demodex* spp. (Fig. 29.18) – cigar-shaped and believed to be normal inhabitants of hair follicles in many species. Occasionally in dogs and rarely in cats, host immunosuppression or immunomodulation allows the population of *Demodex* spp. to expand, and this is associated with local or widespread areas of alopecia. The local form may be non-pruritic and may self-resolve but the generalised form is more severe and is very unlikely to clear without treatment. Affected dogs can be in considerable pain and secondary bacterial infection is not uncommon. Treatment should be carried out with a suitable acaricide, but a cure may not be achieved, particularly when it is not possible to identify or treat the

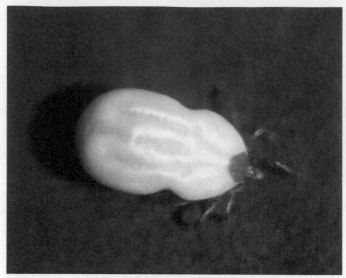

Fig. 29.19 *Ixodes* spp. are the ticks commonly found all over the UK. All *Ixodes* spp. ticks have a groove that runs anterior to the anus. Female engorged tick measures approx. 1 cm

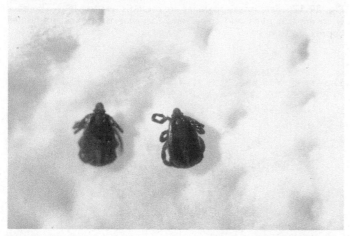

Fig. 29.20 *Rhipicephalus sanguineus* is the predominant tick species in southern Europe and is an important disease vector. Here a male and female are shown side by side; both are quite plain and brown, hence its other name, 'the brown dog tick'. Size varies from 1 to 12 mm

	TABLE 29.3	Common tick species of dogs and cats in Europe	
Tick species	**Approximate geographical location**	**Main infections transmitted**
Ixodes ricinus	Throughout Europe, including the UK	Lyme disease, tick-borne encephalitis (northern Europe)
Ixodes hexagonus	Throughout Europe, including the UK	May be involved in disease transmission but role less well defined than that of *I. ricinus*
Dermacentor reticulatus	Mainland Europe from Germany south. A few distinct foci in the UK. Potential for importation on travelling pets	*Babesia canis*
Rhipicephalus sanguineus	Mainland Europe from southern France south (i.e. the Mediterranean area). Sporadic reports of infestation establishing following the importation of travelling pets carrying the parasite. Establishment in the UK likely only in protected environments such as homes and kennels	*Babesia canis, Ehrlichia canis, Hepatozoon canis*

underlying condition. Some animals improve with treatment but relapses require repeated treatment.

Ticks

Ticks look similar to mites but are the only parasites to possess a hypostome, part of the specialised mouthparts developed for piercing skin, attaching and removing blood from the host. Larval ticks may be only about 1 mm in length, while fully fed female ticks can reach up to 1 cm. Most ticks parasitizing dogs, cats, horses and other pets are 'hard' ticks and possess a scutum or shield on their dorsal surface (Figs. 29.19 and 29.20). In the female this covers just the anterior portion but male ticks are entirely covered by the scutum. There are a number of species of tick but relatively few that infest dogs and cats in the UK (Table 29.3).

Life cycle: All ticks spend part of their life cycle in the environment, as females lay their eggs on the ground in a suitably moist location before dying. Once hatched, larval ticks have to locate a host, attach and feed. Once they have fed for a few days,

depending on the species, they may remain on the same host to develop to the nymphal stage or may drop off to continue their development in the environment.

Most ticks on cats or dogs drop off after both the larval and nymphal stages and, as they thus have to find a separate host to feed on at each stage, they are known as 'three-host' ticks.

As ticks suck blood, a heavy infection can cause anaemia but this occurs rarely in dogs and cats, and ticks are generally most important in these species as vectors of diseases, including Lyme disease and babesiosis. Ticks can also transmit infections to humans, although the source of the ticks is not normally directly from pets; rather, they are derived from wildlife reservoirs. Since the introduction of the PETS travel scheme (www.defra.gov.uk), ticks have become important as a source of non-endemic diseases such as *Babesia canis*. Compulsory acaricidal treatment of dogs and cats prior to their entry into the UK was introduced, but is no longer required. It is important to advise pet owners of the need for adequate tick control throughout their stay in continental Europe. The risk of tick infections can be reduced by avoiding tick-infested areas such as woodland, especially during spring, summer and autumn when ticks are most active. Whenever possible, pets should be checked daily and any ticks removed using, for example, a proprietary tick-removal device. Alternatively, or additionally, ticks can be repelled using pyrethroid-based products and pets can be protected by using a suitable acaricide.

FUNGI

Fungi exist as unicellular yeasts or multi-nuclear mycelia (Fig. 29.21) and most are non-parasitic. Several species of fungi

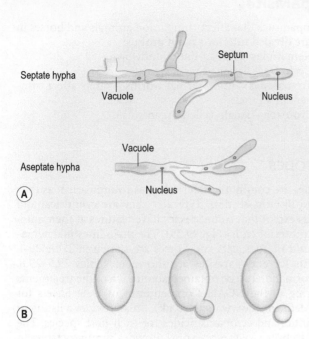

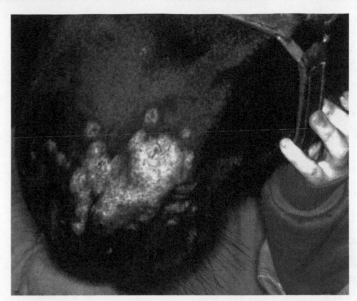

Fig. 29.22 Ringworm lesions may vary from a small area of alopecia to a severe thickened and pruritic lesion. Here lesions on the nose of a horse are caused by *Microsporum gypseum (Courtesy of Mark Craig)*

Fig. 29.21 Fungi appear as (A) mycelia or (B) yeast-like organisms

are parasitic – dermatophytes or ringworm-causing species and the yeasts *Candida albicans* and *Malassezia* spp. in particular.

Ringworm

Ringworm is caused by *Trichophyton* spp. or *Microsporum* spp. Spores are introduced onto abraded skin and then a mycelium begins to develop in hair or keratinised skin. Classically, an area of alopecia develops, which gradually becomes larger in diameter, with infection disappearing as a result of the inflammatory response in the centre, which heals as the infection spreads outwards. Some infections show signs of inflammation or pruritus while others do not (Fig. 29.22). Some species, e.g. *Microsporum canis* infection in cats, have adapted so well to the host that infection can remain inapparent. The simplest way to diagnose infection in cats and dogs is to expose suspect lesions to ultraviolet light, as about 50% of *Microsporum canis* lesions fluoresce under a Wood's lamp. Where fluorescence does not occur, however, it is necessary to collect hair and/or superficial skin samples and examine them directly or submit them for culturing. Samples for direct examination can be placed on a microscope slide, covered with water or Q-ink (which will preferentially stain fungal elements) and a coverslip and then examine for fungal hyphae or arthrospores (Fig. 29.23). The classic medium for dermatophyte culture is Sabouraud's agar but, as dermatophytes can be slow-growing, several media designed to show a rapid colour change in the presence of a dermatophyte have been developed, e.g. dermatophyte test medium (Markey et al. 2013).

Candida albicans

C. albicans is a normal commensal yeast but occasionally overgrows on mucous membranes or even on skin, usually in young or immunocompromised animals. Smears from affected areas show numerous yeasts that must be differentiated from *Malassezia* spp. organisms.

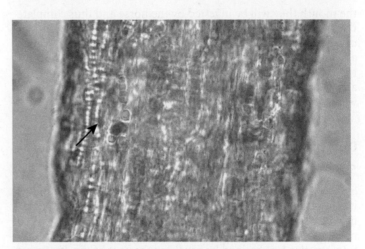

Fig. 29.23 Arthrospore formation (arrowed) in or on hairs that occurs with ringworm infection can be used diagnostically *(Courtesy of Mark Craig)*

Malassezia

Malassezia spp. (Fig. 29.24) can be found on normal skin but the population may grow on some animals to cause an itchy, red dermatitis. The skin may appear greasy and the animal may smell rancid. Swabs or Sellotape strip samples can be collected, stained with Diff-Quik or equivalent and examined for *Malassezia* spp. organisms. Infection occurs more commonly in dogs than cats, and infection occurs more commonly in some breeds of dog, such as the basset hound and West Highland white terrier. Shampooing with a treatment effective against *Malassezia* spp. usually controls the condition (Miller et al. 2012). (For further details see Chapter 31.)

Nematode-related dermatitis

In horses, *Habronema* spp. and *Draschia megastoma* are stomach worms that are transmitted by flies. Flies deposit infective larvae as they feed on secretions or wounds. If the larvae are close to

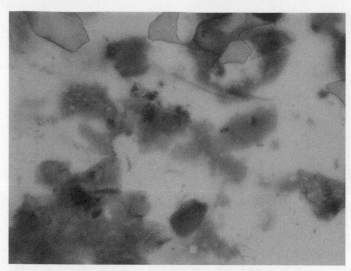

Fig. 29.24 *Malassezia* organisms are bottle-shaped yeasts, some of which may appear to be budding. This slide was stained with methylene blue. Each organism measures 3 μm in length

the mouth they will be ingested by the horse and thus complete the life cycle. Elsewhere the larvae burrow into the skin and cause moist, weeping lesions that are slow to heal and are known as 'summer sores'. The larvae or microfilariae of another nematode, *Onchocerca cervicalis*, can gather in the skin and may be associated with patches of dermatitis with alopecia and scaling, which may be itchy.

DIAGNOSIS OF ECTOPARASITE INFECTION

Specimen collection and examination

Surface parasites can be examined by placing coat brushings into a suitable container and examining with the aid of a magnifying lens or stereo microscope. Take care that any fleas present do not hop away at this stage. Evidence of flea infestation can also be obtained by brushing the coat of the dog or cat over damp absorbent paper. If fleas are present then any flea faeces will fall onto the paper. This then appears as a small black speck surrounded by a halo of red partly digested blood.

Burrowing mites can be collected from scrapings taken from the edge of lesions. Some people like to add a little liquid paraffin to the scalpel blade so that the material attaches to the blade. Alternatively, *Demodex* spp. can sometimes be collected by plucking hairs, since the mites can be found around the hair root. Collected material is placed on to a microscope slide and more liquid paraffin, or a 10% potassium hydroxide (KOH) solution, is added (but the two should not be mixed). Liquid paraffin allows any mites to remain alive, so movement may be seen, while KOH preparations can be left or heated and this assists in removing keratin, making mites more readily visible. However, KOH solution will kill the mites, so movement will not be seen. The preparation should be covered with a coverslip and examined systematically. Alternatively, biopsy samples can be collected for histology, which is particularly useful where the parasites are found deep in the skin. There are additional tests such as blood and skin tests that can be used to help to confirm some parasite infestations including fleas and *S. scabiei*. (For further details see Chapter 31.)

Endoparasites

The endoparasites that affect companion animals and horses in the UK are divided into four main groups:

- **Nematodes** – thread-like roundworms
- **Cestodes** – flattened tapeworms
- **Trematodes** – flukes or flat worms – rarely affect companion animals
- **Protozoa** – single-celled organisms.

NEMATODES

Nematodes are commonly referred to as roundworms, as they are round in cross-section. Typically, they are cylindrical and featureless except that some species have features at their anterior and posterior ends (Fig. 29.25). The main intestinal nematodes found in dogs, cats and horses are shown in Table 29.4. Treatments for endoparasites are shown in Tables 29.5–29.8. More information can be obtained about each of the treatments by referring to the NOAH Compendium of Data Sheets for Animal Medicines (www.noah.co.uk). This provides a listing of anthelmintics and ectoparasiticides for each host species. The ESCCAP website (www.esccap.org) provides summary tables of treatments for companion animals.

Ascarids

The ascarids are found in the small intestine and are the largest roundworms found in dogs, cats and horses.

Toxocara canis. Adult female *T. canis* can measure up to 20 cm in length (Fig. 29.26), are off-white and possess cuticular enlargements at their anterior end known as cervical alae.

Life cycle: Eggs laid by adult female worms are passed in faeces and embryonate in the environment. This occurs in approximately 11 days in optimal conditions and more slowly in cooler weather (Lloyd 1993). The eggs are protected by a thick outer shell and can survive in the environment for extended periods. Survival for over a year has been recorded but this may be reduced by desiccation or exposure to ultraviolet light. Dogs become infected when they ingest eggs from the environment or eat prey that have themselves eaten eggs and are carrying infective larvae in their tissues. Depending on the route of infection (Fig. 29.27) the larvae migrate through the liver and lungs or remain in the intestine to develop into adult worms. Larvae that have migrated may return to the intestine or migrate into tissues, where they remain as somatic larvae. In a bitch, some somatic larvae are reactivated when pregnancy occurs and they migrate across the placenta to the pups from about the 42nd day of pregnancy or, particularly when infection has occurred late in pregnancy, across the mammary gland to infect pups in milk. As a result, pups can carry a large number of egg-laying worms from about 3 weeks of age. When a pup has had a heavy infection the worms are expelled as the pup grows older and subsequent infection will tend to result in somatic larvae and not intestinal infections. The factors that result in adult dogs acquiring patent intestinal infections, however, are not clearly understood and it is estimated that about 10% of adult dogs carry infection, with infection possibly occurring intermittently in a larger proportion of dogs.

A small number of intestinal worms are well tolerated by dogs, as are developing worms or somatic larvae. A heavy

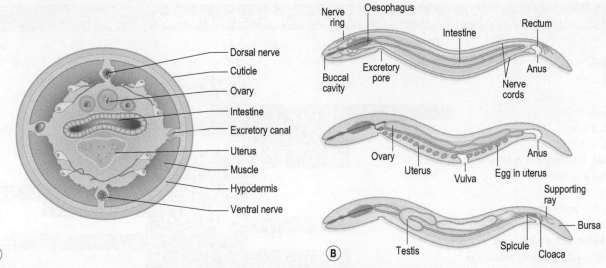

Fig. 29.25 Nematodes. (A) Cross-section through a typical nematode. (B) Longitudinal sections

TABLE 29.4	Major intestinal nematodes of dogs, cats and horses		
Nematode group	**Cat**	**Dog**	**Horse**
Ascarids	Toxocara cati Toxascaris leonina	Toxocara canis Toxascaris leonina	Parascaris equorum
Hookworms	Ancylostoma tubaeforme Uncinaria stenocephala	Ancylostoma caninum Uncinaria stenocephala	
Whipworms		Trichuris vulpis	
Strongyles			Cyathostominae Large strongyles
Pinworms			Oxyuris equi

TABLE 29.5	Anthelmintic agents		
Active ingredient	**Chemical group**	**Mode of action**	**Administration route**
Febantel, fenbendazole	Benzimidazoles	Prevent tubulin construction	Oral
Oxantel, pyrantel	Tetrahydropyrimidines	Neuromuscular paralysis	Oral
Milbemycin oxime, Moxidectin, Selamectin	Macrocyclic lactones	Inhibit GABA-gated chloride channels	Oral or spot on
Nitroscanate	Isothiocyanate	–	Oral
Piperazine	–	Affects neuromuscular transmission	Oral
Praziquantel	Isoquinoline	Damage to parasite tegument and other effects	Oral, spot on

burden of migrating larvae in a puppy however, can cause pneumonia as the worms pass through the lungs. Adult worms interfere with absorption of nutrients and a heavy burden can cause a pup to be cachectic, with an intestine distended by worms. Intestinal worms may cause acute emergencies such as intestinal obstruction or intussusception.

Zoonotic infection: Humans can be infected by accidentally ingesting embryonated eggs from the environment. Clinical signs are seen most commonly in children, although a larger proportion of the population is seropositive, indicating exposure without showing clinical signs. There are two classical disease entities: ocular larva migrans (OLM), associated with larval migration within the eye, and visceral larva migrans (VLM), associated with mass larval migration through, for example, the liver. A third syndrome, known as covert toxocarosis, is associated with ill-defined symptoms including 'flu-like' symptoms. There is evidence of association between *Toxocara* infection and asthma and reduced respiratory function, and *Toxocara* and reduced cognitive ability.

It is very difficult to prevent dogs acquiring infection from the environment when they walk in public places such as parks. Control depends on the prevention of egg output by appropriate anthelmintic treatment of the dog. Treatments are focused on pre-weaned pups and their dams, as bitches can carry patent infections while they are lactating. Weaned pups and adult dogs can then be treated at appropriate intervals. Dogs should be

TABLE 29.6 The spectrum of activity offered by different canine antiparasitic products

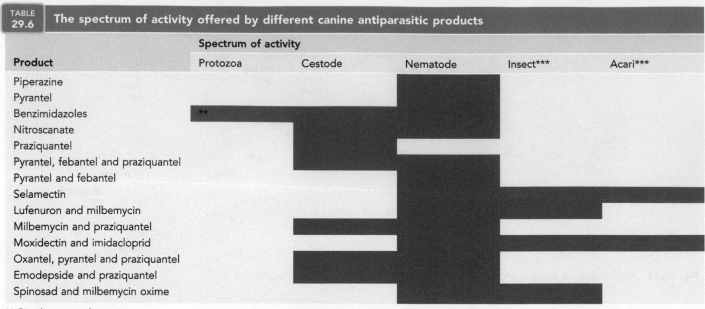

Product	Spectrum of activity				
	Protozoa	Cestode	Nematode	Insect***	Acari***
Piperazine					
Pyrantel					
Benzimidazoles**					
Nitroscanate					
Praziquantel					
Pyrantel, febantel and praziquantel					
Pyrantel and febantel					
Selamectin					
Lufenuron and milbemycin					
Milbemycin and praziquantel					
Moxidectin and imidacloprid					
Oxantel, pyrantel and praziquantel					
Emodepside and praziquantel					
Spinosad and milbemycin oxime					

**Giardia spp. only.
***Some genera only – see individual data sheets for more information.
Note: diagram is based on the data sheet claims for the products.

TABLE 29.7 Diagram of the spectrum of activity offered by different feline antiparasitic products

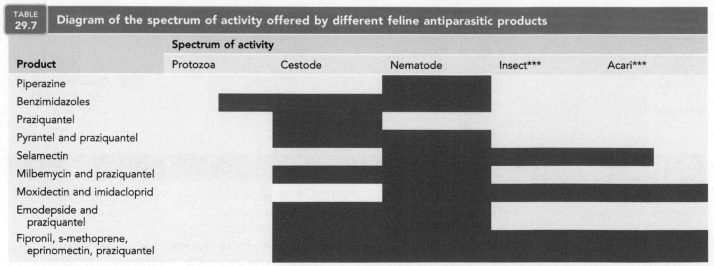

Product	Spectrum of activity				
	Protozoa	Cestode	Nematode	Insect***	Acari***
Piperazine					
Benzimidazoles					
Praziquantel					
Pyrantel and praziquantel					
Selamectin					
Milbemycin and praziquantel					
Moxidectin and imidacloprid					
Emodepside and praziquantel					
Fipronil, s-methoprene, eprinomectin, praziquantel					

Note: diagram is based on the data sheet claims for the products.
***Some genera only – see individual data sheets for more information.

TABLE 29.8 The spectrum of activity offered by different equine antiparasitic products

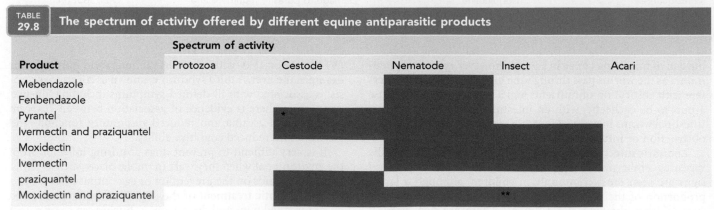

Product	Spectrum of activity				
	Protozoa	Cestode	Nematode	Insect	Acari
Mebendazole					
Fenbendazole					
Pyrantel*					
Ivermectin and praziquantel					
Moxidectin					
Ivermectin					
praziquantel					
Moxidectin and praziquantel			**		

*At double the normal dose rate.
**Bots only.
Note: diagram is based on the data sheet claims for the products.

prevented from defecating in children's play areas and faeces should be picked up.

Toxocara cati. *T. cati* are similar in appearance to *T. canis* but if they are examined under a stereo microscope it may be seen that the cuticular enlargements at the anterior end are like

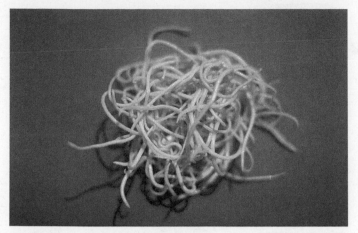

Fig. 29.26 Adult *Toxocara canis* are stout, off-white or pinkish worms when fresh (these are preserved specimens)

arrowheads. The life cycle of *T. cati* is similar to that of *T. canis* except that there is no prenatal migration of larvae across the placenta so kittens first acquire infection from the queen in milk (Fig. 29.28). This means that kittens are probably about 6 weeks old when they begin passing *T. cati* eggs in their faeces.

A small number of worms will be well tolerated by a cat, but a large number may interfere with intestinal function. A large number of larvae following a hepatotracheal migration may cause pneumonia or even death of young kittens. In the past, *T. cati* has not been regarded as as much a zoonotic risk as *T. canis*; however, there is evidence that *T. cati* and *T. canis* should be regarded as equally important zoonoses (Fisher 2003). Cats may acquire infection through ingesting embryonated eggs from the environment or by eating infected paratenic hosts such as mice. Control is normally based on anthelmintic treatment, as prevention of infection is almost impossible unless the animals are maintained in specialised environments. As cats may carry patent infection at any age, anthelmintic treatment should be repeated at regular intervals.

Toxascaris leonina. *T. leonina* can infect both dogs and cats and has a life cycle similar to *T. canis*, but animals are only infected by ingesting eggs or paratenic hosts. Dogs and cats do

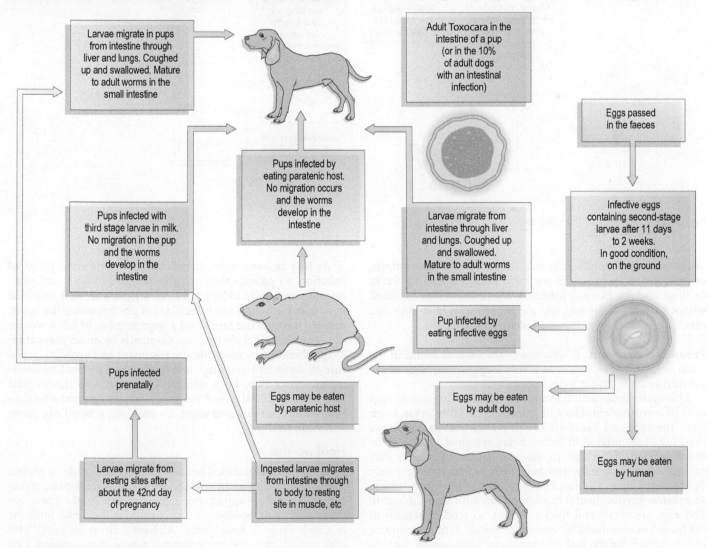

Fig. 29.27 Life cycle of *Toxocara canis*

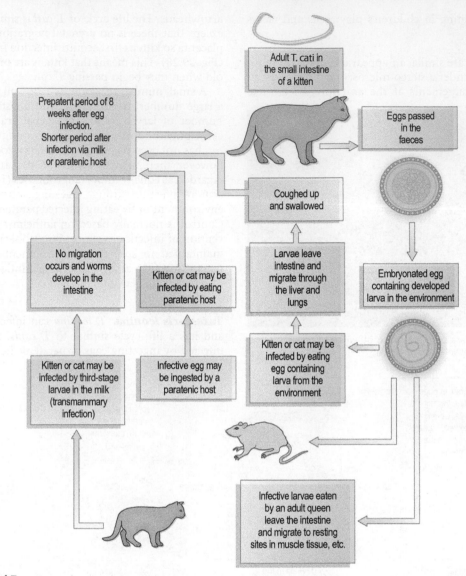

Fig. 29.28   Life cycle of *Toxocara cati*

not acquire a patent infection until they are about three months of age or older, because the prepatent period is about 8 weeks in dogs and 13 in cats. Infection is normally well-tolerated without clinical signs and, like the other ascarids in dogs and cats, *T. leonina* is regarded as a potential zoonosis.

Parascaris equorum. *P. equorum* is the ascarid found in the small intestine of horses. It is a very large worm, with adults measuring up to 40 cm long.

Life cycle: Foals acquire infection from embryonated eggs in their environment. Once ingested the infective larvae hatch from the eggs and penetrate the intestinal wall to undergo a hepatotracheal migration before being coughed up and swallowed, thereby returning to the small intestine, where they mature to adult worms and begin egg-laying approximately 10–12 weeks after infection. Egg output by adult worms is high, so massive environmental contamination with eggs can occur. The eggs are sticky and thickly coated, so tend to remain in the horse's environment for extended periods, acting as a source of reinfection for the foal or a source of infection for foals in subsequent seasons.

As they become older, horses become more recalcitrant to infection, so patent infections are common in foals and yearlings but unusual in older horses. A few worms are well-tolerated but a heavy infection can cause signs of pneumonia as the larvae migrate through the lungs and a large number of adult worms can cause intestinal obstruction. Control is based on prevention of egg shedding by anthelmintic treatment and avoiding exposure of foals and yearlings to heavily contaminated environments. There have been reports of resistance to macrocyclic lactone anthelmintics by *P. equorum* and so treatment effectiveness should be evaluated using, for example, a faecal egg count reduction test.

Hookworms

Hookworms are so-called because the buccal capsule or mouth of the worm is set at an angle to the body of the worm, giving a slightly hooked appearance like a crochet hook. There are many species of hookworm that parasitize the small intestine in a wide range of host species. All have a direct life cycle, with eggs passed into the environment, where they develop into infective larvae. Three species that infect cats or dogs will be

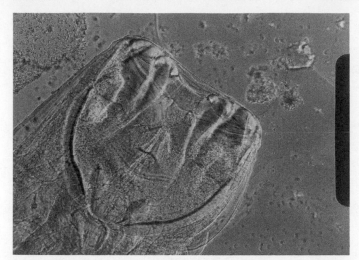

Fig. 29.29 Head end of *Ancylostoma caninum*. Like other hookworms it has a large buccal capsule. *A. caninum* has two pairs each of three teeth

considered in more detail: *Uncinaria stenocephala, Ancylostoma caninum* and *Ancylostoma tubaeforme*. In each case the adult worm measures about 1.5 cm.

Uncinaria stenocephala. *U. stenocephala* is also known as the 'northern hookworm' and is the hookworm that occurs endemically in dogs in the UK. It has a typically large buccal capsule with two cutting plates at the entrance. Dogs are infected when they ingest infective larvae from the environment and the prepatent period is about 3 weeks. The larvae can penetrate skin but in doing so only cause a local dermatitis, unlike other hookworm species where larvae are capable both of penetrating skin and migrating through the animal to culminate in an intestinal infection. Infection is most likely to occur in dogs in kennels such as greyhound or hunt kennels. Dogs carrying a heavy infection may have diarrhoea and there will be some intestinal protein loss. Cats may also carry infection, although they appear to be rarely infected in the UK.

Ancylostoma caninum. *A. caninum* is endemic in continental Europe and has been recorded sporadically in the UK. The buccal capsule has two pairs each of three teeth at the entrance (Fig. 29.29). The larvae in the environment prefer a higher temperature to *U. stenocephala* larvae and so flourish best in warmer climates than the UK. It may be possible for infection to become established in the UK, either in a sheltered kennel environment or in southern England, and the infection may be imported in dogs that have lived in Europe. Dogs are infected by larval penetration through the skin or by ingesting infective larvae (Fig. 29.30). Some larvae fail to develop into adult worms in the intestine, instead remaining as larvae in tissues. Some of these larvae can transfer from the dam to pups in milk. In large numbers, milk-acquired larvae can cause the death of pups by 10 days of age, before the infection has had time to become patent. A low level of intestinal infection is well tolerated but the worms are voracious blood suckers, grasping the intestinal mucosa with their mouths and slashing with the teeth in their buccal capsule, so a heavy infection results in substantial blood loss and subsequent anaemia. Not all the blood is consumed by the worms and large amounts can pass in the faeces, appearing as bloody mucus or blackened blood, which is termed 'melena'.

Over a long term, a smaller number of worms can cause anaemia due to chronic blood loss. Penetrating *A. caninum* can cause dermatitis in dogs and humans and *A. caninum* has caused eosinophilic enteritis in humans.

Ancylostoma tubaeforme. *A. tubaeforme* is a hookworm of cats. It has a buccal capsule with two pairs of three teeth at the entrance to the mouth. It does not appear to be prevalent in the UK but has been reported in cats in mainland Europe and so may be imported in cats entering the UK. *A. tubaeforme* is a blood sucker and can cause anaemia with either a heavy infection or a smaller chronic infection.

Whipworms

Trichuris vulpis. These are known as whipworms, as their anterior end is long and narrow like the lash of a whip and the posterior end broad like a whip handle (Fig. 29.31). The adult worms are found in the large intestine, where the anterior end is buried in the mucosa and the posterior end is free in the lumen. They are found occasionally in the UK, particularly in dogs in kennels. Infections are most likely in southern England, where the climate is most favourable for the development of the infective stages in the environment. Once passed in faeces, the eggs embryonate in the environment, with the larvae remaining within the shell once developed (Fig. 29.32). The larvae are thus protected from environmental conditions and can remain viable for up to one year in favourable conditions. This means that substantial infection can accumulate in the kennel or surroundings of infected dogs. A low-level infection is well tolerated but a heavy infection can result in diarrhoea and metabolic disturbance if untreated. Established infections can be treated using a suitable anthelmintic and thereafter repeat infections can be prevented by moving the animals to uncontaminated surroundings and/or regular anthelmintic treatment. Repeat faecal sampling to monitor the success of any control programme is suggested.

***Strongyloides* species.** Infection with *Strongyloides* spp. is typically seen in young animals. The worms are tiny and hairlike, characterised by an oesophagus that is approximately one-third of the length of the entire worm. *S. westeri* is an important infection in young foals from about 2 weeks of age. Larvae pass from the mare in the milk and develop in the foal's small intestine with a prepatent period of 8–14 days. Infection can be supplemented with larvae ingested directly from the environment and a heavy infection can cause diarrhoea and ill-thrift. As foals become older, patent infections and associated clinical signs become less common. Although less common than infection in horses, occasionally dogs show diarrhoea associated with *Strongyloides* spp. infection.

Strongyles

Cyathostomins. Horses have a large number of species of nematodes that inhabit the large intestine, many of which are about 1 cm in length (Fig. 29.33). There are more than 40 different species but they are grouped together as the cyathostomins (or cyathostomes), also known as the 'small strongyles' or trichonemes. The life cycle is direct, with horses acquiring infection by ingesting third-stage larvae off pasture. The young larvae burrow into the wall of the large intestine, where they may remain in a state of suspended development or hypobiosis for extended periods, or develop and emerge after a short period

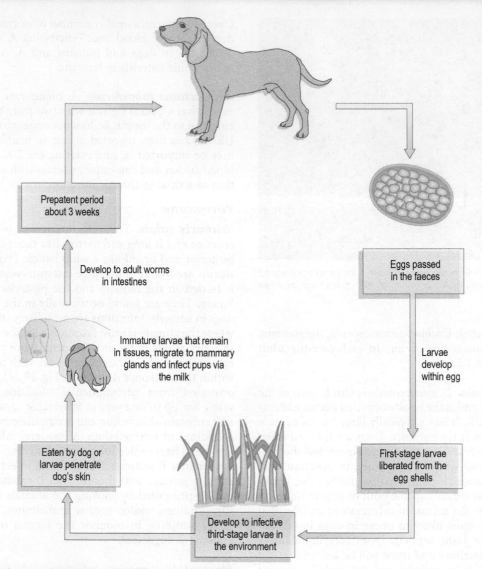

Fig. 29.30 Life cycle of *Ancylostoma caninum*

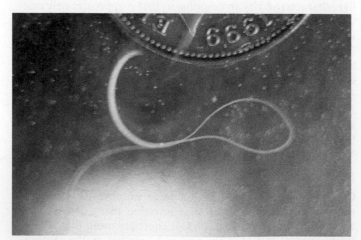

Fig. 29.31 *Trichuris vulpis*, the whipworm, next to a 1p coin to illustrate size

to develop into adults within the lumen of the intestine. The adults are found close to the wall of the intestine, where they feed on the superficial layers of the intestinal mucosa. Adult worms lay typical 'strongyle' eggs that are passed in faeces and develop on pasture.

Low levels of infection are well tolerated but contamination can build up substantially on pasture, and a heavy infection, especially in foals or yearlings, can cause poor condition, anaemia and diarrhoea. An acute syndrome may be seen in spring when thousands of hypobiotic larvae leave the mucosa simultaneously to continue their development. Many may be passed in the faeces and appear as a red layer on the surface of dung. Affected animals show profuse diarrhoea, weight loss and sometimes colic and death. Control depends on reducing the access of horses to larvae on pasture by measures such as avoiding heavily contaminated pasture and dung collection, together with anthelmintic treatment. Over the past decade there has been a move away from reliance on anthelmintic treatment, partly because of increased awareness of the development of anthelmintic resistance towards a combination of monitoring of egg counts and pasture management, with anthelmintic treatment as indicated by season or egg count results.

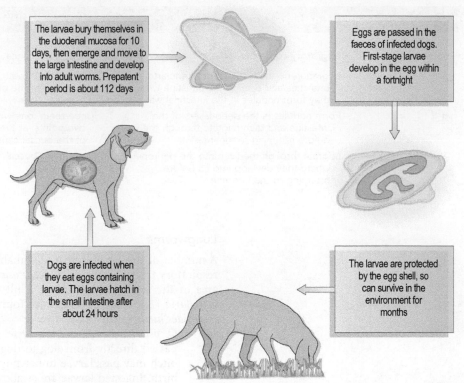

The larvae bury themselves in the duodenal mucosa for 10 days, then emerge and move to the large intestine and develop into adult worms. Prepatent period is about 112 days

Eggs are passed in the faeces of infected dogs. First-stage larvae develop in the egg within a fortnight

Dogs are infected when they eat eggs containing larvae. The larvae hatch in the small intestine after about 24 hours

The larvae are protected by the egg shell, so can survive in the environment for months

Fig. 29.32 Life cycle of *Trichuris vulpis*

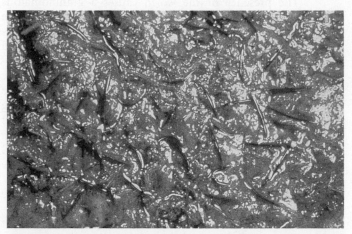

Fig. 29.33 The cyathostomes or small strongyles are small worms that can be present in enormous numbers in the large intestine of a horse (Courtesy of Merial Animal Health)

Large strongyles. Three species of nematode occur in the large intestine but have a migratory life cycle and are larger than the small strongyles, so are known as the large strongyles to differentiate them. The species are *Strongylus vulgaris*, *Strongylus equinus* and *Strongylus edentatus* and the features of each species are shown in Table 29.9 and Figures 29.34–29.36. Infection, particularly with *S. vulgaris* larvae, can cause severe clinical signs. *S. vulgaris* larvae in the cranial mesenteric artery cause considerable pathology, including clot formation and infarction caused by blockage of a branch of the artery and subsequent death of the area of intestine supplied by that artery. The adult worms cause small ulcers as they feed on the large intestinal mucosa. Control is based on pasture management and anthelmintic treatment as described for the cyathostomes. As a cautionary note, care must be taken to ensure that large strongyles are not able to make a 'comeback' by total reliance on faecal egg count monitoring when faecal egg counts may be low for extended periods, providing large strongyles with sufficient time to complete their development in the horse.

Triodontophorus species. *Triodontophorus* spp. are a third group of strongyle nematodes that inhabit the large intestine of the horse. They are differentiated primarily by their feeding habit. They feed as a large group, causing the formation of deep ulcers that may measure several centimetres in diameter.

Pinworms

Oxyuris equi. *O. equi* is the pinworm of horses, so called because the worms look like carpet tacks. The females measure up to 10 cm but the male worms measure only about 1 cm. The worms inhabit the large intestine but unusually the female worms leave the intestine to lay their eggs on the perineum around the anus of the horse. Larvae develop in the egg and horses are reinfected by ingesting eggs containing fully developed larvae. The prepatent period is 5 months. The activity of the female worms on the perineum and the presence of the eggs can cause severe irritation, seen as rubbing and alopecia over the tail head. Infection can be diagnosed by placing a piece of sticky tape across the perineum around the anus and examining it microscopically for eggs. Control is based on anthelmintic treatment, which can be supplemented in heavy infections by washing of the perineal area to remove eggs. This is a species that may be somewhat difficult to remove with anthelmintics, therefore choosing an anthelmintic with *O. equi* as an indication plus monitoring effective removal after treatment is advisable.

TABLE 29.9	Summary of the large strongyles of horses			
Species	Prepatent period (months)	Migratory route of larvae	Adult appearance	Adult length (cm)
Strongylus vulgaris	6–7	Migration up the cranial mesenteric artery and branches and back to the intestine where they form nodules in the intestinal wall	Two rounded teeth at the base of the buccal capsule	1.5–2.5
Strongylus equinus	8–9	Form nodules in the deep layers of the intestine and then migrate through the liver before returning to the intestine	Three teeth, one with two points, at the base of the buccal capsule	2.5–5.0
Strongylus edentatus	10–12	Migrate through the liver into the peritoneum where they develop into L5 before returning to the intestine	No teeth in buccal capsule	2.5–4.5

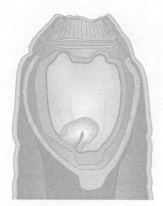

Fig. 29.34 Head of *Strongylus vulgaris*

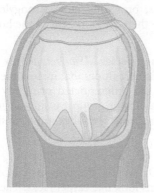

Fig. 29.35 Head of *Strongylus equinus*

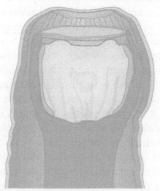

Fig. 29.36 Head of *Strongylus edentatus*

Lungworms

A number of species of nematode inhabit the lungs and upper respiratory tract. In the dog, *Oslerus osleri* is found around the area of the tracheal bifurcation, adult *Crenosoma vulpis* and *Capillaria (Eucoleus) aerophila* are found in the bronchi and *Filaroides hirthi* occur in the alveoli:

- *O. osleri* has a direct life cycle, with first-stage larvae passed directly from dog to dog in saliva. An infected bitch may pass larvae to her pups within a few days of birth. Ingested larvae are swallowed and migrate from the intestine to the lungs, where they ascend the respiratory tree and grow to adults at the base of the trachea. The presence of the worm causes a granulomatous lesion to grow around it, so that the worms become completely enclosed. These nodules may be well tolerated but can be associated with exercise intolerance and coughing, particularly in dogs at exercise.
- *C. vulpis* is known as the fox lungworm as it is endemic in the fox population. Slugs or snails act as intermediate hosts so dogs become infected by eating an infected slug or snail. A heavy infection may be associated with coughing or exercise intolerance.
- *C. (Eucoleus) aerophila* have a similar appearance to *T. vulpis*, but are smaller and are found embedded in the bronchial wall.

Most lungworm infections can be diagnosed by finding larvae in the faeces using the Baermann technique or in bronchoalveolar fluid. The exception is *C. aerophila*, which produces eggs that are not dissimilar to *T. vulpis* eggs, except the polar plugs are smaller and the outer surface is rough. *O. osleri* nodules can sometimes be seen as radio-opaque densities in the trachea. Adult *C. vulpis* may be found in bronchoalveolar fluid, where they appear like pieces of white thread.

- *Aelurostrogylus abstrusus* is the main lungworm in cats. This has an indirect life cycle with a slug or snail as intermediate host. Cats may be infected by eating slugs or snails or possibly small mammals that act as paratenic hosts. Infection may be well tolerated but some cats show respiratory signs, including coughing. Cats can also be infected with *C. aerophila*.
- *Dictyocaulus arnfieldi* is the lung nematode that occurs in the horse. The life cycle is direct, with larvae passed in the faeces and developing to third-stage larvae on pasture. Ingested infective larvae leave the intestine and migrate to the lungs, where the slender adult worms are found in the smaller bronchi. The prepatent period

is about 2 months and the female adult worms lay eggs that have often hatched by the time they are coughed up. Infection in donkeys can be symptomless, while infection in horses can be associated with chronic coughing, sometimes in the absence of a patent infection.

Heartworms

There are two nematodes that inhabit the pulmonary artery and the right side of the heart in the dog – *Angiostrongylus vasorum* and *Dirofilaria immitis*.

- *Angiostrongylus vasorum* occurs in both dogs and foxes in the UK. The first reports in dogs about 20 years ago were limited to Cornwall, South Wales and the southeast of England but it has now been reported in many parts of the UK including Scotland. The adult worms measure only about 2 cm in length, very different from the 30 cm of female *D. immitis*, so there is little problem in differentiating the two species. Dogs are infected when they ingest infected slugs or snails and the larvae leave the intestine and migrate to the pulmonary artery (Fig. 29.37). Female worms lay eggs that are swept into the lung circulation. These hatch and the larvae migrate into the alveoli and are eventually coughed up, swallowed and passed in faeces. A wide range of clinical signs may be seen with some, such as clotting disorders, being related to the presence of worms in the circulatory system and others caused by pulmonary damage. Infection can be diagnosed by finding the characteristic larvae in the faeces using the Baermann technique. Sensitivity is increased by testing three faecal samples collected on consecutive days or in bronchoalveolar fluid. There is now an antigen detection test (Angio Detect™ Test, Idexx) which uses a single serum or plasma sample that may be used as an alternative to detection of larvae.

- *Dirofilaria immitis*, the true heartworm, does not occur in the UK unless a pet already carrying heartworm is imported. At present the northern extremity of the area endemic for heartworm is the south of Switzerland, although the endemic area does appear to be spreading. The adult worms are found in the right side of the heart and the pulmonary artery (Fig. 29.38). Female worms are long and slender, measuring up to 30 cm in length. Instead of eggs they lay larvae, known as microfilariae, which travel in the blood. Infection is transmitted by mosquitoes, which imbibe microfilariae as they feed on blood. The larvae develop to third stage in the mosquito and once mature they leave to infect another final host as the mosquito feeds. At first, the larvae develop in the area where they first penetrated the skin, later entering the circulation and travelling to the heart. The prepatent period for heartworm in dogs is about 6–7 months. Cats can also be infected but they are not such a good host: the prepatent period is extended to about 8 months and many infections never produce microfilariae.

A few heartworms in a dog may be well tolerated but a substantial burden can partially obstruct the pulmonary artery, causing right-sided heart failure.

In addition, dead worms may be swept into the lungs, where they form a focus for inflammatory reactions. Clinical signs associated with infection can be graded as mild, moderate and severe. A dog with severe disease might show low exercise tolerance, marked coughing, weight loss and ascites. Occasionally a large number of worms move suddenly from the pulmonary artery into the right side of the heart, causing an acute condition known as caval syndrome. Infected cats show more diverse signs, which include vomiting and even sudden death.

Adult heartworms may be removed surgically or by anthelmintic treatment but both methods can pose risks to

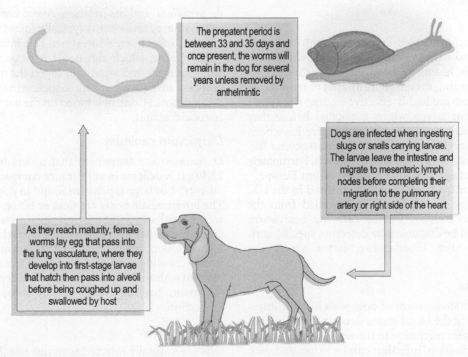

The prepatent period is between 33 and 35 days and once present, the worms will remain in the dog for several years unless removed by anthelmintic

Dogs are infected when ingesting slugs or snails carrying larvae. The larvae leave the intestine and migrate to mesenteric lymph nodes before completing their migration to the pulmonary artery or right side of the heart

As they reach maturity, female worms lay egg that pass into the lung vasculature, where they develop into first-stage larvae that hatch then pass into alveoli before being coughed up and swallowed by host

Fig. 29.37 Life cycle of *Angiostrongylus vasorum*

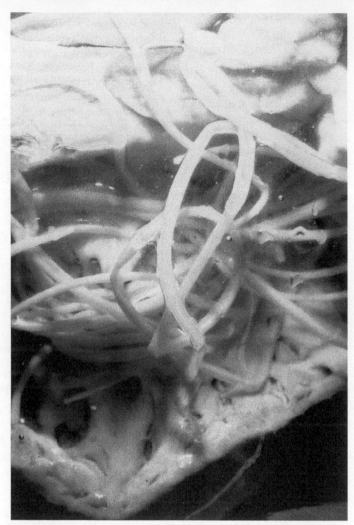

Fig. 29.38 Heartworm (*Dirofilaria immitis*) in situ in an infected dog (*Courtesy of John McGarry*)

the dog or cat. It is recommended that dogs or cats travelling to an area where heartworm is endemic are treated prophylactically with a macrocyclic lactone throughout the season of mosquito activity. These treatments are administered at monthly or 6-monthly intervals and are highly effective against third- and fourth-stage heartworm larvae, which are killed before they begin to migrate towards the heart. Recently there have been some reports from the USA of resistance to macrocyclic lactones and this is currently an area of active research. Fortunately to date there have not been any similar reports from Europe.

Although *D. immitis* infection is not transmitted in the UK, it is possible that dogs or cats that have travelled from the Mediterranean area to the UK will be carrying heartworm infection. Infection can be diagnosed by detecting specific antibodies, antigens or the blood-borne larval stage, the microfilaria.

Oesophageal worms

Spirocerca lupi is a nematode worm of dogs with a beetle intermediate host. In the dog the larval stages develop in the wall of the aorta with subsequent migration to the wall of the oesophagus where the adults develop. Infection can be associated with severe disease including inability to eat and cancerous lesions.

S. lupi is a parasite of Eastern Europe and the Middle East; however, with increased travel it may be introduced to the UK. Infection can be identified by the presence of characteristic eggs in faeces.

CESTODES

Cestodes are flat tapeworms composed of a head or scolex and a chain or strobila of clearly defined segments or proglottids (Fig. 29.39). The adult tapeworm is found in the intestine attached to the intestinal wall by the scolex, which often bears hooks and suckers to assist in making a secure attachment. The segments are produced in a neck region behind the scolex and contain both male and female reproductive tracts, so a single tapeworm can reproduce without need of other tapeworms. As a segment becomes older, signified by its being pushed towards the end of the worm by the younger segments, the eggs inside it develop, until it is almost nothing more than a bag of eggs. Ultimately the attachment to the segment behind breaks down and the segment moves down the intestine with the other intestinal contents to pass through the rectum and into the environment. Segments have a primitive nervous system and are capable of some movement, so may make their own way out of the anus. In the environment the segment is broken down and the eggs are released.

All tapeworms have an intermediate stage of development called the metacestode, the appearance of which varies with tapeworm species. Normally the metacestode is found in a host of a different species from the final host in which the adult tapeworm occurs. The final host is infected when it eats the intermediate host carrying the metacestode. For example, the flea carries the immature cysticercoid stage of *Dipylidium caninum* and dogs and cats are infected when they eat an infected flea. Drugs with cestocidal action are shown in Tables 29.5–29.7.

Anoplocephala perfoliata

A. perfoliata and its relation *Anoplocephala magna* are two squat, stumpy tapeworms typically found around the ileocaecal junction of a horse's intestine. The intermediate host is the oribatid mite, which can occur in large numbers on pasture. Horses are infected when they ingest the mites with grass. Large numbers of tapeworms are associated with an increased incidence of colic. Control is based on the use of anthelmintics with cestocidal action.

Dipylidium caninum

D. caninum is a tapeworm that occurs in dogs and cats (Fig. 29.40). It is delicate in appearance compared to *Taenia* spp., the other type of large tapeworm found in dogs and cats in the UK. The intermediate hosts are fleas or biting lice, and dogs or cats are infected when they ingest an infected louse or flea. The tapeworm causes little harm to the animal unless present in very high numbers, apart from anal irritation associated with segments crawling out of the anus. Occasionally, humans are infected with adult tapeworms. Control depends on anthelmintic treatment, together with flea or louse control to prevent reinfection.

Taenia species

Cats are normally infected with just one *Taenia* species, *Taenia taeniaeformis*. The metacestode stage occurs in rodents and the

TABLE 29.10	*Taenia* species of tapeworms found in the dog				
Species	**Final host**	**Approximate prepatent period (weeks)**		**Intermediate host**	**Intermediate stage – metacestode***
Taenia pisiformis	Dog and fox	6–8		Rabbit	Cysticercus pisiformis Abdomen or liver
Taenia hydatigena	Dog and fox	7–10		Cattle, sheep	Cysticercus tenuicollis Abdomen or liver
Taenia multiceps	Dog	4–6		Sheep, cattle	Coenurus cerebralis Brain and spinal cord
Taenia ovis	Dog and fox	6–8		Sheep and goat	Cysticercus ovis Muscle
Taenia serialis	Dog	–		Rabbit	Coenurus serialis Connective tissue

*The names for these stages are gradually being phased out as it is recognised that they represent simply the immature stage of the tapeworm in the final host, and they are no longer set in italic to denote that they are not regarded as species names.

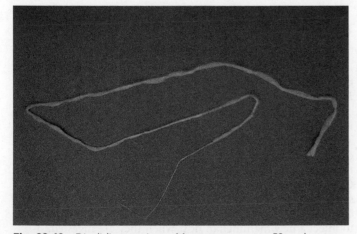

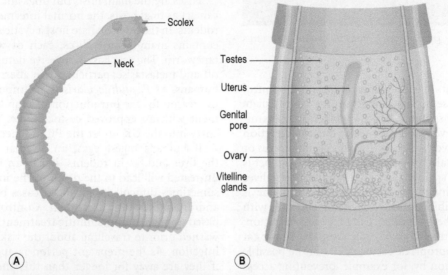

Fig. 29.39 Cestode. (A) Anterior end. (B) Mature segment or proglottid

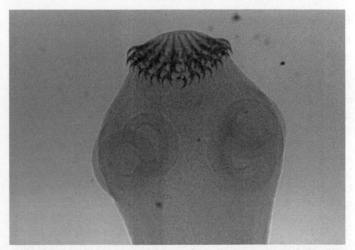

Fig. 29.40 *Dipylidium caninum*. May measure up to 50 cm long

Fig. 29.41 Head of *Taenia* sp. tapeworm

prepatent period in the cat is approximately 47 days. A number of species occur in dogs, with a variety of intermediate hosts, and they are listed in Table 29.10. Without detailed inspection of the shape of the hooks, all *Taenia* tapeworms look the same (Fig. 29.41), although there is some variation in length.

The presence of tapeworms is well tolerated by the host, apart from possibly some anal irritation caused by the presence of segments. Often, however, clinical signs of the metacestode are more severe – sheep with *Coenurus cerebralis* cysts in the brain develop nervous signs known as 'gid', and affected muscle

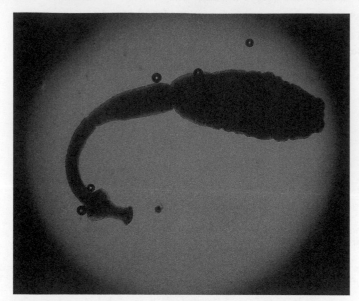

Fig. 29.42 *Echinococcus granulosus.* Entire tapeworm measures about 6 mm

may be devalued as meat. It is therefore important to control *Taenia* tapeworms because of their impact on the intermediate hosts. The eggs of *Taenia* spp. may be seen on faecal egg examination, but this is not a very sensitive technique for detection of cestode eggs. Alternatively, segments may be seen in faeces or on an animal's coat. It is also possible to assess whether a pet is likely to acquire a *Taenia* sp. infection. For example, if a cat lives entirely indoors, eats tinned food and the environment is mouse-free, it is not possible for the cat to become infected with *T. taeniaeformis*. Where there is evidence of tapeworm infection, or a likelihood of the animal acquiring infection, the dog or cat can be treated with an appropriate cestocide. It may be possible to prevent further infection by, for example, preventing access to raw meat, but in some cases where an animal hunts it can be very difficult to prevent re-exposure.

Echinococcus granulosus

E. granulosus (Fig. 29.42) is a minute tapeworm found in the small intestine of dogs and is so small that a dog may carry hundreds or even thousands of worms without any external sign of infection. Each worm measures about 6 mm and consists of only about four segments. The terminal, gravid segment measures about half the length of the worm. The normal intermediate hosts are sheep, although the hydatid cyst, the metacestode stage, can develop in cattle. Infection is widespread across the world and only a few countries, for example Iceland, have managed to eliminate the disease completely. There are two areas of infection in the UK: Wales, particularly the Powys area, together with areas of the midlands of England, and the Hebrides. An eradication programme was conducted in Powys in the 1980s but was not totally successful, as a proportion of lambs carried the metacestode stage in the 1990s after the eradication scheme had been scaled down to an educational programme. A new eradication campaign has recently been initiated by the Welsh Assembly. More details can be found on the Welsh Assembly website (www.gov.wales).

Infection by this cestode is an important zoonosis. If humans eat the eggs passed by a dog then a hydatid cyst may develop in the person's liver, lungs or rarely elsewhere. The cyst can grow to 10 cm or more in diameter and causes pain and debility. Cysts are removed by surgery or anthelmintic treatment. Control depends on regular treatment of dogs in endemic areas with effective cestocides and preventing dogs from having access to sheep carcases or uncooked offal. There is a separate species, *Echinococcus equinus*, that has a dog-to-horse life cycle. It is not believed to be zoonotic.

Echinococcus multilocularis

Like *E. granulosus*, *E. multilocularis* is a very small tapeworm but the final segment comprises slightly less than half the length of the worm compared to *E. granulosus*. *E. multilocularis* does not occur in the UK but the infection is endemic throughout a large part of mainland Europe from France to Germany, Denmark and Sweden in the north and across to Poland in the east. The southern boundary is the southern borders of Switzerland and Austria.

Foxes are the main hosts but dogs and, to a lesser extent, cats can act as final hosts, the normal intermediate host being small rodents. In the intermediate host a cystic structure develops that contains many protoscolices, each of which is an immature tapeworm. The cyst has an invasive nature and parts can break off and metastasise, particularly in aberrant final hosts such as humans. As *E. multilocularis* is an important zoonosis, it was the reason for the introduction of mandatory tapeworm treatment with an approved cestocide, i.e. praziquantel, prior to entry into the UK under the PETS scheme.

If humans ingest eggs, an alveolar cyst may develop in the liver and, as in rodents, it has an invasive nature and if untreated will lead to the death of the individual. Treatment is sometimes difficult in advanced cases but consists of surgery and/or anthelmintic treatment. Control in dogs and cats is based on regular anthelmintic treatment. Pet owners should be warned prior to travelling about the risk of their pet acquiring infection. As the prepatent period is approximately 1 month, if they are away for longer than this and the animal becomes infected it could begin passing segments prior to the cestode treatment on return.

TREMATODES

Trematodes are the flukes, flat worms that parasitize a number of organs including the intestine, bile ducts, blood and lungs of domestic animals. In the UK we are familiar with the liver fluke, *Fasciola hepatica*, which is normally a parasite of sheep and cattle. Horses can be infected but clinical signs associated with infection are rare. Animals on wet ground with standing water are at risk, as these are often suitable locations for the intermediate host, a tiny snail called *Galba* (formerly *Lymnea*) *truncatula*. Eggs passed in the faeces of infected animals develop in the environment and the first stage, the miracidium, infects snails. Eventually, after two more developmental stages, cercariae leave the snail and encyst as metacercariae on grass, ready to infect a new mammalian host when they are ingested.

There are a number of fluke species that occur in cats and dogs but none are endemic in the UK pet population.

PROTOZOA

The protozoa are small, unicellular organisms, some of which are parasites of animals. A major group are the coccidian parasites, which produce oocysts as a result of sexual reproduction.

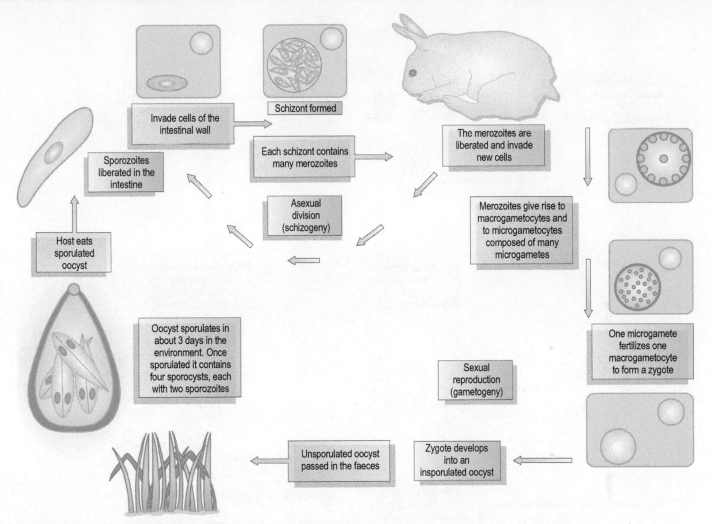

Fig. 29.43 Life cycle of an *Eimeria* spp. coccidium

The coccidian protozoa

Isospora species. A number of *Isospora* species are parasites of the intestine of dogs and cats, but only some, such as *Isospora felis* in cats and *Isospora canis* in dogs, are considered pathogenic. The parasite goes through a complex series of reproductive stages in the dog or cat that terminate in sexual reproduction and the production of oocysts, which are passed in faeces. This is similar to that seen in *Eimeria* spp. (Fig. 29.43). *Isospora* spp. infection may be well tolerated or may result in diarrhoea, particularly in puppies and kittens. The life cycle is direct and hosts are infected when they ingest sporulated oocysts from the environment. Control depends on hygiene, particularly between litters of pups or kittens, as oocysts are robust and will survive in the environment for long periods.

Horses and rabbits may be infected with *Eimeria* spp. (see Fig. 29.43) and infection may result in diarrhoea. One species of *Eimeria* in rabbits affects the liver rather than the intestine.

Some coccidian parasites have a more complex life cycle, with the final host infected by eating an infected intermediate host. These include the agent of equine protozoal myeloencephalitis *Sarcocystis neurona* and other *Sarcocystis* species. The *Sarcocystis* species each have a two-host life cycle and typically for any particular species both hosts are defined, e.g. *Sarcocystis tenella* infects dogs and sheep. The dog is normally little affected by the presence of the intestinal stages but the stages in the sheep occur in muscle tissue and can cause severe illness and even death (Rommel 1985). Equine protozoal myeloencephalitis is a severe nervous disease of horses that is currently the focus of research in the USA.

Toxoplasma gondii. *T. gondii* has a complex life cycle consisting of asexual and sexual reproductive components (Fig. 29.44). The main host is the cat and both stages can occur in the cat, but the asexual reproductive stage can also take place in many other mammals.

Cats are infected by eating infected prey or by ingesting oocysts in faeces. Normally, following infection, sexual reproduction takes place, with the production of oocysts without clinical signs. Oocyst production continues for a period of days and then ceases and thereafter cats are believed not to become reinfected. Other mammals become infected when they ingest sporulated oocysts from a cat's faeces. In these hosts replication takes place in tissues, initially rapidly dividing tachyzoites are formed and then, under the influence of host immunity, slower-dividing bradyzoite cysts.

Like other mammals, humans can become infected. Immunocompromised people and foetuses are most at risk of developing severe disease. A proportion of the adult population are

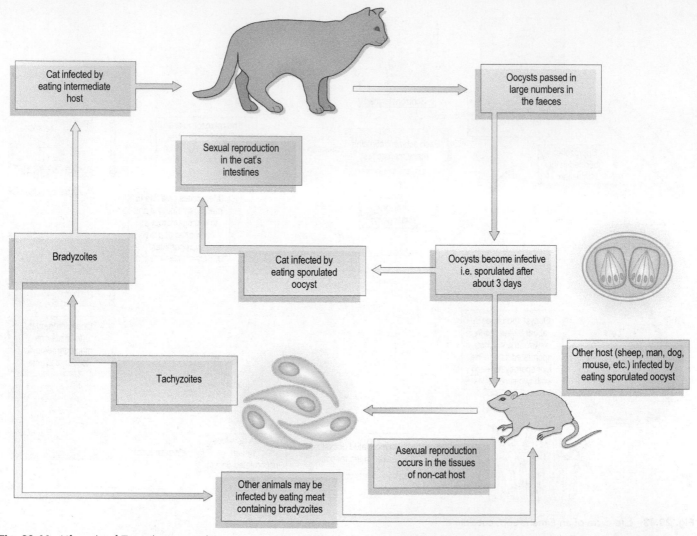

Fig. 29.44 Life cycle of *Toxoplasma gondii*

seropositive, i.e. show evidence of infection, but remain healthy. In immunocompromised individuals, including those whose immunity is suppressed during transplant surgery, the tissue cysts can multiply rapidly. Infection during pregnancy may result in abortion, an affected baby or an infected baby who does not show any clinical signs but may develop them later in life.

Steps to avoid human infection include:

- Wear gloves while gardening and wash hands thoroughly prior to eating
- Cover children's sandpits to prevent cats from using them as litter trays
- Wear gloves when cleaning the cat's litter tray and clean it out daily
- Wash fruit and vegetables prior to eating
- Chop meat separately from vegetables and wash hands after handling raw meat
- Avoid undercooked meat and unpasteurised milk and cheese.

The baby charity Tommys (www.tommys.org) provides advice, including leaflets about human infection and how to avoid it.

Neospora caninum. *N. caninum* was first identified about 40 years ago. It is closely related to *T. gondii* and shows similar tissue cysts associated with asexual reproduction, and sexual reproduction in the intestine of dogs that results in oocyst production. Cattle are the intermediate host and infection can cycle within the cattle population without passing through dogs, causing abortion when foetuses are affected. Occasionally, the tissue stages cause clinical signs in dogs, usually of an ascending paralysis and paresis, together with muscle wasting. Infection can be diagnosed in dogs on the basis of a high antibody titre. Infection in dogs can be treated with a combination of antiprotozoals and is most successful when commenced early in the infection.

Cryptosporidium spp. *Cryptosporidium* spp. are small intestinal protozoan parasites that have a direct life cycle with oocysts passed in faeces. The *Cryptosporidium parvum* host range includes a wide variety of mammalian species including cats, with *Cryptosporidium canis* infecting dogs and *Cryptosporidium felis* infecting cats. Some cats and dogs are subclinical carriers after an initial infection. Diarrhoea associated with infection is most commonly seen in puppies and kittens. The infection may be zoonotic, so care should be taken to avoid transmission to humans, where diarrhoea may be severe particularly in the immunocompromised. The small oocysts (5 μm in diameter) can be visualised in faeces using a variety of methods including

Ziehl-Nielsen staining. There is no specific treatment for dogs or cats and many infections will resolve without treatment.

Giardia spp. *Giardia* spp. are flagellate protozoa that infect the small intestine of many mammalian species, with distinct genotypes or assemblages associated with individual host species. Dogs may be infected with assemblages A–D, cats with A or F and humans with A or B. Infection can cause diarrhoea and increased frequency of defecation, particularly in puppies and kittens. Following infection some animals may remain as carriers and may act as a source of infection for others. The stage in the intestine, the trophozoite, multiplies by binary fission and environmentally resistant cysts are passed in faeces. The infection may be zoonotic, so care should be taken to ensure that humans are not exposed to infection. Infected dogs may be treated with fenbendazole and concomitant strict cleaning and hygiene of their environment will assist in preventing recurrence of the infection.

Babesia spp. *Babesia* spp. are parasites of red blood cells and the presence of the parasite in red blood cells causes breakdown of the cells. Infected animals show bouts of fever and then anaemia, which can be followed by death in some cases. Infection is tick-transmitted and the most prevalent species in Europe, *Babesia canis*, is transmitted by *Rhipicephalus sanguineus* and *Dermacentor* spp. ticks. It does not occur in the UK but there have been reports of dogs returning from Europe with babesiosis. Prompt treatment of clinically affected animals, normally with imidocarb, is essential. Pet owners planning to take their animals on holiday should be informed of the risks associated with tick infestation and how to avoid them. A babesiosis vaccine is available in some European countries. Cats can be infected with *Babesia* spp. but the main species infecting cats occur in Africa and the East but not in the Mediterranean. Cats appear to tolerate infection well until the anaemia becomes very severe, and then they die rapidly. *Babesia equi* occurs in southern Europe and infects horses.

Leishmania spp. *Leishmania* spp. are intracellular parasites of macrophages and the infection is endemic in many of the tropical and subtropical areas of the world, including the Mediterranean. Infection in southern Europe is transmitted by the sandfly, *Phlebotomus* spp. Dogs are the main species infected and disease may develop as long as 5 years after infection. Initial signs vary, but may consist of a skin wound that does not heal. Infected macrophages proliferate in a variety of different organs and clinical signs are related to the organ systems affected. Not every dog that acquires infection will develop disease but a proportion will do so. Presence of infection may be detected using a variety of tests including antibody (IFAT) tests or polymerase chain reaction tests (PCR).

Dogs act as a reservoir for human infection, as leishmaniosis is an important zoonosis. The Mediterranean infection, normally referred to as *L. infantum*, is not as pathogenic in humans as some of the other species; nonetheless, the disease can be severe in the young and immunocompromised. Infected dogs can be treated but a parasitic cure is rarely achieved and so prolonged treatment may be necessary. Repellents and other management strategies such as keeping dogs indoors between dusk and dawn may be helpful in preventing sandflies biting dogs and cats in endemic areas, but total prevention may be difficult to achieve. There is a vaccine for dogs (CaniLeish®) that

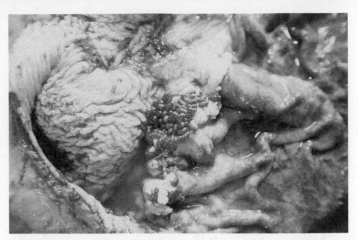

Fig. 29.45 The larvae of *Gastrophilus* sp. or bots attached to the stomach wall of a horse

reduces the risk of disease development following infection. People considering adopting dogs from the Mediterranean area should be aware that the dog may already be infected. Frequency of infection in cats appears to be far less than in dogs. Treatment of leishmaniosis is difficult – most treatments lead, at best, to a resolution of the clinical signs but not elimination of the parasite. This may result in the recurrence of clinical signs if, for example, treatment is stopped.

ARTHROPODS

Bots

Gastrophilus spp. flies are active in the summer and lay their eggs on the hairs of horses. Horses ingest the eggs as they groom and the larvae or bots develop in the stomach or proximal small intestine, depending on the species. The bots are attached to the mucosa (Fig. 29.45) but the following spring when fully developed they pass into the environment and pupate. The adult fly emerges in the summer to complete the life cycle. In the horse they cause some pathology and in addition, the presence of the flies causes disturbance or even panic in horses. The eggs are visible as small white dots on hairs and these can be cut off to prevent ingestion. Horses can also be treated with an ivermectin or other macrocyclic lactones, such as moxidectin, to eliminate bots.

DIAGNOSIS OF ENDOPARASITE INFECTION

Endoparasite infection can be identified by examination of faeces or blood. In many cases the parasite produces eggs with certain identifiable characteristics, which are shown in Figures 29.46–29.48.

Collection of samples

Faeces. Faecal samples should be collected from the animal's rectum or fresh off a cage floor. Old faecal samples from a kennel floor may be contaminated with free-living nematodes, which can confuse identification.

Laboratory analysis – examination of faeces for parasite eggs. The majority of endoparasites produce eggs or larvae

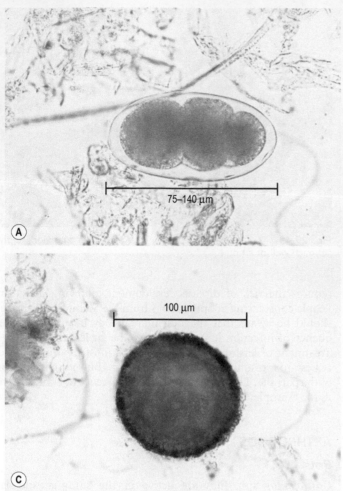

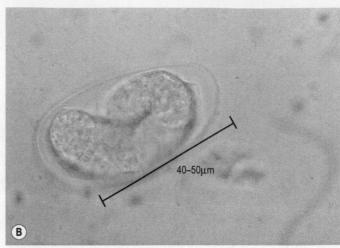

Fig. 29.46 Horse nematode eggs. (A) Strongyle egg. (B) *Strongyloides* sp. egg. (C) *Parascaris equorum* (All courtesy of John McGarry)

which pass out in the host's faeces and there are a variety of techniques that can be used to examine the faeces:

- Where eggs or cysts are abundant, e.g. in ascarid infection, a small piece of faecal material can simply be added to some water on a microscope slide to form an emulsion. The mixture is covered with a coverslip and examined systematically under a microscope
- Two methods, based on the use of fluid of a particular density to separate eggs by floating them from faecal debris, which sinks, are described below. Both use saturated sodium chloride solution as the flotation fluid. The density of 1.0 can be increased to greater than 1.5 using saturated zinc sulphate, which will float both nematode and the heavier trematode eggs. Alternatively, trematode eggs can be sedimented by spinning them down in a centrifuge.

Modified McMaster (quantitative method)

- Place 3 g of faeces in 42 ml water in a beaker or jar, add several glass beads and shake to break up the faecal matter. Cat faeces are notoriously difficult to break up and using lukewarm water and leaving for a few hours in the water will help.
- Pour the mixture through a tea strainer and catch the fluid in a bowl.
- Discard the debris in the tea strainer.
- Fill a 15-ml test tube with the filtrate and centrifuge for 5 minutes at 1500 rpm.

- Discard the supernatant.
- Add a small amount of saturated salt solution (NaCl) to the tube and mix to suspend the pellet from the bottom of the tube. Fill the tube to the 15-ml mark and mix again.
- Remove an aliquot with a pipette and use this to fill one side of a McMaster chamber; repeat to fill the second side of the McMaster slide.
- Dry any excess water off the McMaster slide. Place on to a microscope stage and examine under ×40 magnification.
- Focus on the grid etched on to the upper surface of the slide and work methodically, examining each section of the grid systematically. Any eggs will be in focus at the same time as the grid lines, as will round, black circles, which are air bubbles.
- Count all eggs and oocysts (if different types of egg and/or oocyst are present then each should be counted separately) found on one side of the slide. Repeat the count on the other side of the slide, add the totals together and multiply by 50 to get the number of eggs per gram of faeces.

Faecal flotation (semi-quantitative method)

- Place 3 g of faeces in 42 ml water in a beaker or jar, add several glass beads and shake to break up the faecal matter. Cat faeces are notoriously difficult to break up and using lukewarm water and leaving for a few hours in the water will help.

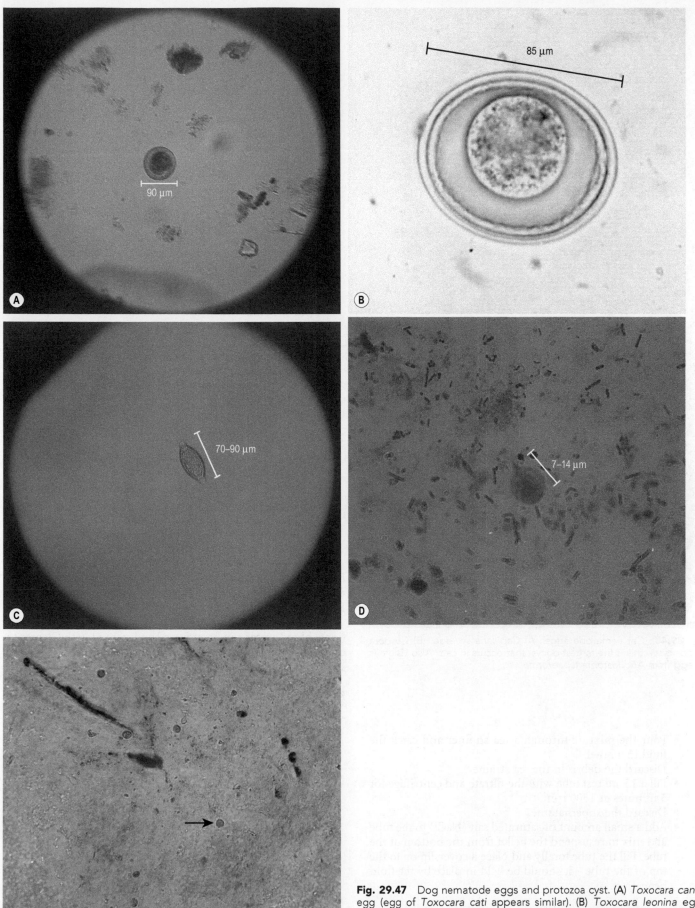

Fig. 29.47 Dog nematode eggs and protozoa cyst. (A) *Toxocara canis* egg (egg of *Toxocara cati* appears similar). (B) *Toxocara leonina* egg (Courtesy of John McGarry). (C) *Trichuris vulpis* egg. Note the prominent plugs at both ends. (D) *Giardia* sp. trophozoite in faeces. (E) *Cryptosporidium* sp. oocyst which stains red with acid-fast stain

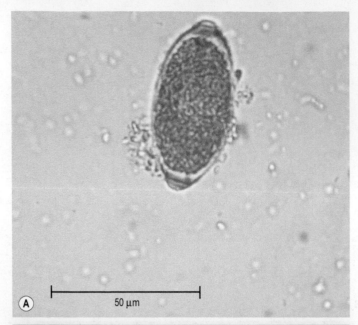

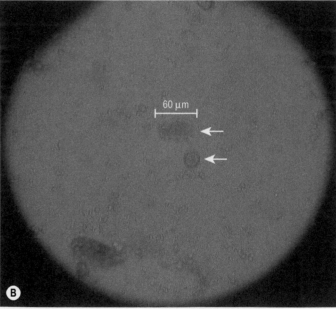

Fig. 29.48 Cat nematode eggs. **(A)** *Capillaria* sp. egg. **(B)** *Isospora felis* oocyst – this is the largest oocyst that occurs in cats. Also visible is an egg from *Ancylostoma tubaeforme*

- Pour the mixture through a tea strainer and catch the fluid in a bowl.
- Discard the debris in the tea strainer.
- Fill a 15-ml test tube with the filtrate and centrifuge for 5 minutes at 1500 rpm.
- Discard the supernatant.
- Add a small amount of saturated salt (NaCl) to the tube and mix to resuspend the pellet from the bottom of the tube. Fill the tube totally and place a coverslip on to the top of the tube – it should be held in place by the fluid beneath it.

- Place into a centrifuge and spin at 1500 rpm for 2 minutes. Gently remove the tube from the centrifuge, pick off the coverslip with a vertical action and place on to a microscope slide.
- Place the slide on to the microscope stage and examine under ×40 magnification.
- Work methodically, examining each section of the coverslip systematically.
- Count all eggs (if different types of egg are present then each should be counted separately) and the number counted equals the number of eggs per gram of faeces.

Baermann technique for detection of larvae in faeces. **Equipment**: a funnel, a metal clamp stand, a short piece of rubber tube, a clip, two strong wires, some muslin, a centrifuge tube, a slide and coverslip, and Lugol's iodine:

- Place the rubber tubing on to the end of the funnel and clamp the funnel into the stand. Place the clip across the end of the rubber tubing so that it forms a watertight seal.
- Fill the funnel with lukewarm water up to about 1 cm of the rim.
- Take a piece of muslin measuring about 15 cm² and thread the two wires through two sides. Place the muslin into the top of the funnel so that the wires are lying across the top of the funnel.
- Place about 10 g of faeces gently on to the muslin, ensuring that it is well covered with water.
- Leave the apparatus overnight and in the morning draw off a centrifuge tube full of fluid from the bottom of the apparatus by unclipping the clip across the rubber tube.
- Allow the tube to stand for about 4 hours or centrifuge at 1500 rpm for 1 minute.
- Remove the supernatant and place the sediment on a microscope slide with a coverslip on the top. A drop of Lugol's iodine can be added, which kills the larvae and stops them moving. It also stains them light brown, which can help to highlight features.

Blood. Blood samples should be collected into ethylenediaminetetraacetic acid (EDTA) as a anticoagulant for microscopic or PCR examination.

Laboratory analysis – examination of blood. A conventional blood smear can be prepared and stained with Giemsa to examine for blood parasites such as *Babesia* spp. or *Leishmania* spp.

Heartworm microfilariae can be identified in blood using the Knott's test:

- The process requires 1 ml of blood, and any excess blood should be conserved so that, if necessary, a sample can be sent to an expert for identification of microfilariae.
- Add 1 ml of blood (heparinised or EDTA) to 9 ml of 2% formaldehyde solution in a centrifuge tube. Mix thoroughly.
- Centrifuge the tube at 1500 rpm for 5 minutes. Discard the supernatant.
- Place the sediment onto a microscope slide, add a drop of methylene blue and mix well.
- Place a coverslip over the preparation and examine systematically.

BIBLIOGRAPHY

Acarus – The University of Bristol's dedicated laboratory for the PCR detection of arthropod-borne infectious diseases in companion animals. Available from: <www.langfordvets.co.uk/diagnostic laboratories/pcr-acarus>.

Curtis, C.F., 2004. Current trends in the treatment of *Sarcoptes*, *Cheyletiella* and *Otodectes* mite infestations in cats and dogs. Vet. Dermatol. 15, 108–114.

Deplazes, P., Fisher, M. (Eds.), 2012. ESCCAP – Toxocara 2012. Vet. Parasitol. special issue.

Dryden, M.W., Rust, M.K., 1994. The cat flea, biology, ecology and control. Vet. Parasitol. 52, 1–19.

Fisher, M., 2003. *Toxocara cati*: an underestimated zoonosis. Trends Parasitol. 19, 167–170.

Holdsworth, P.A., Kramer, L.H., Fisher, M.A., 2015. *Canine leishmaniosis*: an update. Vet. Nurse 6, 150–155.

Holland, C.V., Smith, H.V. (Eds.), 2006. *Toxocara: The Enigmatic Parasite*. CABI Publishing, Wallingford, UK.

Lloyd, S., 1993. *Toxocara canis*: the dog. In: Lewis, J.W., Maizels, R.M. (Eds.), *Toxocara and Toxocariasis*, Clinical, Epidemiological and Molecular

Perspectives. British Society for Parasitology with the Institute of Biology, London.

Markey, B., Leonard, F., Archambault, M., et al., 2013. Clinical Veterinary Microbiology. Mosby Elsevier, London.

Miller, W.H., Griffen, C.E., Campbell, K.L., 2012. Muller and Kirk's Small Animal Dermatology, seventh ed. Elsevier, St. Louis, MO.

Rommel, M., 1985. Sarcocystosis of domestic animals and humans. In Pract. 7, 158–160.

USEFUL WEBSITES

American Heartworm Society: <www.heartworm-society.org>

Details of the Pet Travel Scheme: <www.gov.uk/take-pets-abroad/overview>

Guidelines for parasite control <www.esccap.org>

TestAPet – Veterinary Parasitology Diagnostics: <www.liv.ac.uk/testapet>

Vet and pet owner website about parasites and their control: <esccapuk.org.uk>

RECOMMENDED READING

Jacobs, D.E., 1986. A Colour Atlas of Equine Parasites. Gower Medical, London.

Provides numerous illustrations of the appearance and life cycles of an extensive range of horse parasites.

Macpherson, C.N.L., Meslin, F.X., Wandeler, A.I., 2012. Dogs, Zoonoses and Public Health. CABI Publishing, Wallingford.

Focuses on dog diseases from the perspective of the risk of human disease.

Noah Compendium of Data Sheets for Animal Medicines. National Office of Animal Health, London. <www.noah.co.uk>

Provides data sheets of individual parasiticides.

Taylor, M.A., Coop, R.L., Wall, R.L., 2007. Veterinary Parasitology, third ed. Blackwell Publishing, Oxford.

A thick textbook on parasitology covering all the species. You may also want to the refer to the second edition (1996) for a good basic textbook.

30 Microbiology

HELEN MORETON

KEY POINTS

- Microorganisms are too small to be seen with the naked eye and include bacteria, viruses, fungi, algae and protozoa. The majority of microorganisms are non-pathogenic and are essential for life, e.g. in the breakdown and decay of dead matter.

- Before the symptoms of a disease develop, a pathogenic organism must invade the host, establish itself in the tissues and overcome the host's defence mechanisms.

- Bacteria vary in size and shape and are able to survive away from the host, provided that they do not dry out or encounter extremes of temperature.

- They may be visualised using a light microscope but it is easier to distinguish between different species if biological stains, e.g. Gram's stain, are used to highlight their morphological features.

- Bacterial replication occurs asexually by binary fission and by conjugation, which allows new characteristics to develop as a result of the transfer of genetic material.

- Bacteria can be grown in the laboratory in order to identify them but the culture must be provided with the correct balance of nutrients, water, pH, temperature and gaseous environment.

- Viruses are minute obligate intracellular parasites that can only be seen using an electron microscope.

- Each virus particle or virion consists of either RNA or DNA surrounded by a protein coat. Some viruses also have an envelope around the outside.

- Viral replication occurs inside the host cell and depends on the virus's ability to instruct the cell to start producing virus particles. The new virions burst out of the cell, invade other cells and clinical signs develop.

Introduction

Microbiology is the study of organisms, and other biologically important agents, that are too small to be seen by the naked eye, deriving its name from the Greek words *mikros* ('small'), *bios* ('life') and *logos* ('science'). The organisms are smaller than 1 mm in diameter and are mostly unicellular, i.e. consisting of only one cell, which carries out all the functions necessary for life. A few, such as some fungi, are multicellular.

Microorganisms include:

- **Bacteria** – including the very small forms *Rickettsia*, *Chlamydia* and *Mycoplasma* spp.
- **Viruses**
- **Fungi** – covered in Chapters 29 and 31
- **Algae** – no pathogenic forms affecting animals
- **Protozoa** – covered in Chapter 29.

Microorganisms vary in size from the relatively large protozoa to viruses that can only be seen with an electron microscope (Figs. 30.1 and 30.2). Viruses range in size from about 10–40 nm (nanometres) and differ from other microorganisms in that they have no cellular structure, although they have a wide variety of shapes (Table 30.1).

MICROSCOPES

A light or optical microscope can magnify up to approximately 1500 times without losing resolution (image loses clarity), which means that objects smaller than 0.2 µm (micrometres) cannot be seen in clear detail. As suggested by the name, electron microscopes use an electron beam, which achieves much higher magnification and resolution than light microscopes and distinguishes objects as small as 0.2 nm (250 000 × magnification) (Table 30.2).

Over 10 000 species of bacteria are known, most being less than 10 µm in diameter, while virus particles, virions, range between 10 nm and 400 nm in diameter (see Fig. 30.2).

Visualisation of living bacteria is difficult using bright-field optical microscopy, as they are transparent and often colourless. Contrast-enhancing optical systems can help to elucidate the morphological characteristics of cells (shape, flagellae, etc.), but in order to learn more about their properties bacteria must be differentiated into specific groups for identification purposes. This can be done by the use of biological stains, selective culture media and biochemical tests. Staining procedures involve applying dyes to bacterial smears, which are air-dried and heat-fixed. Gram staining divides bacteria into positive or negative, depending on the thickness of the cell wall, and also helps to show cell shape and typical morphology of groups of cells.

MICROORGANISMS

Microorganisms can be classified according to their method of nutrition:

- **Autotrophs** – manufacture their own food, often by photosynthesis with the aid of chlorophyll
- **Heterotrophs** – obtain their food from the environment. Most microorganisms are this type. They may be:
  - **Saprophytes** – feed on dead material. None are pathogenic
  - **Parasites** – feed on a living organism, which is referred to as the host.

There are three types of parasite:

- **Pathogens** – disease-causing organisms
- **Commensals** – live in or on the host but cause no harm and derive no benefit, e.g. *Staphylococcus intermedius*,

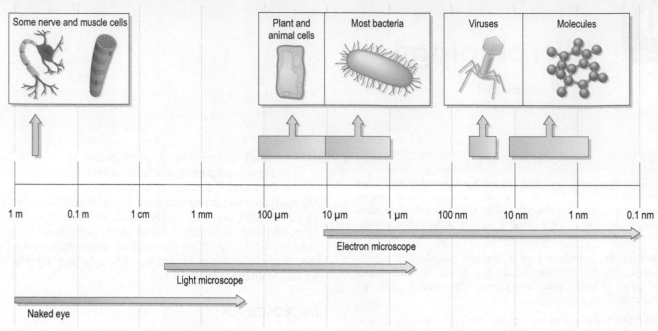

Fig. 30.1 Relative sizes of various types of structure

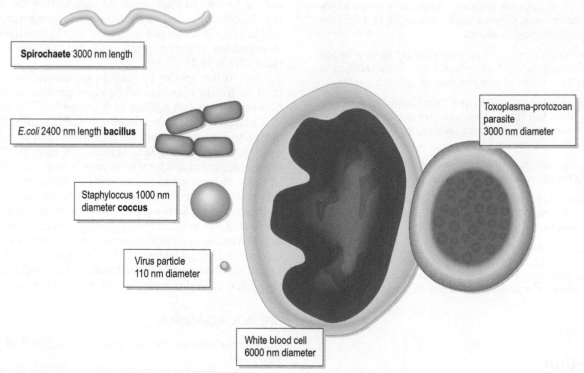

Fig. 30.2 Sizes of common types of pathogenic organism in relation to each other and to a white blood cell

which lives on the skin. May become pathogenic if the balance between the host and the organism is upset

• **Mutualistic or symbiotic organisms** – live in or on the host and both provide a benefit for the host and derive a benefit for themselves, e.g. microbial flora which colonise the caecum of the horse and rabbit, breaking down plant food material for digestion from which the microorganisms gain a source of energy.

When a microorganism invades a host and starts to multiply, it establishes an infection. If the host is susceptible to the infection then disease results.

In order to cause disease, a pathogen must:
• Gain entry into the host
• Establish itself and multiply in the host tissue
• Overcome the normal host body defences for a time
• Damage the host in some way.

TABLE 30.1	Comparison between the characteristics of mammalian cells and those of microorganisms					
Characteristic	Mammals	Bacteria	Viruses	Fungi	Protozoa	Algae
Size	10–100 μm	0.5–<10 μm	200–300 nm	Yeasts 3.8 μm	10–200 μm	0.5–20 μm
Cell arrangement	Multicellular	Unicellular	Non-cellular	Uni- or multicellular	Unicellular	Uni- or multicellular
Cell wall	None	Mainly peptidoglycan	None	Mainly chitin	None	Mainly cellulose
Nucleus	Membrane-bound nucleus	No true membrane-bound nucleus	Absent	Membrane-bound nucleus	Membrane-bound nucleus	Membrane-bound nucleus
Nucleic acids	DNA and RNA	DNA and RNA	DNA or RNA	DNA and RNA	DNA and RNA	DNA and RNA
Reproduction	Cells in tissues asexual; new individuals sexual	Asexual – binary fission	Replicate only within living cell	Asexual and sexual by spores, budding in yeast	Asexual and sexual	Asexual and sexual
Nutrition	Heterotrophic	Mainly heterotrophic, can be saprophytic, parasitic, a few autotrophic	Obligate parasites	Heterotrophic, can be saprophytic or parasitic	Heterotrophic, can be saprophytic or parasitic	Autotrophic
Motility	Some cells are motile, whole individual motile	Some are motile	Non-motile	Non-motile except for certain spore forms	Motile	Some are motile
Toxin production	None	Some form toxins	Some form toxins	Some form toxins	Some form toxins	

TABLE 30.2	Units of measurement of microorganisms		
1 millimetre (mm)	= 10^{-3} metre (m)	= 1/1000 m
1 micrometre (μm)	= 10^{-6} m	= 1/1 000 000 m
1 nanometre (nm)	= 10^{-9} m	= 1/1 000 000 000 m

TABLE 30.3	Routes of infection		
Source of infection	Susceptible organ system	First line of defence
Contaminated food and water	Digestive	Lysozymes in saliva, stomach acid and enzymes
Droplet infection	Respiratory	Mucus, cilia, macrophages
Sexual transmission	Reproductive and urinary	Mucus, acidic, urine flow
Direct contact	Skin	Acid, salty, oily skin. Rapid healing process
Vector organisms	Injected straight to blood	Bypasses the first line of defence

Some microorganisms cause disease by secreting or releasing poisonous substances called **toxins** that disrupt specific physiological processes in the host, while others invade tissue cells and damage or destroy them. Viruses, for example, cause cell damage because they interfere with the normal cell metabolism and many leave the host cell by rupture of the cell membrane. Once they have entered the tissues of the host, some microorganisms are localised and remain at the site of entry; for example, *Staphylococcus intermedius*, which causes skin disease, generally attacks in this way. Others spread through the body (systemic spread), usually via the lymphatic system and blood circulation. Once they have invaded the host, some microorganisms can grow and multiply in any tissues of the body but many are more selective and localise in a particular tissue or organ. If these more demanding organisms do not reach the particular cells in which they can live, they will not produce disease. Viruses in particular often have an affinity for a specific tissue or organ, which is known as **tissue trophism**. A virus is only able to attach to cells that carry a compatible receptor; for example, influenza viruses can only attach to ciliated epithelial cells in the respiratory tract.

Definitions

Infection is the invasion and multiplication of microorganisms in body tissues and may lead to cellular damage. Damage may result from competitive metabolism, intracellular replication, the presence of toxins or by the action of the body's defence mechanisms, such as inflammation and antibody–antigen responses.

An **infectious disease** is one caused by, or capable of being communicated by, the process of infection. If the disease is capable of being transmitted from one animal to another it is described as being **contagious** or **transmissible**.

Pathogens may invade the body in many ways but successful invasion, i.e. one that results in disease, depends on the pathogen avoiding the body's first lines of defence (Table 30.3). See also Chapter 21.

Bacteria

CLASSIFICATION AND NAMING OF BACTERIA

Bacteria are referred to by describing their basic shapes (Fig. 30.3):
- Cylindrical or rod-shaped cells are called **bacilli** (singular: bacillus).
- Some bacilli are curved and these are known as **vibrios**.
- Spherical cells are called **cocci** (singular: coccus). Some cocci exist singly while others remain together in pairs after cell division and are called **diplococci**. Those that remain attached to form chains are called **streptococci** and if they divide randomly and form irregular grape-like clusters they are called **staphylococci**.

- Spiral or helical cells are called **spirilla** (singular: spirillum) if they have a rigid cell wall or **spirochaetes** if the cell wall is flexible.

BACTERIAL CELL STRUCTURE

Bacteria vary in size, e.g. rickettsias, mycoplasmas and chlamydias, which are considerably smaller than a typical bacterium (Table 30.4). Rickettsia and chlamydia both possess a cell wall like other Gram-negative bacteria (Fig. 30.4) but both of these organisms must live inside other cells, i.e. they are obligate intracellular organisms. They are still considerably bigger than viruses, which are also obligate intracellular parasites.

The cell wall and its significance in drug therapy

Like plant cells, most bacteria have a cell wall, but this has a different biochemical structure from the polysaccharide (cellulose) cell wall of plants, being made mainly of a substance called peptidoglycan (sometimes called murein). It maintains cell shape and prevents the cell from bursting. Cell walls vary in thickness and in composition and it is these differences which are a key aid to initial identification using Gram's stain.

The cell wall:
- Resembles a football, i.e. it is elastic but rigid
- Contains several amino acids not found in the proteins of plants and animals so chemotherapeutic agents such as antibiotics can be directed specifically against them without harming the host cell wall.

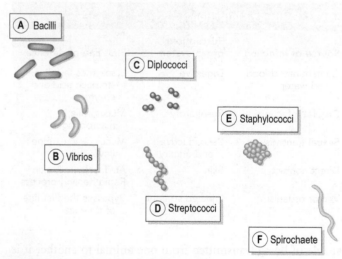

Fig. 30.3 (A–F) Shapes of bacteria

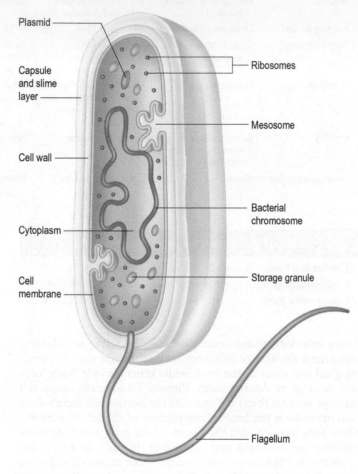

Fig. 30.4 Structure of a bacterial cell, using *Escherichia coli* as an example

	Bacteria			
	Typical bacterium	Rickettsia/Chlamydia	Mycoplasma	Viruses
Size	<5–10 μm	0.8–2 μm	±0.5 μm	10–400 nm
Intracellular parasite	–	+	+	+
Cell wall	+	+	–	–
Plasma membrane	+	+	+	–
Binary fission	+	+	+	–
Filterable through bacteriological filters	–	±	+	+
Possess both DNA and RNA	+	+	+	–
ATP-generating metabolism	+	±	+	–
Ribosomes	+	+	+	–
Sensitive to antibiotics	+	+	?	–
Sensitive to interferon	–	–	–	+

TABLE 30.4 Comparative characteristics of bacteria and viruses

TABLE 30.5	Bacterial diseases of dogs			
Bacterium	**Disease caused**	**Gram's stain**	**Shape**	**Aerobic**
Salmonella spp.	Diarrhoea, etc.	Negative	Rod/bacillus	Yes
Campylobacter spp.	Diarrhoea, etc.	Negative	Curved rods	Yes (but prefer less oxygen than in the air)
Bordetella bronchiseptica	Kennel cough	Negative	Short rods/bacilli	Yes
Leptospira spp.	Leptospirosis	Negative	Helically coiled/spirochaete	Yes
Staphylococcus spp.	Pyoderma	Positive	Cocci	Yes
Clostridium tetani	Tetanus	Positive	Long rods/bacilli	No

TABLE 30.6	Bacterial diseases of horses		
Disease	**Bacterium**	**Tissue affected**	**Comment**
Strangles	*Streptococcus equi*	Upper respiratory tract	Very infectious
Contagious equine metritis	*Taylorella equigenitalis*	Reproductive tract	Notifiable
Summer pneumonia	*Rhodococcus equi*	Lungs	Foals most susceptible
Lyme disease	*Borrelia burgdorferi*	Systemic, joints	Vector-borne – tick

The peptidoglycan of Gram-negative cells has the same fundamental structure as that of Gram-positive cells but only one or two layers linked to the outer membrane by lipoprotein bridges, which anchor it. There are other biochemical differences in the outer layers of the two types of bacteria.

Chemicals that target these differences in cell structure, biochemical composition and metabolism between bacterial and plant or animal cells are frequently used as therapy against bacterial pathogens (see Chapter 19). A common example of this is the antibiotic penicillin, which disrupts the synthesis of new bacterial cell walls during binary fission and hence bursts or lyses the pathogen. Any antibacterial drug that affects the cell wall will be particularly suited to use against Gram-positive organisms.

BACTERIAL DISEASES

Examples of diseases in dogs and horses are shown in Tables 30.5 and 30.6.

Groups of very small bacteria are responsible for a number of diseases in animals, including:

- *Chlamydia* – various strains of *Chlamydia psittaci* (*Chlamydophila psittaci*) are the cause of **psittacosis** in psittacine birds (parrots, parakeets) and mammals. Psittacosis is a zoonotic infection that humans can acquire by inhaling *Chlamydia* in the airborne dust or cage contents of infected birds. **Feline pneumonitis** is also caused by *C. psittaci* and the organism may be the cause of conjunctivitis in the cat. They are transmitted by inhalation of infectious dust and droplets and by ingestion. There is also evidence to suggest that vector-borne infection may occur.
- *Rickettsia* – transmitted by vectors such as the tick, louse, flea and mite from an infected individual; for example, *Haemobartonella felis* (*Mycoplasma haemofelis*) causes **feline infectious anaemia** (**FIA**). Another rickettsial infection is caused by *Ehrlichia* spp. A particularly pathogenic species is *Ehrlichia canis*, endemic in much of France and the Mediterranean basin.

Generally, the identification of *Rickettsia* and *Chlamydia* is more difficult and thus more specialised than that of most bacteria. Diagnosis of infection may be based on demonstration of the organisms themselves or on the demonstration of increased titres of antibodies in paired serum samples. The rickettsiae are smaller than most bacteria and are barely visible under the ordinary light microscope. They can only be cultivated in tissue culture or in the yolk sac of embryonated eggs. Typically, they are rod-shaped.

- *Mycoplasma* – tiny bacteria-like organisms. Unlike other bacteria they do not possess a cell wall. Mycoplasma species have been implicated in complicating respiratory tract infections in a number of species, notably calves and horses (especially young racehorses in training). They include *Mycoplasma felis*, a cause of chronic conjunctivitis in cats. Mycoplasma will grow on agar-based media but, as the bacteria are so fragile, isolation and identification are specialised skills.

PATHOGENICITY

Pathogenicity is the ability of an organism to enter the body, set up disease and cause symptoms. A pathogen is an organism capable of causing disease. A virulent pathogen readily sets up infection and produces severe symptoms.

Virulence may vary between different strains of the same bacterium. Disease is the result of the virulence of the pathogen versus the resistance (defence mechanisms) of the host. In some diseases, symptoms occur because of an overreaction of the host's own defence mechanisms. This can lead to cell damage or an allergic reaction.

Some pathogens will almost always cause serious disease, while others are less pathogenic and cause milder illnesses. Many produce toxic enzymes to assist in the process of invasion and tissue destruction; for example, the enzyme hyaluronidase helps the pathogen to penetrate the tissues of the host by breaking down the 'tissue cement' that holds the cells together. Another enzyme, lecithinase, lyses or disintegrates tissue cells, especially red blood cells.

Virulence is determined by factors such as:

- The ability of the parasite to invade particular cells and tissues and cause damage, i.e. its invasiveness

- Its ability to secrete toxins that disrupt physiological processes in the body, i.e. its toxigenicity
- Its ability to survive in unfavourable conditions.

Invasiveness

- May be assisted by enzymes (which are also toxins) secreted by the bacteria, e.g. collagenase secreted by *Clostridium*; coagulase secreted by *Staphylococcus aureus*; hyaluronidase and protease secreted by *Streptococcus*
- Most bacteria get into the body tissues but some get inside the cells as well, which may assist them in avoiding the immune mechanisms of the host. *Salmonella* species, for example, are facultative intracellular parasites, i.e. they live between the cells but may also get inside them; *Rickettsia* are obligate intracellular parasites, i.e. they have to live inside the cells
- Some bacteria, e.g. *Bacillus anthracis*, have capsules that are antiphagocytic (they imped or prevent the action of the phagocytes)
- Some, e.g. *Escherichia coli*, adhere to the host cells by means of rod-like pili, which prevent them from being swept away by body fluids.

Toxigenicity

Toxins are poisonous substances that have a damaging effect on the cells of the host. The effects of the toxin are not only felt in the affected cells and tissues but also elsewhere in the body as the toxin is transported through the tissues.

Two types of toxin are recognised:

- **Exotoxins** are proteins produced mainly by Gram-positive bacteria during their metabolism. They are released into the surrounding environment as they are produced. This may be into the circulatory system and tissues of the host or, as in food poisoning, into food that is then ingested. Microbial toxins include many of the most potent poisons known to man and may prove lethal even in small quantities. Some examples include those toxins produced by the genus *Clostridium*, which includes *Clostridium tetani*, which causes tetanus, and *Clostridium botulinum*, which causes botulism. Nowadays Botox, a diluted form of the toxin, is used to paralyse the facial muscles to provide a youthful appearance.
  - The body responds to the presence of exotoxins by producing antibodies called antitoxins that neutralise the toxins, rendering them harmless.
  - As they are proteins, exotoxins are destroyed by heat and some chemicals. Chemicals such as formaldehyde are used to treat toxins so that they lose their toxicity but not their ability to elicit an immune response. These treated toxins are called **toxoids** and if they are injected into the body they will stimulate the production of antitoxins. For example, tetanus toxoid is used to provide immunity to tetanus.
- **Endotoxins** are part of the cell wall of certain Gram-negative bacteria and are released only when the cells die and disintegrate. In Gram-negative cells the outer bilayer membrane has the typical phospholipids replaced by lipopolysaccharides, which comprise up to 40% of the surface structure and act as the major somatic antigen of these bacteria. Compared with exotoxins, they are less toxic, cannot be used to form toxoids and are able to withstand heat. Blood-borne endotoxins are responsible for a range of non-specific reactions in the body such as fever. They also make the walls of blood capillaries more permeable, causing blood to leak into the intercellular spaces, sometimes resulting in a serious drop in blood pressure, a condition commonly called endotoxic shock. They are also responsible for the change in capillary blood flow in equine hooves that leads to laminitis.

Toxins are not made exclusively by bacteria. The saprophytic fungus *Aspergillus flavus* produces a toxin called **aflatoxin**. The fungus grows in warm, humid conditions and contaminates a variety of agricultural products such as peanuts, cereals, rice and beans. Aflatoxin has been implicated in the deaths of many farm animals that have been fed on mouldy hay, corn or peanut meal.

Spore formation

To survive unfavourable conditions, such as when the supply of nutrients is inadequate, some species of bacteria produce spores or sporulate. These dormant forms are also called **endospores**. Spore formation is most common in the genus *Clostridium*, which contains the causative agents of tetanus and botulism, and in *Bacillus anthracis*, the causative agent of anthrax. These diseases are zoonotic, most commonly affecting domestic and farm animals. Species susceptibility to each varies; for example, dogs only infrequently suffer from tetanus, while horses are very susceptible and require routine vaccination, as do humans. It is important to note that spore formation is not a method of reproduction: one vegetative bacterial cell produces a single spore, which, after germination, is again just one vegetative cell (Fig. 30.5).

The spore develops within the cell and under the microscope appears as a bright, round or oval structure. Many spore-forming bacteria are inhabitants of the soil but spores can exist almost everywhere, including in dust. They are extremely resistant structures that can remain viable for many years. Cattle have died from anthrax contracted by contact with spores that have remained in soil after the death of an animal there decades before. Spores can survive extremes of heat, pH, desiccation, ultraviolet radiation and exposure to toxic chemicals such as some disinfectants. The reason why spores are so resistant is not completely understood but heat resistance is thought to be due to the fact that a dehydration process occurs during spore formation, which expels most of the water from the spore.

The fact that spores are so hard to destroy is the principal reason for the various sterilisation procedures that are carried out in veterinary practice. Common techniques employed to kill spores include the use of moist heat under pressure and dry heat for at least 2 hours (see Chapter 24).

BACTERIAL REPLICATION

Bacteria reproduce or replicate asexually by simply dividing into two identical daughter cells, a process known as **binary fission** (Fig. 30.6). If their environment is suitable, bacteria can grow and reproduce rapidly. The time interval between successive divisions is called the generation time. Even under optimum conditions the generation time varies:

- *Escherichia coli* – 20 minutes
- *Mycobacterium tuberculosis*, which causes tuberculosis – approximately 18 hours.

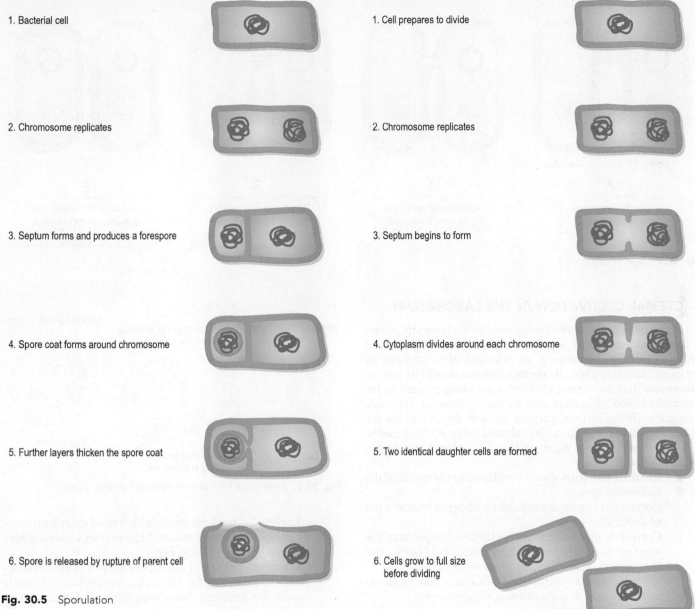

1. Bacterial cell

2. Chromosome replicates

3. Septum forms and produces a forespore

4. Spore coat forms around chromosome

5. Further layers thicken the spore coat

6. Spore is released by rupture of parent cell

Fig. 30.5 Sporulation

1. Cell prepares to divide

2. Chromosome replicates

3. Septum begins to form

4. Cytoplasm divides around each chromosome

5. Two identical daughter cells are formed

6. Cells grow to full size before dividing

Fig. 30.6 Bacterial replication by binary fission

Given appropriate conditions, growth is exponential, i.e. one bacterium produces two, then two produce four, then eight, potentially reaching many millions within 24 hours.

To enable cell replication, the chromosome, i.e. the genetic material, is copied first to form two identical chromosomes. As the parent cell enlarges, the chromosomes separate and the cell membrane grows inwards at the centre of the cell. At the same time, new cell wall material grows inwards to form the septum and this divides the cell into two daughter cells. In some species, e.g. streptococci and staphylococci, the daughter cells remain attached to each other to form the characteristic chains or clusters. In most species the new bacterial cells separate.

Conjugation

Conjugation is rare among Gram-positive bacteria but common among those that are Gram-negative. It is sometimes regarded as a primitive type of sexual reproduction but this is misleading because, unlike sexual reproduction in other organisms, it does not involve the fusion of two gametes to form a single cell.

Frequently, plasmid DNA is transferred from the donor to the recipient but sometimes part of the donor cell chromosome, or even the whole chromosome, is transferred.

Conjugation is important because the recipient acquires new characteristics. For example, one plasmid, the R plasmid, carries genes for resistance to antibiotics, and is the mechanism by which some species can acquire resistance from a similar species. Enterobacteria such as *E. coli* and *Salmonella* spp. are thought to transfer resistance between serotypes in this way.

The process of conjugation involves the passage of DNA from one bacterial cell, the donor, to another, the recipient, while the two cells are in physical contact (Fig. 30.7). The cells are pulled together by a sex pilus, which is formed by the donor cell. Once contact has been made, the pilus retracts so that the surfaces of the donor and recipient are very close to each other. The cell membranes fuse, forming a channel between the two cells to enable transfer to take place.

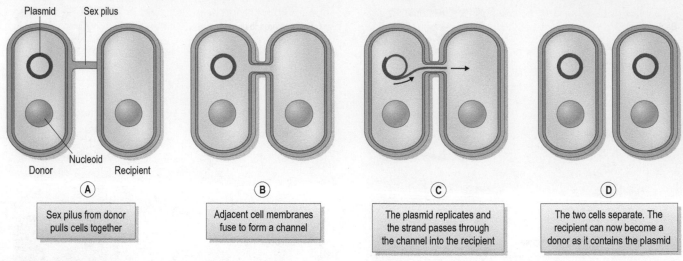

Fig. 30.7 (A–D) Conjugation

BACTERIAL CULTIVATION IN THE LABORATORY

It may be necessary to cultivate bacteria in the laboratory from a sample collected from a patient, e.g. faecal or skin swab, in order to identify the cause of an infection or to perform an antibiotic sensitivity test. By performing the sensitivity test we can ensure that the correct antibiotics are being prescribed for the patient, and ultimately aids in the increase of antibiotic resistance. Unlike viruses, bacteria are not dependent on the presence of host cells and can be cultured using artificial media.

The culture medium must provide the correct balance of:

- Water
- Essential nutrients – vary according to the needs of the individual species
- Correct pH – most mammalian pathogens require a pH of about 7.4
- Correct temperature – the optimum temperature for most pathogens is body temperature, i.e. 37–40°C, and they are described as being normothermic
- Correct gaseous environment – bacteria may be classified according to their gaseous requirements:
  - **Obligate or strict aerobes** – must have oxygen for growth
  - **Obligate anaerobes** – will only grow in the absence of oxygen
  - **Facultative anaerobes** – may grow both in the presence or absence of oxygen
  - **Microaerophiles** – will only grow if the percentage of oxygen is lower than that of atmospheric air.

Culture media consist of two basic types:

- **Liquid broths** – particularly used for bacteria that will grow in fluid
- **Solid or jelly-like nutrient solutions** – based on agar, which is derived from seaweed. Agar can be purchased ready prepared in sterile flat-lidded Petri dishes or can be reconstituted in the lab. The agar provides no nutrients for the bacteria and these are added according to the needs of the species being cultivated.

Solid media can be classified as follows:

- **Simple or basal** – provide all that is needed for basic growth. Simple media are used for nutritionally undemanding species, e.g. *E. coli*

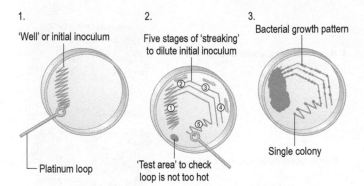

Fig. 30.8 Technique for the inoculation of an agar plate

- **Enriched** – used for bacteria that need extra nutrients, e.g. blood agar used to detect haemolysis, chocolate agar (heated blood), serum, egg
- **Selective** – these will inhibit the growth of some bacteria while selecting for others, e.g. deoxycholate citrate is used for growing *Salmonella* spp.; McConkey's bile lactose agar contains bile salts that encourage the growth of enteric species such as *E. coli*; Sabouraud's medium is used for growing ringworm fungi
- **Biochemical** – used to distinguish between species of bacteria by detecting how they react biochemically, e.g. with different types of sugar or urea.

To produce a bacterial culture:

1. Label the Petri dish with the client's name, the case number or an appropriate lab code to avoid mixing up the samples.
2. Heat a platinum loop in the flame of a Bunsen burner to sterilise it. Cool the loop in the air for few seconds. If it is too hot it will kill the bacterial cells, resulting in no growth.
3. Dip the loop into the sample.
4. Pick up the Petri dish containing the agar with the agar uppermost and smear the material on the loop over a small area to create a well or inoculum (Fig. 30.8).
5. Heat the loop in the flame and allow it to cool. Make three or four short streaks from the well, all in the same direction (see Fig. 30.8). Be careful not to tear the agar.

6. Continue to spread the sample over the agar.
7. Place the lid on the Petri dish and put it into an incubator at 37°C for 18–24 hours.
8. Remove the plate and examine for bacterial growth. If there is no growth reincubate for a further 18–24 hours.

Colonies of bacteria appear as rounded lumps, which are often raised and are distributed along the streak lines. Colonies of different species of bacteria may show individual characteristics, which will be helpful in their identification. To further identify a species of bacteria a smear is made on a glass microscope slide, stained with Gram's stain or methylene blue and examined under the microscope.

To identify the appropriate antibiotic with which to treat a patient it is often quicker and more effective to carry out an antibiotic sensitivity test. In this, discs impregnated with a range of antibiotics are placed on an agar plate that has been smeared with a colony selected from the original culture. The plate is incubated for 18–24 hours and the zones in which bacterial growth has been inhibited by the antibiotic are noted.

Virus

Viruses are subject to debate over whether they really are living organisms as they are incapable of reproduction without a host cell – described as obligate intracellular parasites. A virus particle or virion is little more than a package containing instructions for the re-creation of further virus particles.

Each virus particle is composed of two parts:
- **Nucleic acid** – either RNA or DNA (never both), forming a central core
- A **capsid** (Fig. 30.9) – a protein coat.

Together, these two parts form the nucleocapsid. For some viruses, this is all that comprises an individual virus particle.

Various shapes of virus nucleocapsid have been identified and are illustrated in Figure 30.10:
- Helical
- Icosahedral
- Complex
- Composite – some bacteriophages.

Some viruses have an additional envelope around the outside, often formed of the host cell membrane. Each of the helical or icosahedral shapes of the nucleocapsid could be enveloped or non-enveloped (see Fig. 30.10), giving four possible basic shapes for viruses. In fact, there are no animal viruses (only plant viruses) that are helical and non-enveloped, so cat or dog viruses can be grouped by and large into the other three types. Viruses have been classified together on the basis of structural similarities; for example, the group of viruses causing true

human flu make up the influenza viruses and horse flu is caused by equine influenza virus. Cat flu, unlike equine and human flu, is caused by two viruses, neither of which is an influenza virus.

Viruses are usually both host- and tissue-specific, so that each influenza virus is specific to the host species – an owner is not at risk of catching flu from his or her horse. There is a concern over avian flu (bird 'flu') as it seems to be able to transfer to humans that are in very close contact with infected poultry. Humans cannot at the moment transmit it to other humans, but the possibility of avian flu merging with the human influenza virus in an infected human to produce a transmissible disease is of great concern because of the huge potential for a fatal pandemic as happened in the early part of the 20th century.

VIRAL REPLICATION

Replication of pathogenic viruses takes place inside the host cell, unlike pathogenic bacteria, where reproduction usually takes place outside the host's cells (Fig. 30.11). Enveloped viruses attach to a cell with a suitable receptor, and then the virus envelope merges with the host cell membrane. Alternatively, the host cell is stimulated to engulf the virus particle of a non-enveloped virus and take it into the cell. Once inside the cell, the virus is able to switch the cell's normal metabolism to replication of the virus.

Once a host animal has been infected with a small number of virus particles, there is a time lag before symptoms are seen; this is the incubation period. During this time, the virus reaches the cells with which it has an affinity and initially infects only a small number of cells to increase the number of virus particles. Clinical signs are seen once large numbers of virus particles infect a large number of cells.

There are two types of virus which differ in the period of latency of the infection:
- Replication in the cell may happen immediately, so the cell begins to produce the constituents of new virus particles within hours of infection.
- Retroviral genetic material may join with the host cell's own nucleic acid for an extended period before making any changes to cell metabolism, as in the case of feline influenza virus (FIV) and human immunodeficiency virus (HIV).

Infection may not be apparent for many years after initial disease challenge. New virus particles are then assembled and released from the cell. Depending on the virus, this may leave the host cell intact or may cause its rupture and destruction.

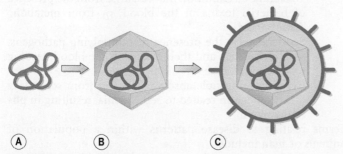

Fig. 30.9 Components of a virion. **(A)** Central core of nucleic acid. **(B)** Surrounding protein coat. **(C)** Some viruses have an outer envelope

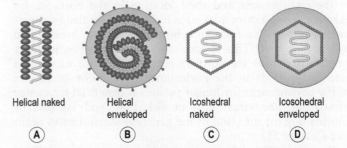

Helical naked   Helical enveloped   Icosahedral naked   Icosohedral enveloped

(A)   **(B)**   **(C)**   **(D)**

Fig. 30.10 Types of viral structure. **(A)** Helical naked. **(B)** Helical enveloped. **(C)** Icosohedral naked. **(D)** Icosohedral enveloped

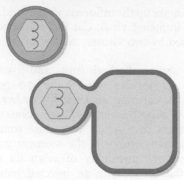

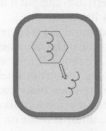

1. The virus attaches to the receptor sites on the host cell membrane and fuses with it

2. The virus enters the host cell and the protein coat (capsid) breaks down to release the viral nucleic acid

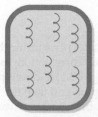

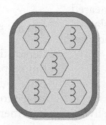

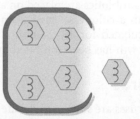

3. The viral nucleic acid replicates (either in the host cell cytoplasm or nucleus) and directs the host cell metabolism to make new virus material

4. The new viruses are assembled

5. They leave the host cell either by budding through or rupture of the cell membrane

Fig. 30.11   The process of replication in an enveloped virus

TABLE 30.7	Some canine viral diseases			
Name of virus	**Disease caused**	**Nucleic acid type**	**Shape of nucleocapsid**	**Enveloped**
Parvovirus	Parvovirus	DNA	Icosahedral	No
Canine adenovirus 1 (CAV-1)	Infectious canine hepatitis	DNA	Icosahedral	No
Canine adenovirus 2 (CAV-2)	Infectious canine tracheobronchitis	DNA	Icosahedral	No
Canine distemper virus	Distemper	RNA	Helical	Yes
Canine parainfluenza virus	Part of kennel cough syndrome	RNA	Helical	Yes
Rabies virus	Rabies	RNA	Helical	Yes

VIRAL TRANSMISSION

Viruses are transmitted from host to host either:

- Directly, e.g. by a cat licking feline calicivirus in nasal secretions off the face of another cat
- Indirectly, e.g. by a dog picking up virus particles from the floor of an inadequately cleaned kennel that has been occupied by a dog with parvovirus infection.

Different viruses have adapted their means of transmission according to their structure, which affects their ability to survive in the environment and their location in the host. So, for example, a respiratory tract virus is often transmitted by sneezing virus particles from one host into the air breathed in by another host. This is ideal for influenza virus, as these enveloped viruses are not very robust so do not survive for extended periods in the environment. An ability to survive in the environment for longer periods is beneficial for canine parvovirus. The virus must be licked up and ingested by another dog for infection of the gastrointestinal tract to occur (see Chapter 21).

Examples of viral diseases in the dog, cat and horse are listed in Tables 30.7–30.9.

Common disease terminology

Terms relating to disease organisms once they are within an animal are:

- **Bacteraemia** – the temporary presence of bacteria in the blood, usually precedes infections such as arthritis, meningitis, etc., without showing clinical signs
- **Viraemia** – viruses in the blood, either free, or associated with cells
- **Toxaemia** – a condition that can arise from the presence of bacterial toxins in the blood, or from metabolic disturbances
- **Septicaemia** – the presence of multiplying pathogens, such as bacteria and their toxins, in the blood, leading to systemic disease
- **Pyaemia** – multiple abscesses formed from secondary foci of infection related to septicaemia, resulting in pus in the blood.

Terms relating to disease patterns within a population of animals or man include:

- **Epidemiology** – the study of relationships of various factors determining the frequency and distribution of

TABLE 30.8 Some feline viral diseases				
Name of virus	**Disease caused**	**Nucleic acid type**	**Shape of nucleocapsid**	**Enveloped**
Feline parvovirus (panleukopenia)	Feline infectious enteritis	DNA	Icosahedral	No
Feline herpesvirus	Feline rhinotracheitis (cat flu)	DNA	Icosahedral	Yes
Feline calicivirus		RNA	Icosahedral	No
Feline coronavirus	Feline infectious peritonitis (FIP)	RNA	Helical	Yes
Feline leukaemia virus	Retrovirus causing feline leukaemia	RNA	Icosahedral	Yes
Feline immunodeficiency virus	Retrovirus	RNA	Icosahedral	Yes
Rabies virus	Rabies	RNA	Helical	Yes

TABLE 30.9 Some equine viral diseases					
Name/type of virus	**Site of infection**	**Disease caused**	**Nucleic acid type**	**Shape of nucleocapsid**	**Enveloped**
Adenovirus	Gastrointestinal tract Respiratory tract	'Scours' Cold/snotty nose	DNA	Icosahedral	No
Rotavirus	Gastrointestinal tract	'Scours'	RNA	Icosahedral	No
Bovine papillomavirus	Skin	Sarcoids	DNA	Icosahedral	No
Arterivirus	Reproductive tract	Equine viral arteritis	RNA	Icosahedral	Yes
Lentivirus	Respiratory	Equine infectious anaemia	RNA	Helical	Yes
Influenza	Respiratory	Equine flu	RNA	Helical	Yes
Equine herpes virus	Several, depending on type	Coital exanthema Rhinopneumonitis Herpes paralysis	DNA	Icosahedral	Yes

diseases in a community. In veterinary science it is how the specific causes of localised outbreaks of infection and other diseases are determined. It is used to monitor the number of cases of disease and to monitor the effectiveness of a control policy as was shown by the 2001 outbreak of foot and mouth disease (FMD) in the UK. It can also predict the likelihood of occurrence of a disease/accident by elucidating the risk factors for the disease associated with the population studied, e.g. the increased risk of heart disease if overweight.

- **Epidemic** (epizootic more specifically refers to an animal disease) – a pronounced increase in the level of infection. Recent examples of epidemics include FMD in the UK, and mumps during 2005 in the unvaccinated 16–24-year-old cohort of students in the UK.

- **Endemic** (enzootic refers to animal disease) – a situation in which a particular disease is present at a low level in a country or area, e.g. myxomatosis in wild rabbits in the UK. FMD is not endemic in the UK, but is in parts of sub-Saharan Africa and South America.
- **Pandemic** – an epidemic which occurs all over the world.
- **Zoonosis** – a disease which can pass from animals to man, e.g. leptospirosis in dogs, cattle and rats; psittacosis in birds; ringworm in many animal species. Sensible routine hygiene precautions and awareness of the existence of such diseases will help to prevent them.
- **Anthroponosis** – a disease which can be passed from man to animals, e.g. it is possible for gorillas and chimpanzees to become infected by measles.

BIBLIOGRAPHY

Aspinall, V., 2014. Clinical Procedures in Veterinary Nursing, third ed. Butterworth-Heinemann, Oxford.

Jawetz, E., Melnick, J.L., Adelberg, E.A., 1991. Medical Microbiology, eighteenth ed. Prentice Hall, Canada.

RECOMMENDED READING

Aspinall, V., 2014. Clinical Procedures in Veterinary Nursing, third ed. Butterworth-Heinemann, Oxford.
 Provides information about the practical aspects of bacteriology.

Ikram, M., Hill, E., 1991. Microbiology for Veterinary Technicians. American Veterinary Publication, Santa Barbara, CA.
 Useful book which provides information at the right level.

31

Laboratory Diagnostic Aids

LORRAINE ALLAN | NICOLA ACKERMAN

KEY POINTS

- Laboratory tests are an invaluable aid to making an accurate diagnosis, assessing the severity of the condition and its response to treatment.

- Health and safety in the laboratory must be observed at all times.

- A wide range of equipment is used in the laboratory and the veterinary nurse must understand how and when it is used and must ensure that it is properly maintained.

- A variety of body tissues and fluids can be sampled to provide an insight into the current health status of the patient.

- The veterinary nurse must know how to collect and preserve the samples and if necessary to dispatch them to a commercial reference laboratory.

- All laboratory tests must be performed correctly following a rigid protocol so that the results are both accurate and comparable to other tests of the same type.

- Accurate records must be kept and passed on to the appropriate veterinary surgeon.

Introduction

The majority of veterinary practices in the UK today are equipped with an 'in house' practice laboratory where a variety of procedures are undertaken, the range and complexity being dependent on various factors, including the equipment available, the expertise of the staff, time and financial constraints. Some procedures, however, are not within the scope of the average practice and commercial reference laboratories are used for these more sophisticated tests, mainly due to a large number of tests required to be carried out daily in order to ensure quality control and assurances. The role of the veterinary nurse may encompass taking the samples, performing the tests, recording the results and sending off samples to a commercial reference laboratory. Furthermore, an increased awareness of the significance of the results is expected, which can have an impact on the nursing care provided to the patient.

(More detailed information on parasitology and microbiology has been provided in Chapters 29 and 30).

Laboratory diagnostic aids are an invaluable tool to the care and welfare of the animal in four main ways:

- **As an aid to making an accurate diagnosis** – although a considerable amount of information can be gained from taking a detailed history and from performing a clinical examination, it might still not be possible to make a precise diagnosis. Further investigative diagnostic procedures, including laboratory tests, may help clarify the situation, enabling the veterinary surgeon to make a definitive diagnosis.

- **To assess the severity of a condition** – this could influence the choice of treatment and the subsequent recovery of the patient, e.g. monitoring blood glucose levels in patients suffering from diabetes mellitus.

- **To assess response to treatment** – on occasion it can be difficult to determine if an animal is responding to treatment solely from its clinical condition. A valuable insight into the patient's progress can be obtained from laboratory tests, e.g. monitoring blood parameters in anaemia.

- **To adjust treatment regimens** – monitoring drug levels can allow adjustment of therapeutic drug doses, e.g. the levels of barbiturate in the treatment of epilepsy.

Health and safety in the laboratory

In common with the rest of a veterinary practice, the laboratory is subject to legislation that attempts to make the workplace as safe an environment as possible (Table 31.1).

COMMON HAZARDS IN THE LABORATORY

A laboratory is potentially a dangerous place with many hazards, i.e. something with the potential to cause harm. The Control of Substances Hazardous to Health (COSHH) Regulations set out to identify hazards and to develop safe protocols to reduce the risks, i.e. something that is likely to cause harm, from these hazards to an absolute minimum and thus creating a safe working environment (see also Chapter 5).

The range of potential hazards in a practice laboratory include:

- Clinical material
- Biological agents
- Chemicals, which may be toxic or corrosive
- Sharp objects
- Toxic fumes
- Eye contaminants
- Zoonoses
- Fire.

Hazard warning signs give clear indications of potential hazards in a variety of situations including the laboratory (see Chapter 5).

To ensure a safe working environment in the laboratory a code of conduct must be followed that encompasses both the local Health and Safety rules and the COSHH regulations:

- Ensure access is only to authorised personnel.
- Provide adequate training and supervision of staff.
- Fully buttoned protective laboratory coats must be worn.

TABLE 31.1	Laboratory health and safety legislation	
Legislation	**Key points**
Health and Safety at Work Act 1974	Applies to all businesses. Sets out specific duties of employer and employee to ensure a safe working environment. Provides protection against risks in the workplace and ensures that all equipment and substances used are handled, stored and transported safely
The Control of Substances Hazardous to Health (COSHH) Regulations 2002	The main legislation covering the control of risks to staff from exposure to harmful substances at work. Includes undertaking risk assessments, drawing up written standard operating procedures (SOPs), monitoring and controlling exposure to harmful substances, and staff training
Control of Pollution (Special Waste) Regulations 1988 Collection and Disposal of Waste Regulations 1992 Environmental Protection Act 1992	The principal regulations that control the correct handling, segregation, storage, transfer and disposal of products, including clinical waste and chemicals, minimising damage to the environment and reducing risks to staff
Reporting of Injuries, Diseases and Dangerous Occurrences (RIDDOR) Regulations 1995	Describe the procedures that must take place if death, serious injury or work-related disease occurs in the workplace. Such occurrences must be reported to the Health and Safety Executive (HSE)
First Aid at Work Act	This regulates first-aid provision and the recording of accidents

- Disposable gloves and, if necessary, eyeglasses and masks must be worn when handling hazardous materials.
- Long hair should always be tied back.
- Smoking, eating, drinking, chewing gum and mouth pipetting are prohibited.
- Hands should be washed when leaving the laboratory using an antibacterial soap and protective coats should be removed.
- The laboratory should be kept clean, neat and tidy.
- The work surfaces must be cleaned and disinfected after use.
- Books and papers should be kept away from the work area and any other source of contamination.
- Labelled containers of suitable disinfectant solutions should be provided for contaminated equipment disinfection.
- Correct disposal of laboratory waste must be observed. Different types of waste must be clearly segregated – infectious, offensive and pharmaceutical. Disposal containers should be clearly marked and colour-coded, to prevent mistakes being made.
- 'Sharps' containers must be provided.
- Hazard warning signs must be displayed as appropriate.
- Appropriate action should be taken in case of spillage and any spills should be contained and disposed of safely. If an infectious agent is involved, thorough disinfection or sterilisation may be required.
- When performing bacteriological procedures, special care must be taken not to contaminate the operative or the environment.
- Bunsen burners must be placed on a heat-resistant mat, must not be left on a working flame in between stages of the procedure and must be turned off immediately when they are no longer required.
- A well-stocked first-aid box must be provided and first-aid equipment, such as eyewash, must be readily available and in working condition. Ideally, a member of staff should be a trained first-aider.
- In case of accident, immediate remedial action should be taken. Medical attention should be sought if necessary. All accidents, no matter how trivial, must be reported to a responsible member of staff and recorded in the accident book, and if of a serious nature should be reported according to the RIDDOR regulations.
- Fire-fighting equipment should be available and an evacuation procedure displayed.
- A senior member of staff should be consulted if any problems are encountered.

Disposal of laboratory waste

The disposal of laboratory waste is controlled by legislation; see Table 31.1 for the specific Acts. The regulations control the correct segregation, storage, transfer and destruction of waste products in the practice including the laboratory. All businesses have a duty of care to ensure that:

- All waste is stored and disposed of responsibly
- Waste is only handled or dealt with by those authorised to do so
- Appropriate records are kept of all waste that is transferred or received.

INFECTIOUS WASTE

The term 'infectious waste' constitutes any veterinary waste containing viable microorganisms or their toxins which are known or reliably believed to cause disease in man or other living organisms. Much of the materials generated within the lab may be classed as infectious waste.

Following a veterinary assessment, waste deemed to be contaminated may include:

- Clinical items (for example swabs, masks and gloves)
- Animal bedding.

Disposal of infectious waste:

- This should be collected and stored in orange-coloured plastic bags for high-temperature incineration only.
- It must be collected by a registered carrier in a designated vehicle, licensed specially for the transport of infectious waste and transferred to a licensed plant for incineration with a waste transfer note.

CONTAMINATED 'SHARPS'

This comprises all sharps contaminated with animal blood or pharmaceuticals (other than cytotoxic or cytostatic). These may include partially and fully discharged sharps, hypodermic needles and other sharp instruments.

Disposal:

- All sharps can be segregated into yellow sharps containers for high-temperature incineration only.
- Contaminated microscope slides, coverslips and capillary tubes should be placed in the yellow sharps bins. Glass vials and blood collection tubes should also be placed in the sharps containers due to the potential for them to break.

CHEMICAL WASTE

There are specific legal requirements about the disposal of waste chemicals when they are discharged into public sewers. All chemical reagents used in the laboratory are subject to COSHH Regulations. Each chemical must be identified and the hazards and risks associated with its use assessed, including its disposal.

DOMESTIC WASTE

This is non-hazardous waste and should be disposed of in black refuse bags. Any confidential paperwork should be shredded prior to disposal.

Routine laboratory equipment

GLASSWARE

Glassware is used to measure and hold reagents and samples, usually liquids. Borosilicate glass (Pyrex) is used as it is harder than ordinary glass and less easily broken.

It is important that all glassware is thoroughly cleaned to remove any contaminated material that might interfere with the accuracy of the tests. New glassware should always be washed before use.

Cleaning glassware

- Rubber gloves should be worn.
- Contaminated glassware should be soaked in an approved disinfectant for 24 hours prior to cleaning.
- Any residues should be removed with the aid of a soft bristle brush. The glassware should then be washed in commercial laboratory detergent, following the manufacturer's instructions, or in an ultrasonic bath.
- The glassware should then be rinsed thoroughly two or three times in distilled/deionised water to remove all traces of the cleaning solution, which could affect the accuracy of results.
- The glassware should be allowed to drain and then dried in a drying cabinet. Bottles should not be dried with their stoppers in place, as the water will not evaporate.
- Once dry, the glassware should be stored in a cupboard or drawer to protect it from dust, grease and possible damage.
- The same method should be adopted to clean plasticware, although cooler water should be used. Organic solvents should be avoided as they could cause damage.
- Pipettes can prove difficult to clean, especially if left, but must be thoroughly cleaned.

MICROSCOPE

A microscope is an essential piece of equipment in any veterinary laboratory. It is advisable to use a monocular or binocular compound light microscope with an inbuilt light source (Fig. 31.1); some older microscopes utilise a mirror and external light source. Table 31.2 explains the function of the parts of the microscope.

A microscope is an expensive precision instrument and should be treated as such:

- In common with all electrical equipment it should be checked regularly for safety.
- Do not site it near a window or sources of heat, moisture or vibration.
- The microscope should be switched off and covered when not in use to avoid contamination from spills and dust.
- The stage should be cleaned with disinfectant wipes.
- The eyepieces and objective lenses should only be cleaned with special lens tissue.
- The oil immersion lens should be cleaned after each use with lens tissue to ensure that the oil does not solidify and damage the lens.
- When moving the microscope, carry it by the limb with one hand under the base.
- If glasses are normally worn, remove them to prevent damage.
- Never move the objective lens and slide towards each other while looking down the microscope, as this could result in breaking the slide and damage to the objective lens.
- Keep spare light bulbs in stock. Do not handle the bulb when replacing it.
- Ensure that the microscope is regularly serviced.

Examination of a blood smear on a microscope slide:

- Switch on the microscope.
- Move the stage approximately 5 cm below the objective lenses.
- Rotate the nosepiece clockwise and click the ×10 objective lens into place.
- Rack up the condenser until its top surface is as high as possible.
- Looking from the side, not down the microscope, adjust the iris diaphragm control lever so that it is at the middle position of its range of movement, i.e. approximately half-open. As the lens power is increased the aperture of the iris diaphragm should be increased to allow more light to be directed up the microscope.
- Place the slide on the mechanical stage and secure it firmly in position.
- Position the area to be viewed over the light source using the mechanical stage control knobs.
- Looking from the side, move the stage towards the lens, by using both the coarse adjustment controls, until it is 4 mm away.
- Looking down the microscope, very carefully and slowly move the stage away from the lens until the image comes into focus.
- Then, adjusting the fine focus, obtain the sharpest possible image. Do not use the fine focus to excess – if you have to do this it means you are not near enough to focus with the coarse focus.

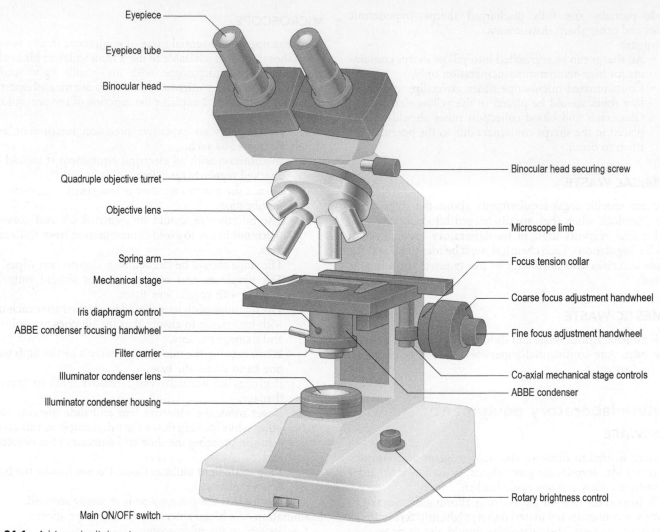

Eyepiece
Eyepiece tube
Binocular head
Quadruple objective turret
Objective lens
Spring arm
Mechanical stage
Iris diaphragm control
ABBE condenser focusing handwheel
Filter carrier
Illuminator condenser lens
Illuminator condenser housing
Main ON/OFF switch
Binocular head securing screw
Microscope limb
Focus tension collar
Coarse focus adjustment handwheel
Fine focus adjustment handwheel
Co-axial mechanical stage controls
ABBE condenser
Rotary brightness control

Fig. 31.1 A binocular light microscope

- To view the specimen under ×40, move the stage away from the ×10 lens and click the ×40 lens clockwise into position.
- Looking from the side, move the stage up towards the lens until the slide is almost touching it.
- Looking down the microscope, focus the slide as previously described.
  - **Note:** the slide will be much closer to the lens when in focus than when using the ×10 lens.
- Next use the oil immersion lens ×100 by moving the stage away from the lens and rotating the nosepiece so that neither the ×40 or ×100 lens are in position.
- Place a small drop of immersion oil on the slide (Fig. 31.3).
- Click the ×100 lens in position.
- Looking from the side, move the stage up towards the ×100 lens until the slide touches the lens.
- Move the stage even closer to the slide; the oil will be seen to spread out from the lens.
- Looking down the microscope, very carefully and slowly focus the slide.
- When focused, the lens must be in the oil.
- It is only practice that will make you proficient in the use of a microscope.

Tips

- Blood and bacterial smears should be examined under ×10, ×40 then ×100 with oil immersion.
- Urine sediments and faeces should be examined under ×10 then ×40.
- Parasite slides should be first examined with the naked eye. If macroscopic, examine under ×5 then ×10. If microscopic, examine under ×10 then ×40.

CENTRIFUGE

This is an important piece of laboratory equipment and is used in many diagnostic tests, including:

- Separation of blood cells from plasma or serum
- Urine sedimentation
- Faecal analysis.

Modern centrifuges are very sophisticated, but all work on the same principle. The samples are contained in special centrifuge tubes and subjected to centrifugal force, which results in the heavier constituents of the suspension settling to the bottom of the tube while the lighter ones settle at the top. This accelerates the process that would occur if the samples were left to settle under the influence of gravity alone.

TABLE 31.2	Parts of the microscope
Part	**Function**
Stage	A flat square platform on which the specimen is placed. A hole in the centre allows light from the condenser to illuminate the specimen. The surface of the stage is covered with chemical resistant vulcanite and can be moved up and down by the coarse and fine adjustment control knobs to focus the specimen
Mechanical stage	This is attached to the stage holding the slide in place and also facilitating movement of the slide in east–west and north–south directions with accuracy
Vernier scales	These are located on both movements of the mechanical scales at right angles to each other and allow relocation of a particular point on the slide. Each scale consists of a main scale divided into millimetres and a Vernier plate with 10 divisions each of 0.9 mm. To read a Vernier scale, observe where the zero mark on the Vernier plate meets the main scale. If it falls between two divisions record the lower one. In Figure 31.2 the zero is between 55 and 56, so 55 is recorded. Next note which of the divisions on the Vernier plate is exactly opposite a division on the main scale. In the example, this is the mark 5. The complete reading is recorded as 55.5. If the zero mark had been exactly opposite 55 the reading would have been 55.0. It is essential that readings from both scales are taken and recorded
Body	This houses the focusing mechanism for the body tube
Body tube	A hollow metal tube that contains no lenses or other optical parts. An eyepiece fits into the upper part and a nosepiece into the lower end
Eyepiece	Contains two lenses: the one closest to the eye is known as the ocular lens and the more distal one is the field lens. Most have a magnifying power of ×10. Its purpose is to magnify the primary image formed by the objective lens. Binocular microscopes have two eyepieces
Nosepiece	Found at the lower end of the body tube with a rotating turret that holds the objective lenses and can be rotated to click a different objective lens into place. It should always be rotated in a clockwise direction so as to move from a lower power to a higher power
Objective lenses	Normally four lenses, each with a different magnification, are housed in the nosepiece. Usually ×4 (scanning), ×10 (low-power), ×40 (high dry) and ×100 (oil immersion)
Condenser	Fitted below the stage and is therefore sometimes called the substage condenser. It consists of two lenses that condense the light from the light source on to the specimen to make it brighter and the image sharper. The position of the condenser and the amount of light passing through the specimen can be adjusted. Remember that when viewed the image will be upside down and reversed
Iris diaphragm	Adjusting the aperture of the iris diaphragm with the iris diaphragm control can regulate the amount of light that passes through the condenser. Below the iris diaphragm there are often glass filters that can alter the wavelength of light passing through the condenser
Limb	This connects the base with the body and supports the stage and condenser. The base houses the light source and on/off switch. Some microscopes have a brightness control which can vary the intensity of light delivered

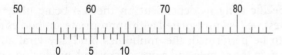

Fig. 31.2 The Vernier scale

Centrifuges contain a rotor or centrifuge head, drive shaft and motor enclosed in the guard bowl. Other features include a timer, speed control, break and safety lock.

Standard centrifuges are of two types according to the type of rotor head:

- **Swing-out head with specimen buckets**, which contain rubber cushions to reduce damage to the centrifuge tubes, suspended vertically from the arms of the rotor. As the rotor turns, the buckets swing out into a horizontal position, falling back to the vertical when the rotor slows down and stops. The sediment is uniformly distributed, allowing the supernatant (liquid) to be easily removed by a pipette.
- **Angle head**, where the tubes are held in a fixed position, usually 25–40° from vertical. The sediment can form at an angle depending on the type of tubes being used. Higher centrifuge speeds can be achieved, however, because of the aerodynamic shape of the rotor.

The microhaematocrit centrifuge is very specialised and is used to measure blood packed cell volume (PCV). It utilises capillary tubes that are held horizontally on a grooved metal or plastic plate.

Care and cleaning of the centrifuge

- Never attempt to open the centrifuge until the head has completely stopped rotating.
- Ensure that the samples are balanced in diametrically opposite buckets by weight, not volume.
- If, with increasing revs, the machine develops excessive vibrations, stop the centrifuge and, when the head has finished rotating, examine the chamber, as the most likely cause is improperly balanced arms.
- Follow the manufacturer's instructions to operate the centrifuge.
- Regularly clean and disinfect the centrifuge.
- Any spillages/breakages should be carefully cleaned away and the chamber disinfected while wearing disposable gloves.
- When using a microhaematocrit centrifuge ensure that the safety plate is fastened over the samples to hold the capillary tubes safely in place. Regularly check the rubber gasket for wear and replace it if necessary.
- Ensure regular servicing and cleaning.

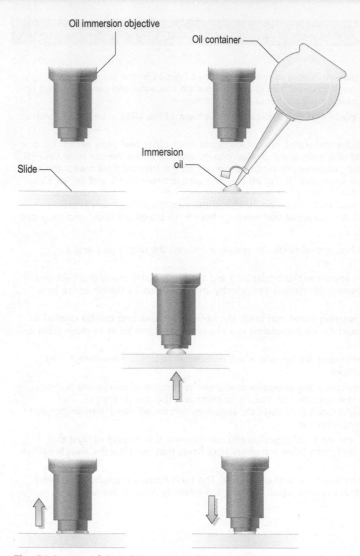

Fig. 31.3 Use of the oil immersion objective

ELECTRONIC ANALYSERS

The majority of veterinary practices have electronic analysers to improve the diagnosis of many conditions, in house. These include biochemistry, haematology, electrolyte, blood gas analysis and hormone analysers, the first two being the most commonly found in practice laboratories.

Care and maintenance

- To avoid damage, position away from vibrations, e.g. produced by centrifuges, or liquids.
- Switch off and cover when not in use, if in accordance to the manufacturer's instructions.
- Use in accordance with the manufacturer's instructions.
- Service regularly.
- Quality control tests against known results should be regularly undertaken. These are in addition to the external quality control tests performed to ensure the accuracy and validity of all tests.

Biochemistry analysers

These are used to measure the levels of various biochemical substances in blood, e.g. glucose, total protein (TP), blood urea nitrogen (BUN), plasma enzymes, fructosamine and hormones.

Most are dry chemistry systems. The sample is placed on a series of slides that results in a colour change reflecting the amount of the substance being tested. The machine reads and interprets the colour change as the level of the substance that is present in the sample. Some biochemistry analysers utilise small wells of fluid rather than slides and are known as wet chemistry systems. Whatever the system, the results are compared with the normal reference range for each parameter measured, which gives valuable information about the clinical condition of the patient (especially prior to anaesthesia), facilitating diagnosis and monitoring.

Haematology analysers

These are used to automatically determine total red and white blood cell counts, differential white blood cell counts, haematocrit and platelet counts, among other parameters. They provide useful information regarding the blood picture of the patient.

Electrolyte analysers

Plasma electrolyte levels provide valuable information that can help in diagnosing diseases such as Addison's disease, monitoring changes caused by dehydration and acid–base balance and also in cases of hypocalcaemia and neoplasia. Parameters commonly measured include sodium, chloride, potassium, bicarbonate, calcium and phosphate. These parameters are more commonly measured as part of the biochemistry or blood gas analyser, rather than in a stand-alone machine.

COMMERCIAL TEST KITS

A number of in-house test kits are available that can be used to diagnose certain viral diseases, determine hormone levels, investigate allergic conditions and blood clotting.

Most utilise the enzyme-linked immunosorbent assay (ELISA) test (see also Chapter 21). The test detects the presence of specific antigens dependent on the test being undertaken. The test well is impregnated with appropriate antibodies for the test to be performed; the antibodies bind any viral antigens present in the sample and a dye is activated, producing a colour change that indicates a positive result.

Test kits in common use in practice include:

- **FeLV ELISA test** – detects viral antigens to feline leukaemia in blood. A coloured spot or line indicates a positive result.
- **FIV ELISA test** – detects viral antigens to feline immunosuppression virus in blood.
- **Parvovirus ELISA test** – detects viral antigens in faeces. Care must be taken in interpreting the results in dogs that have recently been vaccinated with live parvovirus as they can shed the virus for 5–12 days post-vaccination, resulting in a false-positive result.
- **Premate test** – an ELISA test that measures progesterone levels in serum or plasma. It is used to determine the optimum time for mating in the bitch and utilises the fact that blood progesterone levels rise at ovulation. Serial blood samples are taken before ovulation; the test shows a dark pink colour; increased progesterone is indicated by a colour change to pink.
- **Allercept e-screen test** – an ELISA test that detects immunoglobulin E (IgE) in blood. A serum or plasma

sample is required. A positive test suggests that an allergic condition is likely, but further testing at a commercial laboratory will be necessary to determine the specific cause or causes of the allergic condition.

- **Total T₄** – a test that gives a quantitative result for the total thyroxine 4 level within the cat.
- **Species-specific pancreatic lipase test** – the test give a normal or abnormal reading for the pancreatic specific lipase levels in cats and dogs.
- **Heartworm** – in-vitro diagnostic for the semi-quantitative detection of *Dirofilaria immitis* (*D. immitis*) antigen in canine and feline whole blood, serum or plasma.

Other in-house tests include *Giardia*, *Leishmania*, cortisol, bile acids and Lyme disease.

Recording sample details and test reports

This is probably the most important part of laboratory practice. It is vital that the sample can be correctly linked with the patient, the tests required linked with the sample and finally the results of the tests performed linked with those requested and the sample. Provided that each stage of the process is recorded accurately immediately upon completion, this should not be a problem.

PROTOCOL

Immediately the sample has been collected and placed in an already labelled container. It should be labelled either with the details of the owner's name and address and the patient's name or with a reference number that can be computerised. This identifies the sample for all time. The type of sample tube or container that is to be used should be checked prior to the sample being collected. Different tests will require different preservatives.

A laboratory request form should then be completed, even if the tests are to be performed 'in house'. A typical request form should include:

- Practice name and address. This can be omitted if an 'in-house' test is to be performed. Many commercial reference laboratories provide preprinted forms that include a practice reference number.
- The name of the veterinary surgeon to whom the results are to be returned.
- Owner's name and address or reference number.
- Species and breed of the patient. Its name can also be included.
- Age and sex of the patient, including whether the patient is neutered.
- A description of the sample(s).
- A clinical history and provisional diagnosis.
- Details of any medication.
- The tests required.
- The date the sample was taken. Histology samples should be accompanied by a chart indicating the sample sites.
- Any additional information that could help in the interpretation of the results, especially if the sample is sent to a commercial laboratory, e.g. is it a fasted sample, or when were any medications last given.

On receipt at the laboratory, even an internal one, the reference number should be put on the form and all apparatus, e.g. microscope slides, should be labelled with that number. This links the laboratory request form (report forms if used) with the sample, ensuring that no confusion arises, especially if tests are undertaken on multiple samples simultaneously. In most practices the laboratory equipment is directly linked to the practice management system and will automatically link the results to the patient's clinical history.

On completion of the tests, the results should then be reported to the presenting veterinary surgeon. This can be in the form of the laboratory report form or printout, or a communicative to say that the results are available on the patient's clinical history. Commercial reference laboratories can also include an interpretation of the results, which may be emailed (or faxed) to the practice to decrease the turn-around time. In the case of email, in most cases, these will automatically attach to the patient's clinical history via the practice management system.

Notification that the results have been returned should be given to the veterinary surgeon concerned and any other appropriate members of staff and also recorded on the patient's records immediately on receipt if sent by fax. Communicating the results to the client is usually undertaken by the veterinary surgeon but a veterinary nurse, under the direction of a veterinary surgeon, can communicate results if the veterinary surgeon feels it is appropriate.

DISPATCH OF PATHOLOGICAL MATERIAL

In order for the test results to be accurate and meaningful it is essential that the samples sent to an external reference laboratory should arrive in the same condition as when they were sampled, with minimal deterioration. Correct preservation, clearly labelled samples, accurately completed paperwork and correct packaging will ensure this is the case. It is vitally important to clearly label the samples and ensure that the accompanying paperwork is correct.

Samples must be preserved if any delay is expected between sampling and subsequent testing. If preservation is not performed correctly, spoilage of the sample will occur and the results obtained will not reflect the true disease status of the animal.

Causes of spoilage of samples include:

- Haemolysis of blood.
- Clotting of blood – due to absence or insufficiency of anticoagulant, failure to mix the blood sufficiently with the anticoagulant, or too long a time taken when collecting the sample.
- Contamination of the sample – bacterial or gross contamination.
- Death of bacteria – due to using inappropriate preservatives.
- Insufficient volume – this can result from insufficient collection of the sample or leakage of the sample in transit.
- Desiccation – usually of pus or faeces. This may occur if too little of the sample is collected or the sample is collected into a non-airtight container that allows evaporation, especially during hot weather. Plain swabs are especially susceptible.

- Autolysis of tissue samples – digestion of tissue by its own enzymes. This may occur in portions of tissue despatched to an external reference laboratory, especially if the time taken to reach their destination is increased, i.e. over weekends or holiday periods, or if the ambient temperature is increased. It may also occur if a piece of tissue is too large for the fixative solution to penetrate it completely. Post-mortem samples and cadavers should be properly packed to prevent leakage and sent as quickly as possible to the external reference laboratories to prevent autolysis rendering the results useless.
- Fragmentation of preserved tissues – this can result from preserving them in containers that have a narrow neck, making their removal difficult.

It is equally important that the samples are correctly packaged to ensure they are not damaged during transit and that the containers do not break or leak. The containers should be leak-proof, robust, securely fastened and protected from breaking by padding. It should also be ensured that the risk of contamination of the paperwork, other samples, anyone handling the samples in transit or on receipt of the samples should be minimised. This should not make it impossible for the laboratory staff to extricate the samples from the packaging safely.

Samples are usually sent to commercial reference laboratories by courier, but are still sometimes sent in the post.

Pathological specimens pose a potential hazard to members of the public involved in their transport so it is vitally important that they are correctly packaged and correctly labelled according to Post Office regulations. The containers should also conform to United Nations Regulation 602. This protocol should also be followed if despatched by courier or if taken by hand:

- Faeces or liquid samples, such as blood, serum, urine, body fluids and tissue samples, should be placed in an appropriate sealed primary container. This container must not exceed 50 ml unless Post Office–approved multi-specimen packs are used.
- Dry samples such as blood or bacterial smears should be placed in special slide-holding containers. Coat brushings and hair samples can be put into sealed plastic bags or sealed paper envelopes, as the plastic can cause issues in some samples. Skin scrapings can be sent in a sealed container or on a slide in a slide-holding container.
- The sample should then be wrapped in enough absorbent material to absorb all possible leakage in case of damage. This also protects the sample against damage in transit.
- This should then be placed in a sealed leak-proof plastic bag.
- The package must then be placed, along with the request form, into a secondary container: either a plastic clip-down container, a cylindrical lightweight metal container, a strong cardboard box with a full-depth lid or a two-piece polystyrene box with a special grooved join.
- It is recommended that this complete package is then placed and securely sealed in a padded 'Jiffy' bag. This should be labelled on the outside with the words: PATHOLOGICAL SPECIMEN – FRAGILE WITH CARE and the name and address of the laboratory. The package must show the name and address and telephone number of the sender to be contacted in case of leakage, on the reverse side. A biohazard symbol can also be included.
- First class or data post should be used, not parcel post, if the parcel is to be delivered by the Post Office.
- Other packaging systems must be approved by the Post Office.
- Improperly packaged or labelled samples will not be handled by the postal services.

When sending samples by post it is essential that they reach the external reference laboratory as quickly as possible to reduce deterioration of the samples, so send the samples by first class post, data post or courier. Avoid sending the samples over a weekend or a public holiday in the post. Some samples deteriorate faster than others, even though they have been preserved, e.g. bacteriological samples. Also remember that deterioration will be accelerated by high ambient temperatures.

It cannot be emphasised enough how important the correct packaging and despatch is to ensure accurate results.

Blood

Examination of blood samples can provide an invaluable insight into the health status of patients, aiding diagnosis, monitoring response to treatment and the severity of conditions.

COLLECTION OF BLOOD

Collection of a blood sample is normally by venepuncture using a syringe and needle (see also Chapters 12, 13 and 14). It is important that, before the sample is taken, the correct equipment is assembled. The correct gauge of needle should be selected. It should be the largest gauge with the shortest length possible to allow the sample to be taken quickly and reduce damage to the red blood cells. Clippers, a surgical spirit swab, an appropriate disinfectant swab to clean the site and a suitable blood collection bottle should be close at hand.

An alternative method is to use a Vacutainer kit (Fig. 31.4). A Vacutainer is an evacuated tube, i.e. one containing a vacuum. The small tubes have a 3 ml volume but only a 2 ml draw to reduce the pressure on the red blood cells. The tubes are made of glass and are sealed at one end with a rubber bung. The rest of the kit comprises a holder with a double-ended needle (see Fig. 31.4). One end of the needle is inserted into the vein and the other end pierces the bung and the blood is drawn into the Vacutainer, available as plain tubes or containing different anticoagulants.

Syringes are available that have detachable barrels coated with anticoagulant, negating the necessity for sample bottles – these are sold as Monovette. Convertible syringe/evacuated tubes or S-Monovette are also available. These combine the best

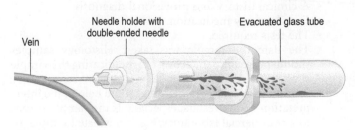

Fig. 31.4 A Vacutainer

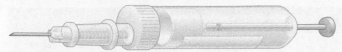

Fig. 31.5 S-Monovette blood collection system

TABLE 31.3	Venepuncture sites
Species	**Vein/site**
Dog and cat	Jugular – ventral aspect of the neck Cephalic – cranial aspect of the radius (only in large dogs) Lateral saphenous – lateral aspect of the hock (in dogs) Medial saphenous – medial aspect of the hind limb (in cats)
Rabbit	Jugular Lateral marginal ear vein – base of pinna Lateral saphenous
Guinea pig	Jugular Lateral marginal ear vein
Rat/mouse/gerbil	Lateral tail vein
Hamster	Jugular under anaesthesia
Ferret	Jugular Cephalic Caudal – ventral aspect of tail
Bird	Jugular Brachial – medial aspect of the elbow Medial metatarsal in larger birds May require anaesthesia
Snakes	Jugular Ventral tail vein Palatine – roof of the mouth Intracardiac under anaesthesia
Lizard	Jugular Cephalic Ventral tail vein
Chelonians	Jugular Dorsal tail vein

features of Vacutainers and blood-collecting syringes and can be used in either mode (Fig. 31.5).

Depending on the species and volume of blood required there are various sites available for venepuncture. The largest accessible vein should always be used (Table 31.3).

Technique

1. Handling and restraint for venepuncture varies with the species involved and the sampling site. Manual restraint is usually adequate for restraining dogs and cats. If the patient is aggressive then a different protocol may be required, e.g. muzzles, wrapping in a towel. If necessary, sedation or anaesthesia may be required, especially with exotic species. It is usually less stressful and safer to anaesthetise most birds prior to blood sampling but large birds such as swans can be blood sampled from the metatarsal vein without causing distress. The application of local anaesthetic gel to the site when taking blood from the marginal ear vein can also make the procedure less stressful.

2. Once suitably restrained by an assistant, the injection site should be clipped, cleaned with an appropriate disinfect-ant and then swabbed with surgical spirit or equivalent to ensure asepsis. All equipment should be assembled and the sample tube labelled with the correct information for identifying the sample.

3. The proximal part of the vein needs to be occluded, which makes the vein easier to visualise and also prevents the blood from returning to the heart – known as 'raising the vein'.

4. The needle should be inserted at a shallow angle while tensing the skin over the site. Once in the vein the plunger is slowly pulled back to ensure the blood is not subjected to excessive pressure, which could damage the red blood cells and also to ensure the vein does not collapse.

5. Once the required volume has been obtained the needle is carefully removed from the vein and the assistant should apply pressure on the injection site to prevent bleeding.

6. The blood sample should then be transferred quickly to the previously selected sample bottle. The needle should be removed prior to filling the sample bottle to reduce damage to the red blood cells.

7. If the sample is transferred to a sample bottle containing anticoagulant the blood should be gently squirted into the bottle and filled to the 'fill line' to ensure that the anticoagulant is diluted correctly; the bottle should then be inverted or rolled to mix the contents. Avoid violent shaking as this can damage the red blood cells. If a serum sample is required there is no need to mix the sample and there is no specified fill line.

8. The pre-labelled sample should then have the time of sampling written on the tube.

9. Any waste should be disposed of appropriately.

Provided the correct protocol is followed the red blood cells will not be damaged and release their haemoglobin and potassium into the plasma. This process of rupture of the red blood cells is called haemolysis. If haemolysis has occurred the plasma or serum will be pink in colour. Haemolysis will ruin all the tests used in haematology except total white blood cell counts and haemoglobin levels, as the number of red blood cells will be diminished. The presence of free haemoglobin will also interfere with biochemical tests. It is therefore essential that haemolysis is avoided.

Tips to avoid haemolysis

- Excessive suction should be avoided when taking the sample.
- The blood should only pass through the needle once to reduce the trauma to the red blood cells, so remove the needle before transferring the blood to the sample bottle.
- Use as wide a gauge of needle as is practicable, with the shortest length, never bend the needle.
- Ensure the skin, needle and syringe are free of water to prevent osmotic damage to the red blood cells.
- Do not shake the sample bottle – roll or invert it to mix the sample.
- The sample should be examined as soon as possible after sampling.
- Store the sample at the correct temperature, cool (4°C) but not freezing.
- Avoid direct sunlight.
- If sending the sample to an external reference laboratory, ensure it is packaged correctly to protect against

TABLE 31.4	Anticoagulants		
Anticoagulant	Test	Tube cap colour	Vacutainer colour
Ethylenediaminetetraacetic acid (EDTA), also known as sequestrene	Routine haematology	Red	Lilac
Sodium fluoride/potassium oxalate	Glucose estimation	Yellow	Grey
Lithium heparin	Biochemistry	Orange	Green/green orange
Sodium citrate	Coagulation profiles	Purple (solid) Green (liquid)	Black
Ammonium/potassium oxalate	Glucose estimation	Turquoise	None
No anticoagulant	Biochemistry	White/colourless Brown for serum gel tubes	Red

careless handling and temperature variations. Ensure it is dispatched as soon as possible.

PRESERVATION OF BLOOD

Blood can be preserved in a number of ways depending on the investigations that are to be undertaken. These include:

- Preventing the blood clotting by using anticoagulants
- Leaving the blood whole and allowing it to clot naturally then removing the serum
- Making blood smears.

Anticoagulants

To perform haematology, the study of the physical characteristics and the number of cells per unit volume in blood, it is essential that the sample is not allowed to clot. To prevent the blood from clotting the inherent clotting process must be disabled by the addition of chemicals immediately on collection of the sample. The clotting process is a complex one that depends on the presence of calcium and a number of enzymes in addition to various clotting factors.

Anticoagulants fall into two categories:

- Those that block calcium – ethylenediaminetetraacetic acid (EDTA), oxalates, citrates and fluorides
- Those that interfere with the enzyme systems – heparin and fluorides.

All the anticoagulants listed in Table 31.4 are available commercially, as ready-prepared sample tubes and the majority as their equivalent Vacutainers.

No one anticoagulant is ideal for every test: each individual anticoagulant has properties that make it better suited for some tests than others. The preference for sodium fluoride/oxalate by some reference laboratories as the anticoagulant of choice for glucose estimation illustrates this point. It reduces the amount of glucose metabolised by the blood cells prior to the glucose estimation, more accurately representing the glucose levels present at the time of sampling. Some reference laboratories will require a serum gel tube that has been spun at a specific time after sampling for glucose measurement. This demonstrates the importance of knowing which tubes (and anticoagulants) are required for certain tests by the laboratory you are sending the sample to.

Serum samples

Serum is plasma, the fluid in which the cellular components of blood are suspended, minus the clotting factors such as fibrinogen. In biochemical examination it is usually serum that is used,

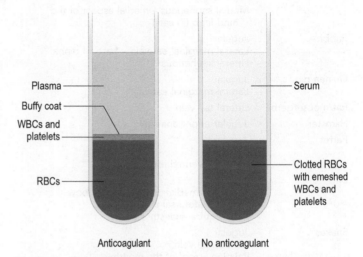

Fig. 31.6 The difference between blood being left to clot naturally or with an anticoagulant

although plasma can be used for most tests except bile acids, insulin and a number of specific serological investigations. It is important that the difference between plasma and serum is appreciated.

If a blood sample is placed in a sample bottle containing an anticoagulant, e.g. EDTA, and allowed to stand, the red blood cells, being the heaviest components, will fall to the bottom of the sample tube. On top of these will lie the white blood cells and platelets forming the 'buffy coat', and above this layer will be the plasma. Inversion of the bottle will result in resuspension of the cellular components (Fig. 31.6). If the blood sample, however, is placed in a sample tube that does not contain an anticoagulant and is left to stand, the red blood cells will clot, enmeshing both the white blood cells and platelets and a fluid will form above the clot, serum. In this case there will not be a distinct buffy coat and inversion of the sample will not result in resuspension of the sample, as the cellular components have clotted.

Serum collection can involve simply collecting the sample into a sample bottle containing no anticoagulant, then leaving the sample to clot, which may take up to 2 hours. The serum is then transferred to a sterile container. Centrifuging the sample may accelerate the process.

Alternatively the sample can be placed in special serum separation bottles. These contain a gel that, when the blood is introduced, allows the sample to clot but separates it from the serum,

TABLE 31.5	Changes in the colour of plasma/serum	
Colour	**Implication**
Pink	Indicates haemolysis has occurred within the body or more usually through faulty collection
Milky appearance	Due to the presence of fat droplets, i.e. lipaemia.
Yellow	Due to the presence of bilirubin. Indicative of severe liver damage or obstruction of the bile duct

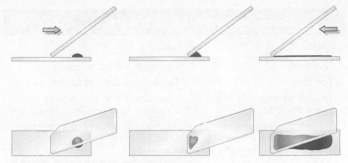

Fig. 31.7 Preparation of a blood smear

which lies above the gel. This prevents haemolysis from interfering with subsequent testing. Separated serum can be stored for a few days at 4°C; if testing is to be delayed longer than this, the sample can be frozen but must be thawed at room temperature and then thoroughly mixed before any tests are performed.

Normal canine and feline plasma and serum are clear and almost colourless to pale yellow in colour. The presence of various substances in the blood can alter this colour and provide valuable information as to the health status of the individual (Table 31.5). Lipaemia can be normal in some animals that have been fed within the previous 3 hours, so blood samples should be taken from fasted animals to reduce the risk of misinterpretation of results. High-protein meals can also interfere with creatinine levels and give a falsely elevated result. Haemolysis interferes with haematological tests and lipaemia with biochemistry analysis.

Blood smears

Smearing blood on to a slide is a common method of preserving blood to examine it for its relative cellular contents, any cellular abnormalities, presence of blood parasites and a rough estimation of the number of platelets. The smear can be left to air-dry but if examination is to be delayed the smear is best fixed by immersing it in 100% methyl alcohol for 1 minute; staining can then be postponed for up to 3 days. Dried smears are very delicate and should be handled with care and carefully packaged if being despatched to an external reference laboratory.

Preparation of a blood smear

1. Gloves must be worn.
2. Take a grease-free microscope slide. All slides should be washed and dried before use.
3. Label the slide with a chinagraph pencil to identify the sample. This should be done on the underside to prevent the labelling from being removed during staining.
4. Place the slide on the bench, against a white background, with its long sides parallel to the edge of the bench.
5. Draw a small sample of fresh or well-mixed EDTA-treated blood into a capillary tube
6. The description that follows is for a right-handed technician (Fig. 31.7). If you are left-handed the directions 'left' and 'right' should be reversed.
7. Place a small drop of blood at the right-hand end of the slide about 1 cm from its edge.
8. Take a 'spreader' in the right hand, holding the long sides between the thumb and index finger, with the spreading edge, which is narrower than the microscope slide, directed downwards. The spreader can be made by cutting the corner off a microscope slide. The narrower edge to the spreader prevents the cells being pushed to the edge of the slide. Ensure that the spreader is not chipped nor has an irregular edge, as this could affect the quality of the smear. Always wipe the edge of the spreader between making smears, as dried blood will produce grooves in subsequent smears.

9. With both elbows resting on the bench, place the spreader in contact with the slide, a little to the left of the drop of blood and parallel to the short side of the slide. Hold the spreader at an angle of 20° to the vertical. A wider angle will result in a thicker smear while a more acute angle produces a thinner smear. Draw the spreader to the right until it makes contact with the blood. Allow the blood to run along the whole edge of the spreader.
10. Once this has occurred, immediately move the spreader to the left-hand end of the slide in a single rapid, smooth, firm action. The blood will be drawn along behind the spreader. Ensure that the edge of the spreader is in contact with the surface of the slide throughout. Never place the spreader to the right of the drop of blood and push the blood across the slide, as this will damage the cells.
11. The faster the spreader is moved the thinner and more even will be the resulting smear. Ideally, the red blood cells should overlap slightly, becoming more separate at the tail. A smear that covers half to two-thirds of the slide is ideal. Usually there are three definable parts to a smear – the head, body and tail.
12. Allow the smear to dry slowly without heating, keeping it horizontal. Heating will distort the cells, making the smear useless. Similarly, exposing the smear to water vapour while it is drying will render the smear of no diagnostic value as haemolysis may occur.
13. It is always advisable to make at least two smears in case one is unsatisfactory.
14. Remember, it takes practice to make a smear of diagnostic quality (Table 31.6).

Staining blood smears. To facilitate examination of the blood cells various stains are employed:

1. **Romanowsky stains**, e.g. Leishman's and Giemsa's stains and rapid stains such as Diff-Quik. This type of stain can be used to:
   - Detect changes in the size, shape and staining of the cells
   - Perform a differential white blood cell count
   - Detect the presence of blood parasites such as *Mycoplasma haemofelis* and *Babesia* spp.
   - Roughly estimate the number of platelets.

TABLE 31.6 Common faults in blood smears	
Fault	**Cause**
Too thick	Too large a drop of blood
Too thin	Too small a drop of blood
Transverse alternate thin and thick bands	Spreading done with a jerky motion, usually due to hesitation
Streaks throughout the length of the smear, especially at the tail	An irregular edge to the spreader Dried blood on the edge of the spreader Dust on the slide or in the blood
'Spots' where blood is absent	Grease on the slide
Very narrow, thick smear	Smear made before the blood has run along the spreading edge One surface of the spreader is lifted during spreading

2. **Supra-vital stains,** e.g. new methylene blue and brilliant cresyl blue. This type of stain can be used to:
   • Perform a reticulocyte count
   • Detect Heinz bodies.

These staining techniques are not routinely carried out in practice.

Technique for Leishman's stain. Always wear gloves as the stain is toxic by ingestion, inhalation and skin contact:

1. Place the labelled slide, smear side uppermost on to a staining rack over a staining bath.
2. Place sufficient concentrated Leishman's stain on the slide to cover it.
3. Leave for 2 minutes.
4. Do not wash off the stain but add twice the stain's volume of buffered distilled water (pH 6.8) and mix well.
5. Leave for 15 minutes.
6. Tip the stain off the slide and wash it well, front and back, with buffered distilled water.
7. Wipe the back of the slide, taking care not to wipe away the label. Prop upright and allow to dry.

Technique for Diff-Quik stain. This is a frequently used staining technique in practice, as it is easy, quick to perform and gives excellent results, comparable with May–Grünwald–Giemsa stain.

1. The staining set consists of three solutions: fixative solution, stain solution I and stain solution II. The blood smear is dipped in each in turn five times for a period of 1 second, i.e. 5 seconds in total.
2. The slide is allowed to drain after each dip.
3. Finally the slide is rinsed with distilled water and allowed to dry.
4. The whole procedure takes approximately 15 seconds.
5. By varying the number of dips in the appropriate solution, different degrees of shading and colour intensity are easily obtained.

It is important that all staining procedures are conducted properly, otherwise the smear may be useless, as the cells cannot be identified with any accuracy nor any abnormalities detected with any certainty. The reasons for the problems will depend

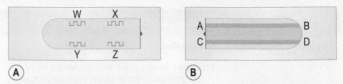

Fig. 31.8 Methods of performing a manual differential white blood cell count. (A) By the four-field meander method. (B) By the strip count method

on the particular staining technique being used but might include incorrect timing, failure to wash the stain off correctly or using stains at the incorrect concentrations.

MICROSCOPIC EXAMINATION OF A BLOOD SMEAR

Blood smears should be examined under ×10, ×40 then ×100 with oil immersion (Fig. 31.3). The slide should be carefully examined and any abnormalities noted (Table 31.7). (For illustrations of individual blood cells see Chapter 6.)

Blood smears can also be used for performing manual differential white blood cell counts. This determines the relative proportions of the different types of white blood cell and can give a valuable insight into the health status of the patient. It is time-consuming and requires a certain degree of expertise and experience to produce accurate results. The technique involves identifying and recording at least 200 white blood cells. The selection of a suitable area to count the cells can be problematic, as the distribution of the white blood cells is not uniform, with accumulation of the white blood cells at the edges and tail of the smear and a disproportionate number of monocytes and eosinophils, the larger blood cells, being found. In the past the 'four-field meander' method was used but this has been superseded with a strip count technique where all the white blood cells lying in one or more longitudinal strips running the complete length of the smear are classified (Fig. 31.8). The results are recorded on a tally chart and, by using a simple calculation, the percentage of each type of white blood cell is determined.

Many practices now carry out **quantitative analysis** of blood using electronic haematology machines, which if used correctly are more accurate and produce the results in a much shorter time frame. **Automated haematology analysers** use a range of different methods in order to perform a comprehensive complete blood count (CBC); these can include a combination of laser flow cytometry, optical fluorescence and laminar flow impedance.

Total red and white blood cell counts can also be performed manually using a **haemocytometer** but, even with practice, the accuracy obtained is not very high and the process is time-consuming. In this test the blood is diluted to a known concentration using special pipettes and the number of cells in a known volume is counted, under the microscope, on the grid etched on the haemocytometer. Different areas of the grid and different diluting fluids are used depending on whether a total red or white blood cell count is to be undertaken. Dacie's fluid is used for a red cell count and Turck's for a white blood cell count.

A **qualitative examination** of a blood smear should always be performed when an automated cell count is performed, as valuable information regarding the health status of the individual may be overlooked and also as part of the quality control

TABLE 31.7	Blood cells					
Cell	**Description**	**% Dog**	**% Cat**	**Size**	**Function**	
Erythrocyte	Biconcave disc; there should be no central pallor; immature cells will be larger than mature cells	37–55	24–45	Dog 7.0 μm Cat 4.5 μm	Carriage of oxygen	
Lymphocyte (small)	Round with a large round purple nucleus which almost fills all the cell, with a pale blue rim of cytoplasm	12–30	20–55	8 μm	Immunity production of antibodies	
Lymphocyte (large)	Similar to small lymphocyte but more oval in shape of the lymphocytes	Variable, approximately 8%	Variable	12–14 μm	As above	
Monocyte	Pleomorphic nucleus (slightly indented oval to horseshoe-shaped) with enlarged knob-like ends. Blue-staining cytoplasm which may contain vacuoles	3–10	1–4	20 μm	Chronic phagocyte	
Neutrophil	Irregular lobed nucleus with pale bluish pink cytoplasm with diffuse indistinct pale granules	60–70	35–75	10–12 μm	Phagocyte	
Immature, juvenile or band neutrophil	Nuclei horseshoe-shaped and not as darkly staining as mature neutrophils	Variable, 0–3	Variable, 0–3			
Eosinophil	Bilobed or segmented nucleus. Numerous reddish pink granules that are rod-shaped in the cat, round in the dog	2–10	2–12	12–14 μm	Increased numbers in parasitic and allergic conditions	
Basophil	Segmented or irregular-shaped nucleus. Blue-grey cytoplasm with dark, bluish granules	Very rare in both dog and cat	0–0.1	10–12 μm	Associated with the release of histamine and heparin	

protocol. The red blood cells should be examined for any abnormalities. The white blood cells should be checked for a 'shift to the left' and the presence of toxic neutrophils. Platelet clumping should also be noted.

Normal values are:

Total red blood cell count
- Dog – 5.5–8.5 × 10^{12}/l
- Cat – 5.0–10.0 × 10^{12}/l

Total white blood cell count
- Dog – 6–17 × 10^9/l
- Cat – 5.5–19.5 × 10^9/l

Abnormalities seen in blood smears

Erythrocyte abnormalities. These include:

a. **Size**
- Anisocytosis – a variation in the size of the red blood cells that is greater than would normally be expected
- Microcyte – an unusually small cell; may be indicative of a bone marrow defect
- Macrocyte – a large cell; usually a juvenile cell.

b. **Shape**
- Crenated – shrinkage of the cells giving a crinkled appearance; seen in old samples or if too high a concentration of anticoagulant has been used
- 'Star' or 'Burr' cells – appear to have blunt processes protruding from their surface; seen in old samples
- Spherocyte – do not have the normal biconcave shape; seen in autoimmune disease.

c. **Colour:**
- Hypochromic – very pale in colour as a result of low levels of haemoglobin

- Polychromasia – irregular areas of blue intermingled with the normal orange-pink colour; seen in immature cells.

d. **Inclusions** – these can be easily confused with stain debris:
- Reticulocyte – presence of dark blue inclusions when stained with supra-vital stains such as new methylene blue stain. Immature red blood cell, still containing residual RNA; seen in increased numbers in anaemia
- Heinz body – round, refractile, blue granular inclusions, again only seen when stained with a supra-vital stain. Formed due to the precipitation of denatured haemoglobin; common in cats. Can result from the action of drugs or infectious agents
- Howell–Jolly body – can be seen with Romanowsky stains as spherical blue-black granules near to the periphery of the cell. These are the remains of the nucleus which is absent in mature erythrocytes. Increased numbers are seen in regenerative anaemias and following splenectomy.

e. **Red cell parasites:**
- *Mycoplasma haemofelis* – the causal agent of feline infectious anaemia. Can usually be detected by Romanowsky stains but more easily seen with acridine orange stain. They are very small coccoid organisms that are found attached to the cell membrane, either singly or in short chains. Easily confused with stain debris. Fresh blood is best used as EDTA can detach the parasites from the cell surface
- *Babesia* – several forms. *Babesia canis* is the commonest form in Europe. Transmitted by ticks. Can be detected

by Romanowsky stains. As there are usually only a few organisms present, a peripheral sample is best taken, e.g. a drop of blood from the ear pinnae. The organism is pear-shaped and usually occurs in pairs, with up to eight or more present. Increasing in incidence in the UK because of the introduction of the PETS travel scheme
- Rouleaux formation is also often seen on blood smears. The red cells stack up behind one another, resembling a stack of coins. This occurs due to spreading the smear too slowly.

Leucocyte abnormalities. These include:
- A **'shift to the left'** describes an increase in the number of immature neutrophils and is indicative of an inflammatory condition.
- **Toxic neutrophils** are seen in severe toxaemic conditions and are characterised by a bluish pink cytoplasm, which is often vacuolated, with dark blue round or angular shaped inclusions known as Döhle bodies.

Abnormal cell counts. Various clinical conditions can cause abnormal blood cell counts (Table 31.8):
1. **Leucocytosis** – an increase in the number of white blood cells above the normal range. Possible causes include:
   - Presence of pathogenic organisms
   - Neoplasia
   - Haemorrhage
   - Steroid hormones
   - Degenerative non-inflammatory disease.
2. **Leucopenia** – a reduction in the number of white blood cells below the normal range. Usually the decrease is limited to one type of leucocyte and can give a useful insight into the health status of the patient. If all the leucocyte types are involved this is known as panleucopenia. Possible causes of leucopenia are:
   - Bone marrow failure
   - Overwhelming infections
   - Viral diseases, e.g. feline viral panleucopenia
   - Cushing's disease.

PACKED CELL VOLUME OR HAEMATOCRIT

Packed cell volume (PCV) is the red blood cell to fluid ratio in the blood. It is expressed as a percentage or litres per litre. A haematocrit (Hct) is not quite the same as a PCV, as the haematocrit is calculated by an automated analyser and not directly measured, but the two terms are used to described the same thing. It is determined by multiplying the red cell count by the mean cell volume (MCV). The haematocrit is slightly more accurate as the PCV includes small amounts of blood plasma trapped between the red cells. An estimated haematocrit as a percentage may be derived by tripling the haemoglobin concentration in g/dl and dropping the units.

Normal PCV ranges are:
- Dog 37–55% (0.37–0.55 l/l)
- Cat 24–45% (0.24–0.45 l/l).

Haemolysis and the use of a liquid coagulant will invalidate the results. Low PCVs are found in anaemia, sedation and anaesthesia and late canine pregnancy. High values are seen in dehydration, which results in haemoconcentration of the other elements within the blood. The PCV is often normally elevated in athletic breeds of dog, e.g. greyhounds, where it may be at the top end of the range. The PCV needs to be read alongside the total protein (TP) level in order to put it into context:
- Increase in PCV and TP = dehydration
- Decrease in PCV and TP = aggressive fluid therapy, haemorrhage
- Decreased PCV and normal TP = possible increased destruction of red blood cells
- Increased PCV and decreased TP = dehydration with protein loss, e.g. haemorrhagic enteritis.

Measurement of packed cell volume

The most common procedure used in practice is the **microhaematocrit method**. This employs the use of capillary 'microhaematocrit' tubes, which are heparinised if fresh blood is used, to prevent clotting. Plain tubes are used with anticoagulated samples.

Using anticoagulated blood:
1. A well-mixed sample is allowed to three-quarters fill a 'haematocrit' tube by capillary action.
2. The outside of the tube is wiped clean and the unfilled end is sealed with a special filler, e.g. Cristaseal.
3. The tube is then placed, sealed end outwards, into a special microhaematocrit centrifuge and spun for approximately 5 minutes at 10 000 rpm.

TABLE 31.8	Interpretation of differential leucocyte and platelet counts	
Cell	**Increased numbers**	**Decreased numbers**
Neutrophil	Neutrophilia caused by inflammation, bacterial infection, stress, fear, excitement, canine pregnancy, regenerative anaemia, neoplasia, necrosis and corticosteroid therapy	Neutropaenia caused by overwhelming infections, virus infections, e.g. FIV, FeLV, poisons, toxaemia, aplastic anaemia, cytotoxic drugs
Lymphocyte	Lymphocytosis caused by stress, strong immune stimulation, lymphocytic leukaemia, transiently following vaccination. Young animals have a higher count than adults	Lymphopaenia caused by viraemias/toxaemias, stress, corticosteroid therapy, Cushing's disease and chylothorax
Eosinophil	Eosinophilia caused by parasitism, allergy, eosinophilic leukaemia, Addison's disease, eosinophilic myositis	Eosinopaenia caused by stress, Cushing's disease and corticosteroid therapy
Monocyte	Monocytosis caused by acute or chronic infection/inflammation involving necrosis, pus, cell debris, internal haemorrhage, haemolytic anaemia and immune-mediated disease	Not significant
Platelets	Thrombocytosis caused by infections, trauma, haemorrhage, splenectomy and some tumours	Thrombocytopaenia caused by autoimmune disease, disseminated intravascular coagulation, aplastic anaemia and chemotherapy

4. The centrifuge must be balanced so a minimum of two samples are spun at the same time at diametrically opposite sides of the centrifuge.
5. The centrifugal process results in the red blood cells concentrating at the bottom of the tube with the white blood cells and platelets – forming a grey/cream layer, the buffy coat – above them. The platelets tend to lie at the top of the buffy coat and can be seen as a thin, cream-coloured layer. The plasma is found above this layer. Gross examination of the plasma can indicate haemolysis, jaundice or lipaemia (Fig. 31.9).
6. The PCV is then read off on a special microhaematocrit reader. Different types of readers are available but all work on a similar principle. The PCV is calculated by dividing the length of the column of red blood cells (a) by the combined length of the red blood cells, buffy coat and plasma (b) then multiplying by 100 to give the result as a percentage (Table 31.9).

The method is rapid, very accurate and relatively easy to perform. It also only requires only a small volume of blood.

HAEMOGLOBIN ESTIMATION

Haemoglobin, packed into the red blood cells, combines reversibly with oxygen and transports it around the body. In order for the body to function properly adequate amounts of haemoglobin are essential. Haemoglobin (Hb) levels are estimated by haematology analysers and are measured in grams per decilitre.

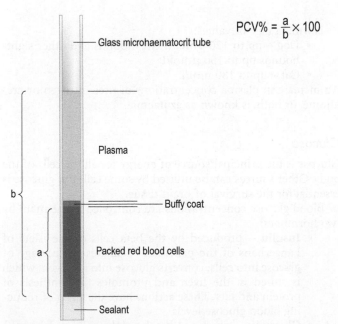

$$PCV\% = \frac{a}{b} \times 100$$

— Glass microhaematocrit tube

Plasma

b

— Buffy coat

a

Packed red blood cells

— Sealant

Fig. 31.9 Packed cell volume

TABLE 31.9	Normal ranges of haematological values			
Species	RBC (10^{12}/l)	WBC (10^9/l)	PCV (%)	Hb (g/dl)
Dog	5.5–8.5	6–17	37–55	12–18
Cat	5.0–10.0	5.5–19.5	24–45	8–15

Normal ranges are:
- Dog 12–18 g/dl
- Cat 8–15 g/dl.

This test is not affected by haemolysis. Haemoglobin levels are decreased in cases of anaemia.

Further information calculable from these tests

'Corpuscular values' can be calculated from the total red blood cell counts, PCV or Hct and haemoglobin contents, or obtained more accurately from haematology analysers.

- **Mean corpuscular volume (MCV)** – indicates the average size of the red blood cells:

$$MCV\,(fl) = \frac{PCV\,(l/l) \times 1000}{Total\ red\ cells\,(10^{12}/l)}$$

(fl = femtolitre: $1\ fl = 10^{-15}\ l$).

- **Mean corpuscular haemoglobin concentration (MCHC)** – indicates the average concentration of haemoglobin per red blood cell:

$$MCHC\,(g/dl) = \frac{Total\ haemoglobin\,(g/dl)}{PCV\,(l/l)}$$

The MCV and MCHC are useful in the evaluation of anaemic conditions. The normal ranges of haematological values are listed in Table 31.9.

SALINE AGGLUTINATION TEST

Saline agglutination tests are exceptionally easy to perform in practice and are used to help in the diagnosis of Immune Mediated Haemolytic Anaemia (IMHA). Mix a drop of blood (fresh whole blood or EDTA) with an equal or slightly larger drop of normal saline on a clean glass slide. Mix thoroughly by tilting the slide back and forth several times. Examine with the naked eye and microscopically. Autoagglutination appears as clumps of cells whereas rouleaux appear as stacks. Autoagglutination should persist after the cells have been washed three times in saline. Its presence is a strong evidence for IMHA and renders a Coombs' test unnecessary.

BLOOD BIOCHEMISTRY

Studying the biochemical parameters of normal substances in the blood can help in the diagnosis of many conditions (Table 31.10). It must be borne in mind that the normal ranges of values of the various determinations will show a degree of variation depending on the analytical system being used.

Blood urea nitrogen (BUN)

Urea is a nitrogenous waste product formed by the liver from the breakdown of amino acids. It is carried in the plasma to the kidneys, where it is excreted in the urine.

Normal range of BUN values will vary depending on analysers used and external reference laboratories having their own reference ranges:
- Dog – 3.0–9.0 mmol/l
- Cat – 5.0–10.0 mmol/l (some researchers give the upper value as 15 mmol/l).

TABLE 31.10	Common blood biochemistry estimations		
Substance	Normal range*	Causes of elevated levels	Causes of depressed levels
Total serum protein	Dog 50–78 g/l Cat 60–82 g/l	Dehydration, chronic and immune-mediated disease, lactation, infection and neoplasia	Renal disease, haemorrhage, malnutrition, malabsorption, hepatic and pancreatic insufficiency. Lower in young animals because of minimal levels of immunoglobulins
Serum albumin	Dog 22–35 g/l Cat 25–39 g/l	Haemoconcentration secondary to dehydration	Chronic liver disease, ascites, tissue oedema, congestive heart failure and renal failure
Cholesterol	Dog 2.7–9.5 mmol/l Cat 1.5–6.0 mmol/l	Diabetes mellitus, hypothyroidism, hyperadrenocorticism, nephritic syndrome and post-feeding sampling	Maldigestion, malabsorption and severe hepatic insufficiency
Total bilirubin	Dog and cat 0–6.8 µmol/l	Haemolytic anaemia, hepatic jaundice, obstruction to bile flow and impaired liver function	Not applicable
Amylase	Dog and cat 400–2000 units/l	Acute pancreatitis but not specific, therefore it is advisable to cross-reference with lipase levels Renal failure and gastrointestinal problems	Not applicable
Calcium	Dog and cat 2.20–2.90 mmol/l	Dehydration, neoplasia, primary hyperparathyroidism, hypoadrenocorticism, renal failure and hypervitaminosis D	Primary hypoparathyroidism, eclampsia, acute pancreatitis, intestinal malabsorption and following bilateral thyroidectomy, antifreeze (ethylene glycol) poisoning
Bile acids	Dog and cat 0–15 µmol/l†	Primary or secondary hepatic disease Biliary obstruction and portosystemic shunt	Intestinal obstruction and severe malabsorption

*May vary depending on analyser.

†Normally a bile acid stimulation test is performed. This involves taking a preprandial (fasting) blood sample then feeding the patient with a fatty meal. A postprandial sample is then taken 2 hours later and the change in the two samples is analysed.

Elevated BUN can be considered under three categories:

a. **Pre-renal**
  - Fever
  - Infection
  - Necrosis
  - Metabolic conditions
  - High-protein diet
  - Chronic heart failure
  - Corticosteroid administration.

b. **Renal** – increased BUN levels are seen in renal failure but approximately 75% of the nephrons have to become non-functional before this occurs

c. **Postrenal**
  - Urethral obstruction
  - Ruptured bladder.

Decreased BUN can occur as a result of:
  - Liver failure
  - Anabolic steroids
  - Portosystemic shunt
  - Low-protein diet, malnourished, anorexia.

Creatinine

This is a metabolite of creatine, which stores energy in muscles. It is freely filtered by the glomeruli of the kidney and the clearance of creatinine from the plasma can be used to provide an approximation of the glomerular filtration rate. Like BUN, it is not a very accurate indicator of kidney function, as approximately 75% of the kidney tissue must be non-functional before elevated levels are seen. The levels of creatinine are not influenced by a high-protein diet.

Normal range of values:
  - Dog – up to 120 µmol/l. Greyhounds and other sight-hounds up to 150 µmol/l
  - Cat – up to 180 mol/l.

An increase in plasma concentrations of urea nitrogen or creatinine, or both, is known as azotaemia.

Glucose

Glucose is the principal source of energy for all the cells of the body. Other sources can be utilised by some cells but glucose is essential for the survival of brain tissue.

Blood glucose concentrations are controlled in the main by two hormones:

  - **Insulin** – produced by the beta cells of the islets of Langerhans of the pancreas. Facilitates the passage of glucose into cells, converts glucose into glycogen, which is stored in the liver, and promotes the synthesis of protein and fats. These actions have the effect of reducing blood glucose levels.
  - **Glucagon** – produced by the alpha cells and has the opposite effects.

Epinephrine (adrenaline) and cortisol also influence blood glucose levels. In the dog and cat glucose is actively reabsorbed in the renal tubules up to the renal threshold of 10–12 mmol/l. If the level of glucose exceeds the renal threshold, glucose will be excreted in the urine, i.e. glucosuria.

Normal ranges of fasting plasma glucose levels:
  - Dog – 3.5–5.5 mmol/l
  - Cat – 3.5–6.5 mmol/l

Elevated blood glucose levels (hyperglycaemia) may be seen in:
- Diabetes mellitus
- Post-feeding sampling
- Stress
- Cushing's disease
- Administration of corticosteroids
- Pancreatitis
- Administration of drugs, e.g. morphine.

Decreased blood glucose levels (hypoglycaemia) may be seen in:
- Neoplasia, e.g. insulinoma, hepatocellular carcinoma
- Hepatic insufficiency
- Hypoadrenocorticism
- Malabsorption
- Starvation
- Neonatal hypoglycaemia in some toy breeds, due to incorrect nutrition and frequency of feeding
- Insulin treatment.

Blood samples for glucose determination can be collected into fluoride and oxalate tubes, as fluoride blocks glycolysis in the red blood cells ensuring that the glucose levels determined at sampling more accurately reflect the glucose levels at the time of testing. The oxalate acts as the anticoagulant. If the biochemical analyser requires the use of heparinised plasma, the sample must be separated immediately to prevent glycolysis occurring. Other sample tubes such as serum gel tubes can be used to measure blood glucose and are preferred by some external reference laboratories for being more accurate. The tube needs to be spun 30 minutes after collection.

Reagent strips, e.g. BM-Test 1-44, can also be used but require whole blood. In general, these are less accurate at high glucose levels. Veterinary species-specific glucometers are the most commonly used method of accessing blood glucose levels, especially in diabetic animals. Lancet devices can be used to collect a peripheral sample from the lip, ear pinnae and pad or from a clipped area of skin.

Many other blood biochemistry estimations can be made with biochemical analysers (see Table 31.10).

Plasma enzymes

Within all cells are enzymes, which are essential for intracellular metabolism. Normally, low levels of these enzymes are found in the plasma but, if a cell dies or is badly damaged, increased amounts of its enzymes are detected. Cells of different tissues contain different enzymes so it would seem feasible to be able to identify the damaged cells by the enzymes found in the plasma. Unfortunately, it is not as simple as this, as one enzyme is seldom specific for one particular tissue, but it is usually possible to localise the damage by looking at a number of different enzymes or, to be more precise, by investigating the isoenzymes involved, which are often specific for a particular tissue.

Results are not expressed as concentrations but as 'activities'. This is a measure of how fast the enzyme can convert substrate to product under standardised assay conditions, and is measured in international units (IU). Reaction temperature can influence the results obtained and is now commonly standardised at 37°C, but results using different temperatures may still be encountered.

- **Alanine aminotransferase (ALT)**, formerly serum glutamic-pyruvic transaminase (SGPT) – in dogs and cats, elevated levels are predominantly specific for hepatocellular damage. Activities of more than 150–200 IU/l

are of clinical significance. In very acute conditions, e.g. acute hepatitis, levels of 5000 IU/l are not uncommon. Levels will also increase in severe muscle damage. Mild increases in ALT are also seen in feline hyperthyroidism
- **Aspartate aminotransferase (AST)**, formerly serum glutamic-oxaloacetic transaminase (SGOT) – this enzyme is widely distributed throughout the body in skeletal and cardiac muscle, liver and red blood cells. Elevated levels are indicative of muscle damage in dogs and cats. Normal levels are below 100 IU/l
- **Alkaline phosphatase (ALP/ALKP)**, formerly serum alkaline phosphatase (SAP) – this is one of the most widely distributed enzymes in the body and has several isoenzymes found in bone (osteoblasts), liver and the intestinal wall. The range of values is quite wide, up to 300 IU/l. It is higher in young animals because of bone development.

It is clear that a plasma enzyme activity result should not be considered in isolation in deciding on a diagnosis.

Hormones

Thyroid. The thyroid produces two important hormones, thyroxine (T_4) and tri-iodothyronine (T_3). These hormones have widespread physiological effects on the body, including controlling the metabolic rate. Abnormal fluctuations in the levels of these hormones can result in the development of various clinical signs and endocrine disorders. The secretion of these hormones is controlled by thyroid-stimulating hormone (TSH) from the anterior pituitary and thyrotrophin-releasing hormone (TRH), produced by the hypothalamus.

Diagnostically T_4 is used to assess thyroid function, as abnormalities show up more readily in this hormone. Normal ranges vary between laboratories but generally fall between 13 and 52 nmol/l.

Increased serum T_4 may be due to:
- Hyperthyroidism
- Young age
- Anti-T_4 antibodies
- Certain drugs
- Oestrus and pregnancy.

Decreased serum T_4 may be due to:
- Hypothyroidism
- Hyperadrenocorticism
- Chronic illness, known as sick euthyroid syndrome, such as renal, liver, or heart failure and diabetes mellitus
- Advanced age
- Drug therapy
- Iodine deficiency.

Serum samples are preferred for testing as this decreases the risk of fibrinogen interfering with the test. T_4 is stable in serum for up to 8 days at room temperature and is unaffected by haemolysis and lipaemia. Tests can be either sent to an external reference laboratory or can be run internally with ELISA SNAP tests to have immediate quantitative results. Additional tests that can be utilised to make confirmation of thyroid disease include TSH, T_3 and free T_4.

Adrenal cortex. The adrenal cortex produces approximately 30 different steroid hormones. The most common disorders affecting the adrenal cortex are hyperadrenocorticism (HAC,

Cushing's disease) or hypoadrenocorticism (Addison's disease). The hormone involved in these conditions is cortisol. A basal plasma or serum cortisol level is not very helpful due to other causes which can affect the cortisol levels, e.g. stress. For this reason dynamic manipulation tests with adrenocorticotropic hormone (ACTH) or dexamethasone are used.

The ACTH stimulation test is used to:

- Screen for primary and secondary Cushing's disease
- Monitor trilostane therapy
- Diagnose primary Addison's disease.

An initial basal cortisol level is performed followed by an intravenous injection of a synthetic form of ACTH. This will stimulate the release of cortisol. A second sample is then taken. The time frame is dependent on the external reference laboratory's protocols and the route of administration of the synthetic ACTH. High post-injection cortisol levels indicate Cushing's while low levels indicate Addison's disease.

Low-dose dexamethasone tests are used to screen for Cushing's. High-dose dexamethasone tests are used to distinguish between animals that have pituitary-dependent Cushing's disease and those that have non-pituitary-dependent Cushing's disease caused by a neoplasm in the adrenal cortex:

- **Low-dose dexamethasone test** – a basal cortisol level is determined. A low dose of dexamethasone (0.01 mg/kg) is then administered intravenously and a second sample is taken 8 hours later to assess the animal's response. In normal animals the release of ACTH will be suppressed by negative feedback and the cortisol levels will be reduced. In animals with Cushing's disease the dexamethasone will not be able to suppress the release of ACTH and the cortical levels will be higher.
- **High-dose dexamethasone test** – a basal cortisol level is determined but on this occasion a high dose of dexamethasone (0.1 mg/kg) is administered intravenously. Subsequent blood samples are taken at 3- and 8-hour intervals to assess the response:
  - Normal – both post-injection samples will be below the basal level
  - Pituitary-dependent – one of the post-injection samples will be below the basal level
  - Non-pituitary-dependent – very little suppression and both post-injection samples above the basal level.

Blood Gas Analysis

Arterial and venous blood gas determination is used to evaluate several elements within a fresh blood sample. These can include pH of the blood, acid–base balance, lactate, glucose, oxygen saturation and electrolytes. Blood gas evaluation is common in equine practice and veterinary hospitals and now more in general practice. 'Bedside monitoring' technology is now widely available, with small, portable, automated units now available for veterinary use (e.g. VetStat, I-STAT). Arterial blood is typically collected from the dorsal metatarsal or femoral artery using a heparinised syringe and 25- or 27-gauge needle. The devices directly measure pH, pCO_2, and pO_2, and calculate H_2CO_3, TCO_2, and haemoglobin saturation. A venous blood sample may be a satisfactory substitute for arterial blood when evaluating only the pH and pCO_2 for respiratory function, but sufficient for electrolytes, ionised calcium and lactate.

Urine

The analysis of urine samples can give a rapid insight into the health status of a patient. It is generally held that the normal dog, cat and horse will produce 1–2 ml/kg of body weight of urine daily:

- **Polyuria** – production of excess urine
- **Oliguria** – reduction of the amount of urine produced
- **Anuria** – absence of urine production
- **Dysuria** – difficulty in passing urine.

COLLECTION AND PRESERVATION OF URINE SAMPLES

Urine is potentially a hazardous substance and protective disposable gloves should be worn during its collection and analysis. Ideally, a sterile sample should be used but this can only be obtained by cystocentesis.

Collection of urine can be achieved by:

- **Free flow voided** – a midstream overnight sample is best for routine urinalysis, as this is the best indicator of the true composition of urine. The first stream of urine is the best sample to collect for lesions low in the urethral tract, e.g. urethral plugs, uroliths and bacteria; however, this fraction is the most likely to be contaminated. End stream is the best to collect for examination for prostatic disease or for haemorrhage or sediment that might have collected on the floor of the bladder. The practicalities of obtaining the last two types of sample are difficult. In the case of dogs, a well-cleaned container should be used to collect the sample, and it should then be transferred to a sterile container. Commercial sterile collection kits are available, e.g. Uripet. Cats are more problematic but again commercial kits are available, which involve using a litter tray with an inert substrate from which the urine can be obtained.
- **Manual expression** – this is convenient provided the bladder contains sufficient urine to be isolated manually on palpation of the abdomen. If strong resistance is encountered, care must be taken to prevent undue pressure rupturing the bladder. This is especially true when dealing with male cats with a potential urinary obstruction.
- **Catheterisation** – involves the passage of a tube aseptically into the urethra to collect urine directly from the bladder (see Chapter 17). There is always the potential for introduction of bacteria from the urethra into the bladder and nosocomial infections, so correct aseptic techniques should be utilised.
- **Cystocentesis** – involves the passage of a needle through the abdominal wall and into the bladder. This will provide the best sample for culture of bacterial growth and antibiotic sensitivity.

Preservation

Ideally, examination of the urine sample should be performed as soon as possible after collection, i.e. within an hour. If the sample is left, bacteria present in the sample will cause decomposition of the urea and the production of ammonia. This, being alkaline, will elevate the pH of the sample, which in turn will facilitate the precipitation of phosphates, which will interfere with subsequent testing. If testing is to be delayed, the sample should be refrigerated, not frozen.

Chemical preservatives can be used if refrigeration is not available, including formalin or thymol, but most commonly used in practice is boric acid. This will preserve and prevent the multiplication of bacteria for up to 4 days and will also preserve cells and urinary casts. It is commercially available in red-capped specimen containers.

PHYSICAL PROPERTIES OF URINE

The physical properties should be observed initially, including colour, odour, turbidity, pH and specific gravity.

Colour

The pigment urochrome is responsible for the colour of normal urine. It is normally yellow and the depth of colour indicates the concentration of the urine. There may be considerable variation in the depth of colour from almost colourless to a darkish brown. This variation depends on numerous factors, including concentration, diet, species, breed and exercise regimen.

Abnormal colours can be due to:
- Presence of blood, haemoglobin or myoglobin – impart a red or pink colour to the urine
- Bile pigments – colour the urine orange
- Drugs
- Food.

Rabbit urine colour ranges from light yellow to orange and even red with brown colouration. Certain pigments may cause a reddish appearance and can be confused with haematuria.

Odour

Normal urine has a sourish odour. Ammonia can be detected in stale urine. Ammonia in freshly passed urine may be due to the presence of urease-producing bacteria, which are commonly involved in cystitis. Male animals, notably cats, produce very strong-smelling urine. This is important in territorial scent marking. Animals suffering from diabetes mellitus can produce a sweet and fruity, pear-drop-smelling urine because of the presence of ketone bodies, e.g. acetone and acetoacetic acid, if the animal is unstable. This can also be smelt on the breath of such ketoacidotic animals.

Turbidity (cloudiness)

Urine is normally clear; however, if the urine is allowed to stand it will become turbid because of phosphate precipitation. Rabbit urine is normally turbid because of the presence of calcium carbonate. Abnormal turbidity can arise from the presence of mucus, pus and vaginal or prostatic secretions.

pH

This is the expression of the hydrogen ion concentration in a volume of liquid. A pH above 7.0 is alkaline while a pH below 7.0 is acidic. False results may occur if the sample is not kept cool and covered. Urine pH is affected by diet: carnivorous animals have acid urine while animals that eat a vegetarian diet have alkaline urine.

Normal pH:
- Dog pH 5.2–6.8
- Cat pH 6.0–7.0.

Acidic urine may be due to pyrexia, acidosis, high-protein diets, starvation, diabetes mellitus and muscle catabolism.

Alkaline urine may be due to urinary retention or infection, alkalosis, a high-vegetable-content diet or certain drugs.

The pH can be determined by pH papers, multireagent dip sticks or electrode pH meters, which are the most accurate and reliable.

Specific gravity

This is the density of a known volume of a fluid, i.e. urine compared with an equal volume of distilled water. Distilled water has a specific gravity of 1.000.

Normal specific gravity:
- Dog – 1.015–1.045
- Cat – 1.020–1.040.

The specific gravity of urine varies considerably even in the same individual and a single measurement should not be taken as conclusive.

Elevated specific gravity may be due to dehydration or lack of fluid intake.

Lowered levels are seen in diabetes insipidus, chronic renal failure or various causes of polydipsia.

Measurement of specific gravity. An accurate measurement of specific gravity can be made by the use of a refractometer (Fig. 31.10). This is an optical instrument that assesses the refractive index of fluids: the higher the refractive index the higher the concentration of urine, i.e. the specific gravity. This method requires only a small volume of urine and is quick and easy to perform.

It is essential that the refractometer is initially calibrated with distilled water before the specific gravity reading is taken. A few drops of distilled water are placed on the face of the prism and the cover plate is gently closed. The refractometer is held up to the light and the scale is brought into focus by turning the eyepiece. If the boundary line does not coincide with the 1.000 line, adjustments are made with a small screwdriver to the scale adjustment knob until the boundary line does coincide with the 1.000 line.

The water is then cleaned away with a soft piece of tissue and a few drops of urine, at room temperature, are applied to the prism surface. The specific gravity is then read off on the appropriate scale. If the reading goes off the scale, this means that the urine is very concentrated; the sample should then be diluted

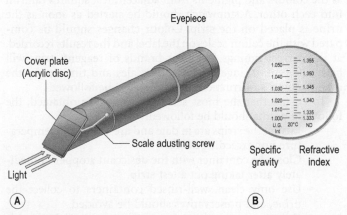

Fig. 31.10 (A) A refractometer. (B) Scale visible inside the eyepiece, which must be calibrated before use

TABLE 31.11	Urinalysis	
Substance	**Normal parameters**	**Causes of elevated values**
Protein	A trace reading for protein, which equates to 0.3 g/l, is of no clinical significance	Pre-renal, e.g. haemolytic anaemia, azotaemia, multiple myeloma and congestive heart failure Renal, e.g. acute and chronic renal failure, pyelonephritis and amyloidosis, protein losing nephropathies Post-renal, e.g. cystitis, urolithiasis, prostatitis and vaginitis
Blood	Any positive result is significant other than a bitch in pro-oestrus	Cystitis, associated infection of the urinary tract, urolithiasis and acute nephritis
Glucose	The presence of glucose in urine, glucosuria, is always significant	Diabetes mellitus, chronic liver damage, Cushing's disease and hyperthyroidism
Ketones pH Bilirubin Urobilinogen	Any levels are significant Dogs: 5–7 Cat: 7–9 Trace Trace/small amounts	Diabetes mellitus, starvation and liver damage Changes can be due to diet, time of eating, bacterial infections, cystitis, alkalosis, pharmaceutical agents Liver disease, haemolytic or obstructive jaundice Liver dysfunction

with an equal volume of distilled water and the reading retaken. Multiplying the scale reading after the decimal point by 2 will give the correct final specific gravity of the sample. Different refractometers have different scale layouts displayed and the manufacturer's instructions should be consulted to ensure that the correct scale is read.

A refractometer can also be used to measure the refractive index of other liquids and enables the plasma (total) protein level to be ascertained. Urine specific gravity should never be measured by dipstick methods because most are designed for human use and are not accurate.

Chemical tests

Many substances can interfere with the chemical testing of urine, giving rise to erroneous results, e.g. concurrent medication. It should also be borne in mind that the majority of commercial strips are designed for measuring human parameters. Test strips are available which test for varying numbers of chemical substances in the urine (Table 31.11). Commercial urine test strips can be used to test for pH, protein, glucose, ketone bodies, urobilinogen, bilirubin, haemoglobin and blood in urine.

Use urine that is fresh, uncentrifuged and thoroughly mixed. The test strip must be laid flat on a piece of absorbent paper, and urine should be gently pipetted onto each individual test square. The test strip should never be dipped into the sample as the colours and pigments from adjacent test squares can run into each other. A stopwatch should be started as soon as the urine is placed on the strip. Colour changes should be compared with the colour scales on the label and the results recorded, at the correct timings. Different brands of reagent strips will have different arrangements of the scales and timings, so the manufacturer's instructions should always be followed.

To ensure that the most accurate results are obtained, the following points should be followed:

- Ensure the strips are in date and are stored at a temperature not exceeding 30°C.
- Close the container with the desiccant stopper immediately after taking out a test strip.
- Use only clean, well-rinsed containers to collect the urine, and preservatives should be avoided.
- Do not expose the urine sample to sunlight as this induces oxidation of bilirubin and urobilinogen, which

can lead to artificially low results for these two parameters.
- False positives for blood and glucose can result from residues of strongly oxidising disinfectants in the collecting container.
- Excessive amounts of ascorbic acid can also interfere with some of the tests, but this is unlikely to be encountered in dogs and cats.

Blood and blood pigments

If dog or cat urine is coloured red it may be due to the presence of blood, haemoglobin or myoglobin:

- **Haematuria** is the presence of whole blood in the urine.
- **Haemoglobinuria** is the presence of free haemoglobin in the urine and may result from haemolytic anaemia, leptospirosis, poisoning and autoimmune disease.

To differentiate between the two, microscopic examination or centrifugation of the sample should be undertaken. With centrifugation methods the supernatant of the sample can be placed on the commercial test strip. If it is positive it will be haemoglobin as red blood cells will be in the sediment of the sample.

- **Myoglobinuria** is the presence of myoglobin in the urine and is usually seen in muscle-wasting disease, e.g. myasthenia gravis, or in horses suffering from exertional rhabdomyolysis (ER).

MICROSCOPIC EXAMINATION OF URINE

This provides useful information on various disease processes that might be present. All samples should be examined before being spun in a centrifuge as some casts and cells can be destroyed by the spinning process.

Preparation of a wet preparation

1. Place a portion of a well-mixed fresh urine sample into a centrifuge tube and spin at 1500 rpm for 5 minutes, or at the manufacturer's setting for urine samples. Ensure that two samples are spun. Use an Eppendorf shaped tube.
2. Remove the supernatant liquid, leaving the sediment with a small amount of supernatant in the tube.
3. Resuspend the sediment by flicking the bottom of the tube.

4. An unstained wet preparation can be made with one of the spun samples, and the other should be used for staining. A stain is added to facilitate examination of the sample. Stains such as 0.5% new methylene blue, or preferably Sedi-Stain, can be added to ease examination. Add 2 drops to the sample and mix well.

5. Pipette a drop of the suspension on to a clean, labelled microscope slide and carefully place a coverslip on top of the sample.

6. Examine the slide systematically under low power, ×10 then ×40. Only a small amount of light is needed so the iris diaphragm should be partially closed.

7. To make a dry preparation, all the supernatant is decanted and a small drop of the sediment is placed on a microscope slide, covered by a coverslip and examined.

Various microscopic components can be identified in a urinary sediment including the following:

Epithelial cells. Flat, irregular squamous cells. Small numbers are normally present.

Transitional cells. Small, round polyhedral cells. Indicate cystitis or pyelonephritis. Higher numbers are detected in catheterised samples, because of trauma to the urethra and bladder.

Tubular epithelial cells. Small, cuboidal epithelial cells. Indicative of renal tubule damage. Can be confused with white blood cells.

Leucocytes. Usually neutrophils. The presence of large numbers is known as pyuria and suggests inflammation of the urogenital tract or pyelonephritis.

Red blood cells. Large numbers are indicative of bleeding into the urogenital tract.

Casts. These are precipitated protein, which tend to form in the distal convoluted tubules and collecting ducts of the nephrons because of the acidic conditions in these regions (Fig. 31.11).

All the casts have a basis of protein that is moulded into the shape of the tubules. They are short cylinders, usually with one rounded and one broken end, although on occasion both ends may be rounded.

Other materials may be incorporated into the basic protein matrix, resulting in different types of casts:

- **Hyaline casts** – clear, refractile, colourless and cylindrical in shape. An increase in numbers is found in mild inflammation of the tubules, poor circulation and pyrexia.
- **Cellular casts** – a variety of cells may be incorporated into the casts:
  - Erythrocytes – indicative of haemorrhage into the tubules
  - Leucocytes – indicate an inflammatory reaction
  - Epithelial cells – indicate acute renal failure.
- **Granular casts** – these are hyaline casts containing granules that are remnants of degenerating leucocytes or epithelial cells. The presence of large numbers of these casts are associated with renal failure, especially in the dog.
- **Waxy casts** – these are more opaque and wider than hyaline casts, with square rather than rounded ends. They are found in chronic degenerative renal tubular damage.

Casts, being relatively large structures, tend to be found at the edges of the coverslip if small square coverslips are used. Larger rectangular coverslips should be used in order to prevent this. They may be confused with hairs, fibres or mucus strands but these are thinner and longer than casts and are usually twisted strands. They are usually products of the lower urinary tract. They tend to dissolve in alkaline urine and easily break up on centrifugation.

Spermatozoa. Commonly found in urine samples from entire male dogs.

Bacteria, fungi and yeasts. May be found as contaminants and their presence is only significant if accompanied by large numbers of leucocytes.

Crystals. The presence of crystals can be associated with various clinical conditions, e.g. urolithiasis, cystitis and haematuria, but they can also be detected in apparently normal animals. Crystals are more likely to be found if freshly collected urine is allowed to stand.

The presence of increased numbers of crystals depends on the pH, concentration of the urine and the solubility of the salts in the urine. Various conditions can influence crystal production, including genetic predisposition, bacterial infection, diet, concurrent illnesses and breed, e.g. Dalmatians excrete uric acid in their urine, hence the relatively high incidence of uric acid crystals in their urine (Table 31.12). Other less common crystals include silica, xanthine, bilirubin and crystals caused by drugs.

Occasionally, urinary crystals clump together to form **calculi or stones**. Calculi in the bladder are known as **cystic calculi**. Those found in the urethra are known as **uroliths**. Chemical analysis of the calculi will identify the crystal and facilitate treatment and control of the condition, usually by adjusting the pH of the urine and reducing supersaturation of the urine.

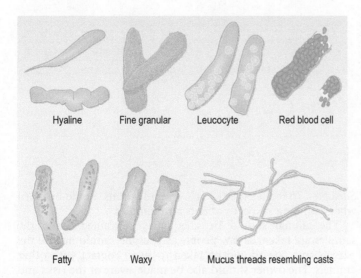

Hyaline   Fine granular   Leucocyte   Red blood cell

Fatty   Waxy   Mucus threads resembling casts

Fig. 31.11 Types of casts that may be found in urine

Table 31.12	Common urinary crystals	

Appearance	Name/composition	pH of urine in which crystals are deposited
Struvite	Magnesium ammonium phosphate. Also known as triple phosphate or struvite crystals. Coffin-lid-shaped	Alkaline, but can occur at any pH
Cystine	Cystine. Large, flat hexagonal crystals	Acidic, but can occur at any pH
Calcium oxalate	Calcium oxalate dihydrate. Envelope-shaped, octahedral/pyramidal in shape. Calcium oxalate monohydrate are dumbbell shaped and seen in antifreeze poisoning cases	Acidic, but can occur at any pH

Skin and hair

Laboratory tests can prove invaluable in the diagnosis of many skin conditions. It is important, when handling animals with skin disease, to avoid transmission of the condition to humans (zoonosis) and cross-contamination of other patients. Examples of potential zoonoses include ringworm, *Cheyletiella* and *Sarcoptes*. To reduce the risk, gloves and aprons should be worn when handling suspect patients and samples.

The animal should be adequately restrained while the samples are taken, as few people as possible should handle the patient and care should be taken to avoid contact with other animals. The owner should also be made aware of the risks and precautions that need to be taken to reduce them.

Table 31.12	Common urinary crystals—cont'd		
Appearance		**Name/composition**	**pH of urine in which crystals are deposited**

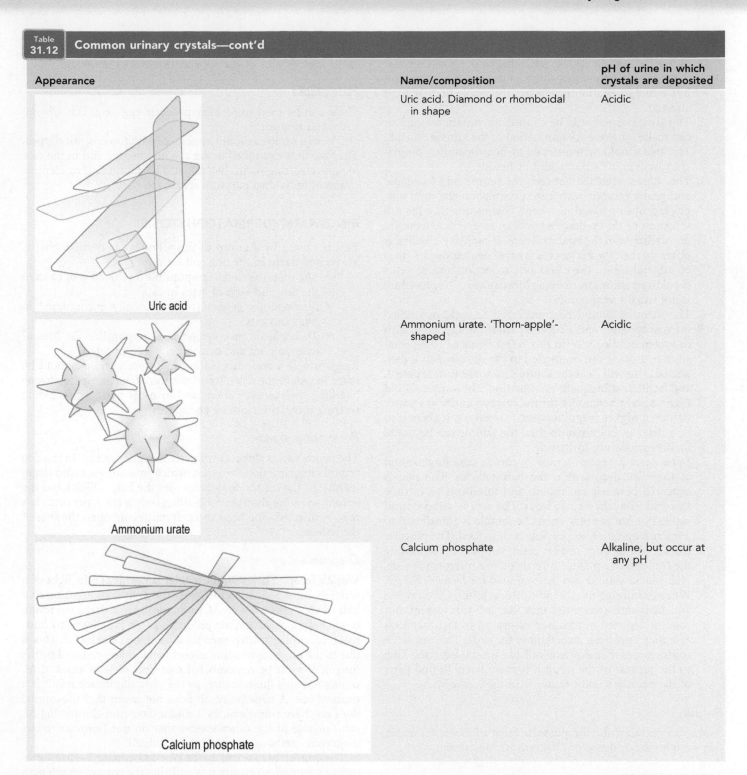

Uric acid		Uric acid. Diamond or rhomboidal in shape	Acidic
Ammonium urate		Ammonium urate. 'Thorn-apple'-shaped	Acidic
Calcium phosphate		Calcium phosphate	Alkaline, but occur at any pH

SAMPLING TECHNIQUES

It is important that the correct sampling protocol is employed when investigating skin problems. These techniques include:

Skin scrapings

This is an easy technique to perform and is routinely performed in practice to identify parasitic skin conditions. It can used to detect burrowing mites such as *Sarcoptes scabei*, *Notedres cati* and *Trixacarus caviae* (see Chapter 29). Identification of

Sarcoptes spp. can be difficult on skin scrapings, so it is more routine to use blood test to identify antibodies against the parasite. Deeper scrapings will reveal *Demodex* spp. Superficial scrapings may also detect *Malassezia* yeasts, which can also be found with the use of tape impressions.

Technique

1. The area to be scraped should be selected carefully and several sites sampled. Any erythematous (reddened) papules or scaly areas should be investigated, especially

the lateral aspect of the pinna, the elbows and the carpal region if *Sarcoptes* is suspected. *Notedres* is found mainly on the head of the cat, especially below the ears. *Demodex* tends in the early stages to be concentrated on the head but as the infestation progresses the whole body may be affected.

2. The sample site should be clipped, as contaminating hair can make subsequent examination of the sample difficult. The area should be moistened by liquid paraffin, propylene glycol or 10% potassium hydroxide.

3. The skin is stretched between the thumb and forefinger and gently scraped with a sterile scalpel blade until pin-prick drops of blood are seen. This means that the full thickness of the epidermis has been sampled, as there are no capillaries in the epidermis and if capillary bleeding is observed then the dermis must have been exposed. A drop of mineral oil on the blade aids collection and prevents the skin scrapings from being blown away. The procedure is not usually very painful.

4. The material should be transferred to a clean, labelled microscope slide and a coverslip carefully applied using a mounted needle. Prior to this, a few drops of 10% potassium hydroxide can be applied to the slide, which is then heated. This will clear the sample, i.e. make it transparent, and facilitate subsequent examination. The sample should then be examined under the microscope under low power ×10 then higher magnification if necessary. If there is to be a delay in examination then the sample can be stored in 10% potassium hydroxide.

5. *Demodex* spp. require a more vigorous sampling method as they live deep within the hair follicles. The skin is squeezed between the thumb and forefinger to extrude material from the hair follicles. The area is scraped until capillary ooze appears, then the sample is transferred to a microscope slide, as previously described. The pustular lesions of *Demodex* can be easily sampled by expressing the contents of a pustule directly on to a microscope slide. Hair plucks should also be examined for *Demodex* spp.

6. When examining microscopic ectoparasites, e.g. *Sarcoptes* and *Demodex*, remember that they are transparent, not solid as depicted in idealised diagrams. In fact they look as if they have been etched on to the slide. This can cause confusion, as they may not look like what is expected. Due to the process of the scrap it is more likely to find parts of the parasite's body, rather than the whole body.

Swabs

Swabs can be taken for the pustular form of *Demodex* or ear wax samples for evidence of *Otodectes* or *Malassezia*.

Tape impression

This technique can be used to detect superficial parasites, surface bacteria and fungi. It is very useful for the identification of *Cheyletiella* spp. and *Malassezia*. A strip of clear, colourless adhesive tape is placed on the sample site then pulled away and transferred to a microscope slide for subsequent microscopic examination.

Hair brushings

This technique is used to detect surface ectoparasites. The animal is placed on a white background and the coat is brushed through with a fine-toothed comb to collect superficial debris. This can then be examined with a hand lens or under the microscope for evidence of surface ectoparasites or their eggs.

Hair plucks

These can be used to identify parasitic eggs, e.g. lice, *Cheyletiella*, and ringworm.

The hair samples should be plucked with forceps, not clipped. They are then examined under the microscope and in the case of suspected ringworm they can also be cultured. (For identification of individual parasites see Chapter 29.)

RINGWORM (DERMATOPHYTOSIS)

This is caused by a group of fungi known as dermatophytes. Those important in the dog and cat are:

- *Microsporum canis* – responsible for 70–80% of cases in the dog and 90% of cases in cats
- *Microsporum gypseum* – occasionally encountered in dogs and cats
- *Trichophyton mentagrophytes* – responsible for 20% of cases in dogs and occasionally seen in cats.

Ringworm is a zoonosis, so adequate precautions should be taken to reduce the risk of transmission of the disease to anyone handling the suspect patient and to other animals, including wearing protective clothing and gloves.

Presenting signs

The major sign is alopecia with crusting and scaling. In the dog typical circular lesions are seen, which may coalesce into larger lesions. In the cat the fungus invades the hair follicles and the lesions are more discrete. Sometimes only a few hairs or a claw may be infected. The head and extremities are often the sites of the lesions.

Diagnosis

Wood's lamp. This is an ultraviolet lamp that emits light of a wavelength of 365–366 nm. When the light is directed on to a hair or claw affected with *M. canis*, ideally in a darkened room, it will emit a characteristic yellowish green (apple green) fluorescence, similar to that seen on a luminous clock dial. This is due to the presence of a fluorescent metabolite produced by the fungus. It must be remembered that only 60% of cases of *M. canis* show this fluorescence, so the only significant result is a positive one. A negative result does not mean that the animal does not have ringworm, as it might have non-fluorescing *M. canis* or one of the other species that do not fluoresce; other diagnostic methods will need to be utilised.

It is important to warm up the Wood's lamp for 5–10 minutes before it is used, to ensure it is emitting the correct wavelength of light and also to allow sufficient time when viewing an area to allow the fluorescence to develop. The examination should be undertaken in a darkened room to aid recognition of the fluorescence. The animal should be screened thoroughly, including the nails. The eyes of the operator and the patient should not be exposed to ultraviolet light unnecessarily, as it can damage the eyes. Other substances, such as cotton fibres, skin scales and petroleum jelly, can also fluoresce and give false-positive results, but their fluorescence is bluish-white. It takes experience to be able to correctly diagnose *M. canis* infections by this technique.

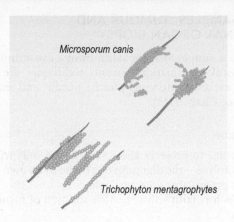

Microsporum canis

Trichophyton mentagrophytes

Fig. 31.12 Fungal spores or arthroconidia along a hair shaft

Microscopic examination. Suspect hairs should be plucked, not clipped, from the edge of the lesion. If the animal is being examined under a Wood's lamp then select the fluorescing hairs. The hairs should be transferred to a clean microscope slide and 10% potassium hydroxide and 1–2 drops of lactophenol cotton blue stain added. A coverslip should be applied and the sample gently heated to clear it. The dye enhances the visibility of the spores. Some dermatologists simply suspend the hair samples in mineral oil.

The specimen is examined under low and then high power. It can be useful to examine a normal hair for comparison. Infected hairs appear broken and damaged. The cortex and cuticle are irregular and have a fuzzy outline because of the presence of the branching hyphae and arthroconidia (spores). The arthroconidia of *M. canis* are small, bead-like and form a dense mosaic pattern on the outside (ectothrix) of the hair shaft. Those of *T. mentagrophytes* are larger and occur as sparse chains (Fig. 31.12). Those of *M. gypseum* are much larger, less numerous and in chains. Care should be taken not to confuse the melanin pigment found within the hair shaft with the fungal growth. The microscopic characteristics of the arthroconidia can be used to identify the ringworm species.

This is probably the most reliable method of diagnosing a dermatophyte infection. Hair samples are plucked as described previously and placed directly on to Sabouraud's dextrose agar or on to dermatophyte test medium (DTM), which contains an indicator system to detect dermatophyte species. In a positive culture the DTM changes colour from yellow to red; this should occur within 3–5 days. The colonies should be checked daily. Non-pathogenic fungi may produce false positives if the incubation period is prolonged. Samples on Sabouraud's dextrose agar should be incubated at room temperature (25–27°C) for 10–14 days, but on occasion this may take as long as 4 weeks.

Colony characteristics:

- *M. canis* – flat, with a white, silky centre and a bright yellow edge. The reverse side is yellow.
- *M. gypseum* – flat, brown, with a powdery irregular fringe. The reverse side is yellow brown.
- *T. mentagrophytes* – flat, granular, tan-coloured or heaped, white, cottony appearance. The reverse side is yellow-red.

Microscopic examination of the arthroconidia will confirm the species identification. The easiest way of transferring the arthroconidia to a microscope slide is by attaching a short length of tape to the end of a spatula or swab and pressing it against the surface of the fungal colony, then applying the tape sticky side down to the surface of the slide. It can then be stained with lactophenol cotton blue stain and examined under the microscope. The arthroconidia of *M. canis* are thick-walled, boat-shaped and have spines at the terminal end that may resemble a knob. Those of *T. mentagrophytes* are cigar-shaped and thin-walled, and the accompanying hyphae are spiral.

YEASTS

The most common species to affect dogs and cats are:

- *Malassezia* **spp.** – can be cultured, by clipping the hair away from the sample site and pressing a culture plate containing a malt-extract-agar-based medium on to the skin for 10 seconds. The plates are then cultured at 32°C for 3 days, when white glistening colonies will be seen and a colony count per square centimetre of skin can be made.
- *Candida albicans* – this is a Gram-positive, yeast-like fungus but is best stained with lactophenol cotton blue, when it appears as oval cells showing replication by budding. It will grow on all routine bacteriological media. On blood agar at 37°C small grey colonies appear after 2–3 days. On Sabouraud's dextrose agar, large, cream-coloured colonies develop that have a yeasty odour.

Body tissues and fluids

Various fluids and tissues can be analysed to monitor the health of the patient.

CEREBROSPINAL FLUID

Examination of cerebrospinal fluid (CSF) can be very useful in diagnosing some neurological conditions. In the dog and cat the normal sampling site is the cisterna magna at the articulation between the atlas and the occipital bone. This technique is similar to the one used for administering contrast material for myelography (see Chapter 32). Occasionally, the lumbosacral space is used.

Technique

1. The animal must be anaesthetised to prevent it moving during the procedure and placed in lateral recumbency with the neck flexed.
2. Strict asepsis must be observed to prevent the introduction of bacteria and contamination of the sample.
3. The site should be prepared as for a surgical procedure.
4. A 20–22 FG spinal needle is carefully inserted and advanced into the subarachnoid space until a sudden decrease in resistance is felt and CSF wells up in the needle hub.
5. CSF is allowed to drip into an EDTA and a plain container. The first few drops are discarded, as they often contain mild blood contamination. Suction should not be applied. It is possible to collect 1 ml/5 kg body weight safely.

SYNOVIAL FLUID

This is collected by **arthrocentesis** from a joint to investigate any joint problems, including arthritis. Depending on the temperament and the degree of pain, a local or general anaesthetic may need to be administered. Aseptic procedures should be observed. Only a relatively small volume of fluid will be obtained and should be initially collected into a plain sample bottle.

THORACIC FLUID

Normally the thoracic fluid only contains sufficient fluid to lubricate the thoracic organs and the parietal pleura. Certain clinical conditions can result in accumulation of fluid, of different types, in the thorax, e.g. hydrothorax, pyothorax, haemothorax. The collection of fluid from the thorax, thoracocentesis, can help to determine the nature of the fluid and aid in the diagnosis. Collection is performed aseptically into EDTA and plain tubes (see also Chapter 23).

ABDOMINAL FLUID

In certain clinical conditions, fluid accumulates in the abdomen, i.e. ascites, and can be collected by abdominocentesis. Examination of any abdominal fluid can prove useful in the identification of peritonitis or a ruptured bladder, or splenic bleed. Aseptic collection is usually performed at the most dependent part of the ventral midline of the abdomen in the standing animal. Some of the sample is transferred to an EDTA tube for cytology while the rest is placed in plain sample tubes for biochemistry or bacteriology. Free fluid can be identified with ultrasonography of the abdomen, and radiography will demonstrate a 'whited-out' image. The presence of erythrocytes will indicate a bleed into the cavity, haemoabdomen, and origin of the bleed will need to be made. Uroabdomen is the accumulation of urine in the peritoneal and/or retroperitoneal spaces. Leakage of urine can originate from the bladder, urethra, ureters and kidneys. Diagnostic peritoneal lavage and abdominocentesis usually show a creatinine level greater than 2:1 with serum creatinine.

If fluid cannot be obtained on aspiration, **diagnostic peritoneal lavage** can be performed by instilling a small volume (approximately 20 ml/kg) of warmed isotonic crystalloid into the abdomen, agitating the abdomen and then re-aspirating this fluid. The sample should be assessed for the presence of neutrophils (and other leucocytes) with intracellular bacteria. If motile organisms are observed when examining your sample microscopically, this is a good indication that a sample of intestinal contents may have accidentally been taken.

Further possible tests include:

- **Bile** where biliary tract rupture is suspected.
- **Creatinine** and **potassium** if the effusion is thought to be a uroabdomen; creatinine levels in a peritoneal sample that are higher than serum concentrations indicate uroperitoneum.
- **Glucose** and **lactate** should be measured; where their values are less than 2.8 mmol/l and greater than 5.5 mmol/l respectively the inflammation is likely to be septic.
- **Culture** is indicated where a bacterial infection is suspected, and should include an anaerobic culture.

In cats with feline infectious peritonitis, the effusion usually has a high protein content (greater than 35g/l) with a high globulin-to-albumin ratio. There is a variably high cellularity mainly composed of lymphocytes.

TISSUE SAMPLES, TUMOUR AND ABDOMINAL ORGAN BIOPSY

A biopsy is a sample of tissue taken from a live animal for histopathological examination. Various techniques are available including excision, incision, punch, needle and endoscopic biopsies (see Chapter 23).

Preservation

It is important to preserve specimens, as the cells will rapidly undergo autolysis – the digestion of a tissue by its own enzymes. Various preservatives are available:

- **10% formalin** – this is a 40% solution of formaldehyde gas.
- **10% formol saline** – made by diluting formalin in a saline solution. It is the solution most commonly used.
- **10% neutral buffered formalin** – also a 10% solution of formalin but buffered to protect against changes in pH and tends to be used in anatomical display specimens.
- **Alcohol** – may be used but causes excessive shrinkage and hardness.

Formalin in its various formulations is a hazardous substance as it gives off formaldehyde, a gas that is irritant to the eyes and mucous membranes. It is important that Health and Safety and COSHH regulations are followed and protective clothing is used, including protective glasses, when handling these substances. Ensure any procedures are carried out in a well-ventilated room. Formalin is a strong antiseptic and disinfectant that will preserve tissues by 'fixing' or hardening them.

Important facts to consider when preserving tissues are:

- It takes a long time for formalin to penetrate tissues so ensure the tissue samples are thin wedges.
- Use plenty of formalin, i.e. at least 10 times the volume of tissue to be fixed.
- Try and take a sample from the junction between healthy and diseased tissue, especially with tumours and excision biopsies. The presence or absence of a capsule can help to determine if the tumour is benign or malignant, which will influence the prognosis.
- Use wide-necked sample bottles that allow easy removal of the fixed sample.
- Label the container to identify the specimen.
- Ensure that the sample bottles are robust and not easily broken, and are sealable to prevent leakage.
- Do not send whole organs but small representative samples.
- Body fluids can be preserved by making a fixed smear or by adding a drop of formol saline to 1 ml of fluid. This will preserve the morphology of any cells present.
- Samples should not be frozen, as this damages the cells.

TOXICOLOGICAL EXAMINATION

Toxicological samples should be sent to a commercial laboratory for analysis. It is always advisable to ensure that the laboratory is able to perform the tests that are required and the precise nature of the samples required. Usually, from live animals these are blood, faeces, urine and vomit. Samples from dead animals should include blood, urine, stomach and intestinal contents, liver and kidney.

Protocol

- Specimens should be collected free from contaminants, e.g. bedding. If they are contaminated, then a sample of the contamination should be sent in a separate container.
- Each sample should be placed in a separate sterile, labelled container.
- Unless samples are to be examined histologically, samples should be frozen and dispatched with ice.
- The samples should be sealed and an identical unused container should be sent to the laboratory.
- Preservatives should be avoided. If necessary, alcohol should be used and a sample from the same supply should be sent, as a control, in a separate container.
- Accurate records must be kept, as evidence may be needed for possible litigation.

VIROLOGICAL SAMPLES

Obviously, the ideal method of virus identification is the isolation and growth of the virus in tissue culture. This is, however, time-consuming, expensive and, as the number of viruses is so vast, only research institutes can offer this service. Some of the common viral diseases can now be diagnosed in practice by ELISA tests. These do not involve growing the virus but employ the reaction between an antibody and a specific antigen to indicate the presence of the virus.

It is important when sending virological samples to ascertain which particular type of sample the laboratory requires. These may be blood, nasopharyngeal aspirates, bronchoalveolar lavage samples, swabs, faeces, body fluids, organ smears and ocular discharges. The sample required will depend on the viral disease being investigated, as will the method of sampling and despatch.

FAECAL SAMPLES

Faecal samples are an excellent insight into the health and functioning of the gastrointestinal system. These samples can be used to aid in a diagnosis of endoparasites, viral disease and gastrointestinal disease (e.g. malabsorption, maldigestion, presence of blood).

Collection of faeces

A faecal sample can be either collected directly from the rectum, or those that have been passed. A pre-labelled sample pot should be used, and specific faecal sample pots can be utilised. These contain a spatula attached to the inside of the lid to aid in collection. Some bacteria and viruses can be intermittently 'shed' into the faeces. In these cases a 3-day pooled sample is required. A small portion of faeces is collected and placed in the sample pot for 3 consecutive days. The collected samples are then thoroughly mixed together before any tests are performed.

Examination of faeces

The contents of the faeces will be a direct result of the diet that the animal consumes. When submitting a sample for analysis it is important to note the animal's diet on the laboratory submission form. If occult faecal blood needs to be analysed, a white-meat-only diet needs to be fed for 48 hours prior to sampling.

Examination of the faecal sample can be divided into gross or macroscopic examination, where the overall appearance is assessed – consistency, odour, colour, mucus and in some cases parasites. Microscopic examination is utilised to detect parasites, bacterial or yeast infections and assessment of impaired digestion or absorption of the digestive system. Details of identification of parasite eggs (modified McMasters) and larvae (Baermann technique) can be found in Chapter 29.

Normal equine physiological values

The majority of laboratory diagnostic procedures for horses are carried out using the same protocols as in small animals. Here is a brief outline of normal equine physiological values. Please refer to the texts listed in the Bibliography for more extensive details.

HAEMATOLOGICAL NORMAL VALUES

Total red blood cell count

- Hot-blooded breeds – 6.8–12.9×10^{12}/l
- Cold-blooded breeds – 5.5–9.5×10^{12}/l
- Foals can vary from an initial 8.2–11.0×10^{12}/l at birth, declining to 7.4–10.6 by 7 days of age, then rising to 8.9–12.7×10^{12}/l by the time they are 4 months of age.

Total white blood cell count

- Hot-blooded breeds – 5.4–14.3×10^{9}/l
- Cold-blooded breeds – 6.0–12.0×10^{9}/l
- Foals can vary from an initial 4.9–11.7×10^{9}/l at birth, rising to 6.3–11.6×10^{9}/l at 7 days, then to 6.2–14.2×10^{9}/l by the time they are 4 months of age.

PCV

- Hot-blooded breeds – 32–53%
- Cold-blooded breeds – 8–14%
- Foals – 32–46%.

Haemoglobin

- Hot-blooded breeds – 11–19 g/dl
- Cold-blooded breeds – 8–14 g/dl
- Foals – 12.0–16.66 g/dl at birth, declining to 10.7–15.8 at 7 days, then rising again to 11.6–17.2 by the time they are 4 months old.

BIOCHEMICAL ADULT NORMAL VALUES

- Total serum protein – 5.8–7.7 g/dl
- Serum albumin – 2.3–3.6 g/dl
- Cholesterol – 1.94–3.88 mmol/l
- Total bilirubin – 0.5–2.3 µmol/l
- Glucose – 4.9–6.2 mmol/l
- Creatinine – 80–177 µmol/l
- Urea – 2 4.5 mmol/l
- Alkaline phosphatase – 86–285 IU/l
- Aspartate aminotransferase – 138–409 IU/l
- Creatine kinase – 119–287 IU/l.

The values in foals vary with age.

NORMAL URINE PARAMETERS

Normal urine production

- Adults 1.24 ml/kg/h
- Foals 6.17 ml/kg/h.

Normal pH

- Adults 7.0–9.0
- Foals 5.5–8.0.

Normal specific gravity

- Adults 1.020–1.050
- Foals 1.004–1.008.

URINARY CRYSTALS

Calcium carbonate crystals are the most commonly seen, although struvite and calcium oxalate crystals can be found.

BIBLIOGRAPHY

Bush, B.M., 1975. Veterinary Laboratory Manual. Heinemann, London.

Bush, B.M., 1991. Interpretation of Laboratory Results for Small Animal Clinicians. Blackwell Science, Oxford.

Corley, K., Stephen, J. (Eds.), 2008. The Equine Hospital Manual. Blackwell Publishing, Oxford.

Feldman, B.F., Zinkl, J.G., Jain, N.C. (Eds.), 2000. Schalm's Veterinary Hematology, fifth ed. Lippincott Williams and Wilkins, Baltimore.

Kerr, M.G., 2002. Veterinary Laboratory Medicine, second ed. Blackwell Science, Oxford.

Kramer, J.W., 2000. Normal Hematology of the Horse. In: Feldman, B.F., et al. (Eds.), Schalm's

Veterinary Hematology, fifth ed. Lippincott Williams and Wilkins, Baltimore.

Villiers, E., Blackwood, L. (Eds.), 2005. Manual of Canine and Feline Clinical Pathology, second ed. BSAVA, Gloucester.

RECOMMENDED READING

BVA Poster. Good practice guide to handling veterinary waste. Available from: <www.bva.co.uk>.
Well worth a visit.

Papasouliotis, K., 2002. Atlas of Canine Haematology. Nova Professional Media, Oxford.
A super little book that describes normal blood cell morphology in the dog and includes many colour photographs. It also includes normal ranges of values, haematological definitions and tech-

niques. Other titles in the range cover feline and equine haematology. They are also quite reasonably priced.

Pratt, P.W. (Ed.), 1992. Laboratory Procedures for Veterinary Technicians, second ed. American Veterinary Publications, Santa Barbara, CA.
Although aimed at the American market, this is a very useful book. It describes a wide range of laboratory procedures in a simple descriptive manner

and is well illustrated throughout. It also contains information on large animals, including horses.

Villiers, E., Blackwood, L. (Eds.), 2005. Manual of Canine and Feline Clinical Pathology, second ed. BSAVA, Gloucester.
This is a comprehensive guide to laboratory diagnostic practice which is beautifully illustrated throughout.

Principles of Diagnostic Imaging

SUZANNE EASTON

- The production of an image of an affected area of the body is a useful diagnostic tool and can be achieved by radiography, ultrasound, nuclear scintigraphy, computed tomography and magnetic resonance imaging.

- Radiography is the most common method and makes use of the fact that X-rays, which are part of the electromagnetic spectrum, will create a permanent image on radiographic film.

- X-rays are produced by an X-ray tube as a result of fast-moving electrons released from the cathode colliding with a tungsten anode or target.

- The exposure used to produce a diagnostic image is controlled by the milliamperage (mA), which affects the number of electrons produced from the cathode and thus the quantity of the X-rays produced, and the kilovoltage (kV), which affects the speed at which the electrons move from the cathode to the anode and thus the force with which they hit the anode. This affects the penetrating power or quality of the X-rays produced.

- The X-ray beam may be absorbed by the tissues of the patient, pass straight through to reach the film or be deflected in a different direction with a loss of energy. This deflected radiation is known as scatter.

- Scattered radiation is the main danger of radiography and can be reduced by the use of a grid, accurate collimation, reducing the thickness of the tissue and reducing the voltage as much as possible.

- The Ionizing Radiation Regulations 1999 detail all the measures that must be taken to reduce the dangers of radiation and ensure the safety of personnel within a veterinary practice.

- The latent image formed by the passage of X-rays through the patient to the film is made into a radiographic image

by the developing process. This may be achieved by using developing and fixing chemicals within developing tanks or within an automatic processor, via a digital imaging processor.

- Correct and accurate positioning of the patient, alongside accurate exposure factors, will produce an image from which a diagnosis can be made.

- Contrast media, which may be either negative (i.e. gas) or positive (i.e. barium or iodine preparations), can be used to highlight soft tissues not otherwise visible on plain radiographs.

- Ultrasound uses high-frequency sound waves that are sent into the body by a transducer and, when reflected from interfaces between the tissues, are collected by the transducer and an image forms on a computer screen. It can be used to demonstrate soft tissues, which are not always clearly visible on radiographs, and is painless and non-invasive.

- Computed tomography and nuclear scintigraphy use radiation to create an image, which thus presents safety problems, while magnetic resonance imaging uses a combination of a strong magnetic field and radio waves, so safety is less of an issue.

- Endoscopy is a type of medical examination in which an instrument called an endoscope is passed into an area of the body (e.g. the bladder or intestine). The endoscope usually has a fiberoptic camera, which allows a greatly magnified image to be projected onto a video screen, to be viewed by the operator. Many endoscopes also allow the operator to retrieve a small sample (biopsy) of the area being examined, in order to more closely view the tissue under a microscope.

Introduction

There is no doubt that diagnosis is made easier by the production of 'pictures' of the affected area within the body, and nowadays we take it for granted that we are able to do this in several ways. Radiography has been available for many years and is the method used by the majority of veterinary practices.

In recent years, veterinary surgeons have become increasingly experienced in the use of ultrasound for both large and small animals and it has the advantage of being non-invasive and much safer for personnel involved in the process. Other less common techniques include computed tomography (CT) and magnetic resonance imaging (MRI) scans, though their use is becoming more frequent.

Each technique has its advantages and disadvantages, and in order for veterinary nurses to be able to make a contribution to the procedure it is important that they have a thorough understanding of the underpinning physical principles and the practical aspects involved in creating a useful diagnostic image.

Principles of radiography

PHYSICS FOR RADIOGRAPHY

All solids, liquids and gases are composed of elements, or materials that cannot be broken down into something else. The details of all elements known are recorded in the periodic table, which gives full details of every element.

Every element is made up of atoms (Fig. 32.1). These atoms contain a nucleus, composed of neutrons and protons, surrounded by orbiting electrons. Protons are always positively charged; neutrons are neutral and have no charge. The orbiting electrons are always negatively charged (Table 32.1). The electrons orbit the nucleus in shells. Each shell can hold a certain number of electrons. The shell nearest the nucleus will always fill first, working outwards until all the electrons are contained in a shell. If a shell is not completely full it will be the outermost

shell and this will be where any interactions take place. For the atom to be stable the outermost shell should be full. The number of electrons should be equal to the number of protons. The number of protons is unique to each element.

In radiography the electrons are used in various ways in the production of X-rays and play an important role in the interactions of X-rays within the body.

The electromagnetic spectrum

X-rays are part of the electromagnetic spectrum; this is composed of energy waves. Contained within the electromagnetic spectrum are radio waves, ultraviolet light, visible light and cosmic rays, as well as X-rays and gamma rays (Fig. 32.2).

Every wave has a different wavelength and frequency. The wavelength is the distance from the peak of one wave to the peak of the next. The frequency is the number of peaks passing a set point every second. Frequency is measured in hertz (Hz). 1 Hz is equal to 1 cycle per second. X-rays have a short wavelength and high frequency.

When electromagnetic radiation is emitted, whether it is from the sun or an X-ray tube, the intensity will decrease as the distance from the source increases. This is known as the **inverse square law**; this is useful in radiation protection. The further away from the X-ray tube you can get, the lower the intensity of X-rays reaching the body and causing damage.

Electrical energy

The production of X-rays is dependent on the provision of electrical energy to the X-ray tube. An electric charge is produced as the electrons of an atom move from the outer shell of one atom to the outer shell of the adjacent atom. This can be done in three main ways:

- **Friction** – electrons build up as two objects are rubbed together
- **Contact** – if two suitable materials make contact, electrons will flow
- **Induction** – this uses the electrical field of a charged object to create a charge in a previously uncharged object.

An electric charge will always move from negative to positive. Like charges will repel each other, and unlike charges will attract each other. If electrons are able to move easily through the

TABLE 32.1	Details of the particles within an atom		
Particle	Position	Charge	Symbol
Proton	In nucleus	Positive	+
Neutron	In nucleus	Neutral	0
Electron	Orbiting nucleus	Negative	–

An atom

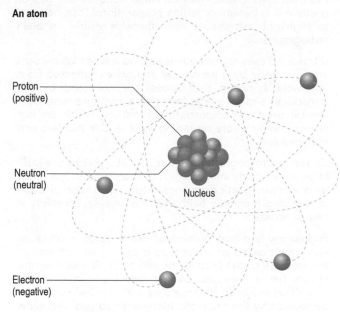

Proton (positive)

Neutron (neutral)

Nucleus

Electron (negative)

Fig. 32.1 Structure of an atom

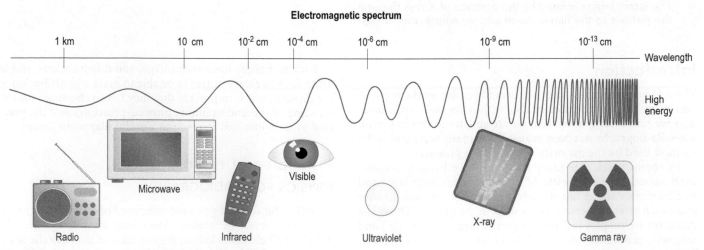

Electromagnetic spectrum

1 km   10 cm 10^{-2} cm 10^{-4} cm 10^{-6} cm 10^{-9} cm 10^{-13} cm   Wavelength

High energy

Radio   Microwave   Infrared   Visible   Ultraviolet   X-ray   Gamma ray

Fig. 32.2 The electromagnetic spectrum

atoms of a material then the material is a conductor. If the electrons cannot move freely or easily then the material is an insulator. All electrical charges have a potential energy and when released, and the electrons move through a material, the energy generated can be used. This electrical potential is measured in volts (V).

An electric current is formed when electrons flow through a conductor. If the electrons flow in one direction, then a direct current (DC) is generated. If the electrons go in alternating directions, then an alternating current (AC) is formed.

X-RAY TUBE CONSTRUCTION

Tube structure

The X-ray tube produces the X-rays and is composed of a Pyrex tube surrounding the anode and cathode (Fig. 32.3). The tube contains a vacuum to prevent unwanted interactions during the production of the X-rays. The anode and cathode both have a high-tension electrical supply, providing the direct current necessary to generate X-rays. The Pyrex tube is surrounded by oil to prevent the build-up of heat, and lead to prevent X-rays from passing straight out of the tube. The entire structure is surrounded by a lead case, within which is a small window directly under the anode to allow the primary beam to exit the tube. The window has a small aluminium filter to remove any low-energy, undesirable X-rays from the primary beam, improving its quality.

The cathode

The cathode is the negative part of the X-ray tube (see Fig. 32.3). The cathode is made up of the filament and focusing cup. The **filament** is a very small piece of wire and is heated to produce electrons in a similar way to the heating filament in a toaster. The filament is made of tungsten, which has a very high melting point. In dual-focus X-ray tubes the cathode has two filament wires. If broad focus is selected, the longer (0.4–1.3 mm) of the two wires will be used; if fine focus is selected the shorter (0.1–0.4 mm) wire will be selected.

The **focusing cup** surrounds the filament wire. The function of the focusing cup is to stream the electrons in a narrow band towards the anode when an exposure is made. The electrons are negatively charged, as is the focusing cup. The focusing cup will repel the electrons to the centre, ensuring that they flow in a narrow band and do not spread out. This ensures that the electrons fall within the target of the anode and do not extend beyond its boundaries.

The anode

The anode is the positive part of the X-ray tube (see Fig. 32.3). The anode may be stationary or rotating, depending on whether it remains in one place or rotates during exposure. Stationary anodes are usually found in dental machines and smaller portable machines. In general machines the anode rotates. This allows for the production of high-quality X-rays in a very short period of time, with reduced damage when compared to stationary anodes using similar exposure factors.

The anode conducts electrons away from the tube to the generator, provides support for the target and removes excess heat from the tube. The process of X-ray production results in 99% heat and 1% actual X-rays. The heat must be removed to prevent the anode from melting.

The **target** is the area that the electrons strike. In a rotating tube this is a disc around the entire circle of the target disc. As the target rotates, so the area that the electrons strike changes, increasing the area that the electrons can strike and increasing the lifespan of the tube. If the anode is stationary the whole surface is the target.

The target is made of tungsten alloy embedded in a copper anode. In some tubes the target is supported on molybdenum or graphite to make tube rotation easier. The area actually hit by the electrons is called the **focal spot** and this is the source of the radiation emitted from the X-ray tube. The effective focal spot that is emitted from the tube will alter depending on the angle of the target. This angle is usually between 7° and 20° to the vertical. As the angle of the target increases, so the effective size of the focal spot increases.

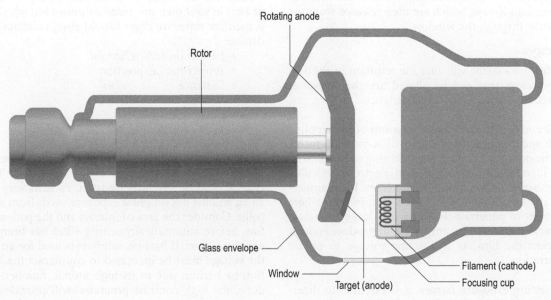

Fig. 32.3 X-ray tube structure

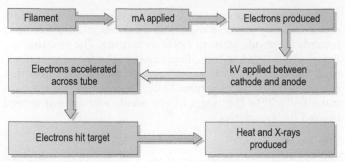

Fig. 32.4   The production of X-rays. Flow diagram from Easton 2002, page 44

X-RAY PRODUCTION

The production of X-rays takes place as the exposure button is fully depressed. In two-stage exposure buttons, the first stage 'preps' the machine, heating the cathode and starting the rotation of the anode; the second stage produces the X-rays, enabling the exposure to be made (Fig. 32.4). The exposure will be terminated immediately if finger pressure on the button is released:

- During the **first stage** the filament at the cathode is heated and the milliamperage selected determines the amount of heating. The higher the milliamperage, the higher the heat and the more electrons produced. Heating releases electrons from the surface of the filament wire. The electrons collect in the focusing cup. These electrons contain electrical potential and, when a charge is applied, will flow from negative to positive (i.e. cathode to anode).
- During the **second stage**, a potential difference is applied between the cathode and anode, ensuring that the electrons flow to the anode. This is achieved by applying a kilovoltage selected when setting the exposure factors. The higher the kilovoltage selected, the faster the electrons will move towards the target, resulting in higher-energy X-rays. The electrons are accelerated from the cathode to the anode and as they strike the target they are stopped. This sudden braking results in the electrons changing into X-rays, which are then released from the X-ray tube through the window.

Exposure factors

The exposure factors selected will alter the resultant image dramatically. The factors that can be altered are the amperage (mA), time (seconds), voltage (kV) and distance.

Amperage. The amperage controls the amount of heat applied to the cathode and changes the quantity of X-rays produced, which affects the density or degree of blackening of the film. As the amperage increases, so the number of electrons and ultimately the number of X-rays produced increases. If the amperage is inadequate the film will appear grey, even in areas where there is no patient to penetrate. In some very large animals it may be necessary to increase the amperage, to produce enough X-rays to blacken the film, as well as the voltage, to ensure adequate penetration.

Time. When setting exposure factors, it is essential to determine a period of time (in seconds) over which to allow the production of X-rays to take place. In the ideal world the time should be as short as possible. This allows limited time for patient movement to occur as even breathing or heart movements can produce blurring on the radiographic image:

Milliamp seconds or mAs – in most machines the amperage and time are combined to provide one exposure factor known as the mAs. When setting the mAs, the time should be as low as possible and the amperage should be as high as possible, i.e. mA × time(s) = mAs.

Voltage. The voltage alters the speed at which the electrons accelerate across the tube and strike the target. The faster the electrons move the higher the energy or penetrating power of the resultant X-rays. The voltage of the beam affects the contrast of the image, i.e. the difference between black and white. If a patient is very small, a low voltage is needed so that the X-rays do not overpenetrate and cause the image to be very dark.

Distance. The focal distance of the film is the distance (usually measured in centimetres) from the target (or source of the X-rays) to the film, and changing it has an effect on the image created. It is usually around 100 cm and should remain constant, as altering it between patients will cause confusion. As the distance increases, so the intensity of the X-ray beam reaching the patient decreases, resulting in underexposed films. This is expressed as the inverse square law.

If a new table or X-ray tube support is purchased and the distance has to be altered, then the mAs must be adjusted to allow for the change. This can be calculated using the following equation:

$$\text{Old mAs} \times (\text{new distance}^2/\text{old distance}^2) = \text{new mAs}.$$

Exposure charts

Exposure charts should be kept wherever possible. The use and provision of an exposure chart is outlined in the Ionizing Radiation Regulations 1999 (see Chapter 5) and by referring to it you should achieve accurate, reproducible exposures and reduce the need for repeat exposure because of incorrect exposure setting. The chart may be taken from a purpose-designed book or kept in your own pre-ruled columns; but whichever method is used the exposure chart should always contain the following details:

- Patient breed/size/weight
- Projection, i.e. position
- Distance
- Voltage
- mAs
- Film–screen combination
- Grid (if used).

If there is more than one X-ray tube or grid in use, then specific details should be given to avoid confusion. The exposure chart should be regularly updated. Patients vary in size and a 15 kg bulldog has different exposure needs from a 15 kg border collie. Consider the area of interest and the patient's conformation before automatically setting what has been listed in the exposure chart. If barium sulphate is used for an examination, the voltage must be increased to counteract the X-ray absorption by barium due to its high atomic number. If this is not done, the high contrast generated will provide a suboptimal image.

Effects of radiation

PROPERTIES OF X-RAYS

X-rays are part of the electromagnetic spectrum and have a wide range of properties which may affect their use:

- **Direction of travel** – X-rays will always travel in straight lines, giving a true representation of the patient or objects they pass through. The only time they can change direction is if they collide with an atom, which may degrade the image.
- **Ionisation** – X-rays can interact with tissues and cause ionisation, which occurs when atoms become positively charged through the loss of an electron in the outer shell. This fact is used to form the image on the film, and is the effect that causes absorption of the X-rays within the body. However, ionisation can cause damage to cells, including burns and the induction of cancer, and is the reason for the need for radiation protection.
- **Penetration** – X-rays are able to pass through most types of solid matter and this is used in radiography to form an image on a film. If the amount of matter is increased, the X-rays will eventually be absorbed and stopped. The denser the object the more easily the X-rays will be stopped. This property is used in radiation protection.
- **Divergence** – as the X-ray beam travels from the target it will lose intensity and will also spread out, following the inverse square law. This is used in radiation protection to reduce the risk, and should be considered when setting the focal film distance, to ensure consistent radiographs.
- **Absorption** – as the X-rays pass through the patient they may be stopped or slowed down by the tissues in the patient. If a tissue is very dense, e.g. bone, then the X-rays will be stopped – the tissue is described as being **radiopaque**. If a tissue is much less dense, e.g. lung, it will not stop the X-rays and they will pass through – the tissue is described as being **radiolucent**. The amount of absorption depends on the atomic number of the tissue. The higher the atomic number the more absorption that will occur. For example, bone is mainly composed of calcium and has a higher atomic number than lung tissue, which is composed of a high proportion of air; bone absorbs more X-rays than lung tissue and appears white on the radiograph while lung tissue appears black (Fig. 32.5).
- **Photographic effect** – X-rays interact with the silver halides within the X-ray film to form an image. They also cause certain phosphors to emit light or fluoresce, the principle used in intensifying screens. Within radiographic film, the more X-rays that strike the silver halide crystals the greater the reaction and the whiter the appearance on the processed radiograph.

Scattered radiation

Scattered radiation or 'scatter' is the reduction in energy of the primary beam and movement of X-rays in a different direction after interaction with matter. It may have a detrimental effect on the resultant image as it darkens the film causing 'fogging' and is also a major factor in the need for radiation protection. As the X-rays have lost energy they are more likely to be

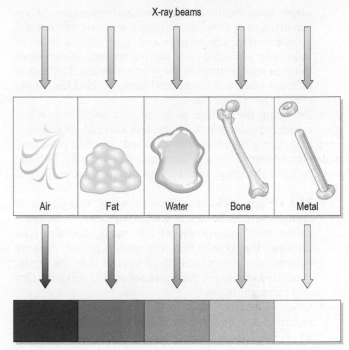

X-ray beams

Air   Fat   Water   Bone   Metal

Fig. 32.5 Difference in absorption shown by different types of tissue

absorbed than the primary beam which passes straight through with minimal absorption.

Sources of scattered radiation. Scatter is caused whenever X-rays interact with matter and this increases:

- As the patient or the region under investigation gets thicker – i.e. the thicker the body part the more chance there is for the X-rays to interact with the electrons within the patient and result in scatter
- If the collimator is not used effectively – the larger the area irradiated the more chance there is of the X-ray photons interacting and being scattered
- With the use of higher voltages – these produce X-rays with higher energy, which will have detrimental effects on the image. This scattered radiation is also more likely to travel in a forward direction and reach the film, causing fogging.

Control of scattered radiation. Scattered radiation should be minimised to increase radiation protection and to prevent it from affecting the film and degrading the image. This can be done in a number of ways:

- If the **thickness of a patient** is very large the area under examination can be compressed to reduce the amount of tissue that the X-rays have to pass through, reducing the chances for interaction to occur. This is especially useful in abdominal radiography of the larger patient. A compression band placed across the abdomen will reduce the thickness, improving contrast and reducing scatter.
- **Collimation of the primary beam** will reduce the area exposed to radiation, which improves safety, reduces the volume of tissue exposed and reduces scatter. Collimation will improve image quality and contrast. It is achieved through the use of a collimator or light beam

diaphragm, usually on the tube head mounting. This is constructed of a box containing a series of mirrors and a light source. The mirrors and light allow a beam of light to be projected on to the patient, which represents the area and position of the primary beam. The area of primary beam can be reduced using beveled lead leaves within the collimator.

- **Reducing the voltage** as much as possible, while still achieving a diagnostic image, will also reduce scatter.

As well as reducing the amount of scattered radiation produced, it is also important to reduce the amount reaching the film and thus decreasing the image quality. This can be achieved in two ways:

- **The air gap technique** – useful when imaging large animals such as horses, as scatter will result in magnification and 'unsharpness' of the image. The aim is to increase the object film distance (i.e. the distance between the patient and the film), so that the scatter generated within the patient is not able to reach the film and form an image.
- **Grids** – efficient tools in the reduction of scattered radiation reaching the film. They are able to remove 85–95% of all scattered radiation, depending on the type used. A grid is constructed of alternating strips of a material able to absorb radiation, e.g. lead, and a radiolucent interspace, usually aluminium or carbon plastic fibres (Fig. 32.6). The interspacer allows the primary

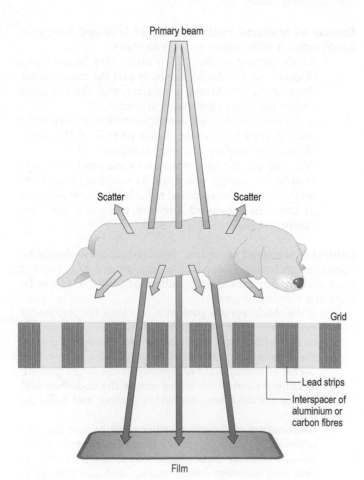

Fig. 32.6 Function of a grid

beam to pass through to the film but any scattered radiation hitting the lead strips will be absorbed, preventing it from reaching the film and causing fogging. The lead strips will also absorb some of the primary beam and the exposure factors must be increased to compensate for this.

The grid has a grid ratio, i.e. the ratio of the height of the lead strips to the distance between them. This is used to calculate the grid factor, i.e. the amount by which the mAs must be increased to compensate for the effects of the grid. The grid factor is usually between 2 and 6 and will be marked on the grid.

New mAs (when using a grid) = old mAs (without a grid)

× grid factor.

The grid must be placed between the patient and the film.
There are a number of different types of grid:

- **Parallel grid** – this is the most common type in use in veterinary practice and is usually stationary, i.e. it does not move. It is the easiest to use and as long as the grid is at 90° to the primary beam and straight it will produce a good result.
- **Potter–Bucky grids** – parallel grids are sometimes integrated into the X-ray table and move rapidly from side to side with the aid of a small motor. This movement eliminates the very fine lines usually visible when a stationary grid is used.

RADIATION SAFETY

Radiation can be harmful to those working with it and the use of radiation to form a diagnosis should be minimised. The risk of exposure to radiation should be balanced by the benefits of forming a diagnosis. All examinations must be clinically justified and the safety of the radiographer and anyone else around should always be the first priority.

The effects of radiation

X-rays will interact with the tissues within the human body, causing ionisation in which the tissue molecules can be broken or damaged. This process may cause the cells to damage each other, or the X-ray itself may damage the cells or DNA within the body. The body is capable of repairing the damage, but sometimes it may be so severe that repair is impossible and the cells will die. Rapidly dividing and developing cells are most susceptible and most likely to be damaged, e.g. hair, nails, the cells of young people or developing foetuses. The most common effect of damage is called a **stochastic effect**. This can happen with any level of radiation but the incidence increases as the level of exposure increases and it results in damage and mutation to the cells.

Safety legislation

The use of ionising radiation is carefully controlled in the UK and is laid down in guidelines governed by the Ionizing Radiation Regulations 1999 (IRR) (see also Chapter 5). These regulations indicate all procedures that should be adhered to when using sources of radiation, how exposure to patients should be minimised, and the measures radiographers and employers should take to ensure optimal safety at all times. The ALARP principle, i.e. 'as low as reasonably practicable', is the basis for these regulations and should be remembered at all times.

TABLE 32.2	Methods by which the dangers of radiation may be reduced in practice
Method of reduction	**How it works**
Avoid the primary beam	The primary beam is the most intense part of the X-ray beam. If you must stay in the room, you should be at least 2 m away. The primary beam should never be directed at the lead screen within the room or at the door. Even when wearing lead gloves, hands should never be placed in the primary beam.
Avoid manual restraint	Patients should not be manually restrained unless there is no alternative. With the use of modern drugs for sedation or anaesthesia, pads and the use of positioning aids, a diagnostic image can be produced in most patients without the need for personnel to hold them.
Lead protection	Lead aprons and thyroid shields should be used whenever an individual needs to remain in the X-ray room. Lead aprons will only protect effectively against scattered radiation and the 2 m rule should be remembered. Attempts should always be made to leave the room or use a lead screen to hide behind rather than remaining in the room during exposure.
Restricting access	Always ensure that the doors to the X-ray room are closed. This will prevent people wandering into the room, disturbing the patient and potentially being exposed to radiation. By closing the doors any scattered radiation will be contained within the room. The controlled area should always have a red warning light on when the X-ray machine is in use.

If these regulations are not followed individuals may be prosecuted.

Radiation protection in practice

In practice radiation protection involves reducing the dose used to produce the radiograph and the dose to staff. Within a practice the radiation protection supervisor (RPS) will ensure that local rules described in the IRR are adhered to and that the regulations are implemented. They are helped by a radiation protection advisor (RPA), who is from outside the practice and who will set up the local rules and ensure that the practice maintains a high standard of safety.

Basic measures to reduce dose include suitable collimation at all times and the use of intensifying screens, eliminating the need for high exposure factors. The dose to staff should be reduced as much as possible and there are a number of very easy ways this can be achieved (Table 32.2).

Dosimetry

All individuals exposed to radiation should be monitored by the use of dosimeters, which measure the dose of radiation received by the body. Every radiographic procedure will result in a dose being received by the patient and potentially by the radiographer if they remain in the room. The staff dose should be monitored and recorded through the use of monitoring devices, in the form of either badges containing film or thermoluminescent dosimeters. These should always be worn on the trunk of the body, under any lead protection, and should be looked after according to the supplier's instructions. They should be returned to the supplier at regular intervals so that the dose received can be read and recorded. If an individual has received more than the maximum permissible dose, it may be recommended that that person is taken off radiography work for a few months and changes may need to be made to the practice. It is unlikely that a veterinary nurse will ever reach this dose level.

Recording the image

The image created by the X-rays passing through the patient and reaching the film must be able to be recorded for diagnostic use and stored for many years. Recording the image requires the use of film and intensifying screens.

RADIOGRAPHIC FILM

Radiographic film is sensitive to both light and X-rays. The film is used to receive X-rays that have passed through the patient and convert them into a latent image. This is then converted into a visible or radiographic image during processing. The film is also sensitive to light, which may reach the film intentionally from the intensifying screens or unintentionally from exposure to daylight.

X-ray film is made up of a number of layers, all providing a vital role in the composition and function of the film (Fig. 32.7). It may be described as being either duplitised or single-sided. In duplitised film the layers are duplicated on either side of the polyester base, which increases its efficiency, resulting in a lower radiation dose to the patient. Single-sided film has an active side and a protective, counterbalanced side to prevent curling (Table 32.3).

Care and storage of X-ray film

X-ray film should be stored for the minimum amount of time and not beyond the expiry date. Stock should be rotated so that the oldest is used first. Ideally, small orders should be placed frequently to maintain optimal film quality.

All films should be handled carefully and stored vertically to prevent pressure marks occurring. These appear as black crescents if created during handling and black lines if created during storage.

The room used for film storage should be well-ventilated, with a temperature within the range given on the film box by the manufacturers. It is not ideal to store the film in the same room as open processing chemicals or anywhere that may be exposed to radiation.

Forming the radiographic image

The radiographic image is the visible image formed from the latent image by processing. Processing involves a chain reaction that starts when the film is exposed to light and/or X-rays. The film contains silver halide crystals that are sensitive to light and X-rays. In conventional film the silver halide is usually silver bromide. The manufacturers usually introduce a spot called the sensitivity speck that assists in the processing. Within the emulsion the silver and bromide ions form a lattice that becomes

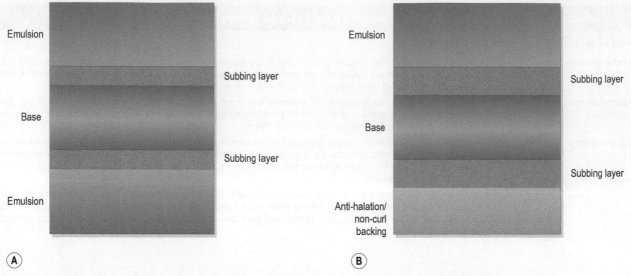

Fig. 32.7 Film structure. (A) Cross-section through duplitised film. (B) Cross-section through single-sided film

TABLE 32.3	Structure of radiographic film	
Layer	**Film type**	**Structure and function**
Base	Single-sided Duplitised	Made of polyester Clear plastic to allow transmission of light Flexible to allow handling Does not react to chemicals
Subbing layer	Single-sided Duplitised	Provides adhesive to attach the emulsion to the base layer
Emulsion	Single-sided – one emulsion layer Duplitised – two emulsion layers on either side of the base	Composed of gelatin impregnated with silver halide crystals. Silver halides react with X-rays and light to form the latent image Liquid gelatin is used for easy application, semi-solid during processing to allow chemical penetration and solid after processing for storage
Supercoat	Single sided – one supercoat Duplitised – two supercoat layers	Thin layer of gelatin that protects the emulsion during and after processing
Anti-curl layer	Single-sided	Duplitised film has equal amounts of emulsion on both sides of the base that absorb liquid and swell equally during processing so curling is not a problem Single-sided film has an anti-curl layer to balance the curling effects of the swollen emulsion. This prevents damage to the film

charged as the silver loses an electron, enabling it to bond with the bromine. During exposure the X-rays and light will cause a reaction that makes the silver migrate towards the sensitivity speck and the bromine to be released. The more silver that moves and the more bromine that is given off, the blacker the final radiograph will appear. Areas where the X-rays or light do not reach at all will have no reaction.

Film speed

Film speed is defined as the sensitivity of the film to light or radiation and is related to the density, i.e. degree of blackening of the image. Film speed is dependent on the size of the silver halide crystals in the emulsion and the thickness of the emulsion. Fast films require less exposure than slow films to produce the same density of film. As the film speed increases, so the density of the image increases. If the same density of image is required then it is the mAs that must be changed if the film speed is changed, i.e. if a faster film is used, reduce the mAs to

produce a similar diagnostic image. However, fast films produce an image with poorer definition, while slow films, which require a longer exposure, produce a more highly defined image. Slower films are used for extremity radiography, e.g. feet carpus, to ensure that the necessary bone detail is shown.

INTENSIFYING SCREENS

Intensifying screens are designed to fluoresce, i.e. emit light, when exposed to X-rays. As the film is sensitive to both X-rays and light, use of an intensifying screen allows for a lower X-ray exposure to be used to form a diagnostic image.

Intensifying screens are contained within a cassette. In cassettes where duplitised films are used there are two separate screens, one on either side of the cassette. In single-sided cassettes there is one intensifying screen on the back of the cassette. The film is sandwiched between the intensifying screens or between the intensifying screen and the front of the cassette.

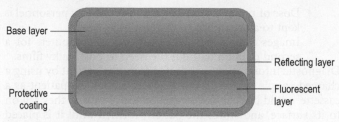

Fig. 32.8 Structure of an intensifying screen

TABLE 32.4	Types of intensifying screen	
Intensifying screen	Speed	Uses
High-resolution	Slow (100)	Fine detail. Needs a higher exposure. Ideal for extremity work
Regular	Medium (400)	General radiography
Fast	Fast (800)	Produces a darker image for given exposure factors Allows for a reduction in exposure time to reduce movement problems

Construction of an intensifying screen

An intensifying screen (Fig. 32.8) is made up of the following layers:

1. **Base (support layer):**
   - Back of intensifying screen
   - Supports the intensifying screen
   - Made of cardboard or polyester
   - Moisture-resistant
   - Flexible
   - Does not interfere with the passage of X-rays through to the phosphor layer and film.

2. **Reflecting layer:**
   - Made of magnesium oxide or titanium dioxide
   - Redirects stray light emitted from the intensifying screen to improve image quality
   - Increases effectiveness of the intensifying screen.

3. **Fluorescent phosphor layer:**
   - Active part of the intensifying screen
   - Layer of tiny phosphor crystals suspended in a binder of polyurethane
   - Phosphor crystals are either rare earth or calcium tungstate
   - Crystals held together and protected from moisture
   - Dye to absorb stray light.

4. **Protective coating:**
   - Outer layer of the intensifying screen
   - Protects the phosphor layer against abrasions, moisture and staining
   - Reduces static
   - Will survive routine cleaning
   - Extends around the back of the screen to prevent curling.

Luminescence

When the phosphor grain is bombarded by X-rays, fluorescence, i.e. the emission of light, and phosphorescence, i.e. the afterglow, occur. Fluorescence occurs when the X-rays pass through the phosphor layer. The interaction excites the phosphor crystals and they emit ultraviolet and visible light. The visible light is used to form the image on the radiographic film. The phosphor will emit hundreds of light photons for every X-ray photon that strikes it. Rare earth intensifying screens will convert 15–20% of all X-rays to light, while the calcium tungstate used in more old-fashioned types of screen will convert approximately 4% of all X-rays to light. This conversion ensures a reduction in the exposure needed to form a diagnostic image on the film, which in turn reduces the dose to the patient and to the staff.

FILM–SCREEN COMBINATIONS

To ensure that the light emitted from an intensifying screen is utilised fully, the wavelength or colour of the light emitted from the intensifying screen must match the light sensitivity of the film. Calcium tungstate intensifying screens will emit blue light, so the film must be sensitive to blue light and these films are described as being **monochromatic**. Rare earth screens usually emit green light, although some types emit blue light, and so the film used should be sensitive to both blue and green light. This is known as **orthochromatic** film. If the film sensitivity is not matched to the light emitted by the screen the beneficial effects of the intensifying screen will be reduced.

Intensifying screen speed

The speed of an intensifying screen describes the relative exposure needed by different types of screen to produce images of a similar density (Table 32.4). The faster the screen the lower the exposure needed to form an image. The screen speed is determined by the **size of the phosphor grain**, the **thickness of the intensifying screen layer** and the **presence or absence of a reflective layer**.

Single screens

Single screens function in exactly the same way as double intensifying screens but have half the intensifying factor. They were developed for use in human mammography and are ideal for extremity work, where the demonstration of fine detail is essential. It should be ensured that the light emission from the intensifying screen matches the film sensitivity and also that the film emulsion is in close contact with the intensifying screen.

Film–screen contact

If a sharp image is to be achieved there must be good contact between the film and the screen. Damaged or old cassettes may have curved screens, which will result in blurring of the image where there is reduced contact. This is due to the divergence in the beam between being emitted from the intensifying screen and reaching the film. Cassettes that produce a blurred image should be checked and replaced if necessary.

Care of intensifying screens

Screens should be carefully cleaned on a regular basis. Dirt will show up as bright, white specks on the processed radiograph because the light is blocked from reaching the film after emission by the dirt and dust. Cotton wool should never be used to clean an intensifying screen, and a preparatory screen cleaner should be used whenever possible. The intensifying screen should not be saturated with liquid and all cleaning movements should be gentle. The cassette should be dried thoroughly by standing it on its end before it is used again.

Radiographic cassettes

Intensifying screens are contained within a protective cassette, and the film is sandwiched between the screens. The cassette ensures that light cannot reach the film and ensures good film–screen contact at all times.

Each cassette is made up of the following parts:

1. **Front:**
   - Uniform thickness
   - Conforms to BS4304/1968
   - Aluminium equivalent of less than 0.2 mm
   - Made from plastic or carbon
   - Lightweight
   - Low absorption of the primary beam, i.e. allows most of it to pass through to the film inside.

2. **Back:**
   - Similar material to the front
   - Lead strips to protect the film from back scatter
   - Foam pad under the intensifying screen to hold the film in place and ensure film–screen contact.

3. **Closure:**
   - Strong closing mechanism
   - Usually a clip or plastic locking bar
   - Good closure ensures light proofing and film–screen contact.

Care of cassettes
- Always treat them gently – they are expensive to replace.
- Do not drop them.
- They are relatively heavy so only carry a few at a time.
- Avoid excessive dampness and water exposure.
- Store upright to prevent bending and damage.
- Use a numbering system to identify damaged or dirty cassettes.

DIGITAL IMAGING

Digital imaging is becoming standard place in veterinary practice. It should be emphasised that the image is still formed by X-rays, so an X-ray machine is still used and radiation safety or personnel must still be considered.

Digital imaging has a number of benefits:
- Digital sensors are used to form an image without the need for radiographic film
- Immediate image display
- High-quality images
- Images may be enhanced to overcome any incorrect exposure factors
- Images may be altered to show different windows and the windows can be varied to show, for example, just bone, just soft tissue or both

- Dose of radiation to patient and veterinary personnel is kept to a minimum
- Images can be emailed to other vets' computers for a second opinion without the need to post bulky films.

Diagnostic information is collected from the patient by using a charged couple device, which is placed under the patient as a cassette would be. The device detects the X-rays as they fall on to its surface, and stores the pattern formed until it is placed into the reader. The data is then analysed by a computer and converted into an image, which is viewed on a monitor.

All images are stored on the hard drive of the machine, though a backup on an external hard drive is recommended. If a hard copy is required, the image can be reproduced on a film laser printer to produce a radiograph, which can then be viewed in the normal way.

Film processing
PROCESSING CYCLE

After a film has been exposed, a **latent image** is present on the film, but to turn this into a visible or **radiographic image** the film must be processed. Regardless of whether this is done manually or by an automatic processor, the cycle is the same (Fig. 32.9).

1. Developer

This is always the first stage:
- In the developer solution there are two active developing agents, hydroquinone and phenindone, both of which reduce exposed silver bromide crystals to metallic silver, which is deposited on the film and appears black. Unexposed silver bromide crystals will not be affected by the developer solution.
- The developer also contains a preservative to slow oxidation and a lid should always be kept on the developer solution to help reduce oxidation as much as possible.
- An accelerator maintains the pH of the developer. The pH is usually 9.6–10.0, i.e. it is alkaline.
- Chemical fogging is reduced using a restrainer, which will improve the selectivity of the developer, ensuring that a minimal number of unexposed silver halide crystals are reduced.
- As the developer is used, calcium sludge builds up, reducing the effectiveness of the developer. To reduce this a sequestering agent is added.

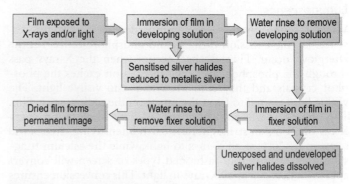

Fig. 32.9 Processing cycle from Easton 2002, page 73

- All the chemicals are dissolved in a solvent. In this case the solvent is water, as it is readily available and cheap. The water will also dissolve all the by-products of processing. The emulsion is softened by water and this allows the developer to penetrate the film surface more easily.

2. Wash

Between the developer and the fixer stages excess developer must be removed from the film surface. In manual processing this is done by rinsing the film in the small wash tank between the developer and the fixer tanks. In an automatic processor, developer is removed by squeegee rollers and there is usually no intermediate wash.

3. Fixer

This stops development and forms a permanent image on the film. The solution converts unexposed silver bromide into a form that can be washed off the film. This is known as conversion:

- The fixer contains a fixing agent that will diffuse into the emulsion and react with the unexposed silver bromide crystals that remain on the film after development. The fixing agent is usually ammonium thiosulphate, which changes the unexposed areas of the film from a milky white colour to transparent.
- The fixing agent is dissolved in a solvent, usually water, which allows the chemical to pass into the film emulsion.
- An acidifier stops development. This neutralises the alkaline developer and prevents further development and dichroic fog.
- Sodium acetate is used as a buffer to maintain the pH to within 0.2 of the manufacturer's predetermined levels.
- Decomposition of the fixer is prevented using sodium sulphite.
- Damage to the film is prevented by the addition of a hardener to the fixer solution, which also helps it to dry efficiently.
- The hardener produces insoluble compounds that form sludge on the bottom of the tank. This sludge formation is reduced and prevented using an antisludging agent, usually boric acid.

4. Wash

The processed film then passes through a wash tank. If the film is being manually processed, this usually consists of running water for at least 10 minutes. In an automatic processor another set of rollers takes the film through a tank of water for about 10–20 seconds. The wash prevents the continuing action of the processing chemicals and deterioration of the image quality during storage.

5. Drying

The final stage of processing is to dry the film, allowing it to be viewed and stored. During the processing cycle the film absorbs water and this makes the emulsion 'mushy'. If the emulsion were not dried this layer would be easily removed and would decrease the image quality. In an automatic processor, drying takes about 25 seconds and is usually preceded by squeegee rollers, which remove as much excess water as possible from the surface of the

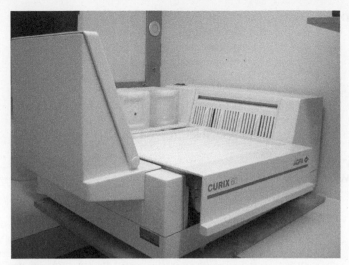

Fig. 32.10 An automatic processor

film. The film is then dried using hot air at 50–60°C blown on to the film. In a manual system the film has to be hung up in a clean, dry environment and steps must be taken to prevent hairs or dirt coming into contact with the film.

AUTOMATIC PROCESSORS

Automatic processors carry the film through a number of tanks using a series of rollers (Fig. 32.10). The dry-to-dry time is usually 2–4 minutes, depending on the type of processor, compared with a minimum of 50 minutes with a manual processor and drying cabinet.

The film enters the processor through a film feed system. This grasps the film and takes it into the developer roller through a guide roller. The film passes through a number of rollers, all of which press the processing chemical into the emulsion, ensuring even and adequate coverage. To eliminate the need for a gear system the tanks are varying depths, so that the time spent in each tank is correct for the solution it contains. The developer tank is usually the deepest; the wash tank is the shallowest and the film spends the shortest time here.

The water used within the processor helps to maintain a constant temperature. If the temperature fluctuates, image quality will be low and inconsistent. Water is also used in the wash tank – usually cold, as warmer water will encourage the growth of algae, which is not ideal.

All processing chemicals should be collected in special containers and sent to a specialist company for disposal. If this is not possible, processing chemicals can be disposed of down a normal drain but care must be taken to ensure dilution and adherence to local bye-laws regarding drainage. The disposal of processing chemicals is controlled by the Deposit of Poisonous Waste Act 1972.

Care of an automatic processor

An automatic processor should be looked after carefully. Before planning a maintenance regimen it is important to read the manufacturer's instructions as machines vary. A cleaning regimen should be implemented to ensure it is always functioning to the highest level possible.

Daily care

- Pass an old film through an automatic processor before use to pick up any debris on the rollers.
- Check levels of chemicals in tanks.
- Check operating temperature.
- Remove any visible chemical deposits.
- Remove lid to allow circulation of air when not in use.
- Wipe any rollers above the solution levels.
- Insert antifungal tablet to wash tanks at the end of the day.

Weekly care

- Repeat daily programme.
- Drain and scrub the wash tanks.
- Remove top rollers and clean.
- Remove wash, developer and fixer rollers and clean thoroughly with running water.
- Check movement on all sets of rollers by manually turning the roller.
- Check that chemicals are being replenished by the machine's system.
- Clean the drier rollers with a damp cloth.
- Record all maintenance performed.

Monthly care

- Repeat daily and weekly programme.
- Strip entire processor down to the basics and clean all tanks and rollers with a sponge and running water.
- Close drain valves.
- Check movement of rollers.
- Replace all chemicals (unless using an automixer).

REPLENISHMENT

The chemicals used within a processor will become tired and less active as time progresses. To ensure that the machine is working at optimum levels, the processing chemicals should be replaced on a regular basis. At least every 6 weeks all the chemicals should be replaced with fresh solutions. As the developer and fixer work, they produce by-products, which will dilute the concentration of the processing chemicals over time. Developer solution will also oxidise in air and this further reduces its activity.

In an automatic processor the chemicals are replaced each time a film enters the machine. A small amount of solution, depending on the film size, will be removed automatically and replaced by fresh chemicals. Within the machine is either a reservoir or a series of small bottles to store a small reserve of chemical.

Maximum efficiency can be achieved by the use of an automixer which mixes stores and dispenses developer and fixer into the processor whenever required. This is ideal in situations where the throughput is large and is much cleaner and safer than the use of small bottles or a reservoir in the processor itself.

SILVER RECOVERY

During the fixing stage, metallic silver is produced and this can be recovered and recycled. There are a number of methods of recovering the silver in fixer. If used fixer is collected for disposal by a specialised firm then this process is already in place but if the fixer is disposed of down the drain then a small silver recovery unit may be installed to remove the silver before disposal. A specialist firm can then recycle the silver collected. Films also contain metallic silver that can be recycled. The process of silver recovery is not expensive and the collection and recycling charges are usually covered by the value of the silver recovered.

THE DARKROOM

With the use of automatic processors that function in daylight and most veterinary practices now using digital radiography, the need for a darkroom is decreasing. However, many practices store film, load cassettes or keep the processor in the darkroom, so when setting one up there are several factors to be considered:

- The room should be easily accessible to all areas of the practice and should be large enough to allow safe movement when the lights are switched off.
- It should not be damp or humid, as this will affect the films, and it should have a reliable source of electricity and running water.
- Films and chemicals should not be stored in the same area, as the chemicals may cause fogging of the films. The darkroom should not be exposed to radiation in any way, especially if this is where film is stored.
- The whole room should be painted a light colour to reflect as much light as possible into the room.
- The surfaces should be washable to allow easy removal of spillages.
- The room should be well-ventilated to ensure the comfort of staff and prevent deterioration of the film quality.
- A method should be in place to prevent anyone entering when the room is in use and causing possible light fogging of the film, e.g. a warning light on the outside, a double-door system or a lock (but make sure the door can be opened from the outside in an emergency).

Safelights

A safelight is needed in the darkroom to prevent white light fogging the film during handling prior to processing while still allowing the radiographer to move safely around the room.

Safelights usually have a red filter but vary according to the colour sensitivity of the film. White light is a combination of red, blue and green light. A red filter allows only red light through, so if the film is sensitive to blue or green light it will be unaffected.

The safelight should be at least 2 m from the work surface and should have no more than a 15-watt bulb. There are two types:

- **Direct safelight** – sometimes known as a beehive safelight; directs light downwards on to work surfaces
- **Indirect safelight** – projects light upwards on to the ceiling; it is then reflected back down into the room.

Radiographic quality and image interpretation

DESCRIBING AND VIEWING AN IMAGE

Radiographs should always be positioned, viewed and described in a systematic and conventional manner.

There are a number of rules to remember when you are viewing a processed radiograph:

- A radiograph should be viewed on a proper viewing box – not against a window or strip light.
- A lateral radiograph should always be viewed with the head to the left, the tail to the right.
- Ventrodorsal and dorsoventral radiographs should be viewed as if you are shaking hands with them, i.e. the left of the animal is on your right.
- An extremity should be viewed so that the proximal end of the region is at the top of the viewing box, or computer screen.
- Correct anatomical descriptions should be used whenever possible.
- Try to describe the image so that it could be seen in the mind of someone who is not able to see the radiograph.
- Use familiar objects to describe the appearance and size of areas seen on the radiograph, e.g. walnut-sized, pea-sized, appearance of a bunch of grapes.

ASSESSING THE RADIOGRAPH

When assessing the quality of a processed radiograph, consider the following points. If all these headings are examined and analysed, then low-quality, non-diagnostic radiographs will not be passed for scrutinisation:

- Correct and visible identification
- Anatomical markers and legends correct and visible
- Area under examination shown
- Correct projection taken
- Suitable exposure factors used for area under examination
- Adequate contrast, density and sharpness
- Suitable collimation, accurate but not too tight
- Artefacts (lead, collar, mud, wet coat, contrast medium)
- Anatomical variants or pathology that may need an alteration of exposure factors
- Good overall image quality
- Need for further projections or repeat radiographs.

A radiograph should be assessed using the following criteria:

- **Latitude** – describes the range of exposures that will ensure that a diagnostic image is possible. If a film has wide latitude there is a greater range of exposure factors that will produce a diagnostic image. Films with wide latitude will have a longer grey scale than films with narrow latitude.
- **Density** – describes the amount of blackening seen on a radiographic film. This degree of blackening is related to the specific gravity and the atomic number of the subject under examination. If the subject area has a high atomic number, e.g. the bone in the pelvis of a large dog, then the X-rays' photons will interact with the tissue and very few X-rays will reach the radiographic film, creating a white image. If the area under examination is air-filled, and thus has a low specific gravity and atomic number, there will be less interaction with the X-ray photons and more will reach the film, resulting in more blackening of the film (Table 32.5).
- **Contrast** – the difference in density, i.e. degree of blackening, between two adjacent structures. If the image has lots of grey but very little black and white, it is described

TABLE 32.5	Appearance of tissues on a radiograph related to their specific gravity and atomic number		
Tissue	Specific gravity	Atomic number	Appearance on radiograph
Bone	High	High	White
Water/muscle	Medium/high	High	Grey
Fat	Low/medium	Low	Grey
Air	Low	Low	Black

as being a low-contrast image or a 'flat-film'. If there is little grey but lots of black and white, the image is said to be a high-contrast image (Fig. 32.11), often described as 'soot and whitewash'.

Contrast is influenced by a number of factors:

- **Tissue specific gravity and atomic number** – an increase in atomic number and specific gravity will result in more X-ray photons being absorbed. A higher voltage will ensure adequate penetration and an overall increase in contrast.
- **Voltage** – low voltage will produce an image with high contrast (very black and white); as the voltage increases so the amount of contrast increases, providing a greater range of greys and less black and white.
- **Object shape and thickness** – if an area is very thin it will absorb fewer X-rays and will lead to an image with minimal contrast, e.g. in abdominal radiographs of very small cats. The resultant image may demonstrate a grey abdomen with no definition of the internal organs because of the limited contrast.
- **Film fogging** – fogging results in an overall greyness and a reduction in contrast and may be due to poor film storage, incorrect processing, scattered radiation or exposure to light.

Most common film faults

Film faults occur when the different radiographic techniques or protocols are not followed. They appear for many reasons and a number of remedial actions can be taken to eliminate the fault(s). Good training and effective practice procedures will reduce film faults and the need for repeated radiographs and ultimately increase radiation safety (Table 32.6).

Positioning

GENERAL PRINCIPLES

The following principles should be followed to ensure that the maximum benefit is gained from accurate positioning:

- All radiographs must have a clinical indication and be requested by a qualified veterinary surgeon.
- Radiation safety must be understood and adhered to at all times.
- Standard projections should be performed whenever possible to allow interpretation and diagnosis.
- If possible, at least two views at 90° to each other should be taken of all extremities and other regions.
- Careful positioning, centring and collimation should always be carried out.
- If positioning will compromise the patient's condition, then alternative methods of diagnosis should be used.

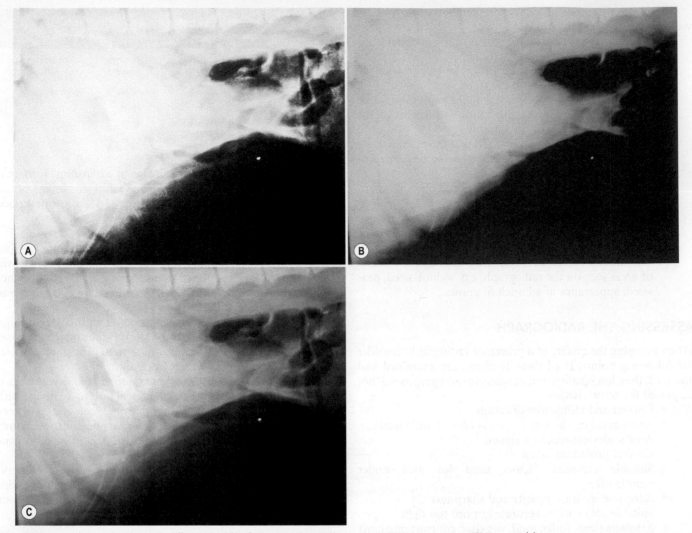

Fig. 32.11 Radiographs showing different levels of contrast. (A) High contrast. (B) Low contrast. (C) Acceptable

TABLE 32.6	Most common film faults		
Image problem	**Description**	**Reason**	**Solution**
Image is too dark	Film is overexposed	Voltage and/or mAs too high	Reduce exposure factors
	Background is blackened as well as the image	Film has been fogged by light or radiation	Eliminate light or radiation source
		Overdevelopment caused by increased developer temperature or increased time	Check temperature of processing chemicals and the time that film remains in solution
Image is too pale	Exposed parts of background are black	The film is underexposed as it has not received enough X-rays	Increase exposure factors
	Exposed parts of the background are pale as well	The film is underdeveloped	Ensure that developer is fresh, warm enough and that the film is in solution for enough time
Film is yellow/brown	May have powdery deposits over the surface	Film is not fixed or washed properly	Check time in fixer and wash stages
			Replace chemicals if exhausted

- Identification labels should be present to prevent the loss of films, left/right markers should be utilised.

RESTRAINT

To prevent production of low-quality, non-diagnostic images, all animals should be restrained. This can be in the form of chemical restraint or through the use of pads, sandbags or ties.

Chemical restraint

Spine, skull, pharynx, some contrast procedures, hip examinations and most fracture investigations should not be carried out unless the animal is anaesthetised. If it is not possible to anaesthetise the animal, then heavy sedation can be used, but accurate diagnostic images may be difficult to produce. In the case of severely dyspnoeic patients, most will tolerate sedation and this will ensure that a diagnostic radiograph with limited stress to the patient is achieved.

In veterinary medicine, the patient cannot be relied upon to remain in position or to stay on the table so most radiographs will be carried out under chemical restraint. Manual positioning is not recommended (unless it is clinically essential) because it usually relies on the veterinary surgeon restraining the patient, putting them in danger of exceeding the maximum permissible dose of radiation over a period of time.

Positioning aids

These should be available for all examinations. They should be radiolucent so that they do not show up on the final radiograph. Always check any new positioning aids introduced into the practice. Care should be taken when using sandbags, which are radiopaque, to prevent them from obscuring any of the area of interest.

The list of available aids below is intended as an outline, and individuals may have personal favourites:

- **Radiolucent foam or plastic troughs** for dorsoventral or ventrodorsal projections.
- A selection of **radiolucent foam wedges and blocks**. These should be in a variety of shapes and sizes.
- A selection of **long, floppy sandbags**.
- **Hobbles or bandages**. These can be used to tie limbs out of the way or to hold the mouth open during examination of the tympanic bullae. They should not be used unless the animal is anaesthetised.
- **Positioning blocks and film holders** are essential for equine examinations.
- A **rope head collar** is used when imaging the equine head to prevent any metal buckles from being seen.

MARKERS AND LEGENDS

All films should have anatomical markers that indicate the limb, the recumbency or the side of the patient. Left and right markers should be placed so that they fall just inside the primary beam and will form a permanent indication of the orientation of the patient. In equine work, the lateral aspect of the distal extremities should be marked so that lesions can be orientated. The most common form of marker is a metal clip that slides over the edge of the cassette, or plastic tablets with lead letters or markers embedded in the plastic.

Where film are still being utilised they should have a permanent label incorporating the:

- Animal's and owner's names, preferable a case/client reference number
- Date of examination.

This can be achieved using lead tape or a light marker that exposes the film with the details, after exposure but before processing.

Terminology

The term used to describe the projection describes the path of the primary beam through the patient; the side struck by the X-ray beam first is first in the description and the side through which the beam exits is second. For example dorsoventral means that the beam enters through the dorsal side and leaves the body through the ventral side (Table 32.7, Fig. 32.12).

BVA/KC HIP DYSPLASIA AND ELBOW SCORING SCHEMES

For both of these schemes there are protocols available from the British Veterinary Association and the Kennel Club, which should be followed closely to produce a diagnostic image. All animals must be over 1 year of age, be either tattooed or microchipped, and should be registered with the Kennel Club; though not essential. The films should have no identification other than the Kennel Club number (for those animals not registered with the Kennel Club, either their identification number used at the practice, other registering body or breed club may be used), the date and a left and right marker and this should be put on the film prior to processing, preferably during exposure, e.g. using lead tape. When digital images have been taken the above information needs to be added to the image. The images can then be submitted as DICOM files, one dog per disc. Images

TABLE 32.7	Terminology used to describe radiographic positions	
Full description	Abbreviation	Direction of X-ray beam or description of area
Left	L	
Right	R	
Dorsal	D	Front of lower limbs below the carpus or tarsus or upper surface of main trunk
Ventral	V	Underside of animal
Cranial	Cr	Front of lower limbs above the carpus or tarsus
Caudal	Cd	Back of lower limbs below the carpus or tarsus
Rostral	R	Towards the nose
Medial	M	Towards the centre or inside of leg
Lateral	L	Outer side of body or legs
Proximal	Pr	The end of an extremity or bone that is closest to the body
Distal	Di	The end of an extremity or bone that is furthest away from the body
Palmar	Pa or P	Undersurface of the lower forelimb below the carpus – opposite to dorsal surface
Plantar	Pl	Undersurface of lower hind limb below the tarsus – opposite to dorsal surface
Oblique	O	
Lesion orientated oblique	LOO	An oblique projection to skyline a lesion

Fig. 32.12 Standard radiographic terminology

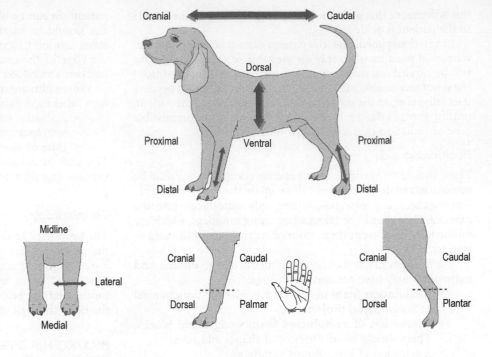

Fig. 32.13 Positioning for ventrodorsal abdomen

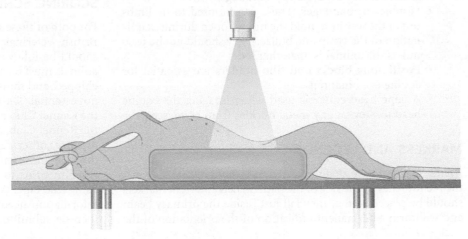

can also be printed from the original DICOM file and submitted as a dry laser image or on high quality photographic paper. When submitted as hard copies the image must include a millimetre scale at the time of radiography and have a size variation of no more than 10% from the actual size of the dog.

SMALL ANIMAL POSITIONING

Thorax

Right lateral. The patient should be placed in right lateral recumbency with the fore limbs extended and held in place by sandbags. A pad should be placed under the sternum to reduce rotation. The primary beam should be centred on the caudal border of the scapula, midway between the skin surfaces. Collimation should include, cranially the front of the shoulder (thoracic inlet), and caudally the diaphragm. Exposure should be made on full inspiration to give maximum inflation of the lungs.

Dorsoventral. The patient should be placed in sternal recumbency using a trough. Use sandbags to hold the fore limbs in

position and the head may need to be supported with a pad. The primary beam is centred on the highest point of the scapulae, on the midline. Collimation should include the front of the shoulder cranially, and the diaphragm caudally. Exposure should be made on full inspiration.

Abdomen

Right lateral recumbency. The patient should be placed in right lateral recumbency with the fore limbs extended and held in place by sandbags. A pad should be placed under the sternum to reduce rotation. Centring should be cranial to the last rib at the 11th/12th intercostal space, midway between the skin surfaces. Collimation should include, cranially the entire diaphragm and caudally the hip. Exposure should be made on full expiration to allow maximum space for the organs in the abdominal cavity.

Ventrodorsal abdomen. The patient should be placed in dorsal recumbency in a trough if needed. The fore limbs and hind limbs should be held in position by sandbags or ties and the head may need to be supported by a pad (Fig. 32.13). The primary beam is centred to the 11th/12th intercostal space, or the umbilicus, on the midline. Collimation should include, cranially the entire liver, and caudally the top of the pelvic region. Exposure should be made on full expiration.

Head and neck

Ventrodorsal skull. The patient is placed in dorsal recumbency and the neck is extended. A foam pad is placed under the neck to ensure that the hard palate is parallel to the cassette. Centre on the midline on a point halfway along the interpupillary line to include the area of interest (Fig. 32.14).

Dorsoventral intraoral view. This position is used to view the nasal chambers. The patient is supported in sternal recumbency with the neck extended. A sandbag is placed over the neck to prevent rotation. A non-screen film is placed corner first as far as possible into the mouth, above the endotracheal tube. The primary beam is centred on a line midway between the external nares and a line joining the eyes (Fig. 32.15). An anatomical marker should be included.

Nasopharynx. The patient is placed in lateral recumbency. A pad supports the skull in a true lateral position and a pad is placed under the neck. The forelegs are pulled caudally against the wall of the thorax to prevent the muscle mass of the shoulder from obscuring the image. Centre on the mid-cervical area to include the pharynx and thoracic inlet. The patient should be extubated prior to exposure.

Distal extremities

Mediolateral. The patient is placed with the side to be imaged nearest the cassette. The opposing limb is placed and supported on the flank (fore limbs pulled caudally, hind limbs pulled cranially). The limb should be parallel with the cassette; a pad may be necessary to prevent rotation (Fig. 32.16). Stifles and elbows should be flexed. Centring is at the level of the joint or mid-shaft. Collimation should include a joint above and below the long bone or a small area above and below the joint under investigation.

Dorsopalmar/plantar and caudocranial, i.e. below the level of the carpus or tarsus. The patient is placed in sternal or dorsal recumbency so that the limb under investigation is parallel with the cassette. The opposing limb may need to be lifted to rotate the limb under investigation so that it is straight (Fig. 32.17). Centring is at the level of the joint or mid-shaft.

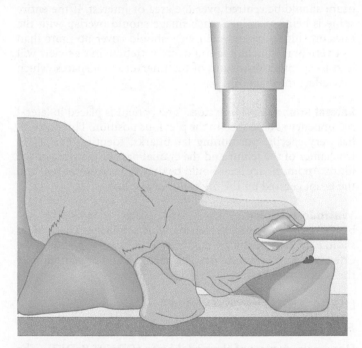

Fig. 32.14 Positioning for a ventrodorsal skull

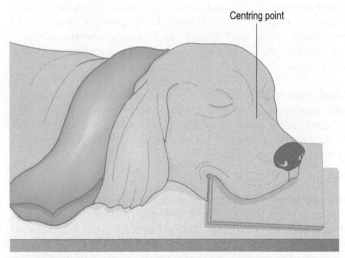

Centring point

Fig. 32.15 Positioning for a dorsoventral intraoral view

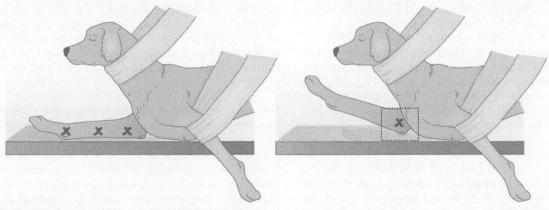

Fig. 32.16 Positioning for a mediolateral view of a distal extremity

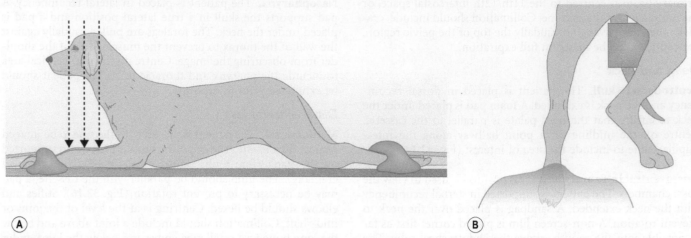

Fig. 32.17 Positioning for **(A)** craniocaudal view of the distal fore limb and **(B)** dorsoplantar view of the distal hind limb

Collimation should include the entire bone for long bones and the joint plus a small area above and below for joints.

Shoulder

Lateral. The animal is placed in lateral recumbency with the area under investigation nearest to the film. The upper limb should be extended caudally and secured in position. The limb under examination should be extended cranially and secured in place. The neck should be extended. The primary beam should be centred at the level of and caudal to the lateral tuberosity. Collimation should include the entire joint and surrounding soft tissues.

Caudocranial. The patient is placed on its back and supported with sandbags; the thorax may need to be rotated slightly. The affected limb is drawn cranially, fully extended and secured with a tie. The beam should be centred level with the acromion process of the scapula.

Pelvis

Ventrodorsal. The patient is placed in dorsal recumbency and supported in a trough. The fore limbs may need to be tied in an extended position (Fig. 32.18). The hind limbs are extended and internally rotated so that the femurs lie parallel to each other and the patellae are centred over the stifle joint. The legs should be supported and secured with sandbags or ties over the stifles and hocks as required. Centre on the midline, level with the greater trochanters. Collimation should include the upper third of the femur and the wings of the ilium.

This extended hip position is required for the KC/BVA hip dysplasia scheme and radiographs will be returned if the animal is not straight – look at the vertebral column and check that the obturator foramina are of equal size.

In patients that may have a damaged pelvis, e.g. as the result of a road traffic accident, the limbs should not be extended but should be allowed to flex into a 'frog legs' position.

Spine

Lateral. The patient should be placed in lateral recumbency. The spine should be supported with foam pads so that it is parallel with the tabletop. Pads should be placed under the sternum and between the limbs to prevent rotation. For the

cervical spine the fore limbs should be pulled caudally. The beam should be centred over the area of interest. If the entire spine is being examined, each image should overlap with the ones on either side and each view should cover no more than 3–4 vertebrae – including too many vertebrae in one view will lead to apparent distortion of the intervertebral spaces, which may affect the diagnosis.

Lateral lumbosacral junction. The patient is placed in lateral recumbency as described in the previous position. This position has very specific positioning landmarks. Identify the greater trochanter of the femur and the cranial part of the wing of the ilium. An imaginary line should be drawn between the two and the beam centred on the midpoint of the line.

Ventrodorsal spine. The patient is placed in dorsal recumbency, supported in a trough or with sandbags. The patient should be as straight as possible. The hind legs should be extended to prevent rotation. The beam should be centred over the region of interest.

LARGE ANIMAL POSITIONING

Foot

Dorsopalmar view of the pedal bone (DPr60°-PaDiO). The foot should be clean and trimmed with the shoes removed. The frog should be packed with soap or play dough or other similar material to remove gas shadows. The film is placed in a film holder and the foot placed on top of this. The primary beam is centred below the coronary band on the midline of the foot with a downward angle of 60° (see Chapter 8). Collimation should include the edges of the hoof wall and the toe and heel of the foot.

Dorsopalmar view of the navicular bone (DPr60°-PaDiO). The foot should be clean and trimmed, with the shoes removed. The frog should be packed to remove gas shadows. The film is placed in a film holder and the foot is placed on top of this. The primary beam is centred just above the coronary band on the midline of the foot, with a downward angle of 60° (Fig. 32.19A). Collimation should be large enough to include all of the navicular bone.

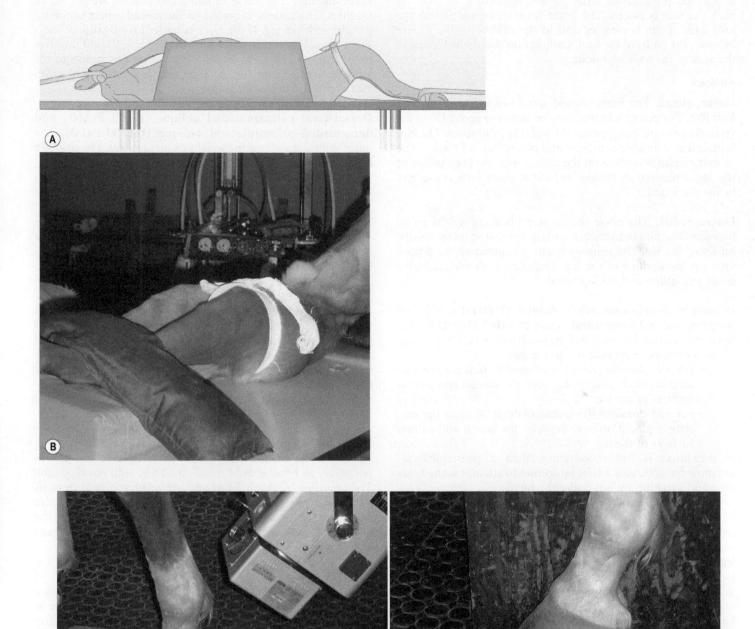

Fig. 32.19 Radiography of the equine foot. (A) Position to show the navicular bone. (B) Position for a lateral view

Lateromedial view of the pedal bone and navicular bone. The foot is prepared as for the dorsopalmar projection. The foot is placed on a block to ensure that it is high enough off the ground, and the horse should take weight on the foot (Fig. 32.19B). If laminitis is suspected, a lead strip with its top end level with the coronary band should be placed down the midline of the hoof wall. The beam is projected horizontally, parallel

with the floor and centred at the level of the coronary band to include the heel and toe. Collimation should include the weight-bearing surface of the foot.

Palmaroproximal–dorsodistal oblique of the navicular bone (Pa45°P-DDiO). The foot is cleaned dand trimmed and the frog is packed to remove any gas shadows. The foot is placed on a film-holder containing the film. The foot is placed as far back as possible without the horse taking a step forward. This removes the fetlock from the area of interest. The X-ray beam is directed proximal to distal 30–40°, depending on how far back the foot is placed. The beam is centred parallel with the long axis of the horse's leg and in the middle of the groove between the bulbs of the heel. Collimation should be limited to the area of the navicular bone.

Fetlock

Dorsopalmar. The horse should stand bearing weight on all four feet. The primary beam is angled down to about 15° to the vertical to ensure that it passes through the joint space. The film is placed in a suitable container and placed behind the leg. The primary beam is centred on the fetlock joint on the midline of the leg. Collimation should include a small area above and below the joint.

Lateromedial. The horse should stand bearing weight on all four feet. The film in a suitable container is placed on the medial aspect of the leg. The primary beam is centred on the fetlock joint on the midline of the leg. Collimation should include a small area above and below the joint.

Dorsolateral–palmaromedial oblique (D45°L-PaMO) and dorsomedial–palmarolateral oblique (D45°M-PaLO). The horse should stand bearing weight on all four feet. The primary beam is directed perpendicular to the leg:

- For the dorsolateral–palmaromedial oblique the cassette is placed midway between the medial and palmar surfaces of the leg.
- For the dorsomedial–palmarolateral oblique the cassette is placed midway between the lateral and palmar surfaces of the leg.

If the horse is not cooperating, then a palmarolateral–dorsomedial oblique is a safer projection to attempt as the X-ray tube and machine are not under the horse.

Cannon and splint bones

Dorsopalmar. The horse should stand bearing weight on all four feet. The film is placed in a film box or holder behind the leg. The beam is centred on the middle of the cannon bone along the midline of the leg. Collimation should include the joints above and below the cannon bone.

Lateromedial. The horse should stand bearing weight on all four feet. The cassette is placed on the medial aspect of the leg parallel with the leg. The X-ray beam is centred on the centre of the cannon bone, parallel with the film. Collimation should include the joints above and below the cannon bone.

Dorsolateral–palmaromedial oblique (D45°L-PaMO) and dorsomedial–palmarolateral oblique (D45°M-PaLO). The horse should stand bearing weight on all four feet. The primary beam is directed perpendicular to the leg. For the dorsolateral–palmaromedial oblique the cassette is placed midway between the medial and palmar surfaces of the leg.

Hock and carpus

Dorsopalmar. The horse should stand bearing weight on all four feet. The film is placed in a film box or holder behind the leg. The beam is centred on the middle of the joint passing along the midline of the leg. Collimation should include the joint and a small area above and below.

Lateromedial. The horse should stand bearing weight on all four feet. The cassette is placed on the medial aspect of the leg parallel with the leg. If the hock is under investigation, then a slight angulation downwards (15° to the vertical) will improve image quality. The X-ray beam is centred on the middle of the joint, parallel with the film. Collimation should include a small area above and below the joint.

Dorsolateral–palmaromedial oblique (D45°L-PaMO) and dorsomedial–palmarolateral oblique (D45°M-PaLO). The horse should stand bearing weight on all four feet. The primary beam is directed perpendicular to the leg:

- For the dorsolateral–palmaromedial oblique the cassette is placed midway between the medial and palmar surfaces of the leg.
- For the dorsomedial–palmarolateral oblique the cassette is placed midway between the lateral and palmar surfaces of the leg.

The X-ray beam is centred on the middle of the joint.

Elbow

Craniocaudal. The horse should stand bearing weight on all four feet. The limb under examination is extended forwards slightly to move it away from the chest wall. A cassette is placed behind the leg, as high as possible. A slight angulation may be needed cranially to demonstrate the entire joint. The primary beam is centred on the distal margin of the humerus. Collimation should include a small amount of the radius and the humerus.

Lateral. The film should be placed in a bag on a drip stand. The leg under examination should be as close to the film as possible. The horse should stand on all feet with equal weight. The opposing foreleg is lifted and extended and held in position. The person holding the leg should wear suitable protective clothing. The primary beam is centred on the joint on the medial aspect. Collimation should include the distal humerus and proximal radius (Fig. 32.20).

Shoulder

Lateral. The film should be placed in a bag on a drip stand, a grid should be used. The leg under examination should be as close to the film as possible. The horse should stand on all feet with equal weight. The opposing foreleg is lifted and extended and held in position. Raising the leg will place the trachea over the joint, which will improve the image quality. The person holding the leg should wear suitable protective clothing. The primary beam is centred on the joint on the medial aspect. Collimation should include the proximal humerus and the soft tissues surrounding the joint.

Stifle

Lateromedial. The horse should stand bearing weight on all four feet. The area around the stifle should be touched so that the horse is aware of contact before a cassette is inserted. A cassette is placed on the medial side of the horse's leg and rotated up as high as possible. The individual holding the cassette should wear suitable lead protection and stand as far away from the primary beam as possible. The long edge of the cassette

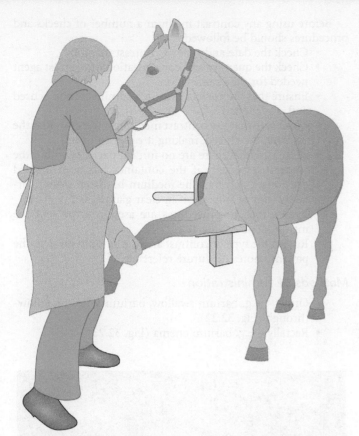

Fig. 32.20 Positioning to show a lateral view of the elbow of a horse

should be visible on the cranial edge of the leg. The primary beam should be perpendicular to the leg. The beam should be centred at the base of the patella. Collimation should include the joint and surrounding soft tissue but the caudal area does not need to be included.

Caudocranial. The horse should stand bearing weight on all four feet. The area around the stifle should be touched so that the horse is aware of contact before a cassette is inserted. A cassette is placed on the cranial aspect of the horse's leg and rotated up as high as possible. The individual holding the cassette should wear suitable lead protection and stand as far away from the primary beam as possible. The long edge of the cassette should be visible on the lateral edge of the leg. The primary beam should be angled downwards about 10° to the vertical so that it passes through the joint space. The beam should be centred at the base of the patella. Collimation should include the joint and surrounding soft tissue.

Skull

Lateromedial skull and sinuses. A film should be placed in a bag on a drip stand. The horse should have a rope head collar as the buckles on a conventional collar will show on the radiograph. The horse is walked into position so that the side under investigation is closest to the film. The head is supported with a gloved hand (the person holding the head must wear suitable lead protection). The primary beam is centred at the base of the facial crest perpendicular to the head and film. Collimation should include all of the maxilla, the frontal sinuses and the first cheek tooth.

Contrast radiography

TYPES OF CONTRAST MEDIUM

Contrast media are substances that, when administered to the body, will enhance areas where radiographic contrast is low. In areas such as the gastrointestinal tract, the urogenital system and the vascular system the difference in contrast between adjacent structures is very low, and so they will not always be distinguishable on a radiograph. The selected contrast medium has a higher atomic number than soft tissue and will therefore prevent more of the X-rays passing through the patient and ultimately reaching the film. The affected area appears white on the radiograph, highlighting it, or increasing the contrast between it and surrounding areas.

Contrast media must:
- Be easy to administer and cause minimal discomfort or distress to the patient
- Be non-toxic
- Be a stable compound that will not alter when introduced into the patient
- Allow good, clear demonstration of the area of interest
- Be eliminated from the body as completely as possible in the shortest possible time
- Not cause further damage to the patient or be carcinogenic
- Be cost-effective.

Negative contrast media

These use gas that absorbs very little of the X-ray beam, making the area of interest appear blacker on the film. Common gases used are:
- Air – e.g. double-contrast cystogram (bladder)
- Carbon dioxide (CO_2) – e.g. barium meals
- Oxygen (O_2) – e.g. arthrograms (joints).

Negative contrast may also be seen in some injuries where gas has formed or entered an area and its presence can be used to aid diagnosis, e.g. perforations or in surgical emphysema.

Positive contrast media

These have a higher atomic number than soft tissues so X-rays are absorbed and the area under investigation appears white.

Common positive contrast media include the following:

Barium sulphate suspension. Barium sulphate (e.g. Baritop) has an atomic number of 56 and is used for barium swallows and meals. It is used to demonstrate the gastrointestinal tract because it does not react with the acid in the stomach. Other substances tend to 'clump' within the stomach, giving a strange appearance that may be mistaken for pathology. Barium sulphate is also very cheap and non-toxic. It should not be given in cases where a perforation is suspected as it can cause severe adhesions within the peritoneal cavity if it escapes from the confines of the intestine.

Iodine-based solutions. Iodine-based contrast media have an atomic number of 35 and include the water-soluble organic compounds, e.g. Omnipaque and Conray, and the non-soluble organic compounds, e.g. Lipiodol. Iodine on its own is toxic but when joined to other substances can be used within the body.

The amount of iodine within a certain type of medium is expressed in milligrams per millilitre (mg/ml); for example, Omnipaque 300 contains 300 mg of iodine per millilitre. The composition of each type of contrast medium alters the way in which it reacts within the patient to produce a diagnostic image. Contrast media can be either ionic or non-ionic. Non-ionic contrast media, e.g. Omnipaque, produce fewer reactions and are more suitable for smaller or very ill patients and in the subarachnoid or spinal areas.

Reactions to iodine-based contrast media may be:

- **Allergic (anaphylactic effects)** – this type of reaction varies from mild urticaria (skin rash), to full anaphylaxis and cardiopulmonary arrest. Whenever iodine-based contrast media are injected, the patient should be anaesthetised to control the effects of a reaction.
- **Chemotoxic effects** – as the dose is increased the chances of a severe reaction will increase. The type of reaction varies from patient to patient. Very sick or very young patients will be more susceptible than the average otherwise healthy patient. Effects include cerebral oedema, red blood cell damage, convulsions and renal function impairment.
- **Osmotic effects** – pain may be experienced because of the osmolar shift of fluid within the tissues of the body during the introduction of contrast medium, especially when given intravenously.

Double contrast

This involves the use of both positive and negative contrast media, and is used to highlight the lining epithelia of hollow structures such as the bladder, stomach and rectum. The organ is emptied as much as possible and a small amount of positive contrast medium is introduced. The patient may need to be turned to coat the lining, and air is then introduced to dilate the organ (Fig. 32.21).

USE OF CONTRAST MEDIUM

All types of contrast medium are prescription only medicines (POM) and should only be used for the diagnosis or treatment of the prescribed patient, under the cascade regulations.

Before using any contrast medium a number of checks and procedures should be followed:

- Check the date and type of contrast medium.
- Check the quantity and concentration of contrast agent needed for the examination.
- Ensure that the correct route for administration is used and is prepared.
- Make sure that the contrast medium is warm so that the viscosity is reduced, making it easier to inject.
- Make sure that there are no foreign particles within the contrast, especially if the container has been opened previously, and that the medium has been stored correctly (out of sunlight if in clear glass vials).
- Ensure that all procedures are aseptic to prevent the introduction of infection.
- Record the type of contrast and the amount given in the patient's notes for future reference.

Methods of administration

- Orally – e.g. barium swallow, barium series or follow-through (Fig. 32.22)
- Rectally – e.g. barium enema (Fig. 32.23)

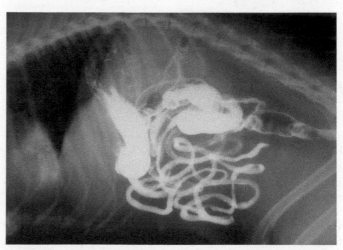

Fig. 32.22 Lateral view of the canine abdomen 2 hours after administration of a barium meal. *(Reproduced by kind permission of Richard Aspinall.)*

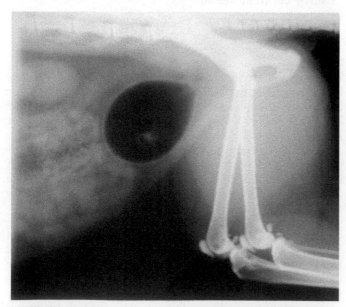

Fig. 32.21 Lateral view of the canine bladder using double-contrast technique. Note the presence of a space-filling defect in the lumen of the bladder. *(Reproduced by kind permission of Richard Aspinall.)*

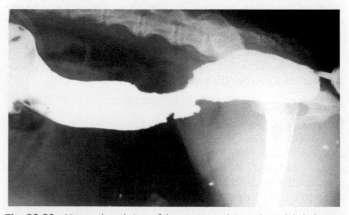

Fig. 32.23 Ventrodorsal view of the canine pelvis and caudal abdomen to demonstrate the administration of a barium enema. Note the space-occupying lesion in the descending colon. *(Reproduced by kind permission of Richard Aspinall.)*

- Intravenously – e.g. intravenous urography, mesenteric portal venography (Fig. 32.24)
- Mechanically – e.g. sinogram, cystogram, myelogram (Fig. 32.25).

Patients should be correctly prepared before administration and this may depend on the contrast medium being used:

- Starvation – may be recommended prior to a barium meal or swallow. If the patient is to be given a general anaesthetic for any other type of procedure, starvation will be necessary.
- Enema – usually recommended prior to a barium enema or prior to intravenous urography, as a full rectum may affect the position of the ureters.

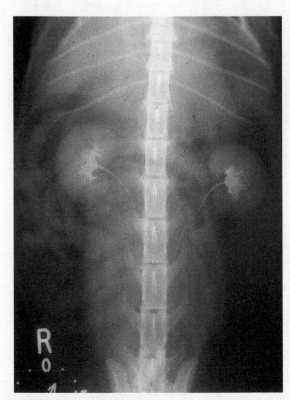

Fig. 32.24 Ventrodorsal view of the canine abdomen and pelvis to demonstrate the technique of intravenous urography. The radiograph was taken 9 minutes after administration of the contrast medium and shows the highlighted kidneys, ureters and bladder. *(Reproduced by kind permission of Richard Aspinall.)*

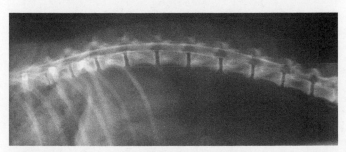

Fig. 32.25 Lateral view of the canine thoracic and lumbar spine to demonstrate the administration of contrast medium to perform a myelogram. Note the contrast medium running along the subarachnoid space of the spine. *(Reproduced by kind permission of Richard Aspinall.)*

- General anaesthesia – for ease of administration and positioning, anaesthesia is essential for most procedures, apart from barium studies of the gastrointestinal tract.
- Plain radiographs – patients should always have preliminary radiographs taken before contrast is introduced to identify any pathology that may prevent the examination from being effective. They are also useful for comparison with the contrast radiographs.

Contrast techniques

These are listed in Table 32.8.

Alternative imaging techniques

ULTRASOUND

Diagnostic ultrasound uses sound waves to provide a diagnostic image of the internal organs of a patient. The sound waves have a frequency, which is measured in hertz (Hz). The sound waves used in ultrasound are above the range of our hearing as they are supersonic and are usually between 1 and 10 megahertz (MHz)

A number of terms are used in ultrasonography:

- **Acoustic window** – the area through which the ultrasound waves will be applied. It should be as close as possible to the area under investigation
- **Acoustic impedance** – the degree of resistance to the passage of ultrasound waves
- **Acoustic interface** – the junction between two tissues of different acoustic impedance
- **Echoes** – the returning ultrasound waves picked up by the transducer and converted into the image on the screen: the brightness of the echo is determined by the acoustic impedance of the acoustic interface
- **Hyperechoic or echogenic** – bright white echoes between highly reflective interfaces, e.g. bone, gas and collagen
- **Hypoechoic or echo-poor** – sparse echoes appearing grey representing intermediate reflection or transmission of the ultrasound waves, e.g. soft tissue
- **Anechoic or echolucent** – absence of echoes so appears black, e.g. fluid.

Ultrasound interactions

The ultrasound image is formed by the reflection of the ultrasound waves within the body. As the wave travels through the patient and tissues it becomes **attenuated**, and the intensity of the wave is reduced. The most common form of attenuation is absorption. The friction caused by the vibration of the molecules within the tissues of the body will cause this absorption to occur. Other causes of attenuation are scattering, reflection, refraction, diffraction, interference and divergence.

The transducer

The ultrasound transducer is the hand held probe used during examinations and it is able to convert electrical energy to mechanical energy from the ultrasound beam and vice-versa (Fig. 32.26). The active part of the transducer is the piezoelectric crystal, which is usually made of lead zirconate titanate. It has a specific thickness for the best resolution possible, which varies depending on the wavelength produced by the crystal.

TABLE 32.8   Indications for and methods of using contrast media

Examination type	Indications	Area demonstrated	Contrast medium used	Quantity	Method of administration	Preliminary radiographs	Projections and time after administration
Barium swallow	Regurgitation, retching, dysphagia, suspected foreign body	Oesophagus	Barium sulphate	Dogs 5–10 ml Cats up to 5 ml	Oral	Lateral thorax	Lateral thorax immediately after administration
Barium meal and follow-through	Vomiting	Stomach and small intestine	Barium sulphate	Dogs 1–3 ml/kg Cats 2–5 ml/kg	Oral. May need stomach tube	Lateral and ventrodorsal abdomen	Immediate. Four views of the abdomen then ventrodorsal and right lateral abdomen every 30 min until stomach is empty
Barium enema	Melaena, chronic diarrhoea, tenesmus	Large bowel	Barium sulphate, plus air if double-contrast examination required	10 ml/kg mixed with water 50:50	Foley catheter inserted into rectum – allow contrast to enter using the effects of gravity	Ventrodorsal and right lateral abdomen	Right and left lateral abdominal radiographs plus ventrodorsal abdomen
Intravenous urography	Incontinence, persistent haematuria, pyelonephritis, trauma	Kidneys and ureters	Ionic contrast medium (Conray 420)	1 ml/kg	Intravenously as a bolus	Right lateral and ventrodorsal abdomen	Immediate. Follow up with 5 min – ventrodorsal abdomen; 10 min – lateral abdomen; 15 min – caudal abdomen. May be followed by a vaginourethrogram
Male urethrogram	Incontinence, dysuria, persistent haematuria, trauma, bladder position	Bladder, urethra and prostate	Ionic contrast medium (Urografin 150)	2 ml/kg	Foley catheter inserted into penile urethra	Right lateral caudal abdomen to include urethra	Same position as preliminary film radiograph taken as contrast is injected
Female urethrogram	Incontinence, dysuria, persistent haematuria, trauma, position of bladder	Bladder, urethra and vagina	Ionic contrast medium (Urografin 150)	1 ml/kg to fill urethra and vagina	Foley catheter inserted into vestibule of vagina and secured to prevent leakage using Allis tissue forceps	Right lateral caudal abdomen to include urethra	Same position as preliminary film, radiograph taken as contrast is injected
Cystogram	Dysuria, persistent haematuria, trauma, position of bladder	Bladder	Ionic contrast medium (Urografin 150) Air	10 ml/kg for cystogram, then fill with air until bladder feels distended for a pneumocystogram	Bladder catheterised and urine removed; contrast and/or air introduced until resistance is felt	Right lateral caudal abdomen to include urethra	Same position as preliminary film Radiograph taken immediately after contrast and/or air is introduced
Myelogram	Spinal pain, paraplegia, quadriplegia, ataxia, trauma	Spinal column	Non-ionic contrast medium (Omnipaque 300)	0.3 ml/kg as a slow bolus	Cisternal puncture or lumbar puncture	Lateral and ventrodorsal of area of interest	Lateral radiographs of entire spine Ventrodorsal of areas of interest
Arthrography	Joint pain degeneration of articular surfaces	Joints, mainly the shoulder	Non-ionic contrast medium (Omnipaque 300)	1–1.5 ml	Injected directly into the joint space	Two projections of joint	Two projections of joint
Sinography	Demonstrate sinus tract path	Sinus tract or fistula	Ionic contrast medium (Urografin 150)	Until backflow or resistance is felt	Foley catheter inserted into opening of sinus or fistula and secured in place using Allis tissue forceps	Two projections of area of interest	Two projections of area of interest

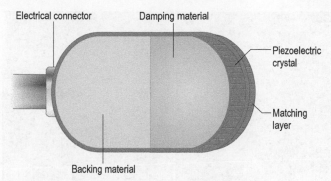

Fig. 32.26 Cross-section through a transducer

The crystal will expand and contract along its shortest side as the electrical signal applied across it alternates. This electrical signal is converted into an ultrasound beam. The beam passes into the patient and is reflected back from the tissues to the transducer. The reflected echoes are detected by the transducer and converted back into an electrical signal to allow the formation of an image on a monitor. Behind the crystal is a damping material, which improves resolution. This is supported on a backing material.

Operational display modes

The ultrasound image may be displayed on the screen in one of the following ways:

1. **A mode – amplitude mode:**
   - Echoes appear on the monitor as a series of blips
   - Used to demonstrate the depth of differences in tissues (interfaces) and their separation
   - Equipment is cheaper.
2. **B mode – brightness mode**
   This is the most common type:
   - Shown in real time; the operator moves the transducer around and shows an image on the monitor as it happens
   - The intensity of the echo is demonstrated as a bright dot on the monitor
   - A composite image will be shown either in a rectangular format or sector view depending on the transducer type.
3. **M-mode – moving mode:**
   - Used mainly for cardiac examinations
   - Produces an image similar to that of an A-mode examination but adds in a time element
   - Being replaced by Doppler imaging and dedicated echocardiography units.

Patient preparation

Careful patient preparation is essential to produce diagnostic images. The area under examination is clipped to remove any hair, and spirit is used to remove any excess oil or debris on the skin surface. A coupling gel is placed between the skin surface and the transducer to ensure good contact between the tissues and the transducer. Ultrasound waves do not travel well through air so the gel is used to ensure that the transducer is always in complete contact with the skin surface. The patient may need to be restrained and in some cases sedation may be needed; however, ultrasound is a completely painless and non-invasive technique.

Ultrasound has a number of advantages:
- Does not use radiation
- Produces real-time images
- Can be used without sedation
- Minimal patient preparation needed
- Non-invasive procedure that gives good visualisation of the abdominal organs.

However, there are a number of disadvantages:
- Cannot be used in areas containing large amounts of air, as ultrasound does not travel well through air.
- Accurate reporting of images is only possible by the operator, though a detailed report can be made by the operator and images recorded, transferred to a digital format or printed.
- Accuracy is dependent on operator experience.

Areas suitable for examination

Ultrasound is ideal for:
- Abdominal organs
- Heart
- Thyroid
- Larynx
- Tendons
- Ligaments
- Soft-tissue masses.

NUCLEAR MEDICINE

This technique is sometimes known as **nuclear scintigraphy**, and is used mainly in the equine field for examination of the bones and in cats for the examination of possible thyroid problems. Other areas of examination are possible and are used in specific cases.

Nuclear medicine will demonstrate the function of a tissue or organ and will show where a problem is but will not provide a specific diagnosis. It involves the use of radioactively labelled drugs or radiopharmaceuticals, which are given intravenously and are taken up by specific tissues depending on their chemical nature.

A number of terms are used in nuclear medicine:
- **Radionuclide** – an atom that disintegrates emitting gamma radiation
- **Radiopharmaceutical** – a medicinal product that is used in the examination technique
- **Half-life** – the time taken for the radioactivity to decay to half its original value. It should be long enough to allow examination but not remain unnecessarily after the examination.

Care should be taken whenever radioisotopes are used, and it should be understood that all substances produced by the patient may be radioactive. Shoes should be changed before examination in case of patient urination, and all urine should be collected and prevented from entering the drainage system. The patient should be isolated for at least 24 hours after examination to ensure that radiation levels are within safe limits. Contact with patients should be minimal within 24 hours of the examination.

Administration of the radioisotope

A radioisotope is attached to the radiopharmaceutical, whose type is determined by the body system under examination. If bone is to be examined then the radiopharmaceutical is

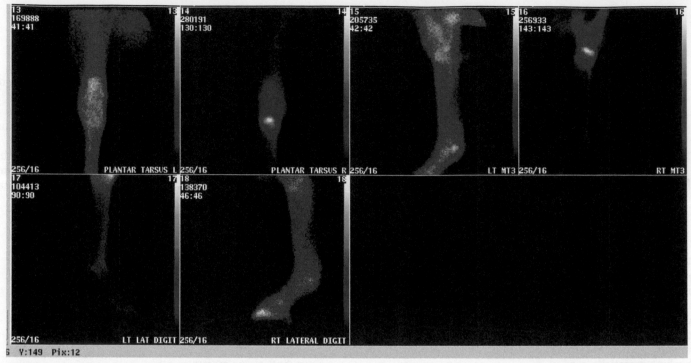

Fig. 32.27   This horse was presented with a persistent lameness that was only resolved by high leg nerve blocks. Radiography failed to identify any obvious pathology, but the gamma scan (shown here) confirmed that the problem was in the region of the third tarsal bone. Subsequent radiology and surgical arthroscopic investigation confirmed a fracture of this bone. *(Reproduced by kind permission of Derek Knottenbelt.)*

methylene diphosphonate and this is attached to technetium-99m (^{99m}TcMDP). Iodine is used for thyroid imaging. The radiopharmaceutical is given intravenously and will be carried to the region under examination and then emit radiation. This is detected using a **gamma camera** or **scintillation detector** placed outside the patient in the region of interest.

Data collection

The patient is placed in front of the gamma camera, which detects any gamma radiation emitted. In a normal patient the gamma radiation emitted will demonstrate a normal distribution and will be symmetrical. Any areas that are not symmetrical or evenly distributed with the isotope are interpreted as being abnormal.

The gamma camera sends signals via a crystal that emits light, and a photomultiplier tube to a computer system where acquisition, processing and storage of the data will take place. All images (Fig. 32.27) will be displayed on a TV monitor and can be manipulated and analysed. Printing can be performed on a conventional printer.

COMPUTED TOMOGRAPHY

This is also called CT or CAT (computer-aided tomography) scanning, and uses an X-ray tube mounted opposite a detector. The tube emits X-rays in a fan shape that passes through the patient to reach the detector (Fig. 32.28). The X-ray tube and the detector move around the patient throughout the examination. In modern machines this is in a spiral movement. The detector then converts the X-rays into a signal that can be used by the computer system to form an image.

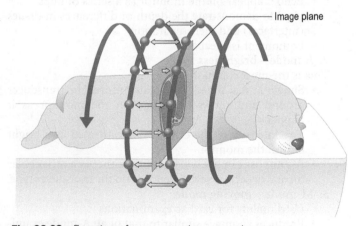

Fig. 32.28   Function of a computed tomography scanner

CT is ideal for demonstration of all organs within the body, especially the skeletal and central nervous systems, and for the demonstration of tumours. It can be used in any area to supplement the findings of a normal radiological examination.

Patient preparation and safety

As this examination takes time, the patient must be anaesthetised. A scout will be performed to provide a scan for planning and positioning. This is the most time-consuming part of the examination. Any individual remaining in the room during the scan must wear a lead apron and adhere to normal radiation safety procedures and, if possible, the patient should be on its own in the room for the very short time it takes to perform the

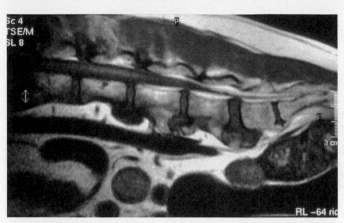

Fig. 32.29 Magnetic resonance imaging scan of the spinal cord

scan. Monitoring can be performed throughout the examination so that the patient is not left unattended.

MAGNETIC RESONANCE IMAGING

Magnetic resonance imaging or MRI is the most modern method of diagnostic imaging and does not use ionising radiation. It was originally invented to unravel the atomic structure of chemical compounds, but is now used to produce an image by mapping the location of the protons of the body tissues. This technique is ideal for demonstrating the central nervous system (Fig. 32.29) and the spinal column and for soft tissues within joints; however, it is less sensitive to calcified areas than CT scans.

Patient preparation

During an MRI scan the patient is exposed to a large magnetic field and for this reason all collars, leads and other metallic objects should be removed. An alternative method of diagnostic imaging should be used for any patients with implants or pacemakers. The scan is very noisy and takes time, so patients should be anaesthetised to reduce the distress caused by noise and having to keep still for the entire scan. Specialised equipment is required and no metallic objects should be taken into the scanner room.

An MRI scan takes place as follows:

1. The anaesthetised patient is placed on the table.
2. A scout image is produced to plan the scan.
3. The patient is then placed within the magnet, which has strength of between 0.2 and 2 tesla (T). The earth's magnetic field is 0.000 06 T.
4. The hydrogen protons of the body align with the magnet as the patient enters the scanner. A radio frequency pulse is applied to the patient, which makes the protons 'flip' as they absorb the energy.

5. After the radio pulse is turned off the protons return to their original positions and emit any excess energy.
6. This energy is received by the scanner and is used to reconstruct an image, which appears on a screen in a similar format to that of a CT scan.

The magnet and detector surround a long tunnel, through which the anaesthetised patient moves very slowly. Scanning times are longer than those for CT scans.

ENDOSCOPY

An endoscope consists of:

* A rigid or flexible tube.
* A light delivery system to illuminate the organ or object under inspection. The light source is normally outside the body and the light is typically directed via an optical fibre system.
* A lens system transmitting the image from the objective lens to the viewer, typically a relay lens system in the case of rigid endoscopes or a bundle of fiberoptics in the case of a fiberscope.
* An eyepiece. Modern instruments may be videoscopes, with no eyepiece – a camera transmits the image to a screen for image capture.
* An additional channel to allow entry of medical instruments or manipulators.

Endoscopy can be split into different areas of study dependent on what area is being imaged.

* The gastrointestinal tract (GI tract):
  * Oesophagus, stomach and duodenum (esophagogastroduodenoscopy)
  * Small intestine (enteroscopy)
  * Large intestine/colon (colonoscopy, sigmoidoscopy)
  * Magnification endoscopy
  * Rectum (rectoscopy) and anus (anoscopy), both also referred to as proctoscopy.
* The respiratory tract
  * The nose (rhinoscopy)
  * The lower respiratory tract (bronchoscopy).
* The ear (otoscope)
* The urinary tract (cystoscopy)
* Normally closed body cavities (through a small incision):
  * The abdominal or pelvic cavity (laparoscopy)
  * The interior of a joint (arthroscopy)
  * Organs of the chest (thoracoscopy and mediastinoscopy).

Cleaning and disinfection of the endoscope after use is essential; in human medicine there are stringent guidelines regarding the decontamination and disinfection of endoscopes. Practices should have protocols in place to ensure competent decontamination and disinfection after each use.

BIBLIOGRAPHY

Ball, J., Price, T., 1995. Chesney's Radiographic Imaging, sixth ed. Blackwell Scientific, Oxford.

Barr, F., Kirberger, R. (Eds.), 2006. BSAVA Manual of Canine and Feline Musculoskeletal Imaging. BSAVA Publications, Gloucester.

Bushberg, J., Seibert, J., Leidholdt, E., et al., 1994. The Essential Physics of Medical Imaging. Lippincott Williams & Wilkins, Philadelphia, PA.

Bushong, S., 1997. Radiological Science for Technologists, sixth ed. Mosby, St Louis, MO.

Easton, S., 2002. Practical Radiography for Veterinary Nurses. Butterworth-Heinemann, Oxford.

Fauber, T., 2000. Radiographic Imaging and Exposure. Mosby, St Louis, MO.

Holloway, A., McConnell, F., 2013. BSAVA Manual of Canine and Feline Radiography and Radiology:

A Foundation Manual. BSAVA Publications, Gloucester.

Mendenhall, A., Cantwell, H., 1988. Equine Radiographic Procedures. Lee & Febiger, Philadelphia, PA.

O'Brein, R., Barr, F. (Eds.), 2009. BSAVA Manual of Abdominal Imaging. BSAVA Publications, Gloucester.

O'Meara, B., O'Neill, H., Fraser, B., 2010. Applications of nuclear scintigraphy in the investigation of equine lameness: Part 2. Thoroughbred Racehorse Companion Anim. 15 (1), 1–4.

RECOMMENDED READING

Bushong, S., 2012. Radiological Science for Technologists, tenth ed. Mosby, St Louis, MO.

This book is everything you need to know about radiographic physics. It covers all topics with clear and self-explanatory diagrams, broken down into small topic areas for easy reading.

Easton, S., 2014. Diagnostic imaging. In: Aspinall, V. (Ed.), Clinical Procedures in Veterinary Nursing. Butterworth-Heinemann, Oxford, pp. 201–228.

This text provides a step-by-step guide to radiographic procedures. Each radiographic procedure is described in stages with the theory behind the procedure provided.

Fauber, T., 2013. Radiographic Imaging and Exposure, fourth ed. Mosby, St Louis, MO.

Explains in detail exactly what happens when you alter exposure factors and processing conditions. There are lots of very clear diagrams and radiographs showing how exposure manipulation and equipment care and use can alter the image.

Lee, R. (Ed.), 1995. Manual of Small Animal Diagnostic Imaging. British Small Animal Veterinary Association, Gloucester.

Although this book is aimed at radiology and diagnosis it provides very clear diagrams and explanations on how positioning should be carried out. It looks at each radiographic projection in detail, with positioning and then detailed discussion on what can be seen on the resultant radiograph.

Management and Care of Exotic Species

BEVERLY SHINGLETON | SARAH COTTINGHAM

KEY POINTS

- More and more people are keeping various species of exotic pets, which have very different husbandry requirements from each other and from the more usual pets such as cats and dogs.

- The order of small mammals include Rodentia, Lagomorpha and Carnivora, which are omnivorous, herbivorous and carnivorous and are commonly kept in groups in cages, either indoors or outdoors.

- Reptiles include snakes, lizards and chelonians, i.e. tortoises and terrapins. They are all cold-blooded and as such are totally dependent on their environment for their health and welfare. It is vital that the owner fully understands their husbandry requirements if they are not to suffer and die.

- Many species of bird are kept, in cages or in aviaries. They encompass several different classes of bird, each of which has differing needs in terms of diet and enclosure.

- It is essential that both the pet keeper and the veterinary nurse understand the husbandry requirements of these animals so that they can live a long, healthy life and experience high levels of welfare. If they should be admitted to the veterinary surgery they can be housed and managed appropriately for their species requirements.

Introduction

As more and more people elect to keep exotic species as 'pets', the veterinary nurse must be aware of the animal's specific needs in relation to their biology, husbandry, general and veterinary care. Nurses need to be able to rise to the challenges these animals bring, and it must be highlighted that the principles applied to nursing a sick or injured dog and cat are not necessarily transferable to a small mammal, rodent, reptile or bird.

This chapter aims to provide sound practical details on how to care effectively for those usual and sometimes unusual pets that are presented for treatment in veterinary practice.

The range of animals covered includes:

- Small mammals – guinea pigs, rabbits, gerbils, mice, rats, hamsters and ferrets
- Reptiles – snakes, lizards, chelonians (shelled reptiles)
- Birds – budgies, canaries, finches, parrots, quail, etc.

Keeping exotic small mammals as pets can be just as rewarding as keeping dogs and cats and they can provide companionship and company in a similar way. When choosing any species of exotic animal as a pet there are advantages and disadvantages that need to be considered before purchasing the animal:

- How much time will their daily routine take?
- Will the animal need specialist veterinary care?
- Will the owner need specialist knowledge to care for the animal correctly?
- Is the animal suitable for children, adults and as a family pet?
- What level of interaction does the owner require from the pet?
- How much is it going to cost to look after the animal?

The veterinary nurse is frequently asked to give advice on pet selection. The advantages and disadvantages of exotic pet ownership are shown in Table 33.1.

Animal husbandry

SMALL MAMMALS

Housing

Housing is obviously one of the most important factors in correct management. Housing requirements are species specific and the ethology and behaviour of the species should be understood and reflected in the choice of housing and management style. When considering owning any small animal, the following factors should be taken into account when selecting the most appropriate environment to meet all of the animal's requirements:

- Correct levels of light/hours of daylight
- Correct temperature/humidity/ventilation
- Space to exercise and express normal behaviour
- Companionship – consider the ratio of male to females, group living requirements and solitary species requirements
- Enclosure substrate/bedding material
- Sleeping area/core territory
- Enclosure style suitable for the individual species' behaviour and physiology
- Safety/security requirements of enclosure
- Adequate and appropriate environmental and behavioural stimulation
- Siting/position of enclosure.

Each species has a different behaviour pattern and therefore has different housing requirements, and these should be reflected in the husbandry and environment (Tables 33.2 and 33.3). These will be discussed in more detail in the following sections.

TABLE 33.1	The advantages and disadvantages of keeping exotic pets	
Pet	Advantages	Disadvantages
Small mammals	Relatively cheap to buy animal Initial set-up is also relatively cheap Daily management costs are low Animals require less time for daily management, e.g. hamsters, gerbils and rats do not need walking; smaller short-haired mammals do not need grooming Small mammals are good for children to learn animal management and responsible pet ownership Parent and child are able to learn to handle pet together Children should always be supervised with animals and taught correct care and consideration As most small, exotic mammals are relatively short-lived, the child has the chance to learn about grief process when the pet dies	Animal is often medically neglected due to misunderstanding/ignorance of illnesses by owners. Many owners resent veterinary costs as the animal was cheap to purchase initially Animals often left in cage/enclosure without adequate husbandry As animal is in enclosure and often away from main household activity, pets often not checked, or cared for, for long periods of time Children's small hands are often unable to hold animal correctly, leading to animal being dropped and injured. Scared pets then tend to bite and scratch in anticipation of being handled Situation spirals, children become nervous of handling the pet, and the pet becomes more aggressive, culminating in the animal not being handled and then becoming neglected Often difficult to find veterinary surgeon that treats exotic animals. Many veterinary surgeons still view small mammals as non-treatable or 'specialist' Natural behaviour (many exotic mammals are prey species) and husbandry needs often neglected through incorrect advice and lack of knowledge of species requirements Pets often inappropriately chosen for children, e.g. many rodents are nocturnal and will be active and noisy at night, and not appreciate being handled during daytime sleeping periods
Reptiles	Keeping reptiles provides an unusual and stimulating challenge. Wide variety available	Specialist knowledge of reptiles and chelonians is needed Ignorance leads to poor husbandry and inadequate housing, which results in disease and death Some species of lizard and snake grow very large and have a poor temperament, which makes them unmanageable, leading to abandonment or euthanasia Hidden costs are heating, specialist feeding and lighting requirements Some people do not understand the need to feed dead rodents or have live invertebrates as food in the house As many reptiles carry zoonotic diseases, hygiene is very important Many small reptile species purchased for young children can live in excess of 15 years – by then the novelty may have worn off!
Birds	Many species have been kept in captivity for hundreds of years and are well established as companions. Interesting, can be exhibited and readily breed in captivity Housing requirements are well documented and a range of housing is available	Some psittacines, especially the parrot family, can be challenging and suffer behavioural problems if they lack sufficient company and stimulus Many of the larger bird species are a huge monetary investment and security must be considered, as valuable birds are often stolen from aviaries Some of the housing on the market is too small and provides inadequate space for flying Aviaries can be expensive and need correct positioning and adequate space

Environmental and behavioural enrichment. All caged animals should be kept in enclosures that allow them to interact with their environment and to display as many natural behaviour patterns as they would do if they were living unconfined in the wild. Environmental enrichment is not necessarily about providing a replica of the natural environment but about providing the animal with a variety of activities which allow natural behaviour to be expressed, e.g. foraging for hidden food rather than being given food in a bowl. Enrichment also allows the animal to 'do something' rather than have large amounts of time with nothing to do, which the animal may then fill with abnormal boredom-induced behaviours that are often repetitive and stereotypical. Figures 33.1–33.9 provide photographic examples related to a number of commonly kept small exotic species. Environmental enrichment does not need to be expensive – boxes, cardboard rolls and chewable containers all provide small mammals with variety and stimulation. Some of the material may just be used for gnawing and chewing, so ensuring that it is not toxic is important.

Suggestions for environmental and behavioural enrichment include:

- Changing the feeding methods and routine – keeps the animal busy and rewards it for its efforts

- Provision of appropriate toys, which can be given for short periods and rotated so that they retain some novelty factor
- Provision of a variety and style of hiding places
- For species that climb, hanging toys are well received
- Species such as ferrets and rabbits can be walked on harnesses, ensuring that the surroundings are safe and predator free
- Provision of communal and individual sleeping areas where social species are housed together will allow choice
- Changing the layout of a cage or enclosure increases exploratory behaviour for inquisitive species
- Ensuring company is available – make sure that if the species is sociable or group living, that there is company and there is an appropriate balance between the sexes if territorial issues are likely to occur
- Providing an indoor and outdoor area so that the animal can choose and control where in the environment it chooses to be
- Providing the animal with choice and therefore a degree of control over its environment, which will reduce stress

Text continued on p. 700

TABLE 33.2 Housing materials that can be used for cages/enclosures for small exotic animals

	Rats	Ferrets	Guinea pigs	Hamsters	Gerbils	Mice	Rabbits
Material suitable for construction of enclosure	Wire mesh and wood/metal-framed cage (see Figs. 33.5, 33.6)	Wire mesh and wood-frame cage and wooden/plastic sleeping enclosure	Plastic and wire-topped cage	Glass aquarium with multi-levels. Metal mesh lid. Plastic-based cage with metal	Glass aquarium with multi-levels. Metal mesh lid	Glass aquarium with multi-levels. Metal mesh lid. Plastic-based cage with metal	Wooden hutch including wooden frame and wire mesh; must ensure wood is hard to resist chewing. New type of enclosure designed by 'Omlet' is made from smooth plastic material and therefore the surfaces do not absorb moisture, unlike traditional wooden hutches that are often porous to liquid, making then hard to clean and disinfect
Construction requirements for indoor/outdoor enclosure	Not necessary	Wooden/metal frame with wire mesh sides. Chew- and escape-proof. Rest area must be waterproof and draught proof. Access to sleeping zone via a 'peep hole'. Concrete base for outdoor run – easily cleaned and known escapable	Wooden frame and wire mesh, with two wooden sides and hiding area. Include a solid roof for predator protection. Movable outside enclosure for continued grazing. Rest area must be waterproof and draught-proof. (Rabbit hutch style is suitable or new Eglu™-style enclosure.) Access to sleeping zone via a 'peep hole'	Not necessary	Not necessary	Not necessary	The rest area must be waterproof and draught-proof. The Eglu™ design has a special, twin-wall construction which insulates it against the outside temperature, so in the summer it is cool inside and in the winter the environment stays warm. Access to sleeping zone via 'pop hole'. Often traditionally wooden frame and wire mesh, with two wooden sides and hiding area. Include a solid roof for predator protection. The wire base should be dug into the ground to prevent tunnelling and escaping; alternatively, the Eglu™ run is made from steel weld mesh and features Omlet's unique anti-tunnel skirt to prevent predators digging in (see Fig. 33.8). If an outdoor enclosure does have a mesh base, it also means that the rabbit cannot have tunnels built into the ground for added enrichment

Continued

TABLE 33.2	Housing materials that can be used for cages/enclosures for small exotic animals—cont'd						
	Rats	Ferrets	Guinea pigs	Hamsters	Gerbils	Mice	Rabbits
Suitable environment substrate	Wood shavings not generally recommended as can be rough on feet and the dust can cause problems to the respiratory system. Newspaper lining with paper-based products covering the surface. Not digging or tunnelling animals, therefore do not require depth of substrate	Newspaper flooring, wood chip flooring for outside pen, paper-based products can be used for indoor pen floor covering	Wood shavings	Wood shavings not generally recommended as can be rough on feet and the dust can cause problems to the respiratory system. Paper-based product are safest/ shredded paper. Non-irritating to the feet and nose and they are designed to break down if ingested without causing impactions	Wood shavings not generally recommended as can be rough on feet and the dust can cause problems to the respiratory system. Paper-based product or dry peat (5–10 cm depth for burrowing). Provision of a sand bath	Wood shavings not generally recommended as can be rough on feet and the dust can cause problems to the respiratory system. Paper-based product and dry peat. Allow depth suitable for tunnelling and digging	Newspaper lining for insulation and absorption of urine, wood shavings, straw or hay for substrate. 'Built-in' 'removable' bedding trays allow easy cleaning and removal of substrate. Peat box for digging
Rest area/ bedding material	Plastic or wooden boxes or tubes lined with shredded paper or shredded tissue	Wooden boxes, non-chewable plastic beds lined with towels or material for bedding. Can also use hay	Separate rest area if housed in a hutch. If housed in pen, cardboard or wooden boxes lined with paper-based product and hay	Shredded paper, hay or specialist hamster bedding	Shredded paper, hay or tissue	Shredded paper, hay or tissue	Hay for deep bedding providing warmth and draught reduction, shredded paper for long-haired rabbits, e.g. Angora rabbits
Provision of latrine	Not necessary	Provide litter trays, several for multi-housed animals. Wooden pellets can be used as litter material	Not necessary	Not necessary	Not necessary	Not necessary	Provide litter tray if training a house rabbit

TABLE 33.3 Suitable environmental enrichment and feeding facilities for small exotic animals

	Rats	Ferrets	Guinea pigs	Hamsters	Gerbils	Mice	Rabbits
Suitable environmental enrichment	Ropes for rats to climb, plastic tubing, material hammocks for playing and sleeping in. Plastic tubes to climb through, boxes to chew and hide in (see Figs. 33.5, 33.6)	Plastic drainage pipes, tunnels, wooden stumps, non-chewable toys. Material hammocks for laying and sleeping in (see Fig. 33.7)	Scatter feeding hard food, fruit-tree wood for chewing and playing, large flower pots and drain pipes for hiding in (see Fig. 33.12). Various grass, herbs and weeds for grazing; mental stimulation and exercise. Hay balls	Fruit-tree wood and cardboard boxes to chew, toilet role inners for tunnels, wheel for choice of exercise. Scatter feeding or hiding food for enrichment	Fruit-tree wood and cardboard boxes to chew, toilet role inners for tunnels, wheel for choice of exercise. Multi layered cage for interest and to add space. Scatter feeding or hiding food for enrichment. Sand bath for personal grooming	Fruit-tree wood and cardboard boxes to chew, toilet role inners for tunnels, wheel for choice of exercise. Multi layered cage for interest and to add space. Small ropes for climbing, millet spays hanging for enrichment. Scatter feeding or hiding food for enrichment	Large plastic tunnels dug into the ground to simulate shallow warren (see Fig. 33.3) tunnels and provide protection, mounds of soil for viewpoints, large boxes to hide in and chew. Boxes filled with meadow hay and herbs to chew and eat. Indoor and outdoor rabbits should also have a peat box provided if they do not have access to digging facilities (see Fig. 33.8)
Feeding facilities and enrichment	Scatter feeding or food in a bowl, can also hide food in tunnels to increase activity and exploration behaviour. Water can be placed in a bottle, multiple sites if communal living	If housed communally, more than one feeding and drinking station should be provided. Water bottles rather than bowls. Hide dry food in tunnels to allow natural exploration behaviour	Plastic water bottle, change water daily as added vitamin C degrades when in contact with metal dripper. Ceramic feed bowls for hard food, but scatter feed is better for mental stimulation. Also use hay balls for enrichment	Water bottle and feeding bowls, or scatter feeding for environmental stimulation	Water bottle or bowls, feeding bowls, or scatter feeding for environmental stimulation	Water bottle or bowls, feeding bowls, or scatter feeding for environmental stimulation	Water bottle or bowls, feeding bowls, or scatter feeding for environmental stimulation. Also use hay balls for enrichment (see Fig. 33.9). Placing fresh herbs and vegetables mixed in hay inside closed boxes allows rabbits to chew and rip while gaining a food source

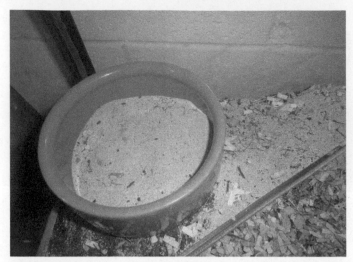

Fig. 33.1   Sand bath for small rodents (*Photo courtesy of Plumpton College Sussex.*)

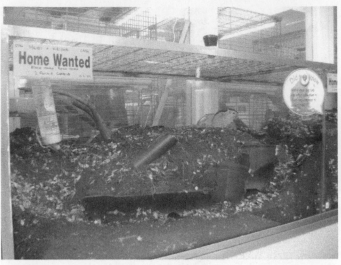

Fig. 33.2   Gerbil enclosure allowing expression of natural tunnelling behaviour (*Photo courtesy of Raystede Centre for Animal Welfare.*)

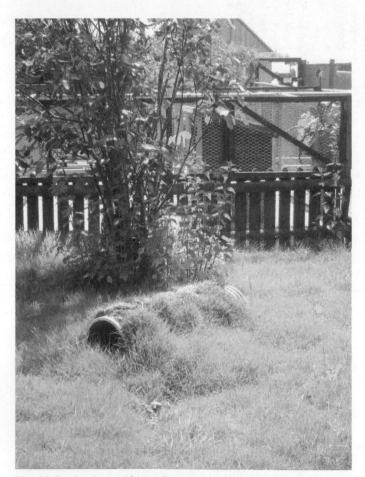

Fig. 33.3   Outdoor rabbit enclosure with built-in tunnels for hiding in (*Photo courtesy of Raystede Centre for Animal Welfare.*)

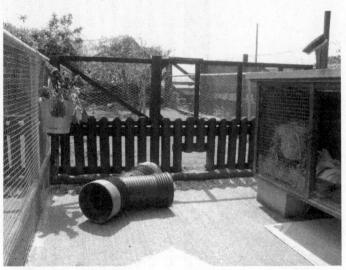

Fig. 33.4   Outdoor rabbit enclosure with traditional wooden hutch and 'pop-hole' into penned area with built-in tunnels (*Photo courtesy of Raystede Centre for Animal Welfare.*)

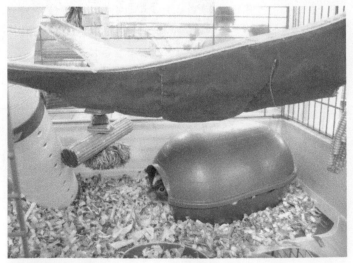

Fig. 33.5   Rat enclosure with various toys and shredded paper substrate (*Photo courtesy of Raystede Centre for Animal Welfare.*)

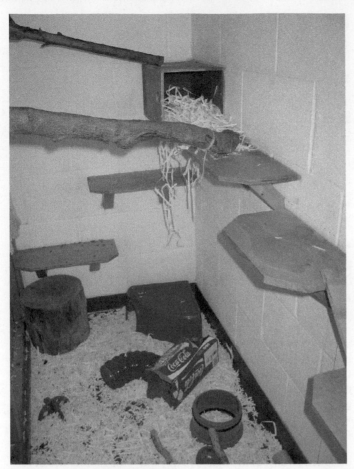

Fig. 33.6 Rat enclosure with arboreal steps allowing for 3D movement *(Photo courtesy of Plumpton College, Sussex.)*

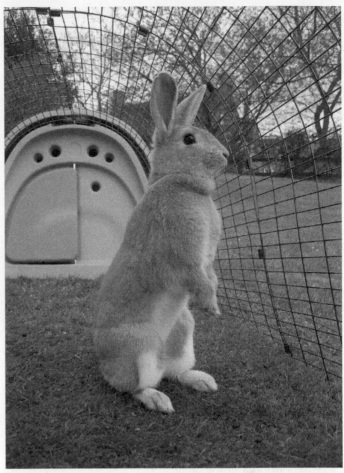

Fig. 33.8 Rabbit showing the natural tendency to stand upright, demonstrating the importance of providing sufficient height allowance in a cage – in this case the rabbit is in an Eglu™ enclosure *(Photo courtesy of Omlet™.)*

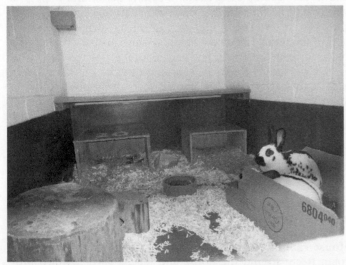

Fig. 33.7 Rabbits 'playing' in a soil box which allows for the expression of natural digging behaviour in a restricted environment *(Photo courtesy of Plumpton College Sussex.)*

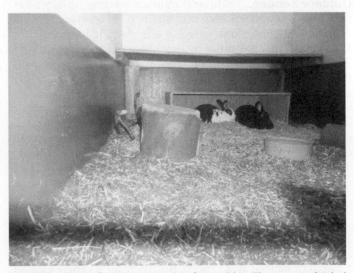

Fig. 33.9 Type of enclosure suitable for a rabbit. The cage is divided into the living quarters lined with short straw mix and the sleeping quarters lined with softer hay *(Photo courtesy of Plumpton College, Sussex.)*

– provide the animal with choice between hiding or being visible; hot areas and colder areas; sun or shade.

Rabbits

It is estimated that over a million rabbits are kept as domestic pets in the UK and that they are the third most popular species of pet in the UK. They are also one of the species most commonly given for rehoming (Magnus 2009). Rabbits are active, energetic and often playful and would naturally exist in a social network where the many eyes and ears would be of mutual benefit to the group when avoiding predators is required. The animals live communally in underground areas known as warrens that are a complex system of tunnels dug out of the earth. As they are a prey species, their social structure and behavioural repertoire is tailored towards survival. Rabbits spend a large amount of time, an estimated 70% while outside the warren (Magnus 2009), selectively grazing on grass, vegetation and plant fibres. They are crepuscular animals and are primarily active outside the warren during the hours of dawn and dusk, when the temperatures are normally cooler and there may be less danger from predators. The domestic rabbit (*Oryctolagus cuniculus*) is a lagomorph descended from the wild rabbit originally found in modern Spain (Ballard and Cheek 2010). The design of the domestic rabbits' housing should reflect their physical and behavioural needs and allow them to live as naturally as possible. Rabbits were originally domesticated for meat and fur, but in the last few decades have become popular pets. Over the last few decades, rabbit housing and management have changed dramatically.

It is now common to house rabbits in two ways:
- Outdoor hutch and run
- Indoors as a house rabbit.

Both methods have their merits, but whatever method is chosen it must satisfy the general requirements shown in Table 33.2.

Outdoor housing. Traditional outdoor housing usually takes the form of a wooden cage with a wire door covering half the front and a solid door covering the sleeping quarters (see Fig. 33.9). The cage must be draught-proof, waterproof and vermin-proof. It is important to ensure that the cage protects the rabbit from extreme temperature, flying insects, predators and environmental dangers. The doors should have good safety locks that are fox-proof and not easily opened by scratching or being pushed by an animal. The internal structure of the hutch should have two areas, one for feeding and moving about and a second for sleeping and as a safe hiding place:
- The feeding area should contain a water bottle, food and an ad lib hay supply.
- The sleeping area should contain plenty of hay for warmth and bedding material with a solid door for privacy (see Table 33.2).

This type of cage housing is only recommended for overnight safety and the rabbit should be free to roam during the day in a fenced or penned area (Fig. 33.10). There are a variety of pens available and the common factors of all designs should include hiding places that double as shelters from the rain and heat, and two opaque sides (four open sides will make the rabbit feel vulnerable and nervous). Rabbits will require shade at temperatures above 27°C (80°F) as they can suffer from heat stress at high temperatures. Tunnels and tubing sunk into the ground will allow natural hiding behaviour (see Fig. 33.3), shelter and

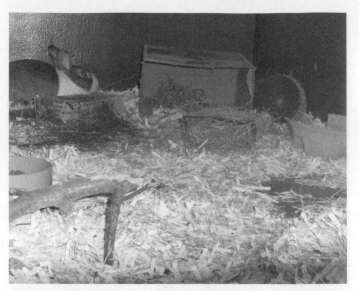

Fig. 33.10   Rabbit pen showing enrichment

a cool environment during hotter periods. Food and water must be available at all times and ideally placed in an open and sheltered position to allow the rabbit to choose where it prefers to eat. An outdoor run would ideally have access to vegetation allowing selective browsing and free choice of food selection. Objects for scent marking can also be provided as rabbits will mark their territories with their chin glands.

Recently there has been a new rabbit/guinea pig enclosure designed known as the Eglu™. The Eglu™ for rabbits was developed in conjunction with leading animal behaviourists, Dr Anne McBride and Emma Magnus. It has two connected areas – the house and a secure outside run. The Eglu™ and run provides a living environment that the manufacturer describes as 'near to nature' (see Fig. 33.8). The security of the enclosure allows the rabbit to exercise and follow its natural biological rhythms by performing and expressing natural behaviour when the need arises. The ability to control its own environment allows the animal to make choices which usually results in a more contented pet with few behavioural problems.

Rabbits should always be kept in groups or a minimum of a pair, as they are social prey animals that have evolved to live in colonies for safety and will not be able to perform normal interactive social behaviour if housed as single pets. If the owner does not wish to breed then the group should consist of compatible single sex, either 'bucks' (male rabbits) or 'does' (female rabbits), although several bucks kept together may fight. Groups of both male and female entire rabbits may show marking and urine-spraying behaviour (Ballard and Cheek 2010). Due to potential fighting of entire rabbits, it is often advised that both males and females should be neutered.

House rabbits. Rabbits may be kept indoors and allowed to roam freely around the house and fenced garden which provides exercise and stimulation for the rabbit. They should be provided with a low cage in which to hide and sleep and can easily be trained to use a litter tray. Rabbits should be safely confined at night to ensure that they are unable to cause any damage to themselves while unsupervised; again, a small cage with a sleeping section, bedding, food and water should be placed in a non-draughty location. It is important to be aware that rabbits will chew electrical wiring and cables, so care must be taken to prevent electrocution. It is also important to ensure that house plants are not in a chewable proximity as many are toxic to rabbits. If an owner decides to keep a rabbit as a house pet, the species requirement for grass/high-fibre forage and exercise outside should not be forgotten and ideally not substituted for a purely indoor environment. If outside access is not possible, then vegetation and fibre forage should be provided for the house rabbit. The animals should also have the provision of mental and physical stimulation as rabbits enjoy gnawing and chewing and a range of safe toys should be available for 'playtime'. Care must be taken to ensure that house rabbits are safely managed with family or visiting pets.

Housing rabbits within the veterinary practice. Separate accommodation should be provided for rabbits as they are a prey species and will suffer from stress if housed with predator species such as dogs, cats and ferrets. Even the smell of these animals, especially ferrets, can cause immense distress to the rabbit. Always provide a box for the rabbit to hide in while in the cage, or elect to leave them in their carrier boxes with the door open inside the cage. Covering the front of the cage with a clean blanket can also reduce stress, as can covering the basket when transporting them within the practice. This will also give them the added feeling of security. Do not place the rabbit in a carrier on the floor as the smell of predators can be very strong and the smell from dogs being walked passed will be highly stressful for a prey species while trapped in a situation they cannot escape from.

Guinea pigs

Domestic Guinea pigs (*Cavia porcellus*) are considered rodents, but are in a suborder known as hystricomorphic rodents, which also includes chinchillas and degus (Ballard and Cheek 2010). Guinea pigs are highly social animals with a well-developed social system, so are easily housed in same-sex groups if raised or introduced at a young age. The traditional rabbit hutch is acceptable for night-time housing, as are large, purpose-built plastic and wire cages. A cage with a top is not necessary as they are not known for jumping or climbing. The sides of the tray should be 8–10 inches high (Ballard and Cheek 2010). The floor space should be a minimum of 0.9 m² per adult (Meredith and Johnson-Delany 2010). Guinea pigs also need access to an outdoor run for exercise and provision of fresh grass and vegetation. If using a tray type of enclosure outdoors, a lid will be necessary to protect animals from local cats. Like rabbits, guinea pigs require hiding places, objects to chew, and items such as cardboard tubes to provide environmental enrichment (see Table 33.3). Any cage designed for guinea pigs should have plenty of ventilation to reduce the build-up of ammonia levels. They tend to be messier that rabbits and will defecate throughout the cage. They are not easily litter trained, and for this reason, house guinea pigs are less manageable than house rabbits. Guinea pigs have easily damaged toes, so a solid floor is preferable to a wire mesh. The cage should be situated out of direct sunlight, as they are susceptible to hyperthermia (Table 33.4) but are quite comfortable at 21°C (70°F) (Ballard and Cheek 2010). Again, the cages should be kept out of draughts and away from central heating. Guinea pigs are neophobic animals and have a strong preference for routine and familiar foods. This being so, a range of foods should be introduced to young guinea pigs, as they are unlikely to try new foods

as adults (Ballard and Cheek 2010). For this reason, they should also be gently and well handled as youngsters.

Ferrets. Ferrets are extremely active acrobatic animals and they need plenty of space, exercise and mental stimulation. They can be housed either indoors or outdoors. The most important aspect in their housing is to ensure that the enclosure is 'ferret proof', i.e. it is free of holes and escape proof. This should also be taken into account when housing them in the veterinary practice. Ferret housing should include the provision of a dark, quiet sleeping zone that can be furnished with soft bedding material such as old sheets and towels. This will allow ferrets to feel secure and perform their natural hiding behaviour. It will also protect outdoor ferrets from extreme heat and cold. Ferrets cannot sweat and are therefore at risk of hyperthermia if the enclosure is inappropriately situated. More than one sleep zone is necessary for multiple-housed animals. Solid toys, tunnels and hiding places should be provided for environmental enrichment; ensure that any toys cannot be consumed as gastrointestinal obstruction is commonly seen in young ferrets (Ballard and Cheek 2010). Ferrets can be housed in wooden/wire cages (Fig. 33.11) with a solid floor but everything must be easily cleaned. They enjoy climbing on multi-level platforms and resting stations at various heights. Litter trays should be provided in several positions throughout the enclosure for elimination ensuring that the sides are low enough for them to access them easily.

Mice, hamsters and gerbils

Gerbils (*Meriones unguiculatus*) and mice (*Mus musculus*) naturally live in colonies, so are much happier kept in family units. Syrian hamsters (*Mesocricetus auratus*) are, however, naturally solitary animals, and will fight to the death if kept with another hamster. The small Chinese and Russian hamsters can be kept in groups, providing they are introduced when young, e.g. littermates or when sexually immature.

Mice, hamsters and gerbils are easily housed in aquarium tanks but there must be plenty of ventilation via a metal mesh lid to ensure that there is no build-up of ammonia from urea breakdown which can contribute to respiratory problems (Figs. 33.12 and 33.2). A solid floor enables easy cleaning and prevents damage to small feet and legs. A tank design is preferable to cages with metal bars as they are able to accommodate a deep layer of substrate in which to burrow and dig. Gerbils in particular enjoy deep substrate in which they can burrow, dig and create a complex network of tunnels. Mice are less inclined to burrow on such a large scale but enjoy cages with plastic tunnels. Both species enjoy having multilayered enclosures with steps or ropes connecting the areas and plenty of cardboard boxes to hide in and to gnaw.

Mice produce pungent-smelling urine and should be cleaned out every 2–3 days; gerbils smell less and can be cleaned less often; hamster cages need fully cleaning about once a month. All three species enjoy chewing and cardboard, small boxes and toilet roll tubes all make excellent shredding material and help to keep their teeth worn down.

Cages with different platforms and objects to supply environmental enrichment can provide plenty of interest and exercise. Hamster balls are not recommended as once inside, the animal has very little control over the action or direction of the ball. Hamsters will naturally want to move forward but the impact of hitting other objects and the vibration produced

TABLE 33.4 Optimum, minimum and maximum housing temperatures (where applicable) and siting and size of accommodation for small mammals

	Rabbits	Guinea pigs	Ferrets	Gerbils	Hamsters	Rats and mice
Optimum temperature	Prefer cooler temperatures	18–26°C	15–21°C	15–21°C	19–23°C	15–27°C
Minimum temperature	4°C	18°C	Below −7°C a heat lamp is required		Below 5°C hamsters start to enter hibernation	
Maximum temperature	28°C+ may cause heatstroke	26–30°C may cause heatstroke	32°C			30°C+ may cause heatstroke
Minimum size of accommodation	Run – minimum 1.5 m² for one rabbit, increase by half for second rabbit. Hutch – 0.3 m² for one animal, and 0.2 m² per animal if several. Rabbits should be able to stand up in enclosure and move around easily (see Fig. 33.10)	1.5 m × 1.5 m × 25 cm high for outdoor run. Hutch – 30 cm height, 0.2 m² floor area per guinea pig	1.5 m long × 0.75 m deep × 1 m high (suitable for three ferrets)	45 cm × 30 cm × 25 cm high for two–three gerbils	45 cm × 30 cm × 25 cm high for one hamster	50 cm × 30 × 50 cm high for one rat. 30 cm × 20 cm × 20 cm high for 4 mice
Siting of housing/ external enclosure	Wind-free area, with outdoor area having access to light for production of vitamin D and interesting activities for mental stimulation. Rabbits need to feel secure, so siting in a safe area where they do not feel vulnerable is essential	Wind-free area, with outdoor area having access to light and environmental stimulation. The run will need to be easily moved for continued grazing	Wind-free area, with outdoor area having access to light and environmental stimulation. Indoor area must be dry, draught-proof and heated if temperature is too cold	Place the cage in a safe area, not able to be knocked off tables or ledges. Also place where cats are unable to climb on the lid. Position cage for good ventilation but no draughts, and out of direct sunlight, but still allowing a good source of natural light	Place the cage in a safe area, not able to be knocked off tables or ledges. Also place where cats are unable to climb on the lid. Position cage for good ventilation but no draughts, and out of direct sunlight, but still allowing a good source of natural light	Rats – place the cage in a draught- and damp-free area. Good source of natural light should be available, but not direct sunlight to cause hyperthermia. Mice – place the cage in a safe area, not able to be knocked off tables or ledges. Also place where cats are unable to climb on the lid. Position cage for good ventilation but no draughts, and out of direct sunlight, but still allowing a good source of natural light

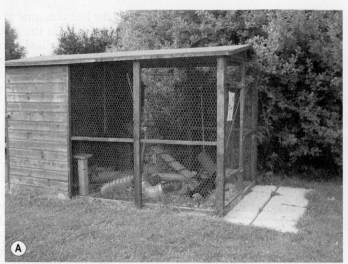
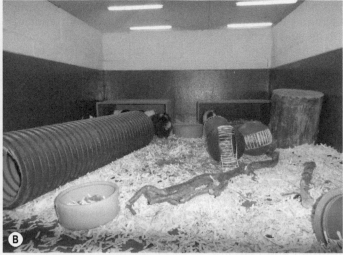

Fig. 33.11 (A) An outdoor ferret cage that provides fresh air, entertainment and exercise *(Photo courtesy of Plumpton College, Sussex.)* (B) A Guinea pig enclosure showing enrichment and substrates *(Photo courtesy of Plumpton College, Sussex.)*

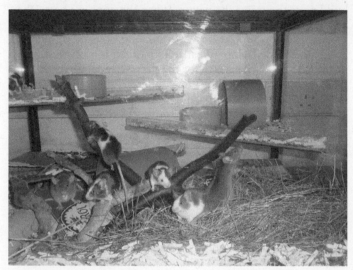

Fig. 33.12 A multilayered aquarium type of cage suitable for a colony of mice. It includes numerous boxes, ladders and tunnels for mental stimulation *(Photo courtesy of Plumpton College, Sussex.)*

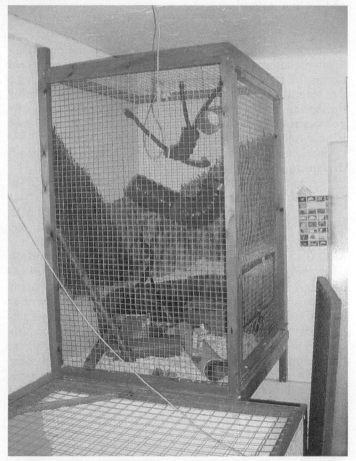

Fig. 33.13 A wooden and wire rat cage. It provides vertical and horizontal exercise and has numerous toys and tunnels for entertainment. The cage also has a bedding area containing hay *(Photo courtesy of Plumpton College, Sussex.)*

may be stressful to such a small prey species. If hamster balls are used for exercising, ensure that they are kept away from stairs and other animals that may wish to play with them. Circular running wheels are more appropriate as the animal has a choice whether to use it and for how long. Sleeping zones are important and wooden or non-chewable plastic houses stuffed full of shredded paper or tissue are often used. Cotton towels should be avoided as a bedding substrate as the animal's feet/legs can get entangled in the thread and cause constriction resulting in loss of feet/limbs (Ballard and Cheek 2010). Gerbils also enjoy sand baths and a shallow bowl filled with sand should be provided for dry bathing (see Fig. 33.1).

Rats

The domestic rat (*Rattus norvegicus*) is a highly sociable and intelligent animal, and makes an excellent small pet for a more interactive pet-owner relationship. They are classed as rodents and the males are referred to as bucks and the females as does. Rats enjoy climbing and gnawing, therefore their enclosure needs to reflect both of these factors. Rats can be kept in large wire cages that allow vertical and horizontal movement and fulfil their need to exercise. The enclosure needs to be situated in a dry, draught-free area with access to natural light. It is important to provide a high level of enrichment which could include items to climb on and chew (Figs. 33.13 and 33.6). Tree branches, ropes and tubes are all ideal for creating a stimulating environment. Plastic tunnels are useful for both running through and sleeping in. Rats enjoy comfortable bedding areas where they can curl up and sleep. The sleeping areas can be any solid type of box with a lid (see Fig. 33.5). The temperature should be between 18°C and 27°C (64°F and 80°F), with a humidity from 50–70% (Bament 2014). These environmental factors will help to prevent heat stress and dermatology problems (Bament 2014). Rats should be kept in pairs or groups due to their highly social nature. In the wild, female rats tend show a hierarchical behaviour, forming colonies of up to six individuals (Bament 2014). Female rats will also help to raise the offspring of other females within their colony (Bament 2014). Due to the fact that they are nocturnal, positioning of the cage should be considered to ensure minimum disturbance from night-time activities.

Nutrition and Feeding

Small mammals have different nutritional requirements. Table 33.5 shows a summary of appropriate nutritional requirements and feeding methods.

Breeding

Breeding small mammals is usually easy, rapid and may result in large numbers of offspring. Most small mammals will breed during the spring and summer and slow down or stop when the day length shortens. This pattern of repeated oestrus during the spring and summer is described as being **seasonally polyoestrous**. Non-seasonally polyoestrous animals will breed all year round regardless of the season (Table 33.6).

Small mammals may be either induced or spontaneous ovulators:

- **Induced ovulation** – the female ovulates as a result of the stimulation of coitus, e.g. ferret, rabbit
- **Spontaneous ovulation** – the female ovulates at a fixed time during the reproductive cycle, e.g. guinea pig, gerbil, rats.

Most female mammals display a behaviour known as lordosis when they are receptive to the male, i.e. the animal flattens its back and raises the pelvis, indicating readiness to mate. Many of the small mammals display more individual behaviour around breeding and gestation periods. Groups of female rats have also been known to spontaneously and synchronously come into oestrus after 72 hours of being exposed to male rat pheromones. This is known as the 'Whitten effect' (Bament 2010). In addition to this ovulation effect, rats may also experience the 'Bruce effect'. This is when pregnant females in the early stages of gestation abort and reabsorb the embryo and return to oestrus in the presence of the pheromones from a new male (Bament 2010).

Rabbits

Rabbits are seasonally polyoestrous and are induced ovulators. The doe may become aggressive towards the buck during mating, therefore supervision is advised. Kits are born in the nest and it is normal behaviour for the doe to pull hair from her dewlap, sides and abdomen to line and soften the nest. This behaviour normally takes place a few days or hours before parturition. The young kits are altricial when born – they are blind, furless and totally dependent on the doe (unlike the young of hares that are born with their eyes open and fully furred). The doe only feeds her young (kits) for about 3–5 minutes once a

day and within this short feeding period the kits consume up to 20% of their body weight. The kits are 'held up' in the nest for 3 weeks with lactation peaking at this point (Ballard and Cheek 2010). At about 2 weeks of age the kits start to consume solid food and cecotrophy starts at about 3 weeks of age (Ballard and Cheek 2010). The process of weaning is complete by about 5–6 weeks (Ballard and Cheek 2010).

Guinea pigs

It is recommended that sows are bred before they reach 7 months of age as at approximately 1 year, the fibrocartilaginous sutures of the pubic symphysis in the pelvis fuse and are no longer able to relax and stretch during parturition and dystocia will occur during labour. Guinea pigs are continuously polyoestrus (every 15–17 days); they are nonseasonal and spontaneous ovulators with oestrus lasting for approximately 12 hours (Bament 2012). The sow will show signs of lordosis and the boar will 'purr' over the female (Bament 2012). It is possible to confirm pregnancy by palpation or ultrasound 2–3 weeks after mating (Bament 2012). Guinea pigs do not build nests to receive the young. When the pups are born, they are fully furred with their eyes open, i.e. they are precocial. Within a few hours after birth they are able to stand, and although they will start to eat solid food within 24 hours they are unable to survive alone for the first 5 days and would normally consume milk for up to 3 weeks. Guinea pig sows will also 'top and tail' the pups after feeding. Groups of sows can often be seen suckling unrelated pups and this altruistic social behaviour is thought to increase the pups' survival chances (Meredith and Johnson-Delaney 2010).

Ferrets

Jills are seasonally polyoestrus and come into season in the spring and late summer and are induced ovulators (Bament 2013). While in season, the female's genital area will be swollen and remain so for up to 3 weeks, until she is mated or artificial hormones are used to suppress the oestrus (Bament 2013). If the jill is not mated or brought out of season, then the levels of oestrogen will remain high and this can cause fatal bone marrow suppression (Bament 2013). The aggressive mating behaviour and biting from the hob during copulation is the trigger for spontaneous ovulation (Bament 2013). Once the female is mated, the vulval swelling decreases and pregnancy can be diagnosed by palpation after 10 days. The kits (a young ferret less than 4 months old) are born altricial and are completely dependent on the jill for survival (Bament 2013).

Hamsters, mice and gerbils

Small rodents are seasonally polyoestrus and are spontaneous ovulators. The offspring of these species are born hairless, deaf, blind and completely reliant on the mother, i.e. they are altricial. The mother feeds her young and will wean at the appropriate time. Gerbils form monogamous pairs that should ideally be introduced before the animals become sexually mature. Once a pair have been mated, they should not be separated and no attempt to introduce a different partner should be made. An introduction at this stage will be very likely to end in fighting and possibly death (Ballard and Cheek 2010). The weaning ages for hamsters, mice and gerbils are 20–25 days, 21–28 days and 21–30 days, respectively (Ballard and Cheek 2010).

Very little human interference is necessary once parturition of the small mammals is complete. If the young are rejected,

TABLE 33.5	Nutritional requirements and feeding methods						
	Rabbits	**Guinea pigs**	**Ferrets**	**Hamsters**	**Rats**	**Gerbils**	**Mice**
Classification by diet	Herbivore	Herbivore	Carnivore	Omnivore	Omnivore	Omnivore	Omnivore
Cophrophagia or caecotrophy	Caecotrophs excreted and eaten at night. They contain high levels of vitamin B and K, and twice the protein and half the fibre of hard faeces. Caecotrophs are eaten directly from the anus many times a day	Caecotrophs are eaten as with rabbit		Caecotrophs are eaten	Caecotrophs are eaten	Caecotrophs are eaten	Caecotrophs are eaten
Special dietary needs	The digestive tract of the rabbit is designed for high fibre, and low protein, necessary for normal peristalsis, correct absorption of vitamins and prevention of dental disease. Vitamin D and calcium are necessary for development and maintenance of bones and teeth	Guinea pigs cannot synthesise vitamin C (ascorbic acid) as they do not have the necessary enzyme L-gluconolactone oxidase. Fresh green food must be given daily. Water may be supplemented with vitamin C at a dose of 10 mg/kg daily, or 1 g/l water (change daily). Pregnant sows – 30 mg/kg daily	Strict carnivores designed to eat their prey whole. Ferrets need a diet high in fat and protein, minimal fibre and carbohydrate	In the wild they will eat invertebrates and insects. Require a small proportion of animal-derived protein, e.g. cooked chicken	In the wild they will eat invertebrates and insects. Require a small proportion of animal-derived protein, e.g. cooked chicken	In the wild they will eat invertebrates and insects. Require a small proportion of animal-derived protein, e.g. cooked chicken	In the wild they will eat invertebrates and insects. Require a small proportion of animal-derived protein, e.g. cooked chicken
Foods to be avoided	Kale and spinach – may cause goitre; succulent fruit and vegetables, e.g. lettuce, may cause diarrhoea. Sugary foods	Fruits or sugary foods	Sweet sugary foods, grains	High-fat seeds, e.g. sunflower seeds, should not be fed regularly, as may exacerbate the onset of osteoporosis	High-fat seeds, e.g. sunflower seeds should not be fed regularly as rats are prone to obesity		
Diet	Ad-lib hay – high in fibre should be the main food source with a variety of vegetables. Grazing in the garden will provide much of the vegetation needed. Complementary dried feeds can be fed in addition	Grass, ad-lib hay, fresh leafy vegetables, complete food in small amounts compared to other food sources	Dead chicks, mice and rats. Raw eggs. Specially prepared dry ferret food	Can be fed a commercial complete food mix. Can also be fed table scraps	Can be fed a commercial complete food mix. Can also be fed table scraps. Rats may benefit from small pieces of cat food	Can be fed a commercial complete food mix. Can also be fed table scraps	Can be fed a commercial complete food mix. Can also be fed table scraps
Required nutritional values (Adult)	Recommended nutritional values for complete mix – fibre 16%; protein 16%	Protein 18–20%; fibre 10%	If complete dried food: fat 20%; protein 30–35%; fibre 20–25%	Minimum of: protein 16%; fat 4–5%	Minimum of: protein 16%; fat 4–5%. Pregnant females may require protein levels up to 20%	Minimum of: protein 16%; fat 4–5%. Pregnant females may require protein levels up to 20%	Minimum of: protein 16%; fat 4–5%
(Young)			Fat 20%; protein 35%				

TABLE 33.6	Significant information required for breeding small mammals						
	Rabbits	**Guinea pigs**	**Ferrets**	**Gerbils**	**Mice**	**Rats**	**Hamsters**
Sexual maturity	Small breeds 4–5 months Medium breeds 4–6 months Large breeds 5–8 months	(M) 3 months (F) 2 months	6–12 months	(M) 9–18 weeks (F) 9–12 weeks	6 weeks	4–5 weeks	(M) 8 weeks (F) 6 weeks
Ovulation	10 h after coitus	Spontaneous	30–40 h post-coitus				
Gestation period	30–32 days	59–72 days	41–43 days	23–26 days	19–21 days	21–23 days	15–18 days
Litter size	4–5 kits (small breeds) 8–12 kits (larger breeds)	1–13 (2–4 is usual) pups/young	1–18 kits, average 8	3–8 pups	7–11 pups	6–13 pups	5–10 pups
Normal birth weight	Varies for breed of rabbit	45–115 g	6–12 g	2.5–3.5 g	1–1.5 g	4–6 g	1.5–3 g
Weaning age	By 28 days full weaning should have occurred	21 days	6–8 weeks	21–28 days	18–21 days	21 days	19–21 days

which may occur if the nest is disturbed by the male or by a human, then bottle-feeding and hand-rearing is possible. The exception is young ferrets who are very difficult to hand-rear when orphaned. Cannibalism of young may occur in mice and hamsters, but rarely gerbils. This may be in response to the nest or mother being disturbed. Hamsters are also able to transfer their offspring via their cheek pouches, but the young may end up suffocating during the procedure (Ballard and Cheek 2010). For this reason, little contact should be made by humans once parturition has occurred. The enclosure should be fully prepared for the litter before birth and adequate food provided so as not to disturb the mother and new offspring after birth.

Common diseases and clinical conditions

Common diseases and clinical conditions of small mammals are shown in Tables 33.7–33.11.

REPTILES

The reptile species kept as exotic pets include various types of lizards and snakes and the shelled reptiles or chelonia, i.e. tortoises and terrapins (Table 33.11). They are a diverse group of animals and the large number of species available for sale and being presented for treatment in veterinary practice means that the veterinary nurse must have a good understanding of their basic housing, nutritional and breeding needs.

Housing

Reptiles are ectothermic or cold-blooded and it is important to remember that their health and well-being depend entirely on the environment in which we place them. If we get it wrong, it can lead to stress, which in turn can cause immunosuppression, ill health and death.

Reptiles are housed in **vivaria**, which are available in a variety of shapes, sizes and construction materials. Figures 33.14 and 33.15 show different types of set-up.

When selecting accommodation for a reptile or chelonian the following must be considered:
- Natural history of the species. The nurse must know the species' country of origin and from this must understand:

- The need to house the reptile in a temperate, desert or tropical environment
- The reptile's activity pattern, i.e. nocturnal, crepuscular or diurnal
- The reptile's requirements for a terrestrial, arboreal, aquatic or semi-aquatic set-up.
- The size, shape and materials used in vivarium construction (Table 33.12)
- Any animal accommodation should:
  - Be durable
  - Be safe and secure
  - Be easy to clean
  - Have ease of access.
- Tortoise species should be housed separately and not mixed as they have varying environmental needs and separate housing is better for health and disease monitoring.

Durability. It is not unusual for animal accommodation to cost more than the creature to be housed and, as reptile and chelonian accommodation is specialised, prices can be high. For the accommodation to last as long as possible, to ensure human and animal safety and to maintain hygiene standards, the materials and the design of the vivarium must be robust, practical and able to withstand the required levels of heat and humidity, and the possibility of destruction by the reptile.

Security. This is a major consideration, as all animals need to be secure and safe. Some reptiles are excellent escape artists, and neighbours are never pleased to hear that there is a 14-foot reticulated python 'on the loose'. Vivarium locks should be used and all vents and joints should be sealed and securely placed. All materials should be free of rough, sharp or jagged edges to prevent injury to the reptile and the handler. If the chelonian has access to outside housing, it must be escape and predator proof.

Ease of cleaning. Materials used in the construction of the vivarium should have a smooth surface, be impervious and be easy to clean. Many reptiles live in a hot, humid environment, which makes ideal conditions for pathogens to grow and multiply. To ensure good health, the ability to clean the animal's accommodation effectively is of the utmost importance.

TABLE 33.7	Common diseases and clinical conditions of gerbils, hamsters and rats					
	Disease	**Causal agent**	**Symptoms**	**Age of animals affected/ incubation period**	**Treatment**	**Prognosis**
Hamsters	Constipation	Inappropriate diet, often due to lack of moisture in food	Swollen abdomen, pain and anorexia	Often in hamsters of 2 weeks old, just as the weaning process starts	Change diet to include green vegetables and fruit, severe cases may need an enema	Good response
Hamsters	Bacterial pneumonia	*Pasteurella pnemotropica* and *Streptococcus* spp., stressful environment can predispose animals to infection	Oculonasal discharge, anorexia, dyspnoea	Any age	Supportive treatment, warmth, antibiotics	Good response
Hamster	Impacted cheeks	Food adhering to cheeks	Swollen cheeks	Any age	Emptied and flushed with water	Good response
Mice, hamsters	Viral pneumonia	Sendai virus – parainfluenza virus type 1	Asymptomatic in adults	Any age		May cause death in younger animals
Gerbils	Swollen sebaceous glands	Infection	Inflammation of large ventral abdominal sebaceous gland	Any age	Corticosteroids and antibiotics, may need surgery, or debridement in severe cases of infection	Good response
Hamsters, gerbils, rats	Dental problems/ malocclusion	Insufficient wear on teeth caused by poor diet, and malocclusion often occurs as a result of bar chewing. Malocclusion is also most common inherited disease in rabbits – change in skull and jaw length	Malocclusion of teeth, problems possible with both incisors and check teeth. Teeth continue to grow and overlap causing anorexia, and drooling. In severe cases – oral lesions and teeth growing into gums	Any age	Regular clipping and food that will wear teeth down and objects to chew	Good response
Gerbils, hamsters, rats	Neoplasia	Spontaneous in gerbils over 2 years old	Tumours commonly found on ovaries, skin (squamous cell carcinomas), sebaceous glands, kidney and adrenal glands. In rats, common tumour sites are mammary, abdomen and shoulders	Over 2 years old. More common in males of the hamster species	No treatment for many tumours. Ovariohysterectomy or ovariectomy may be indicated as prevention of mammary tumours in rats (Bament 2014)	High mortality rate
Gerbils, hamsters, rats	Tyzzer's disease – intracellular bacterium, can only be confirmed via post-mortem	*Clostridium piliforme* Caused by poor sanitation or deprivation of food or water, overcrowding, heavy parasitic load or illness (Bament 2014)	Lethargy, anorexia, loss of weight, piloerection	Weanlings are often affected. 10 days incubation period	Antibiotics are largely unsuccessful, but supportive therapy. Intravenous fluid therapy (IVFT), and rehydration solutions can be given	Usually poor

Continued

TABLE 33.7	Common diseases and clinical conditions of gerbils, hamsters and rats—cont'd				
	Disease	Causal agent	Symptoms	Age of animals affected/incubation period	Treatment	Prognosis
Rats	Chromodacryorrhoea or 'red tears'	Normally an indication of poor health, illness or stress. Increase in the normal production of lipid and porphyrin pigment in the eye (Bament 2014). Rats are normally fastideous groomers, and staining indicates a deviation from this behaviour	The fur around the eyes and nose will appear stained with red pigment which often can be mistaken for blood. The staining can be diagnosed as pigment by using a UV light to check for fluoresce (Bament 2014)	Any age can be affected	Underlying cause to be treated and supportive care, nursing and therapy to be provided	Depends on underlying cause
Rats	Respiratory conditions	Often husbandry related, build-up of ammonia due to poor ventilation, multiple infectious agents including: Mycoplasma pulmonis, Streptococcus pneumoniae, cilia-associated respiratory bacillus and Sendai virus. As these agents often occur at the same time, they are known as 'murine respiratory disease complex (Bament 2014)	Based on clinical signs, include mild to severe dyspnoea to pneumonia and death. Open mouth breathing is a poor sign as rats are obligate nasal breathers. Nasal discharge, weight loss, porphyrin-staining around the eyes, head tilt (Meredith and Johnson-Delany 2010)	Any age	May require life-long therapy, antibiotics for mixed infections, NSAIDs, bronchodilators and mucolytics. Dust-free bedding and well ventilated enclosures (Meredith and Johnson-Delany 2010)	Poor to good depending on severity
Gerbils, hamsters,	Wet tail	Multifactorial, factors include stress, possibly diet. E. coli and Campylobacter have both been isolated from samples	Severe watery diarrhoea causing staining around the anus, lethargy, anorexia, abdominal pain causing huddled appearance	Any age	Antibiotics, but are often unsuccessful, but supportive therapy, fluid therapy, and rehydration/electrolyte solutions can be given	Usually high mortality rate
Gerbils	Salmonellosis	S. enteritidid and S. typhimurium have both been isolated as possible pathogens	Moderate to severe diarrhoea, staring coat dehydration and weight loss	There is often no incubation period seen as patient often dies very quickly	Not recommended as it is a zoonotic disease and recovered patients often then become carriers	High mortality rate

TABLE 33.8	Common diseases and clinical conditions of guinea pigs				
Disease	Causal agent	Symptoms	Age of animals affected/ incubation period	Treatment	Prognosis
Salmonellosis	*S. enteritidid* and *S. typhimurium* have both been isolated as possible pathogens	Moderate to severe diarrhoea, staring coat dehydration and weight loss. Causes septicaemia and abortions in Guinea pigs	There is often no incubation period seen as patient often dies very quickly	Not recommended as it is a zoonotic disease and recovered patients often then become carriers	High mortality rate. Sudden deaths in guinea pigs
Mites	*Trixacarus caviae* – a sarcoptid mite	Pruritus	Any age	Ivermectin (not licensed for rodents)	Good response
Barbering/alopecia	Hair loss with no obvious disease is often caused by other guinea pigs or self-inflicted due to boredom	Loss of hair from body with no pruritus	Any age, seen in female guinea pigs late in pregnancy	Separate animals if specific interactions are problematic, increase environmental enrichment.	Good response
Scurvy (hypovitaminosis C)	Lack of vitamin C in diet – management and husbandry related. Guinea pigs are unable to manufacture vitamin C and therefore need to have it provided in their diet. Vitamin C denatures easily under warm, humid conditions and direct sunlight. Old greens and vegetables may also have reduced vitamin contents	Depressed, weak and lethargic, weight loss, anorexia, anaemia, bleeding gums, gingivitis, reduced immune system and poor skin condition/healing, pain, reluctance to walk, swollen painful joints	Various factors can affect vitamin C metabolism and usage, including life stage, pregnancy, stress, activity and environment	Supplement with 100 mg/kg vitamin C if showing symptoms	

Ease of access. It is imperative to be able to gain access to the reptile and its environment. You should not have to be a contortionist to get into the animal's accommodation, and the design of the vivarium and its furnishings should allow safe handling and safe cleaning.

Shape and size. Reptiles come in a variety of shapes and sizes and the chosen accommodation should reflect their physical needs. Terrestrial or ground-dwelling species require a horizontal vivarium (Fig. 33.15A); arboreal or tree-dwelling animals require a taller vivarium (Fig. 33.15B); and the burrowing species require a deep base to hold a depth of substrate. Desert-type species require a dry, arid set-up (Fig. 33.15D).

Tortoises are best maintained in an indoor enclosure ideally with an open-topped structure (table-top enclosure) (Fig. 33.15C) – this ensures good ventilation. Adequate heating and full-spectrum ultraviolet B (UVB) lighting must be provided with a range of substrates to stimulate digging behaviours. Hay, peat and bark mulch are all good options (Bennett and Jessop 2010). Access to water is essential for drinking and humidity and at a depth that will allow the tortoise to syphon water through the nostril and mouth.

Semi-aquatic chelonian require adequate space for ambulatory exercise, burrowing and soaking. Coconut fibre and compressed peat hold moisture and provide a good substrate medium (Bennett and Jessop 2010).

Substrate. Table 33.12 lists the common substrates. This is the medium that sits in the bottom of the vivarium to absorb faeces and urine and, in the case of burrowing animals, allows them to display their natural behaviour. One would normally select a substrate that is both comparable with the animal's natural habitat and aesthetically pleasing. It is not uncommon for reptiles to ingest substrate which can lead to impaction of the gut.

Foreign body ingestion is a common presentation, especially in pet lizards kept on inappropriate substrate. Both wood chip and sand are common culprits and can be accidentally ingested as the reptile attempts to pick up its food. Substrate intentionally ingested can occur, especially if dietary calcium levels are low (Eatwell 2010).

Cage furnishings. Furnishings are important as they:
- Provide the reptile with exercise opportunities
- Prevent boredom and behaviour problems
- Provide the reptile with security (somewhere to hide)
- Make the vivarium visually interesting.

Hides. One of the main provisions should be a series of hides. These make the reptile feel safe and secure, and reduce stress. As a guide, and to reduce stress, when a snake or lizard is in the hide it should be able to touch three sides. Most chelonians require some form of hide.

Branches. Textured branches that can support the weight of the reptile are needed for climbing and basking.

Text continued on p. 719

TABLE 33.9	Common diseases and clinical conditions of rabbits				
Disease	**Causal agent**	**Symptoms**	**Age of animals affected/ incubation period**	**Treatment**	**Prognosis**
Pododermatitis	Caused by pressure, and are often predisposed by genetically reduced amount of hair on the plantar surfaces. Also caused by wire-floored cages, poor hygiene and heavy weight of larger rabbits	Decubital ulcers on plantar surfaces of hind feet. Appearance of superficial ulcers and scabs, may become abscess if progress.	Any age, larger-sized rabbits, and those with less fur on plantar surface	Topical antibiotic application and bandages changed at a regular interval. Re-evaluate cage flooring	Good response to long-term treatment
Pasteurellosis	*Pasteurella multocida* bacterium	Respiratory disease, sneezing or snuffles, mucopurulent nasal discharge, conjunctivitis, skin abscesses, inner ear infection, pyometra, pneumonia or scepticaemia	Seen in older animals and those kept in large colonies or breeding rabbitries	Supportive therapy depending on symptoms. Antibiotics can be used for a month, but symptoms will return when drugs are stopped. Flush nares and nasolacrimal duct	Virtually impossible to rid animal of infection as very resilient. Euthanasia when symptoms causing distress or untreatable with supportive treatment
Coccidiosis	Hepatotrophic or enteric species of *Eimeria*. Vitamin E may increase coccidiosis	Diarrhoea, may cause fatal hepatic failure, icterus, hepatomegaly, and anorexia	Often seen in younger animals, especially weanlings	Treatment with sulpha drugs and reduced stress and increase in hygiene levels	Good prognosis
Gastric trichobezoars	Fur accumulation in gut possibly due to excessive grooming (possibly stress related) or diet lacking in fibre	Fur accumulation in stomach, causing blockage of the narrow pyloric lumen, leading to gut obstruction, gut dilation and anorexia.		High-fibre diets for prevention. Trichobezoars can be broken down using proteolytic enzymes, e.g. papain or bromelain (from health-food shops). Liquid paraffin is also of use	100% if not treated, otherwise good prognosis if diagnosed and treated quickly
Necrobacillosis (Schmorl's disease)	*Fusobacterium necrophorum*, associated with poor hygiene, skin abrasions and dental disease	Bacteria may cause ulceration and necrosis of skin, particularly on the face, neck and plantar areas of feet, and septicaemia	Not age-specific	Improve hygiene, debride wounds, treat with topical and oral antibiotics	Good prognosis
Myiasis (fly strike)	Due to diarrhoea (diet-related, infection, parasitic), obesity preventing grooming and cleaning (Gosden). Poor husbandry causing faeces-infected environment. Poor management of rabbit fur/ lack of grooming. Fly eggs developing into maggots	Eggs are usually layered around the perineum area of the rabbit. They then develop into maggots and eat the skin and tissue of the animal causing lesions	Not age-specific, related to animal's gut health and husbandry	Remove maggots, clean area (under sedation), Antibiotics, IVFT, wound management. Prevent with use fly repellent. Reduce green vegetables in diet. Weight loss program if necessary	Prognosis dependent on severity of skin lesions and severity of infection. Rabbits are often in very poor condition when presented for treatment. If severe, euthanasia may be advised on welfare grounds

	Cause	Clinical signs	Age	Treatment	Notes
Gastric stasis syndrome	Caused by a change in gastric motility and function, resulting in reabsorption of liquid from stomach content due to: high-carbohydrate/low-fibre diet, stress, lack of exercise, possibly ingestion of hair	Anorexia, decreased stool (faecal pellet) production, large gas-filled stomach with dough-like contents		Laxatives, paraffin oil, pineapple for bromelin (used as protein digestive enzymes). Oral rehydration – soften stomach contents, including water, fruit juices, vegetable puree, Critical Care formulae. IV/ S/C fluids. Metoclopramide to stimulate gut motility. Possibly surgical intervention if non-responsive to medical	Reduced in rabbits undergoing surgery. Patients often die due to hepatic lipidosis in surgical cases
Rabbit calicivirus disease – viral haemorrhagic disease	Caused by calicivirus, spread via faecal – oral route, via conjunctiva, nasal passages or damaged tissue, and via fomites	Acute onset, incubation 1–2 days. May show signs of depression, lethargy, anorexia, tachypnea, cyanosis, diarrhoea and constipation. Often appears asymptomatic and rabbit found dead due to such rapid onset	Older than 2 months	No suitable treatment available. Vaccination 12 monthly as prevention.	Highly infectious and high morbidity rates of 70–80% and high mortality rates of 100%
Encephalomyelitis – head tilt and ataxia	Caused by vestibular dysfunction, central (cerebellum) and peripheral (bacterial inner ear infection – otitis interna), peripheral nerve disease. Hyperaesthesia may indicate central nerve disease, and seizures and rolling may indicate brain lesions. Pasteurella multocida bacterial infection may also causes head tilt. Caused by Encephalitozoon cuniculi (protozoal disease): signs are trauma, heat stroke	Clinical indicators include neurological signs: head tilt, nystagmus, tremors, paresis, paralysis and seizures	Any age, transmitted between rabbits, carriers may be asymptomatic	Treatment is dependent on diagnosis. Otitis media and interna should be treated with antibiotics for 4 weeks or longer, possibly flushing ear canal while under GA. If encephalitozoonosis is diagnosed, steroids to reduce inflammation, antibiotics to treat bacterial infection and sedatives to control seizures (Quesenberry and Carpenter 2003). Anthelmintics for E. cuniculi	
Myxomatosis	Myxoma virus of the pox family. Transmitted via arthropod bite, usually the rabbit flea, but can also be mosquitoes, flies and mites (Benato and Eatwell 2011). Direct contact with infected rabbits and infected fomites (Benato and Eatwell 2011)	Clinical signs depend on virulence of strain and genus of rabbit species infected. Wild rabbits may exhibit benign skin tumours at base of ear – if inoculation entry point. Domestic rabbits can exhibit a variety of clinical signs. There are two classical forms of the disease, nodular and respiratory, with nodular being the most common (Benato and Eatwell 2011) The clinical signs include: severe immunosuppression, lethargy, fever, anorexia, skin haemorrhage, swelling and oedema of the lips, nares, eyelids and genital area. Raised skin nodules and mucopurulent blepharoconjunctivitis (Benato and Eatwell 2011).		Vaccination annually as prevention. Treatment is possible only if strain of virus is mild, then supportive nursing care and antibacterial therapy should be implemented. To help in prevention of myxomatosis transmission, buy hay/straw from myxomatosis-free suppliers, fit fly screens to hutches, stop wild rabbits entering garden, use products to deter mosquitoes.	High mortality rate

Continued

TABLE 33.9 Common diseases and clinical conditions of rabbits—cont'd

Disease	Causal agent	Symptoms	Age of animals affected/ incubation period	Treatment	Prognosis
		The respiratory form (non-myxomatosis form) causes peracute haemorrhagic pneumonia and skin lesions are less obvious (Benato and Eatwell 2011). The rabbit develops secondary infection usually due to gram-negative bacteria causing mucopurulent oculonasal discharges, pneumonia and eventually death (Benato and Eatwell 2011). There is also a third atypical form that affects vaccinated rabbits, where cutaneous signs develop and tend to heal spontaneously (Benato and Eatwell 2011)			
Rabbit ear mite	*Psoroptes cuniculi* (ear mites)	Clinical signs include severe otitis externa, crusting and exudate	Not age-related	Antibiotics to reduce secondary bacterial infection. Topical ear treatment, ivermectin	Good response
Abscesses	Abscesses are walled-off pockets containing bacteria	Commonly occur in the skin (secondary to injury or surgery), head, neck and secondary to dental disease (Hansen 2002). Clinical signs include swellings, pain in area of abscess, possible anorexia	Not age-specific, often due to injury or after surgery, foreign bodies – any factor which can cause localised bacterial infection	Sedation/GA to probe and clean abscess, debride necrotic tissue, pack wound cavity to prevent healing too quickly and trapping bacteria. Oral or systemic antibiotics, should be used, can also use antibiotic-impregnated beads within the wound	Abscess may burst, expelling pus externally, or bacteria may escape capsule and settle around body causing new abscesses – 'seeding' (Hansen 2002); antibiotics will not penetrate multiple abscesses that cannot be treated surgically, therefore euthanasia advised.
Uterine cancer	80% female rabbits develop uterine cancer. Adenocarcinoma – malignant tumour of the glandular tissue that metastasises, often to the lungs	Clinical signs of advanced uterine cancer include: anaemia, decreased lethargy, swollen cystic mammary glands, weight loss, dyspnoea and increased aggression	Most common in does aged 5–6 years	Spay females after 5–6 months of age	If diagnosis is made before metastasises, possible to spay with successful recovery; otherwise, euthanasia or morbidity of affected rabbits is high
Dental problems/ malocclusion	Insufficient wear on teeth caused by poor diet, and malocclusion. Often occurs as a result of bar chewing, tooth loss or due to trauma. Malocclusion is also most common inherited disease in rabbits – change in skull and jaw length from crossing breeds with different head/jaw length and size	Malocclusion of teeth, problems possible with both incisors and cheek teeth. Teeth continue to grow and overlap causing anorexia, and drooling. Lastly, in severe cases – oral lesions and teeth growing into gums	Any age	Regular tooth trimming with appropriate power dental bur or extractions where necessary (Ballard and Cheek 2010) and food that will wear teeth down and objects to chew in the enclosure. Do not breed from animals which have poor mouth conformation	Good response, but continued care and monitoring of the teeth required

TABLE 33.9

| TABLE 33.10 | Common diseases and clinical conditions of ferrets | | | | |

Disease	Causal agent	Symptoms	Age of animals affected/ incubation period	Treatment	Prognosis
Canine distemper	Distemper virus	Mucopurulent ocular nasal discharge, crusty eyelids and facial lesions. Hyperkeratosis of footpads. Possibly anorexic and may be ataxic or show signs of nystagmus. Pyrexia – 40.6–41.1°C	Any age. Incubation period is 7–9 days	Can be vaccinated against using canine vaccine – Vaxitas D	100% fatal in ferrets, and if contracted, the ferret should be euthanised
Influenza	Ferrets are susceptible to several strains of the virus	Influenza causes upper respiratory disease, with symptoms including anorexia, listlessness and nasal discharge	Any age of ferret	Antibiotics may be needed if secondary infection is involved. Often recovers without the need for drugs	100% fatal in kits
Aleutian disease (AD)	Parvovirus. Immune-mediated and may also cause some immunodepression	Black tarry faeces, recurrent fevers, weight loss, behaviour changes – possibly increase in aggression or hyperaesthesia, thyroiditis, paralysis followed by death. Carriers may be asymptomatic	Any age	No specific relief, supportive therapy and antibiotics	Can be fatal
Ear mites	*Otodectes cynotis*	Black sticky discharge in one or both ears	Any age	Clean ears daily and Ivomec injections, one injection repeated in 2 weeks (not to be used in pregnant females). Can also use ear drops with active ingredient gamma BHC	Good response to treatment and prevention
Prolonged oestrus	Female ferrets are polyoestrous and induced ovulators. When in oestrus and not mated they continue to have high circulating oestrogen levels which causes bone marrow suppression	Anaemia and reduced white blood cell production	Sexually mature entire females	Spay at 6–8 months of age if not intended for breeding. Hormone injections control oestrus. Use of vasectomised hob for coitus and completing oestrus cycle	Life-threatening if not treated

| TABLE 33.11 | Common reptilian species kept as pets in the UK | | | |

Species	Country of origin	Food	Reproductive data	Additional comments
SNAKES				
Boas				
Common boa (*Boa constrictor constrictor*)	Central and South America from Mexico to northern Argentina	Depends on the size of the snake – rodents (mice, rats, gerbils, rabbits); chicks (day-old); birds. Males tend to be more prone to periods of seasonally induced non-feeding	Live bearers, i.e. ovoviviparous; 20–60 in a litter. Young approx. 35–60 cm in length. Males sexually mature at approximately 2 years of age. Females average 3 years of age	Heavy-bodied species. Average life span 20 years. Average length 2–3 m but can grow larger. Require temperature range of 28–32°C. Humidity 50–70%. (50% is average room humidity.) Provide with a large ceramic water bowl, as this species likes to soak

Continued

TABLE 33.11	Common reptilian species kept as pets in the UK—cont'd			
Species	**Country of origin**	**Food**	**Reproductive data**	**Additional comments**
Pythons				
Royal python (*Python regius*)	Africa	Depends on the size of the snake – rodents, rabbits, birds, chicks	Oviparous; lays average 6–8 eggs; incubation can last 40–80 average 50 days and young measure 40 cm Males sexually mature within 2 years Females sexually mature 3 years, but body weight can influence the above	Various colour morphs now available. Short, stocky snake that reaches about 1.2 m in length. Females tend to be larger Life span 20–30 plus years. Although usually good-natured, can refuse to eat for periods of time – making it unsuitable for the novice. If threatened will go into a ball. Vivarium temperature range 25–33°C Humidity 60–65%
Burmese python (*Python moluris bivittatus*)	Southeast Asia	Range of rodents rabbits, birds, piglets	Oviparous; Sexual maturity 18 month–4 years. Size and weight are influencing factors Can lay up to 100 eggs (more realistically, 20–30). Incubation temperature 30°C and can last 60–80 days. Young measure 40 cm	Various colour morphs available including Albino or golden Burmese have bright yellow markings on a white background. Very large snake – grows up to 6–7 m. Grows rapidly and reaches 3–4 m in 2 years Temperature range 31–33°C. Humidity 70–80%. Because of potential size, longevity 25 years plus, feeding and space requirements, not recommended as a pet
Reticulated python (*Python reticulatus*)	Southeast Asia	As above	Similar to Burmese python	Very large snake – grows up to 9 m. Not best-tempered snake and because of size and aggressive nature not recommended as a pet
Colubrids				
Corn snake (*Elaphe guttata*) – rat snake family	North America	Depends on the size of the snake: rodents, birds chicks Males require less frequent feeding than females (Rendle and Cracknell 2012)	Oviparous: breed snake from 2 years old. Lays 12 plus eggs 1 month after mating. Incubate at 28°C for ~60–70 days	Many colour mutations. Good pet for novice keeper. Good temperament, grows to 1 m, easy to manage and eats readily in captivity Require temperatures 24–28°C 50–60% humidity Life span 20 years plus
King snake (*Lampropeltis getulus*)	North America	As above	Oviparous: breed from 2 years of age. Usually produce two clutches in each breeding season Clutch size 5–20 – subspecies vary. Incubate at 28°C for 60 days	Adults can grow to 2 m but average length 1 m. Colour variations available usually black with yellow or white markings. Relatively easy to keep in captivity. Best kept on its own, as they have cannibalistic tendencies Temperature 24–28°C 30–50% humidity Life span 20 years plus
Garter snakes				
Common garter snake (*Thamnophis sirtalis*)	North and Central America	Earthworms, fish, small rodents, pinkies In captivity they are mainly fed rodents, a diet that is thought to shorten their life span (Rendle and Cracknell 2012) Supplementation of food with vitamin and mineral powder advised	Ovoviviparous: clutch size 10–20; gestation period 4–5 months	Active snake and requires relatively large accommodation relative to size Life span 10–15 years Temperature range 24–28°C. Small snake: grows to 0.5–1 m males smaller. Humidity 60–75% Care when feeding fish, as this must be blanched for 2 min to kill antivitamin, which causes thiamine deficiency

TABLE 33.11	Common reptilian species kept as pets in the UK—cont'd			
Species	**Country of origin**	**Food**	**Reproductive data**	**Additional comments**
LIZARDS				
Geckos				
Leopard gecko (*Eublepharus macularius*)	India, Afghanistan and Vietnam	Insects, (crickets, hoppers, locusts, silkworms) Waxworms are highly palatable and geckos will become addicted to these, refusing other food items offered. Vitamin and mineral powder supplementation required	Oviparous. Female can lay up to five clutches per season. Eggs are laid in pairs in moistened sand, vermiculite or peat, and have soft, leathery shells. Best removed and placed in an incubator. Temperature of 27–29°C produces females, 32–33°C will produce males. If eggs stuck together do not attempt to separate. Incubate for 6–8 weeks	A variety of colour morphs and patterns available. Good beginner's lizard – does well in captivity; friendly, easy to keep. Crepuscular Life span 20 years plus. Temperature. daytime basking area 26–30°C 20–21°C at the cool end. Night-time temp no lower than 20°C. Evidence supports that low intensity 2% UVB light benefits these species and aids in calcium metabolism and general well-being. Male geckos are very territorial and will fight, so best kept on their own or with females at a ratio of 1 to 4 If handled roughly or threatened will cause tail to autoamputate (autotomy)
Fat-tailed gecko (*Hemitheconyx caudicinctus*)	Northeast Africa			
Day gecko (*Phelsuma cepediana*)		Insectivores eating crickets, hoppers, locusts, silkworms. Also offer fruit puree baby food, nectar mixes. Vitamin and mineral supplementation is advisable	Oviparous: very similar to leopard geckos except that eggs have hard shells	Diurnal lizard lively and quick, need tall, well-planted vivarium and access to UVB light. Very colourful. Both sexes can be territorial and need a large vivarium so they can retreat to their own area. Life span 6–8 years but can span to 20 years Temperate 27–31°C Night-time drop to 25°C Humidity 50–85% Tail Autotomy and skin slough can occur if incorrectly handled
Agamas				
Water dragon (*Physignathus cocincinus*)	Southeast Asia	Insects, crickets, locusts, small rodents, pinkies, some fruit and vegetable matter	Oviparous: Sexual maturity 2 years plus. Female can lay up to 5–15 eggs and can lay a second clutch 3–4 months later. Eggs laid in damp sand or vermiculite and should be removed and placed in an incubator at 28–30°C. Hatch in approx. 60 days. Hatchling size 15 cm	Diurnal Requires good ultraviolet UVB and florescent lighting. Tall vivarium, as arboreal. Need high daytime temperature 28.9–31.1°C, night-time temperatures of between 23.9–26.7°C Life span 10–15 years
Uromastyx or dab lizard (*Uromastyx acanthinurus*)	Northwest Africa, Southwest Asia	Collard greens, dandelions, leafy salad, grated roots vegetables ie. Carrots, lentils, seeds as given to small psittacine birds including safflower seeds occasional insect as a treat once a month Vitamin and mineral supplement	Oviparous. Sexually mature 18–24 months of age; in the wild 4 years Gestation average 4 weeks. Lay 10–12 eggs. Incubate eggs 60–80 days at 33–34°C Provide a laying box in the vivarium mix of sand and moss	Diurnal Average life span 15–20 years but possible 30 years Temperature 45°C in the basking area, dropping to approximately 30°C in the cooler area. Providing a temperature gradient for lizard to thermoregulate. Night temperature can drop as low as 16°C Require good UVB lighting; 12–14-hour light cycle Nasal salt glands excrete excess sodium

Continued

TABLE 33.11	Common reptilian species kept as pets in the UK—cont'd			
Species	**Country of origin**	**Food**	**Reproductive data**	**Additional comments**
Chameleons				
Veiled Chameleon (*Chamaeleo calyptratus*) Panther chameleon (*Chamaeleo pardalis*)	Yemen, in the southwestern region of the Saudi Arabian peninsula Madagascar	Insectivores offer gut-loaded insects such as crickets, mealworms, waxworms, silkworms. Veiled chameleons also enjoy blossoms and leaves such as hibiscus, romaine lettuce and dandelions Panther: Insectivorous: crickets, hoppers, locusts, silkworms, waxworms. Make sure you feed gut-loaded insects with vitamin and mineral supplement advised	Sexual maturity is reached between 4–8 months but only recommend breeding from a healthy female in good body condition, weighing about 65–90 g. Early breeding before she has reached 1 year old often leads dystocia and premature death. Veiled chameleons lay clutches of 30 to 60 oval eggs 20 to 30 days after mating Female veiled chameleons can retain sperm and may produce a second clutch 90 to 120 days after the first, even if not mated again Provide a laying box with moist substrate such as vermiculite Incubation period 165–200 days at 27°C Panther: Gestation is 20 to 30 days approximately 10 to 15 days after mating, the female can fast until she lays eggs. Average clutch is 20 eggs but can range from 10 to 40. Incubation in a sealed container with damp vermiculite for 8 to 12 months at a temperature range 18–27°C degrees, Humidity should be approximately 80–90%	Life span: Females 3–5 years; male 4–6 years. Veiled: May live up to 6–7 years Panther: 5–7 years Fascinating species. Arboreal and require tall vivarium. Can suffer from stress if housing is incorrect. Veiled: Maintain a temperature gradient of 20–35°C using an overhead radiant heat source. Provide a 5–8°C drop in temperature at night Maintain 40–60% relative humidity. Panther: Temperature 24–32°C with a basking spot that reaches 35°C. Cage temperature may drop to 18–21°C at night Humidity 60–80%. As most species will not drink from water bowl, provide water either by misting the plants every 4–8 hours or use an automatic watering system. Highly territorial, so best kept on their own or one male with females, but fighting may still occur
Iguanas				
Green iguana (*Iguana iguana*)	Central America to northern regions of South America	Herbivores offer wide variety of dark, leafy greens should make up the majority of the adult diet. Offer a variety including collard greens, kale, romaine, dandelion greens. Mix greens with other chopped or grated vegetables like squash, sweet potato, broccoli, peas, and carrots Fruit should make up no more than 5% of the diet and should include papaya, melon Occasional treats may consist of non-toxic flower blossoms such as hibiscus Vitamin and mineral supplementation essential as they suffer from MBD	Oviparous: 20–40 eggs per clutch; hatch after 10–15 weeks	Very large lizard Life span 15–20 years; 100–200 cm in length. Needs tall vivarium and males can be very aggressive. Temperature 27–31°C the basking spot should reach 33–35°C Require a UVB light Humidity and water provide a large sturdy bathing area as they often soak in their water bowl and can defecate in their water. Lguanas should be misted daily with warm water Due to size and demands of the animal, not an ideal pet

TABLE 33.11	Common reptilian species kept as pets in the UK—cont'd				
Species	**Country of origin**	**Food**	**Reproductive data**	**Additional comments**
Monitors/tegus				
Savannah monitor (*Varanus exanthematicus*)	Savannahs of Eastern and southern Africa	Carnivore. In the wild monitors are scavengers In captivity feed a range of gut-loaded insects such as large crickets, large mealworms, silkworms, cooked eggs and chicks. Rodents such as mice or rats may be offered, but these lizards are prone to obesity and care should be taken not too overfeed and adults only require feeding 2–3 times per week	Oviparous – limited. Most sourced in the UK are wild caught or captive farmed. Captive breeding requires specialist facilities that will encourage many complex behaviours, such as mating, nest digging and egg laying and seems to be limited to the most experienced keeper	Life span 5–10 plus years Very large, heavy-bodied lizard; can grow to 1–1.5 m. Temperature 29–32°C with a basking of 34–38°C with a night-time drop of 23–26°C Daily access to fresh drinking water as well as access to a larger soaking area allows lizard to bathe 1–2 times weekly for several hours. Humidity 40–50% relative humidity, can mist the cage
Skinks				
Blue-tongued skink (*Tiliqua gigas*)	Australasia	Blue-tongued skinks are omnivores. Need a wide variety of foods: The bulk of the diet (45–60%) should consist of greens such as dark, leafy greens like kale, dandelion and collard greens. Also offer a protein source such as gut-loaded crickets, mealworms, snails, and the occasional pinky. Some skinks may also accept earthworms. Feed adults every 1–2 days. Vitamin and mineral supplements should be added to meals	Viviparous: blue-tongued skinks are usually sexually mature by 2–3 years of age Litter size 5–10. Gestation period varies according to background temperature usually between 6 months to 1 year	Life span 20 plus years Adults reach 30–38 cm in length Generally good-natured and can make good pets. Males can become aggressive during breeding season Temperature range 21–29°C and a basking spot of 33–38°C Will need access to UVB lighting Humidity: 30% relative humidity Fresh drinking water should always be easily accessible
CHELONIA				
Mediterranean tortoises				
Spur-thighed tortoise (Greek) (*Testudo graeca*)	Several sub species that makes taxonomy complex. Range around Spain, Morocco, Algeria, Tunisia, Turkey, Iran, Israel	Herbivores and feed a high fibre, low fat and protein diet supplemented with vitamin and mineral powders. All species can eat a wide range of weeds and green vegetation, such as dandelions, sow thistle, plantains, vetch, mallows, clovers, groundsel Hibiscus flowers Fruits should make up no more than 5% of diet, and salad-based diets kept to a minimum and used when other plant sources limited. Cuttlefish should be provided as tortoise will eat this and aid with addition calcium and beak health	All species are Oviparous and females must be in good health: gestation period 30 days to 3 years. Females can retain sperm. Female can be observed digging several holes. Lay between 5–10 eggs Incubate 28–32°C Hatch 8–12 weeks temperature dependant	With the exception of Horsfield's tortoise (*Testudo horsfieldii*), which is not truly a Mediterranean tortoise, all are protected under CITES legislation and are classified as appendix II. This means that they require DEFRA licence via an article 10 certificate in order to be bought, sold or traded Note: Egyptian tortoise (*Testudo kleinmanni*) is illegal to trade and subject to intense conservation efforts (Jessop and Bennett 2010) All species live in excess of 80-plus years Housing: it's recommended to keep tortoises in a tortoise table with appropriate heating and UVB lighting

Continued

TABLE 33.11	Common reptilian species kept as pets in the UK—cont'd			
Species	**Country of origin**	**Food**	**Reproductive data**	**Additional comments**
Hermann's tortoise (*Testudo hermanni*)	Two subspecies: western Hermann's range from Spain through the south of France to western Italy	As above	Nests before finally laying 3–12 eggs. Depending on temperature and species, eggs need to be incubated for 7–20 weeks at 30–34°C. Sex can be determined by temperature – higher produces females, lower produces males	
Marginated tortoise (*Testudo marginata*)	Greece and its islands			
Horsfield's tortoise (*Testudo horsfieldii*)	Two subspecies: between them range is Iran, Afghanistan, Kazakhstan	As above	Female lay between 2–5 eggs in a clutch, incubated on moist vermiculite at 30°C at 80% humidity. Hatchling should appear within 80–100 days	Escape artists will attempt the great escape by digging and climb out of the garden Do not tolerate damp conditions
East and West African terrestrial chelonian				
Bell's hinge-back tortoise (*Kinixys belliana*)	Five subspecies identified. Wide range in tropical and subtropical Africa and occurs in savannah habitats	Needs a balanced diet of 50% vegetables and fruit and 50% meat. Foods range from salad leaves, tomato, cucumber, fruits such as banana, melon, peach, grapes and other soft fruits. Invertebrates such as mealworms, earthworms, cricket. Dog or cat food. Supplement diet with vitamins and minerals	Clutches of 1–3 eggs	These have a hinge across the rear portion of the carapace, which slopes down steeply from the middle of the fifth vertebra. Newly hatched young show no sign of a hinge. As they are a tropical species they do not hibernate – keep at temperature of 30°C plus
Leopard tortoise (*Geochelone pardalis*)	The leopard tortoise's range extends from Sudan through to Ethiopia and throughout southern Africa. There are two identified subspecies, *G p pardalis* and *G p babcocki*.	Graze on grasses and vegetation. They require a high-fibre diet rich in calcium–fruit should be no more than about 5% of the overall diet	Clutches of 5–20 eggs laid in nests dug by female. Can take 6–18 months to hatch depending on temperature	Leopard tortoises live between 50 and 100 years in the wild. Large specimens can weigh up to 36 kg with an average 10–15 kg, shell length between 40 and 50 cm. Require high temperatures – 30–35°C. Good UVB lighting Do not hibernate
North American species				
American box turtle (tortoise) (*Terrapene carolina*)	Four subspecies and range from south-eastern, eastern and southwestern USA	Omnivores, eat a mixture of meats and vegetable matter approximately 60–70% of the adult diet should be made up of vegetables. Feed invertebrates, fruits and leafy vegetables small quantities of low fat dog or cat food, plus vitamin and mineral supplementation	Mating occurs post-hibernation. Lays clutches of 2–7 eggs. Eggs need high humidity	Life span in captivity with good care 50–60 years. Grow to 11–20 cm in length The daytime temperature gradient should range from 24–29°C with a 50 night-time temperature drop Box turtles require a relative humidity of 60–80%. This can be achieved by frequent misting of the enclosure. They require access to water for bathing and an area of dry land for basking and burrowing. UVB lighting required. Will hibernate for short period but must be in good health

TABLE 33.11	Common reptilian species kept as pets in the UK—cont'd			
Species	**Country of origin**	**Food**	**Reproductive data**	**Additional comments**
South American tortoises				
Red-footed tortoise (*Geochelone carbonaria*)	Tropical South America	Red-footed tortoises are omnivores. They will eat carrion and invertebrates such as slugs and snails. 75% of the diet should consist of dark leafy greens mix with small quantities of chopped vegetables and fruits. They enjoy banana, mango, and papaya. Animal protein can be provided by offering soaking dried dog food, pinkies and cleansed earthworms, vitamin/mineral supplement added to diet.	Lays clutches of 5–13 eggs. Eggs require high humidity. If ideal conditions maintained, hatching takes about 4 months	Life span 25–35 years but higher is possible. Temperature 26–29°C and a basking spot that reaches 32°C with a 50 night-time temperature drop. They require full spectrum UVB lighting. As they come from areas of high humidity they can easily dehydrate so need daily bathing. Do not hibernate. Maturity reached at about 15 years or when animal reaches 20–30 cm in length
Indian star tortoise (*Geochelone elegans*)	Arid lands – India, Pakistan and Sri Lanka	Diet high in fibre, low in protein, high in calcium and low in phosphorus. Like to graze. Offer dried grass (readi-grass or just-grass) softened with water and mixed with grated vegetables Weeds such as dandelion, wild rocket, plantain, sow thistle and hibiscus flowers. Vitamin and mineral supplementation is required	See information for Leopard tortoise	Very attractive tortoise with a beautifully patterned shell Daytime temps of 28–30°C, with a basking spot to reach mid 30°C; night temperature drop to 20°C; require good full-spectrum UVB lighting Indian stars like to bathe in warm water and enjoy frequent misting
Turtles and terrapins (American)				
Red-eared terrapin (*Trachemys scripta elegans*)	Eastern USA to Mexico	Omnivores eat a wide range of meat, fish, invertebrates, pinkies, dried cat food, some vegetable matter. Vitamin and mineral supplements	Captive-farmed in country of origin and lay up to 12 eggs	Life span ranges from 15–25 plus years, aquatic but need access to land and basking area 28–30°C. Water temperature 24–30°C. Now a real problem in the UK, having been released into ponds and rivers, where they are having an effect on native species. Can carry salmonella. Grow up to 30 cm
Alligator snapping turtle (*Macrochelys temminckii*)	Southeast USA	Meat, small rodents, invertebrates, fish and some vegetable matter Requires vitamin and mineral supplement	Lay up to 50 eggs per clutch	Very large, heavy-bodied chelonian with a dubious temperament, so must be handled with care. Do not hibernate

Stones. Make sure that stones or large, heavy objects in the vivarium have a flat, smooth base to prevent them from rolling onto the reptile and causing injury.

Feeding equipment. Large, heavy ceramic bowls provide drinking water and a bathing facility.

Basking and swimming areas. Aquatic and semi-aquatic species, e.g. terrapins and box tortoises, need an area in which to swim (Fig. 33.16) and an area in which to bask – this should take up approximately one-third of the tank, leaving the rest as water. There should also be a filtration system to prevent the water becoming stagnant and polluted – if the water is not filtered it must be changed daily.

Plants. If living, these may provide humidity and a place to hide. They also look nice but are difficult to keep clean. Be warned – lizards will ingest plants and, if these are made of plastic or silk, they can cause intestinal impaction and will not show up on X-ray.

Vivarium conditions. Once a suitable vivarium has been selected there are four main factors to consider:

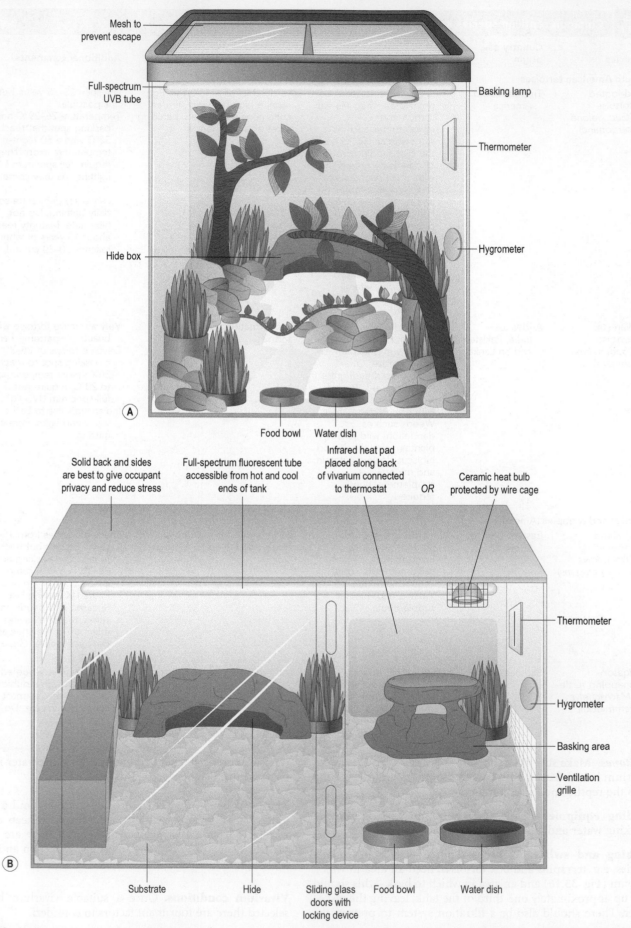

Fig. 33.14 (A) Schematic plan of a typical vivarium for an arboreal species. (B) Schematic plan of a typical vivarium for a terrestrial species

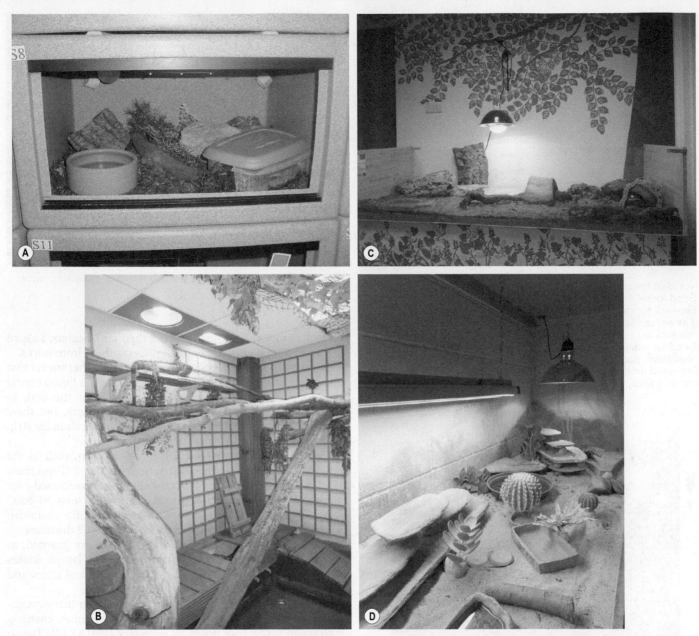

Fig. 33.15 Vivaria. (A) Vivarium suitable for a terrestrial snake. (B) Large walk-in vivarium suitable for a large arboreal lizard such as a green iguana (*Iguana iguana*). (C) Table-top design for a Mediterranean. (D) Desert set-up for two Chuckwallas (*Sauromalus ater*) (*all courtesy of Plumpton College Sussex.*)

1. Ventilation. This is achieved by positioning holes at the back or sides of the cage. To achieve a good through-flow of air and prevent draughts, vents should be placed opposite each other but at different levels, e.g. one at the top and one at the bottom. The holes should not allow the reptile to escape and may need to be covered in wire mesh.

2. Heating. This is essential, and an understanding of reptile biology is important. As ectotherms, reptiles rely on external heat sources to warm up their internal body temperature. All reptiles have a preferred body temperature (PBT) or preferred optimum temperature zone (POTZ), which relates to the optimum temperature that the species requires for its metabolism to function correctly, i.e. movement, feeding, digestion, enzyme activity, reproduction, etc. This temperature must be achieved within the vivarium.

Vivarium temperatures must take into account the species of reptile and its POTZ. Many species require hotter or cooler temperatures depending on the time of year, so the individual species' requirements must be researched, but temperature guidelines are:

- Tropical species – 26.5–37°C (80–98.5°F)
- Temperate species – 24–29.5°C (75–85°F).

The most common forms of heat source are:

- Ceramic
- Tube heaters and cable
- Reflector bulbs with or without UVB content
- Heat mats and rocks*
- Radiant background heating
- Aquarium heaters (as used by fish keepers) – for aquatic and semi-aquatic chelonia. As aquatic species are very

TABLE 33.12	Substrates and materials suitable for vivaria	
Material for vivarium construction	**Substrate**
Melamine chip board*	Peat† and peat substitutes Coco Brick natural sustainable coconut husk
Moulded plastics‡	Wood chip§
Glass tanks¶	Vermiculite†
Marine plywood	Bark chips
Fibreglass‡	Reptile carpet
Plastic tanks (fauna boxes)	Repti/calci sand (for desert species)‖
Small plastic tubs (hatchling snakes)	Newspaper Cypress mulch Gravel Alfalfa pellets Aspen bedding Sphagnum moss†

*Not ideal for species requiring high humidity.
†Good for retaining moisture and humidity.
‡Excellent for cleaning – can be jet-washed.
§If eaten, can cause gut impaction or get stuck in mouth, so should be avoided.
¶Good for aquatic species and species requiring high humidity. Poor insulation, poor security, difficult to attach fittings.
‖Only sand produced specifically for reptiles should be used as others contain silica, which will dehydrate the animal.

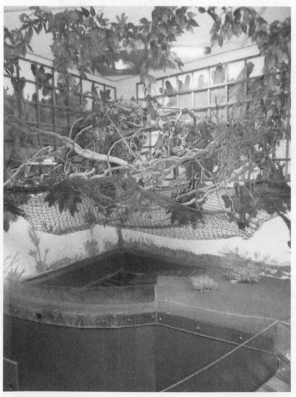

Fig. 33.16 Terrapin enclosure demonstrating provision of swimming and basking areas and above a free-range Panther chameleon (*Furcifer pardalis*) set-up

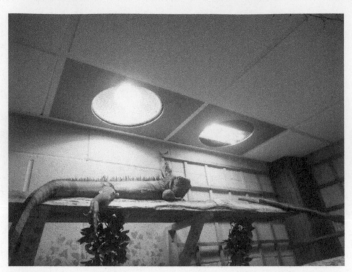

Fig. 33.17 Female green iguana (*Iguana iguana*) basking under a mercury vapour heat lamp

clumsy and frequently break their tank heaters, a guard should be fitted. This also protects them from burns.

Most good tank heaters will be fitted with a thermostat that allows adjustments to the temperature settings. A liquid crystal thermometer can be placed on the outside of the tank to monitor the ambient temperature inside the tank, but these thermometers need replacing yearly as the chemicals in the strip thermometers become exhausted.

For those species that require a basking area, such as the red-eared terrapin (*Trachemys scripta elegans*), a full-spectrum UVB basking lamp with a reflector should be positioned over an area of 'land' and reach temperatures of at least 30–35°C (86–95°F). The provision of such an area allows the chelonian to bask and prevents respiratory disease and shell disorders.

Make sure that all heat and light sources are guarded, as reptiles can suffer serious burns from sitting on lamps. Snakes and lizards have few nerve endings in their ventral scales and will not realise that they are roasting themselves.

The vivarium set-up must allow the reptile to thermoregulate by moving between different temperature zones, enabling it to warm up or cool down as necessary (Fig. 33.17). This is achieved by careful positioning of the heat source(s), creating a temperature gradient between hot and cool spots within the vivarium and allowing the reptile to control its body temperature at different times of the day. The temperature gradient is regulated by the use of thermostats and thermometers – at least two thermometers are required positioned at opposite ends of the enclosure to measure the gradient. Digital thermometers with maximum-minimum function give a good overview of the range of temperatures reached. Thermostats help to regulate temperature and can control daytime and night-time heating, but are not suitable for all types of heating. A useful addition is a digital infrared temperature gun that can be used to accurately assess surface temperatures.

---

*When using heat mats be careful to check placement as some are suitable for inside or outside only; also a reptile can dig underneath a heat mat to cool down and this can result in burns to the animal (Eatwell 2010). Heat rocks look attractive but only serve to provide heat in a focused area and can again lead to burns (Eatwell 2010).

Overheating the reptile can be just as detrimental to its health as underheating. For the POTZ of individual species, refer to specialist books. Sick or injured reptiles will seek out the high ranges of their POTZ to aid their immune system. Drug absorption and utilisation is influenced by the species' POTZ, so when reptiles are receiving medication or anaesthetics the provision of heat is essential.

3. Lighting. There several types of lighting used for reptiles depending on their needs:

- Incandescent bulbs, e.g. light bulbs, coloured light bulbs, halogen lamps
- Fluorescent tubes with UVB and UVA content
- Mercury vapour lamps (high-intensity discharge [HID] lamps)
- Metal halide lamps (HID lamps).

Lighting provides the reptile with a photoperiod, i.e. the amount of light in a normal day, and stimulates natural behaviour, e.g. basking, eating, reproduction. The amount of light depends on the species' native environment and the time of year. For example, a tropical species will require on average a 13-hour day/11-hour night summer cycle and an 11-hour day/13-hour night winter cycle, each lasting 6 months. Temperate climate species should be on a four-season cycle that provides 15 hours of daylight during the summer, 12 hours during the spring and autumn and 9 hours during the winter (Mader et al. 2006).

A **full-spectrum light** is one that mimics the rays produced by the sun and includes UV light. Sunlight produces UV light, which can be separated into UVA, which stimulates behavioural and physiological effects, and UVB, necessary for calcium metabolism and the activation of vitamin D. UVC is not used in reptile husbandry and presents a risk to both reptile and human.

A full-spectrum UV light is important for all diurnal, tropical, subtropical and desert lizards and chelonian, with benefits seen in some snakes, invertebrates and crepuscular reptiles. In an ideal situation we would allow our captive reptiles to bask in natural sunlight outdoors, but the majority of captive reptiles are kept indoors in a controlled environment and we have to supply an artificial light source. The UV requirement of reptiles and chelonian varies according to their wild habitats and behaviour.

UVB lights do not have an infinite life span and, although the white light may still be seen the UVB content is generally exhausted within an average of 6 months of use. For satisfactory vitamin D₃ synthesis the UVB lighting needs to be on for sufficient hours per day and correctly positioned approximately above the reptile. The height should be measured from where the rays will strike the animal, not from the base of the cage as UVB lighting diminishes with distance. The height should be reduced for young animals to maximise UVB utilisation. Replace UVB lights every 3–6 months if young growing stock are kept.

Fluorescent UVB-emitting tubes come in two forms: those that require similar set-ups to the tube lights used in the home, i.e. fixture and ballast controller, and compact fluorescent lamps with internal electronic ballast. They produce limited heat and are available in a range of UVB levels, which makes them very versatile.

Mercury vapour lamps produce heat, light and UVB at a greater intensity and because they get very hot are generally not suitable for smaller enclosures, and distance between reptile and heat source should be carefully monitored to prevent overheating and thermal burns. Their UVB content lasts longer but they cannot be thermostatically controlled.

Metal halide lamps provide high-intensity light with UVB but lower levels of heat which makes them a better choice for smaller vivaria, but they cannot be thermostatically controlled. These bulbs are not routinely used in chelonian habitats (Bennett and Jessop 2010).

A point to factor in when selecting suitable UVB lighting is that UV rays cannot pass through glass or plastic, and efficiency is reduced when passing through wire; therefore UV lights have to be placed inside the enclosure or provide the reptile with access to direct sunlight.

If UVB light is the primary source of heat and light it may not produce sufficient heat to radiate across the vivarium, which may cause the occupant to increase its basking times and result in localised thermal or UV burns (Rendle and Cracknell 2012).

UVB index meters are a very useful way of assessing the output of UVB being emitted by the lighting system.

If full-spectrum lights are used, check the UVB content as they may just contain UVA.

There has been research based on how species use light and shade in the wild and how to re-create this in the captive environment. It is similar to achieving a thermal gradient, i.e. a higher temperature at one end of the vivarium and a lower temperature at the other, but substituting heat for light (Courteney-Smith 2013).

4. Humidity. This is the amount of moisture in the air. The humidity requirements will depend on the natural habitat of the species; for example, a rainforest species will require a higher humidity than a desert species. Most species do well at a relative humidity of 50–70%. The humidity can be increased by frequent spraying of the vivarium using a plant mister, or by placing damp sphagnum moss or tissue paper in a small ice cream tub or plastic sandwich container. Correct humidity is necessary to allow normal ecdysis (shedding of the skin). Decreasing ventilation should not be used as a means of increasing humidity, as this can lead to an increase in fungal disease.

When caring for a reptile within a veterinary practice it is essential to monitor the environment of the patient. Figure 33.18 shows a suggested format for a hospital chart.

Nutrition and feeding

Reptiles present a wide spectrum of nutritional challenges because there is little information about what they eat in the wild and we can only assume, rightly or wrongly, that what we offer the captive reptile goes some way to mimicking its natural diet.

Snakes. All snakes are carnivores and consume a wide variety of prey including mammals, birds, reptiles, amphibians, eggs and fish, but in captivity it is most common to feed rodents. Whatever the food item fed it should be offered whole (Fig. 33.19).

Guidelines:

- Always select a food item that is as near as possible to the animal's wild diet, e.g. offer brown mice rather than white mice.
- Select prey items that the snake can swallow – as a guide, select a prey item that is no larger than the biggest part of the snake's body (Cheek et al. 2010) (Fig. 33.20).
- If offering frozen foods, defrost first. There are various approaches to this – some texts recommend removing the prey item directly from the freezer and submerging

Animal details	**Owner details**
Name	Name
Species and details Sex/age	Address
Preferred temperature zone and humidity	
Diet preference	Tel no.

Date	Temp am/pm B baskirg C cool end AM PM				Humidity % Indicate if sprayed		Food offered Amount (F) Water offered (W)		Food eaten Amount	Urate faeces passed AM and PM **Comment**	Signs of shedding AM and PM **Comment**	Hygiene Spot clean Total clean	Comment signature
	B	C	B	C	AM	PM	F	W 4					

Fig. 33.18 Suggested husbandry sheet to monitor the environment and nutrition of the reptilian patient

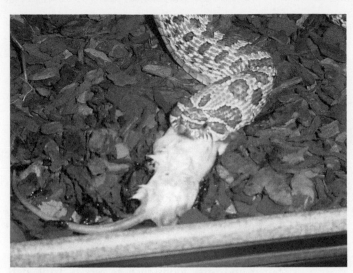

Fig. 33.19 Hognose snake eating a dead mouse

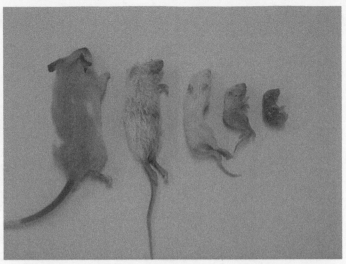

Fig. 33.20 Various sizes of dead rodent prey used to feed snakes and carnivorous lizards

the frozen food item in warm but not boiling water. Once it is completely defrosted and at a roughly mammalian body temperature (Rendle and Cracknell 2012), the item will need to be dried and offered immediately to the snake.

- Alternatively, allow frozen food items to defrost overnight in a fridge in a sealed container away from human foods and once defrosted warm by sealing the food item in a plastic bag, and then immersing the bag into warm but not boiling water until the prey item has reached the correct temperature (Cheek et al. 2010).
- It is best not to leave the frozen prey item to defrost at room temperature as this prolongs the process and can attract flies and cause autolysis (Rendle and Cracknell 2012).
- Offer the warmed dead prey head first, using feeding tongs, as this will keep human smell off the food and will help to prevent the feeder from being bitten.
- It may be necessary to wriggle the food item slightly in front of the snake to stimulate the strike response – this method is especially helpful with reluctant feeders or arboreal species.
- To prevent accidental cannibalism, never feed snakes together. They will try and consume the same prey item.
- To prevent regurgitation, once the snake has accepted its prey item it should be left alone and not handled for 24–48 hours.
- Snakes are opportunistic feeders and do not require feeding every day; they may have periods of fasting.
- It must be noted that due to the lack of energy used for food finding and high fat content of most rodent prey items fed, obesity is rapidly becoming a problem in captive snakes.
- Frequency of feeding will depend on the age of the snake and the species. For example, boids such as Common Boa (*Boa constrictor imperator*) and Rainbow boa (*Epicrates cenchria*) have a slower metabolism than colubrids such as Corn snake (*Pantherophis guttatus guttatus*). As boids reach adulthood, the frequency of feeding should be gradually decreased to one meal every 2–4 weeks – a good rule of thumb is that defecation should occur after every third meal (Raiti 2010).

- Any uneaten prey should be removed from the cage within a few hours of being offered and not left in overnight. Thawed frozen tissue decomposes rapidly after thawing (Wilson 2010).
- There is no need to feed live vertebrate prey in the UK, as most captive snakes will readily eat dead prey; anyone found feeding live vertebrates could be prosecuted under the Animal Welfare Act 2006.
- When feeding raw fish to snakes such as the garter snake, the fish must be blanched in hot water for approximately 10 minutes to destroy the antivitamin thiaminase. This will destroy the B vitamin thiamine and cause a deficiency presenting as convulsions and loss of the righting reflex.

Do not feed a snake:

- Before an anaesthetic
- When it is shedding or moulting
- When it is in brumation (hibernation) or getting ready for brumation.

Lizards. Lizards present more of a challenge when trying to meet their dietary demands and their feeding habits can be classified as:

- Carnivorous – eating whole prey items such as rodents, birds, amphibians and other small lizards (see Fig. 33.20)
- Insectivorous – eating a range of invertebrates such as crickets, locusts, mealworms and waxworms (Fig. 33.21)
- Herbivorous – eating a range of plant, fruit and vegetable matter
- Omnivorous – eating a mixture of both vegetation and animal matter.

Guidelines: first investigate whether the lizard is carnivorous, herbivorous, etc. (see Table 33.11).

1. **Herbivores**, e.g. green iguana (*Iguana iguana*), uromastix (*Uromastyx acanthinurus*)
   - Offer a variety of fresh, leafy vegetables, fruits, etc. to meet the lizard's needs (see Table 33.11), e.g. a green iguana up to 2 years of age must be offered a diet consisting of 80% green leafy matter and 20% fruit and

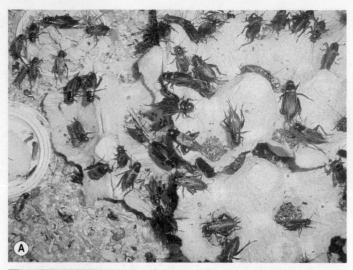

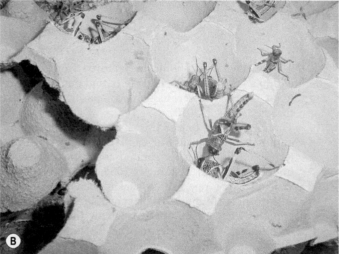

Fig. 33.21 (A) Black crickets suitable for insectivorous lizards; they are more nutritious and easier for the lizard to catch. (B) Locusts are available in various sizes; care must be taken when feeding large locusts as the barbs on their hind limbs can penetrate the mouth or digestive tract

root vegetables; a green iguana over 2 years should be provided with a diet consisting of 95% green leafy matter and 5% fruits and roots.

- Always ensure all foods offered are fresh, free from pesticides and thoroughly washed. If food is taken from the fridge, allow it to reach room temperature before offering it to the lizard.
- Apply necessary supplement to food (see Table 33.11). A range of calcium supplements are available. It is possible to overdose and cause metabolic bone problems and calcification of soft tissues when supplementing with preparations that contain added vitamin D_3 and minerals. The frequency of supplementation depends on the frequency of feeding but, as a general rule, calcium carbonate powder can be added to each meal, whereas powders that contain vitamin D_3 and other supplements should be offered once/twice a week.
- Supplementation of vitamin D_3 should not be used to overcome inadequate provision of UVB lighting – if correctly positioned UVB lighting is provided and replaced at appropriate times, vitamin D_3 synthesis

should be adequate and over-supplementation of vitamin D_3 will harm the lizard.
- All food should be of an appropriate size so that the animal can easily ingest it.
- Take care when offering addictive foods, e.g. banana, as this encourages selective feeding, leading to dietary imbalance.

2. **Insectivores**, e.g. leopard gecko (*Eublepharus macularius*), Chinese water dragon (*Physignathus cocincinus*). These species eat a range of live invertebrate foods (see Fig. 33.21):
   - When selecting foods, make sure they are of appropriate size for the lizard to catch and consume.
   - Before feeding newly purchased live foods, e.g. crickets and locusts, the following steps should be carried out (commonly referred to as gut loading):
     a. Place the live insects in an escape-proof plastic container and offer foods such as cereals, fruit, dark green leafy vegetables and water. To prevent insects from drowning, offer water by soaking cotton wool and placing it in a small dish. Withhold feeding for a minimum of 48 hours to ensure the invertebrates are fully rehydrated and nourished. Keep invertebrates in a warm, well-ventilated room. Many commercially sold invertebrate foods are kept on bran, which is high in phosphorus and contributes further to the poor calcium-to-phosphorus ratio. There are also commercial gut loading products available on the market.
     b. Once live food has been nourished, it is important to dust it with a calcium or vitamin and mineral supplement by shaking it in a pot of supplement. Many invertebrate food species offered have an inverse calcium-to-phosphorus ratio. Ideally, calcium should be offered in the diet at a higher calcium-to-phosphorus ratio, otherwise calcium will be removed from the animal's own stores, causing metabolic bone disease and, in breeding animals, poorly calcified eggs and dystocia. The rules for frequency of supplementation are as for herbivore nutrition.
     c. The food can then be placed in the vivarium.
   - One of the problems associated with dusting live prey is that much of the supplement can fall off the prey before it is consumed and it is difficult to monitor exactly how much of the supplement the lizard ingests. A tip is to chill the live food in a refrigerator for a few minutes. This will slow the insect down and give the reptile an opportunity to catch the prey plus supplement.
   - Feed as many insects as the lizard will eat at once. Do not add too many crickets, etc., to the vivarium, and any uneaten food should be removed as the live food could actually feed on the cage occupants if they get hungry.

3. **Carnivores**, e.g. monitor (*Varanus* spp.), tegu (*Tupinambis* spp.)
   - The reptiles will eat a range of prey items ranging from rodents to other small lizards, which should be offered whole. This reduces the need to supplement unless the animal is ill.
   - Frozen foods must be prepared and offered as described under snake nutrition.

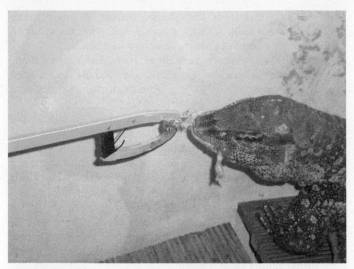

Fig. 33.22 Nile monitor lizard eating a dead rat; note the use of long graspers for the safety of the handler feeding the lizard

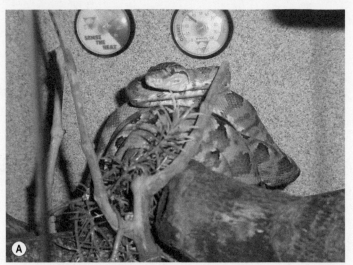

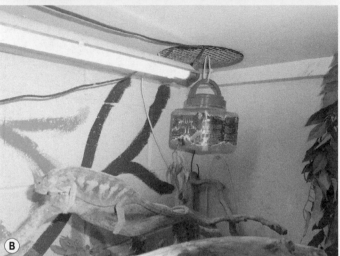

Fig. 33.23 (A) Cooks tree boa (*Corallus caninus*). Tree pythons or boas require daily spraying as they prefer to drink water that has accumulated in their coils. (B) Chameleon enclosure with water dispenser to allow more natural access to water; also observe the positioning of the strip light to give a light shade gradient

- Caution must be taken to prevent injury when offering food to large lizards, especially the monitor family: tongs or graspers must be used (Fig. 33.22).
- Frequency of feeding will depend on the lizard's species age and size. As a guide, smaller or growing lizards should be fed daily; mature or larger species should be fed 2–3 times a week.

4. **Omnivores**, e.g. bearded dragon (*Pogona vitticeps*), skink (*Tiliqua gigas*), plated lizard (*Gerrhosaurus* spp.). This group of lizards will eat a variety of animal and plant matter, so previous information applies.

Feeding summary

- 'Variety is the spice of life' and the reptile should be offered a varied and balanced diet. This is limited for the carnivorous species, but the common boa (*Boa constrictor*) will appreciate a dead gerbil now and again.
- Always feed dead vertebrates. It is inhumane and potentially illegal to feed live ones, and live rodents could actually attack the snake or lizard, inflicting nasty wounds and causing distress to the cage occupant.
- The quality of vertebrate and invertebrate prey will depend on its age, the way it has been fed and its health status.
- It is not acceptable to use wild rodents as food, as they may carry disease and parasites. If collecting wild invertebrates, make sure they are non-toxic and free from pesticides.
- There are a variety of commercially prepared diets on the market and these can make up part of but not the entire diet.
- Non-reptilian foods are not advised because they have been manufactured for animals with different nutritional needs, metabolic processes and stress levels.
- Even if excellent diets are provided for the reptile, if the environmental conditions are incorrect and optimum lighting, humidity and temperature are not available, the lizard or snake will not be able to reach its POTZ and its metabolic processes will be severely compromised, resulting in non-digestion of food or anorexia. Any undigested food in the gut will cause massive bacterial overgrowth, with potentially fatal consequences.

Water. Snakes and lizards require access to clean water at all times:

- For snakes, the water bowl must be large enough to allow the snake to submerge itself in the water. This also helps when the snake is shedding.
- Tropical or arboreal snakes such as the Cooks Tree Boa (*Corallus caninus*) (Fig. 33.23A) or green tree python (*Chondrophython viridis*) require daily misting with lukewarm water. The spray should be a fine mist directed toward the snake's head, allowing it to drink the water as it drips off or collects in its tight coils. Their entire body should be sprayed daily to keep them from becoming too dry, which may result in dysecdysis (difficulty in shedding).
- Non-tropical arboreal species and terrestrial species should only be misted if they are getting ready to shed.
- Some lizards, e.g. arboreal species such as anoles, day geckos and some chameleons, will not drink water from a bowl, preferring to take their water in the form of droplets off a leaf (Fig. 33.23B). Most chameleons need to be 'rained on' daily and some species need to feel the dripping

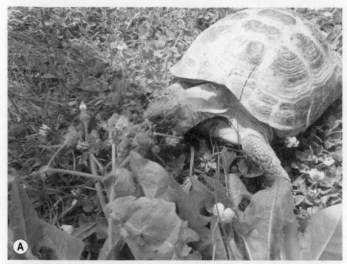

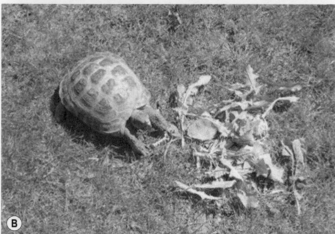

Fig. 33.24 Horsfield's tortoise (*Testudo horsfieldii*) eating a range of weeds and flowers

water before they will attempt to drink. There are several methods:

- Mist the foliage in the vivarium using a handheld spray.
- Set up an elaborate misting system.
- Adapt a drip system so that droplets fall on a leaf or branch – to prevent the substrate from becoming saturated, place a receptacle under the drip tube to collect excess water.
- No water bowl should be so deep that the species is unable to climb out; small pieces of slate can be angled in the bowl to allow small lizards a way into and out of the water.
- If insects are being fed, small stones should be placed in the bottom of the bowl to prevent the insects from drowning and contaminating the water.
- Water containers should be cleaned and water replenished daily, or more often if contaminated with faeces and urates.

Tortoises

Mediterranean tortoises. These common species of tortoise (see Table 33.11) are opportunistic feeders and their natural terrain is sparsely vegetated and infertile. Their natural diet consists of a variety of plant materials – leaves, flowers and fruits (Fig. 33.24).

In captivity the basic diet should consist of low-protein, high-fibre foods with a high mineral and vitamin content, together with a large quantity of calcium carbonate:

- Suitable wild plants – dandelions, sow thistle, clover, plantains, vetch, mallows, hibiscus spp.; edible weed seed can be purchased from specialist tortoise clubs and associations.
- Grass is not digested by the tortoise, so has no nutritional valve except to add bulk and fibre to the diet.
- Green vegetables – e.g. cabbage, watercress, cress, spinach, broccoli. Many cultivated vegetables are high in protein and low in fibre. Most tortoises readily take salad foods such as tomatoes, cucumber and lettuce, but their nutritional value is limited and they should be used to enhance the palatability of the food rather than making up the entire diet. Prepacked mixed salad leaves give the tortoise a range of different leaves and can help the overall nutritional value (Table 33.13).
- Fruits – only small quantities should be fed; ideally, no more than 5% of the total diet should come from fruits, which can be addictive and cause obesity.
- Proprietary foods – dried pelleted foods are available but most are unsuitable to feed and are best avoided as they can lead to nutritional problems.
- Meat products – not recommended, as protein levels in meat are far too high and can lead to severe metabolic and organ problems.
- Dairy products – not recommended: if they are offered the liver may be affected.
- Vitamins and minerals – in the wild diet the levels of vitamins and mineral would be higher than in the diet provided in captivity, so supplementation is necessary:
  - Calcium carbonate should be liberally sprinkled over the diet – it is better to slightly over-supplement than under-supplement. Providing cuttlefish bone for chelonia to gnaw is a good way of getting calcium into the animal and helps to prevent the beak from overgrowing.
  - Vitamin A – a deficiency may lead to swollen eyes and loss of appetite, as the animal cannot see its food.
  - Vitamin D_3 – if this is deficient, calcium absorption from the intestines is affected. If in excess, it can cause excessive calcium uptake and calcification of soft tissues.
- Water – a constant supply of water should be available and a daily bath in 3–4 cm of warm water for 5–10 minutes will allow the tortoise to take in water, via the mouth, nostrils and cloaca. If the bowl of water is too shallow it is usually trampled over and spilled. Tortoises do not have a hard palate, so are unable to lap. Instead, they drop their mouths below the water line and 'siphon up' the water until they have taken in sufficient quantities.

Subadult or adult tortoises. Offer a range of wild plants topped up with a small proportions of salad, dark green leafy vegetables and fruits (see Tables 33.11 and 33.13). Wild plant material should provide at least 75% of the diet, with leafy vegetables and salad making up the remaining 25%. Fruits should be used as a treat, as too large a quantity can cause excessive dilution of dietary protein.

All foods offered should be fit for human consumption, washed and stored in a refrigerator or, in the case of wild plants, freshly picked. Foods should be offered on a flat dish or lid and should be of a size the tortoise can manage, as they prefer to

TABLE 33.13	Calcium-to-phosphorus ratio in some commonly fed vegetables and fruit
Food item	**Ratio cal : phos**
Sweet potato	0.1 : 0.2
Cauliflower florets	1 : 2
Celery stalk*	1.6 : 1
Spinach raw*	2 : 1
Collard greens*	14.5 : 1
Broccoli stems florets chopped	0.7 : 1
Cabbage†	2 : 1
Chinese cabbage (Bok Choy)	2.8 : 1
Dandelions	2.8 : 1
Carrots shredded	0.6 : 1
Parsley chopped	2.4 : 1
Bell peppers	0.5 : 1
Cucumber	0.7 : 1
Lettuce romaine	0 : 8 : 1
Lettuce iceberg‡	1 : 1
Tomatoes	0.2 : 1
Watercress	2 : 1
Apples	0.7 : 1.0
Bananas	0.3 : 1
Grapes	0.8 : 1
Melon (cantaloupe)	0.7 : 1
Strawberries	0.7 : 1
Prickly Pears cactus	2.3 : 2.1
Mango	0.9 : 1

*Oxalates occur in spinach, cabbage, celery, rhubarb, peas and beet greens. They bind to calcium and trace minerals, preventing their absorption from the gut. Although these are high in calcium, they should only be offered less frequently and in smaller amounts (once a fortnight)

†Cabbage, cauliflower, Bok Choy and kale should be fed in small amounts (once a month) as they contain goitrogens that block the production of thyroxine and utilisation of iodine, causing hypothyroidism and goitre

‡Lettuce is considered not an ideal food item for many reptiles, especially tortoises and iguanas, because of its poor nutritional value, but it is no worse or better than many vegetables and better than many fruits. The mixed bag lettuces including wild rocket as sold ready prepared in supermarkets are probably the best choice and should be part of a varied diet.

bite off small pieces of food. Very large pieces of fruit or vegetables can be difficult for the tortoise to eat. All food that is offered on a daily basis should be coated in calcium carbonate powder.

Once the tortoise has had enough it will walk away to rest and digest its food. A note should be made of the amount of food offered and the amount eaten. Water should be available and a bath is the best way of providing it.

Hatchlings. Correct feeding of a hatchling tortoise is of paramount importance, as poor diet can lead to conditions such as lumpy shell, bone and shell deformities and obesity.

Various feeding regimens have been recommended but the main aim is to balance energy, protein and calcium intake and to ensure that the hatchling has access to the factors involved in calcium metabolism, i.e. heat, UVB and vitamin D:

- **Suggested regimen** – feed the tortoise once a day as this allows for more thorough digestion of previously eaten

meals and may help to slow rapid growth. The amount fed will depend on how much the individual consumes at each feed. Be careful not to overfeed, as this has been reported to encourage rapid growth, which can lead to the development of 'lumpy' shells. Overfed tortoises are unhealthy and can become lethargic.
- **Suggested foods** – offer a wide range of coarse weeds, e.g. dandelion, sow thistle, clover. Note: salad leaves and dark leafy vegetables should be kept to a minimum.
- Supplementation is very important and must be added at every meal – calcium and small quantities of multivitamin and mineral powders can be offered daily. Iceberg lettuce is a poor foodstuff and contains little or no nutritional value and indeed some tortoises can become addicted to it, causing long-term damage and difficulty in changing dietary preference.
- **Water** – the hatchling must be kept hydrated and should be observed drinking while being bathed in a shallow dish of warm water. For the first 10 days of life bathe hatchlings every day in lukewarm water for 15–20 minutes reducing to 2–3 times a week.
- Although this text gave an overview of the needs of the Mediterranean tortoise, the reader must be aware that many other species of chelonian are kept as pets which have very different husbandry and dietary needs. These include the Leopard tortoise (*Stigmochelys (Geochelone) pardalis*), the African spurred tortoise (*Geochelone sulcate*) and the red-footed tortoise (*Chelonoidis carbonaria*).

Turtles and terrapins. Note: Species of terrapin are semi-aquatic, while turtles are totally aquatic. In the USA all shelled reptiles, including tortoises, are called 'turtles'.

Terrapins and turtles range from being totally carnivorous to accepting some plant material in their diet. A range of foods should be offered:

- Pinkies and small mice.
- Invertebrates, such as locusts, silkworms, crickets, snails.
- Crustaceans – crayfish, prawns in their shells.
- Cleansed earthworms (place worms in a tub for 12–24 hours to allow soil to pass through).
- Fish – whitebait, sprats.
- Plant material, such as dark leafy greens, carrots, aquatic plants.
- Calcium and multivitamin and mineral supplements need to be given, especially to young, growing terrapins and turtles.
- Feed terrapins and turtles in a separate enclosure or container to reduce water pollution.
- Quantity and frequency of feeding depend on the size and age of the terrapin. Young terrapins and turtles will require feeding daily, whereas adults should be fed every other day on a variety of foods from the list above.

Breeding

Most reptiles lay eggs and are described as oviparous. Some reptiles give birth to live young and can be described as either ovoviviparous or viviparous:

- **Ovoviviparous** – the egg and foetus are retained within the oviduct and nutritional support is gained through the yolk sac. Once the young are fully developed they hatch inside the female and live young are born.

- **Viviparous** – the foetuses develop in the oviduct and gain nutritional support from a type of placenta.

Most newly hatched reptiles are miniature versions of their parents and are independent, receiving little if any maternal care. Table 33.11 identifies the reproductive patterns of the individual species.

Breeding regimens. To breed reptiles successfully they must be in good health and must be given the correct, balanced diet. Most reptiles have a breeding season and breeding usually follows a change to their environment. A change in temperature, for example, is usually used to stimulate breeding but in some species it is the humidity (rainfall) that has to be altered.

Brumation or hibernation. Most breeding follows a period of dormancy referred to as brumation or hibernation that is brought about by slowly reducing the temperature of the vivarium. The reptile remains at this temperature for a set period depending on the species – approximately 4–12 weeks. At the end of brumation the vivarium temperature is slowly increased until the preferred temperature is reached.

Before brumation a reptile must undergo a period of fasting. If the digestive tract is full, food in the gut may rot, possibly leading to death. The fasting period is variable, e.g. snakes 1 month (Raiti 2010). During brumation the reptile must be constantly monitored (once to twice weekly) for signs of illness such as dehydration, dyspnoea or weight loss (Raiti 2010). If a dramatic weight loss is seen, i.e. more than 10%, the reptile must be taken out of brumation. To keep the animal hydrated, water must be available.

Gestation. Gravid or pregnant reptiles need good nutrition and optimum temperatures for both mother and offspring to thrive and survive. It is difficult to determine the length of gestation accurately but some information is included in Table 33.11. Most ovoviviparous or viviparous species will range from 1.5 to 6 months.

Before laying, an oviparous species will normally shed its skin (ecdysis). Colubrid snakes such as the corn snake (*Elaphe guttata*) may lay 8–14 days after shedding, while pythons can range from 18–26 days after shedding.

Incubation. An oviparous reptile requires a 'nesting site'. This can be created in a container such as an ice cream carton with a small hole in the side, filled with moist sphagnum moss and/or vermiculite. The provision of an area to lay the eggs is very important as inadequate provision can lead to dystocia.

A healthy, fertile reptile egg is white, dry and firm. The shell varies from soft and malleable, as seen in snakes and many lizards, to firmer and less pliable, as seen in chelonian and crocodilia. Incubation periods and temperatures vary according to species (Table 33.11). Most snakes and small lizard species range from 45–70 days; larger lizards (iguanas and monitors) range from 90–130 days. Incubation temperatures range from 26–32°C (79–90°F).

Common diseases and clinical conditions

There are many conditions affecting reptiles that may be presented in a veterinary practice. The majority of them are associated with poor management and nutrition. Details are summarised in Table 33.14.

Post-hibernation anorexia. This is associated with the Mediterranean tortoises, because the climate in the UK is not suitable for these species and because the traditional methods of tortoise keeping are flawed. The majority of the wild-caught tortoises that are still alive in the UK are barely surviving and those that do survive have darker shells that absorb heat more efficiently, which maintains the body temperature closer to its preferred range.

If during hibernation the temperature rises, the tortoise will stir and burn off valuable energy reserves. The by-product of this is urea, which is stored in the kidneys in the form of uric acid or urates. If this continues, by the time the tortoise fully awakens from hibernation its energy stores are depleted. It fails to get the normal glucose boost that enables it to move, bask and find food. The increase in stored urate levels depresses the appetite, resulting in an anorexic tortoise. Normally the activity of basking, eating and drinking post-hibernation will rectify the energy imbalance and allow stored urates to be passed in the form of a creamy white paste, which is voided shortly after hibernation, usually after a bath and a long drink of water.

Post-hibernation anorexia can also be the result of a more gradual build-up of urates in the kidneys brought about by a combination of the tortoise suffering a series of poor summers and hibernation in which energy levels are slowly being reduced and urate levels increased. A healthy adult tortoise can be expected to lose about 1% of its body weight during each month of hibernation. Post-hibernation anorexia can be prevented by allowing only healthy tortoises to hibernate, which can be assessed using the Jackson ratio (Fig. 33.25). The use of this ratio should be limited to those tortoises of an average build and is best suited to *Testudo hermanni* (Hermann's tortoise) and *Testudo graeca* (spur-thighed Greek tortoise). It is not suitable for use in the *Testudo marginata* (marginated tortoise) and *Testudo horsfieldii* (Horsfield's tortoise) as their body shape does not match with the original data used to formulate this ratio and will cause inaccurate results.

The ratio is measured by plotting on a graph the weight of the tortoise in grams against the length of the carapace in millimetres. Care should be taken to measure the carapace in a straight line rather than over the curve of the shell. Any animal falling into the 'dangerously low' area should be kept warm and awake all winter. An alternative method that many chelonian societies support is the bone-density ratio. This is achieved by accurately weighing the tortoise in grams and measuring its length in centimetres. To gain the bone-density ratio, the tortoise's weight in grams is dividing by the tortoise's total straight shell length cubed:

$$\text{Bone-density ratio} = \text{Weight in grams}/(\text{Length in cm})^3$$

If the tortoise is healthy and bone-density ratio is in the range 0.20–0.25, the tortoise may be hibernated.

During hibernation the temperature should be kept between 4°C and 5°C (39°F and 41°F) – if it rises the tortoise will begin to wake up. When the tortoise awakens after normal hibernation, the first step is to warm the tortoise and the second is to consider its fluid balance and then feeding.

BIRDS

Birds can make interesting companions, and a wide variety of species are commonly kept as cage or aviary birds (Table 33.15).

Text continued on p. 740

TABLE 33.14	Common diseases and clinical conditions of reptiles		
Disease	**Causal agent**	**Signs**	**Treatment**	**Additional information**

LIZARDS AND SNAKES

Disease	Causal agent	Signs	Treatment	Additional information
Stomatitis (mouth rot)	Seen in both lizards and snakes. Normally caused by poor husbandry and injury to rostal (nasal) area due to fighting or running against glass front of vivarium. Bacteria, viruses and fungi invade site and set up an infection	Decrease in appetite, swollen jaw, fluid build-up on the gum, oral exudate. If not treated the infection will rapidly spread and pus will be seen. If untreated can lead to osteomyelitis of the jawbone	Clean mouth with dilute povidone-iodine 2.5–5% solution applied daily to affected area. Analgesia, Bacteriology swab taken to determine pathogen. Topical antibiotics. If severe the reptile will require an anaesthetic and debridement of area. Parenteral fluids and systemic antibiotics may be given	Look at hygiene and husbandry – environmental conditions, overcrowding. X-ray may be taken to rule out osteomyelitis
Necrotic dermatitis (scale rot)	Seen in snakes. Usually due to poor environmental conditions such as: • Vivarium temperature too low • Poor ventilation • Too much moisture in the cage • Ectoparasites	Small blisters usually appear on the ventral surface that can become infected. If left can become necrotic	Transfer reptile to a clean dry vivarium with a relative humidity of 60–70%; change substrate daily (newspaper ideal). Systemic and topical antibiotics used with analgesia and rehydration therapy. Wound must be cleaned at least once or twice a day using dilute povidone-iodine	If reptile very sick it will require supportive therapy. Environment must be corrected before patient returns to it
Burns	Unguarded heat source hot rocks, heat pads	Signs depend on severity of burn: superficial – pain, erythema, discoloration of scales or loss of scales, wrinkling of scales, blisters and exudate. Deep – present as massive tissue damage that may slough and require surgical debridement	Treatment will depend on severity of the burn and general condition of the reptile. Wet-to-dry bandaging may be necessary (Raiti 2010). Analgesia, parenteral fluid therapy to replace lost body fluid and electrolytes. Apply topical antibiotics silver sulfadizine (Raiti 2010) or systemic if required. Surgery to debride damaged tissue	Healing by granulation can take a month to a year. Each time reptile sheds some improvement to the wound should be seen. Scarring seen, with loss of regular scale pattern. Area around scar may shed incompletely and may require soaking and manual removal. Ensure all heat sources are guarded or thermostatically controlled
Dystocia (egg binding) – snakes	Obstructive – foetal-maternal; non-obstructive – poor husbandry, poor nutrition. Lack of physical activity due to captive environment Lack of nesting sites	Oviparous species: seen as a caudally located mass or able to palpate in thicker-set species (large pythons); viviparous snakes are more difficult as foetuses are malleable, which makes them difficult to locate. Prolonged straining or cloacal prolapse demonstrates unsuccessful parturition. Ultrasound can be useful in identifying the presence of foetuses in viviparous snakes	Intervention should be considered necessary 48h after the cessation of the incomplete parturition or oviposition (egg-laying). Techniques include: • Decompression by transcutaneous aspiration of the distal eggs, followed by warmed water soaks for several hours prior to oxytocin administration (Raiti 2010), caution must be taken not to contaminate the coelomic cavity with egg yolk Manual manipulation under anaesthetic if the above is unsuccessful • Surgery: If above fails a salpingotomy (making an incision into the oviduct) can be performed and eggs/foetus can be removed	Oxytocin or related drugs must not be used if a snake has an obstructive dystocia Responses to oxytocin is quite variable in snakes (Raiti 2010)

Continued

TABLE 33.14	Common diseases and clinical conditions of reptiles—cont'd			
Disease	**Causal agent**	**Signs**	**Treatment**	**Additional information**
Dystocia (egg binding) – lizards	Obstructive – foetal-maternal; non-obstructive – (behavioural) poor husbandry, poor nutrition. Lack of physical activity due to captive environment. Lack of suitable nesting sites common in lizards	Although anorexia is a common sign in the reproducing lizard, the lizard that is not eating and is displaying lethargy, cachexia, and loss of muscle and fat tissue from pelvic girdle, limbs and tail base suggests further investigation	Following diagnosis via radiography or ultrasound. If dystocia due to behavioural reasons giving calcium gluconate followed by oxytocin can lead to oviposition (Eatwell 2010) If obstructive dystocia prompt treatment is necessary, analgesia, fluid therapy, prior to any surgical procedure.. Surgery – salpingotomy or salpingectomy or ovariosalpingectomy. Lizards do not tolerate prolonged periods of dystocia, which can cause death within several days	Many lizards, including iguanas, can produce a clutch of eggs without a male present. Good pre- and postoperative care is essential for the survival of lizards or snakes undergoing surgery Follicular stasis lizards Can be seen in lone females and is caused by a lack of stimuli to ovulate Infection and abscessation of follicles is possible and they can rupture leading to yolk coelomitis (Eatwell 2010) Surgical intervention is recommended
Endoparasites	Mainly seen in wild-caught or farmed species, but can affect any captive snake and lizard. Numerous and varied infestations, although some are self-limiting as to complete their life cycle they need an intermediate host that captivity does not provide. The following have been seen in snakes and lizards: • Protozoans, flagellates • Coccidia • Trematodes and Cestodes • Nematodes Pentastomids	Some infestations go unnoticed until disease or loss of a reptile occurs. Signs: eggs or oocyst are seen in faecal smears. Reptile appears listless, failure to thrive, dull, inappetent, weight loss. Visual signs of the parasite in adult form	Anthelmintic drugs usually given orally once or twice a year. Good hygiene protocols, and do not feed wild-caught foods	Suggested drugs: metronidazole for flagellates; febendazole (Panacur) or ivermectin for nematodes Praziquantel Tematodes and cestodes

Ectoparasites	Mainly seen in wild-caught or farmed species, but can affect any captive snake and lizard: • Ticks – Ixodes spp. • Mites – Ophionyssus natricis (mainly seen in snakes and some lizards) Both are parasitic and feed off animal's blood	Ticks – because of their size relatively easy to spot, but can blend in with scales; tend to favour areas near recess of ear, skin folds of the vent (lizards), cavities such as the nostrils or labial pits in some snakes. Mites – generally smaller than ticks and hide under scales. Colour varies from tan, reddish brown to black depending on engorgement. Common sites include between and under scales, especially around the eyes, under the chin, cloaca, axillae and inguinal regions. Other signs include the snake rubbing against furnishings in cage, spending much time soaking in the water bowl all in an attempt to rid themselves of the mite and associated irritation. The owner may notice mites in the cage, floating in the water or crawling on to their skin. The mite causes the reptile to appear dull and listless. In severe cases can become depressed, anorexic and very sick	Ticks – care must be taken to remove all mouthparts, as any remaining parts can lead to formation of an abscess. Mites – when dealing with a lizard or snake, hygiene is essential to prevent the spread of mites to other patients. One female mite can produce 90–100 eggs in crevices in the cage. Ivermectin and fipronil are both alcohol-based and therefore flammable. If treating the eye area with fipronil, place on a cotton wool bud and carefully apply to the scales around the eye. It has been recommended that, if spraying head (snakes), you should place ophthalmic ointment on spectacle. Ticks – manual removal techniques as used to remove ticks from domestic animals. Mites – many suggested. Reptile and vivarium must be isolated and vivarium totally cleaned to remove all life stages of the mite, including egg, larvae, nymphs and adults. Attention should be paid to corners, crevices, lips and all furnishings. The reptile should not be replaced until the vivarium has received a total clean. Treatment of the reptile: Ivermectin can be used. Fipronil can be used topically on the reptile and also to treat the vivarium). Keep sprayed animal in a well-ventilated cage for 2–3. Also ensure reptile has access post-treatment to a high-humidity hide box to compensate for possible increase in cutaneous water loss. Treatment of the vivarium: burn any disposable or easily replaceable furnishings. Spray non-disposable items and vivarium with fipronil, paying special attention to cracks and crevices. Repeat treatment on animal and vivarium this will help to kill second- and third-generation mites
Thiamine (vitamin B$_1$) deficiency	Mainly seen in fish-eating snakes such as garter snakes. When these are fed thawed frozen fish, an enzyme called thiaminase, present in raw fish, destroys thiamine (vitamin B$_1$) leading to deficiency disease	Neurological signs such as incoordination, convulsions, loss of the righting reflex	Treatment is administration of vitamin B$_1$ by injection or stomach tube. Dietary correction is essential and all raw fish must be blanched/poached before feeding (ideally taking water temperature to 80°C for 5–10 min): this will kill the antivitamin thiaminase Fish-eating snakes should be encouraged to take other foodstuffs, e.g. pinkies, earthworms
Respiratory disease	• Bacterial invasion, viruses, fungi • Poor husbandry • Inadequate nutrition • Poor ventilation • Draughts • Low temperature • Endoparasites • Rhinitis (inflammation of the nasal cavity)	• Dyspnoea • Abnormal elevation of the head • Open-mouth breathing • Wheezing • Nasal discharge • Problems during sloughing • Debilitation • Severe cases – cyanotic membranes	Very sick animals will require hospitalisation and much supportive therapy, such as fluids and assistance with feeding. A pulmonary wash to collect material for cytology microbial culture and sensitivity will aid in identification of pathogen and necessary treatment. Parenteral fluids, antimicrobial therapy is recommended, nebulised antibiotics. Treat endoparasites and any other suspected cause. The environment must be re-evaluated and changes made Less common in lizards. The patient should be maintained at the higher end of its POTZ to stimulate immunogenetics (Raiti 2010); humidity must be kept at the animal's normal range. Coupage: 'chest physiotherapy' and holding the snake to allow mucous to move anteriorly has been shown to have some success. Parenteral vitamin supplements (especially water-soluble ones) have been beneficial in some cases. In severe cases prognosis is guarded and aggressive therapy is recommended

Continued

TABLE 33.14 Common diseases and clinical conditions of reptiles—cont'd

Disease	Causal agent	Signs	Treatment	Additional information
Autotomy (tail loss)	Occurs as a defence mechanism in many species of lizard, geckos, green iguana, water dragons. The tail will keep wriggling to hold the predator's attention while 'lunch escapes'. In captive reptiles, usually caused by rough handling, grasping the tail or stress	Loss of tail and, if it occurs in the surgery because of poor handling, a distressed owner and embarrassed staff!	In time the tail will grow back (5–8 weeks) but it is never the same and is generally less impressive. Minimal intervention needed just daily bathing in povidone-iodine solution will prevent infection until regrowth is established. If tail is sutured back on it will not regrow	The vertebrae have lines of weakness that split with powerful muscular contractions allowing the tail to separate from the body. Food invertebrates if left in with lizard can feast on tail wound.
Dysecdysis (difficulty with sloughing or shedding)	Dysecdysis should be considered as a sign of a problem not the primary problem. Main causes can be attributed to poor environmental conditions: • Low temperature • Low humidity • No water bowl or bowl too small so the snake is prevented from bathing • Insufficient cage furnishings, i.e. logs or rocks for rubbing to initiate shedding • Poor nutrition Underlying systemic disease	Retained flaky, dry skin over body, limbs and digits, also spectacles (snakes). If not treated, retained slough can cause infection or act as tourniquets around small limbs, tail tips and digits	The skin must be hydrated, so increase humidity in the vivarium and make sure the snake has access to a large water bowl for soaking. The snake can be placed in a bag (a pillowcase or duvet cover works well) with wet towels. The snake or lizard can rub against the towels and the moisture should help to soften the skin, allowing it to be shed. If pieces are retained, gently remove them. In snakes, if the spectacle (eye caps) are retained after soaking, leave the snake to see if they are removed during the next shed. In severe cases anaesthesia is recommended and the spectacle removed surgically. Before the patient is discharged the owner must be made aware of the need to improve environmental conditions	This is a cycle that continues throughout the reptile's life. Snakes shed their skin as one single piece whereas lizards, with the exception of geckos, shed in pieces. Frequency of shedding depends on age and health status. Duration of the shedding process is between 7 and 14 days (snakes). Signs – snakes: • Skin lacks lustre and shine • Eyes appear cloudy • Snake will often refuse food to hide or sit for long periods of time in the water bowl (best not to handle) • Very vulnerable at this stage as vision impaired and may strike if handled • Dulling over is followed 3–4-day period where skin and eyes appear clear • When ready to shed, snake will move about cage rubbing its nose against rough objects to break skin. It will then slither out of the skin • The shed should be in one complete piece – check that spectacles and tail tip are included

CHELONIA

Condition	Cause	Clinical signs	Treatment	Notes
Metabolic bone disease (nutritional secondary hyperparathyroidism). Not just limited to chelonia – also seen in lizards. Especially herbivore and insectivorous species	Poor environmental conditions including inadequate heating and provision of good UVB. Diet high in protein or high in phosphorus and lacking in calcium or vitamin D_3	• Hypocalcaemia • Soft shell • Shell deformities • Overgrown rhamphotheca (beak) and nails • Abnormal gait and movement • Demineralisation of bones on x-ray	Correct the nutritional imbalances and environmental factors such as heat and access to good UVB	Can take on many forms according to life stage; each will be discussed separately. For more detail on specific signs and problems, see separate sections below
Hypocalcaemia – common cause of death in UK-bred tortoises	Main cause is diet lacking in calcium but also associated with lack of vitamin D, high phosphorus diets and lack of good-quality UVB and inadequate heating	**Hatchlings – acute problem** • Soft spongy shell • Edges of the mouth fail to harden, inappetence • If not treated, shell haemorrhages, lungs collapse and death • If diet too rich in protein pyramidal growth of scutes on the carapace **Juvenile tortoise – chronic problem** • Shell deformities rather than softness • Overall flattened appearance to the shell • Dip in the rear of the carapace • Scutes raised and shell feels soft and spongy • Carapace can appear too small for the chelonia • Edge of the carapace may curl dorsally • Reduced overall weight gain and growth • Deformed beak and overgrown nails • Problems with walking because of plastron deformities around the hind limbs • X-ray shows poor mineralisation of bone **Adult imported tortoise – chronic problem** • Poor shell growth, shape and hardness • Claws are curved or bent rather than straight • Beak overgrown • Shell damage prolonged, poor healing or may not heal • Poor locomotion – animal tends to rub plastron against the ground; in more severe cases is unable to propel itself forward • Predispose to other disease because of depressed immune system (see text)	Depends on the signs and progression of the disease. Hatchlings – Mild cases, especially if being offered a high-protein diet, increase calcium uptake and slow growth (see feeding section main text) Moderate cases (shell is only partially soft or severe cases that are still bright and able to move – aggressive dietary and environmental management necessary: increase calcium, vitamin D_3 and UVB and heat access. Be warned: this condition can take months to rectify Cases that are debilitated – will require the following suggested treatment: Vitamin D_3 400 IU IM once and calcium gluconate at a rate of 23 mg/kg orally q12hrs for the first week supported by calcium rich diet. Second week if significant bone loss and or little response to treatment (including resistance to diet changes) a second parenteral doses of vitamin D_3 may be administered and oral calcium continued (Jessop and Bennett 2010). In severe or unresponsive case calcitonin may be used (Jessop and Bennett 2010). Debilitated animals will be weak and may suffer from demineralisation of the jaw and find eating difficult gavage or tube feeding will be necessary. Also fluid therapy and analgesia will support recovery. If condition is very severe and some of the more terminal signs are present, euthanasia should be considered Juvenile tortoise – Dietary correction and environmental factors Adult tortoise – Dietary and environmental management Overgrown beak will need to be clipped and shaped Unfortunately, once deformities are established little can be done to alter this	Juvenile tortoise – If excess protein intake is a cause of the problem then the kidney and liver may be affected. Flattening of the shell can cause respiratory problems, as expansion of the lungs is hindered. Unfortunately once the deformities are established little can be done to alter this

Continued

TABLE 33.14	Common diseases and clinical conditions of reptiles—cont'd			
Disease	Causal agent	Signs	Treatment	Additional information
Hypovitaminosis A	Lack of dietary vitamin A. Possible problems with vitamin A metabolism and utilisation from ingested sources. Problem seen in tortoises and terrapins	The main function of vitamin A is to maintain the integrity of the skin and epithelium, especially that lining the respiratory tract and eye tissues. If deficient you may see: • Flaky skin • Poor wound healing and secondary infection • Anorexia • Lethargy • Weight loss • Swollen eyelids • Irritation around the eyes. Solid purulent matter underneath the eye lids if not treated • Respiratory problems • Renal and liver problems • Chronic condition can cause thickening of the skin	Injection of vitamin A 14 days apart. Changes to dietary regime include foodstuffs rich in vitamin A, such as dark leafy greens, yellow or orange fruits and vegetables, for carnivorous species whole mice and fish, as the prey's liver will act as a good source of vitamin A. Liquid cod liver oil is rich in vitamin A and readily accepted by most turtles (Jessop and Bennett 2010). Add multivitamin supplement to the diet every other day for 2 weeks, then reduce to twice weekly for a month. In mild cases the addition of multivitamin supplement to the diet every 2–3 days may suffice, along with appropriate dietary management. If the chelonian is anorexic and debilitated then tube feeding and fluid support will be required. Eye infections will need to be treated with the appropriate antibiotics, as will respiratory infections	If any eye infection does not clear up with treatment, hypovitaminosis A should be considered. Care must be taken not to overdose with vitamin A, as this can cause further problems
Upper respiratory tract disease (runny nose syndrome) – common problem in UK tortoises	Common problem in tortoises, with multifactorial aetiology Some pathogens associated with this problem are: • Mycoplasma • Herpes virus Ranavirus Paramyxovirus Tortoises can act as latent carriers, not showing signs but able to pass on the disease to others. For this reason, mixing tortoises from different geographical regions must be discouraged General health of the tortoise is a factor to be considered: poor diet and husbandry can lead to a susceptible immune system	A secondary bacterial infection usually intensifies the clinical signs: • Clear watery discharge from the nostrils • Occasionally sneezing • If disease progresses to the lungs, breathing becomes audible and very noisy • Open mouth and laboured breathing, lethargy, depression, anorexia	Culture and sensitivity cytology and PCR to identify pathogen. Severe cases will require supportive therapy such as fluid therapy, supplementary heat and lots of nursing care. Assisted feeding, parenteral antibiotics, nasal drops.	A healthy tortoise should not have a wet nose. Hypovitaminosis must also be considered here. Vitamin A supplements can be considered. This is a highly contagious disease and the patient should be isolated. Remember – chelonia do not possess a diaphragm and are unable to cough and swallow excess mucus produced in the lungs. This can cause these types of infection to progress and cause pneumonia. Tip – when administering nasal drops to chelonia, use a small syringe and catheter or extend head, squirt drops in the mouth and simultaneously let go of the head. As the head retracts back into the carapace it will force the fluid from the mouth down the nostrils. Terrapins seen with this disease may float on one side if one lung is more affected than the other

Infectious stomatitis (mouth rot)	Common condition seen in the Mediterranean tortoise, especially if in poor condition post-hibernation. Associated with bacterial infection (Gram-negative, commonly *Pseudomonas* spp.) or viruses such as herpes virus	Early signs are often overlooked: • Reddening inside the mouth • Blistering, which commonly occurs inside lower jaw under tongue • As problem progresses, tongue becomes swollen, mouth fills with mucus and a discharge resembling cottage cheese is seen • Osteomyelitis if infection attacks jaw bone • Inappetence • Death if not treated	Mild cases – topical applications of Betadine gargle and mouthwash can be applied once a day to the affected area. More severe cases will require antibiotic treatment. Swabs can be taken to identify pathogen and treatment. Check for fungal invasion, e.g. *Candida*. Severe cases – aggressive antibiotic treatment and supportive therapy to prevent dehydration	Even if treatment is successful in severe cases where osteomyelitis is seen, the problem can reoccur
Shell rot Also see shell trauma	This problem can be seen in all chelonia. Can be due to fungal or bacterial infection, normally anaerobic Gram-negative. The fungus or bacteria gain entry as a result of shell trauma. Other contributing factors include: • Poor hygiene in both terrestrial and aquatic chelonia • High humidity • Low temperature • Lack of UV light • Inadequate diet • Overcrowding • Lack of basking sites in terrapins and turtles	Discoloration, especially around areas of shell damage. Aquatic and semi-aquatic shell appears paler. Dry flaking of shell or soft tissue. Bacterial infections – affected areas appear wet and there is an obnoxious odour, with blood and purulent discharge. Fungal infections – appear dryer and less smelly than bacterial infections. Infection can spread under scutes and lead to a deep infection with much tissue damage	Debride all infected shell until healthy tissue is seen. For at least 4–6 weeks, the area should be scrubbed for at least 5 min daily using a tooth- or nailbrush, with antibacterial scrub such as chlorhexidine or povidone-iodine. Swabs may need to be taken for culture and sensitivity and antibiotic treatment administered. If abscesses form, these must be flushed out and topical antibiotic or systemic treatments given. Deep or extensive lesions may need to be cleaned and dressed daily. If recommended use wet to dry antimicrobial dressings. 'Dry docking' (forced basking) of aquatic or semi aquatic chelonian can be considered but may cause some distress to the patient but will aid healing. It should be noted that healing may take weeks or, in extreme cases, years. The shell can be considered free from disease when it is smooth, dry and free from odour and discharge. The animal may be permanently scarred. The very sick chelonian will need supportive therapy, including assisted feeding and fluid therapy and analgesia	A common cause of trauma to the shell is oversexed males butting each other or males continually ramming the rear end of females – it is advisable to keep sexes separate. Environmental condition and diet must also be corrected before patient is discharged During hospitalisation, provision of heat* hygiene and nursing support are essential for the recovery. If untreated, septicaemia will ensue and subsequent death. Suggested antimicrobial treatments include: • Fungal infections – oral ketoconazole (20 mg/kg/d) • Bacterial infections – amikacin (Amikin paediatric) 10 mg/kg every other day for 3 days
Endoparasites	Large grey ascarids – *Angusticaecum* spp. Small, thread-like oxyurid-type nematodes *Strongyloides* *Capillaria*	Healthy tortoise shows few physical signs apart from seeing them passed in faeces. Heavy infestations, weight loss, diarrhoea, lethargy. Faecal smear/floatation will show presence of eggs. Death in hatchlings with large infestations	Oral dosage of anthelmintics: fenbendazole (Panacur). Or use Panacur granules or paste in food	Worming should be carried out on a regular basis, especially if groups of tortoises are kept together or kept in small areas. Mediterranean tortoises should be wormed prior to hibernation. It is advisable to keep hatchlings away from pasture grazed by adults, as this is a source of infection

Continued

TABLE 33.14	Common diseases and clinical conditions of reptiles—cont'd			
Disease	**Causal agent**	**Signs**	**Treatment**	**Additional information**
Ear abscess	Seen in tortoises, terrapins and box turtles. Bacterial infections of the middle ear gain entry via mouth and travel along Eustachian tube. Poor husbandry, suboptimal temperatures and hygiene, especially poor water filtration. In aquatic species vitamin A deficiency. Depressed immune system	Large, painful swellings over ear drum (normal slightly concave). Head tilting and circling	Surgery to incise the abscess, remove pus and flush cavity. Antimicrobial therapy given by injection. Vitamin A supplementation	Husbandry and diet will need to be re-evaluated. Healthy tortoises do not get abscesses
Trauma	Trauma to the shell is often caused by the chelonian being dropped or manhandled by young children, chewed by a dog (especially if young or suffering from hypocalcaemia) or coming in contact with the lawn mower or strimmer	Damage to shell. Shock makes the tortoise lethargic and lowers blood pressure. Haemorrhage – external is easy to identify; internal more problematic, so need to observe behaviour and other parameters such as mucous membrane colour. Exposure of coelomic cavity can cause internal organ damage, and lung damage is quite common. Secondary infection should be considered	Stem haemorrhage. Treat shock, give analgesia, fluid therapy. X-rays may be required to establish extent of damage. When patient stabilised, flush wounds using antibacterial scrub, remove debris. Antibiotics and anti-inflammatory drugs prevent infection and aid shock. Repair lung damage and consider other internal injuries. Tissue fluid will seep from wounds for a few days. Once this stops, shell repair can be performed. As with shell rot lesions once debrided should be left open to granulate and daily topical antimicrobial applied (Jessop and Bennett 2010). Resin repair patches, which can be left in place for 6–12 months depending on health status of tortoise prior to injury. Very severe damage can be repaired using orthopaedic techniques	A damaged shell can take 1–2 years to heal. Chelonia that are recovering from a fractured shell should not be allowed to hibernate. Extensive trauma to the shell may never fill completely. In adult chelonia, patches can be left in place indefinitely. In young animals, to allow for growth, patches must be removed after 6 months

Condition	Cause/Signs	Treatment	
Penile prolapse	The penis protrudes from the cloaca for a prolonged period. Mainly seen in juvenile tortoises that have become sexually active and spend most of the day with the penis extruded	The penis can be manually replaced but usually this is only a temporary remedy. The aim is to prevent it becoming infected. Keep the penis clean and lubricated (KY Jelly and povidone-iodine). The condition will settle down in time. If penis suffers injury or becomes infected, it is important to treat the infection and keep the penis clean and lubricated as before. With the addition of systemic antibiotics the penis can be manually replaced once the inflammation has subsided. In severe infections some or all of the organ may have to be removed	It is important not to replace a dirty or infected penis. If the penis continues to prolapse then it may necessitate the need for a purse-string suture around the cloaca, which can be removed in a few days
Dystocia	Poor environmental conditions: • Lack of laying sites • Temperature too low for tortoise to lay eggs • Overcrowding: tortoise feels stressed • Poor diet, especially lack of calcium Virtually impossible to detect without use of a radiograph but signs that may suggest problem include: • Restlessness • Gestation period exceeded • Depression • Anorexia • Straining • Cloacal swelling	Injection of oxytocin (2 IU/kg–10 IU/kg IM) once or twice at 90-minute intervals. During this time the tortoise must be kept at its POTZ and given access to a suitable laying area or placed in a bath of warm water – along with the administration of calcium has proved very beneficial in helping tortoises expel their eggs. Surgical intervention must only be considered if: • Above therapy has failed • Eggs stuck or cracked in the pelvis. If surgery is to be undertaken, a plastronotomy and celiotomy followed by a salpingotomy will have to be performed	In comparison to snakes and lizards, chelonia respond well to oxytocin injections. Problems are more commonly seen in tortoises that are due to lay in the autumn. A tortoise should not be allowed to hibernate with eggs inside her, as this will only make matters worse as the eggs become larger and more calcified, making removal more difficult

Many of the problems identified in the Mediterranean tortoise are due to the fact it is not well adapted to the UK climate: tortoises are kept in suboptimal temperatures and as a result suffer from immunosuppression.

*Sick chelonia will need to be hospitalised and kept at temperatures at the higher range of their POTZ; this will encourage metabolism of drug therapy and stimulate their own metabolism.

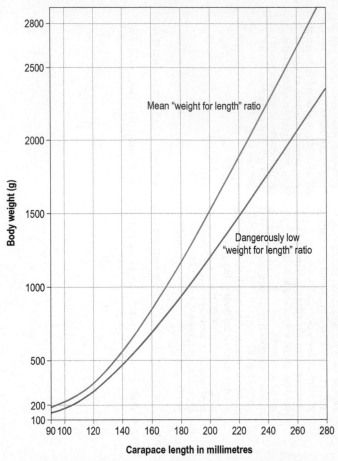

Fig. 33.25 Growth of healthy Mediterranean tortoises using the Jackson ratio. Note that this ratio can only be applied to *Testudo graeca* (Mediterranean spur-thighed tortoise) and *Testudo hermanni* (Hermann's tortoise). This graph is not suitable for *Testudo horsfieldii* (Horsfield's tortoise) or *Testudo marginata* (marginated tortoise)

- **Psittacine birds** include parrots, macaws, cockatoos, budgerigars, cockatiels and lories.
- **Passerine birds** include canary finches and common hill mynah.

Housing

Accommodation for birds kept in captivity should be designed to allow the birds to be maintained in good health and to allow them to exhibit their natural behaviour of flying. The main types of accommodation used to house birds are aviaries and cages.

The design and size depend on the numbers and species of bird but whatever type of accommodation is selected, once the bird is in situ as a minimum it must be able to stretch out both wings fully in all directions. Accommodation should also allow the keeper to carry out general husbandry procedures, including monitoring, feeding, catching, cleaning, etc., with minimum disturbance to the birds.

Aviaries. Aviaries are divided into indoor and outdoor sections. The outdoor area or flight usually has a timber frame covered in wire mesh while the indoor area provides shelter and is normally a solid timber house with a window for light and a door for access.

When choosing an aviary consider the following:

- **Size** – depends on the ground space available, the species and the number of birds to be housed. Overstocking should be avoided, but generally 'the bigger the better' – too small an aviary will make access and cleaning difficult.
- **Shape** – there are a variety of very ornate aviary designs on the market but although these look good they are usually very impractical, favouring design features over the practical needs of the bird. The best advice is keep it simple – rectangular or square shapes work well.

TABLE 33.15	Commonly kept species of cage and aviary birds			
Species	**Origin**	**Captive diet**		**General information**
ORDER PSITTACIFORMES				
Budgerigar (*Melopsittacus undulatus*)	Australia	Over time psittacine who are mainly fed a seed-based diet are likely to develop calcium and vitamin A deficiency. Therefore feed a good-quality proprietary seed mixture (canary seed and millet). Offer a range of green food, watercress, chickweed, groundsel. They need a dietary source of iodine and calcium		Can be kept on own or in groups. Males tend to be more vocal. Can be aggressive toward other smaller birds, e.g. canaries or small finches
Peach-faced lovebird (*Agapornis roseicollis*)	Southwest Africa	Feed proprietary complete formulated pellets (50% of diet). Alternatively good-quality canary mix, sunflowers, safflower seeds, pine nuts, both with daily servings of fruit and vegetables. Hawthorn berries		Keep in pairs or small groups. Can be very aggressive to other species. Enjoy stripping bark from branches of non-poisonous trees
Cockatiel (*Nymphicus hollandicus*)	Australia	Proprietary complete formulated pellets with seed mixtures – saffron, safflower, white/red millet, canary and hemp seed, linseed, niger seed, wheat, groats. Fruits, apples, green vegetables lettuce, root vegetables, raw carrot strips. Chickweed		Good aviary or cage bird. Can talk and mimic. Lives up to 10–25 years
Rosella (*Platycercus eximius*)	Australia	Similar to cockatiel diet		Keep in pairs. Aggressive toward other birds. Very vocal. Good breeders. Need to be kept in large aviary

TABLE 33.15	Commonly kept species of cage and aviary birds—cont'd			
Species	**Origin**	**Captive diet**		**General information**
African grey parrot (*Psittacus erithacus*)	Central Africa	Proprietary complete formulated pellets with additional seed mixtures – saffron, safflower, white/red millet, canary seed, wheat, oats, maize, peanuts, pine nuts, hemp. Fruits (almost any non-citrus). Green vegetables. Root vegetables, raw carrot, celery, spinach, beetroot, peas, beans and lightly cooked corn on the cob. Sprouted seeds. Vitamin mineral supplement		One of the best-talking parrots. Intelligent and sensitive and therefore prone to feather plucking if bored. Needs lots of attention and stimulation. Loves to shower in spray from plant mister. Benefits from low level UVB light 2%
ORDER PASSERIFORMES, WHICH INCLUDES THE PERCHING BIRDS				
Canary (*Serinus canaria*)	Canary Islands	Granivores: good-quality seed mixture – canary millet, rape maw, grass seed, hemp with additional vitamin and mineral supplementation. Uncontaminated green stuff		Good for both cage and aviaries. Males will sing especially if on own or competition from neighbour. Nervous bird – needs careful handling
Zebra finch (*Taeniopygia poephila guttata*)	Australia	Good quality seed mixture – canary millet, rape maw, grass seed, hemp with additional vitamin and mineral supplementation. Supplement with greens and do not remove seed husks, need access to grit		Adaptable, hardy, sociable and easily tamed. Good for both aviary and cage set-ups
Cut-throat finch (*Amadina fasciata*)	Africa	Insects, mixed seeds small amounts of uncontaminated green stuff. Soft foods, e.g. insectivorous mixtures for waxbills with additional vitamin and mineral supplementation		Suitable for both aviary and cage. Can be kept in mixed aviary and good for those with limited experience
Hill mynah (*Gracula religiosa*)	India, Southeast Asia, Indonesia	Soft bill. Chopped fruit. Insectivorous mixture. Mynah food. Large insects such as mealworms		Great powers of mimicry. Well-balanced diet essential with adequate vitamin and mineral supplementation. Need sunlight and without access have been known to have seizures. Messy birds which will need perches and floor cleaned daily. Need heated aviary as prone to chills and respiratory problems
ORDER COLUMBIFORMES – PIGEONS AND DOVES				
Diamond dove (*Geopelia cuneata*)	Australia	Seeds and grains according to size of bird. Chick crumb. Green foods in small amounts		Lively little birds that live well in mixed aviaries or cages. Enjoy the sun and can be seen sunbathing
ORDER GALLIFORMES – DOMESTIC FOWL, PHEASANTS AND QUAIL				
Chinese painted quail (*Excalfactoria chinensis*)	India and southern China	Small seeds. Chick crumb. Finely chopped green food. Occasional mealworm		Ground-dwelling species. If in cage with flight birds, protect water and food bowls from soiling. Do not place food and water bowls at the sides of their accommodation, as they like to run along the perimeter. Cock birds will fight
ORDER STRIGIFORMES – NOCTURNAL BIRDS OF PREY – THE OWLS				
European eagle owl (*Bubo bubo*)	Europe	Meat, dead rats, quail, day-old chicks, rabbit		Large but attractive bird
Barn owl (*Tyto alba*)	Europe	Meat, dead rats, quail, day-old chicks, rabbit		Commonly kept in captivity
ORDER FALCONIFORMES – DIURNAL BIRDS OF PREY – HAWKS AND FALCONS				
Harris hawk (*Circus* spp.)	South to Central America	Meat, dead rats, quail, day-old chicks, rabbit		Usually kept in captivity for hunting or flying displays

Choose a design that allows the bird to display its natural behaviour.

- **Siting** – check with the local planning office to see if planning permission is required. For security and to reduce stress, site the aviary away from roads and public access. The aviary should be southwest-facing, but whatever the position the selected site should be sheltered, not exposed to extremes of weather and away from overhanging trees. Hedges make good windbreaks.

- **Materials** – these must be durable, safe and economic. Most flight areas are made of a timber, treated with an animal-safe preservative and stainless steel or powder-coated wire with a gauge suited to the size of the bird. Birds can be very destructive, especially the larger parrots, which will chew wooden frames and bite wire mesh. For these birds a 16–18-gauge mesh (Stanford 2010) and a metal framework are recommended.

One-third of the aviary should be solid sided and have a solid roof (Jones and Dodd 2012). This will protect the birds from

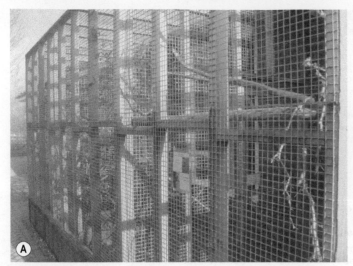

Fig. 33.26A Outside aviary

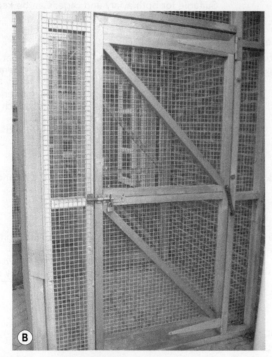

Fig. 33.26B Double-entry doors to prevent escape of birds

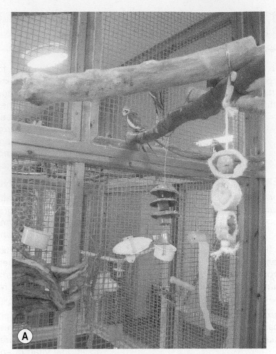

Fig. 33.27A Indoor area of aviary showing enrichment

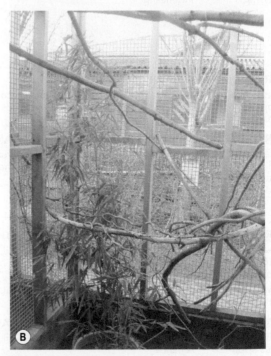

Fig. 33.27B Outside flight area with natural planting

the elements and contamination from wild birds – a salient point considering the threat from avian influenza.

A concrete base and brick surround make the ideal footing for the aviary, provide ease of cleaning and prevent rodents entering the aviary. Access should be via a double door system to prevent escape (Fig. 33.26).

The indoor area is usually a house made of timber and providing shelter. Supplementary heating and lighting can be used to help birds over the winter. Some bird keepers, especially those with extensive collections, utilise large brick-built buildings or sheds. The building is subdivided into smaller aviary units and each one provides the housed birds with access to an outdoor flight. Adjoining aviaries should have double wire partitions to prevent the birds from pecking their neighbours (Fig. 33.27).

Furnishings. These are put into the aviary and are used to prevent boredom and subsequent behavioural problems.

- **Perches** – the outside flight area should have at least two perches, one at either end, but more can be added. Branches make the best perches as they are natural, readily available, cheap and easily replaced when soiled. Only pick branches from deciduous trees – willow and fruit trees are the best choice. Some woods are unsuitable, e.g. yew, laburnum, oak and rhododendron, as they are poisonous if eaten.

Make sure that the wood has not been recently sprayed or chemically treated and that all branches are scrubbed prior to use to remove soiling from wild birds.

- The perch size depends on the species of bird but a range of thicknesses and textures help to exercise the feet – the perch should be of a suitable size to allow the bird to grip without the toes overlapping. Inside the house, at least one perch should be positioned just above the level of those in the flight. This encourages the birds to roost in the most secure part of the aviary. To prevent accidents, perches should be robust and placed securely in the aviary. To prevent contamination from faecal matter perches should be placed away from food and water bowls.
- **Food and water bowls** – must be correctly positioned for birds of all sizes to gain easy access.
- **Toys** – there are various proprietary toys available, e.g. ropes, swings and wooden blocks. These should be used in moderation as too many can turn the aviary or cage into an obstacle course, preventing flight, and may over-stimulate the birds so that they become depressed.
- **Baths** – bathing is a natural activity and should be encouraged as it stimulates the bird to preen and keeps its plumage clean. Maintenance of the plumage is important for flight and for conservation of body temperature. All species love bathing and this is also seen in wild birds. Raptors, including owls, will bathe if given the opportunity and both budgerigars and parrots love having a fine mist directed from a garden hose or plant sprayer on to their plumage, mimicking the rains that would fall in their native rainforests.
  - Birds will actively fly into the spray and enjoy preening themselves afterwards. The size and depth of the bird bath must relate to the species, e.g. for small birds fill the bath with no more than 1–2 cm of water; for larger species fill with 3–4 cm of water.
  - Smaller parrots, e.g. budgerigars, like to bathe in damp foliage; wet lettuce leaves left on the bottom of the cage usually suffice (Jones and Dodd 2012).
  - Lighting:
    - Psittaciformes such as parrots need access to unfiltered sunlight or artificial full-spectrum UV light (Jones and Dodd 2012). This will stimulate the metabolism of vitamin D and preening behaviour.
  - **Note:** Chicks should not be bathed, as the down feathers of many species give little protection.

Cages. Cages may be made from wire (Fig. 33.28) or wire and wood (Fig. 33.29) and can range from basic to elaborate in design. Remember that the bird must be able to stretch out both wings fully in all directions. Cages make a good base for birds that are allowed free range of the home and can be used for feeding, drinking and resting.

Consider the following:

- Wire cages are not suitable for nervous or timid birds as they are too open and the birds feel exposed and stressed.
- Box-type cages must have good ventilation and be well lit.
- Cages must be positioned away from draughts, windows and heaters.

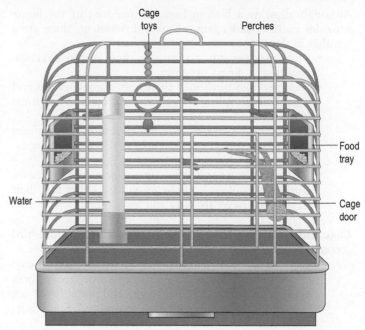

Fig. 33.28 A typical cage suitable for smaller species of bird

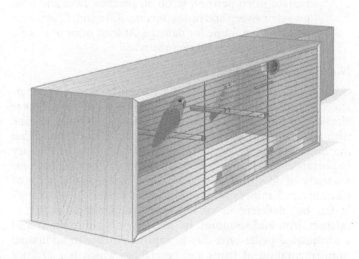

Fig. 33.29 A wooden box-type cage suitable for breeding small species of bird

- Some birds enjoy being in areas of high activity where they receive lots of attention, while others seem to prefer more privacy and solitude.
- A pet bird should never be kept in the kitchen as there are risks from cooking fumes.
- Aerosols, plug-in air fresheners, smoke, excess dust and paint fumes are potentially toxic (Jones and Dodd 2012).
- Perches and furnishings should be provided. The dowelling or rigid perches often sold with cages are not suitable (see Aviaries, discussed previously).
- Food and water receptacles must be fastened securely to the sides of the cage.

Although allowing a bird to have the freedom of the house provides exercise and environmental enrichment, there are a number of dangers:

- They may eat house plants or chew electrical cables, resulting in illness or injury.
- Unsupervised birds may chew and swallow carpet and other similar fabrics, resulting in crop and intestinal impactions.
- Free-flying birds are more vulnerable to injury from ceiling fans, cookers, aquaria and attack by other domestic pets.
- Birds may escape through open doors and windows. Bird owners often have the misguided belief that their bird would never fly away and leave them.

Cage and aviary hygiene. To prevent disease and vermin, bird accommodation must be kept scrupulously clean:

- Cages clean water receptacles and food bowls every day; check perches for soiling and replace or clean them using a mild detergent. Rinse, dry and place them back in the cage. Every week, give the accommodation a thorough cleaning.
- Aviaries clean food and water bowls every day, scrub soiled perches, rake soil or gravel substrate and sweep concrete to remove debris and faecal matter. Every week, replace worn perches, scrub all perches, rake and hose gravel or sweep and hose concrete. Rake soil. Check wire and wooden frame for damage. At least once or twice a year change and replace substrate.

Nutrition and feeding

Good health and performance is achieved by providing a balanced palatable diet that is appropriate to the species. This is vital in the bird, as the shape of the beak is designed to cope with a certain type of food and if the wrong food is provided the bird may be physically unable to eat it. It is of primary importance for all bird owners to encourage their birds to eat a variety of foodstuffs as diets can be lacking in a range of vitamins and minerals. Traditional seed-based diets are high in fats but deficient in vitamins such as A and E as well as calcium, iron and selenium. In the USA it is common to feed a formulated pellet-type diet to captive birds with additional supplementation of fruits and vegetables, which is a practice that has not become widely adopted in the UK among pet bird keepers but does provide a good alternative diet with many benefits.

When feeding caged birds, some consideration must be given to their different feeding, social, and migratory behaviours and the limitations of their accommodation.

Guidelines. Birds represent a large group of varied species so for nutritional purposes they can be classified as follows:

- **Seed-eating birds**. Psittacines – e.g. cockatoos, cockatiels, budgerigars, lovebirds, macaws and parrots. Passerines – finches, doves and canaries
  - These eat predominantly a mixture of seeds or seeds and nuts. The size of the seed or nut must be appropriate to the size of the bird – there is no point in feeding a budgie on Brazil nuts but a large parrot would love them. Many smaller cage birds such as budgies are fed exclusively on commercial diets with little variety. This is not ideal and can have long-term effects on their longevity and health.

Suggested additions to their diet include fruit, leafy vegetables fit for human consumption and safe non-toxic plants, e.g. chickweed, groundsel and dandelion or opt for a formulated pelleted diet.

- Any vitamin and mineral supplements offered to birds has to be specifically designed for them.
- **Parrot diets** – are rapidly evolving and now current recommendations are to feed an extruded pellet diet and to supplement with fruit and vegetables (Jones and Dodd 2012). These diets help to prevent selective feeding, but as there are a variety of diets on the market and nutritional value varies some still require supplementation. If the parrot is resistant to change in diet then there are alternative foods that can be offered that provide a good substitute to complete seed mixes; these include soaked pulses (e.g. chickpeas, haricot beans, black-eyed peas, and mung beans) until they have sprouted, rinsing them thoroughly and regularly throughout soaking and then mixing them with 'meaty yellow' and leafy green vegetables. This provides a better source of protein as well as carbohydrate and vitamins and minerals (Jones and Dodd 2012).
  - Seeds and nuts should only make up 10% of the entire diet (Jones and Dodd 2012).
  - Foods to avoid include dairy products, high-fat or sugary foods such as chocolate, and avocado.
- Fruit and/or insect eaters (softbills), e.g. mynah birds, turacos, starlings. These feed on soft foods such as fruits, vegetables, proprietary soft bill mixes, insects and meat (Fig. 33.30).
- Frugivorous birds – mainly eat fleshy fruits and berries.
- **Nectar feeders** or predominantly nectar feeders – i.e. they eat nectar and fruit, e.g. zosterops, sugarbirds, sunbirds, hummingbirds. These eat artificial nectar mixtures, insects, small mealworms, flies, insectivorous mixture, chopped ripe fruits and soaked/chopped raisins. Design of the feeder must satisfy the species; for example, hummingbirds have long tongues that are inserted deep into certain flowers to reach the nectar.
- **Raptors (birds of prey)** – eaters of meat such as dead rodents and birds, e.g. owls, hawks and eagles (Fig. 33.31).

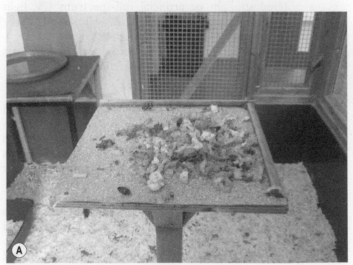

Fig. 33.30A Food prepared for white-cheeked Turacos (*Tauraco leucotis*) that contains fruit, vegetables, soft bill mix, mealworms and a vitamin/mineral supplement

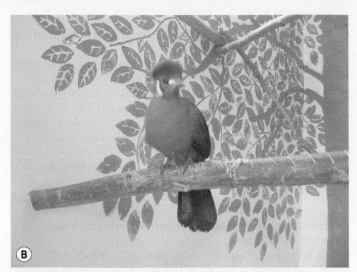

Fig. 33.30B White-cheeked Turacos (*Tauraco leucotis*)

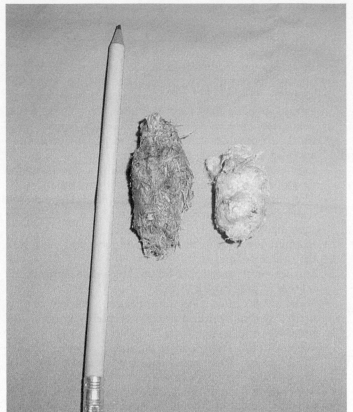

Fig. 33.32 Casts from an owl

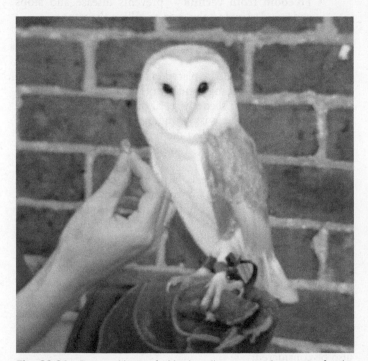

Fig. 33.31 Barn owl being fed by handler. A gauntlet is worn for the safety of the handler

Depending on the species, these birds will consume anything from dead day-old chicks and dead rodents to rabbit, meats and quail. To keep their beaks trim and provide minerals, bones must be offered, and many raptors will enjoy picking the meat off a rabbit skull. Raptors regurgitate to produce casts or pellets, which consist of undigested fur, feathers and bone (Fig. 33.32).

Water is an essential part of the diet; birds should not be allowed to go more than 2 hours without access to water, which is used to soak seeds in the crop and enables enzymes in the proventriculus of the stomach to work.

General feeding tips

- Nuts and seeds have a high fat and protein content and are very palatable. Overfeeding of them can lead to obesity

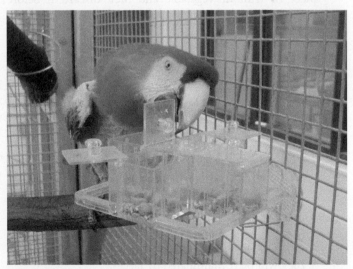

Fig. 33.33 Observe the feeding system used to stimulate a parrot suffering from boredom and demonstrating feather trauma. The parrot is being fed a proprietary complete diet

and selective feeding. They also have low levels of carotene and iodine and provide little calcium – they usually have an inverse calcium-to-phosphorus ratio.
- Complete diets are available that claim to prevent selective feeding and promote general health and well-being in captive birds. Although not necessarily well received by birds on initial introduction, with perseverance they can be a very beneficial diet to many of the parrot family (Fig. 33.33).

- Avocados and apple seeds have been reported to be toxic to birds.
- Hummingbirds require vitamin D and calcium supplements.
- Birds can get addicted to sunflower seeds, leading to obesity and death.
- As birds do not have teeth they need grit within their gizzard to grind their food; therefore, always ensure that seed eaters have access to good-quality quartz grit.
- Cuttlefish provides calcium and phosphorus in the diet and also helps to keep the beak trim.
- Iodine is essential in birds, especially budgerigars, for development and maintenance of the thyroid gland.
- There are a variety of bird seeds available; the type chosen depends on the condition of the bird, e.g. breeding or showing.
- Examine seeds for quality and plumpness and make sure they are dust-free.
- Smaller birds require ad-lib feeding while larger birds require feeding once a day.
- Tonic mixes can be given to seed eaters, especially to help them stay healthy over the winter and when coming into breeding condition.
- When offering fresh food, make sure it is fit for human consumption, fresh and washed to remove traces of chemicals.
- Millet sprays are a useful addition to the diet and can provide extra nutrients during moulting or to stimulate sick birds to eat.
- Birds are messy eaters and will often take a bite out of a piece of fruit or vegetable and then discard it before moving on to the next food item.

Practical feeding. Pellets, seeds and nuts are generally offered in bowls that are attached to the side of the aviary or cage. The positioning of the food receptacle depends on the species being fed:

- Quail and ground-dwelling birds are fed on the floor of the aviary.
- Fresh foods can be placed on a platform in the cage or aviary (see Fig. 33.30).
- As birds are wasteful and will often discard food on to the floor of the aviary, hygiene is very important and all uneaten food must be removed daily.
- Seed husks remaining on the top of the feed container must be removed by blowing them away to allow the birds access to the seeds underneath.
- Remember not to place food bowls under perches, as they will be contaminated by faeces.
- Water is best offered in a gravity-fed bottle or in water hoppers.
- Water receptacles should be small to prevent birds using them as a bath.

Breeding

Over the years, interest in breeding birds has grown, which has resulted in the availability of a wide variety of captive-bred species and colour variations. Breeding is a specialised subject and within this text only a brief outline of breeding procedures and protocols is provided (Table 33.16).

Depending on the species, breeding may be a straightforward procedure with the birds readily breeding and producing healthy offspring, e.g. budgerigars, zebra finches and cockatiels, or it may be more complicated and specialised, e.g. some of the larger parrots.

Before any bird will successfully breed some fundamental requirements must be observed:

- You must have a male and female – this may sound obvious but many birds are not sexually dimorphic and sex must be determined surgically or via DNA polymerase chain reaction (PCR) testing or endoscopic examination (Jones and Dodd 2012).
- Accommodation and environment must be conducive to breeding.
- The correct diet must be fed.

Accommodation and environment. If birds are to be bred in an **aviary** the following must be considered:

- **Siting** – the birds must be given privacy and a stress-free environment. Plants in the aviary will provide ground-dwelling birds, such as pheasants, with hiding areas.
- **Freedom from vermin** – prevents disease and stops rodents destroying the eggs or killing the young.
- **Sheltered flight area** – plastic sheeting on the roof and sides provides protection for nesting birds and fledglings.
- **Nest boxes** should be placed in the aviary before the birds come into breeding condition (Fig. 33.26). Boxes of different sizes and securely set at different heights must be available – if the aviary contains mixed species, this will allow the birds to select the box most suitable for them.

If birds are to be bred in a **cage**, the following must be considered:

- Make sure the cage is large enough for the birds to exercise, as this will improve fitness and fertility.
- Line the cage with plain paper or newspaper rather than sandpaper, as both are more absorbent and cost-effective. Many hen birds are destructive and will often chew the lining paper.
- Nest boxes must be positioned according to the species being housed, but remember to leave enough space for the birds to move in and out of the nest. Budgerigar nest boxes are quite large and are best positioned on the outside of the cage.

Whether housed in indoor cages or aviaries, light and heat must also be considered:

- If the birds are housed in a cage, supplementary heating can be provided in the form of room heating, or for those housed in aviaries or in large indoor flights via tubular heaters. These heaters can be attached to the sides of the accommodation. Supplementary heating can help those birds who breed during the colder months to rear their young and sustain their own body condition, and also reduce the risk of egg binding.
- As most birds tend to breed during the warmer parts of the year and are stimulated by daylight length, controlling the provision of artificial light may stimulate the birds to breed. It also provides them with a longer period to feed, thus increasing body condition and general health. Lighting is best supplied by UVB lights fitted with timers.

Diet. Successful breeding and rearing of young uses a large amount of energy so the bird's diet must be of sufficient quality

TABLE 33.16	Breeding information for the more commonly kept species of caged bird				
Species	Sexing	Clutch size	Incubation period and rearing period	Additional information	
Budgerigar (*Melopsittacus undulatus*)	Cere colour – cock blue or purple; hen brown	4–6 eggs	Incubation 18 days by female. After rearing period, chicks emerge from nest at 35 days and independent by day 42	Easy to breed various colour mutations. Social birds so prefer to breed in groups. Altricial young	
African grey parrot (*Psittacus erithacus*)	Difficult to sex but male may have darker wings; female is smaller	2–4 eggs	Incubation 28–29 days by female. Rearing period approx. 84 days after hatching	May not breed until their fourth year. After that will readily breed and have a long reproductive life. Males will feed young in nest. After fledging fed by both male and female. Sometimes poor parents and hand-rearing is necessary. Altricial young	
Peach-faced lovebirds (*Agapornis roseicollis*)	Monomorphic – need to be surgically sexed	5 eggs	Incubation 28 days. Young fledge approx. 40–42 days after hatching	Various colour mutations. Hens carry nesting materials to line nest. Eggs white. Hatchlings fed by male for extended period. Altricial young	
Cockatiels (*Nymphicus hollandicus*)	Difficult to sex until first moult at approx. 6 months Females plumage duller, especially facial markings, than male. Females have barring on under surface of the tail feathers	5+ eggs	Incubation 18–21 days. Rearing period to fledging is 30–35 days	Both parents incubate eggs. Colour variations available. Breed easily in captivity. To prevent breeding remove nest boxes especially over winter when young vulnerable to cold. Altricial young	
Canary (*Serinus canaria*)	No clear distinction between male and female, although male sings during breeding season	4 eggs	Incubation period 14 days by hen. Rearing period 14 days	Altricial young	
Zebra finch (*Taeniopygia* (*poephilia*) *guttata*)	Females have paler beaks and usually lack chest and flank markings of the males	6 eggs	Incubation period 12 days by hen. Rearing period – chicks start to leave nest 18 days after hatching	Fledglings will eat independently 14 days after leaving. Prolific breeders: need to limit clutches to three per year. Move nests and nesting material to prevent continuous nest building. Altricial young	
Hill mynah (*Gracula religiosa*)	No visible distinction between sexes	2–4 eggs, green blue with brown spots	Incubation period 14–15 days by both parents. Fledge at 4–5 weeks, independent at 8 weeks	Supply cockatiel or starling nest boxes all year. In breeding season supply twigs, leaves, straw, hay and hemp fibres as nesting materials. Altricial young	
Diamond dove (*Geopelia cuneata*)	Both sexes have red eye rings but those of males are thicker during breeding season. Males have more spots on wings than females	2 eggs	Incubation period 13 days, with both parents involved in the process. After rearing period the chicks may leave nest as early as 13 days post hatching	Good parents and care for young. Altricial young	
Chinese painted quail (*Excalfactoria chinensis*)	Hens have brownish overall colour and lack the cock's bluish plumage	6 eggs	Incubation period 18 days	Precocial young are virtually able to live independently after hatching providing temperature, etc. is correct. They are not fed by parents	

NB. Incubation and rearing periods may vary.

and quantity. Various species of parrot and soft bills can be stimulated into breeding condition by increasing protein levels, and it has been shown to be of value in improving reproductive performance. A poor-quality diet will cause poor reproductive performance, egg binding and reduced numbers of offspring.

Egg laying and incubation. Signs that a hen is about to lay her eggs include:
- Spending longer periods on the nest or in the nest box, and the cock bird will often join her
- Hen's vent may appear slightly swollen
- Change in the amount and smell of hen's droppings.

The frequency of laying varies according to species. For instance, finches lay every day, while budgerigars and many of the parrot family lay every other day. To prevent eggs developing at different rates, the hen will often not incubate her eggs until at least three eggs have been laid. This behaviour can alarm the novice breeder but intervention could lead to the hen abandoning her nest. During incubation the sitting bird will turn the eggs daily to prevent the embryo from sticking to the inside of the shell.

Incubation periods vary according to species (see Table 33.16):

1. **Natural incubation** – eggs are incubated by either the hen alone, e.g. budgerigars, or shared between the hen and cock bird, e.g. cockatiels. In wading birds such as coots and moor hens it is the male who takes sole responsibility for incubation.
2. **Artificial incubation** – eggs are incubated in a specially designed avian incubator. There are various models available and features vary but it is advisable to purchase one that will automatically turn the eggs as this is not only time saving but reduces heat loss every time the incubator is opened. Heat is a key factor in successful hatching and a fluctuation of 0.5°C can have quite damaging effects on the viability of the eggs. As a guide incubation temperatures range from 36.9–37.5°C (98.5–99.5°F) with a relative humidity of 40–55% depending on species.

Rearing chicks. When first hatched, chicks can be classified according to their stage of development:

- **Altricial** – blind, bald and totally dependent on the parents, e.g. budgerigars, finches
- **Precocial** – capable of living an independent life, e.g. quail, ducklings.

They may also be grouped according to when they leave the nest:

- **Nidifugous** – capable of leaving the nest soon after hatching, e.g. ducklings and goslings
- **Nidiculous** – remain in the nest until they are feathered and ready to fly, e.g. budgerigar, cockatiel, parrots.

If eggs have been incubated by the parents, then they will care for and feed the young. If they have been hatched using artificial means, then the hatchlings should be moved to a brooder and kept in a controlled environment until they are weaned and feathered. During the rearing period the accommodation and nest boxes or brooder must be kept very clean. If droppings and uneaten food remain, the nestlings' feet can become encrusted in debris, preventing them from walking and leading to disease.

Avian disease

Some bird diseases are extremely difficult to identify so if signs continue for more than 24 hours a veterinary surgeon must be consulted (Table 33.17).

General signs of ill health in a bird include:

- Lethargy
- Bird's feathers ruffled and 'puffed up'
- Sleeping with both feet on perch – especially parrots
- Sitting on the bottom of the cage
- Poor appetite
- Regurgitating food
- Loose, watery or abnormally coloured droppings
- Increased thirst
- Discharge from nostrils and eyes
- Abnormal breathing – laboured, noisy, exaggerated tail movements
- Heavy moult.

Other more specific signs include blood in the droppings, a prominent breast bone indicating severe loss of weight, gasping for breath with the beak open, uncoordinated movements and paralysis.

When dealing with an ill bird you should isolate the bird from other birds and humans as soon as possible. The isolation cage should be positioned in a quiet, well-ventilated room and have three solid sides. There should be an infrared or ceramic heat lamp to keep the cage at a temperature of at least 32°C (89.6°F). If appropriate, offer food that is easily digestible and water that is lukewarm.

Welfare of captive exotic animals

PAIN AND DISTRESS

All the exotic species that are kept as pets are capable of feeling pain and distress and in some cases if this is not identified and is allowed to continue it may lead to the death of the animal. Even the close proximity of the human owner may be a source of distress and it is important to realise that, unlike dogs and cats, many of these exotic species do not enjoy being handled.

Definitions of pain and distress include:

- **Pain** – an unpleasant sensory and emotional experience associated with actual or potential tissue damage. This physical phenomenon may be classified as mild, moderate or substantial or depending on the duration of the pain may be described as being acute or chronic.
- **Discomfort** – milder than pain and may be nothing more than an inconvenience.
- **Distress** – often shortened to 'stress'. This is a psychological phenomenon and may be associated with pain. 'Stressors' include isolation (in social species), maternal separation, overcrowding, noise or lack of privacy.

It is often difficult to decide whether an animal is in pain or distress and veterinary nurses are commonly told that 'it must be very difficult to do your job because animals cannot tell you what is wrong'; however, animals cannot lie or exaggerate their situation, so the presented picture is the true one.

There are three ways of assessing the situation:

- **Subjective assessment** – using your 'gut instinct' where there are no measurable factors. If you would expect an injury or disease to cause pain in humans then it probably causes pain in other species – always remember postoperative pain.
- **Clinical assessment** – certain clinical signs will indicate pain, e.g. raised pulse rate or respiratory rate, raised temperature, loss of weight caused by loss of appetite or dehydration. These are quantifiable, e.g. the higher the pulse rate the greater the degree of pain.
- **Behavioural assessment** – in order to assess whether an animal is behaving abnormally you must first know what is normal for that species, e.g. is it normal for a bird to sit fluffed up on its perch with its eyes shut, for a rabbit to scream or for a mouse to sit separately from the rest of its cage mates?

Pain and distress can be reduced by:

- **Correct handling** – learn the recommended method and do it correctly the first time. Make sure that any equipment you may need is available and in good working order and, if you are likely to need assistance, make sure that help is at hand.
- **Providing a high standard of animal husbandry**, i.e. appropriate housing, environment and diet.
- **Making changes to the environment to reduce pain**, e.g. confine a bird with a broken wing to a small cage so that it cannot fly.

Text continued on p. 754

TABLE 33.17	Common diseases and clinical conditions of birds			
Species	**Causal agent**	**Symptoms**	**Diagnosis and treatment**	**Additional information**
ECTOPARASITES				
Scaly leg and scaly face mite (cnemidocoptic mange) Budgerigars, crossbills, Passeriformes; canaries; occasionally in domestic poultry	Cnemidocoptes spp.	Common in budgerigar. Appears as grey white encrustations around the cere, beak, eyes, feet and legs. Seen on legs of crossbills and appears as foot lesions on canaries and other passerines	Examine a scraping of affected area. Ivermectin at 200–400 µg/kg, PO or by injection, is generally effective. The treatment is usually repeated in 2 wk	May infest cloaca. Mite lives and feeds on bird's beak, surrounding areas and legs. It burrows and feeds off the bird, if untreated leading to infection, rotting skin and osteomyelitis. Hygiene and isolation as mite rapidly spreads. Remember – this drug can remain in the system for prolonged periods so care not to overdose
Red mite (greyish agile mite) Seen in domestic poultry	Dermanyssus spp.	Bird sits restlessly on the perch. Constantly pecking and scratching at itself. If you shine a torch into the cage at night you will see the mite. Zoonotic – humans can develop a rash caused by the mite	Mite-infested birds may be treated with pyrethrin sprays, 5% carbaryl powder, or ivermectin	Mite lives in the dark crevices and seams of the bird's accommodation and emerges from its hiding place at night to attack and suck the blood of the sleeping bird. It is particularly difficult to treat and destroy by just disinfecting as the mite can live up to 5 months without food and reproduce at a rate of 2600 eggs per 2 months life span
Other				
ENDOPARASITES				

Tapeworm (cestodes)
Roundworms (nematodes)
	Large number of different species involved	Thin, anorexic and generally lethargic birds. Diarrhoea. Screen droppings/crop smears for worm eggs	Faecal floatation to identify eggs.
			Crop tube and worm using liquid medication, or place drops in water. Use veterinary prescribed anthelmintics:
			Tapeworms –
			  • Fenbendazole
			  • Praziquantel
			Roundworms –
			  • Levamisole
			  • Fenbendazole
			  • Ivermectin
				Tapeworms – worm eggs found in an intermediate host, i.e. the food they ingested infects birds. The adult worms then develop in the bird's intestine and eggs are shed in the droppings. Intermediate host ingest the worm eggs and the cycle starts again
				Roundworms – worm eggs are passed out in the bird's droppings and are passed onto other birds by contaminating food, eggs, adhere to feathers, and feet Fenbendazole is toxic to finches. Levamisole can be toxic and deaths seen in budgerigars, pigeons and lovebirds

ENTERIC DISEASE				
Enteritis All species	Escherichia coli Campylobacter spp. Change in diet	Anorexia. Change in appearance to droppings yellow-green, watery. Bird listless and quiet	Histology and culture of infected tissue. Antibiotics or sulphonamides. Supportive therapy, i.e. fluid therapy	Watery green droppings suggest reduced food intake and excess bile secretion

Trichomoniasis
All species
	Trichomonas gallinae	Sometimes acute death, white or yellow cheesy-looking plaques, ulcers and/or nodules inside of the mouth and throat, diarrhoea, inappetence, weight loss, lethargy dyspnoea	Microscopic examination to identify parasite
			Treatment:
			  • Metronidazole
			  • Carnidazole
			  • Dimetridazole
			Good hygiene and supportive therapy
				Also called 'canker' in pigeons and 'frounce' in raptors. Infections via direct contact, generally in food

Continued

TABLE 33.17	Common diseases and clinical conditions of birds—cont'd			
Species	**Causal agent**	**Symptoms**	**Diagnosis and treatment**	**Additional information**
Salmonellosis All species Caused by: poor hygiene, rodent infestation, wild birds, and poor quarantine	*Salmonella* spp.	Including: • Blood-stained droppings • Slimy droppings • Smelly droppings • Swelling of wings or joints • Passage of undigested food • Paralysis	Antibiotics, good hygiene, supportive therapy	Zoonosis causing enteric signs, i.e. diarrhoea and vomiting
RESPIRATORY DISEASE				

Ornithosis Psitticosis Chlamydiosis Mainly seen in:
• Psittacine birds
  – cockatiels, lovebirds, budgerigars, parrots
• Columbiformes
  – doves
• Anseriformes
  – ducks, geese and swans
	Chlamydia psittaci	Affected bird may sit huddled up on perch, wheezing, gasping for breath, open beak and exaggerated tail movements. Respiratory signs, nasal, ocular discharge, ruffled feathers, shivering. Enteritis	Recommend PCR testing on 3–5-day-old pooled dropping sample (Stanford 2010) for diagnosis. Isolate affected bird. Keep bird warm and supportive therapy. Antibiotics, e.g. enrofloxacin; tetracyclines, chlorotetracyclines medication must be sustained for a minimum of 35–45 days as pathogen can exist dormant in cells for some time.	Zoonosis causing flu-like signs, diarrhoea, shivering, pyrexia, and headaches. Never share food or allow a bird to take food from your mouth. Always wash hands after handling a bird. Disease passed on via droppings and discharges. Humans inhale causative agent. Strict hygiene protocols. Mainly seen in imported birds or smuggled birds not correctly quarantined. Most imported birds are routinely treated against *Chlamydia*. Chlorotetracyclines are bactericidal and require prolonged use

Avian mycoplasmosis All species	*Mycoplasma* spp.	Upper respiratory infection sneezing, sinusitis, blepharitis	Laboratory diagnosis of causative organism. Use various antimicrobial drugs, e.g. tetracyclines, enrofloxacin not penicillins	Seen where groups of birds kept confined and with poor ventilation
Viscerotropic Velogenic Newcastle's disease (fowl pest) – notifiable disease Affects all avians	Paramyxovirus	Variable: listlessness, green slimy droppings, depression, anorexia, weight loss, sneezing, nasal discharge, dyspnoea, conjunctivitis, ataxia, head bobbing, unilateral or bilateral wing and leg paralysis	Virus isolation. Histopathology	Highly infectious – all affected and in-contact livestock must be destroyed. Affects egg production. Major reason for avian quarantine. Vaccine available for poultry
NUTRITIONAL DISORDERS				
Iodine deficiency Seen in Budgerigars	Iodine-deficient diet	Loss or change in voice, respiratory problems due to pressure from enlarged thyroid on trachea. Bird often has difficulty breathing and makes a characteristic 'click' sound. To aid respiration, bird can be observed sitting with head raised. Crop dilation as seed unable to pass into the thyroid gland into the proventriculus	Iodine supplementation. Improve diet and add iodine to drinking water	Not commonly seen because of use of packaged seeds that have been supplemented. Iodine deficiency affects thyroid hormone production, which then stimulates an increase in thyroid-stimulating hormone (TSH) from the anterior pituitary. Raised levels of TSH cause hyperplasia (enlargement) of the thyroid gland (goitre)

Vitamin A deficiency — Common in all species	Vitamin-A-deficient diet. Lack of fresh vegetables and fruit in diet. Overuse of sunflower seeds in the diet	Generally ill bird, lethargic, weight loss and signs of respiratory problems such as wheezing, dyspnoea and sneezing. Nasal discharge. Eyes appear swollen, with signs of conjunctivitis	Change diet, with addition of dark green vegetables and carrots. Vitamin A therapy	Psittacine birds that have been fed on an all-seed diet will not readily accept fresh fruits and vegetables, but the owner must be persuaded to persevere with this change in diet
Calcium, phosphorus and vitamin D deficiency — Psittacines and those birds fed on an exclusively seed diet	High seed and nut diet, especially peanuts and sunflower seeds	Variety of skeletal problems and poor growth. Egg binding and soft shells. General signs will depend on age and duration of problem. Poor appetite, lethargy, weakness, poor feather growth, soft droppings. Bird unable to perch properly, wings held in abnormal position; in severe cases bird appears to have a hunched back. Muscle spasms and twitching. Death	Severe cases, give intravenous calcium borogluconate and intramuscular diazepam. Improve diet plus calcium supplementation	Vitamin D activated by ultraviolet light on the skin influences the uptake and usage of dietary calcium and phosphorus
FEATHER PROBLEMS				
Feather plucking — Feather destructive syndrome	Self-mutilation due to boredom, stress, isolation, changes in routine, over-preening during breeding season. Poor husbandry and nutrition, hormonal imbalance	Plumage on body is damaged and bald areas apart from head. Clinical history examination to rule out other feather disorders	Once established, this is very difficult to stop. Enrich cage, and bird's life. Education of the owner on how to deal with bird. Fitting of an collar to prevent mutilation. Drug therapy and UVB 2% light	Rule out ectoparasites by careful examination of plumage. Frequently seen in parrots. Placing another bird in the cage may seem a good idea but evidence has shown that behaviour can be passed on to new occupant
Feather cysts — Certain breeds of canary; other domestic species	Genetic or due to damage to developing feather follicle or excess preening	Large, bulging swellings seen in region of the carpus (wings) but can be seen in other parts of the body – contains the remains of the undeveloped feather	Surgical removal	The wall of the follicles can become thickened and a cheesy exudates forms within it
Loss of feather condition	Various pathogens and conditions that can affect the integrity of the feathers and dermis; Ectoparasites; Bullying; Feather plucking; Poor environmental conditions, especially low humidity and nutrition	Baldness; Intense irritation; Damage to feathers		Rule out ectoparasites. Moulting is a natural occurrence and frequency depends on species and environmental conditions. Moulting is a stressful process for the bird and nutritional demands are high, so increased nutrition and supplementation must be considered. Broken feathers will not normally regrow until the next moult. It can take 4–6 weeks for new feathers to grow

Continued

TABLE 33.17	Common diseases and clinical conditions of birds—cont'd			
Species	**Causal agent**	**Symptoms**	**Diagnosis and treatment**	**Additional information**
Psittacine beak and feather disease Various psittacines species, especially cockatoos	Viral: circo virus	Poor feather condition and abnormal plumage. Feathers appear small and club-like, fret lines in the vane, curled feathers. Feather loss. Feathers remain in blood-filled sheath. Beak also abnormal appearance, shiny, elongated, flaky and fault lines. Change in feather coloration	PCR test of blood sample or feather pulp (Stanford 2010) Fatal Supportive therapy may be considered but because of its virulence and threat to bird populations, any suspected cases must be quarantined and diagnosis made rapidly Avian interferon has been demonstrated to be effective (Stanford 2010)	Transmission of virus via faeces, feathers and dust
Regurgitation All species	Many causes, including: • Behavioural response • Proventriculus • Dilatation disease • Ingestion of foreign body • Infections, e.g. yeast, candidiasis, Trichomonas, Megabacterium • Reaction to drug therapy • Ingestion of toxins, e.g. plants, insecticides • Neoplasm • Parasites • Crop stasis/necrosis • Crop impaction	Food regurgitated. Other signs depend on causative agent. Physical examination of the bird to eliminate foreign body. Check oral cavity. Palpate crop, abdomen and cloaca palpated. Faecal examination, bacteriology and blood tests to identify pathogen. Endoscopy to identify and remove foreign body	Depending on diagnosis: fluid therapy and supportive care; tube feeding Ingluviotomy to remove foreign matter.	Regurgitation occurs during courtship, feeding of nestlings and weaning. Pet birds may also adopt an object or family member and regurgitate as a method of courtship or feeding

OTHER CONDITIONS

Condition / Species	Causes / Clinical signs	Treatment
Egg binding All species, particularly budgerigars and cockatiels	Multifactorial: • Size of egg • First clutch • Calcium/vitamin D deficiency • Obesity • Oviduct torsion, infection and neoplasia • Poor environmental conditions • Age of bird As egg laying imminent, bird appears depressed, lethargic, abdominal distension, unsteadiness on perch, squatting, straining and diarrhoea blood present. *Note:* Clinical signs can vary depending on the site of the egg	Treatment varies according to position of egg, but it is important to remove the egg as soon as possible. This may be via drug therapy, 5% calcium gluconate either oral or parental route Manual manipulation under anaesthesia. Aspirate egg contents using hypodermic needle transabdominally collapse egg and expel shell assist with by gentle flushing of warm saline (Stanford 2010) Surgery. Keep bird warm (30–32°C) and UVB lighting Bird will be very distressed and it is important to keep patient warm and quiet and in a darkened room Review diet and husbandry care
Articular gout Poultry, waterfowl, raptors and psittacine birds, especially budgerigars, conures and lovebirds	Associated with renal disease or damage occurs when uric acid and urates are deposited in the legs or wing joints Swollen painful joints. Bird exhibiting shifting lameness, and hanging on side of cage to take weight off painful joints. Loss of condition Diagnosis urine dipstick, blood test (uric acid not urea) radiograph and endoscopy (Stanford 2010)	No specific treatment: only able to manage the signs, e.g. by restricting high-protein foodstuffs in diet and maintaining good state of hydration. Drug therapy to reduce uric acid production in the liver. Allopurinol may be useful as a treatment (Stanford 2010) Water consumption can be improved by adding fruits and vegetables in the diet. Nodules of the uric acid also called tophi are creamy white in colour. They are normally seen on the intertarsals and joints of the feet. Prognosis is poor
Bumble foot Poultry, birds of prey, occasionally psittacine birds	Common microorganisms isolated: • *Staphylococcus aureus* • *Escherichia coli* • *Proteus* spp. Septic condition of the foot leading to abscessation. Microorganism gains entry via a penetrating wound underneath the foot. Infection leads to swelling and pus-filled areas. Infection can track as far as hock. As bird is in discomfort, it can be observed resting against sides of cage	Radiographs to assess extent of damage. Swab taken of area for culture and sensitivity will indicate appropriate antibiotics. Foot may be bandaged changing 7–10 days and bird kept on padded perches of varying widths In severe case under a general anaesthetic debride infected area Antimicrobial treatment Linked with vitamin A deficiency, poor hygiene and perches all the same width. Also high incidence in heavy, inactive birds limited to one size of perch. Initial penetrating wound can be caused by claws growing into foot. If left untreated, area can become gangrenous

- **Attending to wounds and infection** as soon as possible to minimise suffering.
- **Using therapeutic agents** to reduce pain if appropriate, e.g. analgesics and anaesthetics.
- **Be prepared to use euthanasia as a means of relieving suffering** if treatment is likely to cause pain or is unlikely to be successful. Euthanasia by definition is painless and very quick when performed competently and should not be overlooked as a possible course of action.

The welfare of animals should be viewed holistically, i.e. look at every aspect that affects the animal, from its environment and diet to the type of owner, which might include age and experience, employment, whether they smoke, whether they have children, where they live, etc. All these factors and many more will affect the welfare of the animal and should be taken into account when identifying problems.

There are three main areas that must be constantly reviewed by the veterinary nurse and clients should be advised upon:

- Appropriate husbandry, i.e. diet, housing, environment and their management
- Appropriate psychological and behavioural needs to avoid the development of stereotypical and other behaviour problems
- Basic health requirements of the species.

The welfare of exotic animals is also of extreme importance within the veterinary practice and as most nurses and veterinary surgeons see these animals less often, inevitably we know less about their veterinary needs and their responses to anaesthetic and analgesic drugs. Their preoperative and postoperative care is often the responsibility of the nurse, who must be aware of both normal behaviour and the significance of abnormal behaviour.

SMALL MAMMALS

With the exception of the ferret, most small mammals show little evidence of pain. These are all prey species so in the wild, if they were to show pain, they would make themselves vulnerable and obvious to predators, who would then kill them. They rarely vocalise unless handled roughly, although rabbits will scream or become actively aggressive, as would a cat or dog. Table 33.18 describes both normal and abnormal behaviour patterns.

Pain should be assessed and monitored and recorded on hospital sheets at regular intervals, e.g. every 2–3 hours. This should include details of:

- Appetite – what was eaten and quantity
- Urination – quantity and appearance
- Defecation – appearance
- Caecotrophy – able to eat caecotrophs
- Demeanour – bright, lethargic, aggressive
- Activity levels – movement around cage/enclosure
- Body position – hunched, tight, relaxed
- Pupils – dilated or constricted
- Grinding teeth – salivation
- Condition of coat – 'staring' coat/piloerection.

REPTILES

Reptiles are very easily stressed and feel pain. Although pain management in reptiles continues to be an area for further advancement, it should be stressed that reptiles can display pain and the use of analgesia is recommended. Table 33.19 describes both normal and abnormal behaviours that may indicate pain in reptiles.

TABLE 33.18	Normal behaviour and abnormal behaviour as an indicator of pain and distress in small mammals					
	Rabbits	**Guinea pigs**	**Ferrets**	**Gerbils**	**Mice**	**Rats**
Normal behaviour	Active, inquisitive, eating/foraging regularly. Coprophagia performed at night. Body posture relaxed and will often lie stretched out	Active, inquisitive, eating/foraging regularly. Coprophagia performed at night. Normal vocalisation, chunter, chutt, whistles and whines. Only rodent that normally vocalises	Active, inquisitive, sniffing ground and playing. Relaxed body posture	Active, inquisitive, eating/foraging regularly. Interacting with cage mates	Active, inquisitive, eating/ foraging regularly. Interacting with cage mates	Active, inquisitive, eating/ foraging regularly. Interacting with cage mates
Indication of pain/ abnormal behaviour	Hunched body posture, very still and inactive. High-pitched scream if in extreme pain or fear (usually only when attacked by predator). Anorexia. Teeth grinding, indicating pain. Will salivate if oral discomfort. Often more difficult to handle. Hiding at back of cage. Postoperatively, rabbits often interfere with wound/sutures	Hunched body posture, very still and inactive. If scared or in pain, guinea pigs will emit a very high-pitched scream. Anorexia. Teeth grinding, indicating pain. Will salivate if in oral discomfort. Hiding at back of cage	High-pitched scream, associated with fear rather than pain. May become more aggressive if in pain. Will often interfere with wound/sutures if operation site painful	May bite if handled. Fur often looks 'staring'. Quiet hunched body posture; if in communal groups, will avoid contact with other gerbils. Often ostracised by colony, may be thrown out of housing area	May bite if handled. Fur often looks 'staring'. Quiet hunched body posture; if in communal groups, will avoid contact with other mice	Quiet, reduction in exploratory behaviour. Will often interfere with wound/ sutures if operation site painful

TABLE 33.19	Normal and abnormal behaviour as an indicator of pain in reptiles and birds			
	Snakes	**Lizards**	**Chelonia**	**Birds**
Normal behaviour	Hiding under furnishings or curled round branch, or basking, slowly moving round cage. Docile species accept disturbance from handler when cleaning and maintaining accommodation. Non-aggressive toward handler. Normal ecdysis. Accepting food and eating regularly. Passing normal urine and faecal matter	Lively, seen basking and moving around the accommodation. Accepting food. Docile species handled with ease. Accepts being kept in accommodation	Active, walking with shell lifted off the ground. Eating, passing urates and faecal matter. Non-aggressive, basking and thermoregulation. Quickly retreats into shell if threatened or approached. Strength in limbs	Plump and plumage in good condition and feathers held flat against the bird's body. Sits steadily on perch, greets known human companions. Able to carry out free flight. Normal relaxed respiration. Droppings appear normal white urates and brown or black faecal matter
Abnormal	Restless and moving around accommodation. Agitated by normal routine, i.e. feeding, handling and cleaning. Striking at handler. Abnormal posture head and neck raised and mouth gaping and exaggerated breathing. Contortions and twisting of body. Constantly rubbing body against furnishings. Flaccid and lethargic, problems shedding. Watery faecal matter	Quiet species may become more lively or lively species subdued. Docile species becomes aggressive and refuses food. Constantly knocking into vivarium doors, especially glass. Aggression toward fellow occupants. Not actively basking or not moving away from hot spot. Head raised and open-mouthed breathing. Flaccid and lethargic. Dark, dull colour, especially in chameleons. Iguanas males – head bobbing and knocking tail against doors and walls	Failure to retract head into shell. Limp and flaccid limbs. Slow-moving. Remains under hot spot or hidden away. Not eating. Open-mouthed breathing	Hunched or abnormal appearance on perch. Sits with eyes closed. Head under wing. Feathers ruffled and exaggerated breathing. Feather plucking, and aggression toward familiar human companions

Hospitalised reptiles

Sick reptiles should be placed in secure hospital vivaria, ideally made from fibreglass or moulded plastic with correct controlled heating and lighting. They should be kept in a separate room away from other domestic animals and, if a lizard is very stressed and banging against the front of the vivarium, a non-reflective covering can be placed over the glass front, allowing the nurse to observe the patient without disturbing it.

For short-term holding a plastic fauna container resting on a heat mat may suffice.

Tortoises may be housed in an open-topped style enclosure with appropriate heating, lighting and UV lamps (Lewis et al. 2012).

Factors that can cause distress in reptiles

- Poor environmental conditions and positioning of the animal's enclosure or vivarium (see Housing, discussed previously).
- Over-handling – there is little evidence to show that reptiles enjoy constant handling and if it is incorrectly carried out some species of lizards, e.g. geckos, can carry out autotomy (tail loss). Snakes are easily bruised and can suffer spinal injuries, especially in the occipital area. **Note:** Bruising may take several weeks to show in cold-blooded species and can be a cause of death.
- Inadequate nutrition (see Nutrition, discussed previously).
- Overcrowding and fighting – many lizards are territorial and males will fight to defend their territory or to claim females. Geckos, bearded dragons and water dragons are a few examples of lizards that are very territorial and must be kept either on their own or with females.

Juvenile male tortoises are exceedingly 'oversexed' and bachelor groups will constantly try and mate one another, resulting in bite wounds to the legs and shell trauma as they constantly ram into one another. If a male and female are kept together the female will be constantly harassed by the male's amorous advances.

- Poor husbandry and illness.
- Wild-caught species not adjusting to a captive environment.
- Prolonged transportation.

It may take weeks or months for the results of stress to become obvious and animals that have sustained long periods of stress will have a diminished immune response.

BIRDS

Table 33.19 shows both normal and abnormal behaviour in caged and aviary birds.

Hospitalised birds

As most birds spend most of their time above human eye-level, i.e. in aviaries or on cage perches, it makes sense to accommodate these birds in the veterinary surgery at high levels, e.g. on high shelves or in hanging cages, which will make the bird feel less threatened and reduces stress. They should be accommodated away from predator animals and excessive noise and kept in subdued light.

Suitable accommodation will depend on the species being hospitalised. Some species may be able to remain in their own accommodation whereas other species such as poultry and peafowl can be housed in dog and cat kennels (Lewis et al. 2012).

Unless the patient needs to be confined, remember to restrict movement. The cage should be large enough to allow the bird to extend its wings in all directions (Lewis et al. 2012).

When handling a bird it will feel much happier if it can perch on your finger, but there is the risk of escape so steps must be taken to prevent this. Restraining a bird just around the wings causes it much distress and it will attempt to flap.

Factors that can cause distress in birds

- Siting of cages and aviaries – some birds are gregarious and enjoy being in a busy area and, if deprived of human or other bird contact, can become depressed and display behavioural abnormalities. To other species this would cause much distress and health problems.
- Overcrowding and bullying.
- Overbreeding.
- Poor nutrition.
- Poor environmental hygiene.
- Disease and illness.

BIBLIOGRAPHY

Ballard, B., Cheek, R. (Eds.), 2010. Exotic Animal Medicine for the Veterinary Technician, second ed. Blackwell, Iowa, USA.

Bament, W., 2012. A vet nurse's guide guinea pigs, behaviour housing and anatomy. Veterinary Nursing Times, September (9).

Bament, W., 2013. Ferret handling, nutrition and common health problems. Veterinary Nursing Times, November, p. 22.

Bament, W., 2014. Rats – a vet nurse's guide to their behaviour and husbandry needs. Veterinary Nursing Times CPD, April, pp. 29–31.

Bartlett, P.B., Griswold, B., Bartlett, R.D., 2010. Reptiles, Amphibians, and Invertebrates: An Identification and Care Guide, second ed. Barron's Educational Series, Hauppauge, NY.

Benato, L., Eatwell, K., 2011. Myxomatosis care in pet rabbits. Veterinary Times, August, pp. 18–20.

Bennett, T., Jessop, M., 2010. Turtles and tortoises. In: Meredith, A., Johnson-Delaney, C. (Eds.), BSAVA Manual of Exotic Pets, fifth ed. British Small Animal Veterinary Association, Quedgeley pp. 249–272.

Cheek, R., Richards, S., Crane, M., 2010. Snakes. In: Ballard, B., Cheek, R. (Eds.), Exotic Animal Medicine for the Veterinary Technician, second ed. Blackwell, Iowa, USA.

Chitty, J., Raftery, A., 2013. Essentials of Tortoise Medicine and Surgery. John Wiley and Sons Ltd Chichester.

Coles, B.H., 1997. Avian Medicine and Surgery, second ed. Blackwell Science, Oxford.

Courteney-Smith, J., 2013. Light and Shade. <http://www.arcadia-reptile.com/files/2013/01/004_PRK_Mar13.pdf>.

Divers, S.J., 1997. Medical and surgical treatment of reptile dystocias. In: 21st Annual Waltham/Ohio State University Symposium (for the Treatment of Animal Diseases). Lecture Notes. College of Veterinary Medicine, Ohio State University and Waltham USA Inc., Vernon, CA, pp. 75–81.

Eatwell, K., 2010. Lizards. In: Meredith, A., Johnson-Delaney, C. (Eds.), BSAVA Manual of Exotic Pets, fifth revised ed. British Small Animal Veterinary Association, Gloucester.

Girling, S., Raiti, P. (Eds.), 2004. BSAVA Manual of Reptiles, second ed. British Small Animal Veterinary Association, Cheltenham.

Girling, S.J., 2013. Veterinary Nursing of Exotic Pets, second ed. Wiley Blackwell.

Harcourt-Brown, N., Chitty, J. (Eds.), 2005. BSAVA Manual of Psittacine Birds, second ed. British Small Animal Veterinary Association, Cheltenham.

Hedley, J., 2013. Sick reptiles: diagnostics on a budget. Veterinary Times, November 11, pp. 31–32.

Hedley, J., 2014. What every practitioner should know about lizards. Veterinary Times, October 20, pp. 11–13.

Hoby, S., Wenker, C., Robert, N., et al., 2010. Nutritional metabolic bone disease in juvenile veiled chameleons (Chamaeleo calyptratus) and its prevention. J. Nutr. 140 (11), 1923–1931.

Jones, R., Dodd, C., 2012. Birds: biology and husbandry. In: Varga, M., Lumbis, R.Gott, L. (Eds.), BSAVA Manual of Exotic Pet and Wildlife Nursing. British Small Animal Veterinary Association, Gloucester.

Lewis, W., Stanton, L., Flack, S., 2012. The hospital ward. In: Varga, M., Lumbis, R., Gott, L. (Eds.), BSAVA Manual of Exotic Pet and Wildlife Nursing. British Small Animal Veterinary Association, Gloucester, pp. 110–127.

Longley, M., Longley, L., 2008. Caring for Mediterranean tortoises. Veterinary Times, July 21, pp. 26–27.

Longley, M., Longley, L., 2009. Tricky tortoise husbandry tips. Veterinary Times, June 29, pp. 18–19.

Mader, D.R., Divers, S.J., 2013. Current Therapy in Reptile Medicine and Surgery. Elsevier, St. Louis, MO.

Mader, D.R., et al., 2006. Reptile Medicine and Surgery, second ed. Saunders Elsevier, St. Louis, MO.

Magnus, E., 2009. Understanding rabbits part one: what makes a rabbit a rabbit? Veterinary Nursing Times (4), 1 April.

Meredith, A., Johnson-Delaney, C. (Eds.), 2010. BSAVA Manual of Exotic Pets, fifth ed. British Small Animal Veterinary Association, Gloucester.

Quesenberry, K.E., Carpenter, J.W., 2004. Ferrets, Rabbits and Rodents – Clinical Medicine and Surgery, second ed. W B Saunders, St. Louis, MO.

Raiti, P., 2010. Snakes. In: Meredith, A., Johnson-Delaney, C. (Eds.), BSAVA Manual of Exotic Pets, fifth, revised ed. British Small Animal Veterinary Association, Gloucester, pp. 294–314.

Rendle, M., Cracknell, J., 2012. Reptiles: biology and husbandry. In: Varga, M., Lumbis, R.Gott, L. (Eds.), BSAVA Manual of Exotic Pet and Wildlife Nursing. British Small Animal Veterinary Association, Gloucester, pp. 80–108.

Stanford, M., 2010. Cage and aviary birds. In: Meredith, A., Johnson-Delaney, C. (Eds.), BSAVA Manual of Exotic Pets, fifth ed. British Small Animal Veterinary Association, Gloucester, pp. 167–187.

Tully, T.N., Dorrestein, G.M., Jones, A.K., 2009. Handbook of Avian Medicine, second ed. WB Saunders, Philadelphia.

Varga, M., Lumbis, R., Gott, L., 2012. BSAVA Exotic Pet and Wildlife Nursing. British Small Animal Veterinary Association, Gloucester.

Wilson, B., 2010. Lizards. In: Ballard, B., Cheek, R. (Eds.), Exotic Animal Medicine for the Veterinary Technician, second ed. Blackwell, Iowa, USA.

WEBSITES USED

<http://lafeber.com/vet/>: The resource for exotic animal veterinary professionals. Pollock, C., Lafeber Company veterinary consultant. February 25, 2011; reviewed and updated May 30, 2012.

<http://www.reptilesmagazine.com/Reptile-Magazines/Reptiles-Magazine/February-2010/Breeding-Savannah-Monitors/>

<http://www.tortoiseclub.org/index.php>: Tortoise Club. Originally founded in Norfolk by Mr. Leonard Coe in 2002 to improve tortoise welfare in captivity.

<http://www.tortoiseclub.org/CareSheets/General_Tortoise/Waking_Mediterranean_Tortoises_after_hibernation.pdf>

<http://www.tortoiseclub.org/CareSheets/General_Tortoise/Beginners_Guide_Mediterranean_Hatchlings.pdf>

USEFUL WEBSITES

<http://www.tortoisetrust.org/>

<http://www.thetortoisetable.org.uk/site/tortoise_home_1.asp>

<http://www.tortoiselady.co.uk/>

RECOMMENDED READING

Aspinall, V., 2014. Clinical Procedures in Veterinary Nursing, third ed. Butterworth-Heinemann., Oxford.

Excellent chapter on handling and restraint in exotic species.

Girling, S.J., Raiti, P., 2004. BSAVA Manual of Reptiles. second ed. British Small Animal Veterinary Association, (BSAVA) Quedgeley, Gloucester GL2 2AB.

Longley, L.A., 2008. Anaesthesia of Exotic Pets. Saunders Elsevier, London.

Good for nursing and anaesthesia of exotic animals.

Meredith, A., Johnson-Delaney, C., 2010. BSAVA Manual of Exotic Pets, fifth ed. British Small Animal Veterinary Association, Gloucester.

Both manuals provide a wide range of information on the subject.

Quesenberry, K.E., Carpenter, J.W., 2012. Ferrets, Rabbits and Rodents – Clinical Medicine and Surgery, third ed. W B Saunders, St Louis, MO.

Excellent book covering anatomy and physiology, husbandry and clinical conditions.

Richardson, V.C.G., 1997. Diseases of Small Rodents. Blackwell Science, Oxford.

Good coverage of small 'furries'.

34

Management and Care of Injured Wildlife

LUCY KELLS | LOUISE MINSHELL

KEY POINTS

- Wild animals are creatures that live their lives entirely separate from humans, which means that prolonged contact, as happens during hospitalisation, is extremely stressful to them.

- Any attempt to restrain and handle a wild animal will be seen as a threat, so they can be difficult and sometimes dangerous to handle.

- Design of accommodation and diet must mimic as closely as possible what the animal would naturally receive in the wild and any changes necessary to fit in with veterinary practice must be, within reason, as small as possible.

- The aim of veterinary treatment and aftercare is eventually to rehabilitate and release the animal back into the wild. If it is safe to do so, the animal should be released to the same area from where it was taken, or as close by as possible. This is especially important for adult animals, as they will already have established territories.

- The animal must not be kept captive for any longer than is necessary and care must be taken to ensure that it does not become too used to the presence of human beings, which might be dangerous when it returns to a wild existence.

- Before an animal is released it must be capable of surviving in the wild. If an animal will never be able to fend for itself, euthanasia should be considered.

- All aspects of wildlife management are covered by the Wildlife and Countryside Act 1981.

- It should also be remembered that wild animals are rarely suitable patients for the average veterinary surgery. It is therefore almost always better to stabilise the patient, providing first aid only, prior to transfer to a specialist wildlife hospital.

Introduction

The care of sick, injured and orphaned wildlife provides the veterinary nurse with a large variety of species whose needs differ greatly from any group of animals normally presented within a veterinary practice. Wildlife casualties do not appreciate the type of care and comfort given to domestic animals and may even suffer as a result of it. Stress to the casualty is the biggest problem facing wildlife carers and this must constantly be taken into consideration.

The aim of this chapter is to provide advice on the basic care of the most common wildlife casualties based on their natural behaviour and habitat. It will also tell you how to deal with requests for help from members of the public, including how to recognise when an animal is in need of help and when it should be left alone.

Wildlife can be difficult to handle, as they are wild creatures that live in a world where humans are seen as a threat. The first thought of any carer should be how the animal's distress can be minimised and the second should be how soon could it be released back into the wild.

Wild mammals

GENERAL GUIDELINES

Rescue and transportation

On being approached, a wild animal will do one of three things – it will freeze, run or, if cornered, defend itself. Before attempting to catch any animal, assess the situation carefully. The animal should be observed for the way it is behaving and moving and a plan should be worked out for its capture.

Do *NOT* attempt to handle larger mammals such as a badger, otter, deer or fox without sedation, anaesthesia or the appropriate training and experience from working in a wildlife hospital. They can all inflict severe injuries on humans. Always call a wildlife centre for help with large wild mammals.

Any additional help should be organised and then the approach, capture and confinement must be carried out swiftly and firmly but kindly. One of the most important pieces of equipment is a blanket or towel. If a solid transport container is not available, then a cover should be provided over wire baskets. There is nothing more likely to cause stress and injury to an animal than for it to be put into a container it can see out of but from which it cannot escape.

The container should always be lined – newspaper and a towel or a blanket for larger casualties is ideal for providing warmth, absorbency, a place to hide and something to grip on to during transportation. The container should allow enough room for the animal to stand and turn around. If using a cardboard box it must be made secure to prevent the animal from escaping. Containers with grill-type doors must be covered to keep the animal in the dark. Badly injured individuals or those in shock may need an immediate heat source and Snuggle Pads are ideal for use during transportation. A well-wrapped hot-water bottle will suffice until the casualty is livelier.

Admitting a wildlife casualty

It is extremely important to record the following details to gain a complete history and enable successful rehabilitation and release. Many veterinary surgeries sadly fail to do this for their wild patients, and this means we cannot return adults to their territories. For an adult fox, for instance, this could mean death in the wild, if released into the wrong territory.

Many wild animals have specialised or specific requirements for release sites and taking accurate initial details of a casualty can assist in this process. On admittance follow the **5 W's** – 'who, what, where, when, why':

WHO – Who found it and what is their contact number if more information is needed?

WHAT – What species is it?

WHERE – Where was it found? (*Exactly* where?)

WHEN – When did it happen/when was it found and captured?

WHY – the circumstances, what is known (or surmised), and has the patient been given any first aid, treatment or food?

On arrival the injured animal should go through a standard admissions procedure which should include:

Examination prior to handling:

- Obtain a full history of the patient (as above).
- Observe the patient in the box or cage it was brought in, assess state of shock, mentation, observe its ability to stand and move about.
- Observe the patient by handling. Make sure your method is safe, correct, and appropriate to the species and its injuries, and be positive and minimal with your handling to avoid stress to the patient and injury to yourself.
- Protect it and yourself and be prepared for the unexpected. Cover the patient's head, as darkness is calming, avoid direct eye contact and beware of beaks, talons and wings. A patient that appears quiet may become aggressive while handling, especially if in pain.
- Check the box it was transported in – look at droppings and any other residues that may assist diagnosis, such as blood.
- Examine the animal's body condition – weight, level of hydration, muscle coverage – all these will give an indication of the condition the animal is in compared to what it should be, relevant to species and age.
- Always wear and use the appropriate safety and handling equipment for each casualty.
- Pass this information on to the veterinary surgeon for patient assessment and treatment, if necessary, prior to transfer to a wildlife hospital.
- Place into a cage or box suitable for the species and size of patient. Provide warmth if required and keep the patient in a quiet area of the surgery.
- If the patient has a viable chance to recover and be released – organise referral to a wildlife hospital for further rehabilitation.

Remember:

- **Often in wildlife casualties, especially birds, pain is not exhibited; this is a natural response to avoid harm by a predator.**
- **Just because it does not show pain does not mean it is not suffering, so the patient should be treated as if in pain, and analgesia should always be considered.**

A record card or hospital chart should then be completed and remain with the casualty throughout its stay.

If the animal is in shock or particularly distressed, then extra care should be taken at the time of examination to establish if any lifesaving treatment is required, or whether the animal can be saved. If the casualty has been transported in a sensible manner it should be able to cope with the initial examination providing it does not take too long.

It is not necessary to routinely treat for fleas or worms; this should only be done if parasites are present. External and internal parasite treatment can be used safely when needed. In specific species, references such as the British Small Animal Veterinary Association (BSAVA) Exotic Formulary should be checked prior to administration of any medications. As the majority of these will be off license, veterinary prescription will be required. Routine vitamin injections on admission are also unnecessary but long-term patients may benefit from supplements to compensate for the lack of a natural diet.

Housing

Individual housing requirements will be discussed in the sections on specific species but there are a few general guidelines:

- Each wildlife casualty should be housed according to its needs, its natural behaviour and habitat
- Wildlife needs a place to hide and their reaction once placed in a cage or pen will be to find a suitable place out of sight
- Bedding should be put at the back of the accommodation. Unlike birds, which may flap around the cage as it is opened, mammals may remain hidden away.

Heat provision should be carefully considered. Giving wildlife casualties heat that they do not need means that they will have to be weaned off it before they can be released. Remember that these are wild animals that live out in the cold, wet and windy weather. Warm bedding is all that is required. Flexible heat mats and microwavable heat pads should be well wrapped to provide a gentle heat, but they cannot be regulated and provide a constant temperature, and it should also be remembered that wild animals may chew anything in their cage, including electric cables. Bedding must also be kept away from the heat source in case the casualty becomes too warm and needs to move away from it. Those too sick to move away from heat to cool themselves must be carefully monitored to avoid overheating.

To wean an animal off heat, gradually turn the heat supply down and then off during the day, when temperatures are warmer. Once this has been achieved the process should be repeated for night-time heating.

Feeding

Wildlife species may be:

- Diurnal – active during the day
- Nocturnal – active at night
- Crepuscular – active at dawn and dusk.

Their period of natural activity must be taken into account when providing food. A nocturnal creature that is asleep all day cannot be expected to eat breakfast; dinner is far more appropriate. An uneaten meal given early in the morning may cause concern when really the animal has been fed at the incorrect time. Some animals do not eat purely because they are in captivity. One of the main problems when dealing with wildlife is knowing what to feed (Table 34.1).

Orphaned mammals

A basic rule of thumb – if you can approach and/or pick up any wildlife it probably needs help. Exceptions to this rule are baby animals. Fledgling birds, baby deer (fawns) and baby hare

TABLE 34.1	Emergency wildlife feeding for veterinary practices	

PLEASE NOTE: These are diets to use in emergency only. Wild animals cannot stay on these diets for long before being taken to a wildlife hospital for specialist food and care

If opening a packet for rehydration fluid to make for use in your surgery, keep the excess and freeze it into ice-cube trays, ready to use if wildlife needs it

Homemade rehydration fluid can be made by mixing: 1 tablespoon of sugar and 1 teaspoon of salt, with 1 litre of warm water. Water should have been boiled and allowed to cool to body temperature

Species	Wild diet	Alternative food
Swift/swallow/house martin/cuckoo	Flying insects	Give fluid by dripping tiny drops of water or rehydration solution onto side of beak or mouth. These are specialist feeders, and should be taken to a wildlife hospital as soon as possible
Garden birds (Blackbird, blackcap, tit, dunnock, thrush, goldcrest, wagtail, warbler, robin, woodpecker, wren etc.)	Insect eaters	Wild bird seed and mealworms to adults, or tiny pieces of cat food/dog food to babies
Garden birds (Sparrow, bullfinch, linnet, chaffinch, siskin, greenfinch, goldfinch, hawfinch etc.)	Seed eaters	Budgie seed or finch mix to adults, or tiny pieces of cat food/dog food to babies
Adult pigeons and doves	Seed eaters	Wild bird seed (Note: Wood pigeons rarely eat in captivity and may need crop feeding – monitor closely)
Baby pigeons and doves	Fed by parents a regurgitated partially digested seed, known as 'pigeon milk'	If squeaking, you can defrost (but do not cook) some frozen peas and give a few by pushing them gently into the mouth every 2–3 hours. Only about 3 or 4 peas at a time and stop if the bird is not squeaking for more or the crop (the fleshy bag under the bird's beak) looks or feels full. If you are confident enough to try crop feeding them (the correct method of feeding) you can use natural flavour complan, short term. Pigeons/doves cannot be reared on this though and must receive the correct crop feeding food as soon as possible (Tropican or Kaytee exact) at a wildlife hospital
Gulls	At sea, freshly caught fish. Town gulls eat anything, worms and grubs	Tinned cat or dog food, sprats floating in water. Offer the same to babies, but hand feed with forceps if not feeding themselves
Corvids (crows, magpies, jackdaws etc.)	Insects, grubs, worms, eggs, small birds, mammals, seed, grain, berries, nuts, fruit, carrion	Small chunks of cat or dog food. Offer the same to babies, but hand feed with forceps if not feeding themselves
Adult water birds (ducks, geese, swan etc.)	Insects, worms and grubs, aquatic plants, grain and graze on grass	Bird seed and chopped grass floated in a bowl of water. Brown bread pieces in water
Ducklings/goslings/cygnets	Same diet as parents	Offer finely chopped grass floated in a shallow bowl of water. Finely broken up pieces of brown bread in water
Coots, moorhens	Insects and larvae, worms, water weeds, grains	Mashed cat food. Chopped sprats in water, cress in water, maggots and mealworms
Coot and moorhen chicks	Fed by parent initially, then same diet as parents	For very young chicks, brush rehydration fluid onto side of beak and feed soaked porridge oats blended to a fine paste and fed to the chick from a blunted cocktail stick. You will need to feed the bird about 1ml every couple of hours and so this method will be time consuming. Recommended to get to a wildlife hospital as soon as possible. For older chicks, offer same diet as parents would eat, but cut or mash it finely
Game birds (pheasant, partridge)	Insects and larvae, worms, grains	Wild bird seed and mealworms
Game bird chicks	Fed by parent initially, then same diet as parents	For very young chicks, brush rehydration fluid onto side of beak and feed soaked porridge oats blended to a fine paste and fed to the chick from a blunted cocktail stick. You will need to feed the bird about 1ml every couple of hours and so this method will be time consuming. Recommended to get to a wildlife hospital as soon as possible. For older chicks, offer same diet as parents would eat
Heron	Fish, frogs	Sprats floated in water
Raptors (buzzard, kestrel, owl, hawk)	Small birds and mammals. Buzzards will also eat carrion	Mice and day-old chicks. If none available – brush rehydration fluid onto side of beak carefully (avoiding the feet!). Keep in a darkened box and get to a wildlife hospital as soon as possible
Little owl	Insects, voles, mice	Mealworms, crickets, day old mice. If none available – brush rehydration fluid onto side of beak carefully (avoiding the feet!). Keep in a darkened box and get to a wildlife hospital as soon as possible

Continued

TABLE 34.1	Emergency wildlife feeding for veterinary practices—cont'd

Offer fresh water to adult birds only – baby birds can drown very easily if too much fluid is given. They will get sufficient moisture through their food

Species	Wild diet	Alternative food
Snakes	Small mammals and frogs	A bowl of fresh water. Mice. If none available – keep in a secure box and get to a wildlife hospital as soon as possible
Other reptiles/amphibians	Wild diet depends upon species	A bowl of fresh water. Live mealworms
Adult rabbit/hare	Grass, dandelions, clover, hay	A bowl of fresh water. Fresh grass, dandelions, clover, hay
Baby hare	Fed by parent once a day and same diet as parents	Rehydration fluid for first feed, then feed kitten milk formula. Feed as much as they will take, twice a day. Also offer a bowl of fresh water and fresh grass, dandelions, clover and hay
Baby rabbits (eyes open)	Fed by parent initially, then same diet as parents	Rehydration fluid for first feed, then feed kitten milk formula. Feed as much as they will take, twice a day. Also offer a bowl of fresh water and fresh grass, dandelions, clover and hay
Baby rabbits (eyes closed)	Fed by parent initially, then same diet as parents	Rehydration fluid for first feed, then feed kitten milk formula. Feed as much as they will take, twice a day
Adult squirrel/rodent	Nuts, buds, foliage, berries, fruit, grains, seeds	A bowl of fresh water. Unsalted nuts and seeds, fruit, broken digestive biscuits, brown bread
Baby squirrel/rodent	Fed by parent	Rehydration fluid for first feed, then puppy milk formula. Baby squirrels are fed with a syringe, baby rodents should be fed using a paintbrush or clean make-up applicator sponge.
Adult weasel/stoat	Small mammals	A bowl of fresh water. Cat or dog food
Baby weasel/stoat	Fed by parent	Rehydration fluid for first feed, then puppy milk formula. Offer same diet as adults in addition to this, as some will start eating solids even before their eyes open
Adult and juvenile hedgehogs over 300 g	Earthworms, insects, eggs, grubs	A bowl of fresh water. Cat or dog food. Hedgehog store-bought diets
Hoglets under 100 g	Fed by parent	Rehydration fluid for first feed, then puppy milk formula
Hoglets 100–300 g	Fed by parent	A bowl of fresh water. Cat or dog food. Hedgehog store-bought diets. If not feeding themselves, they may need rehydration fluid for first feed, then puppy milk formula
Fox	Rabbits, rodents, earthworms, edible rubbish, carrion, birds, berries, fruit	A bowl of fresh water. Dog food or cat food
Fox cub (eyes open)	Brought food from parents	A bowl of fresh water. Dog food or cat food. If not eating this, try tinned puppy food mixed with puppy milk formula. May still need a bottle of puppy milk formula, depending on its age
Fox cub (eyes closed)	Fed by parent	Rehydration fluid for first feed, then puppy milk formula
Badger	Earthworms, grubs, beetles, fruit	A bowl of fresh water. Dog food or cat food
Badger cub (eyes open)	Brought food from parents	A bowl of fresh water. Dog food or cat food. If not eating this, try tinned puppy food mixed with puppy milk formula, scrambled egg, Weetabix or a human baby cereal. May still need a bottle of puppy milk formula, depending on its age
Badger cub (eyes closed)	Fed by parent	Rehydration fluid for first feed, then puppy milk formula, call a wildlife rescue centre as soon as possible
Bat	Flying insects	Chopped mealworms or maggots. If none available, give fluid only by dripping tiny drops of water or rehydration solution onto side of mouth. These are specialist feeders, call a wildlife rescue centre as soon as possible
Baby bat	Fed by parent	Rehydration fluid for first feed, then puppy milk formula, both fed using a paintbrush or clean make-up applicator sponge. call a wildlife rescue centre or local bat group as soon as possible
Adult deer – minimum handling and keep quiet!	Shrubs, brambles, grass, fruit, flowers, berries	Offer a bowl of fresh water, and some fruit tree branches for them to eat the leaves, hay, root vegetables, apples, brambles, rose flowers and leaves, deer pellets or lamb nuts. Call a wildlife rescue centre as soon as possible
Deer fawns – minimum handling and keep quiet!	Fed by parent	Rehydration fluid for first feed, then lamb milk replacer. These are specialist feeders, call a wildlife rescue centre as soon as possible

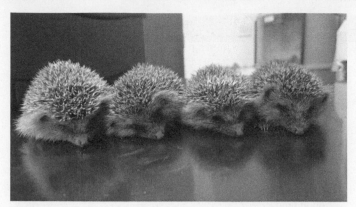

Fig. 34.1 Young animals should be marked so that they can be identified easily

(leverets) are definite exceptions. The adults leave these babies hidden in undergrowth (or sometimes out in the open) for up to 8 hours at a time. If the babies are touched or moved the parent may well abandon them. If you are in doubt about whether or not to intervene, contact your local wildlife centre who will ensure that the animal is discreetly monitored to see if the mother returns.

For genuine confirmed orphans, most of the time the animal will be in a poor state upon arrival, as members of the public often neglect to provide warmth and often try to feed the wrong thing to them, with the best intentions of course.

You would be surprised how many ducklings have been fed milk by well-meaning members of the public. Sadly so many people also insist on force feeding water to animals before they bring them to us – often almost drowning them in the process.

Mammals have often already been fed cow's milk, which, as most of you will know, can kill species other than cows.

It is best to assume the worst and make the first feed you give any wild animal orphan rehydration solution. This will not only rehydrate the animal, but will also allow the stomach to empty and prepare for the correct feeds to be given.

Individuals in a litter of orphans must be identified in some way for their individual progress to be monitored, e.g. with nail polish or Tipp-Ex on fur or feathers on different areas of their bodies so they are easily recognised (Fig. 34.1). The identification mark and weight should be recorded, together with an approximate age and details of condition.

It is essential that a feeding record is completed and a check kept on weight gain. Most orphaned mammals will lose weight to begin with as they adjust to the new feeding routine. The production of urine and faeces should also be monitored in order to pick up on any problems quickly. The Comments column should record any concerns or observations that other carers need to know. It is better if just one person rears the orphan as both the orphan and the carer become used to the way the animal prefers to be fed and the orphan may find it difficult to settle with different carers.

If the orphan mammal has its eyes closed, it must be stimulated to urinate and defecate before and after feeding. The orphan must be warm and comfortable before settling down to a feed – full bladders do not help. In the wild the mother would do this by licking around the genital area. Use cotton wool moistened with warm water, baby oil or Vaseline and gently tickle around the genital area. Urine should start to drip immediately but remember, for newly admitted orphans, they may

not pass urine as they may still be dehydrated. Faeces will also be produced but not at every session. The area should be dried thoroughly and Vaseline or baby oil applied to help prevent soreness and provide protection against moisture. If the orphan becomes sore it will be necessary to bathe and dry the area thoroughly and apply the Vaseline or baby oil again. Once toileting is complete the orphan should be weighed – it is important that the routine of toilet, weigh and feed is kept up.

When feeding, use an appropriate milk formula such as Esbilac or Royal Canin BabyDog. Surprisingly, some puppy and kitten milks are not always suitable for wild orphan mammals, due to the fat and protein ratios often being incorrect for different species. You can always call your local wildlife hospital for advice on which formula is best to use.

If you intend to stabilise the animal prior to transfer to a wildlife hospital the same day, it is best to *only* give rehydration solution *once* the animal is warm enough. Then arrange transfer to the wildlife centre as soon as possible. The correct milk formula to use often changes, due to wildlife rehabbers sharing their experience and success with different foods. It is always worth checking with a local centre before starting a milk formula for any mammal to find out what they are using. This saves the animal being given too many different foods in a short period of time and getting diarrhoea (Box 34.1).

Powdered formula milk should be mixed well to ensure that all the powder has dissolved. The milk should be offered warm; powdered formulas are best made up with boiled water and left to cool. This formula will last for 24 hours, so smaller amounts can be dispensed from it and reheated as needed. The milk should be kept warm throughout the feed by putting the bottle or container of formula into and out of another container of hot water as required. It can be helpful to add probiotics to the first feed of the day.

One-millilitre syringes are ideal for feeding smaller orphans such as squirrels: a measured amount is given a drop at a time and if administered correctly the feeder has total control of the flow of the milk. During feeding the position of the orphan should be such that it can 'paddle' with its forelimbs just as it would at the mother's nipple. Hold the orphan in a towel to

TABLE 34.2	Hazards to hedgehogs	
Hazard	**Symptoms**	**Notes**
Gardens – strimmers, mowers, forks and spades, ponds	Severe cuts, impaled on fork prongs, drowning, exhaustion	Hedgehogs can swim, but not for long
Litter – plastic can or bottle rings, jars/cans, glass	Neck wounds, plastic rings around the neck, suffocation, cuts, constriction injuries, starvation if trapped	Must keep in to monitor, the skin can break down and become necrotic at construction sites.
Poisoning	Jumpy, sensitive to slightest of sounds, stretched out and reluctant to curl. Bleeding gums or from external orifices. Dark faeces	Could be metaldehyde (slug bait), rat poison other garden pesticides
Bonfires	Burns, smoke inhalation	Spines will melt in intense heat and skin and spines will slough off in time
Entangled – fruit netting/football goal nets/tennis nets	Cuts, ligatures, exhaustion, dehydration, starvation	Hedgehogs can push forward through netting but often get stuck and cannot withdraw because of the way the spines grow. Must keep in to monitor. If released without keeping in for a few days to monitor, the skin can break down and become necrotic
Trapped – cattle grid/drain/footings	Exhaustion, dehydration, starvation, cut and sore feet and worn nails from scrabbling to escape	Need to admit them for a few weeks to allow their nails to regrow

keep it warm, then as the feed is slowly dispensed keep an eye on the speed the milk is going down the syringe, whether the orphan is swallowing and that there is no build-up of milk in the mouth. The delivery of milk should synchronise with the orphan's sucking and swallowing. Just as you would with orphan puppies and kittens in your practice, take care to avoid going too quickly with milk formula, or you can risk aspiration pneumonia, which can be fatal for tiny orphans.

When feeding is completed, clean and dry the orphan's face, toilet the orphan, and weigh it again before it is put back to bed. Any milk that is left over should be thrown away and the syringe both washed and sterilised or thrown away. All containers used for the milk should be washed and sterilised ready for the next feed. Hands must be washed before and after each feed and in between different litters or single orphans. The volume taken by each individual and the new weights should be entered on the feeding record.

Successful hand feeding depends on the age and size of the orphan and the level of patience and dedication of the carer. It is not a job to be rushed – and this is another reason why it is best to only stabilise the animal and transfer to a wildlife hospital, as our busy practices do not often allow us the time needed to rear these animals successfully.

If an orphan becomes unwell or develops diarrhoea the milk feeds should be replaced by a rehydrating solution for 24 hours, then half rehydrating solution to half milk until the orphan recovers and is back on to its usual feed.

It can be helpful to have a soft toy available as a substitute 'mum', particularly for single orphans to snuggle up.

HEDGEHOGS (*ERINACEUS EUROPAEUS*)

Hedgehogs are the wild mammal most commonly brought into a veterinary surgery and seasonal changes affect the reasons and the number of admissions (Table 34.2). Hedgehogs inhabit parks and gardens, farmland, waste ground and hedgerows, where they forage for earthworms, grubs and beetles. They may also take small mammals and eggs. Their eyesight is poor and they use their sense of smell to detect prey.

Hedgehogs are solitary creatures, seeking out the company of others only for mating. Once mating has taken place the male plays no part in the rearing of the hoglets and does not stay with the female. Two litters of three to five hoglets are produced each year, the first in May–June and the second in August–September.

Hedgehogs are nocturnal, so activity during the day is unusual and may suggest ill health. This is not always the case though, as pregnant females may come out during this time to gather nesting materials in preparation for birth.

The hedgehog has a unique defence mechanism in that it is able to roll into a spiky ball, which protects it from danger. It can remain in this position for hours.

Hibernation

Hedgehogs hibernate in winter to avoid the problem of lack of food; it is pointless to waste valuable energy endlessly searching for food in frozen ground. Instead, the hedgehog retreats to its hibernaculum (winter nest) and goes to sleep until conditions improve. People think that hedgehogs hibernate from autumn through the winter until the spring, but this is not so. Hedgehogs react to the environmental temperature and, when the temperature at ground level drops below 5°C for a prolonged period, the hedgehog goes into hibernation. In recent years this has been between January and March. The hedgehog slows its system down almost to a standstill, the body temperature cools and breathing and heart rate slow. A hibernating hedgehog may only take a breath every 4 minutes, which can be worrying if a hibernating hedgehog is admitted to a veterinary surgery. Never assume a hedgehog is dead unless it is warmed up at winter time. They can give the appearance of being dead, when in fact they are still hibernating. If a hedgehog is presented that is tightly curled but appears not to be breathing, it should be warmed up gently and slowly in absolute quiet. Hedgehogs may wake up during hibernation for short periods of activity when the weather is milder, so if a hedgehog is spotted out and about in the middle of winter it is not necessarily in difficulty. Small hedgehogs may be presented in late autumn and early winter, the finder thinking that they are too small to survive. This is due to the increasing public awareness about hibernation and the fact that a hedgehog needs to be a minimum of 600 g to survive hibernation. Overenthusiastic autumn garden tidying may result in injured hedgehogs through digging, bonfires and strimming (Fig. 34.2).

Late litters of hoglets do not always have the time to put on sufficient fat to carry them through the winter. An acceptable weight for a hoglet to be released is 600 g and those that are lighter will have to be kept until they reach the acceptable weight, and then released. If temperatures are mild and dry, after October hedgehogs can be released throughout the autumn and early winter period – there is little point in imprisoning a hedgehog in a cage for months on end. If the winter is very cold, hedgehogs may have to be kept in during this time but as soon as the target weight is reached and the conditions in the wild are right, the hedgehog can be released.

Capture and transportation

Hedgehogs are the easiest of wildlife mammals to catch. On approach the hedgehog will either scuttle away or, more often, freeze and curl into a tight ball. Before picking up a hedgehog,

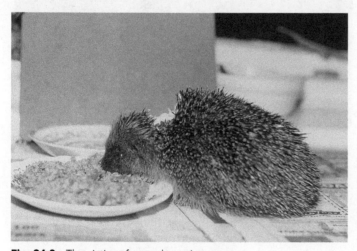

Fig. 34.2 The victim of a garden strimmer

some form of hand protection should be worn. Gardening gloves are ideal, or a towel folded to make several layers will protect from sharp spines. Pick the hedgehog up carefully but firmly, put it into an appropriate container and place it securely in the vehicle so that it does not move around during transportation.

Hedgehogs rarely bite as they are rolled into a ball but it should be assumed that they will. An injured animal may not curl up and if the hedgehog has just frozen it should roll up as soon as it is touched. A hedgehog may also exhibit aggression by thrusting its head upwards with its spines raised and making a wheezing, huffing noise, which may often be misdiagnosed as a respiratory problem.

Examination and handling

Hedgehogs are presented as casualties for a variety of reasons (Table 34.3) and should receive a full examination on arrival. Before handling a hedgehog, put on a pair of gloves, as this will protect you from the spines, and the fact that they can often have ringworm. Before removing the hedgehog from the container, observe it. If it is rolled into a ball this is a good sign as it is a naturally defensive position; however, it makes examination difficult and access to the underside of the animal is impossible.

Before attempting to unroll the hedgehog, check if any of the limbs are poking out – this could suggest limb or spinal injuries. Pick up the hedgehog and look at the condition of its skin and spines; look for wounds, maggots, fly eggs and parasites (Table 34.4).

A healthy hedgehog has a rounded shape; a tapered hedgehog is a thin hedgehog. Infection can be sometimes detected by smell, but its source may be hard to find unless the hedgehog is unrolled.

To unroll the hedgehog, gently stroke its rump and have patience. This is best done in a quiet room, as any loud noises or even vibrations from people walking in and out will make the hog curl up again. Allow it to uncurl fully and watch it walking, making note of any lameness or other issues. Then you can gently slide your fingers underneath the hog and hold it by its back legs so that the front feet are on the table and

TABLE 34.3	Reasons for admission of hedgehog casualties	
Reason for admission	**Injury/symptom**	**Notes**
Road traffic accident	Concussion Cuts/bruises Fractures: limb/pelvis/jaw/spine	A curled hedgehog with legs sticking out indicates a spinal, pelvic or limb fracture/injury. Females with fractured pelvis must be euthanised due to lack of knowing if they will give birth normally in the wild.
Extreme weather – prolonged hot spells	Heat exhaustion, dehydration, emaciation	Hot weather causes ground to dry out so no food or water
Animal attacks	Wounds, fractures	Most commonly by dogs
Out during the day	Lethargic, half curled out in the open	Could be a sign the hedgehog is blind and unable to tell night from day. Also may indicate a sign of possible illness or injury (unless it is an active pregnant female gathering nesting materials)
'Pop off' syndrome (orbicularis muscle prolapse)	The circular muscle used for curling slips up over the pelvis	Can be pulled back down under anaesthetic
'Balloon syndrome' (subcutaneous emphysema)	Build-up of air under the skin, causing balloon effect	Where a wound or maxilla injury has drawn in air under the skin during the action of curling and uncurling/or an injury to the respiratory system that leaks air
Orphan	Too young to leave the nest; no parent present	May have been taken from the nest by dog or cat

TABLE 34.4	Hedgehog parasites			
Parasite	Symptoms	Treatment	Notes	
Hedgehog flea	Easily visible between the spines	Pyrethrum spray in well-ventilated situations	A very exposed habitat between spines means this flea is unique to hedgehogs	
Tick	Easily visible, usually around ears and eyes in clusters, singly all over the body. Heavy infestations will include tiny 'pip-like' larval stages	Removal is best achieved with a tick lasso or forceps.	In heavy infestations on a stressed hedgehog removal by hand is unhelpful. Ivermectin is effective	
Mites	Spine and fur loss, crusty/flaky skin	Ivermectin	Isolate the patient	
Ringworm	Crusty around follicles, small crusty lesions	Appropriate wash, such as Imaverol, made up to a 1:50 solution with water and added to a spray bottle	Isolate the patient. Spray the hog all over, every 3 days, until it has had four sprays	

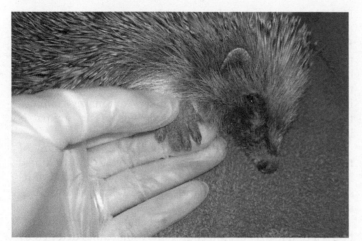

Fig. 34.3 This hedgehog's claws were worn down while the animal was trapped

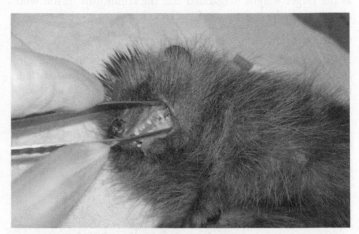

Fig. 34.4 A hedgehog with bad teeth

the back feet directly above. This will provide the opportunity to see the underside; however, touching the hedgehog, particularly on the head or face, will provoke it into curling up again. This method is not fool proof and some individuals will need to be anaesthetised.

Check the following:

- **Length of the claws** – hedgehogs dig and scratch around for their food, which keeps their claws trimmed. Long claws could suggest that the hog has not been using the limb or foot normally. Worn claws may suggest it has been trapped somewhere or the ground is very dry and food is scarce (Fig. 34.3).
- **Teeth** – check for missing and worn teeth. If present the hedgehog may be old or the poor condition of the mouth may be the reason for not feeding. Sadly with raised public awareness of the plight of the hedgehog, more people are feeding them in the wild, often with inappropriate foods, causing tooth decay and gum disease (Fig. 34.4).
- **Abscesses** – if present these are often from old fractures or bites. A fractured limb that is also abscessed is a very poor prognosis for saving that limb.
- **Body temperature** – hedgehogs that are hibernating may only breathe once or twice a minute and feel very cold to the touch. If they are underweight, ill or injured, then they must be warmed up slowly to bring them back out of hibernation safely. Hedgehogs that are found

semi-curled and lying on one side are very sick and/or cold. The underside of the hedgehog should be felt to see if it is warm and the animal tested for dehydration. These individuals will need to be warmed up and given fluids before more investigations are carried out.

- **Faeces** – good indication of the health of the hedgehog. A normal stool is formed and brown, but they can sometimes pass green stools. A green stool does not necessarily indicate a problem, though. Hedgehogs have a fast gut transit time (only 8–12 hours). Many things can cause changes in this, such as lack of food. Baby hedgehogs will always pass a lime-green coloured stool and this is perfectly normal. If the faeces has blood or mucus in it, or you are concerned, then it is very simple to examine a faecal smear under the microscope. On-going treatment will depend on what is found during the examination.
- **Movement** – if a leg injury is suspected it can be difficult to assess how much the normal movement has been affected. The hedgehog will naturally curl or freeze, making movement observation very difficult. If the hedgehog is examined as described above it can allow you to assess for any issues with the way it walks. Limb fractures, if not open or infected, can be successfully splinted or operated on by the vet. Infected or open fractured limbs can be amputated, but considerations must be taken whether it is the right thing to do to a wild animal. Hedgehogs must *never* have front legs amputated, as they will be unable to walk properly and

unable to dig for their food in the wild, and will die. Hind leg amputations are controversial, as many wildlife hospitals have observed serious ear infections on the same side as a missing hind leg, due to the hedgehog's inability to groom itself after amputation.

Once the examination is complete all observations should be recorded on the record card.

Housing

Taking into account the hedgehog's natural behaviour and habitat, a hospital cage similar in size to that used to house a cat is adequate and will provide enough room for bedding, food, water and an area in which to move around. The cage should be lined with newspaper. Bedding in the form of hand-shredded newspaper or a large towel should be placed in one of the far corners of the cage away from the door to enable the hedgehog to make a nest. Paper from a shredding machine is not suitable as it is too coarse and very thin and may become tangled around the legs. The hedgehog will naturally move to the back of the cage once placed inside and head for cover. As the hedgehog makes its nest it will turn around, combing the nesting material into shape.

It may be necessary to cover the cage door with a towel, to allow the hedgehog to settle. Active hedgehogs may pace along the frontage and dig, bite and scratch at the door. This is the time to review the case: a hedgehog that will not settle and continually 'paces' will need further investigation, which will be discussed at a later point in this chapter. If the hedgehog is stressed, pacing and active alternative housing needs to be considered, such as providing a bed-box to hide in, as otherwise this behaviour will lead to injury, distress and ultimately a longer stay in hospital.

Heat – for cold hedgehogs or those unable to maintain their own body temperature, a heat pad or Snuggle Pad is ideal. Hedgehogs must be allowed to hide, so must be covered with their bedding if they are not able to burrow into it themselves.

Feeding

Adult hedgehogs are nocturnal and should be fed later in the day than diurnal species. Feed as close to dusk as you can unless a special feeding regimen is being followed. The average hedgehog should be fed approximately one-third of a standard tin of cat or dog food per night. If the hedgehog eats all that it is offered and appears agitated, a little more should be given until an appropriate amount is reached. Similarly, if food is being left, then reduce the amount offered.

If food is not eaten, check that the hedgehog is warm. Hedgehogs that are thin, sick or on medication may have little or no appetite, so small tempting meals should be offered on an ad-lib basis. The food can be warmed up to increase the smell and warmed liquid pet food such as Royal Canin Convalescence Support or Liquivite poured over the food may also help. Those recovering from serious illness or hedgehogs that are very thin will need a 'little and often' regimen and will benefit from a diet such as Hills a/d or Royal Canin Convalescence Support. Specific hedgehog diets can also be offered, such as those from Ark Wildlife or Spikes world.

Fresh water should always be provided and placed in a non-tip bowl to minimise the risk of spillage. Food is best offered on a saucer and the hedgehog will forage in and through

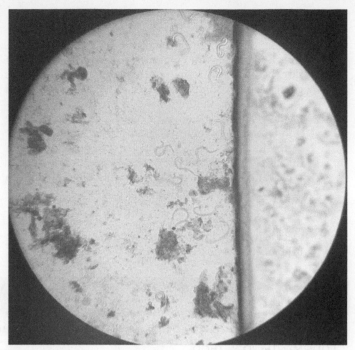

Fig. 34.5 Lungworm larvae

the food and will push it over the sides, so the dish should be placed in the middle of the accommodation.

Pacers

These are hedgehogs that will not settle and are constantly 'on the go', pacing the cage frontage or the entire boundary. This is absolutely not normal behaviour for a hedgehog and could indicate a variety of problems, such as pain, blindness or an internal parasite issue such as fluke. If the hedgehog has been examined and no cause is obvious for the behaviour, then a faecal smear should be examined under the microscope (Fig. 34.5). Hedgehogs frequently have parasites that can be easily spotted in faecal samples. These are easily cured by using a variety of drugs. It is important to note here that fenbendazole is totally ineffective in hedgehogs, yet is still widely prescribed by veterinary surgeries to hogs.

The technique to use to perform a faecal smear, the drugs that are recommended and the doses required for the hedgehog are available to download for your surgery by visiting www.valewildlife.org.uk and clicking the rehabbers area of the website.

Orphaned hoglets

Before attempting to hand-rear orphaned hedgehogs, make sure they really are orphans. The female hedgehog will leave her young to find food and if a nest of hoglets is found it is assumed that they have been abandoned. If the hoglets seem content and sleeping, leave them alone and return to check them later. If they appear unsettled, cold or are emitting a high-pitched sound, indicating hunger, or the nest has clearly been destroyed then they will have to be picked up. A cardboard box full of warm material is adequate for transportation but if the hoglets are cold they will need a heat source, e.g. a Snuggle Pad.

On admission a general examination should also include:

- Weigh the hoglet
- Check the skin for general condition and wounds. Check for fly eggs and maggots; concentrate on folds of skin, behind the ears, in mouth, armpits and around the genital area. Clumps of fly eggs may also be found lodged between the spines and in the softer furry areas of the hedgehog. Removal of eggs is best achieved using pointed metal tweezers, or a nit or flea comb for those in the fur. You can also make use of a hospital suction machine if you have one available, as these make the removal of fly eggs and maggots much easier from in between the hedgehog's spines
- Check body temperature
- Test for dehydration
- Decide its age – this will determine the feeding regimen (Table 34.5).

Once examination is complete the hoglets should be housed according to age and how warm they feel – older hoglets may just need warm bedding, very young ones will need a Snuggle Pad or heat pad.

Feeding. This should be completed as follows (see Table 34.5):

- Stimulate the hoglet to urinate and defecate before and after feeding, if it has its eyes closed. If the eyes are open, this is not necessary.
- Record results on the record sheet – the faeces of young hoglets on an all-milk formula diet are often light green and segmented. As the hoglet is weaned the faeces will change to a browner, more formed stool.
- Weigh the hoglet.
- Once the orphan is warm, give a first feed of rehydration formula and contact a local wildlife hospital to ascertain when you can transfer the orphan to them.

TABLE 34.5	Hedgehog (hoglet) orphans This is a rough guide; each individual is different

Make sure all feeds are prepared fresh daily. **Give rehydration solution for first feed after admission.**

EQUIPMENT AND METHOD:

- 1-ml syringe and soft teat into side of mouth – do not flood the mouth
- Hogs suckle lying on their stomachs
- If eyes closed, toilet before and after syringe feeding by vibrating cotton wool (dipped in baby oil to protect the skin) over the genitals in a head to tail direction. Ensure all urine is removed as it will burn the skin if left
- Weaning starts when first tooth buds show
- Faeces may be a dark green for first few feeds but then will turn a light green colour
- Bloated abdomen can be fatal – try rehydration fluids for next couple of feeds
- Diarrhoea can be fatal – give rehydration fluids instead of milk formula for next 1 or 2 feeds, then give half water/half formula for the next feed, then back to just formula, if faeces go back to normal. If diarrhoea persists try giving probiotics

Age/Weight	Notes	Feeding	
		Food/quantity	Intervals
New-born/4–20 g 	No prickles, fur or teeth, deaf and blind. At 2 hours old the first set of white soft prickles come through	0.5–1 ml milk formula	Every 1½ hours daytime and up to 3 hourly at night
3 days/20–30 g 	Brown prickles begin to push through	0.5–2 ml milk formula	Every 2 hours daytime and once in the middle of the night
7 days/30–50 g 	Can curl into a ball (8 days)	2–3 ml milk formula	Every 2–3 hours daytime
14 days/50–80 g 	Eyes open, ears also start to open	3–4 ml milk formula Also put some formula mixed with Hills a/d or Royal Canin BabyDog/BabyCat mousse in a dish and encourage to lap	4 hourly intervals from 6am to 12am

TABLE 34.5	Hedgehog (hoglet) orphans This is a rough guide; each individual is different—cont'd		
Age/Weight	**Notes**	**Feeding**	
21–28 days/85–170 g 	Should now be lapping from a dish. Introduce some solids. Lower teeth start to push through at about 3 weeks	4–7 ml milk formula Also put some formula mixed with Hills a/d or Royal Canin BabyDog/BabyCat mousse in a dish and encourage to lap	Feed by syringe only 2–3 times a day, and reduce if eating solids well
6 weeks/170–200g 	Only syringe feed if not eating well enough for themselves	Start reducing formula mixed in the food once eating well	
8 weeks/250 g plus 	Independent	Mashed kitten/puppy food	
300 g plus 		Add kitten biscuits to food	

- If the hoglet is going to remain in your care for a time, feed using puppy formula and a 1-ml syringe.

Weaning. The weaning process can begin once the hoglets start to open their eyes. The aim is gradually to reduce the milk feed and introduce solid food. Start with a diet such as Hills a/d or Royal Canin BabyDog mousse. Cover the bottom of a flat dish with food, which should be mixed with the milk formula until the meal is sloppy. Place the hoglets around the food dish and watch to see if they begin to eat by themselves. This is a messy business to start with as the hoglets will walk on to the plate and lick and bite at the food around them. If they show no interest in lapping at the mixture, then milk feeds should be continued, but still offer the sloppy mixture at each feed until they do start eating it. Once the hoglets have finished feeding they may need to be cleaned, as they will get covered in the food.

As the hoglets grow, gradually change the sloppy food to kitten or puppy food, mashed with a fork with the milk formula poured over it. Reduce the milk formula each day until they are eventually on just plain tinned cat or dog food. The hoglets should be fully weaned by around 6 weeks old.

Mother hedgehogs and their babies

Occasionally a pregnant hedgehog is presented and this may only be discovered when newly born hoglets are discovered during cleaning out. It is a good idea to check for signs of pregnancy or lactation in any female hedgehogs that are admitted during the summer months. Mothers and babies must be left alone to reduce the risk of cannibalism by the mother. Do not be tempted to touch or move the babies unless the mother is not sitting with them, and even then it is important to wear latex gloves and be brief, just to check that the hoglets are not cold and have been abandoned. Cleaning of the cage should not be done for a few days. Remove easy to access soiled paper carefully and keep food and water topped up. Regular checks should be made to listen for sounds of distressed hoglets and also to make sure that they are in the nest and have not been left out in the cold. If there are any problems, the hoglets should be removed and hand-reared.

Nursing females should be given an increased amount of food, and the babies can be removed from her to be housed separately when they are about 5–6 weeks old.

BADGERS (*MELES MELES*)

Badgers live in social groups in a network of tunnels and chambers called a sett. They are nocturnal and if they are seen during the day there may be a problem (Table 34.6).

Badgers are usually found injured on roads or caught in wire fences or netting. They are rarely seen when ill. The only time you might see a sick or injured badger in circumstances other than a road traffic accident is if it is an older animal driven away

TABLE 34.6	Reasons for the presentation of badgers as wildlife casualties	
Reason	**Injury/symptom**	**Notes**
Road traffic accident (RTA)	Concussion, cuts and bruising, fractures to legs/pelvis/spine/jaw	Females with fractured pelvis must be euthanised due to lack of knowing if they will give birth normally in the wild.
Prolonged hot and dry weather	Dehydration, emaciation, exhaustion	This weather affects the food and water supply.
Territorial wounds	Wounds around the neck, ears and rump	Usually infected and often fly-blown. Remember to check if teeth are worn, indicating an elderly animal.
Out during the day	Out in the open, no attempt to move, lethargic, staggering	Could have fled from an RTA or be a victim of a territorial attack or extreme weather.
Traps/snares	Injuries to limbs, neck or abdomen	Do not cut them free and release. They must be kept in to monitor for skin breakdown at the site the skin was constricted.
Entangled – football goal nets, tennis nets	Cuts, ligatures, exhaustion, dehydration	Do not cut them free and release. They must be kept in to monitor for skin breakdown at the site the skin was constricted.
Orphan	Very young, out alone, no parent present	

from its sett, i.e. no longer a viable member of the group – badgers do not care for their elderly. In these cases, you may find that the badger has a badly bitten neck and rump and worn teeth, displaying signs of old age. Often it is better to euthanise in these cases, as the badger has reached the end of its life in the wild and will not be accepted back in the sett.

If an injured badger is found between January and April, check if it is female and if there are signs that she has young, e.g. heavy, drooping nipples or if she is still lactating. If you see any of these signs there are probably young nearby. Badger cubs always need specialist care, as they must be hand-reared in groups. Always contact your local wildlife hospital or badger group if you find yourself in this situation.

Badgers eat earthworms, insects, fruit, seeds, eggs, beetles and insect larvae; they may sometimes raid beehives for honey and larvae, and may even eat small mammals such as hedgehogs when there is a lack of other food.

The badger's sense of smell is very good. They have good hearing but their eyesight is poor.

Badgers mate from 2 years of age onwards, at any time of the year. After mating, badgers exhibit what is known as delayed implantation. They keep the fertilised eggs in the womb in a state of suspended development until they implant at the end of December. One litter of young is produced annually and the cubs are born early in the year, usually between January and March.

The average litter size is two or three.

Badgers do not hibernate but may stay underground during the coldest spells.

As with all other wildlife, badgers are likely to have parasites but in general these are few in number and are unlikely to be a problem unless the animal is in poor condition, sick or orphaned (Table 34.7).

Tuberculosis

A badger infected with tuberculosis (TB) will usually have no physical signs of the disease. As there is a risk of spread to other species, including humans, the utmost care should be taken with all badger casualties and orphans. Gloves should be worn at all times and isolation or barrier nursing for all admitted badgers should be continued right through to transfer to a wildlife hospital or release if deemed appropriate. Cubs from different rescue sites should not be introduced to each other

TABLE 34.7	Badger parasites	
Parasite	**Treatment**	**Notes**
Badger flea	Fipronil	Treat only if infested
Badger louse	Fipronil	Treat only if infested
Ticks	Remove with tick hooks. Fipronil	

until they have been tested for TB. All badgers that test positive for TB should be euthanised.

All adult casualties, once recovered, should be returned to where they were found but TB testing is not necessary, as the badger is taken, treated and released back into the same area, so the situation in that area has not been altered.

Capture and transportation

Badgers are very dangerous, strong animals, and they should be treated with great care – their bite is fast and often with little warning. They are also sensible creatures, avoiding confrontation unless provoked.

Rescue in the wild can be difficult – if your casualty has a head injury, retrieval may be fairly easy; if it has a back or rear end injury it will require more thought. Prepare the carrying basket in advance – a crush-type cage lined with a blanket is ideal. The reactions of a badger with a head injury should be tested by offering a biting stick or similar object at arm's length. If there is no reaction then push the head down with a large towel on the non-leading hand and grasp the scruff. Once the badger is restrained it should be lifted into the basket. Remove your hands as quickly as possible while closing the lid tightly. Secure the basket and cover it with a blanket to place the casualty in the dark.

Badgers that have a rear-end injury will be active at the biting end and the same procedure to test the reactions should be followed – the aim of the biting stick is that the badger will bite on it rather than the rescuer and give you some idea of the mentation of the animal before attempts to pick it up. Care must be taken, as the badger is able to shrug its shoulders, curl up and twist its body causing the scruff to 'disappear', leaving the rescuer nothing to grasp. If the badger is able to move then the carrier (end and top opening are best) should be

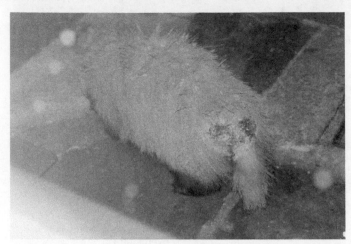

Fig. 34.6 Territorial bite wounds around the tail of a badger

placed on the ground and covered apart from the entrance hole. Badgers will naturally go for a dark hiding place and in most cases with a little encouragement they can be lured into the basket.

It may be necessary to use a grasper or dog-catcher, but avoid them if you can, as badgers will often spin when restrained with a grasper. Time and care must be taken to catch the badger and never be afraid to ask a wildlife centre or the Royal Society for the Prevention of Cruelty to Animals (RSPCA) to help if you are at all concerned.

Examination and handling

Examination can be straightforward if the badger is concussed. Never let your guard down though, as badgers can seem quiet, but will move very fast if provoked. Do not to rely on the scruff as a means of restraint, as it requires a firm grip that cannot be sustained for a thorough examination. Cover the badger's head with a thick towel and have several people on hand to help restrain the animal for as much of the examination as possible. If the badger moves or struggles in the slightest, do not try to examine it further without considering sedation or general anaesthetic, as this is much safer for staff and causes less stress to the animal. A crush cage can be used to sedate the badger if needed.

Examine the badger, paying particular attention to the teeth. An old badger that is thin with long claws indicating that it does little digging for food, with worn and missing teeth, all means that it is near to the end of its life and should not be released back to the wild. Check the neck and rump for bite wounds, often sustained as a result of a territorial dispute with another badger. They are usually infected and often fly-blown. Elderly badgers with rump wounds should be euthanised (Fig. 34.6).

Housing

Suitable accommodation in a veterinary practice is similar to that used for a medium-sized dog. It should be located in the quietest area and the front of the cage should be covered to reduce the light – badgers are nocturnal and excessive light is distressing to them. Line the cage with a thick layer of newspaper and place bedding, e.g. hand-shredded newspaper, hay or blankets, at the back in one corner. There should be sufficient for the badger to bury itself in. Badgers will sleep all day and

wake in the early evening. They can be destructive in a captive situation and 'trashed' accommodation is to be expected. By morning all the lining paper and bedding will be in a heap in one corner with the badger fast asleep underneath it.

A noisy practice is not a good place for a badger to spend any length of time and it should be transferred to more appropriate facilities at a wildlife hospital as soon as possible.

Heat – the best heat source for a badger is a heat lamp unless the accommodation itself is heated. Heat pads with wires will be chewed and the microwavable Snuggle Pads will not last long against the claws or teeth of a badger.

Feeding

Use strong metal food bowls – ceramic food bowls are heavy and may be used but may be broken by the patient and plastic will be chewed and destroyed. Put a non-tip water bowl in the corner of the cage.

As badgers are nocturnal they should be fed late in the day unless they are on a special feeding regimen. They will eat most varieties of cat or dog food. During eating the food will be 'dug out' of the food bowl, although this is rarely seen except in cubs, as the secretive nature of the badger does not allow for an audience.

On the first night and even for a few days the badger may refuse to eat and will simply curl up and go to sleep. Unless the badger is emaciated or dehydrated, it should not be force-fed food or fluids.

For recovering sick adult badgers, Hills a/d, Royal Canin BabyDog or the like are a good first food to try. It may be possible to very carefully trickle food into or near the mouth from a 60-ml syringe, but only while the badger is debilitated, and even then great care must be taken to avoid getting bitten. It is far safer to offer food in a bowl and contact a wildlife hospital if the badger is not eating. As the badger gains strength, small meals of dog or cat food can be offered alongside until the badger is on a normal adult diet.

Cleaning

A hospitalised badger must be thoroughly cleaned out every day. Make up one corner of the hospital cage with a deep bed and, wearing gloves, slowly remove the bedding the badger is hiding under. The badger realises he is being exposed, sees a pile of bedding he can hide in and scuttles across to it, allowing the corner he has just left to be cleaned. Always keep an eye on the pile of the bedding in case the badger decides to come out.

An alternative way is to move the badger to a ready made-up cage.

Orphaned badger cubs

A badger cub out on its own in the day indicates a problem (Table 34.8). Most cubs start to appear above ground at about 2 months old and until this time they are in the sett. Younger cubs may have come above ground if their mother has not returned. Once a cub this young is found in difficulty, the area should be searched for others and for an injured adult. Sometimes tiny cubs are found as a result of a collapsed sett or one that has been dug out by humans. It is well worth contacting your local badger group for assistance, as they will often know the locations of setts and can help to search. Details of your local badger group can easily be found by searching online, as every county in the UK has them.

Make sure all feeds are prepared fresh daily. **Give rehydration solution for first feed after admission.**

EQUIPMENT AND METHOD:

- Use a baby bottle, insert teat in mouth, directed towards roof of mouth, and massage throat gently to encourage swallowing
- If eyes closed, toilet before and after syringe feeding by vibrating cotton wool (dipped in baby oil to protect the skin) over the genitals in a head-to-tail direction. Ensure all urine is removed as it will burn the skin if left
- May be difficult to get feeding initially, as a hungry cub may latch onto a teat, clenches its jaws, hunch its shoulders not sucking. Wait for cub to relax if clenches onto teat
- **Feed about 25–50 ml/kg per feed**
- Bloated abdomen can be fatal – try rehydration fluids for next couple of feeds
- Diarrhoea can be fatal – give rehydration fluids instead of milk formula for next 1 or 2 feeds, then give half water/half formula for the next feed, then back to just formula, if faeces go back to normal. If diarrhoea persists try giving probiotics

Age	Notes	Feeding	
		Food/quantity	Intervals
7–14 days old	Eyes and ears closed. Fine white and grey fur, with a white stripe on the head	5–15 ml	2-hour intervals. 4-hour intervals overnight
2–4 weeks	Ears starting to stand up a little. Eyes show signs of opening	20–30 ml	4-hour intervals, last feed 12am, first feed 6am
4–6 weeks	Eyes and ears open	40–60 ml	4-hour intervals, last feed 12am, first feed 6am. May want to 'practise' with solids now, though cub unlikely to balance well enough on its own to eat properly yet
6–8 weeks	Weaning starts	80–150 ml	Bottle feed 3 to 4 times a day. Offer mashed puppy food and scrambled egg mixed with formula in cage
8–12 weeks	Becoming more independent	100–200 ml. Start to reduce bottle feeding	Bottle feed twice a day. If eating solids well consider stopping
About 12–15 weeks	Must go with other cubs as soon as possible and not be kept alone	They should be fully weaned now. (In the wild they would get milk from their mother for much longer, but as we are giving them complete puppy food, weaning them earlier is preferred to prevent imprinting on humans.)	Only bottle feed once a day and stop as soon as possible

Handling and transportation. Even cute and cuddly looking cubs can bite and they should be approached with care. The cub may snarl and jump and the fur will stand on end, the cub is trying to make itself look larger as a defence mechanism. Wear thick gloves and use a towel or blanket for capturing cubs. A cold sickly cub must be warmed up and a Snuggle Pad or incubator is ideal for this.

Examination. Make a thorough examination, including:
- Check the skin for parasites (see Table 34.7). Badger cubs often have fleas and lice and flea preparation can be used on arrival. Ticks may also be found and may be removed.
- Check the body temperature.
- Check for dehydration – may need an oral rehydrating fluid, intravenous or subcutaneous fluids.
- Weigh the cub.
- Attempt to assess the age.

Housing. A secure hospital cage should be used and it should be realised that even a baby badger is very strong. The cub should be housed in a quiet area of the surgery, and organisation made to transfer it to a wildlife hospital as soon as possible. A Snuggle Pad may be required for very young or sick cubs; older ones may just need warm bedding, but this should be monitored.

Feeding. The cub must be stimulated to urinate and defecate before and after feeding, if it has its eyes closed. If the eyes are open, this is not necessary. The faeces of badger cubs are often yellow and rather like scrambled egg, but change to browner more solid stools as the cub is weaned. The cub should then be weighed and all the information should be recorded. The amount of food and the feeding times will vary depending on the animal's age. Seek advice from a wildlife hospital to help you work out an approximate age and how often to feed the cub (see Table 34.8).

Feed the cub puppy milk formula with a kitten or puppy bottle for very young cubs and a human baby bottle for older ones. Bottle-feeding badger cubs can be difficult. Initially the cub will not suck at the bottle but will hunch its shoulders as it grips the teat with its teeth or clamps its mouth shut, and then it will maintain this position. The only way to succeed is by patience and it can take time. Often reverting to a syringe and carefully drip the milk feed in this way to instigate feeding and then try the bottle again for the next feed. Once the badger has taken to the bottle, feeding becomes much easier. A baby badger with its eyes open should be offered soft food in addition to bottle feeds. The sooner any orphaned animal is weaned the better, as it allows humans to be more 'hands-off' and keep the animal as wild as possible without risk of imprinting.

Weaning starts with soft food, e.g. tinned puppy food mixed with the milk formula, scrambled egg, or a human baby cereal. Badgers can be slow to wean and at first the cub may not accept solid food, but persevere and offer it again at the next feed. Once the cub is eating by itself, more meat-based foods can be added and the diet can become a more solid one. Keep a check on the badger's weight, and providing it is increasing, then bottle feeds can be reduced and then stopped.

Tuberculosis and badger cubs. Each badger cub must be tested for TB three times during its rearing and rehabilitation.

Only a cub with three negative tests can be released back into the wild. Badgers are social animals and should not be reared singly; however, cubs from different litters should not be housed together until they have been tested at least once for TB with negative results. If cubs are housed together before a negative result is obtained and then one tests positive, the lives of the whole group are in question. The first test should be carried out as soon after admission as possible, another during the middle part of their care and the last test as near to release date as possible.

FOXES (*VULPES VULPES*)

There are two types of fox living alongside us these days, the rural fox and the urban fox, and although they are the same species they are very different, and one should never be released in the other's territory. Releasing an adult urban fox into what one may think is a 'better' area in a rural environment will be a death sentence to that animal as they will not find food:
- The rural fox eats a more natural diet consisting of small mammals, birds, worms, beetles and fruit.
- The urban fox results from humans' development of land, trapping wildlife in small areas and forcing them to adapt to a new way of life. Many are presented as road traffic casualties and victims of sarcoptic mange (Table 34.9). The urban fox may forage in rubbish bins, pick up food dropped from bird tables and eat discarded take-away food, as well as small mammals, birds, fruit and insects.

The fox's eye is adapted to movement and they have very good vision to spot moving prey. The fox has excellent hearing and also relies on sound to locate and catch its prey. Although foxes are mainly active at night, it is not unusual to see them out during the day, particularly in quiet areas in the warm sunshine. Cubs are born annually in March and their average litter size is four to five cubs.

Sarcoptic mange

The most severe problem is that of sarcoptic mange, caused by the mite *Sarcoptes scabiei* (see also Chapter 29). The mite burrows into the skin and multiplies rapidly, resulting in loss of most of the fur, which takes about 4 months. The fox loses weight and many die. The lesions ooze fluid, which dries to form a crust that is full of mites. Mange is intensely irritant and the fox will scratch and gnaw at itself, even sometimes chewing its own tail off. As the fox moves around and curls up with other foxes, bits of crust fall off and other foxes become infected. Caught early enough, the condition can be treated; untreated the fox will die. Sarcoptic mange is a zoonosis, so care must be taken when dealing with infected patients.

Other parasites

Foxes can also have fleas and ticks. Adult foxes do not usually have many issues with internal parasites, but in young cubs worms can be a problem and can be treated with a complete puppy worming tablet.

Capture and transportation

The carrying basket should be prepared in advance: a crush cage with top and end openings is ideal. A fox with a head injury can be lifted as described for badgers. Make sure that you use a biting stick to test the animal's reactions and wear thick gloves

TABLE 34.9	Reasons for the admission of foxes as wildlife casualties	
Reason for admission	Injury/symptom	Notes
Road traffic accident	Concussion, cuts and bruising, fractures: leg/spine/jaw/pelvis	Females with fractured pelvis must be euthanised due to lack of knowing if they will give birth normally in the wild.
Sarcoptic mange	Bald patches around rump and tail initially, crusty skin, sores	
Trap/snare/trapped in netting or fencing	Injuries to limbs, particularly feet	Mouth should be checked as the fox will gnaw at the snare to free itself; may even chew off a limb. Do not cut them free and release. They must be kept in to monitor for skin breakdown at the site the skin was constricted.
Fences	General leg damage caused by hanging by one leg and constant struggling. Sometimes irreparable. Exhaustion	Happens when fox tries to clear a fence and does not quite manage it, often hanging and struggling for some time. Do not cut them free and release. They must be kept in to monitor for skin breakdown at the site the skin was constricted.
Leptospirosis	Jaundice	Euthanasia
Parvo virus	Dribbling, vomiting, diarrhoea	Euthanasia or supportive care if not too far gone by the time it is found.
Orphan	Alone, distressed, calling	Ask lots of questions to ascertain if it is a 'true' orphan or picked up in error.

or gauntlets to handle it. When the fox is injured but mobile there is no point in chasing it for miles. The person who contacted you may be able to monitor and feed the fox and so lure it into an area or shed where it is more easily caught or where a humane trap can be set.

In situations where the fox is trapped, or in dense undergrowth, or is not able to be confined in any other way, then a grasper or dog-catcher will have to be used. Once secured, put it into the basket in the usual way. Cover immediately. Foxes will bite and leap around to escape and they will rarely be lured into a carrier resembling a dark, safe, hole as a badger will.

Examination

When examining a fox it may need to be sedated, which can be achieved with the aid of a crush cage. If the fox is concussed the examination can be carried out easily but it must be remembered that it may come round quickly so a muzzle should be used. The material type muzzles are good as you can put them on the animal upside down, so that the underside of the muzzle will cover the animal's eyes.

Foxes can sustain horrific infected injuries in the wild, and we often only get adults brought in when they are beyond saving. Once they become septicaemic and jaundiced it is often too late to save them.

With fresh injuries, an assessment should be made as to the length of captivity needed to treat them and if the injury is treatable without unnecessary handling of the fox. An upper limit of 6 weeks for rehabilitation of an adult is not unreasonable.

Housing

Foxes do not make good captive patients and they may suffer high levels of stress, throwing themselves around and constantly scratching and biting at the wire in an attempt to escape. A kennel with a secure door and a blanket covering the front is the best short-term option, but as soon as possible the fox should be transferred to somewhere with more appropriate facilities, such as a wildlife hospital.

The fox should be given adequate bedding to enable it to hide, e.g. hay, which should be placed in one of the back corners of the cage. This will help to calm the fox – an empty pen will only fuel its anxiety and increase the manic search for a way out. A large cardboard box facing away from the door provides a good place to hide. The fox will be more active at night and the cage will have been reorganised by the morning. Plastic dog beds are not a good idea as they will be eaten.

Heat – the only practical heat source is a heat lamp, unless it is in heated accommodation. Any heat pad with a wire would be destroyed once the fox had warmed up and become more active.

Feeding

Stainless steel food bowls are best as ceramic ones may be broken and plastic ones will be chewed beyond use. Place a non-tip water bowl in a corner to help prevent it from being tipped over. Patients should have access to water at all times and, unless on a special feeding regimen, food is given at the end of the day.

Foxes eat a variety of foods, e.g. tinned cat and dog food, day-old chicks, mice, rabbit and dog mixer biscuit. Warming the food may persuade those foxes that are reluctant to eat initially. A sick fox that is recovering should be offered food ad lib – small portions to start with, increasing the amount as appropriate and eventually reducing the amount of feeds to one meal in the evening.

Cleaning

The fox should be removed from the cage when it is being cleaned and ideally it should be moved to a ready-prepared cage to avoid over-handling, which causes stress. Unlike a badger, a fox will not tolerate its cage being cleaned around it and it will throw itself around in an attempt to escape. If a spare cage is not available then the fox should be put into a secure basket and covered while cleaning is carried out.

Orphaned fox cubs

Fox cubs are born between January and March. For the first couple of weeks their eyes are closed and they remain in the den or 'earth', with both parents going for food and returning to feed them. Often the vixen will move the cubs from the birthing earth to a new earth to avoid predators smelling where the cubs are. She carries each cub in her mouth, moving them one by one. If disturbed she may drop a cub, but would generally come back for it, so you should leave them well alone until you can be sure she is not going to return.

Once the cubs are slightly bigger and their eyes start to open, they become more vocal and adventurous, and may start to emerge from the earth, calling for the vixen. This is the point at which most fox cubs are found by people in their gardens, and this is the time we need to be most careful with our advice. Many of the fox cubs that are picked up and brought to us are perfectly okay; it is just that they are starting to explore and are getting hungry. If you receive a call about a fox cub which seems perfectly healthy, but is out of the earth and crying, then it is probably fine. It is only if it starts to appear thin or dehydrated or is in mortal danger (side of a road, by a river, soaking wet in the rain etc.) that we should intervene. A search around the area may lead to facts that will help with your decision. Consider the following:

- If a group of fox cubs are seen without an adult, the situation should be monitored.
- A group of cubs that appear contented, asleep or playing together should be left alone and checked later from a distance, so as not to disturb the mother, who may be trying to return.
- If more than one cub is present or there is a group, but they are calling or appear to be in distress, then something may well have happened to the mother and they may need to be rescued.
- If the cubs are dispersed over the area rather than together, are cold, lethargic or wet, in a dangerous place or if there are signs of a disturbance, then they should be picked up.
- If a lone cub is found, out in the open, calling or appears to be distressed, it should be monitored for a couple of hours, then picked up if no mother returns.
- If a cub is found in an exposed area that still has its eyes closed, then it is under 2 weeks old and at that age is not able to thermoregulate and will soon become cold and eventually die, so should be rescued.
- Some situations can be difficult to make the right decision whether to intervene or not, and calling a wildlife hospital for advice is a good idea in these cases.

Capture and transportation. Once the orphan or orphans have been rescued they must be approached and handled carefully. Cubs with their eyes closed will offer little resistance but an older cub will be defensive and will spit and bite. Thick gloves will help but if none are available a jumper, coat or car rug will do just as well. Holding the cub by its scruff with a hand supporting its bottom is an acceptable method of picking up a cub. When the mother moves them from place to place she carries them in her mouth by the scruff and in this position the cub will often hang still and not struggle.

Examination. A thorough examination should be carried out, including:

- Checking through the fur and skin for wounds
- Checking for parasites – often fox cubs have ticks
- Checking body temperature – they may need supplementary heat
- Testing for dehydration
- Weighing the cub
- Assessing the age

- If there is more than one cub, decide upon a means of identifying each one. Microchipping or marking with nail polish or Tipp-Ex onto the fur are good methods.

Housing. The cub or cubs should be housed according to age and condition. A hospital cage will provide suitable accommodation but must be covered to provide a dark environment and should be situated in a quiet area. The very young or those that are sick will need supplementary heating. Those who are cold or wet will need gentle heat initially and then warm bedding. Older cubs will need only warm bedding. Single young cubs should be provided with a soft toy as a substitute 'mum', but older cubs should not have soft toys as they will tear them up and may try to eat them. As the cubs grow they can be moved to larger accommodation and eventually to an outside run with a box to hide in. It is important to keep talking and handling to a minimum when dealing with cubs, as they can become easily imprinted on humans if care is not taken.

Feeding. The cubs must be stimulated to urinate and defecate before and after being fed, if they have their eyes closed. Faeces of young cubs are orangey yellow and will turn brown as they are weaned onto solid food. Once toileting is complete each cub should be weighed and all the information recorded.

Feeding of very young cubs can be achieved with a 1-ml syringe or a puppy feeding bottle. The amount of food and the feeding times will vary depending on the animal's age (Table 34.10).

Puppy milk formula should be used for very young cubs. Start feeding with a syringe and move on to a bottle when the cub settles into hand feeding and starts to suck at the syringe – if the bottle is introduced at this time the cubs should take to it well. As the cub grows, and for older cubs, i.e. from about 2 weeks, a human baby bottle can be used. Fox cubs need to be 'burped', just as is done with human babies, as they are enthusiastic feeders and can take in air. The cub's back is rubbed and gently patted until the desired burp is achieved.

When the cub has its eyes open, start weaning with a little mashed tinned puppy food mixed with the milk formula. If the cub shows no interest in the food, carry on with the hand feeding and try again at the next feed. Once the cub is taking the sloppy food well, hand feeding can be gradually reduced. Aim to wean as soon as possible from bottle feeds to reduce the human handling of the cub. Offer mashed puppy food with the milk poured over it. Over the coming days, reduce the milk formula added to the food. Weaning should be completed by 5–6 weeks, by which time the cub will be on a diet of tinned cat or dog food. If available, they can also be given day-old chicks, mice, and rabbit. Cubs must never be reared on their own, and successes are rarely had in a busy veterinary surgery to rehabilitate even a group of cubs. It is very important to transfer them to a wildlife hospital as soon as possible, where they will be put with others and will be released back into the wild in the summer.

RABBITS (*ORYCTOLAGUS CUNICULUS*) AND HARES (*LEPUS CAPENSIS*)

Rabbits and hares are similar in many ways but there are differences that should be taken into consideration when veterinary care is needed (Table 34.11):

TABLE 34.10	Fox cub orphans
	This is a rough guide; each individual is different

Make sure all feeds are prepared fresh daily. **Give rehydration solution for first feed after admission.**

EQUIPMENT AND METHOD:

- Small human baby bottle – do not flood the mouth
- If eyes closed, toilet before and after syringe feeding by vibrating cotton wool (dipped in baby oil to protect the skin) over the genitals in a head-to-tail direction. Ensure all urine is removed as it will burn the skin if left
- Cubs suckle standing up on their hind legs
- As they drink very quickly cubs may get 'trapped wind'. Burping them by rubbing/tapping their backs should ease the condition
- Bloated abdomen can be fatal – try rehydration fluids for next couple of feeds
- Diarrhoea can be fatal – give rehydration fluids instead of milk formula for next 1 or 2 feeds, then give half water/half formula for the next feed, then back to just formula, if faeces go back to normal. If diarrhoea persists try giving probiotics

Age	Notes	Feeding	
		Food/quantity	Intervals
Up to 7 days old	Eyes and ears closed. Ear flaps folded down. Dark brown fur with tiny white tail tip	3–5 ml	2-hour intervals. 3-hour intervals overnight
10 days	Ears starting to stand up a little. Eyes show signs of opening. Dark brown fur, with tiny white tail tip	5–10 ml	3-hour intervals, last feed 12am, first feed 6am. Feed once in the middle of the night
18 days	Eyes will be opening and ears will be almost up	10–15 ml	4 times daily. Allow to lick first solids from finger
About 3 weeks	Eyes open, but still blue. Proper fox coat colours will be starting to show, instead of the dark brown	20–30 ml	Bottle feed 3 times a day, but also offer dish of formula and start to encourage lapping at each feed
About 4 weeks	Weaning starts when all teeth are through	30–40 ml. Offer first solids in their cage – mashed puppy food mixed with formula in a bowl	Bottle feed twice a day, but encouraging lapping formula and puppy food is preferred

TABLE 34.10	Fox cub orphans This is a rough guide; each individual is different—cont'd		
Age	**Notes**	**Feeding**	
About 5 weeks	Eyes start to turn brown	Reduce bottle feeding	Start reducing the formula added to puppy food
6 weeks onwards	Looks like a miniature fox	They should be fully weaned now. (In the wild they would get milk from their mother for much longer, but as we are giving complete puppy food, weaning them earlier is preferred to prevent imprinting on humans.)	Stop formula milk

TABLE 34.11	Reasons for the admission of rabbits and hares as wildlife casualties	
Reason	**Injury/symptom**	**Notes**
Road traffic accident	Concussion, cuts, bruising. Fractures, usually back legs, pelvis, spine	Think seriously if repairing fractures would hinder their ability to run in the wild. They must be perfect to be released. Females with fractured pelvis must be euthanised due to lack of knowing if they will give birth normally in the wild.
Victim of domestic cats	Paralysis, wounds	Mostly rabbits
Myxomatosis	Swelling on the eyes, nose, base of ears and genital area	Die within 2 weeks of catching the virus. Euthanasia
Snares	Injury to neck, abdomen, sometimes limbs	Do not cut them free and release. They must be kept in to monitor for skin breakdown at the site the skin was constricted.
Orphan	See Orphans later in this chapter	

- **Rabbits** – live in large colonies based in a series of linked underground burrows called a warren. Their day is spent underground and they are most active outside the warren at dusk. Young are altricial, i.e. they are hairless and blind and are totally dependent on the mother until they are weaned

- **Hares** – live in scraped out hollows in the ground called forms in open countryside or woodland. They are nocturnal but can be seen at dawn and dusk. Young are precocial, i.e. they are capable of an independent life almost from birth. Hares are becoming increasingly rare because of modern methods of farming.

Myxomatosis

Myxomatosis is a viral disease that was introduced in the 1950s to reduce the rabbit population; it does not seem to affect hares to the same degree. The rabbit flea *Spilopsyllus cuniculi* carries the virus on its blood-sucking mouthparts and passes it from one rabbit to another. A few days after becoming infected the rabbit's eyes begin to discharge a watery substance, the eyelids swell, and swellings appear on the nose, at the base of the ears and around the genital area. These swellings fill with pus and at this stage the rabbit can neither see nor hear and is often seen sitting at the roadside oblivious to its surroundings. Within approximately 2 weeks of catching the virus the rabbit dies.

Capture and transportation

Capture of most rabbit and hare casualties is usually fairly easy if they are a road traffic casualty with severe injuries, have myxomatosis, which debilitates the rabbit, or are cat victims – a rabbit is often brought into the house by the cat. Never grasp the animal by its ears alone. Throw a towel or similar material over it and wrap it up to prevent the rescuer from being scratched. If a box is not available, the animal may be transported by being either held or put in the boot of a car. Rabbits and hares do not generally make any noise but a distressed animal may scream to deter a predator.

Examination

Hares are powerful animals and both rabbits and hares will kick out with all four limbs and must be restrained by two pairs of hands. Remember that they will try to jump away from danger, so hold them securely at all times so they do not fall from the examination table. Cover the casualty's head for as much of the examination as possible:

- In almost all rear-end injuries an X-ray is most helpful in determining the exact problem. Fractured limbs will rarely be able to be treated, as adults will not tolerate long periods of captivity well, so euthanasia should be considered in these cases.
- Where the injuries are cat-inflicted, symptoms may be due to temporary nerve damage and after a few days function may return to the limbs.
- Those cat victims that sustain wounds should be treated and released as soon as possible as prolonged captivity causes fatal stress. Appropriate antibiotics should be administered quickly to combat infection.
- Testing for pain reflex is difficult in wildlife as, in the wild, to react to pain by either noise or movement may alert a predator, so they will hide signs of pain from you.
- Concussed patients can sometimes recover quickly and within 24–48 hours may be released.

Housing

Rabbits and hares do not make good patients and should be housed in quiet, dark accommodation with plenty of bedding, e.g. hay, in which to hide. These animals suffer terribly from stress, so arrange transfer to a wildlife hospital as soon as possible.

Heat – should only be provided in severe cases, as rabbits in particular may suffer if kept too warm.

Feeding

Natural food should be provided, e.g. grass, dandelions, clover, and hay. Food should be left in the cage at all times and the casualty left alone to eat. Always provide a source of fresh water in a non-tip bowl, not a pet rabbit bottle.

Cleaning

As rabbits and hares are very nervous it is better to have a clean, prepared cage ready for transfer. Any further examination, treatment and replacing of food should be done at the same time.

Orphans

Rabbits. Rabbits are born underground and are blind, deaf and without fur, so if very young ones are seen above ground there is a problem. Mechanical diggers and dogs often dig up baby rabbits and the nests are destroyed. Rabbits are weaned at a young age and are often picked up as tiny bunnies, when really they are independent and able to care for themselves. The mother can be pregnant again 12 hours after she gives birth and so the young rabbit kittens are weaned before the next litter is born. The mother will only feed them once every 24 hours.

Hares. Baby hares or leverets are completely different and are born fully furred with their eyes and ears open. They sit motionless in their forms above ground and are often mistakenly picked up as orphans. The mother leaves them all day, returning only once in 24 hours to feed them. Unless they appear weak or injured, they are in direct danger or are wet and cold, they should be left where they are.

Capture and transportation. These orphans are easily picked up and present no danger to the handler. They will need warm bedding during transportation, particularly if they are very young rabbits, but they must be completely covered so that they are in the dark, which will simulate the burrow for rabbits and provide security for leverets.

The initial examination should include:

- Check for wounds – in patients that have been picked up by dogs or cats
- Check the body temperature
- Check for dehydration
- Weigh the orphan
- Assess the age
- If there is more than one, identify the individuals with Tipp-Ex or nail polish onto the fur.

The advice on accommodation and feeding should be suitable for successful rearing of both rabbits and hares (Table 34.12).

Housing. Line a cage with newspaper and a towel. Make a bed of hay at the back and place food near it, as the patient is unlikely to venture away from the back of the cage. Cover the cage to ensure that it is dark and represents the burrow. For hare the dark will help to keep them calm and they will sit in a hollow in the hay, which represents the form.

As the young animals become older, a grass run outdoors will provide more suitable accommodation, but provide a box in which to hide and ensure chicken wire is placed between the run and the ground to prevent them digging out and going free prematurely.

Feeding. Both rabbit and hare mothers leave their young for long periods of time in either the burrow or the form and will only return once or twice a day, allowing them to feed for a few minutes before leaving them again. As the youngsters grow, the mother will return for shorter periods of time until they are weaned. This makes a feeding regimen difficult to formulate; however, one feed at each end of the day, dawn and dusk, seems to work. Overfeeding more often than this is one of the biggest killers of orphan rabbits and hares.

Before feeding it is a good idea to try to stimulate the babies to urinate and defecate in rabbits if the eyes are closed but, as the wild mothers return very infrequently to see to their youngsters, it could be that they do not need to be stimulated as often as other orphaned mammals or that they are able to defecate and urinate unaided. For this reason toileting should not be overdone: if urine is produced immediately then stimulation should be carried on until the youngster is finished but if nothing appears there is no reason to keep trying. Urine from stimulated rabbits tends to spurt out rather than dripping like that of other orphans.

Feed kitten milk formula using a 1-ml syringe and a lot of patience. Orphans should be fed as much as they will take in one sitting and should not be pushed to take more – rabbits in particular become very stressed, so keep the room and yourself as quiet as possible during feeding. The first few feeds will be the most difficult and rabbits will often lose weight over the first few days but once their feeding behaviour settles down they should slowly gain weight. Once their eyes open, have natural greens available (see Table 34.12).

During weaning, a piece of turf with the soil attached can be placed in the accommodation, allowing for nibbling and climbing over. Green food should always be fresh. A shallow container of kitten milk formula and one of water should be

TABLE 34.12	**Rabbit kit (and hare) orphans** **This is a rough guide; each individual is different**

Make sure all feeds are prepared fresh daily. **Give rehydration solution for first feed after admission.**

EQUIPMENT AND METHOD:
- 1-ml syringe (soft teat optional)
- If eyes closed, toilet before and after syringe feeding by vibrating cotton wool (dipped in baby oil to protect the skin) over the genitals in a head-to-tail direction. Ensure all urine is removed as it will burn the skin if left
- Bloated abdomen can be fatal – try rehydration fluids for next couple of feeds
- Diarrhoea can be fatal – give rehydration fluids instead of milk formula for next 1 or 2 feeds, then give half water/half formula for the next feed, then back to just formula, if faeces go back to normal. If diarrhoea persists try giving probiotics
- Not eating can be fatal – monitor intake closely
- They should be released as close as possible to where they were found, at 5–6 weeks old

Weight	Notes	Feeding	
		Quantity	Intervals
Birth (approx. weight 30 g) Rabbit only	Blind, deaf, naked	Feed kitten milk formula by syringe. Whatever amount they will take	Once in morning and once in evening
1 week–10 days Rabbit only	Eyes open around 10 days, covering of velvety fur	Feed kitten milk formula by syringe. Whatever amount they will take	Once in morning and once in evening
2 weeks (rabbit) Baby hare from birth onwards	Now mobile, grooming and digging	Offer natural greens, and offer the milk formula in a bowl for them to lap. If eating well then syringe feeds can start to be reduced	Syringe feed once in morning and once in evening, if not eating well by themselves. Keep in as quiet an area as possible. Neither species will feed well if surrounded by noise and movement
3 weeks	Should be nibbling on solid food; wean off the kitten milk formula feed at dusk	Feed as above, but can add piece of turf with the soil attached in the accommodation, allowing for nibbling and climbing over	Syringe feed once in the evening, if not eating well by themselves
4 weeks onwards	Should be weaned off all kitten milk formula feeds. Eating solid food well now	Feed as above, but stop all kitten formula	May appreciate spending time in a secure outdoor run, if weather is good. Provide a box in which to hide and ensure chicken wire is placed between the run and the ground to prevent them digging out and going free prematurely

placed into the cage, but not in the corners as is done with other mammals as this is often where the orphans will practise their digging.

Little rehabilitation is needed for young rabbits and hares once they are fully weaned. As long as they have not been over handled during the hand-rearing process they should not become tame, and should be released back to the location they were found.

Rabbits and hare are the most difficult orphans to rear and require quiet, patience and time. Sadly this is usually not possible in busy veterinary surgeries, so they should be transferred to a wildlife hospital for rehabilitation once stable.

TABLE 34.13	Reasons for the admission of bats as wildlife casualties	
Reason for admission	**Injury/symptom**	**Notes**
Cat victims	Wounds/ fractures/ holes and tears in the wings	Usually found on the ground, if not deposited at your feet
Entangled, e.g. fruit netting	Cuts/fractures/torn wings	Wounds caused by the struggle to escape
Fly paper	Sticky!	Use bandage adhesive remover spray to remove
Out in the day	Hanging on wall or fence in broad daylight	Often no injuries but benefit from fluids, food and rest for 24–48 hours before release
Orphan	Small and immature, brought in by cat or found on the ground	Sometimes fall from roosts. Contact local bat group or wildlife hospital.
Grounded	On the ground	As a result of trauma or attack. Must have antibiotics.

Young rabbits that are presented with their eyes open should be given the opportunity to go directly on to the first stage of weaning, making sure that kitten milk formula is available in a shallow container. Monitor them closely as some milk feeds by syringe may be needed initially – the older the orphan the more difficult the rearing process.

BATS

Bats are the only flying mammals in the UK. There are 18 species, and some are rarer than others. The species most commonly presented is the tiny common pipistrelle bat *Pipistrellus pipistrellus*. Bats are nocturnal and hunt at night for insects using echolocation. They are also one of the few British mammals that hibernate; they will go into an extended sleep, or torpor, in their roost during this time, but do not build a nest as hedgehogs do. Bats live in a variety of places, referred to as roosts, including the roofs of houses, and the eaves and walls, in barns, stables and churches, under bridges and caves.

Many people fear bats for various reasons, many of which are old wives' tales, but they pose no threat and should be encouraged as they eat many undesirable insects. They are presented for a variety of reasons (Table 34.13), the most common of which is as victims of cats, or in periods of food shortage. In either event, they require specialist help, as they are tricky to feed in captivity.

Don't forget that even though bats are gentle creatures and seldom show aggression they are wild animals and may be frightened or in pain. Most of the UK's bats have such small teeth that a bite will not break the skin. A strain of the rabies virus has, however, been found in a small number of British bats, so although the risk is tiny, you should take precautions to avoid being bitten or scratched.

Capture and transportation

Capture of an injured bat is simple as it is likely to be on the ground and therefore merely requires picking up. Bats that are flying around a room, e.g. having flown inside the house in error, should be allowed to find their own way out. Bats that are flying do not need to be rescued and detained but rescued and released. If all the lights are turned off, all windows and outside doors to the room are opened and the room is left quiet the bat is given the opportunity to make its way out. Chasing it around the room with a net and swatting at it will increase its panic and the chance of injury.

Should the bat be discovered at night and it is not injured and can fly, it should be picked up using gloves or a small towel and taken outside, hung as high as possible and left to fly when it is ready. If it is found during the day then it should be housed in a small box (shoe boxes are ideal for bats), lined with kitchen roll and a face flannel or similar material to enable it to hide. Push a pencil or wooden kebab skewer through one side of the box and out through the other to provide a high hanging place. The box should have small air holes and be taped shut, as bats will easily crawl out of an unsecured shoebox or the smallest of holes. A bat on the ground may be encouraged to crawl into the box.

Examination

First observe the bat in the box – is it active, is there blood on the bedding and is there anything specific that needs closer examination? Wearing latex or thicker gloves the bat should be picked up and supported with the thumb on its back and fingers under its abdomen gently but firmly. The wings should be extended to check for injuries, holes and fractures, one at a time. A bat should never be held by its wings. Check for dehydration, starvation and general bodily condition and record all results.

Housing

A shoebox as described above is sufficient for short-term housing but longer stays need more cleanable accommodation. A plastic tank with a ventilated top is ideal, with a supple twig bent into position to serve as a hanging post. The tank should be lined with kitchen roll and some sort of gauze suspended from under the lid to enable the bat to climb and hide. Cover the plastic tank to provide a dark environment. After treatment, recovery should be completed at a wildlife rescue centre with a suitable flight aviary.

Heat – bats are heterotherms, i.e. they are able to control their body temperature, regulating it to a fixed level or altering it to the ambient temperature. In times of cold weather, rather like the hedgehog, the bat will drop its temperature and enter a torpid state. This saves energy in times when food is difficult to find. When a cold or inactive bat is presented, it should be gently warmed up. A heat mat under one end of the accommodation is preferable.

Feeding

Bats eat flying insects, which they catch using echolocation. In captivity insects or moths may be offered; however, other foods will be taken that are easier to obtain, for example:

- Mealworms fed on bran and then the heads cut off, allowing the bat to suck out the soft insides
- Maggots cut in half

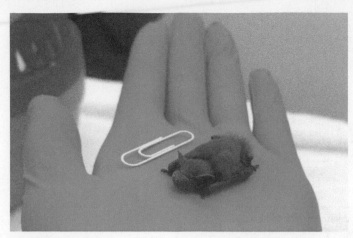

Fig. 34.7 A baby bat

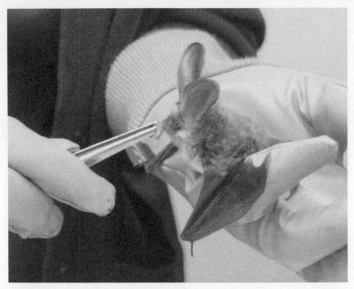

Fig. 34.8 Feeding a bat

- If none of these feeds are easily obtainable for your surgery, then just allow the bat to lick a little rehydration support from a clean make-up applicator or artist's paintbrush and organise transfer to a wildlife hospital as soon as possible.

Offer the bat a little rehydration support from a clean make-up applicator or artist's paintbrush before food is offered and once the bat is warm and fully hydrated it should become more active. Supply water in the housing by using a piece of clean cloth or kitchen paper. Soak it in water and squeeze it out so that it is soggy, then place it on to a jam jar lid or similar flat container. This will enable the bat to lick or suck at the cloth and avoids the risk of it drowning. Food should be offered in a shallow container, e.g. a jam jar lid.

Orphaned bats

Tiny bats sometimes fall from their roosts and where it is not possible to return them, they may have to be hand-reared (Fig. 34.7). Many young bats that are presented are victims of cats and their original roost is unknown. Always liaise with your local bat group, as sometimes they can find the roost and return the bat to its mother.

Examination. On admission a full examination should be carried out:

- Check for general condition and wounds – if the bat is thin the stomach will look indented
- Check for dehydration
- Check body temperature
- Weigh the bat
- Identify the bat if possible (information available from the Bat Conservation Trust www.bats.org.uk).

Record details of the exact location in which the bat was found so that it can be released in the same place.

Housing. Orphan bats should be accommodated in the same way as adults. They are not easy to hand-rear, so consideration should be taken as to whether it may be better to transfer the orphan into the care of a wildlife hospital or licensed bat rehabilitator from a local bat group.

Feeding. It is essential that the orphaned bat is kept warm and that the milk feed is also warm and kept at a constant temperature during feeding. This prevents fermentation of the milk

inside the bat, causing problems. Use puppy milk formula, mixed thoroughly to dissolve it completely, and offer it on an artist's paintbrush or a clean make-up applicator sponge, which allows the bat to suck or lap the milk in tiny quantities. Syringes are not appropriate for these orphans as too much milk is delivered even with the smallest drop. Care must be taken to make sure the milk is taken quickly from the brush or applicator to prevent it from becoming cold.

A new-born bat can weigh very little, depending on the species, and the feeding regimen should be as follows:

- New-born bats – must be fed at 2-hour intervals throughout the day and night
- 1 week old – feed every 2 hours between 6am and midnight
- From 3 weeks old – feed every 3 hours between 6am and midnight.

During weaning increase the interval between feeds. Mealworms can be used as a source of solid food by cutting off their heads and allowing the young bat to suck out the soft insides (Fig. 34.8). Water and small amounts of food should be provided as with adults and replaced regularly to avoid it drying out. A rescue centre or local bat group should be contacted for access to a flight aviary and rehabilitation back to the wild.

DEER

There are six species of deer seen in Britain: the red deer, roe deer, fallow deer, sika deer, Reeves's muntjac and Chinese water deer. The three most often presented as casualties will be dealt with in this chapter.

The majority of deer casualties are the result of road traffic accidents. Deer hit by cars may often be stunned and not injured. They often only require 20–30 minutes to rest and may well run off after this recovery period. Deer in these instances should be moved off the road and monitored. They will not need medical treatment unless they are actually injured. You should leave an injured deer where it is, and should advise the public against attempting to bring them in. A wildlife hospital or the RSPCA can be called to assess or collect the deer if needed. If a member of the public brings a deer in to your

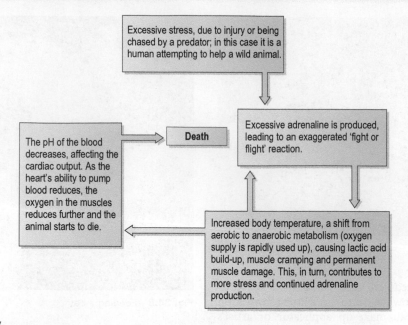

Fig. 34.9 Capture myopathy

TABLE 34.14	Reasons for the admission of deer as wildlife casualties	
Reason for admission	**Injury/symptom**	**Notes**
Road traffic accident (RTA)	Concussion	Most deer casualties presented are RTA victims
	Cuts/bruising/grazes	
	Fractures: limbs/pelvis/spine/jaw	Rarely able to treat, due to long periods of captivity being impossible to manage
Trapped	No physical injuries but have become trapped in an enclosed area and in panic cannot find a way out	No need to admit but may need help in finding a way out by opening a gate, or making an opening through which the deer can pass. Often, if left alone, they will find a way out themselves
Entangled	Hanging on barbed wire/fencing, usually by a limb. Severe tear wounds and fractures	Do not cut them free and release without taking advice from a wildlife hospital. The animal may need observation to check for wound breakdown at the site of the constriction.
Dog victims	Bite/puncture wounds	
Orphans	Sitting alone in long grass	Not necessarily orphaned, need to ask lots of questions to the finder to ascertain if the animal is really an orphan

surgery, get the vet to make an assessment of its injuries and house it securely until a wildlife hospital or the RSPCA can be called to help.

A veterinary practice is not a suitable place to treat or house a deer under any circumstances.

Capture myopathy

Capture myopathy kills deer, and there is no treatment for this condition, only prevention. Capture myopathy causes the deer to produce too much adrenaline, causing an exaggerated fight-or-flight response (Fig. 34.9). The body temperature rises and the increase in adrenaline results in a build-up of lactic acid, cramping and muscle damage. The increased adrenaline causes the metabolism to change from aerobic to anaerobic; the lactic acid builds up causing acidosis. Lactic acid in the bloodstream drops the pH in the body, affecting the heart's output. The heart's ability to pump oxygen to the muscles then deteriorates and they will start to die.

Many deer are brought in unnecessarily, and when this happens it puts unnecessary stress on the animal and prevents

recovery. Most wildlife hospitals will attempt to treat at the site of the injury wherever possible, rather than transport the deer, which causes unnecessary stress.

If the deer is injured, make an assessment of the chances of quick treatment and release. For example, broken limbs in deer are almost impossible to manage, especially in roe deer, and in these cases it is usually kinder to put the animal to sleep rather than attempt heroic surgery on an animal that does not tolerate captivity (Table 34.14):

- **Fallow deer** (*Dama dama*) – main times of activity are dawn and dusk but they may be seen at any time grazing on grass or browsing in deciduous forest on trees and shrubs. Their colouring varies from reddish brown with white spots to a paler brown with spots, and even black or white. The tail is black and white and the rump has distinctive black markings. One fawn is produced in June.
- **Roe deer** (*Capreolus capreolus*) – active at dawn and dusk. They feed on shrubs and the young shoots of trees. The coat is a deep red, which becomes a duller brown

in the winter, the nose is black, there is a white patch on the chin and the rump is cream. Young or kids are born in May–June, often twins.

- **Muntjac deer** (*Muntiacus reevesi*) – the smallest of our deer and an introduced species from Asia. This species is illegal to release without the appropriate licence from Natural England (see relevant legislation below).They are active during the day and at night and are mainly browsers, feeding on shrubs and the leaves of trees. They are sometimes seen grazing. The coat is reddish brown with white around the tail. The male has fang-like teeth protruding from the upper jaw. One fawn is born at any time of the year.

Capture and transportation

Deer are not easy to capture and are equipped with lethal weapons in the form of antlers and sharp hooves. Muntjacs have tusk-like teeth as additional tools for harming humans. If a deer is able to kick, lunge, head-butt and perform other acrobatics that make capture difficult, why is an attempt being made to rescue it? If a deer is injured but can be treated by a vet at the scene, e.g. by giving antibiotics, and then released, there is nothing to be gained by adding to the animal's distress by confining it. The stress of capture and transportation, even a healthy deer, is enough to kill it.

In those deer that are obviously injured the head should be covered as soon as it is safe to do so. Sedation should definitely be considered, as it may be safer to sedate these animals in order to clean wounds, administer antibiotics and even to make transportation safer and less stressful to the animal.

Injured deer that cannot be released but are not candidates for euthanasia on site should be wrapped and transported with a hood over their eyes, with the nose exposed for respiration. Many rescuers tie the legs to help restraint but this is stressful to the deer and unnecessary – wrapping is preferable. The deer should be accompanied and monitored throughout the journey and care should be taken to ensure that it does not overheat in the vehicle.

Road traffic casualties found lying beside a road are usually severely injured or concussed. Any deer hit by a vehicle will, if it is able, run for cover despite having sustained fractures or internal injuries.

The approach to a deer at the roadside should include a rapid assessment of the situation. Consider the position it is in, its reactions, blood on the road, etc., all of which help to identify the injury. Those clearly awake and struggling are likely to need euthanasia on the scene. Those that appear dazed may just have received a blow to the head and be in need of a quiet place to recover.

Road traffic accidents involving deer attract bystanders and often the police are in attendance. There are vehicles, people and noise, all stressful to the casualty, and the rescuer must take charge of the situation and clear the area. Remember that the stress caused by rescuing such casualties may outweigh the possible benefits and that whatever the decision it must be made quickly.

Examination

Assessment and examination must take place at the scene of the rescue and the records must be completed after the casualty has been accommodated. Deer will not tolerate much handling and it is dangerous and exhausting for the rescuers.

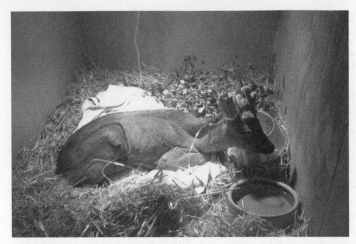

Fig. 34.10 A roe deer patient

Recovered deer must be returned and released where they were found. In the case of road traffic casualties this should be the nearest safe place, so the exact location must be recorded on the patient's notes.

Housing

Housing deer in large practice kennels is not appropriate. Deer must be kept in isolation away from noise and the general buzz of a veterinary practice. Using outside stables or barns or even a strong shed is preferable. A smaller deer may be housed in a large kennel, but it must be dark and well away from disturbance.

Deer will rush around a pen, running into walls, and become very distressed. Absolute quiet and dark is essential for the animal to remain calm and rest. Provide a thick bed of hay and blankets for extra warmth if necessary. Be aware that on entering the pen the deer will attempt to escape and any cleaning, feeding or administering of treatments should be done at the same time, removing the need for constant disturbance (Fig. 34.10).

Heat – a warm bed of straw and blankets is usually enough for an injured deer; however, severely debilitated patients may need supplementary heating. This is best provided using a heat lamp with a protective cover suspended above the animal. Close monitoring is essential and the lamp should be removed as soon as possible.

Feeding

Deer patients are often distressed at being held captive and rarely eat when hospitalised. If they are subjected to the minimum amount of attention and the right food is offered they may feed. Deer are not usually in this situation for long and it is never worth hanging on to an animal that is ready for release just because it has not eaten – the usual reason for inappetence is captivity.

Provide water in a heavy bowl in a corner of the accommodation away from the bedding – this is unlikely to be touched in the first few days. Natural food is always better for the deer, e.g. leaves of deciduous trees, hawthorn, brambles, ivy, and the petals and leaves of roses can be offered. Also try hay, apples and root vegetables, cabbage, lettuce or spring greens and a goat mix from a farm supplier may be eaten.

Cleaning

Cleaning should be undertaken only when necessary. Take the opportunity to do anything else that needs to be done that day at the same time, e.g. injections, wound dressing, etc. Deer are usually short-stay patients and, as they are unlikely to eat or drink initially, the need for cleaning will not arise for the first day or two.

Orphaned deer

Deer are extremely difficult to hand-rear. They are more labour intensive than any other orphaned mammal and are not suitable to hand-rear in a veterinary surgery.

In the wild, does leave their young for long periods of time, often up to 12 hours at a time, usually in long grass or areas of good cover, and often these babies are assumed to be orphaned and are picked up. The doe will usually be close by but will not return to her youngster while the human is present. It should be left where it is and checked on from a distance later. If a deer fawn or kid is presented and circumstances similar to those above are reported, it should be taken back immediately, and unless it is obviously sick or badly injured it should be left alone. Should a young animal be correctly identified as an orphan it should be transported in a large box or wire basket lined with a warm blanket and covered to keep it dark.

Examination. Examination of a very young deer is easier than with an adult but it must not be assumed that the orphan is not distressed. It may be injured or unwell, has lost its mother, has been removed from natural surroundings and will be frightened and may also put up a fight. Make sure that the initial examination is carried out as quickly as possible and that the youngster is then accommodated and left to rest. No attempt should be made at this stage to feed it, unless it needs lifesaving fluids.

A general examination should include:

- Check for wounds, and fly eggs or maggots
- Check for dehydration
- Assess the age – this can be difficult unless evidence of the umbilicus is present
- Check the general body condition
- Contact a wildlife hospital as soon as possible.

An appropriate-sized kennel or large basket should be lined with warm blankets and the orphan should be left to rest. If supplementary heat is needed a Snuggle Pad can be used under the blankets to provide gentle warmth.

Feeding. The first feed should be rehydration fluid once the animal is warm. If the animal cannot be transferred quickly to a wildlife hospital, then commence milk formula feeds. Feed a lamb milk replacer using a lamb or human baby feeding bottle depending on the size of the fawn. The formula should be thoroughly mixed using boiled water cooled to the correct temperature for feeding. Newly admitted orphans are often reluctant to feed and it may take some time. In some cases it may be necessary to stomach tube the fawn until it is ready to suck on the bottle. Three or four feeds per day are adequate for deer fawns and once they have taken to the bottle, feed them until they have had enough at each feed (Fig. 34.11).

Deer need to be stimulated to defecate and urinate and this is best achieved while feeding is under way. Using one hand to hold the bottle, the other hand is used to gently stimulate the genital area with a warm, damp cloth.

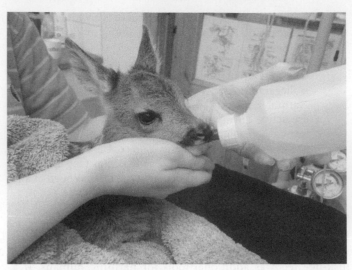

Fig. 34.11 A roe deer fawn

Weaning takes place gradually and from about 1 week of age the fawn will nibble on fresh food, and a tray of soil should be provided along with young shoots and leaves as described in feeding adults. Rose petals and leaves are a popular first food and goat mix and lamb pellets, brambles and hawthorn can also be given. If the fawn is reluctant to take the solid food, try offering sliced apples and carrots, cabbage, lettuce and spring greens, but once the deer is feeding well these should be reduced until natural food and the dried preparations are all that is offered. Weaning should be complete by 10–12 weeks of age and the young deer will need time in an enclosure at a wildlife rehabilitation centre in preparation for release back into the wild.

GREY SQUIRRELS (*SCIURUS CAROLINENSIS*)

The grey squirrel is seen both in urban areas in parks and gardens and in the country, where it often seems to be dicing with death on our roads and this is the reason most are presented as casualties (Table 34.15).

Squirrels are active by day and use their sense of smell and eyesight to survey their surroundings and search for food. They eat nuts, bark, leaves, shoots, acorns, buds and flowers and nest in dreys high up in the trees. Squirrels breed twice a year, and young are born early in the spring and again in the autumn – the average litter size is three to six kittens. They are independent by about 2 months old and are reared exclusively by the female. Squirrels are extremely agile and are able to scale vertical walls, poles and trees, hanging on with sharp claws.

It is illegal to keep or release grey squirrels without the appropriate licence from Natural England (see relevant legislation below).

Capture and transportation

Squirrels are very agile and have a very strong bite that will cause nasty wounds if care is not taken when handling.

Approach the casualty with a pair of thick gloves and a towel. Drop the towel over the squirrel, scoop it up and place both towel and animal into a secure carrier for transportation. For those that are still mobile (usually those with a back or hind leg injury) you may need a net. It must be remembered that a squirrel's teeth are such that they may penetrate the glove, but the towel provides additional protection.

TABLE 34.15	Reasons for the admission of grey squirrels as wildlife casualties		
Reason for admittance	**Injury/symptom**	**Notes**
Road traffic casualty	Concussion Fractures Eye prolapse Cuts/bruising/ grazes	Sometimes impaled on the front grilles of vehicles
	Fractures: pelvis/ spinal/limbs/ jaw	Think seriously if repairing fractures would hinder their ability to run and jump in the wild. They must be perfect to be released. Females with fractured pelvis must be euthanised due to lack of knowing if they will give birth normally in the wild.
Attacks	Bite wounds and scratches	Usually young squirrels. Often by dogs or cats
Orphans	Very young squirrel, no parent present	Often found by a cat or dog, or lying on the ground
Stuck/ frozen in place/ panicked	Up a telegraph pole, on the roof of a house	No rescue needed; usually been frightened up there by a cat or dog. Will come down when safe to do so but may not be until nightfall

Examination

For squirrels that show no obvious sign of injury, examination of the squirrel is a four-handed job. One person should restrain the squirrel and keep the head under control while the second person completes the examination safely. For those with obvious injuries, sedation or anaesthesia may be required for a detailed examination. Always try to keep the head covered to reduce stress.

Housing

The squirrel's ability to bite has already been established, and this must be considered when providing suitable accommodation. Cardboard and thin plastic are not advisable; a small wire kennel with a metal door is ideal. Line the kennel with newspaper and warm bedding; cover it so that the squirrel is in the dark and place it in a quiet room.

Heat – a microwavable Snuggle Pad is excellent to provide heat for seriously sick or injured squirrels as it avoids the use of anything with chewable wires. As soon as the squirrel becomes more active, the heat supply should be removed and replaced with warm bedding. Synthetic fleece is ideal. Towels should be avoided as the loops in the material often get snagged in the animal's claws.

Feeding

Squirrels are rodents, so for adults offer a basic diet of commercial rodent or rat mix. Plain digestive biscuits, fruit and unsalted nuts can be added. Put all food towards the back of the cage, as adult squirrels are very stressed in captivity and unlikely to come towards the front of a cage to eat. Water in a small non-tip bowl should be placed in a back corner of the cage to avoid spillage.

Cleaning

When cleaning, remove the food and water bowls first, but only if it is safe to do so. Then tip the cage up on to its end so the squirrel is at the bottom and the door now at the top. Wearing thick gloves and armed with a towel, transfer the squirrel to a clean, ready-prepared cage. This saves over-handling of a difficult species and ensures that the ordeal is over quickly for the squirrel.

Orphaned squirrels

Always make sure that the squirrel is an orphan before rescuing it. The squirrel's drey is high up in trees, so it is difficult to return orphans to the nest, even if you knew which tree was the right one. The fact that a young squirrel has been found indicates that all is not well. Young squirrels that run up to or onto people are usually orphans, as these are one of the few species that actively seeks help when orphaned. Other examples of young squirrels that may be brought in include young squirrels found in lofts after the parent has been evicted, either by the homeowner or by pest control. If a tree has been cut down with babies in a drey, give time for the parent to return. Female squirrels often use more than one drey, and giving her time to move the babies is important. If after leaving undisturbed for an hour or so no mother returns, then the babies should be brought in.

Hungry orphans will emit a high-pitched and insistent whistle, which may be the reason they are discovered in the first place. A cardboard box filled with warm bedding may be used for transportation and a Snuggle Pad should be provided for very young orphans.

Examination. The orphan should be examined thoroughly, including:

- Check for wounds, bite marks and grazes
- Check the body temperature
- Check for dehydration
- Assess the age of the squirrel
- Weigh the squirrel.

Squirrels are born naked, blind and deaf, so if very young or newly born babies are presented heat should be provided. To identify the orphan as a young squirrel, look for the long tail and if in doubt check the claws, which look as if they have been painted with black nail varnish. Ageing is an inexact science but the eyes open at around 3 weeks and at this stage the fur forms a short but thick covering and the tail is furry but not bushy.

Feeding. Before being fed the squirrel should be stimulated to urinate and defecate and then weighed. The faeces of milk-fed squirrels are tiny yellowy/light brown pellets, which change to darker brown when weaned. Feed using a 1-ml syringe and puppy milk formula (Table 34.16).

Once the eyes open, a little solid food can be introduced. Offer broken digestive biscuits, dry unsweetened breakfast cereals, rusks, fruit and soft unsalted nuts such as walnuts or cashews. Food should be left in the cage and water provided. Reducing the milk feeds can begin when the solid food is being eaten. Weighing is important to monitor the squirrel's progress. Reduce heat in the cage to night time only for a few days and then turn it off completely.

It is important to avoid peanuts, as squirrels in captivity can develop metabolic bone disease if they eat too many peanuts or get an unbalanced diet. Once weaned, the squirrel should move into an aviary or enclosure such as a wildlife

TABLE 34.16	**Squirrel kit orphans** **This is a rough guide; each individual is different**

Make sure all feeds are prepared fresh daily. **Give rehydration solution for first feed after admission.**

EQUIPMENT AND METHOD:

- 1-ml syringe and soft teat
- If eyes closed, toilet before and after syringe feeding by vibrating cotton wool (dipped in baby oil to protect the skin) over the genitals in a head-to-tail direction. Ensure all urine is removed as it will burn the skin if left
- Bloated abdomen can be fatal – try rehydration fluids for next couple of feeds
- Diarrhoea can be fatal – give rehydration fluids instead of milk formula for next 1 or 2 feeds, then give half water/half formula for the next feed, then back to just formula, if faeces go back to normal. If diarrhoea persists try giving probiotics

Weight	Notes	Feeding	
		Quantity	Intervals
Tiny bald squirrels up to 35 g 	Eyes closed	0.5–1 ml	2-hour intervals
35–60 g 	Fuzzy fur starting to show	1–3 ml	2-hour intervals
60–85 g 	Eyes beginning to open. Weaning can begin	3–5 ml	2-hour intervals
86–105 g 	Should be supplementing milk feeds with solid food (unshelled, unsalted nuts – avoid peanuts – rusks, biscuits, unsweetened breakfast cereals, rabbit mix and fruit)	5–7 ml	2.5–3-hour intervals
106–120 g 	Should be eating solid food quite well. Start reducing milk	7–9 ml	4 times daily

rescue centre can offer. If you only have one squirrel kit, it is important to transfer to a wildlife rescue centre sooner, as it will need the company of others as soon as possible.

OTHER SPECIES

Shrews, voles, rats and mice

These animals are frequently brought in for a number of reasons. We shall briefly touch upon some of the reasons for them coming in and what can be done.

They are best housed in a plastic vivarium of appropriate size. Bear in mind to have the tank tall enough so the rat or mouse cannot reach the lid to chew it. Cages with bars are not recommended, as these animals can squeeze into the tiniest of gaps to escape.

Orphaned. If disturbed in a shed or outbuilding, it is best to advise the member of the public to take the babies back, as often the mother will return and move the babies somewhere safer if we give them time.

TABLE 34.16	Squirrel kit orphans This is a rough guide; each individual is different—cont'd		
Weight	**Notes**	**Feeding**	
120–130 g	Watch the squirrel. If eating dry food well, cut milk feeds to twice daily	7–9 ml	2–3 times daily
130–140 g	Observe the squirrel and phase out milk feeds	10 ml maximum	1–2 times daily
After weaning	6–8 weeks old	Stop syringe feeding	Fruit tree sticks and branches with leaves in cage will be appreciated

New-born mice are extremely tiny (the size of kidney beans) and attempting to hand-rear them can be extremely difficult. Often the orphan will suffer, not develop normally and will ultimately die. It may be kinder to see if they are viable before attempting to hand-rear. Babies with a slight covering of fur are much easier to hand-rear and tend to have a far better survival rate.

Poisoning. By the time these animals have been found after consuming poison, it is usually too late for them. Euthanasia is often the kindest option.

Cat attacks. Cats will often capture and bring mice and rats in relatively unharmed. If wounded, they can be given a long-acting antibiotic by the vet and then released, or have wounds treated and given a few days of a palatable oral antibiotic on their food, or directly by mouth. Take care when cleaning them out as they do jump, and may take you by surprise by leaping from their tank.

Trapped in bird feeders. Very much like squirrels, these animals can squeeze into a bird feeder, but cannot get back after eating their fill. The best option is to bring the entire bird feeder in, anaesthetise the animal inside the feeder within an anaesthetic chamber and free them safely while they are asleep. These animals can then go for release once fully awake.

Otters

Otters are very dangerous animals and will bite fingers clean off if handled inappropriately. They are often admitted following territorial battles or after road accidents. Otter cubs are sometimes found after their holt becomes flooded. They are not at all easy to deal with, so it is recommended to seek help and advice from a wildlife hospital as soon as possible.

Reptiles and amphibians

Toads and frogs are frequently brought in after gardening inflicted injuries, such as accidental injury from spades and forks. Depending on the severity of the injury, they often make good recoveries once treated.

Other reptiles, such as snakes, can be brought in due to entanglement in garden netting, or being caught by a cat.

In the UK we only have three species of snake, the adder, the grass snake and the smooth snake. Snakes will not harm you, unless provoked, and even then only one of the species in the UK is venomous, the adder. Although adder venom is rarely fatal to people, the bite should still be taken seriously, and you should seek prompt medical attention.

Adder bites can sometimes be fatal to pets though, recent evidence suggests that the snakes' venom is more potent during March–April after the animals leave hibernation, so extra caution should be taken when walking dogs at this time of year.

The most common species of snake is the grass snake. The grass snake is non-venomous and the only thing you would feel if one did bite you is a small scratch. They will do everything in their power not to bite you, preferring to defend themselves in other ways. One of these ways is to emit a foul garlic-smelling fluid from their anal glands and this smell stays on your hands and clothing for multiple washes.

How do we tell them apart? One of the easiest ways is to look at the eye of the snake (without putting your face too close). Unlike the venomous adder, the smooth snake and grass snake have round pupils. The adder has a more 'feline'-shaped vertical pupil in the eye, a slit shape.

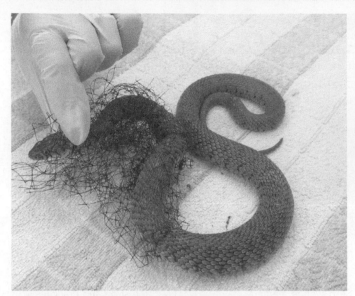

Fig. 34.12 A grass snake caught in netting

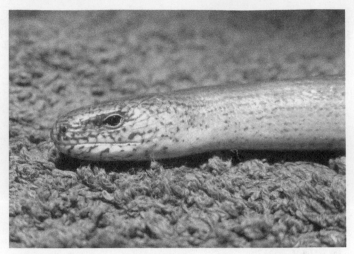

Fig. 34.14 A 'slow worm'

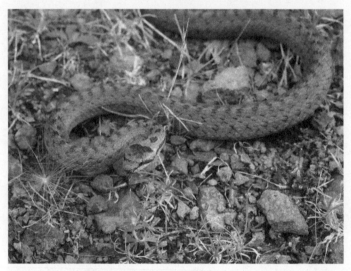

Fig. 34.13 A smooth snake (Photographer: Frank Vassen. To view the terms of the licence visit: https://creativecommons.org/licenses/by/2.0/legalcode. View the original material at: https://www.flickr.com/photos/42244964@N03/4908172087)

Grass snakes are grey/green in colour (Fig. 34.12) and have a yellow/cream/orange collar around the neck. The underside is usually white or pale yellow.

Adders have distinctive dark zigzag markings down the length of their back. They are generally white/pale grey/pale brown but (rarely) they can also be entirely black.

The final species of UK snake is the smooth snake. The smooth snake's appearance is similar to an adder, but without the distinct solid zigzag pattern on its back (Fig. 34.13). The smooth snake is named because it lacks the central ridges on its scales, unlike the adder and grass snake. Due to this difference in their scales they are not as fast moving as other snakes. They are often mistaken for 'slow worms', which are actually not worms or snakes at all – they are legless lizards (Fig. 34.14).

All species of UK snakes are protected under the Wildlife and Countryside Act 1981 and must not be deliberately harmed.

Birds

Birds are admitted as casualties for a variety of reasons, including:

- Road traffic accidents
- Cat and dog attacks – may cause septicaemia, wounds, puncture of the air sacs or feather damage
- Litter – may wind itself around legs and beaks and if the bird is not released it will die
- Oiled birds – from garage waste or polluted water. Oil is removed by washing with detergent but it takes time for the bird's natural oils to return
- Damage caused by fishing line and hooks and the lead weights attached to them – hooks may become fixed in the mouth or oesophagus while lead poisoning may present as loss of weight, lethargy, weakness, the head resting over the back or crooked, green faeces and a change in natural behaviour
- Nestlings (naked/blind or very few feathers) that have fallen from the nest
- Fledglings picked up in error by the public – birds can take anything up to a week to practice flying once they leave the nest, and while this is a very dangerous time for them, they must be left to do this and not brought in unnecessarily. Fledglings are much harder to rear than nestlings as they rarely gape for food and get a lot more stressed in captivity
- Birds that have flown into windows and are concussed.

Birds can also have parasites (Table 34.17). They are not routinely treated for parasites unless a problem is suspected. Good hygiene in the accommodation should prevent their spread and break life cycles. Gapeworm (*Syngamus trachea*) is a roundworm that may be seen in some birds; it causes coughing or sneezing sounds that can resemble breathing difficulties. It is treated by giving fenbendazole.

CAPTURE AND TRANSPORTATION

Any wild adult bird that is easily caught has something wrong with it. Sometimes these casualties have an injury but are still very active, e.g. a duck with an injured leg can still fly and a pigeon with an injured wing can run.

TABLE 34.17	Ectoparasites found on the bird			
Parasite	Appearance	Treatment	Notes
Ticks	Can be white, grey, bluish grey	Remove with tick hook or tick lasso by grasping base of tick near host's skin and twist off	Becoming more common and in greater numbers on birds. Ticks can be life threatening to birds, and they must receive antibiotics after tick removal
Lice/mites	Parasites easily seen on feathers, particularly around the neck	Mite spray for birds	Parasite that chews feathers and skin debris. Plumage looks as if it has been cut
Flat flies	Like a large housefly, but flat for moving under feathers, with feet that grip on to and run along the bird's plumage	Can be removed by hand, but difficult to kill – should be crushed. Use mite spray if the host is infested, but most flat flies leave the body when disturbed	Blood-sucking parasite. Does not bite humans, though we still all hate them!

On approach the bird will either freeze, run or, if cornered, defend itself. Before attempting to catch any bird in the wild, the situation should be carefully assessed. Observe the way that the bird is moving and behaving and work out a plan for its capture. The approach, capture and confinement should be carried out swiftly and firmly.

Capture of most birds is best achieved with a towel, light blanket, coat, car rug, etc. Do not chase the casualty around, as the shock could be fatal. It is much better to lure the bird into a corner, shed or area where there is no escape. Throw the towel over the bird and then gently but firmly scoop it up and place it into a cardboard box or carrier for transportation. Do not remove the towel at this stage as it almost always results in the casualty escaping. If a box or carrying container is not available then the bird should remain loosely but safely contained in its wrap.

Larger more aggressive birds, e.g. birds of prey, can be captured in the same way, but extra care must be taken because talons and beaks are likely to be used as weapons. Most birds, once confined with their heads covered, will not struggle but the rescuer should always be prepared for the unexpected.

Water birds will almost certainly make for the water as their means of escape so rescuers must place themselves between the water and the bird before moving in for the capture. When catching swans and geese it is important to restrain the wings.

The birds use their wings for protection and can be extremely strong. Restrain with one hand around the neck under the head and the other arm enclosing the wings and body. The old saying that a swan can break your arm is untrue but they are very strong birds even so. They are restrained easily by placing them into a large towel or blanket wrapped firmly around them, leaving their head and neck exposed, for transportation safely.

Never use a transparent container for wild bird casualties. If a solid-sided container is not available then cover the basket. The bird will become distressed and may injure itself if it can see out but cannot escape. The container should be lined with newspaper and a towel or a blanket for larger casualties. The bedding provides warmth and absorbency, a place to hide and something to grip on to during transportation.

If using a cardboard box it must be made secure to prevent the casualty from escaping during transportation. Containers with grill-type doors must be covered to keep the casualty in

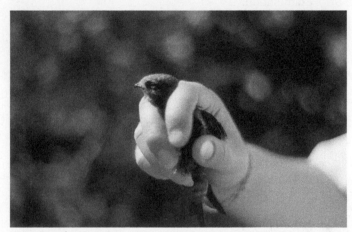

Fig. 34.15 The correct way to restrain a small bird, in this case a young swift

the dark and prevent birds from pushing their beaks through the holes in their attempt to free themselves.

EXAMINATION

Observe the bird before examination. A great deal can be learned by watching the way the bird is moving, e.g. whether it is lame, has any deformities, or wings hanging or sticking up at an odd angle, how it is breathing, the state of its plumage and general behaviour. These are important observations that can be followed up during the examination, and mean less time handling a distressed, struggling patient.

Restraint for examination can be difficult and depends on the size of the bird:

- When restraining small birds, be aware that applying too much pressure to the body can cause asphyxia. The correct method is to create a 'net' with the fingers of your hand to control the wings and allow the head to poke out between the second and third fingers (Fig. 34.15). The underside of the bird and its legs can be examined by turning it over and the wings can be gently extended on each side.
- Some birds, such as members of the crow family and gulls, have strong beaks. For examination, they may

need to have their beaks held by another person to prevent pecking, taking care not to cover the nares or nostrils. Birds rarely inflict more than a sharp pinch, which can be tolerated. Larger water birds such as heron, gannets and gulls, however, can inflict terrible injuries to the eyes and face, so protective goggles are recommended when handling these species. Never tape or put a band around the beak, as in some species (such as gannets) this can cause death from asphyxia. One person should hold the bird while another carries out the examination. Have your assistant never let go of the beak during examination in the case of herons or other long-beaked birds, such as cormorants and gannets. Birds of prey are more likely to strike out with their talons, which can be kept under control by holding the legs between the first two fingers of one hand. If the head is covered the bird is more likely to remain calm. Another person should then make the examination.

- Ducks and game birds are very strong and should also be held by two hands restraining the wings. Swans are best examined on the floor with one person restraining the bird while the other carries out the examination.

A general examination should include checking the following:

- Feet and legs – fractures, wounds, fly eggs and maggots, lesions
- Wings – hanging down or sticking up
- Beak – fractures, splits, top and bottom do not meet or align correctly
- Mouth – general mucous membrane colour, fly eggs, canker (see later in this chapter), smelly breath
- Nares/nostrils – discharge, blockage
- Eyes – discharge, swelling, dilated pupils, unequal pupils, prolapse, haemorrhage
- Crop – torn, impacted
- Keel – sharp keel bone indicates thin bird
- Cloaca – dirty, blocked, fly eggs and maggots, prolapse
- Plumage – should be sleek with no ruffled feathers. Chewed or cut appearance indicates feather mites, abnormal white feathers on a black bird suggest a calcium deficiency
- Respiration – gasping or panting, gurgling, laboured
- Parasites (see Table 34.17)
- Skin – wounds, fly eggs or maggots, feather loss
- Dehydration.

Patient records should include:

- Species (if known, if not then narrow it down to insect eater/bird of prey/seed eater if possible)
- Date
- Details of condition
- Name, address and telephone number of finder
- Details of the exact spot where the casualty was found – this is essential because when the bird recovers it should be returned to the area from where it came
- Any other useful information, e.g. it was lying on its back struggling to stand up. This is important because it may lead to a diagnosis, reducing the need for examination.

Initial treatment for any bird admission:

- Warmth (if needed)
- Darkness
- Quiet

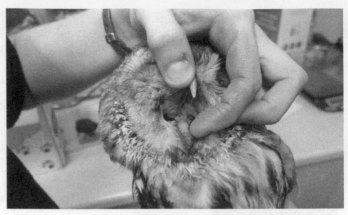

Fig. 34.16 A tawny owl exhibiting symptoms of canker

- Oral rehydration fluids by gavage. There is no need to give routine parasite treatment unless parasites are obvious. Routine vitamin injections are also unnecessary but long-term patients may benefit from supplements to compensate for the lack of a natural diet.
- These birds are wild and must be returned to their natural habitats with as little interference as possible.

COMMON ILLNESSES, INJURIES AND DISEASES IN BIRDS

Trichomoniasis (frounce, trick or canker)

This is a protozoan infection from *Trichomonas gallinae* affecting the throat and mouth. This protozoa causes yellow chalky lesions in the mouth and throat of the bird, thickened saliva and swellings around the eyes. It is seen most commonly in pigeons and doves, but also in birds of prey, finches and corvids. Birds will usually be in a poor condition and emaciated.

Treatment for the protozoan is cardinazone or ronidazole. In your vet practices you can initiate treatment with oral metronidazole. To assess if a canker patient is treatable, you can see if you can get a tube down the bird's throat (Fig. 34.16). If this is not possible it means you cannot treat or even feed the bird.

Spread of this condition is through direct contact, so keep the bird quarantined and use a high level of hygiene with all equipment.

Paramyxovirus

This is a highly contagious viral condition that is seen in feral pigeons. It is also known as Newcastle disease (Fig. 34.17). Symptoms include:

- Watery, green diarrhoea
- Torticollis ('wry neck')
- Tremors
- Paralysis
- Polydipsia.

This disease is notifiable, and euthanasia is recommended. Recovery usually results in later recurrence of the disease, with the virus spreading to other birds.

Avian botulism

This is caused by the bacteria *Clostridium botulinum* and is usually observed in summer when temperatures increase above 23°C and the bacteria thrives. It is usually seen in water

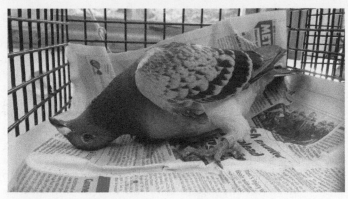

Fig. 34.17 Paramyxovirus in a feral pigeon

birds such as gulls and swans. The bacteria is picked up while the bird is foraging in the silt and mud. Symptoms include:

- Diarrhoea and vomiting
- Ataxia
- Dyspnoea.

Treatment is to withdraw food and water for up to 3 days. The bird is put on a drip, using the medial tarsal vein, and broad-spectrum antibiotics and vitamin B_{12} are administered. Once food is reintroduced after a couple of days, the bird should eat readily. Survival rates with this protocol are high.

Fractures

Fractures can be observed in birds, as in other animals, and are usually to the wing, leg or beak. Birds show little obvious signs of pain and often continue to attempt to fly and walk with fractured limbs. Wing, coracoid and clavicle fractures are common and are often the result of a road traffic accident or flying into windows. The obvious sign is the wing being held drooped against the body lower than the opposite wing, or in the case of the coracoid or clavicle the wing may be held higher and will not flap in the same position as the normal wing. X-rays are advised to assess if the fracture is treatable.

Coracoid and clavicle fractures can sometimes heal with rest, but without specialist surgery the bird only has a slim chance of properly flying again, so euthanasia must be considered for birds that rely upon perfect flight, such as birds of prey.

Fractured wings can be immobilised and splinted by placing them against the body of the bird and bandaging in a figure of eight across the sternum. This may initially affect the bird's balance but it soon learns to accommodate the bandage. Fractures in the wings of birds of prey and migratory birds must seriously be considered candidates for euthanasia, as they will rarely regain full function to live a completely normal life in the wild without specialist surgery or treatment.

The lower legs can be splinted and providing the bird has feeling in its toes, these usually heal very quickly in 1–2 weeks.

Beak repairs can be undertaken using epoxy resin or external fixation. It is important to mention that in many species, if the beak is not perfectly aligned, it will not wear down, and will continue to grow, eventually resulting in an inability to feed – and death. You must be totally sure the beak is aligned before considering release.

Fishing line and hook injuries

Sadly, these are commonplace with water birds. Many birds forage on the riverbed looking for vegetable matter and accidentally ingest hooks or become entangled in fishing lines. The nature of the hook and the soft tissue of the throat lead to penetration of the oesophagus with the hook embedding into the soft tissue, where the hook can remain, especially if the hook is barbed. If the line is still attached this may also be ingested resulting in blockage of the oesophagus, crop or intestine. The hooks can also become embedded in the feet or wings, where removal is easier.

X-ray helps locate the hook for removal. This may be easy if the hook is in the mouth.

Surgery may be required if the hook is located further down the tract. The end of the hook will need to be cut away before the hook is pulled out.

If a bird arrives with line hanging from its beak, put tape around the neck to prevent it travelling further down the throat, as if the bird swallows everything, removal is far more difficult.

Treat with antibiotics to prevent secondary infection developing after removal.

Calcium deficiency

This is seen every year in many species, most commonly in Collared Doves and juvenile crows. Crows will present with white scruffy feathers, which break very easily. They require up to 2 years in an aviary to regrow their feathers. This can be a problem, due to the risk of imprinting or habituating it to a life in captivity. However, crows can live for 10–30 years in the wild, so it is something that can be considered for them, providing they are kept in an aviary with minimal human interference.

Collared Doves are not native to the UK, and need more sunlight than Britain offers. The juveniles cannot metabolise the vitamin D from the sun and calcium in their diets, and will present with the following signs:

- Bowed legs and inability to stand up
- Feathers fully grown, but still 'in pin'
- Weakness, lethargy and often dyspnoea.

In most cases, calcium supplementation administered for a week and then a good-quality diet will allow them to improve quickly and improve the chances of release.

Birds are unable to preen ticks off from around their heads and these ticks transmit deadly bacteria, causing the bird to deteriorate and die. Simply removing the ticks and giving the bird a broad-spectrum antibiotic usually brings fast recoveries.

HOUSING

Each bird should be housed according to its needs, its natural behaviour and its habitat:

- Birds must have sufficient room to stretch their wings and be able to preen.
- Perching birds need the correct size of perch, e.g. a perch for a sparrow could be a twig while a buzzard needs a small branch. Incorrect perch size or lack of a perch may result in difficulties in perching and infections such as bumble foot, which occurs when the claws pierce the underside of the foot. Perch positioning is also important to make best use of the space and to encourage exercise as the bird hops or flies between them.
- Place natural foliage in a cage to provide places to hide. Do not place the cage close to domestic animals or in noisy areas. Some bird species are more susceptible to stress than others and may throw themselves around

when first introduced to a hospital cage. This may be helped by placing a towel over the front.

- Many birds will make for the door as soon as it is opened, in an attempt to escape.
- Sometimes after handling and replacing in the cage a bird may remain flat on the bottom or on its back, 'playing dead'. This is especially common in birds of prey and may take you by surprise when you open the cage to check. Owls, particularly chicks, often sleep lying down.

Heat – the need for heat should be carefully considered. If heat is provided the bird must be weaned off it before release. These are wild birds that naturally live out in cold, wet and windy weather. Heat boxes, brooders, incubators and heat lamps can be regulated and are the best option, but the bird is unable to get away from the heat source so careful monitoring is needed.

FEEDING

The period of major activity, including feeding, in the day varies with the species of bird. Some are diurnal, others nocturnal and a few are crepuscular, i.e. active mainly at dawn and dusk. There will be some patients that are on a special feeding regimen and will not be keeping to their natural hours of activity. Some wild birds may refuse to eat because they are captive.

One of the many problems is knowing what to feed and this is made easier by correct identification of the species. This will then allow you to find out their natural food and if necessary find an acceptable substitute (see Table 34.1).

The shape of a bird's beak will give an idea as to the diet of the bird even if you are unable to identify the species. A robin's beak is small and thin for eating insects; finches and sparrows have shorter, stubbier beaks for cracking seeds; a blackbird's beak is longer for probing soil for earthworms. Every veterinary practice would benefit from a basic bird identification book – those that contain photographs rather than drawings or paintings will make identification much easier.

Casualties that are confined for more than a few days should receive as close to their wild diet as possible, and this is rarely achieved in the average veterinary surgery, thought must be taken whether transfer to a wildlife hospital would be more suitable.

It should also be noted that adult pigeons and doves will rarely eat for themselves when in captivity, especially in a noisy veterinary surgery. These birds may have to be crop fed, and this will be described later in the chapter in the advice for baby pigeons and doves.

CLEANING

Accommodation should be cleaned thoroughly once a day. Handling can be reduced by having clean accommodation ready for the bird to be moved into. Any other tasks such as feeding or treatment should be carried out at the same time to avoid unnecessary distress caused by repeated disturbance. Use a towel to move birds from cage to cage. Food and water containers should not be placed near to or under perches as they will become soiled with faeces.

ORPHANED BIRDS

Orphan birds most commonly result from the death of the parent birds. In other cases, they are not so much orphaned as 'rescued' from their parents in error by well-meaning members of the public. Other reasons include:

- The nest may have been exposed by hedge trimming or tree felling. If it is possible to find a suitable new site for the nest in a neighbouring tree, it is worth a try as the parents may continue to care for their young. If the nest is destroyed, a makeshift nest can be fashioned from a box and can be hung from the tree (out of the reach of cats). Monitor from a distance to see that the parent bird returns. Baby birds are fed pretty constantly throughout daylight hours, so have the home owner observe for a few hours (from a distance) after attempting this to make sure the parents return. If they do not, then the birds must be admitted. It is worth gently advising the member of public who brings these birds in that the felling of trees with nesting birds is only legally permissible between November and January, and violations can result in fines for disturbing nests: £1000 per nest and an additional £1000 per bird or egg. The maximum penalty that can be imposed is a fine up to £5000 and/ or 6 months imprisonment.
- Nests may be built in unused farm machinery or cars, which are then put into use and the nestlings are discovered. In these cases a makeshift nest can be made using a box nearby (as described above) and then have the homeowners observe for a few hours, from a distance, to make sure the parents continue to feed the chicks. If they do not, then the birds must be admitted.
- Ducklings may become separated from their mother – often a single duckling is lost or left behind. Ducks lay their eggs away from water, and then 'walk' the ducklings to the water once they hatch. Often this means crossing busy roads in the process. It is sometimes possible to have people walk ahead and beside her as she does this, preventing cars from running her over as she leads them to water. If one is left behind, and the mother has gone, then this does need to be admitted.
- Birds may have been caught in a storm and are grounded, wet and cold. Even though the parent may still be present, the bird needs more help than the parent can offer.

The most common reason for a young bird being admitted is the fledgling caught by a cat. Up to 275 million animals and birds are caught by domestic cats every year, and only a small percentage of these end up being treated. All birds caught by a cat MUST have antibiotics before release, even if they appear unharmed. The bacteria on a cat's teeth, *Pasteurella multocida*, kills the bird within hours, even with a tiny puncture wound that may not have been noticed. The vet can administer a long-acting antibiotic injection and the bird can be returned to the garden, if the nest site is known. Always advise that the home owner keep the cat in for a few days to ensure that the fledgling gets time to gain strength to fly. If the home owner is unwilling to do this, then the bird should be admitted.

There are two types of fledgling:

- **Altricial** – fledglings remain in the nest and are fed by one or both parents. They are blind, deaf and have few or no feathers or down when they hatch. Examples are blackbirds, thrushes, sparrows, finches, robins, starlings, crows, jackdaws, jays, swallows, swifts, house martins, tits, pigeons, doves, woodpeckers, owls and birds of prey

- **Precocial** – birds that hatch as active chicks, most of which feed themselves. Examples are ducklings, swans, geese and pheasants. Some, e.g. moorhens, are fed by the parents for the first few days, before feeding themselves.

Identification of the species of a baby bird is difficult because there are so many species and the juvenile plumage (if they have any) is different from that of the adult. A good bird book with photographs of both adult and juvenile plumage is essential. Veterinary practices are able to provide initial care and feeding, but then it is usually advisable to pass the fledgling on to a wildlife centre, where it can go with others and will be able to have access to larger aviaries once almost ready for release.

Housing

Accommodation is dependent on the size of the bird. Small garden birds can be placed in old bird cages or the newer design pod carriers for small mammals. For larger species such as swans use a dog kennel.

- Place newspaper in the cage, and perches if it is a perching bird. Perching birds that have been hand-reared in a cage without a perch will develop deformed toes and flat feet as a result.
- Always ensure the cage is covered, to reduce stress.
- For woodpeckers in captivity, place a log vertically in the cage so the bird can hang onto it.
- For swifts, allow them to hang, as they will not perch; place a towel hung over the side of the accommodation and allow them to climb up onto it.

Garden birds. Nestlings must be kept warm until they have feathers and should be provided with an incubator, heat lamp or by placing a Snuggle Pad under the 'nest'. Create a 'nest' in the form of a plastic feeding bowl or similar vessel, lined with kitchen paper. This provides a familiar, temporary home that allows the fledglings to behave normally and it is easy to clean.

Once the bird becomes more active and attempts to leave the nest, low perches can be arranged around the nest pot and a little foliage provided. As the feathers develop the heat can be gradually reduced until it is only provided at night and then turned off completely. As the bird grows, move it to a bird cage lined with paper, which gives more room to move around. The bird will spend more time out of the nest pot and food can be introduced into the cage so that the bird can start to feed itself. Higher perches and more foliage create a natural environment. Once the bird's tail feathers have grown and it is feeding itself, it is time to move it to an aviary for flight practice and muscle building prior to release.

Feeding

There are a variety of diets and ways of administering the food to the fledgling, which depend on the species (see Table 34.1).

Suggested recipe for feeding orphaned birds:
- Baby bird mix: Puppy or kitten food – 1 cup
- Bogena Universal Insect Food (or Sluis) – 1 cup
- Tropican Rearing Mix (or Kaytee Exact) – 1 cup
- Avipro avian probiotic powder – 1 teaspoon
- Powdered Digestive Enzyme – 1 pinch (Pancrex or Probi-zyme)
- Water to mix.

All the ingredients should be mixed well to ensure that there are no lumps, as little birds may choke. The water should be

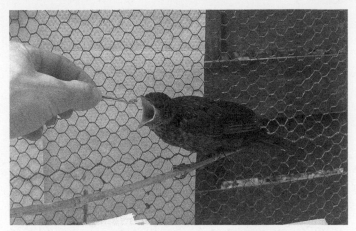

Fig. 34.18 Blackbird fledgling being fed using tweezers

added until the mixture is sloppy – not dripping wet and not too dry. It will dry out over time, so more water may need to be added. Baby bird mix needs to be made up in batches as needed and stored in the refrigerator, it will keep for 24 hours. Small amounts must be taken out prior to feeding, and food should be offered at room temperature.

If you are unable to make this diet, some examples of temporary diets to use in cases of emergency admissions are listed in Table 34.1 at the beginning of the chapter.

Baby birds will not feed if they are cold – if the bird does not open its mouth or gape to begin with, make sure it is warm.

There are a few ways in which to encourage a fledgling to gape:
- By touching the beak
- Tapping the nest pot
- Passing your hand over the nest, which mimics the parent returning to the nest
- Whistling may have heads popping up with the beaks open. The whistle imitates bird song and, although it sounds strange, it really does work.

Once the bird is gaping, small amounts of food can be placed at the back of the mouth using tweezers or a coffee stirrer. Once the fledgling gets used to the food and technique, the bird should readily take food off the tweezers and swallow each time it is offered (Fig. 34.18).

Sometimes new arrivals and some more difficult cases have to be fed by forcibly opening the beak. This must be done by carefully sliding your nail into the gap at the side of the beak and carefully prising it open – the tip of the beak should never be forced open. Once food has been placed in the mouth, the beak often opens ready to receive more – sometimes it takes a bit longer. Nestlings should be fed at least every 30 minutes from dawn until dusk. In the wild they wake up at first light and go to roost at dusk and these times should be adhered to unless the bird is very sick.

Once the birds become more active and are spending more time out of the nest pot, solid food can be introduced. A small flat container of whatever they are used to should be placed in the cage with a shallow container of water. At this time live food can be offered to insect eaters, such as mealworms or maggots. Finch mix can be offered to seed eaters. Hand feeding can then be reduced as the fledglings start to feed themselves.

Food and water containers should be an appropriate size so the birds can drink but not drown and can reach the food easily.

Place the food and water containers in an area that is easily accessible but not on one of the main 'runways', as it will be walked through or flapped in, resulting in the cage and the bird's plumage become soiled.

When first taken into captivity older fledglings are more reluctant to tolerate being hand-fed and they will become distressed and throw themselves around the cage. Restraining the bird gently and offering it food on tweezers may work, as older fledglings will often peck at whatever comes near to them. As it tastes the food it may open its beak and allow itself to be fed. If not, then one half of the cage should be covered to provide a place to hide, the food and water should be placed in this half and the fledgling should be left in peace. It may respond to hand feeding later or may have started to feed itself. The survival rate of fledglings is sadly much lower than nestlings as a result. If the bird will not feed, then specialist help must be obtained quickly from a wildlife hospital.

OTHER SPECIES

Baby pigeons and doves

If squeaking, you can defrost (but do not cook) some frozen peas and give a few by pushing them gently into the mouth every 2–3 hours. Only about 3 or 4 peas at a time and stop if the bird is not squeaking for more or the crop (the fleshy bag under the bird's beak) looks or feels full.

Crop tube feeding. If you are confident enough to try crop feeding them (the correct method of feeding) this is administered using an adapted suitably sized syringe. The food is sucked up into the syringe and must be pushed out again without air bubbles or lumps. Attach a suitable length of a cut section of drip tubing to the end of the syringe. This makes a simple but essential tool for delivering a measured amount of food when crop feeding baby pigeons and doves.

- The correct crop feeding formula for baby pigeons and doves is Kaytee exact or Tropican, but natural flavour complan (for humans) can be used as a very temporary crop feed.
- It lasts for 24 hours once made up, so try to only make up what you need, as you need it. When making it up, be aware that it will thicken a bit after it is made, so make it up and then check the consistency before feeding, adding more pre-boiled water if necessary.
- Smaller babies have 4 parts pre-boiled warm water and 1 part formula (milk consistency).
- Older youngsters have 3 parts pre-boiled warm water and 1 part formula (double cream consistency).
- Feed 1–15 ml 4–6 times a day, depending on the size of the bird.
- Feed the formula warm, but not hot. Check the temperature on your wrist before feeding.
- Tube feeding should be done by two people, as someone will need to keep the bird still for you to be able to correctly place the tube.

Your assistant can then hold the bird securely (allowing its feet to rest on a table top) while you support the head. Open the beak and pass the tube carefully over the tongue and down into the crop. Press the syringe plunger slowly until it is empty, and then withdraw the tube carefully. If any food is seen in the mouth during this procedure, it means the tube is

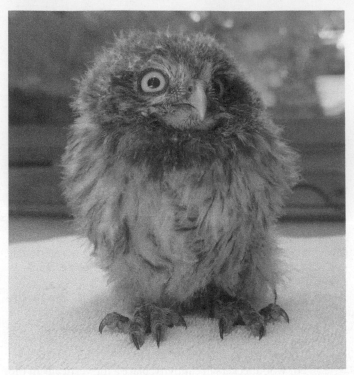

Fig. 34.19 Little owl juvenile

incorrectly positioned. Stop, remove the tube and check the airway is clear before trying again.

Adult pigeons and doves may also need this method of feeding and a rough guideline of amounts to feed is:
- Adult dove – 20 ml
- Adult feral pigeon – 25 ml
- Wood pigeon – 30 ml

Feed 3 times a day if the bird is a good weight, 4 times a day if the bird is underweight, sick or injured.

The crop-feeding technique is not as easy as it sounds, and it may be better to visit your local wildlife hospital to gain hands-on experience before attempting it.

Owls and birds of prey

Housing. Chicks of these species hatch covered in down (Fig. 34.19) and need supplementary heating in the form of a heat lamp or brooder.

The cage should be lined with layers of newspaper and a towel for warmth and should contain a low perch of the correct size for their feet. A mixing or pudding bowl of the appropriate size, lined with warm material, will suit a very young bird that would have naturally come from a nest. Foliage can be used to create hiding places. As the youngster grows, reduce the heat and raise the perches. Birds that are neither newly nor recently hatched will not need supplementary heating unless debilitated.

Feeding. Most birds of prey are fed on mice and day-old chicks. This food should be offered in small pieces using tweezers. When cutting up the chick into pieces to feed the bird, make sure to discard the beak and feet. In cases where a little persuasion is needed, the beak should be touched with the food, or it should be offered from above. If neither method works, then the mouth will have to be opened manually, which can be achieved by carefully prising open the beak at each side.

Once it is open, the food is gently placed at the back of the mouth and the bird should then swallow. This may have to be repeated a few times until the bird starts to grab the food from the tweezers.

Small meals are offered every 2–3 hours. Birds of prey will regurgitate a pellet that contains the indigestible fur, feathers and bone (see also Chapter 33). As the bird grows it should be offered larger pieces of food, which it will stand on and tear with its beak and talons. Eventually it should be given whole food. These birds must be taken to a rescue centre for rehabilitation as soon as possible, as they are easy to imprint on humans and need correct diets, which veterinary surgeries can rarely provide.

Swallows, swifts and house martins

These species of bird are aerial feeders and spend a great portion of their lives in flight. They will not feed themselves from a dish of food and, although swallows and house martins may take advantage of a perch to sit on by the time the hand-rearing process is almost finished, swifts will not. A swift should be provided with something to hang on to; a piece of material such as a tea-towel is ideal so it can grip on to it and climb.

These species are specialist feeders, and it is recommended to only give fluid by dripping tiny drops of water or rehydration solution onto side of beak or mouth. They must be taken to a wildlife hospital soon as possible, as they need an extremely specialised diet, and will die without it.

Precocial fledglings, e.g. swans, ducks, geese, game birds, coots and moorhens

Housing. When these birds first hatch they should be given a heat source to replace their mother. The best kind is a heat lamp or brooder, as these chicks are active and need space to run around and a warm place to huddle together. These chicks will benefit from being provided a substitute 'mum', which could be a soft toy or a stringy mop head – it is unnatural for them to be alone; a substitute 'mum' might make the difference between surviving or not. For single youngsters it is also helpful to provide them with a small mirror, until you are able to transfer them to a wildlife hospital where they can go with others.

At one end of the cage, suspend a heat lamp over warm bedding such as a towel. At the other end place the food and water containers. At this end there should be several layers of newspaper that can be removed one by one to keep the cage clean.

This type of young bird is more susceptible to stress and the accommodation should be partially covered to provide an area in which to hide. Once weaned off the heat lamp, the youngsters can be transferred to a run on grass. Provide a box to hide in. They must be brought inside at night and may need gentle heat for the first few nights or if the temperature drops too low.

Feeding. Some of these babies, e.g. moorhens and pheasants, may need to be fed by hand initially. Most will feed themselves once they have settled in and are left in peace. Food and water should be available from dawn until dusk.

Euthanasia

For any wildlife casualty too severely injured, too sick to recover or too badly imprinted to be able to sustain itself or survive in the wild, euthanasia must be considered. Very often the decision is made to keep the animal alive because it is easier for the human being, although it may be severely disabled or unable to behave normally, e.g. a bird that will never fly. The length of time the casualty is likely to be in captivity and receiving treatment must also be considered, because it will cause immense stress and may result in a certain amount of humanisation, i.e. becoming used to humans, which may be dangerous in the wild.

When treating native wildlife it is very important to ask ourselves whether that animal has a real chance to fully function back in the wild.

Think about that animal's natural behaviour in the wild and think if the injury would hinder that life. Think about how they hunt or search for food, how they need to escape from predators, how they groom themselves, how they possibly need to hold food to eat it, and how they need to travel. A great way of finding this information is on the Internet or an encyclopaedia. Read about the animal's natural lifestyle and it will be much easier to make a decision on its possible release. Again if you are in any doubt, please do call a wildlife centre for advice. Many animals can surprise you with their recoveries if given the right care and treatment, but the prime objective must *always* be to return an animal to the wild. To do this the animal must be released with a chance of survival equivalent to that of other wild animals of the same species.

The alternatives are permanent captivity, which is often unacceptable for the animal due to welfare reasons, or euthanasia. Permanent captivity for disabled wild animals remains a very controversial topic. Birds need to fly, mammals need to roam and to breed. Even the humble hedgehog will roam a massive distance in the wild, up to 70 acres – something that can rarely be provided in the average home garden environment. We must therefore think seriously about the welfare aspects of keeping wild animals captive – they will suffer from huge amounts of stress, be unable to breed or live normal lives, and euthanasia can often be the much kinder option.

The positive aspect of wildlife care

All of us began our careers working with animals to make a difference. Working with wildlife can be even more rewarding; there is no owner to thank you, but the reward you get is to see the animal you have saved go free to live its days in the wild, as it should do (Fig. 34.20).

There are no words to describe the feeling you will get when an animal you have nursed back to health is released. You will be really truly making a difference, really using all the skills you were taught to the utmost to help these creatures go back to the wild.

Do think about volunteering at your local wildlife centre if you enjoy this field of work!

Relevant legislation

The **Wildlife and Countryside Act 1981 (WCA)** is the principal source of information for anyone working in wildlife rescue and rehabilitation. The complete document is available from the Stationery Office, or from their website at www.tso.co.uk.

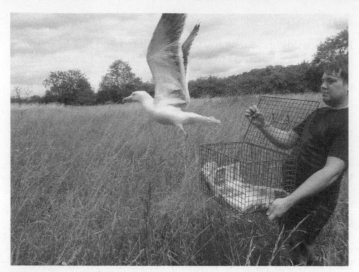

Fig. 34.20 Release

The Act is extensive but the main points in respect to the animals discussed in this chapter are as follows:

- A species that has protection under the Act can only be taken from the wild in order to give it the necessary care it needs to be able to return it to the wild or for humane destruction where appropriate. These creatures should be cared for in a way that ensures their return to the wild, should not be tamed and should be housed appropriately.
- Mammals that do not have protection under the WCA have provision to protect them against cruelty under the **Wild Mammals (Protection) Act 1996**, e.g. it is an offence to 'cruelly kick, beat, impale, burn, drown or crush any wild mammal'.
- Grey squirrels, Canada geese and muntjac deer are non-indigenous species and it is an offence under the WCA to keep or release these species back into the wild or to allow them to escape, although it is permitted to take it

from the wild and euthanise it if it is sick or injured. Many wildlife hospitals have licences for these species that do allow for their treatment and release, though, so it is worth contacting them first to find out.

- All species of bat and their roosts are protected.
- **The Protection of Badgers Act 1992** protects badgers and their setts.
- **The Deer Act 1991** details how and when deer maybe taken from the wild.
- Protection of birds – 'a person cannot kill, injure or take any wild bird, take, damage or destroy the nest of any wild bird that contains chicks or eggs or is being built, or take or destroy any egg of any wild bird'. There are exceptions where birds have no protection or may be taken outside the close season, or may be taken by authorised persons:
  - Game birds have no protection under this Act apart from during the close season, but there are rules governing the way they may be killed or taken. The hunting season for pheasant – 1 October to 1 February; Canada goose and mallard duck – 1 September to 20 February; moorhen – 1 September to 31 January.
  - Part of the Wildlife and Countryside Act 1981 used to include Schedule 2 Part II, which listed 13 'pest' species, e.g. magpie, jay, feral pigeon, that were allowed to be killed or taken by authorised persons at any time. In 1993 this part of the act was removed and was replaced by general licenses allowing the taking of certain 'pest' species by authorised persons. These licenses were designed to protect other wild birds and agricultural interests from damage or pollution and to protect the air, safety and public health. Full details of these licenses and what they refer to can be obtained from the DEFRA website, www.defra.gov.uk/wildlife-country. Licenses are issued by DEFRA annually in England and similar ones can be obtained for Scotland and Wales.

BIBLIOGRAPHY

Best, R., Cooper, J.E., Mullineaux, E. (Eds.), 2003. BSAVA Manual of Wildlife Casualties. British Small Animal Veterinary Association, Gloucester.

Bedford, S., 2013. A Beginner's Guide to Rearing Wild Birds, third ed. CreateSpace Independent Publishing Platform.

Cooper, J.E., Ely, J.T., 1979. First Aid Care of Wild Birds. David & Charles, Newton Abbot.

RECOMMENDED READING

Bedford, S., 2013. A Beginner's Guide to Rearing Wild Birds, third ed. CreateSpace Independent Publishing Platform.
This book covers everything about rearing genuinely orphaned wild birds and giving them that second chance to be wild.

Best, R., Cooper, J.E., Mullineaux, E. (Eds.), 2003. BSAVA Manual of Wildlife Casualties. British Small Animal Veterinary Association, Gloucester.
Provides essential information for dealing with all the injured wildlife that may be presented in the practice. It is written mainly for veterinary surgeons

and therefore focuses on diagnosis and treatment, but also covers care during recovery.

Stocker, L., 2005. Practical Wildlife Care, second ed. Wiley-Blackwell, Oxford.
Guidance on handling, first aid, feeding, treating and releasing wildlife.

Normal Values

(FROM VARIOUS SOURCES)

Dog, cat and horse

TABLE A.1	Normal clinical parameters		
Parameter	**Dog**	**Cat**	**Horse**
Body temperature (°C)	38.3–38.7	38.0–38.5	38.0–38.2
Pulse rate (beats/min)	60–180	110–180	32–44
Respiratory rate (breaths/min)	10–30	20–30	8–12

TABLE A.2	Normal haematological values		
Parameter	**Dog**	**Cat**	**Horse**
Total red blood cell count ($\times 10^{12}$/l)	5.5–8.5	5.0–10.0	7.0
Total white blood cell count ($\times 10^{9}$/l)	6–17	5.5–19.5	8–11
Differential white cell count (%)			
Neutrophils	65–70	45–75	50–60
Eosinophils	2–5	4–12	2–5
Basophils	<1	<1	<1
Monocytes	5	0–4	5–6
Lymphocytes	20–25	20–25	30–40
Thrombocyte count ($\times 10^{9}$/l)	200–500	200–600	113–299
Packed cell volume (%)	37–55	24–45	42
Haemoglobin (g/dl)	12–18	8–15	12.5
Blood pH	7.35–7.45	7.35–7.45	7.35–7.43
Clotting time (min)	2.5	2.5	11.5

TABLE A.3	Normal urine values		
Parameter	**Dog**	**Cat**	**Horse**
pH	5.2–6.8	6.0–7.0	7.5–8.5
Specific gravity	1.015–1.045	1.020–1.040	1.008–1.040
Daily volume (ml/kg body weight)	20–100	10–12	20–50

TABLE A.4	Normal values for blood biochemistry			
Parameter		Dog	Cat	Horse
Total serum protein (g/l)		50–78	60–82	55–71
Serum albumin (g/l)		22–35	25–39	28–36
Cholesterol (mmol/l)		2.7–9.5	1.5–6.0	2.1–3.6
Total bilirubin (μmol/l)		0–6.8	0–6.8	11–48
Calcium (mmol/l)		2.20–2.90	2.20–2.90	2.7–3.2
Blood urea nitrogen (mmol/l)		3.0–9.0	5.0–10.0	4.0–8.0
Creatinine (μmol/l)		Up to 120	Up to 180	86–204
Fasting plasma glucose (mmol/l)		3.5–5.5	3.5–6.5	3.6–6.4

Small mammals

TABLE A.5	Normal clinical parameters for small mammals							
Parameter	Rabbit	Guinea pig	Ferret	Gerbil	Mouse	Rat	Hamster
Weight (g)							
Male	Varies according to breed	900–1200	1000–2000	46–131	20–40	267–500	87–130
Female	Varies according to breed	700–900	600–1000	50–55	22–63	225–325	95–130
Life span	7 years (average)	5–6 years	5–11 years	24–39 mo	12–36 mo	26–40 mo	18–36 mo
Body temperature (°C)	37–39.4	37.2–39.5	37.8–40	38.2	37.1	37.7	37.6
Pulse rate (beats/min)	198–330	240–310	200–300	85–160	427–697	313–493	310–471
Respiratory rate (breaths/min)	35–60	40–80	33–36	85–160	91–216	71–146	38–110

TABLE A.6	Serum biochemical reference values for gerbils, hamsters, mice, rats and guinea pigs				
Value	Gerbil	Hamster	Mouse	Rat	Guinea pig
Total protein (g/dl)	4.6–14.7	5.5–7.2	59–103	5.9–7.8	4.2–6.8
Albumin (g/dl)	1.8–5.8	2.0–4.2	2.5–4.8	3.3–4.6	2.1–3.9
Globulin (g/dl)	0.8–10.0	2.5–4.9	0.6	2.2–3.5	1.7–2.6
Glucose (mg/dl)	47–137	60–160	73–183	74–163	60–125
Cholesterol (mg/dl)	90–141	65–148	59–103	44–138	16–43
Urea nitrogen (mg/dl)	17–30	14–27	18–31	12–22	9.0–31.5
Creatinine (mg/dl)	NA	0.4–1.0	0.48–1.1	0.38–0.8	0.6–2.2
Creatine kinase (IU/l)	NA	366–776	155	111–334	NA
Aspartate aminotransferase (IU/l)	NA	43–134	101–214	54–192	26–68
Alanine aminotransferase (IU/l)	NA	22–63	44–87	52–144	25–59
Alkaline phosphatase (IU/l)	NA	6–14.2	43–71	40–191	55–108
Lactate dehydrogenase (IU/l)	NA	134–360	366	225–275	NA
Total bilirubin (mg/dl)	0.8–1.6	0.24–0.72	0.3–0.8	0.23–0.48	0.0–0.9
Sodium (mEq/l)	143–147	124–147	143–164	142–150	120–152
Potassium (mEq/l)	3.6–5.9	3.9–6.8	6.3–8.0	4.3–6.3	3.8–7.9
Chloride (mEq/l)	93–118	92–103	105–118	100–109	90–115
Phosphorus (mg/dl)	3.7–11.2	4.0–8.2	5.2–9.4	5.3–8.4	3.0–7.6
Calcium (mg/dl)	3.7–6.1	8.4–12.3	4.6–9.6	7.6–12.6	8.2–12.0
Magnesium (mg/dl)	NA	1.9–2.9	1.4–3.1	2.6–3.2	NA

Source: *from Quesenbury, K.E., Carpenter, J.W., 2004. Ferrets, Rabbits and Rodents. Clinical Medicine and Surgery, second ed. W B Saunders, St Louis, MO.*

TABLE A.7 Haematological reference values for gerbils, hamsters, mice, rats and guinea pigs

Parameter	Gerbil	Hamster	Mouse	Rat	Guinea pig
Red blood cells ($\times 10^6$/μl)	7.0–10.0	5–9.2	7.9–10.1	5.4–8.5	3.2–8.0
Haemoglobin (g/dl)	12.1–16.9	14.6–20	11.0–14.5	11.5–16.0	10.0–17.2
Haematocrit (%)	41–52	46–52	37–46	37–49	32–50
Platelets ($\times 10^3$/μl)	400–600	300–570	600–1200	450–885	260–740
White blood cells ($\times 10^3$/μl)	4.3–21.6	5.0–10.0	5.0–13.7	4.0–10.2	5.5–17.5
Neutrophils (%)	5–34	10–42	10–40	6–17	22–48
Lymphocytes (%)	60–95	50–95	55–95	9–34	39–72
Eosinophils (%)	0–4	0–4.5	0–4	0–6	0–7
Monocytes (%)	0–3	0–3	0.1–3.5	0–5	0–1
Basophils (%)	0–1	0–1	0–0.3	0–1.5	0–2.7
Total blood volume (ml/kg)	60–85	65–80	70–80	50–65	NA

Source: from Quesenbury, K.E., Carpenter, J.W., 2004. *Ferrets, Rabbits and Rodents. Clinical Medicine and Surgery,* second ed. W B Saunders, St Louis, MO.

TABLE A.8 Reference ranges for serum biochemistry values in the rabbit

Parameter	Value	Parameter	Value
Serum protein	5.4–8.3 g/dl	Phosphorus	4.0–6.9 mg/dl
Albumin	2.4–4.6 g/dl	Sodium	131–155 mEq/l
Globulin	1.5–2.8 g/dl	Potassium	3.6–6.9 mEq/l
Glucose	75–155 g/dl	Chloride	92–112 mEq/l
Blood urea nitrogen	13–29 mg/dl	Bicarbonate	16–38 mEq/l
Creatinine	0.5–2.5 mg/dl	Amylase	166.5–314.5 U/l
Total bilirubin	0.0–0.7 mg/dl	Alkaline phosphatase	4–16 U/l
Cholesterol	10–80 mg/dl	Alanine aminotransferase	48–80 U/l
Total lipids	243–390 mg/dl	Aspartate aminotransferase	14–113 U/l
Calcium	5.6–12.5 mg/dl	Lactic dehydrogenase	34–129 U/l

Source: from Quesenbury, K.E., Carpenter, J.W., 2004. *Ferrets, Rabbits and Rodents. Clinical Medicine and Surgery,* second ed. W B Saunders, St Louis, MO.

TABLE A.9 Reference ranges for haematological values in the rabbit

Parameter	Value
Erythrocytes	5.1–7.9 $\times 10^6$/μl
Haematocrit	33–50%
Haemoglobin	10.0–17.4 g/dl
Mean corpuscular volume	57.8–66.5 μm³
Mean corpuscular haemoglobin	17.1–23.5 pg
Mean corpuscular haemoglobin concentration	29–37%
Platelets	250–650 $\times 10^3$/μl
Leucocytes	5.2–12.5 $\times 10^3$/μl
Neutrophils	20–75%
Lymphocytes	30–85%
Monocytes	1–4%
Eosinophils	1–4%
Basophils	1–7%

Source: from Quesenbury, K.E., Carpenter, J.W., 2004. *Ferrets, Rabbits and Rodents. Clinical Medicine and Surgery,* second ed. W B Saunders, St Louis, MO.

TABLE A.10 Serum biochemical values in the ferret

Parameter	Albino	Fitch
Total protein (g/dl)	5.1–7.4	5.3–7.2
Albumin (g/dl)	2.6–3.8	3.3–4.1
Glucose (mg/dl)	94–207	62.5–134
Fasting glucose (mg/dl)	–	90–125
Blood urea nitrogen (mg/dl)	10–45	12–43
Creatinine (mg/dl)	0.4–0.9	0.2–0.6
Sodium (mmol/l)	137–162	146–160
Potassium (mmol/l)	4.5–7.7	4.3–5.3
Chloride (mmol/l)	106–125	102–121
Calcium (mg/dl)	8.0–11.8	8.6–10.5
Phosphorus (mg/dl)	4.0–9.1	5.6–8.7
Alanine aminotransferase (U/l)	–	82–289
	–	78–149
Aspartate aminotransferase (U/l)	28–120	57–248
Alkaline phosphatase (U/l)	9–84	30–120
	–	31–66
Bilirubin (mg/dl)	<1.0	0–0.1
Cholesterol (mg/dl)	64–296	119–209
Carbon dioxide (mmol/l)	16.5–28	16–28

Source: from Quesenbury, K.E., Carpenter, J.W., 2004. *Ferrets, Rabbits and Rodents. Clinical Medicine and Surgery,* second ed. W B Saunders, St Louis, MO.

Essential Calculations

PIP MILLARD

This is a summary of all the calculations that may be used in veterinary practice, including:

- Anaesthetic flow rates
- Fluid therapy flow rates
- Percentages of solutions
- Drug dosages
- Calorific requirements
- Radiographic exposures.

Each section provides an explanation of how to approach the calculation, a worked example and then some questions to do on your own with the answers included at the end.

Useful measurements

- 1 kilogram (kg) = 2.2 lb
- 1 kg = 1000 grams (g)
- 1 g = 1000 milligrams (mg)
- 1 mg = 1000 micrograms (μg, mcg)
- 1 litre (l) = 1000 millilitres (ml)
- 1 teaspoon = 5 ml
- 1 metre (m) = 100 centimetres (cm) = 1000 millimetres (mm)
- 1 cm = 10 mm

Anaesthetic flow rates

The formula required to calculate an anaesthetic flow rate is:

Body weight (kg) × Minute volume (ml/min) × Circuit factor.

We must first calculate the minute volume of the patient and in order to do this we need to know the patient's tidal volume and respiratory rate.

1. **Tidal volume** – this is the amount of air which is inhaled or exhaled in each respiration. It is estimated at 10–15 ml/kg:
   - Cats/small dogs = 15 ml/kg
   - Medium/large dogs = 10 ml/kg.
2. **Minute volume** – this is the amount of air passing in and out of the lungs in 1 minute.
   The formula to calculate minute volume is:

   Tidal volume × Respiratory rate.

   If accurate figures are unavailable a minute volume of 200 ml/kg can be used. This is an average minute volume, based on 10 ml/kg tidal volume and 20 breaths per minute respiratory rate.
3. **Circuit factor** – this is the factor by which the minute volume must be increased to prevent rebreathing. These are used to calculate the correct settings for the anaesthetic machine in relation to the particular patient.

Ayre's T-piece	2.5–3 × minute volume
Bain	2.5–3 × minute volume
Magill	1–1.5 × minute volume
Lack	1–1.5 × minute volume
Circle – closed	No circuit factor: calculate using a flow rate of 10 ml/kg
To-and-fro – partial rebreathing	No circuit factor: calculate using a flow rate of 25 ml/kg

EXAMPLE

What is the required anaesthetic flow rate for a 30-kg dog with a respiratory rate of 20 breaths per minute on a Magill circuit?

Body weight × minute volume × circuit factor
30 kg × (10 ml tidal volume × 20 breaths/min) × 1–1.5
30 kg × 200 ml × 1–1.5

Answer: 6000 ml (6 l) to 9000 ml (9 l) per minute

EXAMPLE

Calculate the anaesthetic flow rate required to maintain anaesthesia in a 15-kg dog on a Bain circuit with a respiratory rate of 20 breaths per minute:

Body weight × minute volume × circuit factor
15 kg × (10 ml tidal volume × 20 breaths/min) × 2.5–3
15 kg × 200 ml × 2.5–3

Answer: 7500 ml (7.5 l) to 9000 ml (9l) per minute

QUESTIONS

1. Calculate the gas flow rate for a dog weighing 20 kg when using a Lack system, at a respiratory rate of 20 breaths per minute.

2. A 30-kg dog is anaesthetised and maintained on a Magill circuit. Calculate the flow rate required if the dog is breathing 20 times per minute.

3. Calculate the flow rate for a 5-kg dog on an Ayre's T-piece anaesthetic circuit breathing at a rate of 15 breaths per minute.

4. Calculate the flow rate required for a 35-kg dog maintained on a circle circuit, breathing 15 times per minute.

5. Calculate the flow rate for a 3-kg cat on an Ayre's T-piece anaesthetic circuit with a respiratory rate of 15 breaths per minute.

Fluid therapy flow rates

GIVING SETS

These usually have the number of drops per millilitre stated on the packaging so check before calculating the drip rate. A standard giving set will deliver approximately 15–20 drops/ml. For smaller patients, a paediatric giving set can be used, which gives 60 drops/ml – this faster rate is useful to administer small volumes more accurately. Automated infusion pumps are also available, which can deliver a set amount of fluid over a given period of time.

ESTIMATING FLUID LOSS

There are three main ways to estimate fluid loss:

- Using percentage dehydration of the animal
- Calculating the water deficit from the patient's history
- Using the packed cell volume (PCV).

1. **Percentage dehydration method**

A clinical examination should enable the veterinary surgeon to estimate the percentage by which the patient is dehydrated.

> **EXAMPLE**
>
> A 20-kg dog is found to be 9% dehydrated. Calculate the total fluid deficit for this animal:
>
> 20 kg × % dehydration × 10
> 20 kg × 9% × 10
>
> **Answer:** 1800 ml fluid deficit

2. **Calculating the water deficit from the history**

The volume of fluid required to maintain a healthy animal is calculated at 50–60 ml/kg/24 hours, which compensates for normal fluid losses during the day – these are made up as follows:

Respiratory/cutaneous losses:	20 ml/kg – these are described as inevitable losses
Faecal losses (normal faeces):	10–20 ml/kg
Urinary losses (normal range):	20 ml/kg
Further losses include: Vomit	Approximately 4 ml/kg/vomit

With an accurate history the fluid deficit can be calculated.

> **EXAMPLE**
>
> An 8-kg dog has been anorexic for 3 days and has vomited 3 times daily for the last 2 days. It has not produced urine for 24 hours. Calculate the total fluid deficit for this animal:
>
> | Inevitable water losses: | 20 ml × 8 kg × 3 days
= 480 ml |
> |---|---|
> | Urinary water losses: | 20 ml × 8 kg × 2 days
= 320 ml |
> | Vomiting: | 4 ml × 8 kg × 3 vomits × 2 days
= 192 ml |
>
> **Answer:** Total water deficit: 480 + 320 + 192 = 992 ml

3. **Using the packed cell volume (PCV)**

For every 1% increase in PCV, there is a 10 ml/kg water deficit. In most cases, the patient's normal PCV is unlikely to be known so the following average figures are used:

Dog: 45%
Cat: 37%.

> **EXAMPLE**
>
> A 15-kg dog has a PCV of 54%. Calculate the total fluid deficit:
>
> Body weight (kg) × 10 ml for every 1% increase in PCV
> 15 kg × (54% − 45%) × 10 ml = 15 kg × 9% × 10 ml
>
> **Answer:** 1350 ml fluid deficit

INTRAVENOUS FLUID THERAPY

Once fluid deficit has been calculated it must be added to the daily maintenance fluid requirement – 50–60 ml/kg. This will give the total amount of fluid to be replaced. Ideally, half of the total amount should be replaced in the first 8 hours.

> **EXAMPLE**
>
> A 20-kg dog has a fluid deficit of 1800 ml. A standard giving set delivering 20 drops/ml is used. Calculate the fluid flow rates over 24 hours:
>
> *Maintenance:*
>
> | 50 ml/24 hours × 20 kg | = 1000 ml/24 hours |
> |---|---|
> | 1000 ml ÷ 24 hours | = 41.67 ml/hr |
>
> *Replacing deficit:*
>
> | Half in first 8 hours: | 1800 ml ÷ 2 = 900 ml
900 ÷ 8 hours = 112.5 ml/hr |
> |---|---|
> | Total ml/hr: | *Maintenance + deficit:*
41.67 ml + 112.5 ml/hr = 154.17 ml/hr |
> | Total ml/min: | 154.17 ml ÷ 60 min = 2.57 ml/min |
> | Drops/min: | 2.57 ml × drip factor
2.57 ml × 20 = 51.4 drops/min |
> | Seconds/drop: | 60 seconds ÷ 51.4 drops/min |
>
> **Answer:** 1 drop every 1.17 seconds for first 8 hours
>
> *Replacing deficit:*
>
> | Last 16 hours: | 1800 ml ÷ 2 = 900 ml
900 ÷ 16 h = 56.25 ml/hour |
> |---|---|
> | Total ml/hr: | Maintenance + Deficit
41.67 ml + 56.25 ml = 97.92 ml/hour |
> | Total ml/min: | 97.92 ml ÷ 60 min = 1.63 ml/min |
> | Drops/min: | 1.63 ml × 20 = 32.6 drops/min |
> | Seconds/drop: | 60 seconds ÷ 32.6 drops/min |
>
> **Answer:** 1 drop every 1.84 (2) second for remaining 16 hours

EXAMPLE

A 21-kg dog requires 1000 ml of fluid over a 6-hour period at a rate of 5 ml/kg/hr. A standard giving set is used delivering 20 drops/ml. Calculate the flow rate:

Flow rate: 5 ml × 21 kg = 105 ml/hr
ml/min: 105 ml ÷ 60 min = 1.75 ml/min
Drops/min: 1.75 ml × 20 drops = 35 drops/min
Seconds/drop: 60 s ÷ 35 drops/min

Answer: 1 drop every 1.71 (2) seconds

QUESTIONS

6. A 16-kg dog requires fluids at a rate of 10 ml/kg/hr. A standard giving set is used delivering 15 drops/ml. Calculate the flow rate

7. A 3-kg cat requires a total of 60 ml of fluids at a rate of 5 ml/kg/hr. A paediatric giving set is used. Calculate the flow rate

8. A 20-kg dog with a PCV of 50% requires fluid therapy to replace fluid deficit. A standard giving set delivering 20 drops/ml is used. Calculate the fluid therapy flow rates over 24 hours

9. A 15-kg dog requires 750 ml of fluid over 24 hours. Using a giving set that delivers 15 drops/ml, calculate the flow rate

10. Calculate the fluid rate for a 5-kg cat requiring 125 ml of Hartmann's over 10 hours. A paediatric giving set is used.

Percentage solutions

The percentage of a solution is expressed as the weight (w) of a drug per volume (v) of a solution:

    1 g (w) in 100 ml (v) = 1% solution
    2 g (w) in 100 ml (v) = 2% solution

and so on.
It is, however, more useful to express the percentage in terms of mg/ml when calculating doses:

    2.5% solution   = 2.5 g/100 ml
    ÷ 100   = 0.025 g/ml
    convert g to mg – 1000 mg in 1 g
    so to convert 0.025 g to mg = 25 mg/ml.
    multiply by 1000

FORMULAE FOR CALCULATING VOLUME, PERCENTAGE SOLUTION AND WEIGHT OF A DRUG

$$\text{Volume (ml)} = \frac{\text{weight (g)} \times 100}{\%\ \text{solution}}$$

$$\text{Weight (g)} = \frac{\%\ \text{solution} \times \text{volume (ml)}}{100}$$

$$\%\ \text{solution} = \frac{\text{weight (g)} \times 100}{\text{volume (ml)}}$$

EXAMPLE 1

Calculate the percentage solution that could be made up with 125 mg of glucose and 50 ml of water, using all the glucose and water:

Convert mg to g: 125 mg ÷ 1000 = 0.125 g

Apply formula:

$$\%\ \text{solution} = \frac{\text{Weight (g)} \times 100}{\text{Volume (ml)}}$$

$$= \frac{0.125\ \text{g} \times 100}{50\ \text{ml}}$$

Answer: 0.25%

EXAMPLE 2

A 44-lb dog requires injections every 8 hours at a drug rate of 25 mg/kg/24 hours. The injection is produced as a 5% solution. Calculate the volume of solution to be given at each injection.

(1 kg = 2.2 lb)
Convert 44 lb to kg: 44 ÷ 2.2 = 20 kg
(1 g = 1000 mg)
Convert mg to g: 25 ÷ 1000 = 0.025 g
Total drug required per 24 hours: 20 kg × 0.025 g = 0.5 g/24 hours
Apply formula:

$$\text{Volume} = \frac{\text{Weight (g)} \times 100}{5\%} = 10\ \text{ml}$$

Given every 8 hours, i.e. 3 times per day: 10 ml ÷ 3

Answer: 3.33 ml per injection

EXAMPLE 3

Calculate the amount of glucose required to produce 20 ml of a 2.5% solution:
  Apply formula:

$$\text{Weight (g)} = \frac{\%\ \text{solution} \times \text{volume (ml)}}{100}$$

$$= \frac{2.5\% \times 20\ \text{ml}}{100}$$

Answer: 0.5 g

QUESTIONS

11. An antibiotic is supplied as a 15% suspension. If the dose for a dog is 10 mg/kg, calculate the volume required for a 30-kg Labrador

12. A 20-kg dog is to be given an intravenous injection of a 5% solution. The dose rate of the drug is 15 mg/kg. Calculate the volume of the solution to be given

13. Calculate the percentage solution achieved when mixing 500 mg of a drug in 100 ml of sterile water

14. Calculate the amount of dextrose required to produce 1 litre of a 2.5% solution

15. An 11-lb rabbit requires antibiotic injections twice daily. Calculate the volume required for each injection of a 5% solution at a dose rate of 15 mg/kg.

Drug dosages

In order to calculate a drug dose, the following information is required:

- Body weight of the animal in kilograms
- Daily dose rate – this may need to be divided throughout the day
- Strength of each tablet.

EXAMPLE

A 10-kg dog requires antibiotic tablets for 14 days. The recommended dose is 5 mg/kg every 6 hours. The tablets contain 200 mg antibiotic each. Calculate the number to be dispensed.

Total dose required:	10 kg × 5 mg = 50 mg every 6 hours
Number of tablets required:	50 mg ÷ 200 mg = 0.25 tablet = ¼ tablet every 6 hours
Number of tablets daily:	24 hours ÷ 6 hours = 4
	4 times × ¼ tablet = 1 tablet daily
Total number of tablets dispensed:	1 daily × 14 days

Answer: 14 tablets dispensed

QUESTIONS

16. A cat weighing 4 kg requires antibiotics by mouth as a tablet for 5 days. The recommended dose is 24 mg/kg/24 hours and should ideally be divided into two or three equal doses throughout the day. The tablets are available in the following strengths: 50 mg, 100 mg and 250 mg. Calculate the strength and number dispensed.

17. Antibiotic tablets are to be dispensed to a 4-kg cat at a dose rate of 25 mg/kg/day. The tablets are presented as 50 mg and should be given in divided doses. Calculate the number to be given per day.

18. A 7-kg dog requires tablets at a rate of 1.5 mg/kg twice daily for 7 days. The tablets are available as 10 mg, 15 mg, 50 mg and 150 mg. Calculate the correct tablet size to dispense, the number to dispense and the instructions for dosing.

19. An 8.8-lb rabbit requires oral antibiotics twice daily for 10 days. The dose rate is 5 mg/kg. The tablets are available in 5 mg, 10 mg and 20 mg blister packs. Calculate the total number of tablets to be dispensed and of which strength.

20. A 33-lb dog requires antibiotics for 21 days. The recommended dose is 5 mg/kg every 12 hours. Each capsule is 25 mg. Calculate the number dispensed.

Calorific requirements

Calculating the calorific requirement of a patient involves working out the basal energy requirement (BER) and then multiplying this by the disease factor:

BER × Disease factor = Kilocalories required in 24 hours

BASAL ENERGY REQUIREMENT

For dogs over 5 kg   BER = [30 × body weight (kg)] + 70
For small dogs and cats   BER = 60 × body weight (kg)

DISEASE FACTORS

The disease factor is the proportion of extra kilocalories (kcal) required in certain stressful or disease situations:

Cage rest	1.2
Surgery/trauma	1.3
Multiple surgery/trauma	1.5
Sepsis/neoplasia	1.7
Burns	2.0
Growth	2.0.

EXAMPLE

Calculate the calorific requirement of a 25-kg dog following routine surgery:

Calculate BER:	(30 × Body weight [kg]) + 70
	(30 × 25 kg) + 70 = 820 kcal
Disease factor (surgery):	1.3
Total kcal:	1.3 × 820 kcal

Answer: 1066 kcal required

QUESTIONS

21. Calculate the calorific requirement of a 55-kg great Dane that is hospitalised after parturition with a disease factor of 1.2.

22. Calculate the calorific requirement of a 1-kg kitten who is recovering from severe burns.

23. Calculate the calorific requirement of a 10-kg dog fitted with a nasogastric tube. Then calculate the amount of food required if the energy density of the food is 0.8 kcal/ml.

24. Calculate the calorific requirement of a 32-kg dog. Using your answer, calculate the amount of food required if the food has an energy density of 420 kcal per 100-g tin.

25. Calculate the daily calorific requirement of a 5-kg Yorkshire terrier.

Radiographic exposures

There are a number of different calculations that are encountered in radiography:

- Amperage (in milliamps, mA) and exposure time (mAs)
- Voltage (in kilovolts, kV)
- Film focal distance (FFD)
- Grid factor.

1. mAs

$$\text{mAs} = \text{Amperage (mA)} \times \text{Time (s)}$$

Provided the mAs and mA are given, the exposure time in seconds can be calculated:

$$\text{mAs} \div \text{mA} = \text{time (s)}$$

EXAMPLE

The radiographic exposure required for a dog's chest is 70 kV and 50 mAs. Calculate the exposure time if the machine has an output of 200 mA:

Time (s) = mAs ÷ mA
= 50 mAs ÷ 200 mA.

Answer: 0.25 seconds

2. kV

The rule when calculating voltage is:

If the voltage is raised by 10 kV, then the mAs should be halved
If the voltage is lowered by 10 kV, then the mAs should be doubled.

Thus

60 kV @ 16 mAs
70 kV @ 8 mAs
50 kV @ 32 mAs

are all the same.

EXAMPLE

An exposure for a dog's abdomen has been found to be satisfactory at 75 kV and 40 mAs. Calculate the new mAs if the voltage were increased to 85 kV:
    The kV has been increased by 10 so the mAs should be halved:

40 mAs ÷ 2

Answer: 20 mAs

3. Film focal distance (FFD)

The inverse square law applies when altering the FFD: 'The intensity of the beam varies inversely as the square of the distance from the source', i.e.:

$$\text{New mAs} = \frac{\text{Old mAs} \times \text{New FFD}^2}{\text{Old FFD}^2}$$

EXAMPLE

An exposure is found to be satisfactory for a dog's abdomen at 60 kV, 20 mAs and an FFD of 40 cm. Calculate the new mAs if the FFD were increased to 80 cm:

New mAs = $\dfrac{\text{Old mAs} \times \text{New FFD}^2}{\text{Old FFD}^2}$

$= \dfrac{20 \times 80^2}{40^2}$

$= \dfrac{20 \times 6400}{1600}$

Answer: 80 mAs

4. Grid factor

The grid factor is the amount by which the exposure (mAs) must be increased to compensate for the use of the grid. It is usually written on the grid:

$$\text{New mAs} = \text{Old mAs} \times \text{Grid factor.}$$

EXAMPLE

A radiograph requires an exposure of 20 mAs when taken at an FFD of 90 cm without a grid. Calculate the new mAs if a grid with a grid factor of 4 is used:

Old mAs × Grid factor
20 mAs × 4

Answer: 80 mAs

QUESTIONS

26. If the mAs is 50 and the amperage is 200 mA, calculate the correct exposure time.

27. A dog is radiographed using an FFD of 50 cm with an mAs of 5. A decision is made to increase the FFD to 100 cm to minimise geometric distortion. Calculate the new mAs.

28. A radiograph requires an exposure of 30 mAs without the use of a grid. Calculate the new mAs when a grid is introduced with a grid factor of 3.

29. A radiograph has been taken at 60 kV and 35 mAs. Calculate the new mAs if the voltage were changed to 50 kV.

30. Calculate the mAs for a radiograph with a time of 0.4 s and an mA of 180.

Answers to questions

Now let's see how much you have understood!

1. Calculate the gas flow rate for a dog weighing 20 kg when using a Lack system, at a respiratory rate of 20 breaths per minute:

    Body weight × Minute volume × Circuit factor

    20 kg × (10 ml × 20 breaths per minute) × 1–1.5

    20 kg × 200 ml × 1–1.5

    = 4000 ml (4 l) to 6000 ml (6 l) per minute

2. A 30-kg dog is anaesthetised and maintained on a Magill circuit. Calculate the flow rate required if the dog is breathing 20 times per minute:

    Body weight × Minute volume × Circuit factor

    30 kg × (10 ml × 20 breaths per minute) × 1–1.5

    30 kg × 200 ml × 1–1.5

    = 6000 ml (6 l) to 9000 ml (9 l) per minute

3. Calculate the flow rate for a 5-kg dog on an Ayre's T-piece anaesthetic circuit breathing at a rate of 15 breaths per minute:

Body weight × Minute volume × Circuit factor

5 kg × (15 ml × 15 breaths per minute) × 2.5 – 3

5 kg × 225 ml × 2.5 – 3

= **2812.5 ml (2.8 l) to 3375 ml (3.4 l) per minute**

4. Calculate the flow rate required for a 35-kg dog maintained on a circle circuit, breathing 15 times per minute:

35 kg × 10 ml = **350 ml**

5. Calculate the flow rate for a 3-kg cat on an Ayre's T-piece anaesthetic circuit with a respiratory rate of 25 breaths per minute.

Body weight × Minute volume × Circuit factor

3 kg × (15 ml × 25 breaths/min) × 2.5 – 3

3 kg × 375 ml × 2.5 – 3

= **2812.5 ml (2.8 l) to 3375 ml (3.4 l) per minute**

6. A 16-kg dog requires fluids at a rate of 10 ml/kg/hr. A standard giving set is used delivering 15 drops/ml. Calculate the flow rate:

16 kg × 10 ml = 160 ml/hr

160 ml ÷ 60 min = 2.67 ml/min

2.67 ml × 15 drops = 40.05 drops/min

60 s ÷ 40.05 = **1 drop every 1.5 second**

7. A 3-kg cat requires a total of 60 ml of fluids at a rate of 5 ml/kg/hr. A paediatric giving set is used. Calculate the flow rate:

3 kg × 5 ml = 15 ml/hr

15 ml ÷ 60 min = 0.25 ml/min

0.25 ml × 60 drops = 15 drops/min

60 s ÷ 15 drops = **1 drop every 4 seconds**

8. A 20-kg dog with a PCV of 50% requires fluid therapy to replace fluid deficit. A standard giving set delivering 20 drops/ml is used. Calculate the fluid therapy flow rates over 24 hours:

Body weight (kg) × 10 ml for every 1% increase in PCV

20 kg × (50 – 45%) × 10 ml

20 kg × 5% × 10 ml = 1000 ml fluid deficit/24 hours

Maintenance: ÷ 24 hours	50 ml/24 hours × 20 kg = 1000 ml 1000 ml ÷ 24 hours = 41.67 ml/hr
Replacing deficit: Half in first 8 hours:	1000 ml ÷ 2 ÷ 8 = 62.5 ml/hr
Total ml/hr:	*Maintenance + deficit* 41.67 ml + 62.5 ml/hr = 104.17 ml/hr
Total ml/min:	104.17 ml ÷ 60 min = 1.74 ml/min
Drops/min:	1.74 ml × Drip factor 1.75 ml × 20 = 34.8 drops/min

Seconds/drop: 60 s ÷ 34.8 drops = **1 drop every 1.72 second for first 8 hours**

Replacing deficit:	
Last 16 hours:	1000 ml ÷ 2 ÷ 16 hours = 31.25 ml/hr
Total ml/hr:	*Maintenance + deficit* 41.67 ml + 31.25 ml = 72.92 ml/hr
Total ml/min:	72.92 ml ÷ 60 = 1.22 ml/min
Drops/min:	1.22 ml × 20 = 24.4 drops/min
Seconds/drop:	60 s ÷ 24.4 drops = **1 drop every 2.46 seconds for remaining 16 hours**

9. A 15-kg dog requires 750 ml of fluid over 24 hours. Using a giving set that delivers 15 drops/ml, calculate the flow rate:

750 ml ÷ 24 hours = 31.25 ml/hr

31.25 ml ÷ 60 min = 0.52 ml/min

0.52 ml × 15 drops = 7.8 drops/min

60 s ÷ 7.8 drops = **1 drop every 7.7 seconds**

10. Calculate the fluid rate for a 5-kg cat requiring 125 ml of Hartmann's over 10 hours. A paediatric giving set is used.

125 ml ÷ 10 hours = 12.5 ml/hr

12.5 ml ÷ 60 minutes = 0.21 ml/min

0.21 ml × 60 drops = 12.6 drops/min

60 s ÷ 12.6 drops = **1 drop every 5 seconds**

11. An antibiotic is supplied as a 15% suspension. If the dose for a dog is 10 mg/kg, calculate the volume required for a 30-kg Labrador:

Dose = (30 kg × 10 mg) ÷ 1000 (to convert to grams) = 0.3 g

$$\text{Volume (ml)} = \frac{\text{weight of drug (g)} \times 100}{\% \text{ solution}}$$

$$= \frac{0.3 \times 100}{15}$$

$$= \textbf{2 ml}$$

12. A 20-kg dog is to be given an intravenous injection of a 5% solution. The dose rate of the drug is 15 mg/kg. Calculate the volume of the solution to be given:

$$\text{Dose} = 20 \text{ kg} \times 15 \text{ mg} = \frac{300 \text{ mg}}{1000} = 0.3 \text{ g}$$

$$\text{Volume (ml)} = \frac{\text{weight of drug (g)} \times 100}{\% \text{ solution}}$$

$$= \frac{0.3 \times 100}{5\%}$$

$$= \textbf{6 ml}$$

13. Calculate the percentage solution achieved when mixing 500 mg of a drug in 100 ml of sterile water:

$$\frac{500 \text{ mg}}{1000} = 0.5 \text{ g}$$

$$\% = \frac{\text{weight (g)} \times 100}{\text{volume (ml)}}$$

$$= \frac{0.5 \times 100}{100}$$

$$= 0.5\%$$

14. Calculate the amount of dextrose required to produce 1 litre of a 2.5% solution:

$$\text{Weight (g)} = \frac{\text{Volume (ml)} \times \text{solution}}{100}$$

$$= \frac{0.5 \times 100}{100}$$

$$= \textbf{25 g}$$

15. An 11-lb rabbit requires antibiotic injections twice daily. Calculate the volume required for each injection of a 5% solution at a dose rate of 15 mg/kg.

Convert lb to kg: $11 \text{ lb} \div 2.2 = 5 \text{ kg}$

$5 \text{ kg} \times 15 \text{ mg} = 75 \text{ mg}$

Convert mg to g: $75 \text{ mg} \div 1000 = 0.075 \text{ g}$

$$\text{Volume (ml)} = \frac{\text{Weight of drug (g)} \times 100}{\% \text{ solution}}$$

$$= \frac{0.075 \text{ g} \times 100}{5\%}$$

$$= 1.5 \text{ ml}$$

Divide into 2 doses: $= 1.5 \text{ ml} \div 2 = 0.75 \text{ ml}$

16. A cat weighing 4 kg requires antibiotics by mouth as a tablet for 5 days. The recommended dose is 24 mg/kg/24 hours and should, ideally, be divided into two or three equal doses throughout the day. The tablets are available in the following strengths: 50 mg, 100 mg and 250 mg. Calculate the strength and number dispensed:

Dose/24 hours $= 4 \text{ kg} \times 24 \text{ mg} = 96 \text{ mg}$

Twice-daily dose $= 96 \text{ mg} \div 2 = 48 \text{ mg}$

$= 1 \times 50 \text{ mg tablet}$

Two tablets daily $\times 5$ days $= \textbf{10} \times \textbf{50 mg tablets}$

dispensed

17. Antibiotic tablets are to be dispensed to a 4-kg cat at a dose rate of 25 mg/kg/day. The tablets are presented as 50 mg and should be given in divided doses. Calculate the number to be given per day:

Daily dose $= 4 \text{ kg} \times 25 \text{ mg} = 100 \text{ mg}$

Number of tablets $= 100 \text{ mg}/50 \text{ mg} = 2$

1 tablet to be given twice daily

18. A 7-kg dog requires tablets at a rate of 1.5 mg/kg twice daily for 7 days. The tablets are available as 10 mg, 15 mg, 50 mg and 150 mg. Calculate the correct tablet size to dispense, the number to dispense and the instructions for dosing:

Twice-daily dose $= 7 \text{ kg} \times 1.5 \text{ mg} = 10.5 \text{ mg} = 1 \times$

10 mg tablet

2 tablets $\times 7$ days $= 14$ tablets

14 $\times$ 10 mg tablets dispensed to be given twice daily

19. An 8.8-lb rabbit requires oral antibiotics twice daily for 10 days. The dose rate is 5 mg/kg. The tablets are available in 5 mg, 10 mg and 20 mg blister packs. Calculate the total number of tablets to be dispensed and of which strength.

Convert lb to kg: $8.8 \text{ lb} \div 2.2 = 4 \text{ kg}$

Dose/24 hours: $4 \text{ kg} \times 5 \text{ mg} = 20 \text{ mg}$

Twice-daily dose: $20 \text{ mg} \div 2 = 10 \text{ mg}$

$= 1 \times 10 \text{ mg tablet twice daily}$

Total number dispensed: $(2 \times 10 \text{ kg daily}) \times 10 \text{ days}$

$2 \times 10 = \textbf{20 of the 10 mg tablets}$

20. A 33-lb dog requires antibiotic capsules for 21 days. The recommended dose is 5 mg/kg every 12 hours. Each capsule is 25 mg. Calculate the number dispensed.

Dog's weight (kg) $= 33 \div 2.2 = 15 \text{ kg}$

12-hour dose $= 15 \times 5 \text{ mg} = 75 \text{ mg}$

Number of tablets $= 75 \text{ mg} \div 25 \text{ mg} = 3 \text{ tablets}$

3 tablets every 12 hours $= 6 \text{ tablets/day}$

6 tablets $\times$ 21 days = 126 tablets dispensed

21. Calculate the calorific requirement of a 55-kg great Dane that is hospitalised after parturition with a disease factor of 1.2:

Daily requirement (kcal) $= (30 \times \text{Body weight [kg]}) + 70)$

$\times \text{Disease factor}$

$= ([30 \times 55] + 70) \times 1.2$

$= \textbf{2064 kcal}$

22. Calculate the calorific requirement of a 1-kg kitten who is recovering from severe burns:

Daily requirement (kcal) $= \text{Body weight (kg)} \times 60$

$\times \text{disease factor}$

$= 1 \times 60 \times 2$

$= \textbf{120 kcal}$

23. Calculate the calorific requirement of a 10-kg dog fitted with a nasogastric tube. Then calculate the amount of food required if the energy density of the food is 0.8 kcal/ml:

$$\text{Daily requirement (kcal)} = (\text{Body weight [kg]} \times 30) + 70$$
$$= (10 \text{ kg} \times 30) + 70$$
$$= 370 \text{ kcal}$$

Amount of food required at 0.8 kcal/ml = 370 ÷ 0.8
$$= \textbf{462.5 ml}$$

24. Calculate the calorific requirement of a 32-kg dog. Using your answer, calculate the amount of food required if the food has an energy density of 420 kcal per 100-g tin:

$$\text{Daily requirement (kcal)} = (\text{Body weight (kg)} \times 30) + 70$$
$$= (32 \text{ kg} \times 30) + 70$$
$$= 1030 \text{ kcal}$$

Amount of food required at 420 kcal/100 g = 1030 ÷ 420
$$= 245 \text{ g}$$

Number of tins at 100 g per tin = 245 ÷ 100 tins
$$= \textbf{2.45 tins required}$$

25. Calculate the daily calorific requirement of a 5-kg Yorkshire terrier.

$$\text{Daily requirement (kcal)} = \text{Body weight (kg)} \times 60$$
$$= 5 \text{ kg} \times 60$$
$$= \textbf{300 kcal}$$

26. If the mAs is 50 and the amperage is 200 mA, calculate the correct exposure time:

$$\text{Time (s)} = \frac{\text{mAs}}{\text{mA}}$$
$$= \frac{50 \text{ mAs}}{200}$$
$$= \textbf{0.25 seconds}$$

27. A dog is radiographed using an FFD of 50 cm with an mAs of 5. A decision is made to increase the FFD to 100 cm to minimise geometric distortion. Calculate the new mAs:

$$\text{New mAs} = \frac{\text{Old mAs} \times \text{New FFD}^2}{\text{Old FFD}^2}$$
$$= \frac{5 \times 100^2}{50^2}$$
$$= \frac{5 \times 10000}{2500}$$
$$= 5 \times 4$$
$$= \textbf{20 mAs}$$

28. A radiograph requires an exposure of 30 mAs without the use of a grid. Calculate the new mAs when a grid is introduced with a grid factor of 3:

$$\text{New mAs} = \text{mAs without grid} \times \text{Grid factor}$$
$$= 30 \text{ mAs} \times 3$$
$$= \textbf{90 mAs}$$

29. A radiograph has been taken at 60 kV and 35 mAs. Calculate the new mAs if the voltage were changed to 50 kV:

If the voltage is lowered by 10 kV, then the mAs should be doubled:

$$35 \text{ mAs} \times 2 = \textbf{70 mAs}$$

30. Calculate the mAs for a radiograph with a time of 0.4 seconds and an mA of 180.

$$\text{mAs} = \text{mA} \times \text{s}$$
$$= 180 \text{ mA} \times 0.4 \text{ s}$$
$$= \textbf{72 mAs}$$

Persian cats, brachycephaly in, 256–257
Persistent right aortic arch/vascular ring anomaly, 410*t*
Personal monitoring of radiation exposure, 61
Personal protective equipment, 219
Pet Animals Act 1951, 1983, 63*t*–64*t*
Pet Travel Scheme, 62*t*
Pethidine, 549
Petit mal, 415
Petrissage, 307
pH, of urine, 655
Pharmaceutical adjuvants, 324
Pharmaceuticals, 31–32
  as non-hazardous waste, *e*12
Pharmacodynamics, 321–322, 321*f*
  non-receptor-mediated, 322
  receptor-mediated, 321–322
    affinity and competitiveness, 321–322, 322*f*
    agonist and antagonist effects, 321, 321*f*
    down-regulation and up-regulation, 322
    specificity/potency and efficacy, 322
Pharmacokinetics, 317–321
  drug absorption, 317–318
    administration route and effect on, 317–318, 318*f*
    drug formulation, 318
    tissue perfusion, 318
  drug distribution, 318–319
    factors affecting, 318–319, 319*f*
  drug elimination, 320–321
    factors affecting, 321
    half-life and therapeutic range, 320–321, 320*f*
    hepatic, 321
    renal, 321
  drug metabolism, 319–320
    drug interaction affecting, 319–320
    factors affecting, 319–320
    metabolic system and, 319
    process of, 319
    species variation and, 320
Pharmacology, fundamental, 317–343. *see also* Drugs
  definition of, 317
Pharmacy, management of, 339–340
  key considerations for effective, 340, 341*t*
Pharyngeal packing, for dental procedures, 514, 514*f*
Pharyngostomy tube, in anorexia, 171
Pharynx, 89, 90*f*, 92
  function of, 94*f*
  horse, 140
Phenols, *e*11
Phenothiazines, 547
Phenotype, definitions, 244*b*, 248
Phlebitis, as catheter complications, 493
Phosphofructokinase deficiency, 249
Phosphorus, 358
  dietary, dog and cat, 149–150
    intake, 159
Photographic chemicals, 55, 56*f*, 61
  as hazardous waste, *e*12
Photographic effect, 669
Photophobia, 378
Physical welfare, 3
Physics, or radiography, 665–667, 666*f*, 666*t*
Physiology
  canine and feline, 65–113
  exotic species, 115–133
  horse, 135–144
Physiotherapy
  aim of, 301
  immobilization and disuse effects
    bone, 304
    cartilage, 303
    ligaments and tendons, 304

Physiotherapy (*Continued*)
    muscle, 303–304
    on musculoskeletal tissues, 303–304
    nerves, 304
  indications for, 301
  role of
    owner, 302–303
    veterinary nurse, 302
    veterinary physiotherapist, 302
    veterinary surgeon, 302
  in small animal practice, 301, 302*b*
  team approach in, 301–303, 302*f*
  techniques, 301–315
  therapeutic exercises for, 308–314
    active, 312–313
    assisted, 310–312, 310*f*
    passive, 308–310
  treatments for, 304–308
    massage therapy, 306–308
    thermotherapy, 304–306
Pia mater, 78
Pica, 295
PICCs. *see* Peripherally inserted central catheters (PICCs)
Pigment production, 256
Pineal gland, 83*t*
Pinworms, 611
  Oxyuris equi, 611
Pipistrellus pipistrellus, 780
PIVA. *see* Partial intravenous anaesthesia (PIVA)
Placental development, 107–108, 109*f*
Plain drapes, 469
Planning, 288
Plasma, 84
Plasma enzymes, 653
Plasma (cell) membrane, 65, 241
Plasma proteins, 70, 84
Plasmid, 628*f*
Plastic plain urethral catheter, 409*t*
Platelets, 85
Plenum vaporiser, 537*f*
Pleura, 70, 70*f*
Pleural disorders, 406–407, 407*f*, 407*t*
Plunge method, of gloving, 458
PN. *see* Parenteral nutrition (PN)
Pneumonia, dyspnoea caused by, 405
Pneumothorax, 407*t*, 446
Pododermatitis, in rabbits, 711*t*–712*t*
Poikuria, 291
Poisoning, dyspnoea caused by, 405–406
Polishing, 524–525, 525*f*
Polishing units, 509
Politico-economic factors, nursing care and, 285
Polycystic kidney disorder, feline, genetic screening, 251, 251*f*
Polymerase chain reaction, 250
Polymerised haemoglobin, 485–486, 485*f*
Polypharmacy, 322
Polyploidy, 249
Polyps, in rectum, 442
Polyurethane foam dressings, 372
Polyuria, 291, 654
Portable appliance testing (PAT), 58
Portosystemic shunt, 423, 423*f*
Positioning, in radiographic, 677–685
  aids, 679
  BVA/KC hip dysplasia and elbow scoring schemes, 679–680
  general principles of, 677–678
  large animal, 682–685
  markers and legends, 679, 679*t*, 680*f*
  restraint, 678–679
  small animals, 680–682
Positive punishment, 211
Positive reinforcement
  cats/dogs, 196–197

Positive reinforcement (*Continued*)
  horse, 211
    secondary, 211
Post-anaesthetic myopathy, as anaesthetic complications, 590
Post-anaesthetic neuropathy, as anaesthetic complications, 590
Post-hibernation anorexia, 730, 740*f*
Post-ictal phase, of seizures, 380
Post-neutering clinics, 26
Posterior pituitary gland, 83*t*
Postsurgical clinics, 33–34
Posture
  body, in communication
    cats, 194, 194*f*
    dogs, 191
  neurological examination for, 416*t*
Potassium, 356
  abnormalities of, 482–483, 483*t*
  dietary, dog and cat, 150
Potassium-sparing diuretics, 331
Potentiation, 322, 323*t*
Potter-Bucky grids, 670
Powders, 325*t*–326*t*
Power equipment
  care and maintenance of, 513
  for extraction, 510–511
  general maintenance of, 513, 513*t*
Power of petting, 272–273
Practical animal breeding, 255–266
Practice, 4, 13, 14*f*, 37–49, 43*f*
  ethical considerations, 4, 6*t*
  veterinary, 40, 48*t*
  vision, 44*f*
PRBCs. *see* Packed red blood cells (PRBCs)
Pre-emptive analgesia, 567
Pre-ictal phase, of seizures, 380
Prebiotics, 164
Precaecal digestion, horse, 173–175
Precocial, 748
Precocial fledgling, 793
Pregnancy, 106–108
  changes during, 108
  feeding in, 158–159, 159*t*
  horse, 181, 182*f*
Premate test, 642
Premature beats/missed or dropped beats, 411*t*
Premium pet foods, 155
Prepatent period, 595
Prescriptions, writing, 336–337, 337*t*–338*t*
Preservative, of drug, 324
Pressure relief bandages, 373–374
Preventive analgesia, 567
Primary inertia, 263
Primary layer, of bandage, 373
Primary wound contraction, of wound healing, 427
Probiotics, 164
Proctodeum, 125
Production diet, equine, 180–181
Profession, ethical considerations, 4, 6*t*
Professional accountability, 24–25
Professional periodontal therapy, 518–525
  equipment and instrumentation for, 507–509
  polishing, 524–525, 525*f*
  root planing, 524, 524*f*
  subgingival scaling, 524, 524*f*
  sulcular lavage, 525
  supragingival scaling, 518–524, 523*f*–524*f*
Progestagens, 332
Progesterone, 83*t*, 105
Prognosis, of business health, 37
Prohibited substances in horse feed, 180
Prolactin, 83*t*, 105
Proliferation, of wound healing, 427
Prophase, 243
Prophy paste, 509